# SAUNDERS
# Q & A REVIEW FOR
# NCLEX-RN

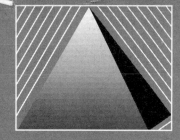

# SAUNDERS
# Q & A
# REVIEW for
# NCLEX-RN

**LINDA ANNE SILVESTRI**, MSN, RN

Assistant Professor of Nursing,
Salve Regina University,
Newport, Rhode Island;
President, Nursing Reviews, Inc., and
Professional Nursing Seminars, Inc.,
Charlestown, Rhode Island

SECOND EDITION

**W.B. SAUNDERS COMPANY**
An Imprint of Elsevier Health Science
Philadelphia London New York St. Louis Sydney Toronto

**W.B. SAUNDERS COMPANY**
*An Imprint of Elsevier Science*

The Curtis Center
Independence Square West
Philadelphia, Pennsylvania 19106

NOTICE:
Pharmacology is an ever-changing field. Standard safety precautions must be followed, but as new research and clinical experience broaden our knowledge, changes in treatment and drug therapy may become necessary or appropriate. Readers are advised to check the most current product information provided by the manufacturer of each drug to be administered to verify the recommended dose, the method and duration of administration, and contraindications. It is the responsibility of the treating appropriately-licensed health care provider, relying on experience and knowledge of the patient, to determine dosages and the best treatment for each individual patient. Neither the publisher nor the editor assumes any liability for any injury and/or damage to persons or property arising from this publication.

The Publisher

*Vice President and Publishing Director, Nursing:* Sally Schrefer
*Senior Editor:* Loren S. Wilson
*Senior Developmental Editor:* Michele D. Hayden
*Project Manager:* Patricia Tannian
*Production Editor:* Steve Hetager
*Book Design Manager:* Gail Morey Hudson
*Cover Designer:* Teresa Breckwoldt

SAUNDERS Q & A REVIEW FOR NCLEX-RN                    ISBN-0-7216-9238-9

Printed in the United States of America

Last digit is the print number:   9   8   7   6   5   4   3   2

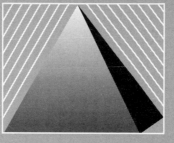

# About the Author

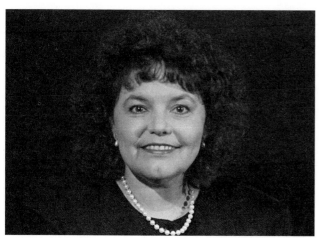

PHOTO BY Laurent W. Valliere.

**Linda Anne Silvestri** received her diploma in nursing at Cooley Dickinson Hospital School of Nursing in Northampton, Massachusetts. Afterward, she worked at Baystate Medical Center in Springfield, Massachusetts. At Baystate Medical Center, she worked in acute medical-surgical units, the intensive care unit, the emergency department, pediatric units, and other acute care units. She later received an associate's degree from Holyoke Community College in Holyoke, Massachusetts, and then received her bachelor of science degree in nursing from American International College in Springfield, Massachusetts.

A native of Springfield, Massachusetts, Linda began her teaching career as an instructor of medical-surgical nursing and leadership-management nursing at Baystate Medical Center School of Nursing in 1981. In 1985, she earned her master of science degree in nursing from Anna Maria College, Paxton, Massachusetts, with a dual major in nursing management and patient education.

Linda relocated to Rhode Island in 1989 and began teaching advanced medical-surgical nursing and psychiatric nursing to RN and LPN students at the Community College of Rhode Island. While she was teaching at the Community College of Rhode Island, a group of students approached Linda, asking her to help them prepare for the NCLEX. On the basis of her experience as a nursing educator and as an NCLEX item writer, she developed a comprehensive review course to prepare nursing graduates for the NCLEX examination.

In 1994, Linda began teaching medical-surgical nursing at Salve Regina University in Newport, Rhode Island. She also prepares nursing students at Salve Regina University for the NCLEX-RN examination. Currently, she is matriculated at the University of Rhode Island in the PhD program in nursing. Linda is also a member of Sigma Theta Tau.

In 1991 Linda established Professional Nursing Seminars, Inc., and in 2000 she established Nursing Reviews, Inc. Both companies are dedicated to conducting NCLEX-RN and NCLEX-PN review courses and to assisting nursing graduates to achieve their goals of becoming registered nurses or licensed practical or vocational nurses.

Today, Linda Silvestri's companies conduct NCLEX review courses throughout New England. She is the successful author of numerous NCLEX-RN and NCLEX-PN review products, including *Saunders Comprehensive Review for NCLEX-RN, Saunders Q & A Review for NCLEX-RN, Saunders Computerized Review for NCLEX-RN, Saunders Instructor's Resource Package for NCLEX-RN, Saunders Comprehensive Review for NCLEX-PN, Saunders Q & A Review for NCLEX-PN,* and *Saunders Instructor's Resource Package for NCLEX-PN.*

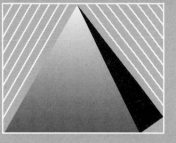

# Contributors

**Jessica Bianco, RN**
Graduate, Department of Nursing, Salve Regina University
Newport, Rhode Island

**Mary Ann Hogan, MSN, RN, CS**
Clinical Assistant Professor, University of Massachusetts
Amherst, Massachusetts

**Jo Ann Barnes Mullaney, PhD, RN, CS**
Professor of Nursing, Salve Regina University
Newport, Rhode Island

**Laurent W. Valliere, BS**
Vice President, Professional Nursing Seminars, Inc.
Charlestown, Rhode Island

*The author and publisher would also like to acknowledge the following individuals for contributions to the first edition of this book:*

**Marianne P. Barba, MS, RN**
Care New England
Coventry, Rhode Island

**Nancy Blasdell, MSN, RN**
Doctoral Student, University of Rhode Island
Kingston, Rhode Island

**Barbara Bono-Snell, MS, RN, CS**
Psychiatric Clinical Nurse Specialist, St. Joseph's Certified
  Home Health Care Agency
Liverpool, New York

**Netta Moncur Bowen, MSN, RN**
Nursing Faculty, Seminole Community College
Sanford, Florida

**Carolyn Pierce Buckelew, RNCS, NC, CHyp**
Nursing Instructor, Charles E. Gregory School of Nursing
Raritan Bay Medical Center
Perth Amboy, New Jersey

**Janis M. Byers, MSN, RNC**
Nursing Faculty, Sewickley Valley Hospital School of Nursing
Sewickley, Pennsylvania

**Penny S. Cass, PhD, RN**
Dean, Division of Nursing, Indiana University—Kokomo
Kokomo, Indiana

**Deborah H. Chatham, MS, RN, CS**
Assistant Professor of Nursing, William Carey College
Gulfport, Mississippi

**Tom Christenbery, MSN, RN**
Assistant Professor of Nursing, Tennessee State University
Nashville, Tennessee

**Anita M. Creamer, MS, RN, CS**
Associate Professor of Nursing, Community College of
  Rhode Island
Warwick, Rhode Island

**Barbara A. Dagastine, MSN, RN**
Associate Professor of Nursing, Hudson Valley
  Community College
Troy, New York

**Jean DeCoffe, MSN, RN**
Assistant Professor of Nursing, Salve Regina University
Newport, Rhode Island

**DeAnna Jan Emory, MS, RN**
Assistant Professor of Nursing, Bacone College
Muskogee, Oklahoma

**Mary E. Farrell, MS, RN, CCRN**
Associate Professor of Nursing, Salem State College
Salem, Massachusetts

**Patsy H. Fasnacht, MSN, RN, CCRN**
Nursing Instructor, Lancaster Institute for Health Education
Lancaster, Pennsylvania

**Dona Ferguson, MSN, RN,C**
Assistant Professor of Nursing
Chair, Nursing and Allied Health
Atlantic Community College
Mays Landing, New Jersey

**Thomas E. Folcarelli, MSN, RN**
Associate Professor of Nursing, Community College of
    Rhode Island
Newport, Rhode Island

**Florence Hayes Gibson, MSN, CNS**
Associate Professor of Nursing, Northeast Louisiana
    University
Monroe, Louisiana

**Alma V. Harkey, MSN, RNC, ACCE**
Instructor of Nursing, Southeast Missouri State University
Cape Girardeau, Missouri

**Joyce Ellen Heil, BSN, CCRN**
Assistant Instructor of Nursing, St. Margaret School of
    Nursing
Pittsburgh, Pennsylvania

**Barbara Hicks, DSN, RN**
Instructor of Nursing, Central Alabama Community College,
Coosa Valley School of Nursing
Sylacauga, Alabama

**Noreen M. Houck, MS, RN**
Assistant Director, Crouse Hospital School of Nursing
Syracuse, New York

**Amy Lawyer Hudson, MSN, RN**
Nursing Faculty, Phillips Community College
University of Arkansas
Helene, Arkansas

**Frances E. Johnson, MS, RNC**
Assistant Professor of Nursing, Andrews University
Berrien Springs, Michigan

**Deborah Klaas, PhD, RN**
Assistant Professor of Nursing, Northern Arizona University
Flagstaff, Arizona

**June Peterson Larson, MS, RN**
Associate Professor of Nursing, University of South Dakota
Vermillion, South Dakota

**Suzanne K. Marnocha, MSN, RN, CCRN**
Assistant Professor of Nursing, University of Wisconsin,
    Oshkosh
Oshkosh, Wisconsin

**Ellen Frances McCarty, PhD, RN, CS**
Co-Chairperson, Department of Nursing
Professor of Nursing, Salve Regina University
Newport, Rhode Island

**Connie M. Metzler, MSN, RN**
Instructor of Nursing, Lancaster Institute for Health
    Education
Lancaster, Pennsylvania

**Patricia A. Miller, MSN, RN**
Formerly Director, School of Nursing, Baystate Medical
    Center School of Nursing
Springfield, Massachusetts

**Kathleen Ann Ohman, MS, EdD, RN**
Associate Professor of Nursing, College of St. Benedict,
    St. John's University
St. Joseph, Minnesota

**Lynda C. Opdyke, MSN, RN**
Facilitator, Academic Affairs, Mercy School of Nursing
Charlotte, North Carolina

**MaeDella Perry, MSN, RN**
Nurse Educator, Medical College of Georgia
Augusta, Georgia

**Lisa A. Ruth-Sahd, MSN, RN, CEN, CCRN**
Nursing Instructor, Lancaster Institute for Health Education
Lancaster, Pennsylvania;
Adjunct Faculty, York College of Pennsylvania
York, Pennsylvania

**Jeanine T. Sequin, MS, RN, CS**
Assistant Professor of Nursing, Keuka College
Keuka Park, New York

**Alberta Elaine Severs, MSN, MA, RN**
Associate Professor of Nursing, Community College of
    Rhode Island
Lincoln, Rhode Island

**Kimberly Sharpe, MS, RN**
Instructor of Nursing, Crouse Hospital School of Nursing
Syracuse, New York

**Susan Sienkiewicz, MA, RN, CS**
Associate Professor of Nursing, Community College of
    Rhode Island
Lincoln, Rhode Island

**Yvonne Marie Smith, MSN, RN, CCRN**
Instructor, Aultman Hospital School of Nursing
Canton, Ohio

**Judith Stamp, MS, RN**
Assistant Professor of Nursing, Hudson Valley
   Community College
Troy, New York

**Yvonne Nazareth Stringfield, EdD, RN**
Associate Professor of Nursing, BSN Program Director
Tennessee State University
Nashville, Tennessee

**Mattie Tolley, MS, RN**
Instructor of Nursing, Southwestern Oklahoma State
   University
Weatherford, Oklahoma

**Johanna M. Tracy, MSN, RN, CS**
Instructor of Nursing, Mercer Medical Center,
Trenton, New Jersey

**Joyce I. Turnbull, MN, RN**
Nursing Lecturer, Clinical Instructor, San Jose State University
San Jose, California

**Paula A. Viau, PhD, RN**
Professor of Nursing, University of Rhode Island
Kingston, Rhode Island

**Carol Warner, MSN, RN, CPN**
Instructor of Nursing, St. Luke's School of Nursing
Bethlehem, Pennsylvania

**Deborah Williams, EdD, RN**
Associate Professor of Nursing, Western Kentucky University
Bowling Green, Kentucky

## REVIEWERS

**Carolyn Banks, MSN, RN**
Nursing Faculty, Pratt Community College
Pratt, Kansas

**Janice Boundy, PhD, RN**
Professor and Coordinator, Saint Francis College of Nursing
Peoria, Illinois

**Michele Bunning, MSN, RN**
Instructor, Good Samaritan Hospital School of Nursing
Cincinnati, Ohio

**Gina Catena, MS, CNM, NP**
Nurse-Midwife, Bay Care Women's Health Services
San Rafael, California

**Mary Ellen Lashley, PhD, RN, CRNP**
Associate Professor, Towson University, Department of
   Nursing
Towson, Maryland

**Caron Martin, MSN, RN**
Assistant Professor, Northern Kentucky University
Department of Nursing
Highland Heights, Kentucky

**Debbie Ocedek, MSN, RN**
Professor, PN/ADN Program, Mott Community College
Flint, Michigan

**Sharon Powell-Laney, MSN, RN**
Coordinator of Nursing, Indiana County Technology Center
Indiana, Pennsylvania

**Anita K. Reed, MSN, RN**
Instructor of Nursing, St. Elizabeth School of Nursing
Lafayette, Indiana

**Christine M. Rosner, PhD, RN**
Lecturer, Division of Nursing, Holy Family College
Philadelphia, Pennsylvania

**Linda S. Smith, DSN, RN**
Assistant Professor, Oregon Health Sciences University
Klamath Falls, Oregon

**Ann D. Sumners, PhD, RN**
Professor, North Georgia College and State University
Department of Nursing
Dahlonega, Georgia

## STUDENT REVIEWERS

**Allison Belisle**
Salve Regina University
Newport, Rhode Island

**Melissa Caporale**
Salve Regina University
Newport, Rhode Island

**Shannon DaCunha**
Salve Regina University
Newport, Rhode Island

**Stephanie G. Ferreira**
Salve Regina University
Newport, Rhode Island

**Natalie Gendron**
Salve Regina University
Newport, Rhode Island

**Jill A. Klein**
Villa Julie College
Stevenson, Maryland

**Lauren C. Rodrigues**
Salve Regina University
Newport, Rhode Island

**Jinae Selvey**
Johns Hopkins University, School of Nursing
Baltimore, Maryland

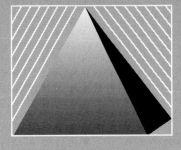

# Preface

*"Success is climbing a mountain,
facing the challenge of obstacles, and
reaching the top of the mountain."*
Linda Anne Silvestri

Welcome to Saunders Pyramid to Success!

*Saunders Q & A Review for NCLEX-RN* is one of a series of products designed to assist you in achieving your goal of becoming a registered nurse. *Saunders Q & A Review for NCLEX-RN* provides you with more than 3500 practice NCLEX-RN test questions based on the 2001 NCLEX-RN test plan.

The new 2001 test plan for NCLEX-RN identifies a framework based on *Client Needs*. These Client Needs categories include Safe, Effective Care Environment; Physiological Integrity; Psychosocial Integrity; and Health Promotion and Maintenance. *Integrated Concepts and Processes* are also identified as a component of the test plan. These include Caring; Communication and Documentation; Cultural Awareness; Nursing Process; Self-Care; and Teaching/Learning. This book has been uniquely designed and includes chapters that describe each specific component of the 2001 NCLEX-RN Test Plan framework and chapters that contain practice questions specific to each component.

## CAT NCLEX-RN TEST PREPARATION

This book begins with information regarding NCLEX-RN preparation. Chapter 1 addresses all of the information related to the 2001 NCLEX-RN test plan and the testing procedures related to the examination. This chapter answers all of the questions that you may have regarding the testing procedures. Chapter 2 discusses the NCLEX-RN from a nonacademic view and emphasizes a holistic approach to your individual test preparation. This chapter identifies the components of a structured study plan and pattern, anxiety-reducing techniques, and personal focus issues. Nursing students want to hear what other students have to say about their experiences with NCLEX-RN. Students seek a view of

what it is really like to take this examination. Chapter 3 is written by a nursing student who recently took the NCLEX-RN. This chapter addresses the issue of what NCLEX-RN is all about, and includes the student's "story of success." Chapter 4, "Test-Taking Strategies," includes all of the important strategies that will assist in teaching you how to read a question, how not to read into a question, and how to use the process of elimination and various other methods to select the correct response from the options presented.

## CLIENT NEEDS

Chapters 5 to 9 address the 2001 NCLEX-RN test plan component *Client Needs*. Chapter 5 describes each category of Client Needs as identified by the test plan and lists the subcategories of each category, the percentage of test questions for each subcategory, and some of the content included on NCLEX-RN. Chapters 6 to 9 contain practice test questions related specifically to each category of Client Needs. Chapter 6 contains questions related to Safe, Effective Care Environment, Chapter 7 contains Physiological Integrity questions, Chapter 8 contains Psychosocial Integrity questions, and Chapter 9 contains Health Promotion and Maintenance questions.

## INTEGRATED CONCEPTS AND PROCESSES

Chapters 10 and 11 address *Integrated Concepts and Processes* as identified in the test plan for NCLEX-RN. Chapter 10 describes each Integrated Concept and Process. Chapter 11 contains practice test questions related specifically to each Integrated Concept and Process, including Caring; Communication and Documentation; Cultural Awareness; Nursing Process; Self-Care; and Teaching/Learning.

## COMPREHENSIVE TEST

A comprehensive test is included at the end of this book. It consists of 300 practice questions representative of the components of the 2001 test plan framework for NCLEX-RN.

## SPECIAL FEATURES OF THE BOOK
### Book Design

The book is designed with a unique two-column format. The left column presents the practice questions and options, and the right column provides the corresponding answers, rationales, test-taking strategies, and references. The two-column format makes the review easier because you do not have to flip through pages in search of answers and rationales.

## Practice Questions
### Multiple Choice

While you are preparing for the NCLEX-RN, it is crucial for you to review practice questions. This book contains 1800 multiple-choice practice questions in NCLEX format. The accompanying software includes all of the multiple-choice questions from the book, plus an additional 1700 questions, for a total of 3500 questions.

### Critical Thinking: Free-Text Entry

Chapters 6, 7, 8, 9, and 11 each contain several *Critical Thinking: Free-Text Entry* questions. This type of question provides you practice in prioritizing, decision making, and critical thinking skills.

## Answer Sections for Practice Questions

Each practice question is followed by the correct answer, rationale, test-taking strategy, question categories, and a reference source. The structure of the answer section is unique and provides the following information for every question.

**Rationale:** The rationale provides you with significant information regarding both correct and incorrect options.

**Test-Taking Strategy:** The test-taking strategy provides you with the logic for selecting the correct option and assists you in selecting an answer to a question on which you must guess. Specific suggestions for review are identified in the test-taking strategy.

**Question Categories:** Each question is identified on the basis of the categories used by the NCLEX-RN test plan. Additional content area categories are provided with each question to assist you in identifying areas in need of review. The categories identified with each question include Level of Cognitive Ability, Client Needs, Integrated Concept/Process, and the specific nursing Content Area. All categories are identified by

their full names so that you do not need to memorize codes or abbreviations.

**Reference Source:** The reference source, including a page number, is provided so that you can easily find the information that you need to review in your undergraduate nursing textbooks.

## NCLEX-RN REVIEW SOFTWARE

Packaged in this book you will find an NCLEX-RN review CD-ROM. This software contains 3500 questions, 1800 from the book and 1700 additional questions. This Windows- and Macintosh-compatible program offers three testing modes for review of the multiple-choice questions.

**Quiz:** Ten randomly chosen questions on Client Needs, Integrated Concept/Process, or specific Content Area. Results are given and review of the answer, rationale, and test-taking strategy is provided after you answer all 10 questions.

**Study:** All questions on Client Needs, Integrated Concept/Process, or specific Content Area. The answer, rationale, and test-taking strategy appear after you answer each question.

**Examination:** One hundred randomly chosen questions from the entire pool of 3500 questions, chosen according to Client Needs, Integrated Concept/Process, or specific Content Areas. Results are given and review is provided after you answer all 100 questions.

The CD-ROM allows you to customize your review and determine your areas of strength and weakness. It also provides you with a wealth of practice test questions while at the same time simulating the NCLEX-RN experience on computer.

## HOW TO USE THIS BOOK

*Saunders Q & A Review for NCLEX-RN* is especially designed to help you with your successful journey to the peak of the Pyramid to Success, becoming a registered nurse. As you begin your journey through this book, you will be introduced to all of the important points regarding the CAT NCLEX-RN examination, the process of testing, and the unique and special tips regarding how to prepare yourself for this important examination. Read the chapter written by the nursing graduate who recently passed NCLEX-RN, and consider what this graduate has to say about the examination. The test-taking strategy chapter will provide you with important strategies that will guide you in selecting the correct option or assist you in guessing the answer. Read this chapter and practice these strategies as you proceed through your journey with this book.

Once you have completed reading the introductory components of this book, it is time to begin the practice questions. As you read through each question and select an answer, be sure to read the rationale and the test-taking strategy. The rationale provides you with the significant information regarding both the correct and incorrect options, and the test-taking strategy provides you with the logic for selecting the correct option. The strategy also identifies the content area that you need to review if you had difficulty with the question. Use the reference source provided so that you can easily find the information that you need to review.

As you work your way through *Saunders Q & A Review for NCLEX-RN* to identify your areas of strength and weakness, you can return to the companion book, *Saunders Comprehensive Review for NCLEX-RN*, to focus your study on these areas. The companion book and its accompanying CD-ROM provide you with a comprehensive review of all areas of the nursing content reflected in the 2001 CAT NCLEX-RN test plan. To determine your readiness for CAT NCLEX-RN, you will use the next step in the Saunders Pyramid to Success, *Saunders Computerized Review for NCLEX-RN*, which is a software program that contains nearly 2000 NCLEX-RN–style questions. The final component of the Saunders Pyramid to Success is *Saunders Instructor's Resource Package for NCLEX-RN*. This manual and CD-ROM accompany the Saunders program of NCLEX-RN review products. Be sure to ask your nursing program director and nursing faculty about the CD-ROM and its use for a review course or for a self-paced review in your school's computer laboratory.

Good luck with your journey through the Pyramid to Success! I wish you continued success throughout your new career as a registered nurse!

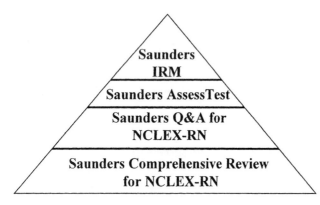

## ACKNOWLEDGMENTS

There are many individuals who in their own ways have contributed to my success in making my professional dreams become a reality.

First, I want to acknowledge my parents, who opened my door of opportunity in education. I thank my mother, Frances Mary, for all of her love, support, and assistance as I continuously worked to achieve my professional goals. I thank my father, Arnold Lawrence, who always provided insightful words of encouragement. My memories of his love and support will always remain in my heart. I also thank my sister, Dianne Elodia, my brother, Lawrence Peter, and my niece, Gina Marie, who were continuously supportive, giving, and helpful during my research and preparation of this publication. I sincerely thank Mary Ann Hogan, MSN, RN, who has always encouraged and supported me through my professional endeavors. Her numerous contributions to this publication are a reflection of her dedication to the profession of nursing and to nursing students. A very special thank you to Sarah Miller, my assistant. She provided continuous support and dedication to my work both in the NCLEX review courses and in preparing the second edition of this book. I want to thank all of my nursing students at the Community College of Rhode Island in Warwick, who approached me in 1991 and persuaded me to assist them in preparing to take the NCLEX-RN examination. Their enthusiasm and inspiration led to the commencement of my professional endeavors in conducting NCLEX-RN review courses for nursing students. I also thank the numerous nursing students who have attended my review courses, for their willingness to share their needs and ideas. Their input has certainly added a special uniqueness to this publication. I thank all of the contributors to this publication who provided practice questions and the many faculty and student reviewers of this publication. A special thank you to Dr. JoAnn Mullaney from Salve Regina University in Newport, Rhode Island, for her numerous and expert contributions to this publication and to Jessica Bianco, RN, for providing a chapter regarding her experiences with NCLEX-RN. I wish to acknowledge all of the nursing faculty who taught in my NCLEX-RN review courses. Their commitment, dedication, and expertise have certainly assisted nursing students in achieving success with the NCLEX-RN. In addition, I want to acknowledge Laurent W. Valliere for his contribution to this publication, for teaching in my NCLEX-RN review courses, and for his commitment and dedication in assisting my nursing students to prepare for NCLEX-RN from a nonacademic point of view. I sincerely acknowledge and thank two very important individuals from Elsevier Science. I thank Loren Wilson, Senior Editor, for all of her assistance throughout the preparation of this edition and for her continuous enthusiasm, support, and expert professional guidance. And I thank Shelly Hayden, Senior Developmental Editor, for her continuous assistance and for keeping me on track. Her expert organizational skills maintained order in all of the work that I submitted for manuscript production. I want to acknowledge all of the staff at Elsevier Science for their tremendous assistance throughout the preparation and production of this publication. A special thank you to all of them. I thank all of the special people in the production department: Steve Hetager, production editor, whose consistent editing assisted in finalizing this publication, Trish Tannian, Project Manager, and Gail

Morey Hudson, Book Design Manager. I sincerely thank Linda Morris, Marketing Manager from the Nursing Marketing Department, whose support, hard work, and special creativity assisted with this publication. I would also like to acknowledge Patricia Mieg, Educational Sales Representative, who encouraged me to submit my ideas and initial work to the W.B. Saunders Company and initiated my meeting with Maura Connor, my former Senior Acquisitions Editor. I want to thank Maura for the professional direction that led me to success as I initially created Saunders Pyramid to Success for NCLEX-RN. I thank Salve Regina University for the opportunity to educate nursing students in the baccalaureate nursing program and for its support during my research and writing of this publication. I would like to especially acknowledge Dr. Louise Murdock and Dr. Ellen McCarty, Co-Chairpersons of the Department of Nursing at Salve Regina University, for their continuous support, academic mentoring, and astute vision regarding the profession of nursing. I wish to acknowledge the University of Rhode Island, College of Nursing, for providing me with the opportunity for professional growth in my nursing education, particularly Dr. Donna Schwartz-Barcott and Dr. Suzie Kim, my academic advisors in the doctoral program at the university. I wish to acknowledge the Community College of Rhode Island, which provided me the opportunity to educate nursing students in the Associate Degree of Nursing Program, and a special thank you to Patricia Miller, MSN, RN, and Michelina McClellan, MS, RN, from Baystate Medical Center, School of Nursing, in Springfield, Massachusetts, who were my very first mentors in nursing education.

Last, a very special thank you to all my nursing students: you light up my life, and your hearts and minds will shape the future of the profession of nursing!

**Linda Anne Silvestri**

To All Future Registered Nurses,

Congratulations to you!

Whether you are a nursing student in a nursing program completing your studies, or a graduate preparing to take the NCLEX-RN examination, you should be very proud and pleased with yourself on your many accomplishments. I know that you are working very hard to become successful and that you have proved to yourself that you indeed can achieve your goals.

I have been teaching nursing students for many years and have been conducting NCLEX-RN review courses since 1991. Preparing to take an examination can be an anxiety-producing experience. A component of achieving success in examinations is possessing the knowledge and experience needed to answer a question correctly. An additional component of becoming successful in these examinations is to become comfortable and confident in the ability to face the challenge of a question and to answer the question correctly. In my experience in working with students, it is evident that students strongly need to review practice questions. The more questions, answers, and rationales with which a student can practice, the more proficient the student becomes with test-taking strategies and the ability to answer a question correctly. One of the things that you need to realize is that when you take an examination consisting of multiple-choice questions, the answer is right there in front of you. You need to use your nursing knowledge and skills and to become proficient in the strategy involved in reading a question and specifically identifying what the question is asking you. Your knowledge, your experience, and the incorporation of test-taking strategies will lead you to success. On NCLEX-RN, the questions require thought and critical analysis. Consistent practice with test questions will assist you in becoming comfortable, confident, and proficient in answering the questions correctly.

I am excited and pleased to be able to provide you with the second editions of *Saunders Pyramid to Success* products. These products will prepare you for your most important professional goal, becoming a registered nurse. Saunders Pyramid to Success products provide you with everything that you need to prepare for NCLEX-RN. These products include material that is required for examination preparation for all nursing students regardless of educational background, specific strengths, areas in need of improvement, or clinical experience during the nursing program.

*Saunders Q & A Review for NCLEX-RN* is designed to provide you with questions specifically representative of the components of the 2001 NCLEX-RN test plan. The framework for the test plan focuses on *Client Needs* and *Integrated Concepts and Processes*. Therefore, chapters representative of this framework are included in this book.

So let's get started and begin our journey through the Pyramid to Success, and welcome to the profession of nursing!

Sincerely,

*Linda Anne Silvestri MSN, RN*

**Linda Anne Silvestri, MSN, RN**

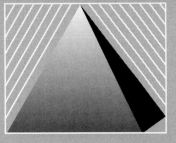

# Contents

# NCLEX-RN Preparation

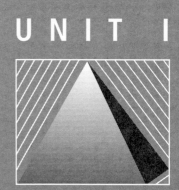

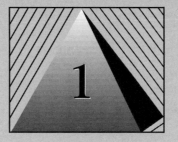

# 1

# NCLEX-RN

## THE PYRAMID TO SUCCESS

Welcome to Saunders *Q & A Review for NCLEX-RN*, the second component of the Pyramid to Success!

At this time, you have completed your first path toward the peak of the Pyramid with the *Saunders Comprehensive Review for NCLEX-RN*. Now it is time to continue that journey to become a registered nurse with the *Saunders Q & A Review for NCLEX-RN!*

As you begin your journey through this book, you will be introduced to all of the important points regarding the NCLEX-RN examination, the process of testing, and the unique and special tips regarding how to prepare yourself for this very important examination. You will read what a nursing graduate who recently passed NCLEX-RN has to say about the examination. All of those important test-taking strategies are detailed. These details will guide you in selecting the correct option or in selecting an answer to a question you must guess at.

*Saunders Q & A Review for NCLEX-RN* contains 3500 NCLEX-RN–style practice questions. The chapters have been developed to provide a description of the components of the NCLEX-RN Test Plan, including the Client Needs and the Integrated Concepts and Processes. In addition, chapters have been prepared to contain practice questions specific to each category of Client Needs and the Integrated Concepts and Processes.

In each chapter that contains practice questions, a rationale, test-taking strategy, and reference source containing a page number are provided with each question. Each question is coded on the basis of the Level of Cognitive Ability, Client Needs category, Integrated Concept and Process, and the content area being tested. The rationale provides you with significant information about both the correct and incorrect options. The test-taking strategy provides you with the logical path to selecting the correct option and identifies

the content area to review, if necessary. The reference source and page number provide easy access to the information that you need to review.

After you complete the *Saunders Q & A Review for NCLEX-RN*, you are ready for the *Saunders Computerized Review for NCLEX-RN*, a computer disk program that contains 1700 NCLEX-RN–style questions to help you determine your readiness for NCLEX-RN.

Let's continue with our journey through the Pyramid to Success!

## THE EXAMINATION PROCESS

An important step in the Pyramid to Success is to become as familiar as possible with the examination process. The challenge of this examination can arouse significant anxiety. Knowing what the examination is all about and knowing what you will encounter during the process of testing will assist in alleviating fear and anxiety. The information contained in this chapter addresses the procedures related to the development of the NCLEX-RN Test Plan, the components of the Test Plan, and the questions most commonly asked by nursing students and graduates preparing to take the NCLEX-RN. This information was adapted from *Test Plan for the National Council Licensure Examination for Registered Nurses*, National Council of State Boards of Nursing, Chicago, 2000, and *The NCLEX Process: Serving as an Anchor for the NCLEX Examination*, National Council of State Boards of Nursing, Chicago, 2000.

## DEVELOPMENT OF THE TEST PLAN

As an initial step in the test development process, the National Council of State Boards of Nursing considers the legal scope of nursing practice as governed by state laws and regulations, including the Nurse Practice Act. The National Council uses these laws to define the areas on NCLEX-RN that will assess the competence of candidates for nurse licensure.

The National Council of State Boards of Nursing also conducts a Practice Analysis study to determine the framework for the Test Plan for NCLEX-RN. Since nursing practice continues to change, this study is conducted every 3 years. The results of this study, most recently conducted in 1999, provided the structure for the new Test Plan, implemented in April 2001.

## PRACTICE ANALYSIS STUDY

The participants of this study include newly licensed registered nurses from all types of basic education programs. The participants are provided a list of nursing activities and are asked about the frequency of performing these specific activities, their impact on maintaining client safety, and the settings in which the activities were performed. The analysis of the data obtained from this study guides the development of a framework for entry-level nurse performance that incorporates specific client needs and the concepts and processes fundamental to the practice of nursing. The NCLEX-RN Test Plan is derived from this framework.

## THE TEST PLAN

The content of NCLEX-RN reflects the activities that a newly licensed entry-level registered nurse must be able to perform in order to provide clients with safe and effective nursing care. The questions are written to address the Levels of Cognitive Ability, Client Needs, and Integrated Concepts and Processes as identified in the Test Plan.

## Levels of Cognitive Ability

The NCLEX-RN examination includes questions at the cognitive levels of knowledge, comprehension, application, and analysis. The majority of the questions are written at the application and analysis levels because the practice of nursing requires critical thinking and complex thought processing. This means that the test taker will be required to analyze and/or apply the information provided in the test question (Box 1-1).

## Client Needs

In the new Test Plan implemented in April 2001, the National Council of State Boards of Nursing has identified a test plan framework based on Client Needs. This framework was selected on the basis of the findings in the Practice Analysis study, and because Client Needs provide a structure for defining nursing actions and competencies across all settings for all clients. The National Council of State Boards of Nursing identifies four major categories of Client Needs. These categories are further divided into subcategories, and the percentage of test questions in each subcategory is identified. Table 1-1 identifies these categories and subcategories and the associated percentages of test questions. Refer to Chapter 5 for a detailed description of the categories of Client Needs and the NCLEX-RN Examination.

---

**BOX 1-1**

### Level of Cognitive Ability

A client with trigeminal neuralgia who is receiving carbamazepine (Tegretol) 400 mg PO daily has a white blood cell (WBC) count of 2800/uL, blood urea nitrogen (BUN) of 17 mg/dL, sodium of 141 mEq/L, and uric acid of 5.0 ng/dL. On the basis of these laboratory values, the nurse determines that the:
1. Sodium level is low, indicating an electrolyte imbalance
2. Uric acid level is elevated, indicating a risk for renal calculi
3. BUN is elevated, indicating nephrotoxicity
4. WBC is low, indicating a blood dyscrasia

**Answer:** 4
This question requires the test taker to analyze each of the laboratory values identified in the question. The test taker needs to know the adverse effects of carbamazepine and the normal laboratory values in order to make an accurate interpretation regarding the client's status.

**Level of Cognitive Ability:** Analysis

---

**TABLE 1-1**

### Client Needs and the Percentage of Test Questions

| | PERCENTAGE (%) |
|---|---|
| **SAFE, EFFECTIVE CARE ENVIRONMENT** | |
| Management of care | 7-13 |
| Safety and infection control | 5-11 |
| | |
| **PHYSIOLOGICAL INTEGRITY** | |
| Basic care and comfort | 7-13 |
| Pharmacological and parenteral therapies | 5-11 |
| Reduction of risk potential | 12-18 |
| Physiological adaptation | 12-18 |
| | |
| **PSYCHOSOCIAL INTEGRITY** | |
| Coping and adaptation | 5-11 |
| Psychosocial adaptation | 5-11 |
| | |
| **HEALTH PROMOTION AND MAINTENANCE** | |
| Growth and development through the life span | 7-13 |
| Prevention and early detection of health problems | 5-11 |

From National Council of State Boards of Nursing (eds.) (2000). *Test plan for the National Council Licensure Examination for Registered Nurses.* Chicago: Author.

## Integrated Concepts and Processes

The National Council of State Boards of Nursing has identified six concepts and processes that are fundamental to the practice of nursing. These concepts and processes are a component of the Test Plan and are incorporated throughout the major categories of Client Needs. Box 1-2 identifies these six concepts and processes. Refer to Chapter 10 for a detailed description of the Integrated Concepts and Processes and the NCLEX-RN Examination.

## ITEM WRITERS

NCLEX-RN item writers are selected by the National Council of State Boards of Nursing following an extensive application process. The item writers are registered nurses who hold a master's degree or a higher degree. Most of the item writers are nursing educators; however, clinical nurse specialists are also selected to participate in this process. These item writers are clinical experts who are currently involved in clinical practice with entry-level registered nurses. Item writers voluntarily submit an application to become an item writer and must meet specific established criteria designated by the National Council in order to be accepted as a participant in the process.

## CAT NCLEX-RN

The term *NCLEX-RN* stands for National Council Licensure Examination for Registered Nurses. The term *CAT* stands for Computerized Adaptive Testing. The CAT NCLEX-RN is a computer-administered examination that the nursing graduate must take and pass in order to practice as a registered nurse. This examination measures the candidate's knowledge, skills, and abilities required to perform safely and competently as a newly licensed entry-level registered nurse.

## COMPUTERIZED ADAPTIVE TESTING (CAT)

The CAT system provides each candidate with a unique examination experience, because the examination adapts to each test taker's skill level. The CAT examination is assembled interactively as the candidate answers

the questions. All of the test questions are stored in a large test bank and are categorized on the basis of the test plan structure and the level of difficulty of the question. With the CAT method of testing, an examination is created and tailored to test the candidate's knowledge and abilities while fulfilling test plan requirements. In this way, the candidate will not waste time answering questions that are far above or below his or her competency level.

When a candidate answers a question on CAT NCLEX-RN, the computer will calculate a competency skill estimate based on the answer that the candidate selected. If the candidate selected a correct answer to a question, the computer scans the test bank and selects a more difficult question. If the candidate selected an incorrect answer, the computer scans the test bank and selects an easier question. This process continues until the Test Plan requirements are met and a reliable pass or fail decision is made.

## THE PROCESS OF REGISTRATION

The initial step in the registration process is that each candidate applies to the State Board of Nursing in the state in which he or she intends to obtain licensure. (The addresses, telephone numbers, and web sites, if available, of Boards of Nursing in all states and territories of the United States are provided at the end of this chapter.) The candidate needs to obtain information from the Board of Nursing regarding the specific registration process, because the process may vary from state to state. It is very important that the candidate follow the registration instructions and complete the registration forms precisely and accurately. Registration forms not properly completed, or not accompanied by the proper fees in the required method of payment, will be returned to the candidate and will delay testing. The initial fee for the application process may vary from state to state. Each Board of Nursing will set its initial license fee according to its own needs. The registration forms will identify the registration and testing service fees. When the Board of Nursing receives the completed registration form, the candidate's eligibility is determined, on the basis of the criteria established by the Board, and the Board authorizes his or her admission to the examination.

Once eligibility to test has been determined by the Board of Nursing in the jurisdiction in which licensure is requested, the valid NCLEX registration is processed, and an Authorization to Test form will be sent to the candidate. The candidate cannot make an appointment until the Board of Nursing declares eligibility and an Authorization to Test form is received. The Authorization to Test form will provide a candidate identification number and an authorization number; these numbers will be needed to make an appointment with the testing center.

---

### BOX 1-2

**Integrated Concepts and Processes**

Caring
Communication and Documentation
Cultural Awareness
Nursing Process
Self-Care
Teaching/Learning

## SPECIAL TESTING CIRCUMSTANCES

A candidate who is requesting special accommodations should contact the Board of Nursing before submitting a registration form. The Board of Nursing will provide the candidate with the procedures for the request. The Board of Nursing must authorize special testing accommodations. Following Board of Nursing approval, the National Council of State Boards reviews the requested accommodations to ensure that the proposed modification does not affect the psychometric properties of NCLEX or cause a security risk. The National Council of State Boards must also approve the accommodations.

## MAKING AN APPOINTMENT TO TEST

The CAT NCLEX-RN examination is administered on a year-round basis. Each candidate will be provided with a list of testing centers and the telephone numbers of these centers. The candidate must note the expiration date on the Authorization to Test form and must schedule and make an appointment before this expiration date. The candidate may take the examination at any approved testing center and does not have to test in the same jurisdiction in which licensure is sought. An eligible candidate taking NCLEX for the first time will be offered an appointment date within 30 days of the telephone call to the testing center. Repeat candidates will be offered an appointment date within 45 days of the telephone call to the testing center. A confirmation notice will not be sent to the candidate; therefore it is important that the candidate note the date and time of the appointment. When the testing center is called, it is also important to verify the address and the directions to the testing center.

## CANCELING OR RESCHEDULING AN APPOINTMENT

If for any reason the candidate needs to cancel or reschedule the appointment to take the examination, he or she must remember that the scheduling change must be made before noon, 2 business days before the scheduled appointment. The original appointment must be canceled before a new appointment can be scheduled.

## LATE ARRIVALS TO THE TESTING CENTER

It is important that the candidate arrive at the testing center 30 minutes before the examination is scheduled. Candidates arriving late for the scheduled testing appointment may be required to forfeit the NCLEX appointment. If it is necessary for an appointment to be forfeited, the candidate will need to reregister for the examination and pay an additional fee. The Board of Nursing will be notified that the candidate will not test.

A few days before the scheduled date of testing, the candidate should take the time to drive to the testing center to determine its exact location, the length of time required to arrive at that destination, and any potential obstacles that might cause a delay, such as road construction, traffic, or parking sites.

## THE TESTING CENTER

The testing center is designed to ensure complete security of the testing process. Strict candidate identification requirements have been established. To be admitted to the testing center, the candidate must bring the Authorization to Test form, along with two forms of identification. Both forms of identification must be signed by the candidate, and one must contain the candidate's photograph. The name on the photograph identification must bear the same name as stated on the Authorization to Test form. Examples of acceptable forms of identification will be included in the information received with the Authorization to Test form. The candidate will be required to sign in and out on the test center log form. Each candidate will be thumbprinted and photographed at the test center, and the photograph will accompany the NCLEX results to confirm the candidate's identity. Personal belongings are not allowed in the testing room. Secure storage will be provided for the candidate; however, storage space is limited, so the candidate must plan accordingly. In addition, the testing center will not assume responsibility for the candidate's personal belongings. The waiting areas are generally small; therefore friends or family members who accompany candidates are not permitted to wait in the testing center while candidates are taking the NCLEX-RN.

Once the candidate has completed the admission process and a brief orientation, the proctor will escort the candidate to the assigned computer. The candidate will be seated at an individual table area with an appropriate work space that includes computer equipment, appropriate lighting, scratch paper, and a pencil. Unauthorized scratch paper may not be brought into or removed from the testing room. Eating, drinking, and smoking are not allowed in the testing room. A video camera is located in the testing room, and all test sessions are videotaped with full sound and motion. Candidates should keep two forms of identification with them at all times. Candidates cannot leave the testing room without the permission of the proctor. If a candidate leaves the testing room for any reason, he or she will be required to show two forms of identification to be readmitted. Candidates must follow the directions given by the test center staff and must remain seated during the examination, except when authorized to leave. If a candidate believes that there is a problem with the computer, needs more scratch paper, or needs the proctor for any reason, he or she must raise a hand to notify the proctor.

## THE COMPUTER

Computer experience is not needed to take the CAT NCLEX-RN examination. A keyboard tutorial is administered to all test takers at the start of the examination. In addition, a proctor is present to assist in explaining the use of the computer to ensure the candidate's full understanding of how to proceed.

## CAT NCLEX-RN TEST QUESTIONS

The examination consists of individual (stand-alone) test questions. In other words, this examination does not present a case situation followed by several test questions that relate to that case situation. With an individual (stand-alone) test question, you can expect that the question will appear on the left-hand side of the screen, with the four options on the right-hand side of the screen, or the question appears across the top of the screen with the four options below (Box 1-3).

Primarily, the test questions will be presented in the form of a multiple-choice question: a question and four options. You may also be presented with a visual or image display and be asked a question about the visual or image. For example, you may be presented with a cardiac rhythm strip and be asked what the nursing action would be if this cardiac rhythm was noted on a client's cardiac monitor. In this example, you would be required to identify the cardiac rhythm and then determine the appropriate nursing action.

Another type of question that you may encounter will require you to use the mouse component of the computer system. For example, you may be presented with a visual that displays an adult client's thorax. In this visual, you may be asked to "point and click" (using the mouse) on the area where the stethoscope would be placed to take an apical pulse rate.

Finally, you may encounter a question known as a free-text entry. In this type of question, you will be asked to type the answer to the question. For example, you may be provided with intake and output figures for a client receiving a continuous bladder irrigation and then be asked to determine the client's true urine output. Once this is determined, you will need to type your answer in the appropriate area as designated on the computer screen.

When a test question is presented on the computer screen, it must be answered or the examination will not move on. This means that you will not be able to skip questions, go back and review questions, or go back and change answers. Students preparing for CAT NCLEX-RN become anxious and frustrated because questions cannot be skipped and returned to at a later time during the examination process. Remember, in a CAT examination, once an answer is recorded, all subsequent questions administered depend, to an extent, on the answer selected for that question. Skipping questions and returning to them later are not compatible with the logical methodology of a computerized adaptive test. Recall the number of times you may have changed a correct answer to an incorrect one on a pencil-and-paper nursing examination during your nursing education. The inability to skip questions or go back to change previous answers will not be a disadvantage to you. Actually, you will not fall into that trap of changing a correct answer to an incorrect one with CAT.

There is no penalty for guessing on CAT NCLEX-RN. Remember, the answer to the question will be right there in front of you. If you need to guess, use your nursing knowledge to its fullest extent, as well as all of the test-taking strategies provided to you in Chapter 4 of this book.

## TESTING TIME

The maximum testing time is 5 hours. This time period includes the tutorial, sample questions, and all rest breaks. There is no minimum amount of examination time. A mandatory 10-minute break will be taken after 2 testing hours, and an optional 10-minute break can be taken at the end of 3.5 hours of testing. The computer screen will notify you of the times for these breaks. You must leave the testing room during breaks. You may leave the room for additional, unscheduled breaks, but no additional testing time will be allowed.

## LENGTH OF THE EXAMINATION

The minimum number of questions that you will need to answer to meet adequate testing in each area of the test plan is 75. Of these 75 questions, 60 of the

---

**BOX 1-3**

**Appearance of an Individual (Stand-Alone) Test Question on the Computer Screen**

| The most appropriate method for feeding an infant with a cleft lip or palate is with the infant('s): | 1. Head in an upright position<br>2. In a lying position<br>3. In a side-lying position<br>4. Prone |
|---|---|

A client is admitted with a diagnosis of myasthenia gravis. Pyridostigmine (Mestinon) is prescribed for the client. A nurse monitors the client, knowing that an adverse effect of this medication is:
1. Muscle cramps
2. Mouth ulcers
3. Depression
4. Unexplained weight gain

questions will be real (scored) questions and 15 of the questions will be tryout (unscored) questions. The maximum number of questions in the test is 265. Fifteen of the total number of questions that you need to answer will be tryout (unscored) questions.

The tryout questions are questions that may be presented as scored questions on future NCLEX-RN examinations. These tryout questions are not identified as such. In other words, you do not know which questions are the tryout (unscored) questions.

## COMPLETING THE EXAMINATION

Once the examination is completed, the candidate will complete a brief computer-delivered questionnaire about the testing experience. After this questionnaire is completed, the test proctor will collect all scratch paper, sign the candidate out, and permit the candidate to leave.

## PROCESSING RESULTS

When a candidate completes the examination, the examination is transmitted electronically to the data center for scoring. The results are then transmitted to the Board of Nursing in the state in which the candidate applied for licensure. The Board of Nursing will mail the results to the candidate. In some states, results may be obtained from the Board of Nursing web site. The candidate should not telephone the Testing Center, the National Council, or the State Board of Nursing for results. The results will not be given to candidates over the telephone.

## INTERSTATE ENDORSEMENT

Because the CAT NCLEX-RN is a national examination, the candidate can apply to take the examination in any state. Once licensure is received, the registered nurse can apply for Interstate Endorsement. The procedures and requirements for Interstate Endorsement may vary from state to state, and these procedures can be obtained from the State Board of Nursing in the state in which endorsement is sought.

## STATE BOARDS OF NURSING

Alabama Board of Nursing
RSA Plaza, Suite 250
770 Washington Avenue
Montgomery, AL 36130-3900
(334) 242-4060
Web Site: http://www.abn.state.al.us/

Alaska Board of Nursing
Dept. of Community & Economic Development
Div. of Occupational Licensing
3601 C Street, Suite 722
Anchorage, AK 99503
(907) 269-8161
Web Site: http://www.dced.state.ak.us/occ/pnur.htm

American Samoa Health Services
Regulatory Board
LBJ Tropical Medical Center
Pago Pago, AS 96799
(684) 633-1222

Arizona State Board of Nursing
1651 E. Morten Avenue, Suite 150
Phoenix, AZ 85020
(602) 331-8111
Web Site: http://www.azboardofnursing.org/

Arkansas State Board of Nursing
University Tower Building
1123 S. University Ave., Suite 800
Little Rock, AR 72204
(501) 686-2700
Web Site: http://www.state.ar.us/nurse

California Board of Registered Nursing
400 R Street, Suite 4030
Sacramento, CA 95814-6239
(916) 322-3350
Web Site: http://www.rn.ca.gov/

Colorado Board of Nursing
1560 Broadway, Suite 880
Denver, CO 80202
(303) 894-2430
Web Site: http://www.dora.state.co.us/nursing/

Commonwealth Board of Nurse Examiners
Public Health Center
P.O. Box 1458
Saipan, MP 96950
(670) 234-8950

Connecticut Board of Examiners for Nursing
Division of Health Systems Regulation
410 Capitol Avenue, MS no. 13 ADJ
P.O. Box 340308
Hartford, CT 06134-0328
(860) 509-7624
Web Site: http://www.state.ct.us/dph/

Delaware Board of Nursing
861 Silver Lake Boulevard
Cannon Building, Suite 203
Dover, DE 19904
(302) 739-4522

District of Columbia Board of Nursing
Department of Health
825 N. Capitol Street, N.E., 2nd Floor
Room 2224
Washington, DC 20002
(202) 442-4778

Florida Board of Nursing
4080 Woodcock Drive, Suite 202
Jacksonville, FL 32207
(904) 858-6940
Web Site: http://www.doh.state.fl.us/mqa/nursing/
rnhome.htm

Georgia Board of Nursing
237 Coliseum Drive
Macon, GA 31217-3858
(912) 207-1640
Web Site: http://www.sos.state.ga.us/ebd-rn/

Guam Board of Nurse Examiners
P.O. Box 2816
1304 East Sunset Boulevard
Barrgada, GU 96913
(671) 475-0251

Hawaii Board of Nursing
Professional and Vocational Licensing Division
P.O. Box 3469
Honolulu, HI 96801
(808) 586-3000
Web Site: http://www.state.hi.us/dcca/pvloffline/

Idaho Board of Nursing
280 N. 8th Street, Suite 210
P.O. Box 83720
Boise, ID 83720
(208) 334-3110
Web Site: http://www.state.id.us/ibn/ibnhome.htm

Illinois Department of Professional Regulation
James R. Thompson Center
100 West Randolph, Suite 9-300
Chicago, IL 60601
(312) 814-2715
Web Site: http://www.dpr.state.il.us/

Indiana State Board of Nursing
Health Professions Bureau
402 W. Washington Street, Room W041
Indianapolis, IN 46204
(317) 232-2960
Web Site: http://www.state.in.us/hbp/isbn/

Iowa Board of Nursing
RiverPoint Business Park
400 S.W. 8th Street
Suite B
Des Moines, IA 50309-4685
(515) 281-3255
Web Site: http://www.state.ia.us/government/nursing/

Kansas State Board of Nursing
Landon State Office Building
900 S.W. Jackson, Suite 551-S
Topeka, KS 66612
(785) 296-4929
Web Site: http://www.ksbn.org

Kentucky Board of Nursing
312 Whittington Parkway, Suite 300
Louisville, KY 40222
(502) 329-7000
Web Site: http://www.kbn.state.ky.us/

Louisiana State Board of Nursing
3510 N. Causeway Boulevard, Suite 501
Metairie, LA 70003
(504) 838-5332
Web Site: http://www.lsbn.state.la.us/

Maine State Board of Nursing
158 State House Station
Augusta, ME 04333
(207) 287-1133
Web Site: http://www.state.me.us/nursingbd/

Maryland Board of Nursing
4140 Patterson Avenue
Baltimore, MD 21215
(410) 585-1900
Web Site: http://dhmh1d.dhmh.state.md.us/mbn/

Massachusetts Board of Registration in Nursing
Commonwealth of Massachusetts
239 Causeway Street
Boston, MA 02114
(617) 727-9961
Web Site: http://www.state.ma.us/reg/boards/rn/

Michigan CIS/Office of Health Services
Ottawa Towers North
611 W. Ottawa, 4th Floor
Lansing, MI 48933
(517) 373-9102
Web Site: http://www.cis.state.mi.us/bhser/
    genover.htm

Minnesota Board of Nursing
2829 University Avenue, SE
Suite 500
Minneapolis, MN 55414
(612) 617-2270
Web Site: http://www.nursingboard.state.mn.us/

Mississippi Board of Nursing
1935 Lakeland Drive, Suite B
Jackson, MS 39216
(601) 987-4188
Web Site: http://www.msbn.state.ms.us/webtest

Missouri State Board of Nursing
3605 Missouri Boulevard
P.O. Box 656
Jefferson City, MO 65102-0656
(573) 751-0681
Web Site: http://www.ecodev.state.mo.us/pr/nursing/

Montana State Board of Nursing
301 South Park
Helena, MT 59620-0513
(406) 444-2071
Web Site: http://www.com.state.mt.us/License/POL/
    index.htm

Nebraska Health and Human Services System
Dept. of Regulation and Licensure, Nursing Section
301 Centennial Mall South, P.O. Box 94986
Lincoln, NE 68509-4986
(402) 471-4376
Web Site: http://www.hhs.state.ne.us/crl/nns.htm

Nevada State Board of Nursing
1755 East Plumb Lane
Suite 260
Reno, NV 89502
(775) 688-2620
Web Site: http://www.nursingboard.state.nv.us

New Hampshire Board of Nursing
78 Regional Drive, Building B
P.O. Box 3898
Concord, NH 03302
(603) 271-2323
Web Site: http://www.state.nh.us/nursing/

New Jersey Board of Nursing
124 Halsey Street, 6th Floor
P.O. Box 45010
Newark, NJ 07101
(973) 504-6586
Web Site: http://www.state.nj.us/lps/ca/medical.htm

New Mexico Board of Nursing
4206 Louisiana Boulevard, NE, Suite A
Albuquerque, NM 87109
(505) 841-8340
Web Site: http://www.state.nm.us/clients/nursing

New York State Board of Nursing
89 Washington Avenue
Education Building
2nd Floor West Wing
Albany, NY 12234
(518) 473-6999
Web Site: http://www.nysed.gov/prof/nurse.htm

North Carolina Board of Nursing
3724 National Drive, Suite 201
Raleigh, NC 27612
(919) 782-3211
Web Site: http://www.ncbon.com/

North Dakota Board of Nursing
919 South 7th Street, Suite 504
Bismarck, ND 58504
(701) 328-9777
Web Site: http://www.ndbon.org/

Ohio Board of Nursing
17 South High Street, Suite 400
Columbus, OH 43215-3413
(614) 466-3947
Web Site: http://www.state.oh.us/nur/

Oklahoma Board of Nursing
2915 N. Classen Boulevard, Suite 524
Oklahoma City, OK 73106
(405) 962-1800

Oregon State Board of Nursing
800 N.E. Oregon Street, Box 25
Suite 465
Portland, OR 97232
(503) 731-4745
Web Site: http://www.osbn.state.or.us/

Pennsylvania State Board of Nursing
124 Pine Street
P.O. Box 2649
Harrisburg, PA 17101
(717) 783-7142
Web Site: http://www.dos.state.pa.us/bpoa/nurbd/
    mainpage.htm

Commonwealth of Puerto Rico
Board of Nurse Examiners
800 Roberto H. Todd Avenue
Room 202, Stop 18
Santurce, PR 00908
(787) 725-8161

Rhode Island Board of Nurse Registration and Nursing
  Education
105 Cannon Building
Three Capitol Hill
Providence, RI 02908
(401) 222-5700
Web Site: http://www.health.state.ri.us

South Carolina State Board of Nursing
110 Centerview Drive
Suite 202
Columbia, SC 29210
(803) 896-4550
Web Site: http://www.llr.state.sc.us/pol/nursing

South Dakota Board of Nursing
4300 South Louise Avenue, Suite C-1
Sioux Falls, SD 57106-3124
(605) 362-2760
Web Site: http://www.state.sd.us/dcr/nursing/

Tennessee State Board of Nursing
426 Fifth Avenue North
1st Floor, Cordell Hull Building
Nashville, TN 37247
(615) 532-5166
Web Site: http://170.142.76.180/bmf-bin/
  BMFproflist.pl

Texas Board of Nurse Examiners
333 Guadalupe, Suite 3-460
Austin, TX 78701
(512) 305-7400
Web Site: http://www.bne.state.tx.us/

Utah State Board of Nursing
Heber M. Wells Building, 4th Floor
160 East 300 South
Salt Lake City, UT 84111
(801) 530-6628
Web Site: http://www.commerce.state.ut.us/

Vermont State Board of Nursing
109 State Street
Montpelier, VT 05609-1106
(802) 828-2396
Web Site: http://vtprofessionals.org/nurses/

Virgin Islands Board of Nurse Licensure
Veterans Drive Station
St. Thomas, VI 00803
(340) 776-7397

Virginia State Board of Nursing
6606 W. Broad Street, 4th Floor
Richmond, VA 23230
(804) 662-9909
Web Site: http://www.dhp.state.va.us/

Washington State Nursing Care
Quality Assurance Commission
Department of Health
1300 Quince Street SE
Olympia, WA 98504-7864
(360) 236-4740
Web Site: http://www.doh.wa.gov/nursing/

West Virginia Board of Examiners for Registered
  Professional Nurses
101 Dee Drive
Charleston, WV 25311
(304) 558-3596
Web Site: http://www.state.wv.us/nurses/rn/

Wisconsin Department of Regulation and Licensing
1400 E. Washington Avenue
P.O. Box 8935
Madison, WI 53708
(608) 266-0145
Web Site: http://www.drl.state.wi.us/

Wyoming State Board of Nursing
2020 Carey Avenue, Suite 110
Cheyenne, WY 82002
(307) 777-7601
Web Site: http://nursing.state.wy.us/

## REFERENCES

Hodgson, B., & Kizior, R. (2001). *Saunders Nursing drug handbook 2001.* Philadelphia: W.B. Saunders.

National Council of State Boards of Nursing (eds.) (2000). *Test plan for the National Council Licensure Examination for Registered Nurses.* Chicago: Author.

National Council of State Boards of Nursing (eds.) (2000). *The NCLEX process: Serving as an anchor for the NCLEX examination.* Chicago: Author.

National Council of State Boards of Nursing. Web Site: http://www.ncsbn.org/files/boards/boardscontact.asp

Smeltzer, S., & Bare, B. (2000) *Brunner & Suddarth's Textbook of medical-surgical nursing* (9th ed.). Philadelphia: Lippincott Williams & Wilkins.

Wong, D. (1999). *Whaley & Wong's Nursing care of infants and children* (6th ed.). St. Louis: Mosby.

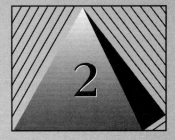

# 2

# Profiles to Success

LAURENT W. VALLIERE, B.S.

Preparing to take the National Council Licensure Examination (NCLEX-RN) can produce a great deal of anxiety in a nursing graduate. You may be thinking that the NCLEX-RN is the most important examination that you will ever have to take and that it reflects the culmination of everything that you have worked so hard for. NCLEX-RN is an important examination, because achieving that nursing license defines the beginning of your career as a registered nurse. A vital ingredient to your success on NCLEX-RN involves avoiding negative thoughts that allow this examination to seem overwhelming and intimidating. Such thoughts will take full control over your destiny.

Nursing graduates preparing for NCLEX-RN must develop a comprehensive plan to prepare for this examination. The most important component in developing a plan is to identify the study patterns that guided you to your nursing degree. It is important to begin your planning by reflecting on all of the personal and academic challenges you experienced during your nursing education. Take time to focus on the thoughts, feelings, and emotions that you experienced before taking an examination while in your nursing program. Examine the methods that you used in preparing for that examination both academically and from the standpoint of how you dealt with the anxiety that parallels the experience of facing an examination.

These factors are very important considerations in preparing for NCLEX-RN. The reason that these factors are so important is that they identify the patterns that worked for you. Think about this for a moment. Your own methods of study must have worked, or you would not be at the point of preparing for NCLEX-RN.

Each individual requires his or her own methods of preparing for an examination. Graduate nurses who have taken NCLEX-RN will probably share their experiences and methods of preparing for this challenge with you. It is very helpful to listen to what they may tell you.

These graduates will provide you with important strategies that they have used. Listen closely to what they have to say, but remember that this examination is all about you. Your identity and what you require in terms of preparation are most important.

Reflect on the methods and strategies that worked for you throughout your nursing program. Do not think that you need to develop new methods and strategies in preparing for NCLEX-RN. Use what has worked for you. Take some time to reflect on these strategies, write them down on a large blank card, sign your name, and write "R.N." after your name. Post this card in a place where you will see it every morning of every day. Commit to your own special strategies. These strategies reflect your profile and identity and will lead you to success!

A frequent concern of graduates preparing for NCLEX-RN relates to deciding whether they should study alone or become a part of a study group. Examining your profile will easily direct you in making this decision. Again, reflect on what has worked for you throughout your nursing program as you prepared for examinations. Remember, your needs are most important. Address your own needs and do not become pressured by peers who are encouraging you to join a study group, if this is not your normal pattern for study. Remember that additional pressure is not what you need at this important time of your life.

Nursing graduates preparing for NCLEX-RN frequently inquire about the best method of preparing for NCLEX-RN. First, remember that you are prepared. In fact, you began preparing for this examination on the first day you entered your nursing program.

The task you are faced with is to review, in a comprehensive manner, all of the nursing content that you learned in your nursing program. It can become totally overwhelming to look at your bookshelf, which is overflowing with the nursing books that you used during nursing school, and your challenge becomes monumental when you look at the boxes of nursing lecture notes that you have accumulated. It is unrealistic to even think that you could read all of those nursing books and lecture notes in preparation for NCLEX-RN. These books and lecture notes should be used as reference sources, if needed, during your preparation for NCLEX-RN.

*Saunders Comprehensive Review for NCLEX-RN* has identified for you all of the important nursing content areas relevant to the examination. During your comprehensive review, you should have noted the areas that may be unfamiliar or unclear. Be sure that you have taken the necessary time to become familiar with these needed areas. Now, progress through the Pyramid to Success and test your knowledge with this book, *Saunders Q & A Review for NCLEX-RN.* You may identify nursing content areas that still require further review. Take the time to review, as you are guided to do in this book.

Your profile to success requires that you develop realistic time goals to prepare for NCLEX-RN. It is essential to take the time to examine your life and all of the commitments that you may have. These commitments may include family, work, and friends. As you develop your goals, remember to plan time for fun and exercise. To achieve success, you require a balance of work time and enjoyment time. If you do not plan for some leisure time, you will become frustrated and perhaps even angry. These sorts of feelings will block your ability to focus and concentrate. Remember that you need time for yourself.

Goal development may be a relatively easy process, because you have probably been juggling your life commitments ever since you entered nursing school. Remember that your goal is to identify a daily time frame and time period for you to use in reviewing and preparing for NCLEX-RN. Open your calendar and identify days on which life commitments will not allow you to spend this time preparing. Block those days off and do not consider them as a part of your review time. Identify the time that is best for you in terms of your ability to concentrate and focus, so that you can accomplish the most in your identified time frame. Be sure that you consider a time that is quiet and free of distractions. Many individuals find that the morning hours are the most productive hours, whereas others find the afternoon and evening hours most productive. Remember that this examination is all about you, and select that time period that will be most conducive to your success.

The place of study is also very important. Select a place that is quiet and comfortable for study and a place where you normally do your studying and preparing. Some individuals prefer to study at home in their own environment; if this is your normal pattern, be sure that you are able to free yourself of distractions during your scheduled preparation time. If you are not able to free yourself of distractions, you may consider spending your preparation time in a library. Reflect on what worked best for you during your nursing program in selecting your place of study.

Selecting the amount of daily preparation time has frequently been a dilemma for many graduates preparing for NCLEX-RN. It is very important to set a realistic time period that can be adhered to on a daily basis. Set a time frame that will provide you with quality time and a time frame that can be achieved. If you set a time frame that is not realistic and cannot be achieved every day, you will become frustrated. This frustration will block your journey toward the peak of the Pyramid to Success.

The best suggestion to you is to spend at least 2 hours daily for NCLEX-RN preparation. Two hours is a realistic time period both in terms of quality time and in terms of a time frame that is achievable. You may find that after 2 hours your ability to focus and concentrate will diminish. You may, however, find that on some days you are able to spend more than the scheduled 2 hours; if you can and feel as though your ability to concentrate and focus is still present, then do so.

Discipline and perseverance will automatically bring control. Control will provide you with the momentum that will sweep you to the peak of the Pyramid to Success.

Discipline yourself to spend time preparing for NCLEX-RN every day. Daily preparation is very important because it maintains a consistent pattern and keeps you in synchrony with the mind flow needed the day you are scheduled to take the NCLEX-RN examination. Some days you may think about skipping your scheduled preparation time because you are not in the mood for study or because you just don't feel like studying.

On these days, practice discipline and persevere. Stand yourself up, shake off those thoughts of skipping a day of preparation, take a deep breath, and get the oxygen flowing throughout your body. Look in the mirror, smile, and say to yourself, "This time is for me, and I can do this!" Look at your card that displays your name with "R.N." after it, and get yourself to that special study place. Remember that discipline and perseverance will bring control!

In the profile to success, academic preparation directs the path to the peak of the Pyramid to Success. However, there are additional factors that will influence successful progression to the peak. These factors include your ability to control anxiety, physical stamina, the amount of rest and relaxation you have, your self-confidence, and the belief in yourself that you will achieve success on NCLEX-RN. You need to take time to think about these important factors and incorporate them into your daily preparation schedule.

Anxiety is a common concern among students preparing to take NCLEX-RN. Some anxiety is a normal feeling and will keep your senses sharp and alert. A great deal of anxiety, however, can block your process of thinking and hamper your ability to focus and concentrate. You have already practiced the task of controlling anxiety when you took examinations in nursing school. Now you need to continue with this practice and incorporate this control on a daily basis.

Each day, before beginning your scheduled preparation time, sit in your quiet special study place, close your eyes, and take a slow, deep breath. Fill your body with oxygen, hold your breath to a count of four, and then exhale slowly through your mouth. Continue with this exercise and repeat it four to six times. This exercise will help relieve your mind of any unnecessary chatter and will deliver oxygen to all of your body tissues and to your brain. On your scheduled day for the NCLEX-RN, after the necessary pretesting procedures, you will be escorted to your test computer. Practice this breathing exercise before beginning the examination. Use this exercise during the examination if you feel yourself becoming anxious and distracted and you are having difficulty focusing or concentrating. Remember that breathing will move the oxygen to your brain!

Physical stamina is an essential component of readiness for NCLEX-RN. Plan to incorporate a balance of exercise with adequate rest and relaxation time in your preparation schedule. It is also important that you maintain healthy eating habits. Begin to practice these healthy habits now, if you haven't already done so. There are a few points to keep in mind each day as you plan your daily meals. Three balanced meals are important, with snacks, such as fruits, included between meals. Remember that food items that contain fat will slow you down, and food items that contain caffeine will cause nervousness and sometimes shakiness. Avoid these items. Healthy foods that are high in carbohydrates work best to supply you with your energy needs. Remember that your brain can work like a muscle: it requires carbohydrates. In addition, be sure that you include those needed fruits and vegetables in your diet.

If you are the type of individual who is not a breakfast eater, work on changing that habit. Practice the habit of eating breakfast now, as you are preparing for NCLEX-RN. Attempt to provide your brain with energy in the morning with some form of carbohydrate food; it will make a difference. On your scheduled day for NCLEX-RN, feed your brain and eat a healthy breakfast. In addition, on this very important day, bring some form of snack, such as fruit or a bagel, for break time, and feed your brain again so that you will have the energy to concentrate, focus, and complete your examination.

Adequate rest, relaxation, and exercise are important in your preparation process. Many graduates preparing for NCLEX-RN have difficulty sleeping, particularly the night before the examination. Begin now to develop methods that will assist you in relaxing your body and mind and allow you to obtain a restful sleep. You may already have developed a particular method to help you sleep. If not, it may be helpful to try the breathing exercise while you lie in bed to eliminate any mind chatter that is present. It is also helpful to visualize your favorite and most peaceful place while you do the breathing exercise. Graduates have also stated that listening to quiet music and relaxation tapes has helped them relax and sleep. Begin to practice some of these helpful methods now, while you are preparing for NCLEX-RN. Identify those that work best for you. The night before your scheduled examination is an important one. Spend time having some fun, get to bed early, and incorporate the relaxation method that you have been using to help you sleep.

Confidence and belief that you have the ability to achieve success will bring your goals to fruition. Reflect on your profile maintained during your nursing education. Your confidence and belief in yourself, along with your academic achievements, have brought you to the status of graduate nurse. Now you are facing one more important challenge.

Can you meet this challenge successfully? Yes, you can! There is no reason to think otherwise, if you have taken all of the necessary steps to ensure that profile to success.

Each morning, place your feet on the floor, stand tall, take a deep breath, and smile. Take both hands and imagine yourself brushing off any negative feelings. Look at your card that bears your name with the letters "R.N." after it, and tell yourself, "Yes, I can do this successfully!"

Believe in yourself, and you will reach the peak of the Pyramid to Success! Congratulations, and I wish you continued success in your career as a registered nurse.

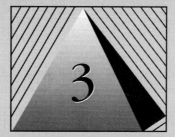

# The NCLEX-RN Examination: From a Student's Perspective

JESSICA BIANCO, R.N.

It's a Sunday morning and it's Graduation Day! The sun is shining through my bedroom blinds. I roll over in bed. Five more minutes until my alarm goes off. For most of the night I have been awake, too excited to sleep. My years of hard work and dedication have brought this joyous day. Today is "my big day." Finally the alarm buzzes, officially signifying the start of the day. I slide out of bed in a dreamlike state and begin to get ready.

As I step out of the house, I notice that there is not a single cloud floating in the deep blue sky. The brilliant sun warming my face comforts me, and the soft, subtle breeze feels refreshing.

Soon thereafter, I join my peers for the graduation procession. They too share my excitement. Before I realize it, the graduation ceremony is over. I ask myself, could it really be over so quickly? My peers and I are smiling, throwing our graduation caps up in the air, screaming, "We did it!"

I feel as though so much weight is lifted off my shoulders. I can't wait to celebrate. I skip up to my large group of family and friends eagerly waiting for me outside. I find my father first. He gives me a big bear hug and plants a kiss on my forehead. He looks me in the eye and says, "Honey, I want you to know that your Mom and I are very proud of you. You have far surpassed our expectations over these past 4 years." Tears well up in my eyes. He gives my hand a squeeze as he continues, "So now that you have graduated from nursing school, when are you going to take the boards?"

I want to scream and think, is that all anyone cares about? Immediately, I feel the weight back on my shoulders.

Sound familiar? If you are able to relate to this scenario, let me first congratulate you on your graduation from nursing school. Second, if you made it this far, take a deep breath and relax. Despite the terrifying rumors you may have heard about the NCLEX-RN

examination, I want to assure you that if you prepare as you need to, you will certainly be successful.

The first major step in preparing for the NCLEX-RN examination is making the commitment to review and study. After 2, 3, or 4 years of college, you know your study habits best. You need to commit to a study plan that complements your own study style, whether it be group studying at the library or studying alone at a desk or special place at home.

I tend to be a procrastinator and knew that I needed to make a commitment to study and discipline myself. A friend from nursing school and I decided to take the examination on the same day. So we communicated, took out a calendar and set up our study schedule, and, as soon as we received our Authorization to Test forms, scheduled an appointment to take the NCLEX-RN examination. Although we were physically separated by nine states, using the "buddy system" was a mental motivator. We communicated every day and encouraged each other to study and stay on track with our study schedule. It was helpful and reassuring to have someone to talk to who could personally identify with the anxieties, fears, and pressures that encompass preparing for and taking the NCLEX-RN examination.

As you well know, there is a vast amount of information to review. Throughout nursing school, I kept my textbooks with the thought that I would use them to study for the NCLEX-RN examination. However, I was overwhelmed when I saw at least 10 textbooks piled up in front of me. I knew that it was impossible to review from these textbooks and that this was not the way to prepare for this examination. So I took these textbooks, moved then to a special area in my special study place, and placed a sign reading "references" on top of the pile of books.

I selected an NCLEX-RN review book to prepare for this examination. I referred to my textbooks if I did not understand the information or was unfamiliar with the content presented in the review book. I reviewed from the *Saunders Pyramid to Success* program. These review resources provide a comprehensive review and thousands of NCLEX-RN–style questions. I believe that the key to success with this examination is to practice as many questions as you can. You will not only master the content but will also develop mastery in test-taking strategies. I spent 2 hours each day reviewing and practicing test questions. As I encountered content that I was unfamiliar with, I took notes. At the end of my 2-hour session, I went to my "reference" pile of textbooks and reviewed these needed areas.

I started my review sessions with the *Saunders Comprehensive Review for NCLEX-RN*. When I finished the questions in that book and on the CD-ROM that accompanied that book, I moved up the Pyramid to Success and reviewed from the *Saunders Q & A Review for NCLEX-RN*. Two weeks before my scheduled testing date, I started the *Saunders Computerized Review for NCLEX-RN*. The questions on this CD-ROM reinforced my knowledge and test-taking abilities and determined my readiness for the NCLEX-RN examination. I was able to identify any final areas that I needed to review.

The day before the NCLEX-RN examination, I put my review books and my pile of textbooks in a closet so that I could not see them. I tried not to think about anything related to nursing. And after all the reviewing that I did, I felt prepared for the challenge. Surprisingly, I was relieved that this important examination was now only a day away. I relaxed, spent time with friends, and made my final preparations for success.

It is important to try to get adequate sleep the night before the examination. I practiced relaxation techniques and deep breathing exercises. After a good night's sleep, I woke up excited and anxious to meet the challenge of this examination and have this day behind me. I ate a healthy breakfast, making sure I steered clear of any fatty foods, knowing that they would slow down my thought processes.

I drove myself to the testing center, knowing my destination exactly because I had done a test drive a few days earlier. I was the first person to arrive at the testing center. In fact, the doors were still locked. As I waited outside, I observed other test takers arriving. I took slow, deep breaths to relax myself. Within a few minutes, the door to my future opened.

I sat in the lobby with eight or nine other individuals of various ages. However, not all of these individuals were at the testing center to take the NCLEX-RN examination. It is important to remember that the testing center administers examinations other than the NCLEX-RN. Hearing individuals who start the test at the same time as you do leaving long before your time of completion can cause anxiety. Remembering that they are most likely taking different examinations is helpful in avoiding anxious feelings related to the need to "speed up and finish."

I entered an office and was asked to have a seat in front of the camera. My identification was checked and my picture was taken. I then followed the proctor into the computer testing room. The room was smaller than I had imagined it would be. There were 25 computers in cubicles lined up in five rows. I was seated at a computer with my picture on the screen. I was given a pencil, scrap paper, and earplugs. The proctor wished me good luck. I took a deep breath, put the earplugs in my ears, and followed the instructions on the computer screen in front of me.

As I began to answer questions, I felt really comfortable and well prepared because of all the practice questions I had done. When I encountered a really difficult question, I remembered that the answer was right there in front of me. I read the question carefully and reviewed the stem of the question, making sure that I understood what the question was asking. It is important to use the process of elimination, and when you get to two possible options, read the question again and use your test-taking strategies to help you. Before I knew it, I had answered question number 75, and the computer shut off. I was incredibly relieved at that moment. I did not have negative feelings about my performance. I felt I had done well.

I drove home smiling. I called my family and friends to tell them how the examination went. My "buddy" called me to let me know that her computer had also shut off after 75 questions.

I felt that waiting for the test results was more difficult than taking the examination. The results arrived by mail approximately 12 days after I took the examination. Some states provide results through the Internet. In fact, I was able to obtain my test result in this way. When I saw my name on the screen next to an R.N. license number, I couldn't believe it. I had to double-check to make sure I was reading correctly!

Passing the NCLEX-RN examination was an extremely rewarding and challenging experience. It is the final step to becoming a registered nurse. Starting your new career will also be exciting. Your learning is never-ending, and exciting new experiences will arise every day, challenging you.

Put effort and pride into all that you have accomplished. Maintain a positive attitude and self-confidence. It is most important to relax and try to keep things in perspective. Believe in yourself and you will accomplish your goals and reach the peak of the Pyramid to Success, just as I did!

Congratulations to you, and I wish you the best in your career as a registered nurse!

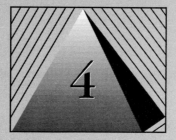

# Test-Taking Strategies

I.
I. Pyramid to Success (Box 4-1)
II. How to Avoid Reading into the Question
  A. Pyramid Points
    1. Identify the case situation from the stem of the question
    2. Identify what the question is asking
    3. Look for the key words
    4. Read every option
    5. Use the process of elimination
    6. As you read the question, avoid asking yourself, "What if . . . ?"
  B. The Case Situation (Box 4-2)
    1. The case situation provides you with the information about a clinical health problem and the information that you need to consider in answering the question
    2. Read all of the information and every word in the case situation
  C. The Stem of the Question (see Box 4-2)
    1. The stem of the question follows the case situation and asks something specific about the case situation
    2. Read the stem carefully, and specifically identify exactly what is being asked
  D. The Options (see Box 4-2)
    1. The options are all of the answers, and you must select one
    2. Read every option carefully, and reread the stem of the question to be sure that you understand what is being asked
    3. Use the process of elimination
    4. Once you have eliminated two incorrect options, reread the stem of the question again to identify specifically what the question is asking, before selecting the correct option
III. Key Words (Box 4-3)
  A. Key words focus your attention on critical ideas in the case situation, the stem, and the options
  B. Key words are important to identify because they will assist in eliminating the incorrect options (Box 4-4)
  C. Some of the key words may indicate that all of the options are correct and that it will be necessary to prioritize to select the correct option
IV. The Client of the Question
  A. Identify the client of the question

---

**BOX 4-1**

**Pyramid to Success**

Read the question and every option thoroughly and carefully!
Ask yourself, "What is the question specifically asking?"
Be alert to key words and true and false response stems!
Eliminate the incorrect options!
Use all of your nursing knowledge, your clinical experiences, and your test-taking skills and strategies to answer the question!

---

**BOX 4-2**

**Case Situation, Stem, and Options**

**Case Situation:** A client arrives in the surgical unit following nasal surgery. The client has nasal packing in place.

**Stem:** A nurse reviews the physician's orders and anticipates that which of the following client positions would be prescribed to reduce swelling?

**Options:**
1. Sims'
2. Prone
3. Supine
4. Semi-Fowler's

---

**BOX 4-3**

**Common Key Words**

Early or late
Best
First
Initial
Immediately
Most likely or least likely
Most appropriate or least appropriate
On the day of
After several days

---

**BOX 4-4**

**Use of Key Words to Eliminate Incorrect Options**

Noting the key words in each of these situations will
assist in directing you to select the correct option:
Which of the following is an *early sign* of shock?
Which of the following is a *late sign* of shock?
*On the day of* surgery, following a transurethral resection of the prostate (TURP), the nurse notes that the
client's urine is bright red in color. Which of the following nursing actions is *most appropriate?*
*After several days,* following a transurethral resection of
the prostate (TURP), the nurse notes that the client's
urine is bright red in color. Which of the following
nursing actions is *most appropriate?*
The *early* signs of shock are quite different from the *late*
signs of shock.
Bright red urine might be expected *on the day of*
surgery following a transurethral resection of the
prostate (TURP), but would not be expected *after
several days.*

---

**BOX 4-5**

**The Issue of the Question**

A pediatric nurse in the ambulatory care unit is caring for
a child after a tonsillectomy. The mother of the child tells a
nurse that the child is complaining of a dry throat and
would like something to relieve the dryness. Which of the
following would the nurse give to the mother for the
child?
1. Cool cherry Kool-Aid
2. A glass of milk
3. Cola with ice
4. Yellow noncitrus Jell-O

**Answer: 4**

**Test-Taking Strategy:** The issue of the question relates to
the foods and fluids that should be avoided following
tonsillectomy. Focusing on the issue and thinking about
the food items that irritate the throat will direct you to
the correct option.

---

**BOX 4-6**

**True Response Stem**

A community health nurse is providing an educational
session to community members regarding dietary measures that will assist in reducing the risk of osteoporosis.
The nurse instructs the community members to increase
dietary intake of which food that would be most helpful
to minimize this risk?
1. Yogurt
2. Turkey
3. Spaghetti
4. Shellfish

**Answer: 1**

**Test-Taking Strategy:** Note the key words *most helpful.*
Recall that in a client with osteoporosis, calcium intake
should be increased. This will assist in directing you to
option 1.

---

B. The client is the person who is the focus of the
question
C. It is important to remember that the client of
the question may not necessarily be the person
with the health problem; in the test question,
the client may be a relative, friend, spouse,
significant other, or another member of the
health care team
D. After identifying the client of the question,
select the option that relates to and most
directly addresses that client
V. The Issue of the Question (Box 4-5)
A. Identify the issue of the question
B. The issue of the question is the specific subject
content that the question is asking about
C. Identifying the issue of the question will assist
in eliminating the incorrect options and direct
you to selecting the correct option
D. The issue of the question can include
1. A medication or intravenous (IV) therapy
2. A side effect of a medication
3. An adverse or toxic effect of a medication
4. A treatment or procedure
5. A complication of a health care problem,
treatment, or procedure
6. A specific nursing action
VI. True or False Response Stems
A. True Response Stem (Box 4-6)
1. True response stems use key words that ask
you to select an option that is true regarding
the case situation in the question
2. Common key words used in a true response stem
a. Most or most appropriate
b. Most likely
c. Most helpful
d. Best
e. Best judgment
f. Initial
g. First

## BOX 4-7

### False Response Stem

A nurse has provided instructions to a client with glaucoma regarding measures that will prevent an increase in intraocular pressure. Which statement, if made by the client, indicates a need for further education?
1. "I should limit my fluid intake to prevent an increase in pressure."
2. "I should eat foods that are high in fiber."
3. "I should avoid lifting objects that weigh more than 20 pounds."
4. "I should move objects by using my feet and pushing them rather than lifting them."

**Answer: 1**

**Test-Taking Strategy:** Note the key words *indicates a need for further education.* These key words indicate that you need to select an option that identifies an incorrect client statement. Recall that an increase in intraocular pressure is a concern. Using principles related to activities that will increase intraocular pressure will direct you to option 1.

## BOX 4-8

### Prioritizing: Maslow's Hierarchy of Needs Theory

A neighborhood nurse is attending a football game at a local high school. One of the high school students falls off the bleachers and sustains an injury to the left arm. The nurse quickly attends to the child and suspects that the child's arm may be broken. Which nursing action would be of highest priority before transferring the child to the emergency room?
1. Tell the child that the arm is probably fractured but not to worry because permanent damage to the arm will not occur
2. Immobilize the arm
3. Ask the child the name of his or her pediatrician so that he or she can be contacted
4. Have someone call the radiology department of the local hospital to let them know that the child will be arriving

**Answer: 2**

**Test-Taking Strategy:** Note the key words *highest priority* in the stem of the question. Use Maslow's Hierarchy of Needs theory to prioritize, remembering that physiological needs come first. Using this guideline will direct you to option 2. Immobilizing the arm is a physiological need and the priority nursing action.

  h. Chief
  i. Immediate
 B. False Response Stem (Box 4-7)
  1. False response stems use key words that ask you to select an option that is NOT true regarding the case situation in the question
  2. Common key words used in a false response stem
   a. Except or not
   b. Least likely
   c. Need for further instructions or education
   d. Lowest priority
   e. Incorrect
   f. Unsafe
VII. Questions that Require Prioritizing
 A. Identify the key words in the question that indicate the need to prioritize
 B. Common key words
  1. Initial
  2. Essential
  3. Vital
  4. Immediate
  5. Highest
  6. Best
  7. Most
  8. Priority
 C. Use Maslow's Hierarchy of Needs theory as a guide to prioritize (Box 4-8)
  1. Physiological needs come FIRST; select an option that addresses a physiological need
  2. When a physiological need is not addressed in the question or noted in one of the

## BOX 4-9

### Prioritizing: Use of the ABCs

A nurse is preparing to suction a client's tracheostomy tube. The nurse gathers the supplies needed for the procedure and prepares to suction the tube. Which of the following is the initial nursing action?
1. Set the suction pressure range at 150 mm Hg
2. Hyperoxygenate the client's lungs
3. Place a catheter into the tracheostomy tube and apply suction while advancing it
4. Insert normal saline solution into the tracheostomy tube after the suction catheter has been inserted

**Answer: 2**

**Test-Taking Strategy:** Note the key word *initial* in the stem of the question. Use the ABCs—airway, breathing, and circulation—as a guide to direct you to the correct option. Recall that suctioning will remove oxygen from the client's system. The correct option addresses airway.

  options, safety needs receive priority; select an option that addresses safety
 D. ABCs: Airway, Breathing, and Circulation (Box 4-9)
  1. Use the ABCs when selecting an option
  2. Remember the order of priority: airway, breathing, and circulation
 E. Nursing Process (Box 4-10)
  1. Guidelines
   a. Use the steps of the Nursing Process to prioritize

---

### BOX 4-10

**Steps of the Nursing Process**

1. Assessment
2. Analysis
3. Planning
4. Implementation
5. Evaluation

Use the Nursing Process to answer questions.
Follow the steps of the Nursing Process to select an option.
The first step of the Nursing Process is assessment.
When the question asks you what the nurse's initial, first, or most appropriate action is, select the option that relates to assessment of the client.

---

### BOX 4-11

**Nursing Process: Assessment**

A client with multiple sclerosis tells a home health care nurse that she is having increasing difficulty in transferring from the bed to a chair. The home health care nurse would initially:

1. Observe the client demonstrating the transfer technique
2. Document the number of falls that the client has had in recent weeks
3. Discuss potential nursing home placement
4. Start a restorative nursing program before an injury occurs

**Answer: 1**

**Test-Taking Strategy:** Use the steps of the Nursing Process to answer this question. Assessment is the first step. Options 2, 3, and 4 identify the implementation step of the nursing process. The initial action is to observe the client demonstrating the transfer technique.

---

### BOX 4-12

**Assessment: Key Words**

Ascertain
Assess
Check
Determine
Find out
Identify
Monitor
Observe
Obtain information

---

### BOX 4-13

**Nursing Process: Analysis**

A nurse is reviewing the laboratory results of an infant suspected of having hypertrophic pyloric stenosis. Which of the following laboratory findings would the nurse most likely expect to note in this infant?

1. A blood pH of 7.50
2. A blood pH of 7.30
3. A blood bicarbonate of 22 mEq/L
4. A blood bicarbonate of 19 mEq/L

**Answer: 1**

**Test-Taking Strategy:** It is necessary to understand the physiology associated with hypertrophic pyloric stenosis and that metabolic alkalosis is likely to occur as a result of vomiting. Next, it is necessary to know which laboratory findings would be noted in this acid-base condition. Analysis of this information will direct you to the correct option.

---

b. Remember that assessment is the first step of the Nursing Process
c. When you are asked to select your first or initial nursing action, follow the steps of the Nursing Process to select the correct option
d. If an option contains the concept of assessment or the collection of client data, select that option

2. Assessment (Box 4-11)
   a. Assessment questions address the process of gathering subjective and objective data relative to the client, confirming the data, and communicating and documenting the data
   b. When answering questions that focus on assessment, look for key words in the options that reflect assessment (Box 4-12)

3. Analysis (Box 4-13)
   a. Analysis questions are the most difficult questions because they require under-standing of the principles of physiological responses and require interpretation of the data based on assessment
   b. Analysis questions require critical thinking and determining the rationale for therapeutic interventions that may be addressed in the case situation
   c. Analysis questions may address the formulation of a nursing diagnosis and the communication and documentation of the results of the process of analysis

4. Planning (Box 4-14)
   a. Planning questions require prioritizing nursing diagnoses, determining goals of care and outcome criteria for goals of care, developing the plan of care, and communicating and documenting the plan of care
   b. Remember that this is a nursing examination and that the answer to the question most likely involves something that is included in the nursing care plan, rather than the medical plan

5. Implementation (Box 4-15)
   a. This exam is about NURSING, so focus

## BOX 4-14

### Nursing Process: Planning

A client is being discharged from the hospital after being treated for infective endocarditis. A nurse includes which most appropriate intervention in the discharge plan of care?
1. Take acetaminophen (Tylenol) if the chest pain worsens
2. Use a firm-bristle toothbrush and floss vigorously to prevent cavities
3. Take antibiotics until the chest pain is fully resolved
4. Notify all health care providers of the history of infective endocarditis before any invasive procedures

**Answer: 4**

**Test-Taking Strategy:** Planning questions include developing the plan of care and determining goals and outcome criteria for goals of care. Focus on the client's diagnosis and the risks associated with this disorder. Note that both the question and the correct option address infective endocarditis.

## BOX 4-15

### Nursing Process: Implementation

A client is being admitted to the hospital after receiving a radium implant for bladder cancer. A nurse would take which priority action in the care of this client?
1. Encourage the client to take frequent rest periods
2. Admit the client to a private room
3. Encourage the family to visit
4. Place the client in reverse isolation

**Answer: 2**

**Test-Taking Strategy:** Implementation questions address the process of organizing and managing care and providing care to achieve established goals. The client who has a radium implant is placed in a private room and has limited visitors. This reduces the exposure of others to the radiation. Frequent rest periods are a helpful general intervention but are not a priority for the client in this situation. Reverse isolation is unnecessary.

## BOX 4-16

### Nursing Process: Evaluation

A home health nurse is reviewing medications with a client receiving colchicine for the treatment of gout. The nurse concludes that the medication is effective if the client reports a decrease in:
1. Blood glucose
2. Blood pressure
3. Joint inflammation
4. Headaches

**Answer: 3**

**Test-Taking Strategy:** This is an evaluation question and contains a true response stem as identified by the words *medication is effective.* In this question, focusing on the client's diagnosis and recalling the pathophysiology associated with gout will direct you to option 3.

d. When you are answering a question, remember that this client is your only assigned client
e. Answer the question as if the situation were textbook and ideal, and the nurse had all the time and resources needed and readily available at the client's bedside
6. Evaluation (Box 4-16)
a. Evaluation questions focus on comparing the actual outcomes of care with the expected outcomes
b. Evaluation questions address evaluating the client's ability to implement self-care, health care team members' ability to implement care, and the process of communicating and documenting evaluation findings
c. Evaluation questions also focus on how the nurse should monitor or make a judgment concerning a client's response to therapy or to a nursing action
d. In an evaluation question, be alert to false response stems, because they are frequently used in evaluation-type questions, and the question may ask for a client statement that indicates either accurate or inaccurate information related to the issue of the question
VIII. Client Needs
A. Safe, Effective Care Environment
1. These questions address the provision that the nurse provides and directs care that will ensure an environment that promotes protecting the client, family or significant others, and other health care personnel
2. Content addressed in these questions relates to the nursing role of coordinating and

on the nursing action rather than on the medical action, unless the question is asking you what prescribed medical action is anticipated
b. Implementation questions address the process of organizing and managing care, counseling and teaching, providing care to achieve established goals, supervising and coordinating care, and communicating and documenting nursing interventions
c. On NCLEX-RN, the only client that you need to be concerned about is the client in the question that you are answering

integrating cost-effective care, supervising and/or collaborating with members of the multidisciplinary health care team, and environmental safety

3. Be alert to safety needs addressed in a question and remember the importance of hand washing, call bells, bed positioning, and the appropriate use of side rails

B. Physiological Integrity

1. These questions address the provision that the nurse promotes physical health and well-being in the client by providing care and comfort, reducing client risk potential, and managing the client's health alterations

2. Content addressed in these questions relates to basic care and comfort, pharmacological and parenteral therapies, reducing the risk of the development of complications, and managing and providing care to clients with acute, chronic, or life-threatening conditions

3. Remember that physiological needs are a priority and are addressed first

4. Use the ABCs—airway, breathing, and circulation—and the steps of the Nursing Process when selecting an option addressing physiological integrity

C. Psychosocial Integrity

1. These questions address the provision that the nurse provides nursing care that supports and promotes the emotional, mental, and social well-being of the client and significant others

2. Content addressed in these questions relates to promoting the client's or significant others' ability to cope, adapt, or problem solve in situations such as illness or stressful events, and providing care to clients with maladaptive behavior or acute or chronic mental illness

3. Communication Questions (Table 4-1)
   a. Identify the use of therapeutic communication techniques
   b. Use of therapeutic communication techniques indicates a CORRECT option
   c. Use of nontherapeutic communication techniques indicates an INCORRECT option
   d. Always focus on the client's feelings first; if an option reflects the client's feelings, select that option as the answer to the question (Box 4-17)

D. Health Promotion and Maintenance

1. These questions address the provision that the nurse provides and directs care that

prevents health problems, provides early detection of health problems, and provides and directs care that incorporates knowledge of expected growth and development principles

2. Content addressed in these questions relates to assisting the client and significant others through the normal stages of growth and development, and assisting the client and significant others to develop health

---

**TABLE 4-1**

Therapeutic and Nontherapeutic Communication Techniques

| Therapeutic | Nontherapeutic |
|---|---|
| Being silent | Giving advice |
| Offering self for assistance | Showing approval or disapproval |
| Showing empathy | Using cliches and false reassurance |
| Focusing | Requesting an explanation: "Why?" |
| Restatement | Devaluing client feelings |
| Validation/clarification | Being defensive |
| Giving information | Focusing on inappropriate issues or persons |
| Dealing with the here and now | Placing the client's issues on "hold" |

Always focus on the client's feelings FIRST!
If an answer reflects the client's feelings, select that answer!

---

**BOX 4-17**

**Focusing on the Client's Feelings**

A client is admitted to the emergency department with an acute anterior wall myocardial infarction. A nurse discusses streptokinase (Streptase) therapy with the client and the spouse. The spouse is concerned about the dangers of this treatment. Which of the following statements by the nurse to the spouse is most appropriate?

1. "Your loved one is very ill. The physician has made the best decision for you."
2. "There is no reason to worry. We use this medication all of the time."
3. "I'm certain you made the correct decision to use this medication."
4. "You have concerns about whether this treatment is the best option."

**Answer: 4**

**Test-Taking Strategy:** Paraphrasing is restating the client or family member's own words. Option 1 denies the person's right to an opinion. Option 2 is offering a false reassurance. In option 3 the nurse is expressing approval, which can be harmful to the client-nurse or family-nurse relationship. Option 4 is the only option that is therapeutic and addresses feelings.

practices that promote wellness and to recognize alterations in health care status

3. Use Teaching/Learning Theory if the question addresses client education, remembering that client motivation and client readiness to learn are the FIRST priority

4. Be alert to false response stems with questions that address health promotion and maintenance

IX. Pyramid Points (Box 4-18)

A. Unfamiliar Content

1. Answer questions by using your nursing knowledge, clinical experiences, and test-taking skills and strategies

2. If the content of the question is unfamiliar and you are unable to answer the question by using your nursing knowledge, look for a global option, similar distracters, or similar words, behaviors, thoughts, or feelings in the question and in one of the options

B. Global Option (Box 4-19)

1. When more than one option appears to be correct, look for a global option

2. A global option is one that is a general statement and may include the ideas of the other options within it

C. Similar Distracters

1. If you don't know the answer, try looking for similar distracters

2. Remember that there is only ONE correct option

3. If two options say the same thing or include the same idea, then NEITHER OF THESE OPTIONS can be correct

4. The answer to the question is the option that is different

D. Similar Words, Behaviors, Thoughts, or Feelings

1. If you do not know the answer, look for a similar word, behavior, thought, or feeling used in the case situation or the stem of the question and in one of the options

2. If you find a word, behavior, thought, or feeling that is used in the case situation or the stem of the question and is repeated in one of the options, that option MAY be the correct one

E. Pharmacology Questions

1. If you are familiar with the medication, use nursing knowledge to answer the question

2. Remember that the question will identify both the generic name and the trade name of the medication

3. If the case situation identifies a diagnosis, then you can make a relationship between the medication and the diagnosis; for example, you can determine that cyclophos-

---

**BOX 4-18**

**Pyramid Points**

▲ If the question asks for an immediate action or response, all options may be correct; therefore base your selection on priorities.

▲ Reword a difficult question, but if you do so, be careful not to change the intent of the question.

▲ Relate the situation to something that you are familiar with and try to visualize the client as you go through the case situation and the question.

▲ If there are words in the case situation or stem of the question that are unfamiliar, try to figure out the meaning in terms of the context of the sentence or break down the word and use medical terminology skills.

▲ If one option includes qualifiers such as *generally, usually, tends to, possibly,* or *may* and other options do not, select that option.

▲ Absolute terms such as *always, never, all, every, none, must,* and *only* tend to make an option incorrect.

▲ With medication calculations, talk yourself through each step and be sure the answer makes sense; recheck the calculation before selecting an option, particularly if the answer seems like an unusual dosage.

Remember, the only client you need to be concerned about is the one in the question you are answering. Answer the question as if the situation were ideal and the nurse had all the time and resources readily available at the client's bedside. Pace yourself, concentrate, and focus on one item at a time; if you find yourself becoming distracted, take a few minutes to breathe deeply and then refocus.

SMILE!
BELIEF!
CONFIDENCE!
CONTROL!
SUCCESS!

---

**BOX 4-19**

**Global Option**

A nurse is developing a plan of care for a client with a diagnosis of Ménière's disease who is being admitted to the hospital. The priority nursing intervention in the plan of care would focus on which of the following?

1. Safety measures
2. Activity limitations
3. Knowledge about medication therapy
4. Food items to avoid

**Answer: 1**

**Test-Taking Strategy:** Focus on the client's disorder, Ménière's disease. All of the options identify a component of the plan of care for this client. Remember that safety is a priority and note that option 1 identifies the global option.

phamide (Cytoxan) is an antineoplastic medication if the question refers to a client with breast cancer taking this particular medication

4. Try to determine the classification of the medication being addressed to assist in answering the question; identifying the classification will assist in determining a medication's action and/or side effects (Cardiazem is a cardiac medication)

5. Use medical terminology and break the name of the medication into parts. For example, Lopressor can be broken down into *Lo* and *pressor*, meaning lowering the blood pressure

6. Look at the prefix and/or suffix of the medication name: *ase* indicates an enzyme, *sone* indicates a corticosteroid; *line* indicates a bronchodilator, and *lol* indicates a beta-blocker

7. General Principles to Remember
   a. Clients are instructed to avoid alcohol with medications
   b. Capsules and sustained-released medications are not to be crushed
   c. The nurse never adjusts or changes the client's medication dosage and never discontinues a medication
   d. Medications are never administered if the order is difficult to read, is unclear, or identifies a medication dose that is not a normal one

## REFERENCES

Clark, M.J. (1999). *Nursing in the community: Dimensions of community health nursing* (3rd ed.). Stamford, Conn.: Appleton & Lange.

Corbett, J. (2000). *Laboratory tests and diagnostic procedures* (5th ed.). Upper Saddle River: N.J.: Prentice-Hall.

Elkin, M., Perry, A., & Potter, P. (2000). *Nursing interventions and clinical skills* (2nd ed.). St. Louis: Mosby.

Fortinash, K., & Holoday-Worret, P. (2000). *Psychiatric mental health nursing* (2nd ed.). St. Louis: Mosby.

Hodgson, B., & Kizior, R. (2001). *Saunders nursing drug handbook 2001.* Philadelphia: W.B. Saunders.

Ignatavicius, D., Workman, M., & Mishler, M. (1999). *Medical-surgical nursing across the health care continuum* (3rd ed.). Philadelphia: W.B. Saunders.

National Council of State Boards of Nursing (eds.) (2000). *Test plan for the National Council Licensure Examination for Registered Nurses.* Chicago: Author.

Potter, P., & Perry, A. (2001). *Fundamentals of nursing* (5th ed.). St. Louis: Mosby.

Riley, J. (2000). *Communication in nursing* (4th ed.). St. Louis: Mosby.

Smeltzer, S., & Bare, B. (2000). *Brunner & Suddarth's Textbook of medical-surgical nursing* (9th ed.). Philadelphia: Lippincott Williams & Wilkins.

Wong, D. (1999). *Whaley & Wong's Nursing care of infants and children* (6th ed.). St. Louis: Mosby.

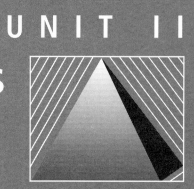

# UNIT II
# Client Needs

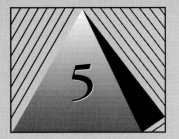

# Client Needs and the NCLEX-RN Test Plan

In the new Test Plan implemented in April 2001, the National Council of State Boards of Nursing has identified a test plan framework based on *Client Needs.* This framework was selected on the basis of the findings in a practice analysis study of newly licensed registered nurses in the United States. This study identified the nursing activities performed by entry-level nurses. Also, the Client Needs categories identified by the National Council of State Boards of Nursing provides a structure for defining nursing actions and competencies across all settings for all clients. The National Council of State Boards of Nursing identifies four major categories of Client Needs. These categories are further divided into subcategories, and the percentage of test questions in each subcategory is identified (Table 5-1).

## SAFE, EFFECTIVE CARE ENVIRONMENT

The Safe, Effective Care Environment category addresses content related to the nurse's role in providing and directing nursing care that promotes the achievement of client outcomes and protects the client, family or significant others, and health care personnel from environmental hazards. The Safe, Effective Care Environment category includes two subcategories: Management of Care and Safety and Infection Control.

The National Council of State Boards of Nursing identifies nursing content related to the subcategories of this Client Needs category (Box 5-1). Management of Care (7% to 13%) addresses content that tests the knowledge, skills, and ability required to provide integrated, cost-effective care to clients by coordinating, supervising, and/or collaborating with members of the multidisciplinary health care team. Safety and Infection Control (5% to 11%) addresses content that tests the knowledge, skills, and ability required to protect clients

| TABLE 5-1 | |
|---|---|
| Client Needs and the Percentage of Test Questions | |
| **SAFE, EFFECTIVE CARE ENVIRONMENT** | **PERCENTAGE (%)** |
| Management of care | 7-13 |
| Safety and infection control | 5-11 |
| | |
| **PHYSIOLOGICAL INTEGRITY** | |
| Basic care and comfort | 7-13 |
| Pharmacological and parenteral therapies | 5-11 |
| Reduction of risk potential | 12-18 |
| Physiological adaptation | 12-18 |
| | |
| **PSYCHOSOCIAL INTEGRITY** | |
| Coping and adaptation | 5-11 |
| Psychosocial adaptation | 5-11 |
| | |
| **HEALTH PROMOTION AND MAINTENANCE** | |
| Growth and development through the life span | 7-13 |
| Prevention and early detection of health problems | 5-11 |

From National Council of State Boards of Nursing (eds.) (2000). *Test plan for the National Council Licensure Examination for Registered Nurses.* Chicago: Author.

and health care personnel from environmental hazards (Box 5-2). Refer to Chapter 6 for practice questions reflective of this Client Needs category.

## PHYSIOLOGICAL INTEGRITY

The Physiological Integrity category addresses content related to the nurse's role in providing care and comfort to promote physical health and well-being, reduce the client's risk potential, and manage the client's health alterations. The Physiological Integrity category includes

---

**BOX 5-1**

### NCLEX-RN Content: Safe, Effective Care Environment

| | |
|---|---|
| **MANAGEMENT OF CARE** | Informed consent |
| Advance directives | Organ donation |
| Advocacy | Referrals |
| Case management | Resource management |
| Client rights | |
| Concepts of management | **SAFETY AND INFECTION CONTROL** |
| Confidentiality | Accident prevention |
| Consultation with members of the health care team | Disaster planning |
| Continuity of care | Error prevention |
| Continuous quality improvement | Handling hazardous and infectious materials |
| Delegation and supervision | Medical and surgical asepsis |
| Establishing priorities | Standard (universal) and other precautions |
| Ethical practice and legal responsibilities | Use of restraints |
| Incident/irregular occurrence/variance reports | |

From National Council of State Boards of Nursing (eds.) (2000). *Test Plan for the National Council Licensure Examination for Registered Nurses.* Chicago: Author.

---

**BOX 5-2**

### Safe, Effective Care Environment Questions

**MANAGEMENT OF CARE**

A registered nurse is delegating activities to a nursing staff. Which activity is least appropriate for a nursing assistant?
1. Assisting a 12-year-old boy who is profoundly developmentally disabled to eat lunch
2. Obtaining frequent oral temperatures on a client
3. Accompanying a 51-year-old man, being discharged to home following a bowel resection 8 days ago, to his transportation
4. Collecting a urine specimen from a 70-year-old woman admitted 3 days ago

**Answer: 1**

**Rationale:** This question addresses the subcategory Management of Care in the Client Needs category of Safe, Effective Care Environment, and specifically addresses content related to delegation. Work that is delegated to others must be done consistent with the individual's level of expertise and licensure or lack of licensure. In this case, the least appropriate activity for a nursing assistant would be assisting with feeding a profoundly developmentally disabled child. The child is likely to have difficulty eating and has a high potential for complications, such as choking and aspiration. The remaining three options do not include situations to indicate that these activities carry any risk.

**SAFETY AND INFECTION CONTROL**

A nurse has given a subcutaneous injection to a client with acquired immunodeficiency syndrome (AIDS). The nurse disposes of the used needle and syringe by:
1. Recapping the needle and discarding the syringe in the disposal unit
2. Placing the uncapped needle and syringe in a labeled, rigid plastic container
3. Breaking the needle before discarding it
4. Placing the uncapped needle and syringe in a labeled cardboard box

**Answer: 2**

**Rationale:** This question addresses the subcategory Safety and Infection Control, in the Client Needs category of Safe, Effective Care Environment, and specifically addresses content related to standard (universal) precautions. Universal precautions include specific guidelines for handling of needles. Needles should not be recapped, bent, broken, or cut after use. They should be disposed of in a labeled, impermeable container specific for this purpose. Needles should not be discarded in cardboard boxes, because they are not impervious. Needles should never be left lying around after use.

---

four subcategories: Basic Care and Comfort, Pharmacological and Parenteral Therapies, Reduction of Risk Potential, and Physiological Adaptation.

The National Council of State Boards of Nursing identifies nursing content related to the subcategories of this Client Needs category (Box 5-3). Basic Care and Comfort (7% to 13%) addresses content that tests the knowledge, skills, and ability required to provide comfort and assistance in the performance of activities of daily living. Pharmacological and Parenteral Therapies (5% to 11%) addresses content that tests the knowledge, skills, and ability required to manage and

**BOX 5-3**

### NCLEX-RN Content: Physiological Integrity

**BASIC CARE AND COMFORT**
Assistive devices
Comfort and palliative care
Comfort interventions: nonpharmacological
Elimination
Mobility and immobility
Nutrition and oral hydration
Personal hygiene
Rest and sleep

**PHARMACOLOGICAL AND PARENTERAL THERAPIES**
Adverse effects and contraindications
Blood and blood products
Central venous access devices
Chemotherapy
Expected effects
Intravenous therapy
Medication administration
Parenteral fluids
Pharmacological actions
Pharmacological agents
Pharmacological interactions
Pharmacological pain management

Side effects
Total parenteral nutrition

**REDUCTION OF RISK POTENTIAL**
Diagnostic tests
Laboratory values
Pathophysiology
Potential for alterations in body systems
Potential for complications of diagnostic tests, procedures, surgery, and health alterations
Therapeutic procedures

**PHYSIOLOGICAL ADAPTATION**
Alterations in body systems
Fluid and electrolyte imbalances
Hemodynamics
Infectious diseases
Medical emergencies
Pathophysiology
Radiation therapy
Respiratory care
Unexpected responses to therapies

From National Council of State Boards of Nursing (eds.) (2000). *Test plan for the National Council Licensure Examination for Registered Nurses.* Chicago: Author.

**BOX 5-4**

### Physiological Integrity Questions

**BASIC CARE AND COMFORT**
A client has been taught to use a walker to aid in mobility following internal fixation of a hip fracture. A nurse determines that the client is using the walker incorrectly if the client:
1. Holds the walker by using the hand grips
2. Leans forward slightly when advancing the walker
3. Advances the walker with reciprocal motion
4. Supports body weight on the hands while advancing the weaker leg

**Answer: 3**

**Rationale:** This question addresses the subcategory Basic Care and Comfort, in the Client Needs category of Physiological Integrity, and addresses content related to the use of an assistive device. The client should use the walker by placing the hands on the hand grips for stability. The client lifts the walker to advance it, and leans forward slightly while moving it. The client walks into the walker, supporting the body weight on the hands while moving the weaker leg. A disadvantage of the walker is that it does not allow for reciprocal walking motion. If the client were to try to use reciprocal motion with a walker, the walker would advance forward one side at a time as the client walks; thus the client would not be supporting the weaker leg with the walker during ambulation.

**PHARMACOLOGICAL AND PARENTERAL THERAPIES**
A nurse is caring for a client who received an allogenic liver transplant. The client is receiving tacrolimus (Prograf) daily. Which of the following indicates to the nurse that the client is experiencing an adverse reaction to the medication?
1. A decrease in urine output
2. Hypotension
3. Profuse sweating
4. Photophobia

**Answer: 1**

**Rationale:** This question addresses the subcategory Pharmacological and Parenteral Therapies, in the Client Needs category of Physiological Integrity, and addresses content related to the adverse effect of a medication. Tacrolimus (Prograf) is an immunosuppressant medication used in the prophylaxis of organ rejection in clients receiving allogenic liver transplants. Frequent side effects include headache, tremor, insomnia, paresthesia, diarrhea, nausea, constipation, vomiting, abdominal pain, and hypertension. Adverse reactions and toxic effects include nephrotoxicity and pleural effusion. Nephrotoxicity is characterized by an increasing serum creatinine level and a decrease in urine output.

*Continued*

## BOX 5-4

**Physiological Integrity Questions—cont'd**

**REDUCTION OF RISK POTENTIAL**
A nurse is caring for a client who is going to have an arthrogram using a contrast medium. Which of the following assessments by the nurse would be of highest priority?
1. Allergy to iodine or shellfish
2. Ability of the client to remain still during the procedure
3. Whether the client has any remaining questions about the procedure
4. Whether the client wishes to void before the procedure

**Answer: 1**

**Rationale:** This question addresses the subcategory Reduction of Risk Potential, in the Client Needs category of Physiological Integrity, and addresses a potential complication of a diagnostic test. Because of the risk of allergy to contrast dye, the nurse places highest priority on assessing whether the client has an allergy to iodine or shellfish. The nurse also reinforces information about the test, tells the client about the need to remain still during the procedure, and encourages the client to void before the procedure for comfort.

**PHYSIOLOGICAL ADAPTATION**
A pregnant client tells a nurse that she felt wetness on her peri-pad and that she found some clear fluid. The nurse immediately inspects the perineum and notes the presence of the umbilical cord. The nurse's initial action is to:
1. Notify the physician
2. Monitor fetal heart rate
3. Transfer the client to the delivery room
4. Place the client in Trendelenburg position

**Answer: 4**

**Rationale:** This question addresses the subcategory Physiological Adaptation, in the Client Needs category of Physiological Integrity, and addresses an acute and life-threatening physical health condition. On inspection of the perineum, if the umbilical cord is noted, the nurse immediately places the client into Trendelenburg position while pushing the presenting part upward to relieve the cord compression. This position is maintained and the physician is notified. The nurse monitors the fetal heart rate. The client is transferred to the delivery room when prescribed by the physician.

## BOX 5-5

**NCLEX-RN Content: Psychosocial Integrity**

**COPING AND ADAPTATION**
Coping mechanisms
End of life
Grief and loss
Mental health concepts
Religious and spiritual influences on health
Sensory/perceptual alterations
Situational role changes
Stress management
Support systems
Therapeutic interactions
Unexpected body image changes

**PSYCHOSOCIAL ADAPTATION**
Behavioral Interventions
Chemical dependency
Child abuse/neglect
Crisis intervention
Domestic violence
Elderly abuse/neglect
Psychopathology
Sexual abuse
Therapeutic milieu

From National Council of State Boards of Nursing (eds.) (2000). *Test plan for the National Council Licensure Examination for Registered Nurses.* Chicago: Author.

provide care related to the administration of medications and parenteral therapies. Reduction of Risk Potential (12% to 18%) addresses content that tests the knowledge, skills, and ability required to reduce the likelihood that clients will develop complications or health problems related to existing conditions, treatments, or procedures. Physiological Adaptation (12% to 18%) addresses content that tests the knowledge, skills, and ability required to manage and provide care to clients with acute, chronic, or life-threatening physical health conditions (Box 5-4). Refer to Chapter 7 for practice questions reflective of this Client Needs category.

## PSYCHOSOCIAL INTEGRITY

The Psychosocial Integrity category addresses content related to the nurse's role in providing and directing nursing care that promotes and supports the emotional, mental, and social well-being of the client and significant others. The Psychosocial Integrity category includes two subcategories: Coping and Adaptation and Psychosocial Adaptation.

The National Council of State Boards of Nursing identifies nursing content related to the subcategories of this Client Needs category (Box 5-5). Coping and Adaptation (5% to 11%) addresses content that tests the knowledge, skills, and ability required to promote the client and/or significant others' ability to cope, adapt, and/or problem solve in situations related to illnesses, disabilities, or stressful events. Psychosocial Adaptation (5% to 11%) addresses content that tests the knowledge, skills, and ability required to manage and provide care to clients with maladaptive behaviors or with acute or chronic mental illnesses (Box 5-6). Refer to Chapter 8 for practice questions reflective of this Client Needs category.

---

### BOX 5-6

#### Psychosocial Integrity Questions

**COPING AND ADAPTATION**
A stillborn was delivered in the birthing suite a few hours ago. After the birth, the family has remained together, holding and touching the baby. Which statement by the nurse would further assist them in their initial period of grief?
  1. "Don't worry, there is nothing you could do to prevent this from happening."
  2. "We need to take the baby from you now so that you can get some sleep."
  3. "What have you named your lovely baby?"
  4. "We will see to it that you have an early discharge so that you don't have to be reminded of this experience."

**Answer: 3**

**Rationale:** This question addresses the subcategory Coping and Adaptation, in the Client Needs category of Psychosocial Integrity, and addresses content related to grief and loss. Nurses should be able to explore measures that assist the family to create memory of a baby so that the existence of the child is confirmed and the parents can complete the grieving process. Option 3 addresses this issue and also demonstrates a caring and empathetic response. Options 1, 2, and 4 are blocks to communication and devalue the parents' feelings.

**PSYCHOSOCIAL ADAPTATION**
A nurse in the mental health clinic is performing an initial assessment of a family with a diagnosis of domestic violence. Which of the following factors would the nurse initially want to include in the assessment?
  1. The family's anger toward the intrusiveness of the nurse
  2. The family's denial of the violent nature of their behavior
  3. The coping style of each family member
  4. The family's current ability to use community resources

**Answer: 3**

**Rationale:** This question addresses the subcategory Psychosocial Adaptation, in the Client Needs category of Psychosocial Integrity, and addresses domestic violence. Note the key word *initially*. The initial family assessment includes a careful history of each family member. Options 1, 2, and 4 address the family. Option 3 addresses each family member.

## HEALTH PROMOTION AND MAINTENANCE

The Health Promotion and Maintenance category addresses content related to the nurse's role in providing and directing nursing care that incorporates the knowledge of expected growth and development principles. The nurse's role in the prevention and/or early detection of health care problems is also a component of this Client Needs category. The Health Promotion and Maintenance category includes two subcategories: Growth and Development Through the Life Span and the Prevention and Early Detection of Health Problems.

The National Council of State Boards of Nursing identifies nursing content related to the subcategories of this Client Needs category (Box 5-7). Growth and Development Through the Life Span (7% to 13%) addresses content that tests the knowledge, skills, and ability required to assist the client and significant others through the normal, expected stages of growth and development, from conception through advanced old age. Prevention and Early Detection of Health Problems (5% to 11%) addresses content that tests the knowledge, skills, and ability required to assist clients to recognize alterations in health and to develop health practices that promote and support wellness (Box 5-8). Refer to Chapter 9 for practice questions reflective of this Client Needs category.

### BOX 5-7

#### NCLEX-RN Content: Health Promotion and Maintenance

**GROWTH AND DEVELOPMENT THROUGH THE LIFE SPAN**
Aging process
Antepartum, intrapartum, and postpartum periods
Developmental stages and transitions
Expected body image changes
Family planning
Family systems
Human sexuality
Newborn

**PREVENTION AND EARLY DETECTION OF HEALTH PROBLEMS**
Disease prevention
Health and wellness
Health promotion programs
Health screening
Immunizations
Lifestyle choices
Techniques of physical assessment

From National Council of State Boards of Nursing (eds.) (2000). *Test plan for the National Council Licensure Examination for Registered Nurses.* Chicago: Author.

## BOX 5-8

### Health Promotion and Maintenance Questions

**GROWTH AND DEVELOPMENT THROUGH THE LIFE SPAN**
A clinic nurse is providing instructions to a client in the third trimester of pregnancy regarding measures to relieve heartburn. The nurse tells the client to:
1. Eat fatty foods only once a day in the morning
2. Avoid milk and hot tea
3. Eat small, frequent meals
4. Use antacids that contain sodium

**Answer: 3**

**Rationale:** This question addresses the subcategory Growth and Development through the Life Span, in the Client Needs category of Health Promotion and Maintenance, and addresses the antepartum period. Measures to provide relief of heartburn include small frequent meals, and avoidance of fatty fried foods, coffee, and cigarettes. Mild antacids can be used if they do not contain aspirin or sodium. Frequent sips of milk, hot tea, or water are helpful. Gum is also helpful in the relief of heartburn.

**PREVENTION AND EARLY DETECTION OF HEALTH PROBLEMS**
A client with atherosclerosis asks a nurse about dietary modifications to lower the risk of heart disease. The nurse encourages the client to eat which of the following foods that will lower this risk?
1. Baked chicken with skin
2. Fresh cantaloupe
3. Broiled cheeseburger
4. Mashed potato with gravy

**Answer: 2**

**Rationale:** This question addresses the subcategory Prevention and Early Detection of Health Problems, in the Client Needs category of Health Promotion and Maintenance, and addresses health and wellness. To lower the risk of heart disease, the diet should be low in saturated fat, with the appropriate number of total calories. The diet should include fewer red meats and more white meat, with the skin removed. Dairy products used should be low in fat, and foods with high amounts of empty calories should be avoided. Fresh fruits and vegetables are naturally low in fat.

## REFERENCES

Hertz, J., Yocom, C., & Gawel, S. (2000). *Linking the NCLEX-RN examination to practice: 1999 practice analysis of newly licensed registered nurses in the United States.* Chicago: National Council of State Boards of Nursing.

Hodgson, B., & Kizior, R. (2001). *Saunders nursing drug handbook 2001.* Philadelphia: W.B. Saunders.

National Council of State Boards of Nursing (eds.) (2000). *Test plan for the National Council Licensure Examination for Registered Nurses.* Chicago: Author.

National Council of State Boards of Nursing (eds.) (2000). *The NCLEX Process: Serving as an anchor for the NCLEX Examination.* Chicago: Author.

National Council of State Boards of Nursing. Web Site: http://www.ncsbn.org/files/boards/boardscontact.asp

Potter, P., & Perry, A. (2001). *Fundamentals of nursing* (5th ed.). St. Louis: Mosby.

Riley, J. (2000). *Communication in nursing* (4th ed.). St. Louis: Mosby.

Smeltzer, S., & Bare, B. (2000). *Brunner & Suddarth's Textbook of medical-surgical nursing* (9th ed.). Philadelphia: Lippincott Williams & Wilkins.

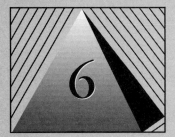

# 6

# Safe, Effective Care Environment

1. A nurse employed in a long-term care facility is planning the client assignments for the shift. Which of the following clients would the nurse most appropriately assign to the nursing assistant (NA)?
   1. A client requiring BID dressing changes
   2. A client requiring frequent ambulation
   3. A client on a bowel management program requiring rectal suppositories and a daily enema
   4. A client with diabetes mellitus requiring daily insulin and reinforcement of dietary measures

**Answer: 2**

*Rationale:* Assignment of tasks needs to be implemented based on the job description of the NA, the level of clinical competence, and state law. Options 1, 3, and 4 involve care that requires the skill of a licensed nurse.

*Test-Taking Strategy:* Use the process of elimination and knowledge regarding tasks that can be safely delegated to the NA. Eliminate options 1, 3, and 4 because these clients require care that needs to be provided by a licensed nurse.

*Level of Cognitive Ability:* Application
*Client Needs:* Safe, Effective Care Environment
*Integrated Concept/Process:* Nursing Process/Planning
*Content Area:* Fundamental Skills

*Reference*
Yoder-Wise, P. (1999). *Leading and managing in nursing* (2nd ed.). St. Louis: Mosby, pp. 310-311.

2. A psychotic client is pacing, agitated, and presenting with aggressive gestures. The client's speech pattern is rapid and the affect is belligerent. Based on these objective data, the immediate priority of care is to:
   1. Provide safety for the client and other clients on the unit
   2. Bring the client to a less stimulating area to calm down and gain control
   3. Provide the clients on the unit with a sense of comfort and safety
   4. Assist the staff in caring for the client in a controlled environment

**Answer: 1**

*Rationale:* If a client is exhibiting signs that indicate loss of control, the nurse's immediate priority is to ensure safety for all clients. Option 1 is the only option that addresses the client and other clients' safety needs. Option 2 addresses the client's needs. Option 3 addresses other clients' needs. Option 4 is not client centered.

*Test-Taking Strategy:* Focus on the data in the question. Note the issue of the question—safety. Option 1 is a global option and addresses the safety of all. Review nursing care for the client who is agitated and out of control if you had difficulty with this question.

*Level of Cognitive Ability:* Application
*Client Needs:* Safe, Effective Care Environment

*Integrated Concept/Process:* Nursing Process/Implementation
*Content Area:* Mental Health

**Reference**
Stuart, G.W., & Laraia, M.T. (1998). *Principles and practice of psychiatric nursing.* (6th ed.). St. Louis: Mosby, p. 626.

---

**3.** A magnetic resonance imaging (MRI) is prescribed for a client with Bell's palsy. Which nursing action is included in the client's plan of care to prepare for this test?
1. Keep the client NPO for 6 hours before the test
2. Remove all metal-containing objects from the client
3. Shave the groin for insertion of a femoral catheter
4. Instruct the client in inhalation techniques for the administration of gas

**Answer: 2**
*Rationale:* In an MRI, radio frequency pulses in a magnetic field are converted into pictures. All metal objects, such as rings, bracelets, hairpins, watches, etc., should be removed. In addition, a history should be taken to ascertain whether the client has any internal metallic devices, such as orthopedic hardware, pacemakers, shrapnel, etc. For an abdominal MRI, the client is usually NPO. NPO status is not necessary for an MRI of the head. The groin may be shaved for an angiogram. Inhalation of gas is not a component of an MRI.

*Test-Taking Strategy:* Focus on the name of the test and the client's diagnosis. Note the relationship between *magnetic* in the question and *metal* in the correct option. If you are unfamiliar with client preparation for an MRI, review this content.

*Level of Cognitive Ability:* Application
*Client Needs:* Safe, Effective Care Environment
*Integrated Concept/Process:* Nursing Process/Planning
*Content Area:* Adult Health/Neurological

**Reference**
Smeltzer, S., & Bare, B. (2000). *Brunner & Suddarth's Textbook of medical-surgical nursing* (9th ed.). Philadelphia: Lippincott Williams & Wilkins, p. 1675.

---

**4.** A physician asks a nurse to discontinue the feeding tube in a client who is in a chronic vegetative state. The physician tells the nurse that the request was made by the client's spouse and children. The nurse understands the legal basis for carrying out the order and first checks the client's record for documentation of:
1. A court approval to discontinue the treatment
2. A written order by the physician to remove the tube
3. Authorization by the family to discontinue the treatment
4. Approval by the institutional Ethics Committee

**Answer: 3**
*Rationale:* The family or a legal guardian can make treatment decisions for the client who is unable to do so. Once the decision is made, the physician writes the order. Generally, the family makes decisions in collaboration with physicians, other health care workers, and other trusted advisors.

*Test-Taking Strategy:* Note the key word *first* to determine the sequence of decision making in this situation. There are no data in the question that indicate the need for court approval. Therefore assessment for family authorization is the nurse's first action. Review these principles if you had difficulty with this question.

*Level of Cognitive Ability:* Application
*Client Needs:* Safe, Effective Care Environment
*Integrated Concept/Process:* Communication and Documentation
*Content Area:* Fundamental Skills

**Reference**
Potter, P., & Perry, A. (2001). *Fundamentals of nursing* (5th ed.). St. Louis: Mosby, p. 436.

**5.** A nurse is assisting a physician with the insertion of a Miller-Abbott tube. The nurse understands that the procedure puts the client at risk for aspiration. The nurse implements which action to decrease the risk of aspiration?
1   Inserting the tube with the balloon inflated
2   Instructing the client to cough when the tube reaches the nasal pharynx
3   Placing the client in a high-Fowler's position
4   Instructing the client to perform a Valsalva maneuver if the impulse to gag and vomit occurs

**Answer: 3**
*Rationale:* The Miller-Abbott tube is a nasoenteric tube that is used to decompress the intestine, as in correcting a bowel obstruction. Initial insertion of the tube is a physician responsibility. The tube is inserted with the balloon deflated in a manner similar to the proper procedure for inserting a nasogastric tube. The client is usually given water to drink to facilitate passage of the tube through the nasopharynx and esophagus. A high-Fowler's position decreases the risk of aspiration if vomiting occurs.

*Test-Taking Strategy:* Focus on the issue, decreasing the risk of aspiration for the client undergoing insertion of a Miller-Abbott tube. Option 1 can be eliminated because a tube could not be inserted if the balloon was inflated. Eliminate option 2 because coughing can cause the tube to be expelled. A Valsalva maneuver is not used if the impulse to gag occurs. Review this procedure if you had difficulty with this question.

*Level of Cognitive Ability:* Application
*Client Needs:* Safe, Effective Care Environment
*Integrated Concept/Process:* Nursing Process/Implementation
*Content Area:* Adult Health/Gastrointestinal

*Reference*
Smeltzer, S., & Bare, B. (2000). *Brunner & Suddarth's Textbook of medical-surgical nursing* (9th ed.). Philadelphia: Lippincott Williams & Wilkins, p. 838.

**6.** A nurse is caring for a client receiving total parenteral nutrition (TPN). The nurse implements which action to decrease the risk of infection?
1   Assessing vital signs at 4-hour intervals
2   Instructing the client to perform a Valsalva maneuver during intravenous tubing changes
3   Administer acetaminophen (Tylenol) before changing the central line dressing
4   Using aseptic technique in handling the TPN solution and tubing

**Answer: 4**
*Rationale:* Clients receiving TPN are at high risk for developing infection. Concentrated glucose solutions are an excellent medium for bacterial growth. Using aseptic technique in handling all equipment and solutions is paramount to prevention. Option 1 will detect signs of an infection but is not associated with prevention. Options 2 and 3 are unrelated to decreasing the risk of infection.

*Test-Taking Strategy:* Note the key words *decrease the risk*. Option 1 relates to early detection of infection, not decreasing the risk. Options 2 and 3 do not relate to the issue of the question. Remember, aseptic technique is critical to prevent infection. Review care of the client receiving TPN if you had difficulty with this question.

*Level of Cognitive Ability:* Application
*Client Needs:* Safe, Effective Care Environment
*Integrated Concept/Process:* Nursing Process/Implementation
*Content Area:* Fundamental Skills

*Reference*
Smeltzer, S., & Bare, B. (2000). *Brunner & Suddarth's Textbook of medical-surgical nursing* (9th ed.). Philadelphia: Lippincott Williams & Wilkins, p. 853.

**7.** A nurse is assisting a home health care client in managing cancer pain. To ensure that the client has adequate and safe pain control, the planning strategy would include:

1    Trying multiple medication modalities for pain relief to get the maximum pain relief effect
2    Starting with low doses of medication and gradually increasing to a dose that relieves pain, not exceeding the maximum daily dose
3    Relying totally on prescription and over-the-counter medications to relieve pain
4    Keeping a baseline level of pain so that the client does not get sedated or addicted

**Answer: 2**
*Rationale:* Safe pain control includes starting with low doses and working up to a dose of medication that relieves the pain. Interventions with multiple medication modalities can be unsafe and ineffective. Option 3 does not take into account other nursing interventions that may relieve pain, such as massage, therapeutic touch, or music. Maintaining a baseline level of pain to avoid sedation or addiction is not appropriate practice, unless the client requests this, and this information has not been provided in the case situation.

*Test-Taking Strategy:* Use the process of elimination and focus on safety issues. Option 1 uses the word *multiple* and option 3 uses the word *totally*. Therefore eliminate these options. Option 4 can be eliminated, because it is inaccurate information. Review safe pain control management if you had difficulty with this question.

*Level of Cognitive Ability:* Application
*Client Needs:* Safe, Effective Care Environment
*Integrated Concept/Process:* Caring
*Content Area:* Adult Health/Oncology

*Reference*
Smeltzer, S., & Bare, B. (2000). *Brunner & Suddarth's Textbook of medical-surgical nursing* (9th ed.). Philadelphia: Lippincott Williams & Wilkins, p. 288.

---

**8.** A nurse provides medication instructions to a home health care client. To ensure safe administration of medication in the home, the nurse:

1    Demonstrates the proper procedure for taking prescribed medications
2    Allows the client to verbalize and demonstrate correct administration procedures
3    Instructs the client that it is OK to double up on medications if a dose has been missed
4    Conducts pill counts on each home visit

**Answer: 2**
*Rationale:* To ensure safe administration of medication, the nurse allows the client to verbalize and demonstrate correct procedure and administration of medications. Demonstrating the proper procedure for the client does not ensure that the client can safely perform this procedure. It is not acceptable to double up on medication, and conducting a pill count on each visit is not realistic or appropriate.

*Test-Taking Strategy:* Use the process of elimination. Options 3 and 4 can be eliminated, because these are not appropriate practices. From the remaining options, note that option 2 is client centered. Review the principles of teaching and learning if you had difficulty with this question.

*Level of Cognitive Ability:* Application
*Client Needs:* Safe, Effective Care Environment
*Integrated Concept/Process:* Teaching/Learning
*Content Area:* Fundamental Skills

*Reference*
Potter, P., & Perry, A. (2001). *Fundamentals of nursing* (5th ed.). St. Louis: Mosby, p. 492.

**9.** A client remains in atrial fibrillation with rapid ventricular response, despite pharmacological intervention. Synchronous cardioversion is scheduled to convert the rapid rhythm. Which of the following is the most important nursing action to ensure safety and prevent complications of this procedure?

1 Sedate the client before cardioversion
2 Ensure that emergency equipment is available
3 Ensure that the defibrillator is set on the synchronous mode
4 Cardiovert at 360 joules

**Answer: 3**

*Rationale:* Cardioversion is similar to defibrillation with two major exceptions. The countershock is synchronized to occur during ventricular depolarization (QRS complex), and less energy is used for the countershock. The rationale for delivering the shock during the QRS complex is to prevent the shock from being delivered during repolarization (T wave), often called the *vulnerable period*. If the shock is delivered during this period, the resulting complication is ventricular fibrillation. It is crucial that the defibrillator be set on the *synchronous* mode for successful cardioversion. Options 1 and 2 will not prevent complications. Cardioversion usually begins with 50 to 100 joules.

*Test-Taking Strategy:* Focus on the issue of the question: ensure safety and prevent complications. Noting the key word *synchronous* in the question will direct you to option 3. Review this procedure if you had difficulty with this question.

*Level of Cognitive Ability:* Application
*Client Needs:* Safe, Effective Care Environment
*Integrated Concept/Process:* Nursing Process/Implementation
*Content Area:* Adult Health/Cardiovascular

*Reference*
Smeltzer, S., & Bare, B. (2000). *Brunner & Suddarth's Textbook of medical-surgical nursing* (9th ed.). Philadelphia: Lippincott Williams & Wilkins, p. 580.

**10.** A client is being treated with heparin sodium therapy for a diagnosis of thrombophlebitis. In planning care, the nurse ensures that which medication is available if the client develops a significant bleeding problem?

1 Fresh frozen plasma
2 Protamine sulfate
3 Streptokinase (Streptase)
4 Vitamin K

**Answer: 2**

*Rationale:* Protamine sulfate is the antidote for heparin sodium. Vitamin K is the antidote for warfarin (Coumadin). Fresh frozen plasma may also be used for bleeding related to warfarin therapy. Streptokinase is a thrombolytic agent, used to dissolve blood clots.

*Test-Taking Strategy:* Specific knowledge regarding the antidote for heparin sodium is required to answer this question. Review the antidotes for commonly administered medications if you had difficulty with this question.

*Level of Cognitive Ability:* Application
*Client Needs:* Safe, Effective Care Environment
*Integrated Concept/Process:* Nursing Process/Planning
*Content Area:* Pharmacology

*Reference*
Hodgson, B., & Kizior, R. (2001). *Saunders Nursing drug handbook 2001.* Philadelphia: W.B. Saunders, p. 650.

**11.** A nurse is teaching a client with cardiomy-opathy about home care safety measures. The nurse addresses which most important measure to ensure client safety?
1    Assessing pain
2    Avoiding over-the-counter medications
3    Administering vasodilators
4    Moving slowly from a sitting to a standing position.

**Answer: 4**
*Rationale:* Orthostatic changes can occur in the client with cardiomyopathy as a result of venous return obstruction. Sudden changes in orthostatics may lead to falls. Vasodilators are not normally prescribed for the client with cardiomyopathy. Options 1 and 2, although important, are not directly related to the issue of safety.

*Test-Taking Strategy:* Note the key words *most important*. Focusing on the issue, home care safety measures, will direct you to option 4. Review client teaching related to cardiomyopathy if you had difficulty with this question.

*Level of Cognitive Ability:* Application
*Client Needs:* Safe, Effective Care Environment
*Integrated Concept/Process:* Self-Care
*Content Area:* Adult Health/Cardiovascular

*Reference*
Smeltzer, S., & Bare, B. (2000). *Brunner & Suddarth's Textbook of medical-surgical nursing* (9th ed.). Philadelphia: Lippincott Williams & Wilkins, p. 645.

**12.** A nurse instructs a client with a diagnosis of valvular disease to use an electric razor for shaving. The nurse tells the client that the importance of its use is that:
1    Any cut may cause infection
2    Electric razors can be disinfected
3    All straight razors contain bacteria
4    Cuts need to be avoided

**Answer: 4**
*Rationale:* Anticoagulants are prescribed for clients with valvular disease to prevent thrombus formation and possible stroke. The importance of using an electric razor is to prevent cuts and possible bleeding. Options 1, 2, and 3 are all unrelated to the issue of bleeding.

*Test-Taking Strategy:* Recalling that a client with valvular disease will be given a course of anticoagulant therapy will assist in answering the question. Note that options 1, 2, and 3 are similar and relate to infection. Option 4 relates to bleeding. Review care of the client with valvular disease if you had difficulty with this question.

*Level of Cognitive Ability:* Application
*Client Needs:* Safe, Effective Care Environment
*Integrated Concept/Process:* Self-Care
*Content Area:* Adult Health/Cardiovascular

*Reference*
Smeltzer, S., & Bare, B. (2000). *Brunner & Suddarth's Textbook of medical-surgical nursing* (9th ed.). Philadelphia: Lippincott Williams & Wilkins, p. 651.

**13.** A nurse is caring for a client during the recovery phase following a myocardial infarction. A cardiac catheterization, using the femoral artery approach, is performed to assess the degree of coronary artery thrombosis. Which nursing action following the procedure is unsafe for the client?

1 Placing the client's bed in the Fowler's position
2 Encouraging the client to increase fluid intake
3 Instructing the client to move the toes when checking circulation, motion, and sensation
4 Resuming prescribed precatheterization medications

**Answer: 1**

*Rationale:* Immediately following a cardiac catheterization with the femoral artery approach, the client should not flex or hyperextend the affected leg to avoid blood vessel occlusion or hemorrhage. Placing the client in the Fowler's position (flexion) increases the risk of occlusion or hemorrhage. Fluids are encouraged to assist in removing the contrast medium from the body. Asking the client to move the toes is done to assess motion, which could be impaired if a hematoma or thrombus were developing. The precatheterization medications are needed to treat acute and chronic conditions.

*Test-Taking Strategy:* Note the key word *unsafe* in the stem of the question. Also note the words *femoral artery approach*. Recalling that flexion or hyperextension is avoided will direct you to option 1. Review postcardiac catheterization care if you had difficulty with this question.

*Level of Cognitive Ability:* Application
*Client Needs:* Safe, Effective Care Environment
*Integrated Concept/Process:* Nursing Process/Implementation
*Content Area:* Adult Health/Cardiovascular

*Reference*
Smeltzer, S., & Bare, B. (2000). *Brunner & Suddarth's Textbook of medical-surgical nursing* (9th ed.). Philadelphia: Lippincott Williams & Wilkins, p. 557.

---

**14.** A nurse plans to carry out a multidisciplinary research project on the effects of immobility on clients' stress levels. The nurse understands that which principle is most important when planning this project?

1 Collaboration with other disciplines is essential to the successful practice of nursing
2 The Corporate Nurse Executive should be consulted, because the project will take nursing time
3 All clients have the right to refuse to participate in research using human subjects
4 The cooperation of the physicians on staff must be ensured for the project to succeed

**Answer: 3**

*Rationale:* The proposed project is research and includes human subjects. Although options 1, 2, and 4 need to be considered, they are all secondary to the overriding principle of the legal and ethical practice of nursing that any client has the right to refuse to participate in research using human subjects.

*Test-Taking Strategy:* Use the process of elimination. Focus on the issue, most important principle. Recalling that the client has the right to refuse to participate in research will direct you to option 3. Review the ethical and legal guidelines related to research if you had difficulty with this question.

*Level of Cognitive Ability:* Application
*Client Needs:* Safe, Effective Care Environment
*Integrated Concept/Process:* Nursing Process/Planning
*Content Area:* Fundamental Skills

*Reference*
Potter, P., & Perry, A. (2001). *Fundamentals of nursing* (5th ed.). St. Louis: Mosby, p. 436.

**15.** A nurse has an order to obtain a sputum culture from a client admitted to the hospital with a diagnosis of pneumonia. The nurse avoids which action when obtaining the specimen?
1   Placing the lid of the culture container face down on the bedside table
2   Obtaining the specimen early in the morning
3   Having the client brush teeth before expectoration
4   Instructing the client to take deep breaths before coughing

**Answer: 1**
*Rationale:* Placing the lid face down on the bedside table contaminates the lid and could result in inaccurate findings. The specimen is obtained early in the morning whenever possible, because increased amounts of sputum collect in the airways during sleep. The client should rinse the mouth or brush the teeth before specimen collection to avoid contaminating the specimen. The client should take deep breaths before expectoration for best sputum production.

*Test-Taking Strategy:* Use the process of elimination, noting the key word *avoids*. Begin by eliminating options 2 and 4, which are helpful in obtaining a specimen of sufficient volume. From the remaining options, use of basic principles of aseptic technique will direct you to option 1. Review the procedure for sputum collection if you had difficulty with this question.

*Level of Cognitive Ability:* Application
*Client Needs:* Safe, Effective Care Environment
*Integrated Concept/Process:* Nursing Process/Implementation
*Content Area:* Fundamental Skills

*Reference*
Monahan, F., & Neighbors, M. (1998). *Medical-surgical nursing: Foundations for clinical practice* (2nd ed.). Philadelphia: W.B. Saunders, p. 546.

**16.** A multidisciplinary health care team is planning care for a client with hyperparathyroidism. The health care team develops which most important outcome for the client?
1   Describes the administration of aluminum hydroxide gel
2   Restricts fluids to 1000 mL per day
3   Walks down the hall for 15 minutes, three times per day
4   Describes the use of loperamide (Imodium)

**Answer: 3**
*Rationale:* Mobility of the client with hyperparathyroidism should be encouraged as much as possible because of the calcium imbalance that occurs in this disorder and the predisposition to the formation of renal calculi. Fluids should not be restricted. Discussing the use of these medications is not the priority in this client.

*Test-Taking Strategy:* Use the process of elimination. Eliminate options 1 and 4 first because they are similar. From the remaining options, recalling that the client is predisposed to the formation of renal calculi will direct you to option 3. If you had difficulty with this question, review care to the client with hyperparathyroidism.

*Level of Cognitive Ability:* Analysis
*Client Needs:* Safe, Effective Care Environment
*Integrated Concept/Process:* Nursing Process/Planning
*Content Area:* Adult Health/Endocrine

*Reference*
Potter, P., & Perry, A. (2001). *Fundamentals of nursing* (5th ed.). St. Louis: Mosby, p. 1052.

**17.** A nurse has inserted a nasogastric tube (NG) into the stomach of a client and prepares to check for accurate tube placement. The nurse avoids which least reliable method for checking tube placement?

**1** Aspirating the tube with a 50-mL syringe to obtain gastric contents

**2** Measuring the pH of gastric aspirate

**3** Placing the end of the tube in water to check for bubbling

**4** Instilling 10 to 20 mL of air into the tube while auscultating over the stomach

**Answer: 3**

*Rationale:* The least reliable method for determining accurate placement of the NG tube is to place the end of the tube in water to observe for bubbling. However, the best method for determining tube placement is to verify placement by x-ray films.

*Test-Taking Strategy:* Use the process of elimination. Note the key words *avoids* and *least reliable.* Visualize this procedure and focus on the issue, accurate tube placement, to direct you to option 3. Review this procedure if you had difficulty with this question.

*Level of Cognitive Ability:* Application
*Client Needs:* Safe, Effective Care Environment
*Integrated Concept/Process:* Nursing Process/Implementation
*Content Area:* Fundamental Skills

*Reference*
Monahan, F., & Neighbors, M. (1998*). Medical-surgical nursing: Foundations for clinical practice* (2nd ed.). Philadelphia: W.B. Saunders, p. 978.

---

**18.** A nurse employed in a preschool agency is planning a staff education program to prevent the spread of an outbreak of an intestinal parasitic disease. The nurse includes which priority intervention in the educational session?

**1** Staff will practice universal precautions when changing diapers and assisting children with toileting

**2** All toileting areas will be cleansed daily with soap and water

**3** Only bottled water will be used for drinking

**4** All food will be cooked before eating

**Answer: 1**

*Rationale:* The fecal-oral route is the mode of transmission of an intestinal parasitic disease. Universal precautions prevent the transmission of infection. Cleaning with soap and water is not as effective as the use of bleach. Water and fresh foods can be vehicles for transmission, but municipal water sources are usually safe. Some fresh foods do not need to be cooked as long as they are washed well and provided that they weren't grown in soil contaminated with human feces.

*Test-Taking Strategy:* Focus on the issue, preventing the spread of infection. Option 1 addresses the issue of the question and is the most global option, addressing universal precautions. Also, note that options 2, 3, and 4 contain the absolute words *all* and *only.* Review measures that will prevent the spread of an intestinal parasitic infection if you had difficulty with this question.

*Level of Cognitive Ability:* Application
*Client Needs:* Safe, Effective Care Environment
*Integrated Concept/Process:* Teaching/Leaning
*Content Area:* Child Health

*Reference*
Ball, J., & Bindler, R. (1999). *Pediatric nursing: Caring for children* (2nd ed.). Stamford, Conn.: Appleton & Lange, p. 403.

**19.** A client has arrived at the labor and delivery unit in active labor. The nursing assessment reveals a history of recurrent genital herpes and the presence of lesions in the genital tract. The nurse plans to:

1    Prepare the client for a cesarean delivery
2    Limit visitors and maintain reverse isolation
3    Prepare the client for a spontaneous vaginal delivery
4    Rupture the membranes artificially, looking for meconium-stained fluid

**Answer: 1**

*Rationale:* A cesarean delivery can reduce the risk of neonatal infection with a mother in labor who has herpetic genital tract lesions. Intact membranes provide another barrier to transmitting the disease to the neonate. There is no need to limit visitors or maintain isolation, although universal precautions should be maintained.

*Test-Taking Strategy:* Use the process of elimination, focusing on the issue, presence of genital herpes lesions. Eliminate options 3 and 4 first because they are similar and would place the neonate in contact with the lesions. From the remaining options, consider the risks to the neonate to direct you to option 1. Review care of the client in labor who has genital herpes lesions if you had difficulty with this question.

*Level of Cognitive Ability:* Application
*Client Needs:* Safe, Effective Care Environment
*Integrated Concept/Process:* Nursing Process/Planning
*Content Area:* Maternity

*Reference*
Lowdermilk, D., Perry, S., & Bobak, I. (2000). *Maternity & women's health care* (7th ed.). St. Louis: Mosby, p. 161.

**20.** A nurse is performing a bladder catheterization and is inserting an indwelling Foley catheter. The nurse understands that which of the following represents an incorrect action when performing this procedure?

1    Inflating the balloon to test patency before catheter insertion
2    Advancing the catheter just until urine appears in the catheter tubing
3    Inflating the balloon with 4 to 5 mL more than the balloon capacity
4    Placing the bag lower than bladder level, with no kinks in the tubing

**Answer: 2**

*Rationale:* The catheter should be advanced for 1 to 2 more inches beyond the point where the flow of urine is first noted. This ensures that the balloon is fully in the bladder before it is inflated. Each of the other options represents correct procedure.

*Test-Taking Strategy:* Use the process of elimination, noting the key word *incorrect*. Visualize the procedure to assist in answering the question. Basic principles related to this procedure will assist in eliminating options 1 and 4. From the remaining options, recall either that the catheter is advanced 1 to 2 more inches, or that extra fluid is needed to fill the lumen that runs between the external port and the balloon at the tip of the catheter. Review this procedure if you had difficulty with this question.

*Level of Cognitive Ability:* Application
*Client Needs:* Safe, Effective Care Environment
*Integrated Concept/Process:* Nursing Process/Implementation
*Content Area:* Fundamental skills

*Reference*
Potter, P., & Perry, A. (2001). *Fundamentals of nursing* (5th ed.). St. Louis: Mosby, p. 1412.

**21.** A moderately depressed client who was admitted to the mental health unit 2 days ago suddenly begins smiling and reporting that the crisis is over. The client says to the nurse, "Call the doctor. I'm finally cured." The nurse interprets this behavior as a cue to modify the treatment plan by:

1    Allowing off-unit privileges prn
2    Suggesting a reduction of medication
3    Allowing increased "in room" activities
4    Increasing the level of suicide precautions

**Answer: 4**

*Rationale:* A client who is moderately depressed and has only been hospitalized 2 days is very unlikely to have such a dramatic cure. When a mood suddenly lifts, it is very likely that the client may have made the decision to harm himself or herself. Suicide precautions are necessary to keep the client safe.

*Test-Taking Strategy:* Use the process of elimination, focusing on the data in the question and recalling that depression does not resolve in two days. Options 1 and 2 support the client's notion that a cure has occurred. Option 3 allows the client to increase isolation. Recalling that safety is of the utmost importance will direct you to option 4. Review care of the client with depression if you had difficulty with this question.

*Level of Cognitive Ability:* Analysis
*Client Needs:* Safe, Effective Care Environment
*Integrated Concept/Process:* Nursing Process/Planning
*Content Area:* Mental Health

*Reference*
Stuart, G.W., & Laraia, M.T. (1998). *Principles and practice of psychiatric nursing.* (6th ed.). St. Louis: Mosby, 352.

**22.** A nurse is planning care for a suicidal client. The nurse implements additional precautions at which of the following times?

1    Day shift
2    Weekdays
3    8 A.M. to 10 A.M.
4    Shift change

**Answer: 4**

*Rationale:* At shift change, many times there are fewer staff members available. The psychiatric nurse and staff should increase precautions for suicidal clients at that time. Weekends are also high-risk times, not weekdays. The night shift also presents a high-risk time.

*Test-Taking Strategy:* Use the process of elimination. Options 1, 2, and 3 are similar and can be eliminated. Remember that the nurse could anticipate that times with less supervision of the client could be times of increased risks. Review care of the suicidal client if you had difficulty with this question.

*Level of Cognitive Ability:* Application
*Client Needs:* Safe, Effective Care Environment
*Integrated Concept/Process:* Nursing Process/Planning
*Content Area:* Mental Health

*Reference*
Stuart, G.W., & Laraia, M.T. (1998). *Principles and practice of psychiatric nursing.* (6th ed.). St. Louis: Mosby, p. 352.

**23.** A nurse is assisting with transferring a client from the operating room table to a stretcher. To provide safety for the client, the nurse:

1 Moves the client rapidly from the table to the stretcher

2 Uncovers the client completely before transferring to the stretcher

3 Secures the client with safety belts after transferring to the stretcher

4 Instructs the client to move himself or herself from the table to the stretcher

**Answer: 3**

*Rationale:* During the transfer of a client after a surgical procedure is complete, the nurse should avoid exposure of the client because of the risk for potential heat loss. Hurried movements and rapid changes in position should be avoided, since these predispose the client to hypotension. At the time of the transfer from the surgery table to the stretcher, the client is still affected by the effects of the anesthesia; therefore the client should not move himself or herself. Safety belts can prevent the client from falling off the stretcher.

*Test-Taking Strategy:* Use the process of elimination and focus on the issue, safety. Options 1 and 2 are unsafe techniques for the client. Note the word *rapidly* in option 1 and the words *uncover the client completely* in option 2. Option 4 is not appropriate because of the effects of the anesthesia. Review care of the postoperative client if you had difficulty with this question.

*Level of Cognitive Ability:* Application
*Client Needs:* Safe, Effective Care Environment
*Integrated Concept/Process:* Nursing Process/Implementation
*Content Area:* Fundamental Skills

*Reference*
Ignatavicius, D., Workman, M., & Mishler, M. (1999). *Medical-surgical nursing across the health care continuum* (3rd ed.). Philadelphia: W.B. Saunders, p. 361.

**24.** A nurse is planning care for a hallucinating and delusional client who has been rescued from a suicide attempt. The nurse plans to:

1 Check the whereabouts of the client every 15 minutes

2 Initiate suicide precautions with 30-minute checks

3 Initiate one-to-one suicide precautions

4 Ask that the client report suicidal thoughts immediately

**Answer: 3**

*Rationale:* One-to-one suicide precautions is required for the client rescued from a suicide attempt. In this situation, additional key information is that the client is delusional and hallucinating. Both of these factors increase the risk of unpredictable behavior or decreased judgment, and make the risk of suicide greater. Options 1, 2, and 4 do not provide the constant supervision necessary for this client.

*Test-Taking Strategy:* Use the process of elimination. Focusing on the data in question will direct you to option 3, the intervention that will provide most supervision. Review suicidal precautions if you had difficulty with this question.

*Level of Cognitive Ability:* Application
*Client Needs:* Safe, Effective Care Environment
*Integrated Concept/Process:* Nursing Process/Planning
*Content Area:* Mental Health

*Reference*
Stuart, G.W., & Laraia, M.T. (1998). *Principles and practice of psychiatric nursing* (6th ed.). St. Louis: Mosby, p. 400.

**25.** A nurse is developing a plan of care for a client receiving anticoagulant agents. The nurse identifies which priority nursing diagnosis for the client?
1    Fluid volume deficit
2    High risk for activity intolerance
3    High risk for injury
4    High risk for infection

**Answer: 3**
*Rationale:* Anticoagulant therapy predisposes the client to injury because of the agent's inhibitory effects on the body's normal blood clotting mechanism. Bruising, bleeding, and hemorrhage may occur in the course of activities of daily living and with other activities. Options 1, 2, and 4 are unrelated to this form of therapy.

*Test-Taking Strategy:* Use the process of elimination. Recalling that anticoagulants present a risk for bleeding will assist in directing you to option 3. If you had difficulty with this question, review the effects of anticoagulants.

*Level of Cognitive Ability:* Analysis
*Client Needs:* Safe, Effective Care Environment
*Integrated Concept/Process:* Nursing Process/Analysis
*Content Area:* Pharmacology

*Reference*
Ignatavicius, D., Workman, M., & Mishler, M. (1999). *Medical-surgical nursing across the health care continuum* (3rd ed.). Philadelphia: W.B. Saunders, p. 874.

**26.** A client being seen in the emergency department with complaints of abdominal pain has a diagnosis of acute abdomen and the cause has not been determined. The nurse would question an order for which of the following at this time?
1    Insertion of a nasogastric tube
2    Insertion of an intravenous (IV) line
3    Administration of a narcotic analgesic
4    Institution of an NPO diet status

**Answer: 3**
*Rationale:* Until the cause of the acute abdomen is determined and a decision about the need for surgery is made, the nurse would question an order to give a narcotic analgesic because it could mask the client's symptoms. The nurse can expect the client to be placed on NPO status and to have an IV line inserted. Insertion of a nasogastric tube may be helpful to provide decompression of the stomach.

*Test-Taking Strategy:* Note the key words *cause has not been determined.* Think about the client's diagnosis and that surgery may be a necessary intervention to direct you to option 3. Review interventions for the client with acute abdomen if you had difficulty with this question.

*Level of Cognitive Ability:* Application
*Client Needs:* Safe, Effective Care Environment
*Integrated Concept/Process:* Communication and Documentation
*Content Area:* Adult Health/Gastrointestinal

*Reference*
Monahan, F., & Neighbors, M. (1998). *Medical-surgical nursing: Foundations for clinical practice* (2nd ed.). Philadelphia: W.B. Saunders, p. 1064.

**27.** A home care nurse is working with a family to assist them in caring for a newborn with congenital tracheoesophageal fistula who is receiving enteral feedings. A woman identifying herself as a family friend telephones the nurse to inquire if there is anything she can do to assist the parents. The best nursing action is to:

1 Request that the friend come to the client's home where she can be taught to administer the feedings
2 Inform the friend to directly contact the family and offer her assistance to them
3 Report the friend's telephone call to the nurse manager for referral to the client's social worker
4 Inform the friend that the family has no need for assistance at this time because the nurse is making daily visits

**Answer: 2**
*Rationale:* A nurse must uphold the client's rights and does not give any information regarding a client's care needs to anyone not directly involved in the client's care. To request that the friend come for teaching is a direct violation of the client's right to privacy. There is no information in the question to indicate that the family desires assistance from the friend. To refer the call to the nurse manager and social worker again assumes that the friend's assistance and involvement is desired by the family. By informing the friend that the nurse is visiting daily is providing information that is considered confidential. Option 2 directly refers the friend to the family.

*Test-Taking Strategy:* Use the process of elimination and focus on the issue, confidentiality and the client's right to privacy. Option 2 is the only option that upholds the client's rights. Review these rights if you had difficulty with this question.

*Level of Cognitive Ability:* Application
*Client Needs:* Safe, Effective Care Environment
*Integrated Concept/Process:* Caring
*Content Area:* Fundamental Skills

*Reference*
Potter, P., & Perry, A. (2001). *Fundamentals of nursing* (5th ed.). St. Louis: Mosby, p. 431.

**28.** A nurse has been assigned to care for a young man recovering at home from a disabling lung infection. While obtaining a nursing history, the nurse learns that the infection is probably the result of human immunodeficiency virus (HIV). The nurse informs the client that he or she is morally opposed to homosexuality and cannot care for him. The nurse then leaves the client's home. Which of the following is true regarding the nurse's actions?

1 The nurse has a duty to protect self from client care situations that are morally repellent
2 The nurse has a legal right to inform the client of any barriers to providing care
3 The nurse has the right to refuse to care for any client without justifying that refusal
4 The nurse has a duty to provide competent care to assigned clients in a nondiscriminatory manner

**Answer: 4**
*Rationale:* The nurse has a duty to provide care to all clients in a nondiscriminatory manner. Personal autonomy does not apply if it interferes with the rights of the client. There is no legal obligation to inform the client of the nurse's personal objections to the client. Refusal to provide care may be acceptable if that refusal does not put the client's safety at risk, and the refusal is primarily associated with religious objections, not personal objection to lifestyle or medical diagnosis. The nurse also has an obligation to observe the principle of nonmaleficence (neither causing nor allowing harm to befall the client).

*Test-Taking Strategy:* Use the process of elimination, thinking about client's rights and ethical and legal responsibilities of the nurse. Note the key words *provide competent care* and *nondiscriminatory* in the correct option. Review client rights if you had difficulty with this question.

*Level of Cognitive Ability:* Analysis
*Client Needs:* Safe, Effective Care Environment
*Integrated Concept/Process:* Caring
*Content Area:* Adult Health/Immune

*Reference*
Potter, P., & Perry, A. (2001). *Fundamentals of nursing* (5th ed.). St. Louis: Mosby, p. 384.

**29.** A nurse is administering heparin sodium (Liquaemin) 5000 units subcutaneously (SC). The nurse plans to:
1 Inject within 2 inches of the umbilicus
2 Massage the injection site following administration
3 Inject via an infusion device
4 Change the needle on the syringe after withdrawing the medication from the vial

**Answer: 4**
*Rationale:* The injection site is located in the abdominal fat layer. It is not injected within 2 inches of the umbilicus or into any scar tissue. The needle is withdrawn rapidly, pressure is applied, and the area is not massaged. Injection sites are rotated. Heparin administered SC does not require an infusion device. After withdrawal of heparin from the vial, the needle is changed before injection to prevent leakage of medication along the needle tract.

*Test-Taking Strategy:* Specific knowledge regarding the administration of SC heparin is required to answer this question. Review this procedure if you had difficulty with this question.

*Level of Cognitive Ability:* Application
*Client Needs:* Safe, Effective Care Environment
*Integrated Concept/Process:* Nursing Process/Planning
*Content Area:* Pharmacology

*Reference*
Hodgson, B., & Kizior, R. (2001). *Saunders Nursing drug handbook 2001.* Philadelphia: W.B. Saunders, p. 489.

**30.** A nurse is caring for a client with cancer. The client tells the nurse that a lawyer will be arriving today to prepare a living will. The client asks the nurse to act as one of the witnesses for the will. The most appropriate nursing action is to:
1 Agree to act as a witness
2 Refuse to help the client
3 Inform the client that a nurse caring for a client cannot serve as a witness to a living will
4 Call the physician

**Answer: 3**
*Rationale:* Living wills address the withdrawal or withholding of life sustaining interventions that unnaturally prolong life. It identifies the person who will make care decisions if the client is unable to take action. It is witnessed and signed by two people who are unrelated to the client. Nurses or employees of a facility in which the client is receiving care, and beneficiaries of the client, must not serve as a witness. There is no reason to call the physician.

*Test-Taking Strategy:* Use the process of elimination. Note the key words *most appropriate action*. Eliminate option 2 because of the word *refuse*. From the remaining options, it is necessary to recall the nurse's role regarding witnessing a legal document. Review the concepts surrounding a living will if you are unfamiliar with them.

*Level of Cognitive Ability:* Application
*Client Needs:* Safe, Effective Care Environment
*Integrated Concept/Process:* Nursing Process/Implementation
*Content Area:* Fundamental Skills

*Reference*
Potter, P., & Perry, A. (2001). *Fundamentals of nursing* (5th ed.). St. Louis: Mosby, p. 436.

**31.** A home health nurse visits a three-year-old with chickenpox. The child's mother tells the nurse that the child keeps scratching the skin at night and asks the nurse what to do. The nurse tells the mother to:
1  Apply generous amounts of a cortisone cream to prevent itching
2  Place soft cotton gloves on the child's hands at night
3  Keep the child in a warm room at night so the covers will not cause the child to scratch
4  Give the child a glass of warm milk at bedtime to help the child to sleep

**Answer: 2**
*Rationale:* Gloves will keep the child from scratching the open lesions from chickenpox. Generous amounts of any topical cream can lead to drug toxicity. A warm room will increase the child's skin temperature and make itching worse. Warm milk will have no effect on itching.

*Test-Taking Strategy:* Use the process of elimination. Eliminate option 3 first because this action will promote scratching and itching. Option 4 should be eliminated next because it is unrelated to scratching. From the remaining options, the words *generous amounts* in option 1 should provide you with the clue that this option is incorrect. Review home care measures for the child with chickenpox if you had difficulty with this question.

*Level of Cognitive Ability:* Application
*Client Needs:* Safe, Effective Care Environment
*Integrated Concept/Process:* Teaching/Learning
*Content Area:* Child Health

*Reference*
Ball, J., & Bindler, R. (1999). *Pediatric nursing: Caring for children* (2nd ed.). Stamford, Conn.: Appleton & Lange, p. 382.

**32.** An elderly client has been identified as a victim of physical abuse. In planning care, the nurse places highest priority on:
1  Obtaining treatment for the abusing family member
2  Adhering to the mandatory abuse reporting laws
3  Notifying the caseworker to intervene in the family situation
4  Removing the client from any immediate danger

**Answer: 4**
*Rationale:* The priority nursing intervention is to remove the abused victim from the abusive environment. Options 1, 2, and 3 may be appropriate interventions, but are not the priority.

*Test-Taking Strategy:* Note the key words *highest priority*. Use Maslow's Hierarchy of Needs theory, remembering that if a physiological need is not present, then safety is the priority. Option 4 is the only option that directly addresses client safety. Review care to the abused elderly client if you had difficulty with this question.

*Level of Cognitive Ability:* Application
*Client Needs:* Safe, Effective Care Environment
*Integrated Concept/Process:* Nursing Process/Planning
*Content Area:* Mental Health

*Reference*
Stuart, G.W., & Laraia, M.T. (1998). *Principles and practice of psychiatric nursing* (6th ed.). St. Louis: Mosby, p. 831.

〈ïg'zɛkjətɪ〕遺囑執行人

**33.** A client diagnosed with leukemia asks the nurse questions about preparing a living will. The nurse informs the client that the initial step in preparing this document is to:

1   Consult with the American Cancer Society
2   Talk to the hospital chaplain
3   Contact a lawyer
4   Discuss the request with the physician

**Answer: 4**

*Rationale:* The client should discuss the request for a living will with the physician. The client should also discuss this desire with the family. Wills should be prepared with legal counsel and should identify the executor of the estate, address distribution and use of property, and the specific plans for burial. Although options 1 and 2 may be helpful, their contact would not be the initial step. The lawyer would be contacted following discussion with the physician and family.

*Test-Taking Strategy:* Use the process of elimination and note the key words *initial step*. Remembering that the physician is the primary care provider will assist in directing you to the correct option. Contacts addressed in options 1, 2, and 3 may follow the discussion with the physician. Review the concepts related to living wills if you had difficulty with this question.

*Level of Cognitive Ability:* Application
*Client Needs:* Safe, Effective Care Environment
*Integrated Concept/Process:* Nursing Process/Implementation
*Content Area:* Fundamental Skills

**Reference**
Potter, P., & Perry, A. (2001). *Fundamentals of nursing* (5th ed.). St. Louis: Mosby, p. 437.

**34.** A client recovering from cardiogenic shock occasionally becomes disoriented. The most appropriate nursing action to ensure safety for this client would be to:

1   Raise the head of the bed to 45 degrees
2   Keep the side rails up at all times and the call light within reach
3   Keep the over-the-bed light on in the client's room
4   Request that only two visitors visit at a time

**Answer: 2**

*Rationale:* Keeping the side rails up prevents the disoriented client from accidentally falling out of bed. Providing the call light to the client provides access to the health care team when assistance is needed. Raising the head of the bed will not ensure safety. Keeping the over-the-bed light on may be disruptive. Limiting visitors will not ensure safety.

*Test-Taking Strategy:* Focus on the issue of safety. Eliminate options 1 and 4 because these actions do not provide for safety for this client. Eliminate option 3 because this option may be disruptive and lead to further disorientation. Review basic safety measures for the disoriented client if you had difficulty with this question.

*Level of Cognitive Ability:* Application
*Client Needs:* Safe, Effective Care Environment
*Integrated Concept/Process:* Nursing Process/Implementation
*Content Area:* Adult Health/Cardiovascular

**Reference**
Potter, P., & Perry, A. (2001). *Fundamentals of nursing* (5th ed.). St. Louis: Mosby, p. 1019.

〈ïg'zɛkjətɪ〕遺囑執行人

**35.** A client with a subarachnoid hemorrhage has been placed on subarachnoid (aneurysm) precautions. The nurse ensures that the client is provided with which of the following?
1    Daily stool softeners
2    Bright lights
3    Television and radio
4    Enemas as needed

**Answer: 1**
*Rationale:* Subarachnoid (aneurysm) precautions include a variety of measures designed to decrease stimuli that could increase the client's intracranial pressure. These include instituting dim lighting and reducing environmental noise and stimuli. Enemas should be avoided, but stool softeners should be provided. Straining at stool is contraindicated because it increases intracranial pressure. Suction equipment and oxygen should be available at the bedside.

*Test-Taking Strategy:* Focus on the client's diagnosis and the need to reduce environmental stimuli and prevent increased intracranial pressure. Options 2 and 3 can be eliminated first because these items will stimulate the client. From the remaining options, eliminate option 4 because enemas will increase intracranial pressure. Review the nursing interventions for the client on aneurysm precautions if you had difficulty with this question.

*Level of Cognitive Ability:* Application
*Client Needs:* Safe, Effective Care Environment
*Integrated Concept/Process:* Nursing Process/Implementation
*Content Area:* Adult Health/Neurological

*Reference*
Monahan, F., & Neighbors, M. (1998). *Medical-surgical nursing: Foundations for clinical practice* (2nd ed.). Philadelphia: W.B. Saunders, p. 816.

**36.** A nurse is about to administer an intravenous dose of tobramycin (Tobrex) when the client complains of vertigo and a ringing in the ears. The nurse most appropriately:
1    Hangs the dose immediately
2    Gives a dose of droperidol (Inapsine) with the tobramycin
3    Holds the dose and calls the physician
4    Checks the client's pupillary responses

**Answer: 3**
*Rationale:* Ringing in the ears and vertigo are two symptoms that may indicate dysfunction of the eighth cranial nerve. Ototoxicity is a toxic effect of therapy with the aminoglycosides, and could result in permanent hearing loss. The nurse should hold the dose and notify the physician. Options 1, 2, and 4 are inappropriate nursing actions.

*Test-Taking Strategy:* Note the key words *most appropriately*. Focusing on the client's complaints and recalling that ototoxicity can occur with this medication will direct you to option 3. Review the toxic effects of this medication if you had difficulty with this question.

*Level of Cognitive Ability:* Application
*Client Needs:* Safe, Effective Care Environment
*Integrated Concept/Process:* Nursing Process/Implementation
*Content Area:* Pharmacology

*Reference*
Hodgson, B., & Kizior, R. (2001). *Saunders Nursing drug handbook 2001.* Philadelphia: W.B. Saunders, p. 998.

**37.** A nurse is preparing to administer amiodarone (Cordarone) intravenously. The nurse ensures that which of the following is in place for the client before administering the medication?
1    Noninvasive blood pressure cuff
2    Oxygen saturation monitor
3    Oxygen therapy
4    Continuous cardiac monitoring

**Answer: 4**
*Rationale:* Amiodarone is an antidysrhythmic used to treat life-threatening ventricular dysrhythmias. The client should have continuous cardiac monitoring in place, and the medication should be infused by intravenous pump. Although options 1, 2, and 3 may be in place for the client, they are not specific items needed for the administration of this medication.

*Test-Taking Strategy:* Use the process of elimination. Recalling that this medication is an antidysrhythmic will direct you to option 4. If this question was difficult, review the classification of this medication and the nursing considerations when administering this medication.

*Level of Cognitive Ability:* Application
*Client Needs:* Safe, Effective Care Environment
*Integrated Concept/Process:* Nursing Process/Implementation
*Content Area:* Pharmacology

*Reference*
Hodgson, B., & Kizior, R. (2001). *Saunders Nursing drug handbook 2001.* Philadelphia: W.B. Saunders, p. 47.

---

**38.** A client is admitted to the hospital for a bowel resection following a diagnosis of a bowel tumor. During the admission assessment, the client tells the nurse that a living will was prepared three years ago. The client asks the nurse if this document is still effective. The most appropriate nursing response is which of the following?
1    "Yes it is."
2    "You will have to ask your lawyer."
3    "It should be reviewed yearly with your physician."
4    "I have no idea."

**Answer: 3**
*Rationale:* The client should discuss the living will with the physician and it should be reviewed annually to ensure that it contains the client's present wishes and desires. Option 1 is incorrect. Option 4 is not at all helpful to the client and is in fact a communication block. Although a lawyer would need to be consulted if the living will needed to be changed, the most appropriate and accurate nursing response would be to inform the client that the living will should be reviewed annually.

*Test-Taking Strategy:* Use the process of elimination. Eliminate options 1 and 4 first because they are nontherapeutic and place the client's question on hold. From the remaining options, it is necessary to know that the document is reviewed annually. Review the concepts related to living wills if you had difficulty with this question.

*Level of Cognitive Ability:* Application
*Client Needs:* Safe, Effective Care Environment
*Integrated Concept/Process:* Communication and Documentation
*Content Area:* Fundamental Skills

*Reference*
Potter, P., & Perry, A. (2001). *Fundamentals of nursing* (5th ed.). St. Louis: Mosby, p. 437.

**39.** A home care nurse visits a client recently discharged from the hospital following an acute myocardial infarction. The client tells the nurse that a living will was prepared and asks the nurse where a copy of the will can be obtained. The nurse tells the client that which area will not have a copy?

**1** Lawyer's office
**2** Physician's office
**3** Medical record at the hospital
**4** Hospital emergency room files

**Answer: 4**

*Rationale:* Copies of a living will should be kept with the medical record, at the physicians office, and in the home of the client. A copy will also be maintained in the lawyer's office. The emergency room does not maintain these documents in their files.

*Test-Taking Strategy:* Use the process of elimination. Note the key word *not*. It would seem reasonable that both a physician and lawyer would hold a copy of this document. It would also seem reasonable that a copy would be maintained in the client's medical record to provide guidance to care providers if a situation arose during hospitalization requiring referral to this document. The client should have a copy in the home because this document identifies the client's wishes. It is not realistic for an emergency room to maintain such documents in their files. Review the concepts related to living wills if you had difficulty with this question.

*Level of Cognitive Ability:* Application
*Client Needs:* Safe, Effective Care Environment
*Integrated Concept/Process:* Nursing Process/Implementation
*Content Area:* Fundamental Skills

*Reference*
Potter, P., & Perry, A. (2001). *Fundamentals of nursing* (5th ed.). St. Louis: Mosby, p. 437.

---

**40.** A nurse is caring for a client immediately following a bronchoscopy. The client received intravenous sedation and a topical anesthetic for the procedure. In order to provide a safe environment for the client at this time, the nurse plans to:

**1** Place a padded tongue blade at the bedside in case of a seizure
**2** Check the bedside to ensure no food or fluid is within the client's reach to prevent aspiration
**3** Connect the client to a bedside ECG to monitor for dysrhythmias
**4** Place a water-seal chest drainage set at the bedside in case of a pneumothorax

**Answer: 2**

*Rationale:* Following this procedure, the client remains NPO until the cough and swallow reflexes have returned, which is usually in 1 to 2 hours. Once the client can swallow, oral intake may begin with ice chips and small sips of water. There are no data in the question that suggest the client is at risk for a seizure. Even though the client is monitored for signs of any distress, seizures would not be anticipated and therefore a padded tongue blade would not be placed at the bedside routinely. A pneumothorax could possibly occur, and the nurse should bear this in mind when monitoring the client for signs of distress. However, a water-seal chest drainage set would not be placed routinely at the bedside. No data are given to support that the client is at increased risk for cardiac dysrhythmias.

*Test-Taking Strategy:* Note the key words *immediately following a bronchoscopy* and *topical anesthetic*. Use the ABCs, airway, breathing, and circulation, to direct you to option 2. Review postprocedure care following this procedure if you had difficulty with this question.

*Level of Cognitive Ability:* Application
*Client Needs:* Safe, Effective Care Environment
*Integrated Concept/Process:* Nursing Process/Planning
*Content Area:* Adult Health/Respiratory

*Reference*
Ignatavicius, D., Workman, M., & Mishler, M. (1999). *Medical-surgical nursing across the health care continuum* (3rd ed.). Philadelphia: W.B. Saunders, p. 559.

**41.** A client with a history of silicosis is admitted with respiratory distress and impending respiratory failure. The nurse plans to have which of the following items readily available at the client's bedside?

1   Chest tube and drainage system
2   Intubation tray
3   Thoracentesis tray
4   Code cart

**Answer: 2**

*Rationale:* The client with impending respiratory failure may need intubation and mechanical ventilation. The nurse ensures that an intubation tray is readily available. The other items are not needed at the client's bedside.

*Test-Taking Strategy:* Focus on the client's diagnosis. Use the ABCs, airway, breathing, and circulation, to direct you to option 2. Review care of the client with impending respiratory failure if you had difficulty with this question.

*Level of Cognitive Ability:* Application
*Client Needs:* Safe, Effective Care Environment
*Integrated Concept/Process:* Nursing Process/Planning
*Content Area:* Adult Health/Respiratory

*Reference*
Ignatavicius, D., Workman, M., & Mishler, M. (1999). *Medical-surgical nursing across the health care continuum* (3rd ed.). Philadelphia: W.B. Saunders, p. 690.

---

**42.** A nurse is administering a first dose of pentamidine (Pentam 300) intravenously to a client. Before administering the first dose, the nurse should place the client:

1   On respiratory precautions
2   In a private room
3   In a supine position
4   In semi-Fowler's position

**Answer: 3**

*Rationale:* Pentamidine can cause severe and sudden hypotension, even with administration of a single dose. The client should be lying down during administration of this medication. The blood pressure is monitored frequently during administration. Options 1 and 2 are unnecessary. Option 4 is incorrect.

*Test-Taking Strategy:* Use the process of elimination. Recalling that the medication causes hypotension will direct you to option 3. Review the nursing considerations related to this medication if you had difficulty with this question.

*Level of Cognitive Ability:* Application
*Client Needs:* Safe, Effective Care Environment
*Integrated Concept/Process:* Nursing Process/Implementation
*Content Area:* Pharmacology

*Reference*
Hodgson, B., & Kizior, R. (2001). *Saunders Nursing drug handbook 2001.* Philadelphia: W.B. Saunders, pp. 801-803.

**43.** A nurse is administering a dose of intravenous hydralazine (Apresoline) to a client. The nurse ensures that which of the following items is in place before injecting the medication?
1. Central line
2. Foley catheter
3. Cardiac monitor
4. Noninvasive blood pressure (BP) cuff

**Answer: 4**
*Rationale:* Hydralazine is an antihypertensive medication used in the management of moderate to severe hypertension. The blood pressure and pulse should be monitored frequently after administration, so a noninvasive blood pressure cuff is the item to have in place. Options 1, 2, and 3 are not necessary.

*Test-Taking Strategy:* Use the process of elimination. The name of the medication "Apresoline" may provide you with the clue that the medication is used to lower the BP. This will direct you to option 4. If this question was difficult, review the action of this medication.

*Level of Cognitive Ability:* Application
*Client Needs:* Safe, Effective Care Environment
*Integrated Concept/Process:* Nursing Process/Implementation
*Content Area:* Pharmacology

*Reference*
Hodgson, B., & Kizior, R. (2001). *Saunders Nursing drug handbook 2001.* Philadelphia: W.B. Saunders, p. 493.

---

**44.** A nurse is preparing to care for a client who has undergone left pneumonectomy. The nurse plans to do which of the following immediately after transfer from the post-anesthesia care unit?
1. Place the IV on a pump
2. Assist the client to sit in the bedside chair
3. Position the client supine
4. Position the client on the left side

**Answer: 1**
*Rationale:* Following pneumonectomy, the fluid status of the client is monitored closely to prevent fluid overload, since the size of the pulmonary vascular bed has been reduced as a result of the pneumonectomy. Complete lateral turning and positioning is avoided. The head of bed should be elevated to promote lung expansion. The client should remain on bed rest in the immediate postoperative period.

*Test-Taking Strategy:* Use the process of elimination. Eliminate options 3 and 4 first, since the client should not lie flat and because lateral positioning is avoided. Eliminate option 2 because the client should not be sitting in a chair immediately after a surgical procedure such as this. Review postoperative care following pneumonectomy if you had difficulty with this question.

*Level of Cognitive Ability:* Application
*Client Needs:* Safe, Effective Care Environment
*Integrated Concept/Process:* Nursing Process/Planning
*Content Area:* Adult Health/Respiratory

*Reference*
Ignatavicius, D., Workman, M., & Mishler, M. (1999). *Medical-surgical nursing across the health care continuum* (3rd ed.). Philadelphia: W.B. Saunders, p. 656.

**45.** A client being seen in the emergency room is being evaluated for possible pleurisy. A nurse is preparing the client for a chest x-ray examination. The nurse plans to:
1  Ask the client to remove a neck chain being worn
2  Ask the client about the time of last food intake
3  Scrub the chest with Betadine
4  Determine whether the client has any metallic implants

**Answer: 1**
*Rationale:* If a chest x-ray examination is prescribed, jewelry or metal objects that might obstruct the x-ray need to be removed. The client does not need to have food or fluid restricted before a chest x-ray procedure, and skin preparation is not required. Notation of metallic implants is required before magnetic resonance imaging (MRI), but a MRI is not used to diagnose pleurisy.

*Test-Taking Strategy:* Use the process of elimination, noting the diagnostic test addressed in the question. Recalling the principles related to client preparation will direct you to option 1. Review this diagnostic test if you had difficulty with this question.

*Level of Cognitive Ability:* Application
*Client Needs:* Safe, Effective Care Environment
*Integrated Concept/Process:* Nursing Process/Planning
*Content Area:* Adult Health/Respiratory

*Reference*
Smeltzer, S., & Bare, B. (2000). *Brunner & Suddarth's Textbook of medical-surgical nursing* (9th ed.). Philadelphia: Lippincott Williams & Wilkins, p. 395.

**46.** A nurse has administered diazepam (Valium) 5 mg intravenously (IV) to a client. The nurse plans to maintain the client on bed rest for at least:
1  30 minutes
2  1 hour
3  3 hours
4  8 hours

**Answer: 3**
*Rationale:* The client should remain in bed for at least 3 hours following a parenteral dose of diazepam. The medication is a centrally acting skeletal muscle relaxant and also has antianxiety, sedative-hypnotic, and anticonvulsant properties. Cardiopulmonary side effects include apnea, hypotension, bradycardia, or cardiac arrest. For this reason, resuscitative equipment is also kept nearby.

*Test-Taking Strategy:* Specific knowledge of the effects of diazepam administered intravenously is needed to answer this question. Review the nursing considerations related to the administration of this medication if you had difficulty with this question.

*Level of Cognitive Ability:* Application
*Client Needs:* Safe, Effective Care Environment
*Integrated Concept/Process:* Nursing Process/Planning
*Content Area:* Pharmacology

*Reference*
Hodgson, B., & Kizior, R. (2001). *Saunders Nursing drug handbook 2001.* Philadelphia: W.B. Saunders, pp. 307, 309.

**47.** A nurse is caring for a hospitalized client who is having a prescribed dosage of clonazepam (Klonopin) adjusted. The nurse plans to:

1. Monitor blood glucose levels
2. Institute seizure precautions
3. Weigh the client daily
4. Observe for ecchymoses

**Answer: 2**

*Rationale:* Clonazepam is a benzodiazepine that is used as an anticonvulsant. During initial therapy and during periods of dosage adjustment, the nurse should initiate seizure precautions for the client. Options 1, 3, and 4 are unrelated to the use of this medication.

*Test-Taking Strategy:* Use the process of elimination. Recalling that this medication is an anticonvulsant will direct you to option 2. Review the nursing considerations related to this medication if you had difficulty with this question.

*Level of Cognitive Ability:* Application
*Client Needs:* Safe, Effective Care Environment
*Integrated Concept/Process:* Nursing Process/Planning
*Content Area:* Pharmacology

*Reference*
Hodgson, B., & Kizior, R. (2001). *Saunders Nursing drug handbook 2001.* Philadelphia: W.B. Saunders, pp. 238-240.

**48.** A nurse is planning to obtain an arterial blood gas (ABG) from a client with chronic obstructive pulmonary disease (COPD). The nurse plans time for which activity after the arterial blood is drawn?

1. Holding a warm compress over the puncture site for 5 minutes
2. Applying pressure to the puncture site by applying a 2 × 2 gauze for 5 minutes
3. Encouraging the client to open and close the hand rapidly for 2 minutes
4. Having the client keep the radial pulse puncture site in a dependent position for 5 minutes

**Answer: 2**

*Rationale:* Applying pressure over the puncture site reduces the risk of hematoma formation and damage to the artery. A cold compress would aid in limiting blood flow. Keeping the extremity still and out of a dependent position will aid in the formation of a clot at the puncture site.

*Test-Taking Strategy:* Use the process of elimination. Focus on the issue, preventing bleeding. Options 1, 3, and 4 promote bleeding. Option 2 aids in the prevention of bleeding into the surrounding tissues. Review nursing responsibilities following ABGs if you had difficulty with this question.

*Level of Cognitive Ability:* Application
*Client Needs:* Safe, Effective Care Environment
*Integrated Concept/Process:* Nursing Process/Planning
*Content Area:* Adult Health/Respiratory

*Reference*
Smeltzer, S., & Bare, B. (2000). *Brunner & Suddarth's Textbook of medical-surgical nursing* (9th ed.). Philadelphia: Lippincott Williams & Wilkins, pp. 238-239.

**49.** A nurse is admitting a client to the nursing unit who has an arteriovenous (AV) fistula in the right arm for hemodialysis. The nurse would best plan to prevent injury to the site by:
1  Putting a large note about the access site on the front of the medical record
2  Applying an allergy bracelet to the right arm, indicating the presence of the fistula
3  Placing a sign at the bedside: "No blood pressure (BP) measurements or venipunctures in the right arm."
4  Telling the client to inform all caregivers who enter the room about the presence of the access site

**Answer: 3**
*Rationale:* There should be no venipunctures or blood pressure measurements in the limb with a hemodialysis access device. This is commonly communicated to all caregivers by placing a sign at the client's bedside. Placing a note on the front of the medical record does not ensure that everyone caring for the client will be aware of the access device. An allergy bracelet is placed on the client with an allergy. The client should not be responsible for informing the caregivers.

*Test-Taking Strategy:* Use the process of elimination, noting the key word *best.* Eliminate option 2, because an allergy bracelet is used for a client with an allergy. Eliminate option 4 next, because this responsibility should not be placed on the client. From the remaining options, note that option 3 best informs those caring for the client of the presence of the fistula. Review care of a client with a fistula if you had difficulty with this question.

*Level of Cognitive Ability:* Application
*Client Needs:* Safe, Effective Care Environment
*Integrated Concept/Process:* Nursing Process/Planning
*Content Area:* Adult Health/Renal

*Reference*
Smeltzer, S., & Bare, B. (2000). *Brunner & Suddarth's Textbook of medical-surgical nursing* (9th ed.). Philadelphia: Lippincott Williams & Wilkins, p. 1124.

**50.** Regular insulin by continuous intravenous (IV) infusion is prescribed for a client with a blood glucose level of 700 mg/dL. The nurse plans to:
1  Infuse the medication via an electronic infusion pump
2  Mix the solution in 5% dextrose
3  Change the solution every 6 hours
4  Titrate the infusion according to the client's urine glucose levels

**Answer: 1**
*Rationale:* Insulin is administered via an infusion pump to prevent inadvertent overdose and subsequent hypoglycemia. Dextrose is added to the IV line once the serum glucose level reaches 250 mg/dL to prevent the occurrence of hypoglycemia. Administering dextrose to a client with a serum glucose level of 700 mg/dL would counteract the beneficial effects of insulin in reducing the glucose level. Glycosuria is not a reliable indicator of the actual serum glucose levels because there are many factors that affect the renal threshold for glucose loss in the urine. There is no reason to change the solution every 6 hours.

*Test-Taking Strategy:* Use the process of elimination. Eliminate option 4, knowing that urine glucose levels do not provide an accurate indication of the client's status. Next, eliminate option 2, knowing that dextrose would not be administered to a client with a blood glucose level of 700 mg/dL. From the remaining options, recalling the complications associated with a continuous infusion of insulin will direct you to option 1. Review nursing care of a client with a continuous IV infusion of insulin if you had difficulty with this question.

*Level of Cognitive Ability:* Application
*Client Needs:* Safe, Effective Care Environment
*Integrated Concept/Process:* Nursing Process/Planning
*Content Area:* Adult Health/Endocrine

*Reference*
Smeltzer, S., & Bare, B. (2000). *Brunner & Suddarth's Textbook of medical-surgical nursing* (9th ed.). Philadelphia: Lippincott Williams & Wilkins, p. 990.

---

**51.** A nurse is developing a plan of care for a client with diabetic ketoacidosis (DKA). The nurse most appropriately includes which intervention in the plan?
1    Maintain side rails in the upright position
2    Ambulate the client every 2 hours
3    Assess for fluid overload
4    Limit family visitation

**Answer: 1**
*Rationale:* The client with DKA may experience a decrease in the level of consciousness (LOC) secondary to acidosis. Safety becomes a priority for any client with a decreased LOC, thus requiring the use of side rails to prevent fall injuries. The client may be too ill to ambulate and will experience fluid loss (dehydration) rather than overload. Family visitation is helpful for both the client and family to assist with psychosocial adaptation.

*Test-Taking Strategy:* Use the process of elimination. Focus on the diagnosis to eliminate options 2 and 4. From the remaining options, recalling that dehydration is an issue in DKA and that mental status changes occur will direct you to option 1. Review care of the client with DKA if you had difficulty with this question.

*Level of Cognitive Ability:* Application
*Client Needs:* Safe, Effective Care Environment
*Integrated Concept/Process:* Nursing Process/Planning
*Content Area:* Adult Health/Endocrine

*Reference*
Smeltzer, S., & Bare, B. (2000). *Brunner & Suddarth's Textbook of medical-surgical nursing* (9th ed.). Philadelphia: Lippincott Williams & Wilkins, p. 100.

---

**52.** A nurse practicing in a Nurse Managed Clinic wants to set up a diabetic teaching seminar. The nurse understands that to meet the needs of the clients, the nurse must first:
1    Assess the clients' functional abilities
2    Ensure that the insurance documentation is up-to-date
3    Discuss the focus of the seminar with the multidisciplinary team
4    Include everyone who comes into the clinic in the teaching sessions

**Answer: 1**
*Rationale:* The focus of Nurse Managed Clinics is on individualized disease prevention and health promotion and maintenance. Therefore the nurse must first assess the clients and their needs to effectively plan the seminar. Options 2, 3, and 4 do not address the needs of the clients.

*Test-Taking Strategy:* Use the process of elimination and the steps of the nursing process. Remember the first step is assessment. Option 1 reflects assessment. Review teaching/learning principles if you had difficulty with this question.

*Level of Cognitive Ability:* Application
*Client Needs:* Safe, Effective Care Environment
*Integrated Concept/Process:* Teaching/Learning
*Content Area:* Fundamental Skills

*Reference*
Smeltzer, S., & Bare, B. (2000). *Brunner & Suddarth's Textbook of medical-surgical nursing* (9th ed.). Philadelphia: Lippincott Williams & Wilkins, p. 41.

**53.** A nurse notes that a postoperative client has not been obtaining relief of pain with the prescribed narcotics, but only while a particular licensed practical nurse (LPN) is assigned to the client. The nurse:

1   Reviews the client's medication administration record and immediately discusses the situation with the nursing supervisor
2   Notifies the physician that the client needs an increase in narcotic dosage
3   Decides to avoid assigning the LPN to the care of clients receiving narcotics
4   Confronts the LPN with the information about the client having pain control problems and asks if the LPN is using the narcotics personally

**Answer: 1**

*Rationale:* In this situation, the nurse has noted an unusual occurrence, but before deciding what action to next take, the nurse needs more data than just suspicion. This can be obtained by reviewing the client's record. State and federal labor and narcotic regulations, as well as institutional policies and procedures, must be followed. It is therefore most appropriate that the nurse discuss the situation with the nursing supervisor before taking further action. The client does not need an increase in narcotics. To avoid assigning the LPN to clients receiving narcotics only ignores the issue. A confrontation is not the most advisable action, because the appropriate administrative authorities need to be consulted first.

*Test-Taking Strategy:* Use the process of elimination and knowledge regarding the roles and responsibilities of the nurse. Option 1 is the only option that includes consultation with an authority figure, the nursing supervisor. Review the nurse's role when substance abuse in another nurse is suspected if you had difficulty with this question.

*Level of Cognitive Ability:* Application
*Client Needs:* Safe, Effective Care Environment
*Integrated Concept/Process:* Nursing Process/Implementation
*Content Area:* Fundamental Skills

*Reference*
Potter, P., & Perry, A. (2001). *Fundamentals of nursing* (5th ed.). St. Louis: Mosby, p. 55.

---

**54.** A medication nurse is supervising a newly hired licensed practical nurse (LPN) during the administration of pyridostigmine (Mestinon) PO to a client with myasthenia gravis. Which observation by the medication nurse would indicate safe practice by the LPN?

1   Asking the client to lie down on his or her right side
2   Instructing the client to void before taking the medication
3   Asking the client to take sips of water
4   Asking the client to look up to the ceiling for 30 seconds

**Answer: 3**

*Rationale:* Myasthenia gravis can affect the client's ability to swallow. The primary assessment is to determine the client's ability to handle PO medications or any oral substance. Options 1 and 4 are not appropriate. In this situation, there is no reason for the client to lie down to swallow medication or to look up to the ceiling. There is no specific reason for the client to void before taking this medication.

*Test-Taking Strategy:* Use the process of elimination. Recalling that myasthenia gravis affects the client's ability to swallow will direct you to option 3. Also, note the relationship between *PO* in the question and *sips of water* in the correct option. If you had difficulty with this question, review nursing care of the client with myasthenia gravis.

*Level of Cognitive Ability:* Analysis
*Client Needs:* Safe, Effective Care Environment
*Integrated Concept/Process:* Nursing Process/Evaluation
*Content Area:* Fundamental Skills

*Reference*
Salerno, E. (1999). *Pharmacology for health professionals.* St. Louis: Mosby, p. 444.

**55.** A client's vital signs have noticeably deteriorated over the past four hours following surgery. A nurse does not recognize the significance of these changes in vital signs and takes no action. The client later requires emergency surgery. The nurse could be prosecuted for inaction according to the definition of which of these?

1 Tort
2 Misdemeanor (misdi minə) 輕罪
3 Common law
4 Statutory law

**Answer: 1**

*Rationale:* A tort is a wrongful act intentionally or unintentionally committed against a person or his or her property. The nurse's inaction in the situation described is consistent with the definition of a tort offense. Option 2 is an offense under criminal law. Option 3 describes case law that has evolved over time via precedents. Option 4 describes laws that are enacted by State, Federal, or local governments.

*Test-Taking Strategy:* Use the process of elimination. Recalling that a tort is a wrongful act will direct you to option 1. Review the definitions related to the various types of laws if you had difficulty with this question.

*Level of Cognitive Ability:* Analysis
*Client Needs:* Safe, Effective Care Environment
*Integrated Concept/Process:* Nursing Process/Analysis
*Content Area:* Fundamental Skills

*Reference*
Potter, P., & Perry, A. (2001). *Fundamentals of nursing* (5th ed.). St. Louis: Mosby, p. 425.

**56.** A well-known individual from the community is admitted to the hospital with a diagnosis of Parkinson's disease. The nurse gives medical information regarding the client's condition to a person assumed to be a family member. Later, the nurse discovers that this person is not a family member and realizes that this is a violation of which legal concept of the nurse-client relationship?

1 Invasion of privacy
2 Lack of experience
3 Teaching/learning principles
4 Performing a focused physical assessment

**Answer: 1**

*Rationale:* Discussing a client's condition without client permission violates a client's rights and places the nurse in legal jeopardy. This action by the nurse is both an invasion of privacy and affects the confidentiality issue with client rights. Options 2, 3, and 4 do not represent violation of the situation presented.

*Test-Taking Strategy:* Use the process of elimination. Focus on the information in the question. The issue of the question is related to sharing information, which constitutes an invasion of privacy. If you had difficulty with this question, review client rights and the situations that involve invasion of privacy.

*Level of Cognitive Ability:* Analysis
*Client Need:* Safe, Effective Care Environment
*Integrated Concept/Process:* Nursing Process/Analysis
*Content Area:* Adult Health/Neurological

*Reference*
Potter, P., & Perry, A. (2001). *Fundamentals of nursing* (5th ed.). St. Louis: Mosby, p. 905.

**57.** A clinic nurse is assessing a client for environmental risk factors related to neurological disorders. The nurse understands that which of the following is least likely associated with neurological disorders?

1   Exposure to fumes, such as paints or bonding agents (glue)
2   Exposure to pesticides
3   Ventilation in the work area
4   Number of windows in the work area

**Answer: 4**

*Rationale:* The nurse would assess for the risk of exposure to neurotoxic fumes and chemicals. These could include paint, bonding agents, pesticides and many more. The nurse also inquires about the adequacy of ventilation in the home, and work area. There are many work spaces (such as factories, insurance companies, and operating rooms) which are adequately ventilated without the use of windows.

*Test-Taking Strategy:* Use the process of elimination. Note the key words *least likely*. Focusing on the issue, environmental risk factors will direct you to option 4. Review environmental risk factors associated with neurological disorders if you had difficulty with this question.

*Level of Cognitive Ability:* Analysis
*Client Needs:* Safe, Effective Care Environment
*Integrated Concept/Process:* Nursing Process/Assessment
*Content Area:* Adult Health/Neurological

*Reference*
Smeltzer, S., & Bare, B. (2000). *Brunner & Suddarth's Textbook of medical-surgical nursing* (9th ed.). Philadelphia: Lippincott Williams & Wilkins, p. 1640.

---

**58.** A nurse performing an initial admission assessment notes that a client has been taking metoclopramide (Reglan) for a prolonged period of time. The nurse would immediately call the physician if which of the following signs or symptoms was then noted by the nurse?

1   Anxiety or irritability
2   Dry mouth relieved with the use of sugar-free hard candy
3   Excessive drowsiness or excitability
4   Uncontrolled rhythmic movements of the face or limbs

**Answer: 4**

*Rationale:* If the client experiences tardive dyskinesia (rhythmic movements of the face or limbs), the nurse should call the physician because these side effects may be irreversible. The medication would be discontinued and no further doses should be given by the nurse. Anxiety, irritability, and dry mouth are milder side effects that do not harm the client. Excitability is not a side effect.

*Test-Taking Strategy:* Use the process of elimination. Note that the question contains the key word *immediately*, which guides you to select the most harmful option. Recalling that this medication causes tardive dyskinesia will direct you to option 4. Review the side effects of this medication and the signs of tardive dyskinesia if you had difficulty with this question.

*Level of Cognitive Ability:* Analysis
*Client Needs:* Safe, Effective Care Environment
*Integrated Concept/Process:* Communication and Documentation
*Content Area:* Pharmacology

*Reference*
Deglin, J., & Vallerand, A. (2001). *Davis's Drug guide for nurses* (7th ed.). Philadelphia: F.A. Davis, p. 634.

**59.** A nurse calls the physician of a client scheduled for a cardiac catheterization because the client has numerous questions regarding the procedure and has requested to speak to the physician. The physician is very upset and arrives at the unit to visit the client after prompting by the nurse. The nurse is outside of the client's room and hears the physician tell the client in a derogatory manner that the nurse "doesn't know anything." Which legal tort has the physician violated?

1 Libel
2 Slander
3 Assault
4 Negligence

**Answer: 2**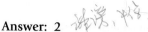
*Rationale:* Defamation takes place when something untrue is said (slander) or written (libel) about a person, resulting in injury to that person's good name and reputation. An assault occurs when a person puts another person in fear of a harmful or an offensive contact. Negligence involves the actions of professionals that fall below the standard of care for a specific professional group.

*Test-Taking Strategy:* Use the process of elimination and eliminate options 3 and 4 first. Recalling that slander constitutes verbal defamation will direct you to option 2. If you had difficulty with this question, review the torts identified in each option.

*Level of Cognitive Ability:* Analysis
*Client Needs:* Safe, Effective Care Environment
*Integrated Concept/Process:* Nursing Process/Analysis
*Content Area:* Fundamental Skills

*Reference*
Harkreader, H. (2000). *Fundamentals of nursing: Caring and clinical judgment.* Philadelphia: W.B. Saunders, pp. 23-24.

---

**60.** A nurse enters a client's room and finds the client sitting on the floor. The nurse performs a thorough assessment and assists the client back to bed. The nurse completes an incident report and notifies the physician of the incident. Which of the following is the next appropriate nursing action regarding the incident?

1 Make a copy of the incident report for the physician
2 Place the incident report in the client's chart
3 Document a complete entry in the client's record concerning the incident
4 Document in the client's record that an incident report has been completed

**Answer: 3**
*Rationale:* The incident report is confidential and privileged information and should not be copied, placed in the chart, or have any reference made to it in the client's record. The incident report is not a substitute for a complete entry in the client's record concerning the incident.

*Test-Taking Strategy:* Use the process of elimination and eliminate options 2 and 4 first because they are similar. Recalling that incident reports should not be copied will direct you to option 3. Review nursing responsibilities related to incident reports if you had difficulty with this question.

*Level of Cognitive Ability:* Application
*Client Needs:* Safe, Effective Care Environment
*Integrated Concept/Process:* Communication and Documentation
*Content Area:* Fundamental Skills

*Reference*
Kozier, B., Erb, G., Berman, A., & Burke, K. (2000). *Fundamentals of nursing: Concepts, process, and practice* (6th ed.). Upper Saddle River, N.J.: Prentice-Hall, p. 66.

**61.** A client had a colon resection. A Levin tube was in place when a regular diet was brought to the client's room. The client did not want to eat solid food and asked that the physician be called. The nurse insisted that the solid food was the correct diet. The client ate and subsequently had additional surgery because of complications. The determination of negligence in this situation is based on:

1  A duty existed and it was breached
2  Not calling the physician
3  The dietary department sending the wrong food
4  The nurse's persistence

**Answer: 1**

*Rationale:* For negligence to be proven, there must be a duty, then a breach of duty; the breach of duty must cause the injury, and damages or injury must be experienced. Options 2, 3, and 4 do not fall under the criteria for negligence. Option 1 is the only option that fits the criteria of negligence.

*Test-Taking Strategy:* Use the process of elimination. Options 2, 3, and 4 do not directly support the issue of negligence because it would be difficult to determine that these elements caused injury. The focus relates to what the nurse is responsible for. Option 1 is a global response to the question. Review the legal elements of nursing practice and criteria for negligence if you had difficulty with this question.

*Level of Cognitive Ability:* Analysis
*Client Needs:* Safe, Effective Care Environment
*Integrated Concept/Process:* Nursing Process/Analysis
*Content Area:* Fundamental Skills

*Reference*
Craven, R., & Hirnle, C. (2000). *Fundamentals of nursing: Human health and function* (3rd ed.). Philadelphia: Lippincott, p. 100.

**62.** A nurse is caring for a child with intussusception. While caring for the child, the child passes a normal brown stool. The most appropriate nursing action is to:

1  Report the passage of a normal brown stool to the physician immediately
2  Prepare the child and the parents for the possibility of surgery
3  Note the child's physical symptoms
4  Prepare the child for hydrostatic reduction

**Answer: 1**

*Rationale:* Passage of a normal brown stool usually indicates that the intussusception has reduced itself. This is immediately reported to the physician, who may chose to alter the diagnostic/therapeutic plan of care. Options 2, 3, and 4 are incorrect actions.

*Test-Taking Strategy:* Use the process of elimination. Note the similarity between the information in the question and the correct option. Also, recalling the physiology associated with intussusception will direct you to option 1. Review care of the child with intussusception if you had difficulty with this question.

*Level of Cognitive Ability:* Application
*Client Needs:* Safe, Effective Care Environment
*Integrated Concept/Process:* Nursing Process/Implementation
*Content Area:* Child Health

*Reference*
Wong, D., & Perry, S. (1998). *Maternal child nursing care.* St. Louis: Mosby, pp. 1429-1430.

**63.** A new nursing graduate is attending an agency orientation regarding the nursing model of practice implemented in the facility. The nurse is told that the nursing model is a primary nursing approach. The nurse understands that which of the following is a characteristic of this type of nursing model of practice?

**1** The nurse manager assigns tasks to the staff members

**2** Critical paths are used in providing client care

**3** A single registered nurse (RN) is responsible for planning and providing individualized nursing care

**4** Nursing staff are led by an RN leader in providing care to a group of clients

**Answer: 3**

*Rationale:*  Primary nursing is concerned with keeping the nurse at the bedside actively involved in direct care while planning goal directed, individualized client care. Option 1 identifies functional nursing. Option 2 identifies a component of case management. Option 4 identifies team nursing.

*Test-Taking Strategy:*  Note that the issue of the question relates to primary nursing. Keep this issue in mind and use the process of elimination. Option 3 is the only option that identifies the concept of a primary approach. Review the various types of nursing delivery systems if you had difficulty with this question.

*Level of Cognitive Ability:*  Comprehension
*Client Needs:*  Safe, Effective Care Environment
*Integrated Concept/Process:*  Nursing Process/Implementation
*Content Area:*  Fundamental Skills

*Reference*
Rocchiccioli, J., & Tilbury, M. (1998). *Clinical leadership in nursing.* Philadelphia: W.B. Saunders, p. 32.

**64.** A client asks the nurse how to become an organ donor. Which of the following would not be a component of the nurse's response?

**1** The donor must be 18 years of age or older

**2** The donation is done by written consent

**3** The family is responsible for making that decision at the time of death

**4** Clients have the right to donate their own organs for transplantation

**Answer: 3**

*Rationale:*  The client has the right to donate her or his own organs for transplantation. Any person 18 years of age or older may become an organ donor by written consent. In the absence of appropriate documentation, a family member or legal guardian may authorize donation of the decedent's organs.

*Test-Taking Strategy:*  Note the key word *not* in the stem of the question. Using the process of elimination and the issues related to client rights will easily direct you to option 3. If you had difficulty with this question, review the procedure for organ donation.

*Level of Cognitive Ability:*  Application
*Client Needs:*  Safe, Effective Care Environment
*Integrated Concept/Process:*  Communication and Documentation
*Content Area:*  Fundamental Skills

*Reference*
Kozier, B., Erb, G., Berman, A., & Burke, K. (2000). *Fundamentals of nursing: Concepts, process, and practice* (6th ed.). Upper Saddle River, N.J.: Prentice-Hall, p. 985.

**65.** A registered nurse (RN) is providing instructions to a licensed practical nurse (LPN) who is preparing to care for a deceased client. The RN notes on the client's record that the client's eyes will be donated. The nurse avoids telling the LPN to do which of the following?

1 Elevate the head of the bed
2 Close the client's eyes
3 Place wet saline gauze pads and an ice pack on the eyes
4 Close the client's eyes and place a dry sterile dressing over the eyes

**Answer: 4**

*Rationale:* When a corneal donor dies, the eyes are closed and gauze pads wet with saline solution are placed over them with a small ice pack. Within 2 to 4 hours, the eyes are enucleated. The cornea is usually transplanted within 24 to 48 hours. The head of the bed should also be elevated.

*Test-Taking Strategy:* Note that the issue relates to donation of the eyes. Also note the key word *avoids* in the stem of the question. Knowledge regarding care to the donor's eyes will direct you to option 4. Review this procedure if you had difficulty with the question.

*Level of Cognitive Ability:* Application
*Client Needs:* Safe, Effective Care Environment
*Integrated Concept/Process:* Teaching/Learning
*Content Area:* Fundamental Skills

*Reference*
Monahan, F., & Neighbors, M. (1998). *Medical-surgical nursing: Foundations for clinical practice* (2nd ed.). Philadelphia: W. B. Saunders, p. 1954.

---

**66.** A clinical nurse manager is planning an inservice educational session for the staff nurses. The topic of the discussion is case management. Which of the following is not a characteristic of case management and would not be included in the discussion?

1 Represents a primary health prevention focus managed by a single case manager
2 Manages client care by managing the client care environment
3 Designed to promote appropriate use of hospital personnel and material resources
4 Maximizes hospital revenues while providing for optimal outcome of client care

**Answer: 1**

*Rationale:* Case management represents an interdisciplinary health care delivery system to promote appropriate use of hospital personnel and material resources to maximize hospital revenues while providing for optimal outcome of care. It manages client care by managing the client care environment.

*Test-Taking Strategy:* Use the process of elimination and knowledge regarding the characteristics of case management. Note the key word *not* in the stem of the question. Also, note the key word *single* in the correct option. Review the characteristics of case management if you had difficulty with this question.

*Level of Cognitive Ability:* Comprehension
*Client Needs:* Safe, Effective Care Environment
*Integrated Concept/Process:* Teaching/Learning
*Content Area:* Fundamental Skills

*Reference*
Rocchiccioli, J., & Tilbury, M. (1998). *Clinical leadership in nursing.* Philadelphia: W.B. Saunders, pp. 38-39

**67.** A registered nurse is delegating activities to the nursing staff. Which activity is least appropriate for the nursing assistant?

1 Assist a 12-year-old boy who is profoundly developmentally disabled to eat lunch

2 Obtain frequent oral temperatures on a client

3 Accompany a 51-year-old man, being discharged to home following a bowel resection 8 days ago, to his transportation

4 Collect a urine specimen from a 70-year-old woman admitted three days ago

**Answer: 1**

*Rationale:* Work that is delegated to others must be done consistent with the individual's level of expertise and licensure or lack of licensure. In this case, the least appropriate activity for a nursing assistant would be assisting with feeding a profoundly developmentally disabled child. The child is likely to have difficulty eating, and therefore has a high potential for complications such as choking and aspiration. The remaining three options do not include situations to indicate that these activities carry any risk.

*Test-Taking Strategy:* Note the key words *least appropriate*. Use the process of elimination. Consider the ABCs, airway, breathing, and circulation, and recall the principles of delegation in answering the question. Review the principles of assignments and delegation if you had difficulty with this question.

*Level of Cognitive Ability:* Application
*Client Needs:* Safe, Effective Care Environment
*Integrated Concept/Process:* Nursing Process/Planning
*Content Area:* Fundamental Skills

*Reference*
Rocchiccioli, J., & Tilbury, M. (1998). *Clinical leadership in nursing.* Philadelphia: W.B. Saunders, p. 140.

**68.** A clinical nurse manager is reviewing the critical paths of the clients on the nursing unit. The nurse manager collaborates with each nurse assigned to the clients and performs a variance analysis. Which of the following would indicate the need for further action and analysis?

1 A client is performing own colostomy care

2 A 1-day postoperative client has a temperature of 98.8° F

3 Purulent drainage is noted from a postoperative wound incision

4 A new diabetic client is preparing own insulin for injection

**Answer: 3**

*Rationale:* Variances are actual deviations or detours from the critical paths. Variances can be either positive or negative, avoidable, or unavoidable and can be caused by a variety of things. Positive variance occurs when the client achieves maximum benefit and is discharged earlier than anticipated. Negative variance occurs when untoward events prevent a timely discharge. Variance analysis occurs continually in order to anticipate and recognize negative variance early so that appropriate action can be taken. Option 3 is the only option that identifies the need for further action.

*Test-Taking Strategy:* Use the process of elimination identifying the negative variance. Options 1, 2, and 4 identify positive outcomes. Option 3 identifies a negative outcome. Review the purpose of variance analysis if you had difficulty with this question.

*Level of Cognitive Ability:* Analysis
*Client Needs:* Safe, Effective Care Environment
*Integrated Concept/Process:* Nursing Process/Evaluation
*Content Area:* Fundamental Skills

*Reference*
Rocchiccioli, J., & Tilbury, M. (1998). *Clinical leadership in nursing.* Philadelphia: W.B. Saunders, p. 42.

**69.** A nurse manager is conducting a conference with the nursing staff regarding concerns and proposals for actions related to the nursing unit. The nurse manager presents his or her own analysis of the problem and proposals for actions to members of the team, and invites the team members to comment and provide input. Which style of leadership is the nurse manager specifically employing?

1 Laissez-faire
2 Authoritarian
3 Situational
4 Participative

**Answer: 4**

*Rationale:* Participative leadership suggests a compromise between the authoritarian and the democratic style. In participative leadership, the manager presents his or her own analysis of problems and proposals for actions to members of the team, inviting critique and comments. The participative leader then analyzes the comments and makes the final decision. A laissez-faire leader abdicates leadership and responsibilities, allowing staff to work without assistance, direction, or supervision. The autocratic style of leadership is task oriented and directive. In the situational leadership style, the style employed depends on the situation and events.

*Test-Taking Strategy:* Knowledge regarding the various types of leadership styles is required to answer this question. Reading the question carefully will assist in directing you to the correct option. If you had difficulty with this question, review the various types of leadership styles.

*Level of Cognitive Ability:* Comprehension
*Client Needs:* Safe, Effective Care Environment
*Integrated Concept/Process:* Nursing Process/Implementation
*Content Area:* Fundamental Skills

*Reference*
Rocchiccioli, J., & Tilbury, M. (1998). *Clinical leadership in nursing.* Philadelphia: W.B. Saunders, p. 104.

---

**70.** A clinic nurse teaches a pregnant client with herpes genitalis about the measures that will be implemented during the pregnancy. Which of the following statements, if made by the client, indicates that teaching was effective?

1 "I must continue to take my acyclovir (Zovirax)."
2 "I need to abstain from sexual intercourse during the entire pregnancy."
3 "I need to take sitz baths four times a day."
4 "I may need a cesarean section if the lesions are present at the time of labor."

**Answer: 4**

*Rationale:* For women with active lesions, either recurrent or primary, at the time of labor, delivery should be cesarean; therefore, option 4 is correct. Acyclovir is used with caution during pregnancy. Clients should be advised to abstain from sexual contact while the lesions are present. If it is an initial infection, they should continue to abstain until they become culture negative because prolonged viral shedding may occur in such cases. Option 3 is incorrect. Keeping the genital area clean and dry will promote healing.

*Test-Taking Strategy:* Use the process of elimination and eliminate option 1 first because of the absolute word *must*. Next, eliminate option 2 because of the word *entire*. Knowing that the genital area should remain clean and dry will assist in eliminating option 3. Review the health care measures related to genital herpes if you had difficulty with this question.

*Level of Cognitive Ability:* Analysis
*Client Needs:* Safe, Effective Care Environment
*Integrated Concept/Process:* Teaching/Learning
*Content Area:* Maternity

*Reference*
Gorrie, T., McKinney, E., & Murray, S. (1998). *Foundations of maternal-newborn nursing* (2nd ed.) Philadelphia: W.B. Saunders, pp. 735-736.

**71.** A nurse has an order to test a client's stools using hemoccult slides. The nurse would question the order if the client was taking which of the following medications that could cause false negative results?

1  Ascorbic acid
2  Colchicine
3  Iodine
4  Acetylsalicylic acid

**Answer: 1**

*Rationale:* Ascorbic acid can interfere with the result of occult blood testing, causing false-negative findings. Colchicine and iodine can cause false-positive results. Acetylsalicylic acid would either have no effect on results or could cause a positive result, since aspirin is irritating to the stomach lining.

*Test-Taking Strategy:* Specific knowledge of the interfering factors with occult blood testing is needed to answer this question accurately. Focus on the key words *false-negative results*. If this question was difficult, review the nursing considerations associated with this test.

*Level of Cognitive Ability:* Application
*Client Needs:* Safe, Effective Care Environment
*Integrated Concept/Process:* Communication and Documentation
*Content Area:* Adult Health/Gastrointestinal

**Reference**
Fischbach, F. (2000). *A manual of laboratory & diagnostic tests* (6th ed.). Philadelphia: Lippincott Williams & Wilkins, p. 293.

**72.** A community health nurse is providing instructions to a group of mothers regarding the safe use of car seats for toddlers. The nurse determines that the mother of a toddler understands the instructions if the mother states which of the following?

1  "The car seat can be placed in a face-forward position when the height of the toddler is 27 inches."
2  "The car seat should never be placed in a face-forward position."
3  "The car seat can be placed in a face-forward position at any time."
4  "The car seat is suitable for a toddler until the toddler reaches the weight of 40 pounds."

**Answer: 4**

*Rationale:* The transition point for switching to the forward-facing position is defined by the manufacturer of the safety seat but is generally at a body weight of 9 kg (20 pounds). The car safety seat should be used until the child weighs at least 40 pounds, regardless of age. Options 1, 2, and 3 are incorrect.

*Test-Taking Strategy:* Use the process of elimination and focus on the issue of the question. Eliminate options 2 and 3 first because of the absolute words *never* and *any*. From the remaining options, use knowledge regarding car safety and the toddler to answer the question. Review these safety principles if you had difficulty with this question.

*Level of Cognitive Ability:* Analysis
*Client Needs:* Safe, Effective Care Environment
*Integrated Concept/Process:* Teaching/Learning
*Content Area:* Child Health

**Reference**
Wong, D. (1999). *Whaley & Wong's Nursing care of infants and children* (6th ed.). St. Louis: Mosby, p. 687.

**73.** A home health nurse is providing instructions to the mother of a toddler regarding safety measures in the home to prevent an accidental burn injury. Which statement, if made by the mother, indicates a need for further instruction?
1   "I need to remain in the kitchen when I prepare meals."
2   "I need to be sure to place my cup of coffee on the counter."
3   "I need to use the back burners for cooking."
4   "I need to turn pot handles inward and to the middle of the stove."

**Answer: 2**
*Rationale:* Toddlers, with their increased mobility and developing of motor skills, can reach hot water or hot objects placed on counters and open fires or burners on stoves above their eye level. Parents should be encouraged to remain in the kitchen when preparing a meal, to use the back burners on the stove, and to turn pot handles inward and toward the middle of the stove. Hot liquids should never be left unattended and the toddler should always be supervised. The mother's statement in option 2 does not indicate an adequate understanding of the principles of safety.

*Test-Taking Strategy:* Use the process of elimination and note the key words *a need for further instruction.* Options 1, 3, and 4 can be easily eliminated because they identify basic safety principles. Recalling that the toddler is in the stage of developing motor skills will assist in directing you to option 2. Review these safety principles if you had difficulty with this question.

*Level of Cognitive Ability:* Analysis
*Client Needs:* Safe, Effective Care Environment
*Integrated Concept/Process:* Teaching/Learning
*Content Area:* Child Health

*Reference*
Wong, D. (1999). *Whaley & Wong's Nursing care of infants and children* (6th ed.). St. Louis: Mosby, p. 691.

---

**74.** A client with a right pleural effusion noted on a chest x-ray film is being prepared for a thoracentesis. The client experiences severe dizziness when sitting upright. The nurse assists the client to which of the following positions for the procedure?
1   Prone, with the head turned to the side supported by a pillow
2   Sims' position, with the head of the bed flat
3   Right side-lying, with the head of bed elevated 45 degrees
4   Left side-lying, with the head of bed elevated 45 degrees

**Answer: 4**
*Rationale:* To facilitate removal of fluid from the chest wall, the client is positioned sitting at the edge of bed leaning over the bedside table with the feet supported on a stool. If the client is unable to sit up, the client is positioned lying in bed on the unaffected side with the head of the bed elevated 30 to 45 degrees. The prone and Sims' positions are inappropriate positions for this procedure.

*Test-Taking Strategy:* Use the process of elimination. Eliminate option 3 first, because if the client was lying on the affected side, it would be very difficult to perform the procedure. Option 2 can be eliminated next because the Sims' position is primarily used for rectal enemas or irrigations. Next, visualize the prone position. In the prone position, the client is lying on the abdomen, which is not an appropriate position for this procedure. Review the procedure for a thoracentesis if you had difficulty with this question.

*Level of Cognitive Ability:* Application
*Client Needs:* Safe, Effective Care Environment
*Integrated Concept/Process:* Nursing Process/Implementation
*Content Area:* Fundamental Skills

*Reference*
Smeltzer, S., & Bare, B. (2000). *Brunner & Suddarth's Textbook of medical-surgical nursing* (9th ed.). Philadelphia: Lippincott Williams & Wilkins, p. 398.

**75.** A physician has written an order to administer methylergonovine (Methergine) to a postpartum client with uterine atony. The nurse would contact the physician to verify the order if which of the following conditions were present in the mother?

1  Excessive lochia
2  Excessive bleeding and saturation of more than 1 peripad per hour
3  Hypertension
4  Difficulty locating the uterine fundus

**Answer: 3**

*Rationale:* Methergine is contraindicated for a hypertensive woman, individuals with severe hepatic or renal disease, and during the third stage of labor. A uterine fundus that is difficult to locate, excessive bleeding, and excessive lochia are clinical manifestations of uterine atony indicating the need for Methergine.

*Test-Taking Strategy:* Use the process of elimination. Eliminate options 1, 2, and 4 because they are similar in that they are all clinical manifestations of uterine atony. If you had difficulty with this question or are unfamiliar with the use of this medication and its contraindications, review this content.

*Level of Cognitive Ability:* Application
*Client Needs:* Safe, Effective Care Environment
*Integrated Concept/Process:* Communication and Documentation
*Content Area:* Maternity

*Reference*
Gorrie, T., McKinney, E., & Murray, S. (1998). *Foundations of maternal-newborn nursing* (2nd ed.). Philadelphia: W.B. Saunders, p. 785.

**76.** A physician's order reads: theophylline timed-release capsules (Slo-bid), 100 mg PO every 6 hours. The medication label reads: 50-mg capsules. The nurse prepares how many capsule(s) to administer one dose?

1  1 capsule
2  2 capsules
3  3 capsules
4  4 capsules

**Answer: 2**

*Rationale:* Use the following formula for calculating medication dosages:

$$\frac{Desired}{Available} \times 1 \text{ Capsule} = \text{Capsule(s) per dose}$$

$$\frac{100 \text{ mg}}{50 \text{ mg}} \times 1 \text{ Capsule} = 2 \text{ Capsules}$$

*Test-Taking Strategy:* Identify the key components of the question and what the question is asking. In this case, the question asks for capsule(s) per dose. Set up the formula knowing that desired dose is 100 mg and available is 50 mg in 1 capsule. Review medication calculations if you had difficulty with this question.

*Level of Cognitive Ability:* Application
*Client Needs:* Safe, Effective Care Environment
*Integrated Concept/Process:* Nursing Process/Planning
*Content Area:* Fundamental Skills

*Reference*
Kee, J., & Marshall, S. (2000). *Clinical calculations: With applications to general and specialty areas* (4th ed.). Philadelphia: W.B. Saunders, p. 78.

**77.** A child with a brain tumor is admitted to the hospital for removal of the tumor. To ensure a safe environment for this child, the nurse includes which of the following in the plan of care?
1   Assisting the child with ambulation at all times
2   Avoiding contact with other children on the nursing unit
3   Initiating seizure precautions
4   Using a wheelchair for out of bed activities

**Answer: 3**
*Rationale:* Seizure precautions should be considered for any child with a brain tumor, both preoperatively and postoperatively. Options 1 and 4 are not required unless functional deficits exist. Option 2 is not necessary.

*Test-Taking Strategy:* Use the process of elimination. Note the key words *safe environment* in the stem of the question. Eliminate options 1 and 4 first because they are similar. Additionally, note the absolute word *all* in option 1. From the remaining options, eliminate option 2, because there is no reason for the child to avoid contact with other children. If you had difficulty with this question, review nursing interventions related to the child with a brain tumor.

*Level of Cognitive Ability:* Application
*Client Needs:* Safe, Effective Care Environment
*Integrated Concept/Process:* Nursing Process/Planning
*Content Area:* Child Health

*Reference*
Ball, J., & Bindler, R. (1999). *Pediatric nursing: Caring for children* (2nd ed.). Stamford, Conn.: Appleton & Lange, p. 568.

**78.** A home care nurse provides instructions to the mother of a child with croup. The mother expresses concern regarding the occurrence of an acute spasmodic episode. The nurse instructs the mother regarding management if an acute episode occurs. Which statement made by the mother indicates a need for further instructions?
1   "I will place a steam vaporizer in the child's room."
2   "I will place the child in a closed bathroom and allow the child to inhale steam from warm running water."
3   "I will place a cool mist humidifier in the child's room."
4   "I will take the child out into the cool, humid night air."

**Answer: 1**
*Rationale:* Steam from warm running water in a closed bathroom and cool mist from a bedside humidifier are effective in reducing mucosal edema. Cool mist humidifiers are recommended over steam vaporizers, which present a danger of scald burns. Taking the child out into the cool humid night air may also relieve mucosal swelling. Remember however, that a cold mist may precipitate bronchospasm and the child needs to be monitored carefully.

*Test-Taking Strategy:* Focus on the issue of the question. The issue of the question is twofold; to reduce mucosal edema and to provide a safe environment. Note the key words *need for further instructions*. Option 1 is the option that would provide an unsafe environment for the child. Review management of acute spasmodic croup if you had difficulty with this question.

*Level of Cognitive Ability:* Analysis
*Client Needs:* Safe, Effective Care Environment
*Integrated Concept/Process:* Teaching/Learning
*Content Area:* Child Health

*Reference*
Wong, D. (1999). *Whaley & Wong's Nursing care of infants and children* (6th ed.). St. Louis: Mosby, p. 1478.

**79.** A nurse is reviewing the results of the rubella screening (titer) with a pregnant 24-year-old client. The test results are positive and the mother asks if it is safe for her toddler to receive the vaccine. The most appropriate nursing response is:

1 "You are still susceptible to rubella, so your toddler should receive the vaccine."
2 "Most children do not receive the vaccine until 5 years of age."
3 "It is not advised for children of pregnant women to be vaccinated during their mother's pregnancy."
4 "Your titer supports your immunity to rubella, and it is safe for your toddler to receive the vaccine at this time."

**Answer: 4**

*Rationale:* All pregnant women should be screened for prior rubella exposure during pregnancy. All children of pregnant women should receive their immunizations according to schedule. Additionally there is no definitive evidence that the rubella vaccine virus is transmitted from person to person. A positive maternal titer further indicates that a significant antibody titer has developed in response to a prior exposure to the rubivirus.

*Test-Taking Strategy:* Knowledge regarding the rubella titer-screening test is required to answer this question. Recalling that a positive titer indicates immunity will easily direct you to option 4. If you had difficulty with this question, review this important screening test.

*Level of Cognitive Ability:* Application
*Client Needs:* Safe, Effective Care Environment
*Integrated Concept/Process:* Nursing Process/Implementation
*Content Area:* Maternity

*Reference*

Olds, S., London, M., & Ladewig, P. (2000). *Maternal-newborn nursing: A family and community-based approach* (6th ed.). Upper Saddle River, N.J.: Prentice-Hall, pp. 941-943.

**80.** Following delivery, the postpartum nurse instructs the client with known cardiac disease to call for the nurse when she needs to get out of bed or when she plans to care for her infant. The nurse informs the mother that this is necessary to:

1 Minimize the potential of postpartum hemorrhage
2 Help the mother assume the parenting role
3 Provide an opportunity for the nurse to teach infant care techniques
4 Avoid maternal/infant injury that may occur because of the potential for syncope or overexertion

**Answer: 4**

*Rationale:* The immediate postpartum period is associated with increased risks for the cardiac client since about 500 mL of additional blood is added to the intravascular volume following placental separation. In addition, hormonal changes and fluid shifts from extravascular tissues to the circulatory system cause additional stress on cardiac functioning. Although options 2 and 3 are appropriate nursing concerns during the postpartum period, the primary concern for the cardiac client is to maintain a safe environment because of the potential for cardiac compromise.

*Test-Taking Strategy:* Focus on the issue of the question as it relates to safety, and use the process of elimination. Option 4 is the only option that relates directly to the issue of safety. Review the physiological manifestations that occur in a cardiac client following delivery and the need to implement safety precautions if you had difficulty with this question.

*Level of Cognitive Ability:* Application
*Client Needs:* Safe, Effective Care Environment
*Integrated Concept/Process:* Teaching/Learning
*Content Area:* Maternity

*Reference*

Gorrie, T., McKinney, E., & Murray, S. (1998). *Foundations of maternal newborn nursing* (2nd ed.). Philadelphia: W. B. Saunders, pp. 722-727.

**81.** A nurse is assessing a client who has just been measured and fitted for crutches. The nurse determines that the client's crutches are fitted correctly if:

1   The elbow is at a 30-degree angle when the hand is on the handgrip
2   The elbow is straight when the hand is on the handgrip
3   The client's axilla is resting on the crutch pad during ambulation
4   The top of the crutch is even with the axilla

**Answer: 1**

*Rationale:* For optimal upper extremity leverage, the elbow should be at approximately 30 degrees of flexion when the hand is resting on the handgrip. The top of the crutch needs to be two to three fingerwidths lower than the axilla. When crutch walking, all weight needs to be on the hands to prevent nerve palsy from pressure on the axilla.

*Test-Taking Strategy:* Use the process of elimination. Options 3 and 4 are similar and can be eliminated first. Visualize the mechanics of crutch walking to assist in selecting from the remaining options. If the weight should be resting on the hands, then there needs to be some flexion to push off from during ambulation. Review crutch walking and the safe and appropriate associated measures if you had difficulty with this question.

*Level of Cognitive Ability:* Analysis
*Client Needs:* Safe, Effective Care Environment
*Integrated Concept/Process:* Nursing Process/Evaluation
*Content Area:* Adult Health/Musculoskeletal

**Reference**
Kozier, B., Erb, G., Berman, A., & Burke, K. (2000). *Fundamentals of nursing: Concepts, process, and practice* (6th ed.). Upper Saddle River, N.J.: Prentice-Hall, p. 1053.

**82.** A physician has written an order for a vest restraint to be applied on a client from 10:00 P.M. to 7:00 A.M. because the client becomes disoriented during the night and is at risk for falls. At 6:30 A.M., the nurse manager makes rounds on all of the clients in the unit. When assessing the client with the vest restraint, which observation would indicate that the nurse who cared for this client performed unsafe care in the use of the restraint?

1   A hitch knot was used to secure the restraint
2   The client's record indicates that the restraint was released every 2 hours
3   The restraint was applied tightly to prevent a fall
4   The call light was placed within reach of the client

**Answer: 3**

*Rationale:* Restraints should never be applied tightly, because it could impair the circulation. The restraint should be applied securely to prevent the client from slipping through the restraint and endangering him/herself. A hitch knot may be used on the client because it can easily be released in an emergency. Restraints, especially limb restraints, must be released every 2 hours (or per agency policy) to inspect the skin for abnormalities. The call light must always be within the client's reach in case the client needs assistance.

*Test-Taking Strategy:* Use the process of elimination and knowledge regarding the safe use of restraints to answer this question. Note the key word *unsafe* in the stem of the question and the word *tightly* in the correct option. Review the principles regarding the safe use of restraints if you had difficulty with this question.

*Level of Cognitive Ability:* Analysis
*Client Needs:* Safe, Effective Care Environment
*Integrated Concept/Process:* Nursing Process/Evaluation
*Content Area:* Fundamental Skills

**Reference**
Leahy, J., & Kizilay, P. (1998). *Foundations of nursing practice: A nursing process approach.* Philadelphia: W.B. Saunders, pp. 398-400.

(nisenateri) 不足に

**83.** A nurse is providing an educational session to a group of students who are enrolled in a certified nursing assistant program. The nurse prepares an instructional list for the students regarding the correct procedure for handwashing. Which instructions does the nurse include on the list?

1　Turn on the water. Allow the warm water to wet the hands. Apply soap to the hands and rub them vigorously. Keep hands pointed downward. Rinse the hands. Dry the hands using a paper towel. Turn the water faucet off with the paper towel.

2　Turn on the water. Allow the warm water to wet the hands. Apply soap to the hands and rub them vigorously. Keep hands pointed upward. Rinse the hands. Dry the hands using a paper towel. Turn the water faucet off with the paper towel.

3　Turn on the water. Allow the warm water to wet the hands. Apply soap to the hands and rub them vigorously. Keep hands pointed downward. Rinse the hands using a paper towel. Turn the water off with the clean hands.

4　Turn on the water. Allow the cold water to wet the hands. Apply soap to the hands and rub them vigorously. Keep hands pointed upward. Rinse the hands using a paper towel and warm water. Turn the water off with the clean hands.

**Answer: 1**

*Rationale:* Warm water should be used for handwashing, because it increases the sudsing action of the soap. Hands should be kept downward to enable the unsanitary material to fall off the skin. The faucet should be turned off by using towels to prevent the hands from getting recontaminated.

*Test-Taking Strategy:* Read each of the options carefully and visualize the correct procedure for handwashing. Recall that care must be taken to avoid recontamination of the hands during and after this procedure. Handwashing is only effective if it is done correctly. Review the procedure for handwashing if you had difficulty with this question.

*Level of Cognitive Ability:* Application
*Client Needs:* Safe, Effective Care Environment
*Integrated Concept/Process:* Teaching/Learning
*Content Area:* Fundamental Skills

*Reference*
Leahy, J., & Kizilay, P. (1998). *Foundations of nursing practice: A nursing process approach.* Philadelphia: W.B. Saunders, pp. 423-424.

---

**84.** A nurse is preparing to suction a client through a tracheostomy tube. Which of the following protective items would the nurse wear to perform this procedure?

1　Gown, mask, and sterile gloves
2　Goggles, mask, and sterile gloves
3　Mask, gown, and a cap
4　Mask, sterile gloves, and a cap

**Answer: 2**

*Rationale:* Standard precautions involves body substance and universal precautions. The nurse should wear a mask and goggles when suctioning the client. Sterile gloves are worn. A mask would offer full protection of the nose and mouth. Goggles would protect the eyes from getting injured. A gown would protect the nurse's uniform and a cap would protect the nurse's hair, but these items are not required for suctioning a client.

*Test-Taking Strategy:* Use the process of elimination. Attempt to visualize the suctioning procedure and the potential exposure of body fluids that this procedure could cause. This should easily direct you to option 2. If you had difficulty with this question, review standard and universal precautions.

*Level of Cognitive Ability:* Application
*Client Needs:* Safe, Effective Care Environment

*Integrated Concept/Process:* Nursing Process/Implementation
*Content Area:* Fundamental Skills

*Reference*
Leahy, J., & Kizilay, P. (1998). *Foundations of nursing practice: A nursing process approach.* Philadelphia: W.B. Saunders, p. 429.

---

85. A nurse is instructing a client how to safely use crutches for ambulating at home. Which measure would the nurse recommend to minimize the risk of falls while ambulating with the crutches?
    1 Use grab bars in the bathtub or shower
    2 Remove scatter rugs in the home
    3 Keep all pets out of the house
    4 Use soft-soled slippers when walking with the crutches

**Answer: 2**
*Rationale:* To reduce the risk of falls, all obstacles should be removed from the home. Not all pets are trip hazards (fish, birds, guinea pigs). Grab bars in the bathtub or shower will not necessarily assist the client while walking with crutches. Shoes with nonslip soles should be worn.

*Test-Taking Strategy:* Use the process of elimination and principles related to safety measures to assist in answering the question. Focus on the issue: minimize the risk of falls, then eliminate option 3 first, because of the word *all.* Visualize the items identified in the remaining options to assist in directing you to option 2. Review home care measures related to safety and ambulation if you had difficulty with this question.

*Level of Cognitive Ability:* Application
*Client Needs:* Safe, Effective Care Environment
*Integrated Concept/Process:* Self-Care
*Content Area:* Fundamental Skills

*Reference*
Craven, R., & Hirnle, C. (2000). *Fundamentals of nursing: Human health and function* (3rd ed.). Philadelphia: Lippincott, p. 777.

---

86. An 85-year-old client is on postoperative day 2 following repair of a fractured hip. The nurse has observed that the client has episodes of extreme agitation. Which of the following nursing interventions would be most appropriate for the nurse to implement to avoid these episodes of agitation?
    1 Walk up behind the client and gently put a hand on the client's shoulder while speaking
    2 Speak to the client at the entrance of the room to avoid any episodes of violence
    3 Speak and move slowly toward the client while assessing the client's needs
    4 Wait until the client's agitation has subsided before approaching the client

**Answer: 3**
*Rationale:* Speaking and moving slowly toward the client will prevent the client from becoming further agitated. Any sudden moves or speaking too quickly may cause the client to have a violent episode. Walking up behind the client may cause the client to become startled and react violently. Remaining at the entrance of the room may make the client feel alienated. If the client's agitation is not addressed, it will only increase. Therefore waiting for the agitation to subside is not an appropriate option.

*Test-Taking Strategy:* It is important to remember the fundamental principles in preventing episodes of agitation or violent episodes. One of the most basic principles is to avoid further agitation. Use the process of elimination and remember to be empathetic to the client while at the same time, avoid actions that would startle the client. These principles will direct you to option 3. Review nursing interventions for the client that is agitated if you had difficulty with this question.

*Level of Cognitive Ability:* Application
*Client Needs:* Safe, Effective Care Environment

*Integrated Concept/Process:* Nursing Process/Implementation
*Content Area:* Fundamental Skills

*Reference*
Leahy, J., & Kizilay, P. (1998). *Foundations of nursing practice: A nursing process approach.* Philadelphia: W.B. Saunders, p. 395.

---

**87.** A 17-year-old client is about to be discharged with her newborn baby. Which statement if made by the client would alert the nurse that further teaching is required regarding child care?
1   "I have locks on all my cabinets that contain my cleaning supplies."
2   "I have a car seat that I will put in the front seat to keep my baby safe."
3   " I will not use the microwave to heat my baby's formula."
4   "I keep all my pots and pans in my lower cabinets."

**Answer: 2**
*Rationale:* A baby car seat should never be placed in the front seat because of the potential for injury on impact. Any cabinets that contain dangerous items that a baby or child could swallow should be locked. Microwaves should never be used to heat formula because it could burn and even scald the baby's mouth. Even though the bottle may feel warm, it could contain hot spots that could severely damage the baby's mouth. It is perfectly safe to leave pots and pans in the lower cabinets for a child to investigate, as long as they are not made of glass, which would harm the baby if broken.

*Test-Taking Strategy:* Note the key words *further teaching is required.* Use the process of elimination, keeping in mind the principles related to child care and safety. If you had difficulty with this question, review these principles.

*Level of Cognitive Ability:* Analysis
*Client Needs:* Safe, Effective Care Environment
*Integrated Concept/Process:* Teaching/Learning
*Content Area:* Child Health

*Reference*
Leahy, J., & Kizilay, P. (1998). *Foundations of nursing practice: A nursing process approach.* Philadelphia: W.B. Saunders, pp. 388-389.

---

**88.** A nurse has administered an injection to a client. After the injection, the nurse accidentally drops the syringe on the floor. Which nursing action is most appropriate in this situation?
1   Carefully pick up the syringe from the floor and gently recap the needle
2   Carefully pick up the syringe from the floor and dispose it in a sharps container
3   Obtain a dust pan and mop to sweep up the syringe
4   Call the housekeeping department to pick up the syringe

**Answer: 2**
*Rationale:* Syringes should never be recapped in any circumstances because of the risk of getting pricked with a contaminated needle. Used syringes should always be placed in a sharps container immediately after use to avoid individuals getting injured. A syringe should not be swept up, because this action poses an additional risk for getting pricked. It is not the responsibility of the housekeeping department to pick up the syringe.

*Test-Taking Strategy:* Use the process of elimination and basic principles related to the safe disposal of syringes to answer the question. Remember that a needle is never recapped and is always disposed of in a sharps container. If you had difficulty with this question, review these safety principles.

*Level of Cognitive Ability:* Application
*Client Needs:* Safe, Effective Care Environment

*Integrated Concept/Process:* Nursing Process/Implementation
*Content Area:* Fundamental Skills

*Reference*
Leahy, J., & Kizilay, P. (1998). *Foundations of nursing practice: A nursing process approach.* Philadelphia: W.B. Saunders, p. 394.

**89.** A nurse is assigned to care for a client who is in traction. The nurse prepares a plan of care for the client and includes which nursing action in the plan?
1  Monitor the weights to be sure that they are resting on a firm surface
2  Check the weights to be sure that they are off the floor
3  Make sure that the knots are at the pulleys
4  Make sure the head of the bed is kept at a 45 to 90 degree angle

**Answer: 2**
*Rationale:* To achieve proper traction, weights need to be free-hanging with knots kept away from the pulleys. Weights are not to be kept resting on a firm surface. The head of the bed is usually kept low to provide countertraction.

*Test-Taking Strategy:* Use the process of elimination. Attempt to visualize the traction, recalling that there must be weight to exert the pull from the traction setup. This concept will assist in eliminating options 1 and 3. Recalling that countertraction is needed will assist in eliminating option 4. Review care of the client in traction if you had difficulty with this question.

*Level of Cognitive Ability:* Application
*Client Needs:* Safe, Effective Care Environment
*Integrated Concept/Process:* Nursing Process/Planning
*Content Area:* Adult Health/Musculoskeletal

*Reference*
Smeltzer, S., & Bare, B. (2000). *Brunner & Suddarth's Textbook of medical-surgical nursing* (9th ed.). Philadelphia: Lippincott Williams & Wilkins, p. 1789.

**90.** A nurse is observing a client using a walker. The nurse determines that the client is using the walker correctly if the client:
1  Puts all four points of the walker flat on the floor, puts weight on the hand pieces, and then walks into it
2  Puts weight on the hand pieces, moves the walker forward, and then walks into it
3  Puts weight on the hand pieces, slides the walker forward, and then walks into it
4  Walks into the walker, puts weight on the hand pieces, and then puts all four points of the walker flat on the floor

**Answer: 1**
*Rationale:* When the client uses a walker, the nurse stands adjacent to the affected side. The client is instructed to put all four points of the walker two feet forward flat on the floor before putting weight on the hand pieces. This will ensure client safety and prevent stress cracks in the walker. The client is then instructed to move the walker forward and walk into it.

*Test-Taking Strategy:* Attempt to visualize each of the options. Options 2 and 3 can be liminated because putting weight on the hand pieces initially would cause an unsafe situation. From the remaining options, recalling that the walker is placed on all four points first, will direct you to option 1. Review this procedure if you had difficulty with this question.

*Level of Cognitive Ability:* Analysis
*Client Needs:* Safe, Effective Care Environment
*Integrated Concept/Process:* Self Care
*Content Area:* Fundamental Skills

*Reference*
Potter, P., & Perry, A. (2001). *Fundamentals of nursing* (5th ed.). St. Louis: Mosby, p. 1007.

**91.** A client is fitted for crutches and the nurse observes the client to evaluate for the correct height of the crutches. The nurse expects to note which of the following?

1　The client is able to rest the axillae on the axillary bars

2　The nurse is able to place two fingers comfortably between the axillae and the axillary bars

3　The client is able to maintain the arms in a straight position when standing with the crutches

4　The nurse is able to place four fingers comfortably between the axillae and the axillary bars

**Answer: 2**

*Rationale:* With the client's elbows flexed 20 to 30 degrees, the shoulders in a relaxed position, and the crutches placed approximately 15 cm (6 inches) anterolateral from the toes, the nurse should be able to place two fingers comfortably between the axillae and the axillary bars. The crutches are adjusted if there is too much or too little space at the axillary area. The client is advised never to rest the axillae on the axillary bars because this could injure the brachial plexus (the nerve in the axillae that supply the arm and shoulder area). The nurse should terminate ambulation and recheck the crutch height if the client complains of numbness or tingling in the hands or arms.

*Test-Taking Strategy:* Focus on the issue, correct height of crutches. Attempt to visualize each of the options. This will direct you to option 2 because the incorrect options are not reasonable and would not provide safety. Review this procedure if you had difficulty with this question.

*Level of Cognitive Ability:* Analysis
*Client Needs:* Safe, Effective Care Environment
*Integrated Concept/Process:* Nursing Process/Evaluation
*Content Area:* Fundamental Skills

*Reference*
Potter, P., & Perry, A. (2001). *Fundamentals of nursing* (5th ed.). St. Louis: Mosby, p. 1008.

---

**92.** A nurse is caring for an adolescent client with conjunctivitis. The nurse provides instructions to the client and tells the adolescent to:

1　Avoid using all eye makeup to prevent possible reinfection

2　Apply warm compresses to lessen irritation

3　Replace contact lenses for use after the infection clears

4　Stay home for 3 days after starting antibiotic eye drops to avoid the spread of infection

**Answer: 3**

*Rationale:* Eye makeup should be replaced, but can still be worn. Cool compresses decrease pain and irritation. Isolation for 24 hours after antibiotics are initiated is necessary. All contact lenses should be replaced.

*Test-Taking Strategy:* Use the process of elimination. Eliminate option 1 because of the absolute word *all*. Recalling the principles related to the effectiveness of antibiotics will assist in eliminating option 4. From the remaining options, recalling the effects related to cool and warm compresses will direct you to option 3. Review home care instructions for the client with conjunctivitis if you had difficulty with this question.

*Level of Cognitive Ability:* Application
*Client Needs:* Safe, Effective Care Environment
*Integrated Concept/Process:* Teaching/Learning
*Content Area:* Child Health

*Reference*
Wong, D. (1999). *Whaley & Wong's Nursing care of infants and children* (6th ed.). St. Louis: Mosby, p. 733.

**93.** A client who has experienced a cerebro-vascular accident has partial hemiplegia of the left leg. The straight leg cane formerly used by the client is not sufficient to provide support. The nurse interprets that the client could benefit from the somewhat greater support and stability provided by a:

1   Quad-cane
2   Wooden crutch
3   Lofstrand crutch
4   Wheelchair

**Answer: 1**

*Rationale:*  A quad-cane may be prescribed for the client requiring greater support and stability than is provided by a straight leg cane. The quad-cane provides a four-point base of support and is indicated for use by clients with partial or complete hemiplegia. Neither crutches nor a wheelchair are indicated for use with a client such as described in this question. A Lofstrand crutch is useful for clients with bilateral weakness.

*Test-Taking Strategy:*  Use the process of elimination. Providing a wheelchair to a client with partial hemiplegia is excessive, and is eliminated first. Wooden crutches are not indicated, because there is no restriction in weight bearing. From the remaining options, recalling that a Lofstrand crutch is useful for bilateral weakness will direct you to option 1. Review the use of assistive devices for ambulation if you had difficulty with this question.

*Level of Cognitive Ability:*  Analysis
*Client Needs:*  Safe, Effective Care Environment
*Integrated Concept/Process:*  Self-Care
*Content Area:*  Adult Health/Neurological

*Reference*
Potter, P., & Perry, A. (2001). *Fundamentals of nursing* (5th ed.). St. Louis: Mosby, p. 1008.

**94.** A client begins to drain small amounts of bright red blood from the tracheostomy tube 24 hours after a supraglottic laryngectomy. The best nursing action is to:

1   Notify the surgeon
2   Increase the frequency of suctioning
3   Add moisture to the oxygen delivery system
4   Document the character and amount of drainage

**Answer: 1**

*Rationale:*  Immediately following laryngectomy, a small amount of bleeding occurs from the tracheostomy that resolves within the first few hours. Otherwise, bleeding that is bright red may be a sign of impending rupture of a vessel. The bleeding in this instance represents a potential life threat and the surgeon is notified to further evaluate the client and suture or repair the bleed. The other options do not address the urgency of the problem. Failure to notify the surgeon places the client at risk.

*Test-Taking Strategy:*  Use the process of elimination. Note the key words *blood* and *24 hours after*. This should indicate that a potential complication exists. Review the complications following laryngectomy if you had difficulty with this question.

*Level of Cognitive Ability:*  Application
*Client Needs:*  Safe, Effective Care Environment
*Integrated Concept/Process:*  Nursing Process/Implementation
*Content Area:*  Adult Health/Respiratory

*Reference*
Smeltzer, S., & Bare, B. (2000). *Brunner & Suddarth's Textbook of medical-surgical nursing* (9th ed.). Philadelphia: Lippincott Williams & Wilkins, p. 417.

**95.** A client has a risk for infection following radical vulvectomy. The nurse avoids which of the following when giving perineal care to this client?
1   Cleanses using warm tap water and a bulb syringe
2   Intermittently exposes the wound to air
3   Provides perineal care after each voiding and bowel movement (BM)
4   Provides prescribed sitz baths after the sutures are removed

**Answer: 1**
*Rationale:* A sterile solution such as normal saline should be used for perineal care using an aseptic syringe or a water pick. This should be done regularly at least twice a day and after each voiding and BM. The wound is intermittently exposed to air to permit drying and prevent maceration. Once sutures are removed, sitz baths may be prescribed to stimulate healing and for the soothing effect.

*Test-Taking Strategy:* Use the process of elimination noting the key word *avoids* and the issue: risk for infection. Using principles of asepsis will direct you to option 1. Review these principles if you had difficulty with this question.

*Level of Cognitive Ability:* Application
*Client Needs:* Safe, Effective Care Environment
*Integrated Concept/Process:* Nursing Process/Implementation
*Content Area:* Fundamental Skills

*Reference*
Monahan, F., & Neighbors, M. (1998). *Medical-surgical nursing: Foundations for clinical practice* (2nd ed.). Philadelphia: W.B. Saunders, p. 1829.

**96.** A nurse prepares to assist a postoperative client to progress from a lying to a sitting position to prepare for ambulation. Which nursing action is most appropriate to maintain the safety of the client?
1   Assist the client to move quickly from the lying position to the sitting position
2   Assess the client for signs of dizziness and hypotension
3   Elevate the head of the bed quickly to assist the client to a sitting position
4   Allow the client to rise from the bed to a standing position unassisted

**Answer: 2**
*Rationale:* Early ambulation should not exceed the client's tolerance. The client should be assessed before sitting. The client is assisted to rise from the lying position to the sitting position gradually until any evidence of dizziness, if present, has subsided. This position can be achieved by raising the head of the bed slowly. After sitting, the client may be assisted to a standing position. The nurse should be at the client's side to provide physical support and encouragement.

*Test-Taking Strategy:* Use the process of elimination. Eliminate options 1 and 3 because of the word *quickly* and option 4 because of the word *unassisted*. Additionally, option 2 is the only option that reflects assessment, the first step of the nursing process. Review safety measures for ambulation if you had difficulty with this question.

*Level of Cognitive Ability:* Application
*Client Needs:* Safe, Effective Care Environment
*Integrated Concept/Process:* Nursing Process/Implementation
*Content Area:* Fundamental Skills

*Reference*
Smeltzer, S., & Bare, B. (2000). *Brunner & Suddarth's Textbook of medical-surgical nursing* (9th ed.). Philadelphia: Lippincott Williams & Wilkins, p. 358.

**97.** A client has an order for a stool culture. The nurse avoids doing which of the following when carrying out this order?

1   Wearing sterile gloves
2   Using a sterile container
3   Refrigerating the specimen
4   Sending the specimen directly to the laboratory

**Answer: 3**

*Rationale:* Storing a stool specimen in a refrigerator is contraindicated because it can retard the growth of organisms. A stool specimen is obtained using sterile gloves and a sterile container. After obtaining the specimen, the stool is sent immediately to the laboratory.

*Test-Taking Strategy:* Note the key word *avoids*. This indicates that the correct option will be a wrong action on the part of the nurse. Recalling that a culture is done to identify organisms will assist you in identifying that options 1, 2, and 4 must be carried out to ensure accuracy of results. Review this procedure if you had difficulty with this question.

*Level of Cognitive Ability:* Application
*Client Needs:* Safe, Effective Care Environment
*Integrated Concept/Process:* Nursing Process/Implementation
*Content Area:* Adult Health/Gastrointestinal

*Reference*
Smeltzer, S., & Bare, B. (2000). *Brunner & Suddarth's Textbook of medical-surgical nursing* (9th ed.). Philadelphia: Lippincott Williams & Wilkins, p. 804.

---

**98.** A client is being transferred to the nursing unit from the post-anesthesia care unit following spinal fusion with Harrington rod insertion. The nurse prepares to transfer the client from the stretcher to the bed by using:

1   A bath blanket and the assistance of 3 people
2   A bath blanket and the assistance of 4 people
3   A slider board and the assistance of 2 people
4   A slider board and the assistance of 4 people

**Answer: 4**

*Rationale:* Following spinal fusion, with or without instrumentation, the client is transferred from the stretcher to the bed using a slider board and the assistance of 4 people. This permits optimal stabilization and support of the spine, while allowing the client to be moved smoothly and gently.

*Test-Taking Strategy:* Use the process of elimination. Think about the level of comfort and stability provided to the client's spine with the amounts of assistance given in each option. Using this approach will assist in eliminating options 1, 2, and 3. Review care of the client following Harrington rod insertion if you had difficulty with this question.

*Level of Cognitive Ability:* Application
*Client Needs:* Safe, Effective Care Environment
*Integrated Concept/Process:* Nursing Process/Planning
*Content Area:* Adult Health/Neurological

*Reference*
Smeltzer, S., & Bare, B. (2000). *Brunner & Suddarth's Textbook of medical-surgical nursing* (9th ed.). Philadelphia: Lippincott Williams & Wilkins, p. 1747.

**99.** A nurse is preparing to nasotracheally suction a client with acquired immunodeficiency syndrome (AIDS) who has had blood-tinged sputum with previous suctioning. The nurse plans to use which of the following items as part of universal precautions for this client?
1    Gloves, mask, and protective eyewear
2    Gloves, gown, and mask
3    Gown, mask, and protective eyewear
4    Gloves, gown, and protective eyewear

**Answer: 1**
*Rationale:* Universal precautions include the use of gloves whenever there is actual or potential contact with blood or body fluids. During procedures that aerosolize blood, the nurse wears a mask and protective eyewear, or a face shield. Impervious gowns are worn in those instances when it is anticipated that there will be contact with a large amount of blood.

*Test-Taking Strategy:* Focus on the data in the question. Note the issue: suctioning, so expect airborne secretions and possibly airborne particles of blood with this procedure. This will direct you to the option that includes mask, protective eyewear, and gloves. If you did not answer this question correctly, review universal precautions.

*Level of Cognitive Ability:* Application
*Client Needs:* Safe, Effective Care Environment
*Integrated Concept/Process:* Nursing Process/Planning
*Content Area:* Adult Health/Immune

*Reference*
Smeltzer, S., & Bare, B. (2000). *Brunner & Suddarth's Textbook of medical-surgical nursing* (9th ed.). Philadelphia: Lippincott Williams & Wilkins, p. 1352.

**100.** A nurse is inserting an indwelling urinary catheter into a male client. As the catheter is inserted into the urethra, urine begins to flow into the tubing. At this point, the nurse:
1    Immediately inflates the balloon
2    Withdraws the catheter approximately 1 inch and inflates the balloon
3    Inserts the catheter until resistance is met and inflates the balloon
4    Inserts the catheter 2.5 to 5 cm and inflates the balloon

**Answer: 4**
*Rationale:* The catheter's balloon is behind the opening at the insertion tip. The catheter is inserted 2.5 to 5 cm after urine begins to flow in order to provide sufficient space to inflate the balloon. Inserting the catheter the extra distance will ensure that the balloon is inflated inside the bladder and not in the urethra. Inflating the balloon in the urethra could produce trauma.

*Test-Taking Strategy:* Visualize the procedure described in the question and the effects of each description in the options to direct you to option 4. Review the procedure for inserting a urinary catheter into a male if you had difficulty with this question.

*Level of Cognitive Ability:* Application
*Client Needs:* Safe, Effective Care Environment
*Integrated Concept/Process:* Nursing Process/Implementation
*Content Area:* Fundamental Skills

*Reference*
Kozier, B., Erb, G., & Blais, K. (1998). *Fundamentals of nursing: Concepts, process, and practice* (5th ed.). Menlo Park, Calif.: Addison-Wesley, pp. 1256-1257.

**101.** A nurse is preparing to administer oxygen to a client with carbon dioxide narcosis who has a history of chronic airflow limitation (CAL). The nurse checks to see that the oxygen flow rate is prescribed at:
1   2 to 3 L/min
2   4 to 5 L/min
3   6 to 8 L/min
4   8 to 10 L/min

**Answer: 1**
*Rationale:* The nurse administers oxygen to the client with carbon dioxide narcosis and CAL very cautiously. This is because the client's respiratory center is insensitive to carbon dioxide levels as the respiratory stimulant. If oxygen is given too freely, the client loses the respiratory drive, and respiratory failure results. Thus, the nurse checks the flow of oxygen to see that it does not exceed 2 to 3 L/min.

*Test-Taking Strategy:* Focus on the client's diagnosis. Recalling the pathophysiology that occurs in CAL will direct you to option 1, the lowest oxygen liter flow. Review the concerns related to the administration of oxygen to a client with CAL if you had difficulty with this question.

*Level of Cognitive Ability:* Application
*Client Needs:* Safe, Effective Care Environment
*Integrated Concept/Process:* Nursing Process/Assessment
*Content Area:* Adult Health/Respiratory

*Reference*
Smeltzer, S., & Bare, B. (2000). *Brunner & Suddarth's Textbook of medical-surgical nursing* (9th ed.). Philadelphia: Lippincott Williams & Wilkins, p. 447.

---

**102.** A client undergoes a subtotal thyroidectomy. The nurse ensures that which priority item is at the client's bedside on arrival from the operating room?
1   An apnea monitor
2   A blood transfusion warmer
3   A suction unit and oxygen
4   An ampule of phytonadione (vitamin K)

**Answer: 3**
*Rationale:* Following thyroidectomy, respiratory distress can occur either from tetany, tissue swelling, or hemorrhage. It is important to have oxygen and suction equipment readily available and in working order if such an emergency were to arise. Apnea is not a problem associated with thyroidectomy, unless the client experienced a respiratory arrest. Blood transfusions can be administered without a warmer if necessary. Vitamin K would not be administered for a client who is hemorrhaging, unless deficiencies in clotting factors warrant its administration.

*Test-Taking Strategy:* Recall the anatomical location of the thyroid gland and its close proximity to the trachea. Use the ABCs, airway, breathing, and circulation, to direct you to option 3. Review postoperative care following thyroidectomy if you had difficulty with this question.

*Level of Cognitive Ability:* Application
*Client Needs:* Safe, Effective Care Environment
*Integrated Concept/Process:* Nursing Process/Planning
*Content Area:* Adult Health/Endocrine

*Reference*
Ignatavicius, D., Workman, M., & Mishler, M. (1999). *Medical-surgical nursing across the health care continuum* (3rd ed.). Philadelphia: W.B. Saunders, p. 1618.

**103.** A nurse places a hospitalized client with active tuberculosis in a private, well-ventilated room. In addition, which of the following critical actions is most appropriate for the nurse to do before entering this client's room?

1 Wash the hands
2 Wash the hands and place a HEPA respirator over the nose and mouth
3 The nurse needs no special precautions, but the client is instructed to cover his or her mouth and nose when coughing or sneezing.
4 Wash the hands and wear a gown and gloves

**Answer: 2**
*Rationale:* The nurse wears a HEPA respirator when caring for a client with active tuberculosis. Hands are always thoroughly washed before and after caring for the client. Option 1 is an incomplete action. Option 3 is an incorrect statement. Option 4 is also inaccurate and incomplete. Gowning is only indicated when there is a possibility of contaminating clothing.

*Test-Taking Strategy:* Use the process of elimination. Noting the client's diagnosis and recalling the need for respiratory precautions will direct you to option 2. Review these respiratory isolation precautions if you had difficulty with this question.

*Level of Cognitive Ability:* Application
*Client Needs:* Safe, Effective Care Environment
*Integrated Concept/Process:* Nursing Process/Implementation
*Content Area:* Adult Health/Respiratory

*Reference*
Ignatavicius, D., Workman, M., & Mishler, M. (1999). *Medical-surgical nursing across the health care continuum* (3rd ed.). Philadelphia: W.B. Saunders, p. 530.

---

**104.** A nurse is assigned to care for a hospitalized toddler. The nurse plans care, knowing that the highest priority should be directed toward:

1 Protecting the toddler from injury
2 Adapting the toddler to the hospital routine
3 Allowing the toddler to participate in play and divisional activities
4 Providing a consistent caregiver

**Answer: 1**
*Rationale:* The toddler is at high risk for injury because of developmental abilities and an unfamiliar environment. While adaptation, diversion, and consistency are important, protection from injury is the highest priority.

*Test-Taking Strategy:* Note the key words *highest priority*. Use Maslow's Hierarchy of Needs theory. Physiological needs come first, followed by safety. Since no physiological needs are addressed, the safety option of preventing injury takes priority. Review care to the hospitalized toddler if you had difficulty with this question.

*Level of Cognitive Ability:* Application
*Client Needs:* Safe, Effective Care Environment
*Integrated Concept/Process:* Nursing Process/Planning
*Content Area:* Child Health

*Reference*
Wong, D. (1999). *Whaley & Wong's Nursing care of infants and children* (6th ed.). St. Louis: Mosby, p. 1242.

**105.** A client is to undergo pleural biopsy at the bedside. Knowing the potential complications of the procedure, the nurse plans to have which of the following items available at the bedside?

1 Chest tube and drainage system
2 Intubation tray
3 Portable chest x-ray machine
4 Morphine sulfate injection

**Answer: 1**
*Rationale:* Complications following pleural biopsy include hemothorax, pneumothorax, and temporary pain from intercostal nerve injury. The nurse has a chest tube and drainage system available at the bedside for use if hemothorax or pneumothorax develops. An intubation tray is not indicated. The client should be premedicated before the procedure, or a local anesthetic is used. A portable chest x-ray machine would be called for to verify placement of a chest tube if one was inserted, but it is unnecessary to have at the bedside before the procedure.

*Test-Taking Strategy:* Note that the client is having a pleural biopsy. Recalling the complications of this procedure will direct you to option 1. If this question was difficult, take a few moments now to review this procedure and its complications.

*Level of Cognitive Ability:* Application
*Client Needs:* Safe, Effective Care Environment
*Integrated Concept/Process:* Nursing Process/Planning
*Content Area:* Adult Health/Respiratory

*Reference*
Ignatavicius, D., Workman, M., & Mishler, M. (1999). *Medical-surgical nursing across the health care continuum* (3rd ed.). Philadelphia: W.B. Saunders, p. 563.

**106.** A nurse is preparing to begin hemodialysis on a client with renal failure. Which measure would the nurse avoid during this procedure?

1 Putting on a mask and giving one to the client to wear during connection to the machine
2 Wearing full protective clothing such as goggles, mask, apron, and gloves
3 Covering the connection site with a bath blanket to enhance extremity warmth
4 Using sterile technique for needle insertion

**Answer: 3**
*Rationale:* Infection is a major concern with hemodialysis. For that reason, the use of sterile technique and the application of a face mask for both the nurse and client are extremely important. It is also imperative that universal precautions be followed, which includes the use of goggles, mask, gloves, and an apron. The connection site should not be covered and it should be visible so that the nurse can assess for bleeding, ischemia, and infection at the site during the hemodialysis procedure.

*Test-Taking Strategy:* Use the process of elimination, noting the key word *avoid*. Note that options 1, 2, and 4 are similar in that they relate to infection control and universal precautions. Review the basic procedure related to hemodialysis if you had difficulty with this question.

*Level of Cognitive Ability:* Application
*Client Needs:* Safe, Effective Care Environment
*Integrated Concept/Process:* Nursing Process/Implementation
*Content Area:* Adult Health/Renal

*Reference*
Smeltzer, S., & Bare, B. (2000). *Brunner & Suddarth's Textbook of medical-surgical nursing* (9th ed.). Philadelphia: Lippincott Williams & Wilkins, p. 1114.

**107.** A nurse is going to suction an adult client with a tracheostomy who has copious amounts of secretions. The nurse does which of the following to perform this procedure safely?
1  Hyperoxygenate the client using a manual resuscitation bag
2  Set the suction pressure range between 160 to 180 mm Hg
3  Occlude the Y-port of the catheter while advancing it into the tracheostomy
4  Apply continuous suction in the airway for up to 15 seconds

**Answer: 1**
*Rationale:* To perform suctioning, the nurse hyperoxygenates the client using a manual resuscitation bag, or the sigh mechanism if the client is on a mechanical ventilator. The safe suction range for an adult is 100 to 120 mm Hg. The nurse advances the catheter into the tracheostomy without occluding the Y-port; suction is never applied while introducing the catheter because it would traumatize mucosa and remove oxygen from the respiratory tract. The nurse uses intermittent suction in the airway for up to 10 to 15 seconds.

*Test-Taking Strategy:* Use the process of elimination and visualize this procedure. Recalling that suction is applied intermittently and on catheter withdrawal only, eliminates options 3 and 4. From the remaining options, use the ABCs—airway, breathing, and circulation—to direct you to option 1. Review this procedure if you had difficulty with this question.

*Level of Cognitive Ability:* Application
*Client Needs:* Safe, Effective Care Environment
*Integrated Concept/Process:* Nursing Process/Implementation
*Content Area:* Adult Health/Respiratory

*Reference*
Smeltzer, S., & Bare, B. (2000). *Brunner & Suddarth's Textbook of medical-surgical nursing* (9th ed.). Philadelphia: Lippincott Williams & Wilkins, p. 502.

---

**108.** A nurse has just collected a sputum specimen by expectoration for a culture on a client who has a productive cough. The nurse plans to implement all of the following nursing interventions. Which nursing action does the nurse identify as the priority?
1  Giving the client mouthwash
2  Checking to see that the sputum basin is clean
3  Sending the sputum specimen to the laboratory immediately
4  Providing tissues for expectoration

**Answer: 3**
*Rationale:* Sputum specimens for culture should be labeled and transported immediately to the laboratory. Identification of the organism is critical in determining the appropriate treatment for the client. If the sputum sample is not transported immediately for culture, organisms will collect and the potential for contamination of the sample exists, which will then alter results. Options 1, 2, and 4 are important but option 3 identifies the priority action.

*Test-Taking Strategy:* Note the key word *priority.* Recalling that microorganisms will multiply in the specimen and that accurate identification of organisms is needed to determine treatment will direct you to option 3. Review the procedure for sputum collection if you had difficulty with this question.

*Level of Cognitive Ability:* Application
*Client Needs:* Safe, Effective Care Environment
*Integrated Concept/Process:* Nursing Process/Planning
*Content Area:* Fundamental Skills

*Reference*
Potter, P., & Perry, A. (2001). *Fundamentals of nursing* (5th ed.). St. Louis: Mosby, p. 1154.

ɪˌreɪdɪoˈnjuːklaɪd 較常使檢查

**109.** A postmyocardial infarction client is scheduled for a multigated acquisition (MUGA) scan. The nurse ensures that which item is in place before the procedure?
1 Signed informed consent
2 Notation of allergies to iodine or shellfish
3 A central venous pressure (CVP) line
4 A Foley catheter

**Answer: 1**
*Rationale:* MUGA is a radionuclide study used to detect myocardial infarction, decreased myocardial blood flow, and left ventricular function. A radioisotope is injected intravenously. Therefore, a signed informed consent is necessary. The procedure does not use radiopaque dye. Therefore, allergies to iodine and shellfish is not a concern. A Foley catheter and CVP line are not required.

*Test-Taking Strategy:* Focus on the procedure. Recalling that the procedure involves injection of a radioisotope will direct you to option 1. Review preparation for this procedure if you had difficulty with this question.

*Level of Cognitive Ability:* Application
*Client Needs:* Safe, Effective Care Environment
*Integrated Concept/Process:* Nursing Process/Implementation
*Content Area:* Adult Health/Cardiovascular

*Reference*
Fischbach, F. (2000). *A manual of laboratory & diagnostic tests* (6th ed.). Philadelphia: Lippincott Williams & Wilkins, p. 698

---

**110.** A nurse is developing a nursing care plan for a client with severe Alzheimer's disease. The nurse identifies which nursing diagnosis as the priority?
1 Impaired communication
2 Disturbance in role performance
3 High risk for injury
4 Social isolation

**Answer: 3**
*Rationale:* Clients who have Alzheimer's disease have significant cognitive impairment and are therefore at high risk for injury. It is critical for the nurse to maintain a safe environment particularly as the client's judgment becomes increasingly impaired. Options 1, 2, and 4 may be appropriate but the highest priority is directed toward safety.

*Test-Taking Strategy:* Use Maslow's Hierarchy of Needs theory. When a physiological need is not addressed, safety needs receive priority. Review care of the client with Alzheimer's disease if you had difficulty with this question.

*Level of Cognitive Ability:* Analysis
*Client Needs:* Safe, Effective Care Environment
*Integrated Concept/Process:* Nursing Process/Analysis
*Content Area:* Adult Health/Neurological

*Reference*
Smeltzer, S., & Bare, B. (2000). *Brunner & Suddarth's Textbook of medical-surgical nursing* (9th ed.). Philadelphia: Lippincott Williams & Wilkins, p. 160.

**111.** A client with a diagnosis of recurrent major depression who is exhibiting psychotic features is admitted to the psychiatric unit. In creating a safe environment for the client, the nurse most importantly develops a plan of care that deals specifically with the client's:

1 Altered thought processes
2 Altered nutrition
3 Self-care deficit
4 Knowledge deficit

**Answer: 1**

*Rationale:* Major depression, recurrent, with psychotic features alerts the nurse that in addition to the criteria that designates the diagnosis of major depression, one must also deal with a client's psychosis. Psychosis is defined as a state in which a person's mental capacity to recognize reality and communicate and relate to others is impaired, thus interfering with the person's capacity to deal with life's demands. Altered thought processes generally indicates a state of increased anxiety in which hallucinations and delusions prevail. Although options 2 and 3 are important, option 1 is specific to the client. Option 4 is not a priority at this time.

*Test-Taking Strategy:* Use the process of elimination focusing on the client's diagnosis and the key word *specifically*. Recall that the client with psychotic features experiences altered thought processes, such as hallucinations and delusions, and that altered thought processes presents a risk related to safety. Review care of the client with major depression and psychosis if you had difficulty with this question.

*Level of Cognitive Ability:* Analysis
*Client Needs:* Safe, Effective Care Environment
*Integrated Concept/Process:* Nursing Process/Analysis
*Content Area:* Mental Health

**Reference**
Stuart, G.W., & Laraia, M.T. (1998). *Principles and practice of psychiatric nursing.* (6th ed.). St. Louis: Mosby, p. 351.

---

**112.** A client is being admitted to the hospital after receiving a radium implant for bladder cancer. The nurse takes which of the following priority actions in the care of this client?

1 Encourages the client to take frequent rest periods
2 Admits the client to a private room
3 Encourages the family to visit
4 Places the client on reverse isolation

**Answer: 2**

*Rationale:* The client who has a radiation implant is placed in a private room, and has limited visitors. This reduces the exposure of others to the radiation. Frequent rest periods are a helpful general intervention, but is not a priority for the client in this situation. Reverse isolation is unnecessary.

*Test-Taking Strategy:* Note the key word *priority* and focus on the issue, radiation implant. Recalling the concepts related to environmental safety and that other individuals should have limited exposure to clients with radium implants will direct you to option 2. Review care of the client with a radiation implant if you had difficulty with this question.

*Level of Cognitive Ability:* Application
*Client Needs:* Safe, Effective Care Environment
*Integrated Concept/Process:* Nursing Process/Implementation
*Content Area:* Adult Health/Oncology

**Reference**
Smeltzer, S., & Bare, B. (2000). *Brunner & Suddarth's Textbook of medical-surgical nursing* (9th ed.). Philadelphia: Lippincott Williams & Wilkins, p. 275.

**113.** A client is to undergo weekly intravesical chemotherapy for bladder cancer for the next 8 weeks. The nurse interprets that the client understands how to manage the urine as a biohazard if the client states to:

1  Disinfect the urine and toilet with bleach for 6 hours following a treatment

2  Have one bathroom strictly set aside for the client's use for the next 2 months

3  Purchase extra bottles of scented disinfectant for daily bathroom cleansing

4  Void into a bedpan and then empty the urine into the toilet

**Answer: 1**

*Rationale:* After intravesical chemotherapy, the client treats the urine as a biohazard. This involves disinfecting the urine and the toilet with household bleach for 6 hours following a treatment. Scented disinfectants are of no particular use. The client does not need to have a separate bathroom for personal use. There is no value in using a bedpan for voiding.

*Test-Taking Strategy:* Use the process of elimination. Option 4 makes no sense and is eliminated first. Since scented disinfectants have no value, option 3 is eliminated next. Knowing that the urine needs special treatment for 6 hours after each treatment directs you to option 1. Also, option 2 is unnecessary and may be unrealistic for a number of clients. Review home care measures for the client receiving intravesical chemotherapy if you had difficulty with this question.

*Level of Cognitive Ability:* Analysis
*Client Needs:* Safe, Effective Care Environment
*Integrated Concept/Process:* Teaching/Learning
*Content Area:* Adult Health/Oncology

*Reference*
Ignatavicius, D., Workman, M., & Mishler, M. (1999). *Medical-surgical nursing across the health care continuum* (3rd ed.). Philadelphia: W.B. Saunders, p. 275.

**114.** A male client who is admitted to the hospital for an unrelated medical problem is diagnosed with urethritis resulting from chlamydial infection. The nursing assistant assigned to the client asks the nurse what measures are necessary to prevent contraction of the infection during care. The nurse tells the assistant that:

1  Enteric precautions should be instituted for the client

2  Contact isolation should be initiated, since the disease is highly contagious

3  Universal precautions are quite sufficient, since the disease is transmitted sexually

4  Gloves and mask should be used when in the client's room

**Answer: 3**

*Rationale:* Chlamydia is a sexually transmitted disease, and is frequently called non-gonococcal urethritis in the male client. It requires no special precautions other than universal precautions. Caregivers cannot acquire the disease during administration of care, and using universal precautions is the only measure that needs to be used.

*Test-Taking Strategy:* Use the process of elimination. Recall that this infection is sexually transmitted. Also, note that option 3 is the global option. If this question was difficult, review transmission of this disorder and universal precautions.

*Level of Cognitive Ability:* Application
*Client Needs:* Safe, Effective Care Environment
*Integrated Concept/Process:* Teaching/Learning
*Content Area:* Fundamental Skills

*Reference*
Smeltzer, S., & Bare, B. (2000). *Brunner & Suddarth's Textbook of medical-surgical nursing* (9th ed.). Philadelphia: Lippincott Williams & Wilkins, p. 1182.

**115.** A client is in extreme pain from scrotal swelling that is caused by epididymitis. The nurse administers a subcutaneous narcotic analgesic in the left arm to relieve the pain. The nurse does which of the following actions next?
1   Tells the client to do range of motion (ROM) exercises with the left arm to absorb the medication into the bloodstream
2   Checks the name bracelet of the client
3   Puts the side rails up on the bed
4   Dims the lights in the room

**Answer: 3**
*Rationale:* The client who receives a narcotic analgesic should immediately have the side rails raised on the bed, to prevent injury once the medication has taken effect. Dimming the light in the room is the next most helpful action. The name bracelet should have been checked before administering the medication. It is unnecessary to do ROM to the site of injection.

*Test-Taking Strategy:* Use the process of elimination. Eliminate option 2 first because this should have been done before administering the medication. Option 1 is not necessary, and is eliminated next. From the remaining options, note the key word *next* to direct you to option 3. As part of protecting the client's safety after administration of a narcotic analgesic, you would put the side rails up first. Review nursing interventions when administering a narcotic analgesic if you had difficulty with this question.

*Level of Cognitive Ability:* Application
*Client Needs:* Safe, Effective Care Environment
*Integrated Concept/Process:* Nursing Process/Implementation
*Content Area:* Pharmacology

*Reference*
Smeltzer, S., & Bare, B. (2000). *Brunner & Suddarth's Textbook of medical-surgical nursing* (9th ed.). Philadelphia: Lippincott Williams & Wilkins, p. 359.

**116.** A nurse is preparing the client's morning NPH insulin dose. The nurse notices a clumpy precipitate inside the insulin vial. The most appropriate nursing action is to:
1   Draw up and administer the dose
2   Shake the vial in an attempt to disperse the clumps
3   Draw the dose from a new vial
4   Warm the bottle under running water to dissolve the clump

**Answer: 3**
*Rationale:* The nurse should always inspect the vial of insulin before use for changes that may signify loss of potency. NPH insulin is normally uniformly cloudy. Clumping, frosting, and precipitates are signs of insulin damage. In this situation, since potency is questionable, it is safer to discard the vial and draw up the dose from a new vial.

*Test-Taking Strategy:* Remember that NPH insulin is cloudy but not clumpy. Noting the key words *most appropriate* will direct you to option 3, the safest action for the client. Remember, when in doubt throw it out. Review the characteristics of NPH insulin if you had difficulty with this question.

*Level of Cognitive Ability:* Application
*Client Needs:* Safe, Effective Care Environment
*Integrated Concept/Process:* Nursing Process/Implementation
*Content Area:* Pharmacology

*Reference*
Ignatavicius, D., Workman, M., & Mishler, M. (1999). *Medical-surgical nursing across the health care continuum* (3rd ed.). Philadelphia: W.B. Saunders, p. 1660.

**117.** A nurse is preparing the bedside for a postoperative parathyroidectomy client. The nurse ensures that which piece of medical equipment is at the client's bedside?
1 Underwater seal chest drainage
2 Tracheotomy set
3 Intermittent gastric suction
4 Cardiac monitor

**Answer: 2**
*Rationale:* Respiratory distress resulting from hemorrhage and swelling and compression of the trachea is a paramount concern for the nurse managing the care of a postoperative parathyroidectomy client. An emergency tracheotomy set is always routinely placed at the bedside of the client with this type of surgery, in anticipation of this potential complication. Options 1, 3, and 4 are not specifically needed with the surgical procedure.

*Test-Taking Strategy:* Use the process of elimination. Think about the location of the surgical incision and what potential problems might occur from that location. This will direct you to option 2. Review postoperative care following parathyroidectomy if you had difficulty with this question.

*Level of Cognitive Ability:* Application
*Client Needs:* Safe, Effective Care Environment
*Integrated Concept/Process:* Nursing Process/Planning
*Content Area:* Adult Health/Endocrine

*Reference*
Ignatavicius, D., Workman, M., & Mishler, M. (1999). *Medical-surgical nursing across the health care continuum* (3rd ed.). Philadelphia: W.B. Saunders, p. 1619.

**118.** A nurse has an order to administer foscarnet (Foscavir) intravenously to a client with acquired immunodeficiency syndrome (AIDS). Before administering this medication, the nurse plans to:
1 Place the solution on a controlled infusion pump
2 Obtain folic acid as an antidote
3 Ensure that liver enzyme levels have been drawn as a baseline
4 Obtain a sputum culture

**Answer: 1**
*Rationale:* Foscarnet is an antiviral agent used to treat cytomegalovirus (CMV) retinitis in clients with AIDS. Because of the potential toxicity of the medication, it is administered with the use of a controlled infusion device. It is very toxic to the kidneys, and serum creatinine levels are measured frequently during therapy. Folic acid is not an antidote to the medication. A sputum culture is not necessary.

*Test-Taking Strategy:* Use the process of elimination. Eliminate option 4 because the medication is usually indicated in the treatment of CMV retinitis, and not respiratory infection. Option 2 is eliminated next, because folic acid is not an antidote. From the remaining options, it is necessary to know that the medication can be very toxic, and cannot be infused too quickly. This will direct you to option 1. Also, recalling that the medication is toxic to the kidneys, not the liver will direct you to the correct option. Review this medication if you had difficulty with this question.

*Level of Cognitive Ability:* Application
*Client Needs:* Safe, Effective Care Environment
*Integrated Concept/Process:* Nursing Process/Planning
*Content Area:* Adult Health/Immune

*Reference*
Hodgson, B., & Kizior, R. (2001). *Saunders Nursing drug handbook 2001.* Philadelphia: W.B. Saunders, p. 447.

**119.** A client who is scheduled for gallbladder surgery is mentally impaired and is unable to communicate. In regard to obtaining permission for the surgical procedure, which nursing intervention would be most appropriate?
1    Ensure that the family has signed the informed consent
2    Ensure that the client has signed the informed consent
3    Inform the family about the advance directive process
4    Inform the family about the process of a living will

**Answer: 1**
*Rationale:* A client must be alert, able to communicate, and competent to sign an informed consent. If the client is unable to, then the family can sign the consent. A living will lists the medical treatment a person chooses to omit or refuse if the person becomes unable to make decisions and is terminally ill. Advanced directives are forms of communication in which persons can give direction on how they would like to be treated when they cannot speak for themselves.

*Test-Taking Strategy:* Focus on the issue, obtaining permission for the surgical procedure. Recalling that an informed consent is required will eliminate options 3 and 4. From the remaining options, noting the words *mentally impaired* will direct you to option 1. Review the process of informed consent if you had difficulty with this question.

*Level of Cognitive Ability:* Application
*Client Needs:* Safe, Effective Care Environment
*Integrated Concept/Process:* Nursing Process/Implementation
*Content Area:* Fundamental Skills

*Reference*
Potter, P., & Perry, A. (2001). *Fundamentals of nursing* (5th ed.). St. Louis: Mosby, p. 431.

**120.** A client diagnosed with tuberculosis (TB) is scheduled to go to the radiology department for a chest x-ray evaluation. Which nursing intervention would be appropriate when preparing to transport the client?
1    Apply a mask to the client
2    Apply a mask and gown to the client
3    Apply a mask, gown, and gloves to the client
4    Notify the x-ray department so that the personnel can be sure to wear a mask when the client arrives

**Answer: 1**
*Rationale:* Clients known or suspected of having TB should wear a mask when out of the room to prevent the spread of the infection to others. A gown or gloves are not necessary.

*Test-Taking Strategy:* Use the process of elimination. Recalling that the route of transmission of TB is airborne will direct you to option 1. Review the transmission associated with TB if you had difficulty with this question.

*Level of Cognitive Ability:* Application
*Client Needs:* Safe, Effective Care Environment
*Integrated Concept/Process:* Nursing Process/Implementation
*Content Area:* Fundamental Skills

*Reference*
Potter, P., & Perry, A. (2001). *Fundamentals of nursing* (5th ed.). St. Louis: Mosby, p. 838.

**121.** A nurse is taking care of a client on contact isolation. After the nursing care has been performed, on leaving the room, which protective item worn during client care, would the nurse remove first?

1   Gloves
2   Mask
3   Eye wear (goggles)
4   Gown

**Answer: 3**

*Rationale:* The nurse removes the goggles first. The nurse unties the gown at the waist and then removes the goggles and discards them. The nurse then removes and discards the mask, unties the neck strings of the gown and allows the gown to fall from the shoulders. The gown is removed without touching the outside of the gown and discarded. The hands are then washed.

*Test-Taking Strategy:* Use the principles of universal precautions and the methods of preventing contamination to answer the question. Attempt to visualize the correct process of removing contaminated clothing and items after caring for a client. Review this procedure if you had difficulty with this question.

*Level of Cognitive Ability:* Application
*Client Needs:* Safe, Effective Care Environment
*Integrated Concept/Process:* Nursing Process/Implementation
*Content Area:* Fundamental Skills

*Reference*
Potter, P., & Perry, A. (2001). *Fundamentals of nursing* (5th ed.). St. Louis: Mosby, p. 858.

**122.** A client requests pain medication and the nurse administers an intramuscular (IM) injection. After administration of the injection, the nurse does which of the following first?

1   Recaps the needle
2   Removes the gloves
3   Washes the hands
4   Places the syringe in the puncture-resistant needle box container

**Answer: 4**

*Rationale:* Following administration of an IM injection, the nurse would massage the site to assist in medication absorption. Then the nurse assists the client to a comfortable position. The uncapped needle is discarded in a puncture-resistant container, gloves are removed, and the hands are washed. A needle is never recapped. Of the options provided, the nurse would perform option 4 first.

*Test-Taking Strategy:* Note the key word *first*. Visualize the procedure and read each option to identify the first action. Review this procedure if you had difficulty with this question.

*Level of Cognitive Ability:* Application
*Client Needs:* Safe, Effective Care Environment
*Integrated Concept/Process:* Nursing Process/Implementation
*Content Area:* Fundamental Skills

*Reference*
Potter, P., & Perry, A. (2001). *Fundamentals of nursing* (5th ed.). St. Louis: Mosby, p. 944.

**123.** A nurse is in the process of giving a client a bed bath. In the middle of the procedure, the unit secretary calls the nurse on the intercom to tell the nurse that there is an emergency phone call. The most appropriate nursing action is to:
1 Leave the client's door open so that client can be monitored and answer the phone call
2 Finish the bath before answering the phone call
3 Immediately walk out of the client's room and answer the phone call
4 Cover the client, place the call light within reach, and answer the phone call

**Answer:** 4

*Rationale:* Since the telephone call is an emergency, the nurse may need to answer it. The other appropriate action is to ask another nurse to accept the call. This, however, is not one of the options. To maintain privacy and safety, the nurse covers the client and places the call light within the client's reach. Additionally, the client's door should be closed or the room curtains pulled around the bathing area.

*Test-Taking Strategy:* Use the process of elimination. Noting the key words *emergency phone call* will assist in eliminating option 2. From the remaining options, recalling the rights of the client and the principles related to safety will direct you to option 4. Review client's rights if you had difficulty with this question.

*Level of Cognitive Ability:* Application
*Client Needs:* Safe, Effective Care Environment
*Integrated Concept/Process:* Nursing Process/Implementation
*Content Area:* Fundamental Skills

*Reference*
Potter, P., & Perry, A. (2001). *Fundamentals of nursing* (5th ed.). St. Louis: Mosby, p. 1035.

---

**124.** A nursing manager is reviewing the purpose for applying restraints with the nursing staff. The nurse manager tells the staff that which of the following is not an indication for the use of a restraint?
1 To prevent falls
2 To restrict movement of a limb
3 To prevent the client from pulling out IV lines and catheters
4 To prevent the violent client from injuring self and others

**Answer:** 1

*Rationale:* Restraints do not necessarily prevent falls. Restraints are devices used to restrict the client's movement in situations when it is necessary to immobilize a limb or other body part. They are applied to prevent self-inflicted injury or from injuring others; from pulling out intravenous lines, catheters, or tubes; or from removing dressings. Restraints also may be used to keep children still and from injuring themselves during treatments and diagnostic procedures. Restraints should not be used as a form of punishment.

*Test-Taking Strategy:* Read each option carefully. Note the key word *not.* Eliminate options 2 and 3 first because they are similar. From the remaining options, recalling the guidelines for the use of restraints will direct you to option 1. Review these guidelines if you had difficulty with this question.

*Level of Cognitive Ability:* Application
*Client Needs:* Safe, Effective Care Environment
*Integrated Concept/Process:* Teaching/Learning
*Content Area:* Fundamental Skills

*Reference*
Potter, P., & Perry, A. (2001). *Fundamentals of nursing* (5th ed.). St. Louis: Mosby, p. 1038.

**125.** A client has an order to receive valproic acid (Depakene) 250 mg once daily. To maximize the client's safety, the nurse schedules administration of the medication:
1   At bedtime
2   Before breakfast
3   After breakfast
4   With lunch

**Answer: 1**
*Rationale:* Valproic acid is an anticonvulsant that causes central nervous system (CNS) depression. For this reason, the side effects include sedation, dizziness, ataxia, and confusion. When the client is taking this medication as a single daily dose, administering it at bedtime negates the risk of injury from sedation and enhances client safety.

*Test-Taking Strategy:* Recalling that this medication is an anticonvulsant with CNS depressant properties and that sedation is a side effect will direct you to option 1. Administration at bedtime allows the sedative effects of the medication to occur at a time when the client is sleeping. Review the side effects of this medication if you had difficulty with this question.

*Level of Cognitive Ability:* Application
*Client Needs:* Safe, Effective Care Environment
*Integrated Concept/Process:* Nursing Process/Planning
*Content Area:* Pharmacology

*Reference*
Hodgson, B., & Kizior, R. (2001). *Saunders Nursing drug handbook 2001.* Philadelphia: W.B. Saunders, p. 1039.

**126.** A client with an acute respiratory infection is admitted to the hospital with a diagnosis of sinus tachycardia. The nurse develops a plan of care for the client and includes which of the following?
1   Providing the client with short, frequent walks
2   Measuring the client's pulse each shift
3   Eliminating sources of caffeine from meal trays
4   Limiting oral and intravenous fluids

**Answer: 3**
*Rationale:* Sinus tachycardia is often caused by fever, physical and emotional stress, heart failure, hypovolemia, certain medications, nicotine, caffeine, and exercise. Exercise and fluid restriction will not alleviate tachycardia. Option 2 will not decrease the heart rate. Additionally the pulse should be taken more frequently than each shift.

*Test-Taking Strategy:* Use the process of elimination, focusing on the client's diagnosis. Recalling the causes of tachycardia will direct you to option 3. Remember, caffeine is a stimulant and will increase the heart rate. Review care of the client with tachycardia if you had difficulty with this question.

*Level of Cognitive Ability:* Application
*Client Needs:* Safe, Effective Care Environment
*Integrated Concept/Process:* Nursing Process/Planning
*Content Area:* Adult Health/Cardiovascular

*Reference*
Smeltzer, S., & Bare, B. (2000). *Brunner & Suddarth's Textbook of medical-surgical nursing* (9th ed.). Philadelphia: Lippincott Williams & Wilkins, p. 570.

**127.** A nurse has an order to obtain a urinalysis from a client with an indwelling urinary catheter. The nurse avoids which of the following, which could contaminate the specimen?
1 Obtaining the specimen from the urinary drainage bag
2 Clamping the tubing of the drainage bag
3 Aspirating a sample from the port on the drainage bag
4 Wiping the port with an alcohol swab before inserting the syringe

**Answer: 1**
*Rationale:* A urine specimen is not taken from the urinary drainage bag. Urine undergoes chemical changes while sitting in the bag and does not necessarily reflect the current client status. In addition, it may become contaminated with bacteria from opening the system.

*Test-Taking Strategy:* Use the process of elimination, focusing on the issue of preventing contamination. Also note the key word *avoids*. Recalling basic principles of asepsis will direct you to option 1. Review this procedure if you had difficulty with this question.

*Level of Cognitive Ability:* Application
*Client Needs:* Safe, Effective Care Environment
*Integrated Concept/Process:* Nursing Process/Implementation
*Content Area:* Fundamental Skills

*Reference*
Potter, P., & Perry, A. (2001). *Fundamentals of nursing* (5th ed.). St. Louis: Mosby, p. 864.

---

**128.** A nursing assistant is caring for an elderly client with cystitis who has an indwelling urinary catheter. The registered nurse provides directions regarding care and ensures that the nursing assistant:
1 Uses soap and water to cleanse the perineal area
2 Keeps the drainage bag above the level of the bladder
3 Loops the tubing under the client's leg
4 Lets the drainage tubing rest under the leg

**Answer: 1**
*Rationale:* Proper care of an indwelling urinary catheter is especially important to prevent prolonged infection or reinfection in the client with cystitis. The perineal area is cleansed thoroughly using mild soap and water at least twice a day and following a bowel movement. The drainage bag is kept below the level of the bladder to prevent urine from being trapped in the bladder, and for the same reason, the drainage tubing is not placed or looped under the client's leg. The tubing must drain freely at all times.

*Test-Taking Strategy:* Use the process of elimination. Eliminate options 3 and 4 first because they are similar. From the remaining options, noting the word *above* in option 2 will assist in eliminating this option. Also, note that option 1 relates to preventing infection. Review care of the client with an indwelling urinary catheter if you had difficulty with this question.

*Level of Cognitive Ability:* Application
*Client Needs:* Safe, Effective Care Environment
*Integrated Concept/Process:* Teaching/Learning
*Content Area:* Fundamental Skills

*Reference*
Potter, P., & Perry, A. (2001). *Fundamentals of nursing* (5th ed.). St. Louis: Mosby, p. 1423.

**129.** A nurse is assigned to care for a woman with preeclampsia. The nurse plans to initiate which action to provide a safe environment?
1  Turn off room lights and draw the window shades
2  Maintain fluid and sodium restrictions
3  Take the vital signs every four hours
4  Encourage visits from family and friends for psychosocial support

**Answer: 1**
*Rationale:* Clients with preeclampsia are at risk of developing eclampsia (convulsions). Bright lights and sudden loud noises may initiate convulsions in this client. A woman with preeclampsia should be placed in a dim lighted, quiet, private room. Visitors should be limited to allow for rest and prevent overstimulation. Clients with preeclampsia have decreased plasma volume and adequate fluid and sodium intake is necessary to maintain fluid volume and tissue perfusion. Vital signs need to be monitored more frequently than every 4 hours when preeclampsia is present.

*Test-Taking Strategy:* Use the process of elimination. Eliminate option 4 because it is not a physiological need. Eliminate option 3 next because vital signs need to be monitored more frequently than every 4 hours. From the remaining options, knowing that seizures may be precipitated by sudden loud noises and bright lights will assist in directing you to option 1. Review care of the client with preeclampsia if you had difficulty with this question.

*Level of Cognitive Ability:* Application
*Client's Needs:* Safe, Effective Care Environment
*Integrated Concept/Process:* Nursing Process/Planning
*Content Area:* Maternity

*Reference*
Lowdermilk, D., Perry, S., & Bobak, I. (2000). *Maternity & women's health care* (7th ed.). St. Louis: Mosby, p. 829.

**130.** A client is scheduled for a bronchoscopy. The nurse plans for which of the following measures as the highest priority item?
1  Restricting the diet to clear liquids on the day of the test
2  Asking the client about allergies to shellfish
3  Obtaining informed consent for an invasive procedure
4  Administration of preprocedure antibiotics prophylactically

**Answer: 3**
*Rationale:* Bronchoscopy requires that informed consent be obtained from the client before the procedure. The client is kept NPO for at least 6 hours before the procedure. It is unnecessary to inquire about allergies to shellfish before this procedure, because contrast dye is not injected. There is also no need for prophylactic antibiotics.

*Test-Taking Strategy:* Use the process of elimination. Recalling that bronchoscopy is an invasive procedure and requires an informed consent will direct you to option 3. If this question was difficult, review preprocedure preparation for bronchoscopy.

*Level of Cognitive Ability:* Application
*Client Needs:* Safe, Effective Care Environment
*Integrated Concept/Process:* Nursing Process/Planning
*Content Area:* Adult Health/Respiratory

*Reference*
Smeltzer, S., & Bare, B. (2000). *Brunner & Suddarth's Textbook of medical-surgical nursing* (9th ed.). Philadelphia: Lippincott Williams & Wilkins, p. 396.

**131.** A nurse has given a subcutaneous injection to the client with acquired immuno-deficiency syndrome (AIDS). The nurse disposes of the used needle and syringe by:

1    Placing the uncapped needle and syringe in a labeled, rigid plastic container
2    Recapping the needle and discarding the syringe in the disposal unit
3    Breaking the needle before discarding it
4    Placing the uncapped needle and syringe in a labeled cardboard box

**Answer: 1**
*Rationale:* Universal precautions include specific guidelines for handling of needles. Needles should not be recapped, bent, broken, or cut after use. They should be disposed of in a labeled, impermeable container specific for this purpose. Needles should not be discarded in cardboard boxes, because they are not impervious. Needles should never be left lying around after use.

*Test-Taking Strategy:* Use the process of elimination and universal precautions. Recalling that a needle should never be recapped or broken will eliminate options 2 and 3. From the remaining options, noting the key words *rigid plastic container* in option 1 will direct you to this option. Review the principles related to needle disposal if you had difficulty with this question.

*Level of Cognitive Ability:* Application
*Client Needs:* Safe, Effective Care Environment
*Integrated Concept/Process:* Nursing Process/Implementation
*Content Area:* Adult Health/Immune

*Reference*
Potter, P., & Perry, A. (2001). *Fundamentals of nursing* (5th ed.). St. Louis: Mosby, p. 1352.

**132.** A nurse is planning care for a client with acute glomerulonephritis. The nurse instructs the nursing assistant to do which of the following in the care of the client?

1    Monitor the temperature every two hours
2    Remove the water pitcher from the bedside
3    Ambulate the client frequently
4    Encourage a diet that is high in protein

**Answer: 2**
*Rationale:* A client with acute glomerulonephritis commonly experiences fluid volume excess and fatigue. Interventions include fluid restriction, as well as monitoring weight and intake and output. The client may be placed on bed rest, or at least encouraged to rest. This is because there is a direct correlation between proteinuria, hematuria, edema, and increased activity levels. The diet is high in calories but low in protein. It is unnecessary to monitor the temperature as frequently as every two hours.

*Test-Taking Strategy:* Use the process of elimination. The question provides no information about the client's actual temperature, so option 1 is eliminated first. Knowing that the client needs rest eliminates option 3. From the remaining options, it is necessary to know either that fluids are restricted or that protein is limited. Review interventions related to this condition if you had difficulty with this question.

*Level of Cognitive Ability:* Application
*Client Needs:* Safe, Effective Care Environment
*Integrated Concept/Process:* Teaching/Learning
*Content Area:* Adult Health/Renal

*Reference*
Smeltzer, S., & Bare, B. (2000). *Brunner & Suddarth's Textbook of medical-surgical nursing* (9th ed.). Philadelphia: Lippincott Williams & Wilkins, p. 1142.

**133.** A nurse is caring for a client with a C6 spinal cord injury during the spinal shock phase. The nurse implements which of the following when preparing the client to sit in a chair?

1   Teach the client to lock the knees during the pivoting stage of the transfer   [pivoting] 枢转动作.

2   Administer a vasodilator in order to improve circulation of the lower limbs

3   Raise the head of the bed slowly to decrease orthostatic hypotensive episodes

4   Apply knee splints to stabilize the joints during transfer

**Answer: 3**

*Rationale:* Spinal shock is often accompanied by vasodilation of the lower limbs, which results in a fall in blood pressure on rising. The client can have dizziness and feel faint. The nurse should provide for a gradual progression in head elevation while monitoring the blood pressure. A vasodilator would exacerbate the problem. Clients with cervical cord injuries cannot lock their knees, and the use of splints would impair the transfer.

*Test-Taking Strategy:* Use the process of elimination. Focusing on the client's diagnosis will assist in eliminating options 1 and 4. From the remaining options, recalling that spinal shock is accompanied by vasodilation will direct you to option 3. Review care of the client with spinal shock if you had difficulty with this question.

*Level of Cognitive Ability:* Application
*Client Needs:* Safe, Effective Care Environment
*Integrated Concept/Process:* Nursing Process/Implementation
*Content Area:* Adult Health/Neurological

*Reference*
Smeltzer, S., & Bare, B. (2000). *Brunner & Suddarth's Textbook of medical-surgical nursing* (9th ed.). Philadelphia: Lippincott Williams & Wilkins, p. 259.

**134.** A nurse notes that a client's lithium level is 3.9 mEq/L. The nurse implements which priority intervention?

1   Determining visual acuity
2   Monitoring intake and output
3   Assisting with ambulation
4   Instituting seizure precautions

**Answer: 4**

*Rationale:* A therapeutic regimen is designed to attain a serum lithium level of 1.0 to 1.5 mEq/L during acute mania, and levels of 0.6 to 1.4 mEq/L for maintenance treatment. A level of 3.9 mEql/L is within the toxic range, and seizures may occur at levels of 3.5 mEq/L and higher. Options 1, 2, and 3 are indicated but are not the priority.

*Test-Taking Strategy:* Use the process of elimination. Focusing on the word *priority* and recalling the manifestations that occur in a toxic level, will direct you to option 4. Review toxicity related to lithium and the manifestations that occur as a result of toxicity if you had difficulty with this question.

*Level of Cognitive Ability:* Application
*Client Needs:* Safe, Effective Care Environment
*Integrated Concept/Process:* Nursing Process/Implementation
*Content Area:* Pharmacology

*Reference*
Hodgson, B., & Kizior, R. (2001). *Saunders Nursing drug handbook 2001.* Philadelphia: W.B. Saunders, pp. 598-600.

**135.** A client with a diagnosis of anorexia nervosa, who is in a state of starvation, is in a two-bed room. A newly admitted client will be assigned to this client's room. Which client would be inappropriate to assign to this two-bed room?

1   A client with pneumonia
2   A client with a fractured leg that is casted
3   A client who can care for self
4   A client who is scheduled for a diagnostic test

**Answer: 1**

*Rationale:* The client in a state of starvation has a compromised immune system. Having a roommate with pneumonia would place the client at risk for infection. Options 2, 3, and 4 are appropriate roommates.

*Test-Taking Strategy:* Use the process of elimination, noting the client's diagnosis and the key words *in a state of starvation.* Note the key word *inappropriate.* Thinking about the physiological risks for this client will direct you to option 1. Review care of the client with anorexia nervosa if you had difficulty with this question.

*Level of Cognitive Ability:* Application
*Client Needs:* Safe, Effective Care Environment
*Integrated Concept/Process:* Nursing Process/Implementation
*Content Area:* Mental Health

*Reference*
Stuart, G.W., & Laraia, M.T. (1998). *Principles and practice of psychiatric nursing.* (6th ed.). St. Louis: Mosby, p. 527.

---

**136.** A child with an undiagnosed exanthema (rash) profusely covering the trunk and sparsely on the extremities is hospitalized. The child was exposed to varicella two weeks ago. The most appropriate nursing intervention is to:

1   Allow the child to play in the playroom until the physician can be contacted
2   Place the child in a private room on strict isolation
3   Immediately admit the child to any available bed
4   Assess the progression of the exanthema and report it to physician

**Answer: 2**

*Rationale:* The child with undiagnosed exanthema needs to be placed on strict isolation. Varicella causes a profuse rash on the trunk with a sparse rash on the extremities. The incubation period is 14 to 21 days. It is important to prevent the spread of this communicable disease by placing the child in isolation until further diagnosis and treatment is made. Options 1 and 3 are inaccurate and option 4 is not the most appropriate intervention.

*Test-Taking Strategy:* Use the process of elimination. Noting the key words *exposed to varicella* will direct you to option 2. This action will prevent exposure to others of this communicable disease. Review care to the child with varicella if you had difficulty with this question.

*Level of Cognitive Ability:* Application
*Client Needs:* Safe, Effective Care Environment
*Integrated Concept/Process:* Nursing Process/Implementation
*Content Area:* Child Health

*Reference*
Wong, D. (1999). *Whaley & Wong's Nursing care of infants and children* (6th ed.). St. Louis: Mosby, pp. 722-723.

**137.** A nurse is observing a second nurse who is performing hemodialysis on a client. The second nurse is drinking coffee and eating a doughnut next to the hemodialysis machine, while talking with the client about the events of the client's week. The first nurse should:
1 Appreciate what a wonderful therapeutic relationship this nurse and client have
2 Get a cup of coffee and join in on the conversation
3 Ask the client if he or she would like a cup of coffee also
4 Ask the nurse to refrain from eating and drinking in that area

**Answer: 4**
*Rationale:* A potential complication with hemodialysis is the acquisition of dialysis-associated hepatitis B. This is a concern for clients (who may carry the virus), client families (at risk from contact with client and with environmental surfaces), and staff (who may acquire the virus from contact with the client's blood). This risk is minimized by the use of universal precautions, appropriate handwashing and sterilization procedures, and the prohibition of eating, drinking, or other hand-to-mouth activity in the hemodialysis unit. The first nurse should ask the second nurse to stop eating and drinking in the work area.

*Test-Taking Strategy:* Use the process of elimination and the principles related to universal precautions. This will easily direct you to option 4. Review infection control measures related to the client receiving hemodialysis if you had difficulty with this question.

*Level of Cognitive Ability:* Application
*Client Needs:* Safe, Effective Care Environment
*Integrated Concept/Process:* Nursing Process/Implementation
*Content Area:* Adult Health/Renal

*Reference*
Smeltzer, S., & Bare, B. (2000). *Brunner & Suddarth's Textbook of medical-surgical nursing* (9th ed.). Philadelphia: Lippincott Williams & Wilkins, p. 1352.

**138.** A nurse is caring for a client who is going to have an arthrogram using a contrast medium. Which of the following preprocedure assessments by the nurse would be of highest priority?
1 Allergy to iodine or shellfish
2 Ability of the client to remain still during the procedure
3 Whether the client has any remaining questions about the procedure
4 Whether the client wishes to void before the procedure

**Answer: 1**
*Rationale:* Because of the risk of allergy to contrast medium, the nurse places highest priority on assessing whether the client has an allergy to iodine or shellfish. The nurse also reinforces information about the test, tells the client about the need to remain still during the procedure, and encourages the client to void before the procedure for comfort.

*Test-Taking Strategy:* Note the key words *highest priority*. This tells you that more than one or all of the options are correct (in fact, they all are). While options 2, 3, and 4 all compete for priority, only option 1 presents a life-threatening situation. Review priority assessments of a client receiving a contrast medium if you had difficulty with this question.

*Level of Cognitive Ability:* Analysis
*Client Needs:* Safe, Effective Care Environment
*Integrated Concept/Process:* Nursing Process/Assessment
*Content Area:* Adult Health/Musculoskeletal

*Reference*
Fischbach, F. (2000). *A manual of laboratory & diagnostic tests* (6th ed.). Philadelphia: Lippincott Williams & Wilkins, pp. 792-793.

**139.** A client with a possible rib fracture has never had a chest x-ray examination. The nurse plans to tell the client which of the following about the procedure?
  1   The x-ray stimulates a small amount of pain
  2   It is necessary to remove jewelry and any other metal objects
  3   The client will be asked to breathe in and out during the x-ray procedure
  4   The x-ray technologist will stand next to the client during the x-ray procedure

**Answer: 2**
*Rationale:* An x-ray film is a photographic image of a part of the body on a special film, which is used to diagnose a wide variety of conditions. The x-ray itself is painless, and any discomfort would arise from repositioning a painful part for filming. The nurse may premedicate a client, if prescribed, who is at risk for pain. Any radiopaque objects such as jewelry or other metal must be removed. The client is asked to breathe in deeply, and then hold the breath while the chest x-ray is taken. To minimize the risk of radiation exposure, the x-ray technologist stands in a separate area protected by a lead wall. The client also wears a lead shield over the gonads.

*Test-Taking Strategy:* Use the process of elimination. Think about the procedure and the associated risks to direct you to option 2. Review the procedure for a chest x-ray examination if you had difficulty with this question.

*Level of Cognitive Ability:* Application
*Client Needs:* Safe, Effective Care Environment
*Integrated Concept/Process:* Nursing Process/Implementation
*Content Area:* Adult Health/Musculoskeletal

*Reference*
Fischbach, F. (2000). *A manual of laboratory & diagnostic tests* (6th ed.). Philadelphia: Lippincott Williams & Wilkins, p. 761.

**140.** A nurse is planning discharge teaching for a client with a spinal cord injury. To provide for a safe environment regarding home care, which of the following would be the priority in the plan of care?
  1   What the physician has indicated needs to be taught
  2   Follow-up laboratory and diagnostic tests
  3   Assisting the client to deal with long-term care placement
  4   Including the significant others in the teaching session

**Answer: 4**
*Rationale:* Involving the client's significant others in discharge teaching is a priority in planning for the client with a spinal cord injury. The client will need the support of the significant others. Knowledge and understanding of what to expect will help both the client and significant others deal with the client's limitations. A physician's order is not necessary for discharge planning and teaching; this is an independent nursing action. Laboratory and diagnostic testing are not priority discharge instructions for this client. Long-term placement is not the only option for a client with spinal cord injury.

*Test-Taking Strategy:* Use the process of elimination. Eliminate option 3 first because long-term placement is not the only option for a client with a spinal cord injury. Eliminate option 1 next because although the physician's orders need to be addressed, teaching is an independent nursing action. From the remaining options, focusing on the client's diagnosis will direct you to option 4. Remember, home care and support will be needed. Review care of the client with a spinal cord injury if you had difficulty with this question.

*Level of Cognitive Ability:* Application
*Client Needs:* Safe, Effective Care Environment

*Integrated Concept/Process:* Self Care
*Content Area:* Adult Health/Neurological

*Reference*
Potter, P., & Perry, A. (2001). *Fundamentals of nursing* (5th ed.). St. Louis: Mosby, p. 480.

---

**141.** A nurse observes a client wringing his hands and looking frightened. The client reports feeling out of control. Which approach by the nurse is most appropriate to maintain a safe environment?

1    Administer the ordered PRN anti-anxiety medication immediately
2    Move the client to a quiet room and talk about his feelings
3    Isolate the client in a "time-out" room
4    Observe the client in an ongoing manner but do not intervene

**Answer: 2**
*Rationale:* The anxiety symptoms demonstrated by this client require some form of intervention. Moving the client to a quiet room decreases environmental stimulus. Talking provides the nurse an opportunity to assess the cause of the client's feelings and to identify appropriate interventions. Isolation is appropriate if a client is a danger to self or others. Medication is used only when other noninvasive approaches have been unsuccessful.

*Test-Taking Strategy:* Use therapeutic communication techniques. Option 2 is the only option that addresses the client's feelings. Remember, the client's feelings are most important. Review therapeutic communication techniques if you had difficulty with this question.

*Level of Cognitive Ability:* Application
*Client Needs:* Safe, Effective Care Environment
*Integrated Concept/Process:* Nursing Process/Implementation
*Content Area:* Mental Health

*Reference*
Stuart, G.W., & Laraia, M.T. (1998). *Principles and practice of psychiatric nursing.* (6th ed.). St. Louis: Mosby, p. 288.

---

**142.** A client with urolithiasis is scheduled for extracorporeal shock wave lithotripsy. The nurse assesses to ensure that which of the following items are in place or maintained before sending the client for the procedure?

1    Signed informed consent, clear liquid restriction, Foley catheter
2    Signed informed consent, NPO status, IV line
3    IV line, clear liquid restriction, Foley catheter
4    IV line, NPO status, Foley catheter

**Answer: 2**
*Rationale:* Extracorporeal shock wave lithotripsy is done with the client under epidural or general anesthesia. The client must sign an informed consent for the procedure and must be NPO for the procedure. The client needs an IV line for the procedure as well. A Foley catheter is not needed.

*Test-Taking Strategy:* Use the process of elimination. Begin to answer this question by eliminating options 3 and 4, since the client must sign an informed consent for this procedure. From the remaining options, recalling that the procedure is done under general anesthesia will direct you to option 2. Review preparation for this procedure if you had difficulty with this question.

*Level of Cognitive Ability:* Application
*Client Needs:* Safe, Effective Care Environment
*Integrated Concept/Process:* Nursing Process/Assessment
*Content Area:* Adult Health/Renal

*Reference*
Ignatavicius, D., Workman, M., & Mishler, M. (1999). *Medical-surgical nursing across the health care continuum* (3rd ed.). Philadelphia: W.B. Saunders, p. 1841.

**143.** A nurse is assisting at a code and the physician is going to defibrillate the client. Of the following items, which is the only one that the nurse does not need to remove from the bedside just before the client is defibrillated?

1    Backboard
2    Oxygen
3    Nitroglycerin patch
4    Ventilator

**Answer: 1**

*Rationale:* Flammable materials and metal devices or liquids (that are capable of carrying electricity) are removed from the client and bed before discharging the paddles of the defibrillator. The nitroglycerin patch has a metallic backing and should be removed.

*Test-Taking Strategy:* Use the process of elimination. Note the key word *not*. Eliminate options 2 and 4 because they are similar. From the remaining options, recall that the backboard is needed to resume cardiopulmonary resuscitation immediately if defibrillation is unsuccessful. Review procedures for defibrillation if you had difficulty with this question.

*Level of Cognitive Ability:* Application
*Client Needs:* Safe, Effective Care Environment
*Integrated Concept/Process:* Nursing Process/Implementation
*Content Area:* Adult Health/Cardiovascular

*Reference*
Ignatavicius, D., Workman, M., & Mishler, M. (1999). *Medical-surgical nursing across the health care continuum* (3rd ed.). Philadelphia: W.B. Saunders, p. 798.

**144.** A nurse is planning the discharge instructions from the emergency department for an adult client who is a victim of family violence. The nurse understands that the discharge plans must include:

1    Instructions to call the police next time the abuse occurs
2    Exploration of the pros and cons of remaining with the abusive family member
3    Specific information regarding "safe havens" or shelters in the client's neighborhood
4    Specific information about self-defense classes

**Answer: 3**

*Rationale:* Any of the options might be included in the discharge plan at some point if long-term therapy or a long-term relationship with the nurse is established. The question refers to an emergency department setting. It is most important to assist victims of abuse with identifying a plan for how to remove self from harmful situations should they arise again. An abused person is usually reluctant to call the police. Teaching the victim to fight back (as in the use of self-defense) is not the best action when dealing with a violent person.

*Test-Taking Strategy:* Use Maslow's Hierarchy of Needs theory. Remember if a physiological need is not present, then safety is the priority. Review care to the victim of abuse if you had difficulty with this question.

*Level of Cognitive Ability:* Application
*Client Needs:* Safe, Effective Care Environment
*Integrated Concept/Process:* Nursing Process/Planning
*Content Area:* Mental Health

*Reference*
Stuart, G.W., & Laraia, M.T. (1998). *Principles and practice of psychiatric nursing.* (6th ed.). St. Louis: Mosby, p. 211.

**145.** A physician is about to defibrillate a client in ventricular fibrillation, and says in a loud voice "CLEAR!" The nurse immediately:

1   Shuts off the IV infusion going into the client's arm
2   Shuts off the mechanical ventilator
3   Steps away from the bed and makes sure all others have done the same
4   Places the conductive gel pads for defibrillation on the client's chest

**Answer: 3**

*Rationale:* For the safety of all personnel, when the defibrillator paddles are being discharged, all personnel must stand back and be clear of all contact with the client or the client's bed. It is the primary responsibility of the person defibrillating to communicate the "clear" message loudly enough for all to hear, and ensure their compliance. All personnel must immediately comply with this command. The gel pads should have been placed on the client's chest before the defibrillator paddles were applied. A ventilator is not in use during a code, rather an Ambu (resuscitation) bag is used. Shutting off the infusion has no useful purpose. Stepping back from the bed prevents the nurse or others from being defibrillated along with the client.

*Test-Taking Strategy:* Use the process of elimination, focusing on the issue, the procedure for defibrillation. Recalling the risks associated with this procedure and noting the word *clear* in the question will direct you to option 3. Review the risks associated with this procedure if you had difficulty with this question.

*Level of Cognitive Ability:* Application
*Client Needs:* Safe, Effective Care Environment
*Integrated Concept/Process:* Nursing Process/Implementation
*Content Area:* Adult Health/Cardiovascular

*Reference*
Ignatavicius, D., Workman, M., & Mishler, M. (1999). *Medical-surgical nursing across the health care continuum* (3rd ed.). Philadelphia: W.B. Saunders, p. 798.

---

**146.** A client with chronic renal failure has an indwelling catheter in the abdomen for peritoneal dialysis. The client spills water on the dressing while bathing. The nurse plans to immediately:

1   Reinforce the dressing
2   Change the dressing
3   Flush the peritoneal dialysis catheter
4   Scrub the catheter with povidone-iodine solution

**Answer: 2**

*Rationale:* Clients with peritoneal dialysis catheters are at high risk for infection. A dressing that is wet is a conduit for bacteria to reach the catheter insertion site. The nurse ensures that the dressing is kept dry at all times. Reinforcing the dressing is not a safe practice to prevent infection in this circumstance. Flushing the catheter is not indicated. Scrubbing the catheter with povidone-iodine solution is done at the time of connection or disconnection of peritoneal dialysis.

*Test-Taking Strategy:* Focus on the issue, that the dressing is wet. The correct option would focus on the dressing, not the catheter. Therefore eliminate options 3 and 4. Knowing that it is better to change a wet dressing than reinforce it, will direct you to option 2. Review care of the client with a peritoneal dialysis catheter if you had difficulty with this question.

*Level of Cognitive Ability:* Application
*Client Needs:* Safe, Effective Care Environment
*Integrated Concept/Process:* Nursing Process/Planning
*Content Area:* Adult Health/Renal

*Reference*
Smeltzer, S., & Bare, B. (2000). *Brunner & Suddarth's Textbook of medical-surgical nursing* (9th ed.). Philadelphia: Lippincott Williams & Wilkins, p. 1121.

**147.** A client is scheduled for elective cardioversion to treat chronic high rate atrial fibrillation. The nurse determines that the client is not yet ready for the procedure after noting that the:

1  Client's digoxin (Lanoxin) has been withheld for the last 48 hours
2  Client has received a dose of midazolam (Versed) intravenously
3  Client is wearing a nasal cannula delivering oxygen at 2 liters per minute
4  Defibrillator has the synchronizer turned on and is set at 50 joules

**Answer: 3**
*Rationale:* Digoxin may be withheld for up to 48 hours before cardioversion, because it increases ventricular irritability and may cause ventricular dysrhythmias post countershock. The client typically receives a dose of an IV sedative or antianxiety agent. The defibrillator is switched to synchronizer mode to time the delivery of the electrical impulse to coincide with the QRS and avoid the T wave, which could cause ventricular fibrillation. Energy level is typically set at 50 to 100 joules. During the procedure, any oxygen is removed temporarily, because oxygen supports combustion, and a fire could result from electrical arcing.

*Test-Taking Strategy:* Use the process of elimination, noting the key word *not*. Think about the procedure and recall the concept related to oxygen combustion to direct you to option 3. Review this procedure if you had difficulty with this question.

*Level of Cognitive Ability:* Analysis
*Client Needs:* Safe, Effective Care Environment
*Integrated Concept/Process:* Nursing Process/Evaluation
*Content Area:* Adult Health/Cardiovascular

*Reference*
Smeltzer, S., & Bare, B. (2000). *Brunner & Suddarth's Textbook of medical-surgical nursing* (9th ed.). Philadelphia: Lippincott Williams & Wilkins, p. 582.

**148.** A nurse is planning activities for a depressed client who was just admitted to the hospital. The nurse plans to:

1  Provide an activity that is quiet and solitary in nature to avoid increased fatigue, such as working on a puzzle or reading a book
2  Plan nothing until the client asks to participate in milieu
3  Offer the client a menu of daily activities and insist the client participate in all of them
4  Provide a structured daily program of activities and encourage the client to participate

**Answer: 4**
*Rationale:* A depressed person often suffers with depressed mood and is often withdrawn. Also, the person experiences difficulty concentrating, loss of interest or pleasure, low energy, fatigue and feelings of worthlessness, and poor self-esteem. The plan of care needs to provide stimulation in a structured environment. Options 1 and 2 are too "restrictive" and offer little or no structure and stimulation. Option 3 is eliminated because of the word *all* in the option.

*Test-Taking Strategy:* Use the process of elimination focusing on the client's diagnosis. Eliminate option 3 first because of the word *all*. From the remaining options, noting the word *structured* in option 4 will direct you to this option. Review care of the client with depression if you had difficulty with this question.

*Level of Cognitive Ability:* Application
*Client Needs:* Safe, Effective Care Environment
*Integrated Concept/Process:* Nursing Process/Planning
*Content Area:* Mental Health

*Reference*
Stuart, G.W., & Laraia, M.T. (1998). *Principles and practice of psychiatric nursing.* (6th ed.). St. Louis: Mosby, p. 376.

**149.** A nurse is caring for an elderly client who had a hip pinned for a fractured hip. In planning nursing care, the nurse avoids which of the following to minimize the chance for further injury?

1  Side rails in the "up" position
2  Use of the night-light in hospital room and bathroom
3  Call bell placed within the client's reach
4  Delays in responding to the call light but telling the client via the intercom that someone will attend to his or her needs

**Answer:  4**

*Rationale:*  Safe nursing actions intended to prevent injury to the client include keeping the side rails up, the bed in low position, use of a night-light, and providing a call bell that is within the client's reach. Responding promptly to the client's use of the call light minimizes the chance that the client will try to get up alone, which could result in a fall. Communicating with the client via an intercom does not meet the client's need to prevent potential injury.

*Test-Taking Strategy:*  Use the process of elimination. Focusing on the issue, preventing injury, and noting the key word *avoids* will direct you to option 4. Communicating with the client via an intercom does not meet the client's need to prevent injury. Review measures to prevent injury if you had difficulty with this question.

*Level of Cognitive Ability:*  Application
*Client Needs:*  Safe, Effective Care Environment
*Integrated Concept/Process:*  Nursing Process/Planning
*Content Area:*  Fundamental Skills

*Reference*
Smeltzer, S., & Bare, B. (2000). *Brunner & Suddarth's Textbook of medical-surgical nursing* (9th ed.). Philadelphia: Lippincott Williams & Wilkins, p. 359.

**150.** A nurse is assisting in the care of a client who is to be cardioverted. The nurse plans to set the defibrillator to which of the following starting energy range levels, depending on the specific physician order?

1  50 to100 joules
2  150 to 200 joules
3  250 to 300 joules
4  350 to 400 joules

**Answer:  1**

*Rationale:*  When a client is cardioverted, the defibrillator is charged to the energy level ordered by the physician. Cardioversion is usually started at 50 to 100 joules. Options 2, 3, and 4 are incorrect.

*Test-Taking Strategy:*  Use the process of elimination. Remember that in instances when cardioversion is used, there is an underlying cardiac rhythm that needs to be converted to a better rhythm, so lower voltages are used. Review this procedure if you had difficulty with this question.

*Level of Cognitive Ability:*  Application
*Client Needs:*  Safe, Effective Care Environment
*Integrated Concept/Process:*  Nursing Process/Planning
*Content Area:*  Adult Health/Cardiovascular

*Reference*
Smeltzer, S., & Bare, B. (2000). *Brunner & Suddarth's Textbook of medical-surgical nursing* (9th ed.). Philadelphia: Lippincott Williams & Wilkins, p. 580.

**151.** A nurse has an order to get the client out of bed to a chair on the first postoperative day following total knee replacement (TKR). The nurse plans to do which of the following to protect the knee joint?

1  Apply a knee immobilizer before getting the client up, and elevate the client's surgical leg while sitting
2  Apply a compression dressing, and put ice on the knee while sitting
3  Lift the client to the bedside chair leaving the continuous passive motion (CPM) machine in place
4  Obtain a walker to minimize weight bearing by the client on the affected leg

**Answer: 1**

*Rationale:* The nurse assists the client to get out of bed on the first postoperative day after putting a knee immobilizer on the affected joint to provide stability. The surgeon orders the weight-bearing limits on the affected leg. The leg is elevated while the client is sitting in the chair to minimize edema. Ice is not used unless prescribed. A compression dressing should already be in place on the wound. A CPM machine is used only while the client is in bed. Ambulation is not started until the second postoperative day.

*Test-Taking Strategy:* Use the process of elimination. Note the relationship between the issue *protect the knee joint* and *knee immobilizer* in option 1. Review postoperative care following TKR if you had difficulty with this question.

*Level of Cognitive Ability:* Application
*Client Needs:* Safe, Effective Care Environment
*Integrated Concept/Process:* Nursing Process/Planning
*Content Area:* Adult Health/Musculoskeletal

*Reference*
Smeltzer, S., & Bare, B. (2000). *Brunner & Suddarth's Textbook of medical-surgical nursing* (9th ed.). Philadelphia: Lippincott Williams & Wilkins, p. 1796.

---

**152.** A client is admitted to the psychiatric unit following a suicide attempt by hanging. The nurse's most important aspect of care is to maintain client safety, and the nurse plans to:

1  Assign a staff member to the client who will remain with the client
2  Place the client in a seclusion room where all potentially dangerous articles are removed
3  Remove the client's clothing and place the client in a hospital gown
4  Request that a peer remain with the client at all times

**Answer: 1**

*Rationale:* Hanging is a serious suicide attempt. The plan of care must reflect the action that will promote the client's safety. Constant observation by a staff member is necessary. It is not a peer's responsibility to safeguard a client. Removing the client's clothing does not maximize all possible safety strategies. Placing the client in seclusion further isolates the client.

*Test-Taking Strategy:* Use the process of elimination, focusing on the issue, suicide attempt. Recalling that one-to-one supervision is necessary will direct you to option 1. Review suicide precautions if you had difficulty with this question.

*Level of Cognitive Ability:* Application
*Client Needs:* Safe, Effective Care Environment
*Integrated Concept/Process:* Nursing Process/Planning
*Content Area:* Mental Health

*Reference*
Stuart, G.W., & Laraia, M.T. (1998). *Principles and practice of psychiatric nursing.* (6th ed.). St. Louis: Mosby, p. 389.

**153.** A nurse receives a telephone call from a male client who states that he wants to kill himself and has a loaded gun on the table. The best nursing intervention is to:
1   Insist that the client give you his name and address so that you can get the police there immediately
2   Keep the client talking and allow the client to ventilate feelings
3   Use therapeutic communications, especially the reflection of feelings
4   Keep the client talking; signal to another staff member to trace the call so that appropriate help can be sent

**Answer: 4**
*Rationale:* In a crisis, the nurse must take an authoritative, active role to promote the client's safety. A loaded gun in the home of the client who verbalizes he wants to kill himself is a *crisis*. The client's safety is of prime concern. Keeping the client on the phone and getting help to the client is the best intervention. Insisting may anger the client and he might hang up. Option 2 lacks the authoritative action stance of securing the client's safety. Using therapeutic communication is important, but overuse of "reflection" may sound uncaring or superficial and is lacking direction and a solution to the immediate problem of the client's safety.

*Test-Taking Strategy:* Use the process of elimination and focus on the crisis, a potential for suicide. The only option that will provide direct help is option 4. Review crisis intervention for a client contemplating suicide if you had difficulty with this question.

*Level of Cognitive Ability:* Application
*Client Needs:* Safe, Effective Care Environment
*Integrated Concept/Process:* Nursing Process/Implementation
*Content Area:* Mental Health

*Reference*
Stuart, G.W., & Laraia, M.T. (1998). *Principles and practice of psychiatric nursing.* (6th ed.). St. Louis: Mosby, p. 237.

**154.** Following initial assessment, the nurse determines the need to place a vest restraint on a client. The client tells the nurse that he does not want the vest restraint applied. The best nursing action is to:
1   Apply the restraint anyway
2   Contact the physician
3   Medicate the client with a sedative then apply the restraint
4   Compromise with the client and use wrist restraints

**Answer: 2**
*Rationale:* The use of restraints needs to be avoided if possible. If the nurse determines that a restraint is necessary, this should be discussed with the family and an order needs to be obtained from the physician. The physician's order protects the nurse from liability. The nurse should explain carefully to the client and family about the reasons that the restraint is necessary, the type of restraint selected, and the anticipated duration of restraint. If the nurse applied a restraint on a client who was refusing it, the nurse could be charged with battery. Compromising with the client is unethical.

*Test-Taking Strategy:* Use the process of elimination and principles and concepts related to ethical and legal issues. Eliminate options 1 and 3 first because they are similar. From the remaining options, eliminate option 4 because it is unethical. Review the legal implications related to the use of restraints if you had difficulty with this question.

*Level of Cognitive Ability:* Application
*Client Needs:* Safe, Effective Care Environment
*Integrated Concept/Process:* Nursing Process/Implementation
*Content Area:* Fundamental Skills

*Reference*
Potter, P., & Perry, A. (2001). *Fundamentals of nursing* (5th ed.). St. Louis: Mosby, p. 1038.

**155.** A client is being discharged and will receive oxygen therapy at home. The nurse is teaching the client and family about oxygen safety measures. Which of the following statements by the client indicates the need for further teaching?
1   "I realize that I should check the oxygen level of the portable tank on a consistent basis."
2   "I will keep my scented candles within 5 feet of my oxygen tank."
3   "I will not sit in front of my woodburning fireplace with my oxygen on."
4   "I will call the physician if I experience any shortness of breath."

**Answer: 2**
*Rationale:* Oxygen is a highly combustible gas, although it will not spontaneously burn or cause an explosion. It can easily cause a fire to ignite in a client's room if it contacts a spark from a cigarette, burning candle, or electrical equipment. Options 1, 3, and 4 are appropriate oxygen safety measures.

*Test-Taking Strategy:* Use the process of elimination noting the key words *need for further teaching.* Recalling that oxygen is a highly combustible gas will direct you to option 2. If you had difficulty with this question, review teaching points related to home care and oxygen.

*Level of Cognitive Ability:* Analysis
*Client Needs:* Safe, Effective Care Environment
*Integrated Concept/Process:* Teaching/Learning
*Content Area:* Fundamental Skills

*Reference*
Potter, P., & Perry, A. (2001). *Fundamentals of nursing* (5th ed.). St. Louis: Mosby, p. 1176.

**156.** A home health nurse visits a client who is to receive intravenous (IV) therapy via an IV pump. The nurse notes that the electrical plug on the wall to be used for the IV pump has only two prongs. Which of the following is the most appropriate action?
1   Use the plug anyway
2   Tape the electrical cord from the IV pump to the floor before plugging it in
3   Run the electrical cord from the IV pump under the carpet before plugging it in
4   Obtain a three-prong grounded plug adapter

**Answer: 4**
*Rationale:* Electrical equipment should be grounded. The third longer prong in an electrical plug is the ground. Theoretically, the ground prong carries any stray electrical current back to the ground, hence its name. The other two prongs carry the power to the piece of electrical equipment. In this situation, the nurse obtains a three-prong grounded plug adapter, attaches it to the cord, and plugs it into the wall. Options 1, 2, and 3 are unsafe actions.

*Test-Taking Strategy:* Use principles of basic electrical safety to direct you to the correct option. Noting the key words *only two prongs* in the question will direct you to option 4. Review these principles if you had difficulty with this question.

*Level of Cognitive Ability:* Application
*Client Needs:* Safe, Effective Care Environment
*Integrated Concept/Process:* Nursing Process/Implementation
*Content Area:* Fundamental Skills

*Reference*
Potter, P., & Perry, A. (2001). *Fundamentals of nursing* (5th ed.). St. Louis: Mosby, p. 1046.

**157.** On an initial home health care visit, the home health nurse assesses the client's environment for potential hazards. Which observation is an indication that the client needs instruction about safety?
1    Skid-resistant small area rugs in the living room
2    Clothes hamper at the end of the hallway
3    Area rugs on the stairs
4    Carpeted stairs secured with carpet tacks

**Answer: 3**
*Rationale:* Area rugs and runners should not be used on stairs. Any carpeting on the stairs should be secured with carpet tacks. Injuries in the home frequently result from objects, including small rugs, on the stairs and floor, wet spots on the floor, and clutter on bedside tables, on closet shelves, on the top of the refrigerator, and on bookshelves. Care should also be taken to ensure that end tables are secure and have stable straight legs. Nonessential items should be placed in drawers to eliminate clutter.

*Test-Taking Strategy:* Focus on the key words *needs instruction about safety*. Using the principles related to home safety will direct you to option 3. Review these principles if you had difficulty with this question.

*Level of Cognitive Ability:* Analysis
*Client Needs:* Safe, Effective Care Environment
*Integrated Concept/Process:* Nursing Process/Assessment
*Content Area:* Fundamental Skills

*Reference*
Potter, P., & Perry, A. (2001). *Fundamentals of nursing* (5th ed.). St. Louis: Mosby, p. 1021.

**158.** A hospitalized client with a history of alcohol abuse tells the nurse, "I am leaving now. I have to go. I don't want any more treatment. I have things that I have to do right away." The client has not been discharged. In fact, the client is scheduled for an important diagnostic test to be performed in 1 hour. After discussing the client's concerns with the client, the client dresses and begins to walk out of the hospital room. The most appropriate nursing action is to:
1    Restrain the client until the physician can be reached
2    Call security to block all exit areas
3    Tell the client that he cannot return to this hospital again if he leaves now
4    Call the nursing supervisor

**Answer: 4**
*Rationale:* A nurse can be charged with false imprisonment if a client is made to wrongfully believe that he or she cannot leave the hospital. Most health care facilities have documents for the client to sign that relate to the client's responsibilities when he or she leaves against medical advice (AMA). The client should be asked to sign this document before leaving. The nurse should request that the client wait to speak to the physician before leaving, but if the client refuses to do so, the nurse cannot hold the client against his will. Restraining the client and calling security to block exits constitutes false imprisonment. Any client has a right to health care and cannot be told otherwise.

*Test-Taking Strategy:* Use the process of elimination. Keeping the concept of false imprisonment in mind, eliminate options 1 and 2 because they are similar. Eliminate option 3, knowing that any client has a right to health. Review the points related to false imprisonment if you had difficulty with this question.

*Level of Cognitive Ability:* Application
*Client Needs:* Safe, Effective Care Environment
*Integrated Concept/Process:* Nursing Process/Implementation
*Content Area:* Fundamental Skills

*Reference*
DeLaune, S., & Ladner, P. (1998). *Fundamentals of nursing: Standards and practice.* Albany, N.Y.: Delmar, p. 233.

**159.** Two nurses are in the cafeteria having lunch in a quiet secluded area. A physical therapist from the physical therapy department joins the nurses. During lunch, the nurses discuss a client who was physically abused. After lunch, the physical therapist provides therapy as prescribed to this physically abused client and asks the client questions about the physical abuse. The client discovers that the nurses told the therapist about the abuse situation and is emotionally harmed. The ramifications associated with the nurses' discussion about the client are most appropriately associated with which of the following?

1    None, because the discussion took place in a quiet secluded area
2    They can be charged with slander
3    They can be charged with libel
4    None, because the physical therapist is involved in the client's care

**Answer: 2**

*Rationale:* Defamation occurs when information is communicated to a third party that causes damage to someone else's reputation either in writing (libel) or verbal (slander). Common examples are discussing information about a client in public areas, or speaking negatively about coworkers. The situation identified in the question can cause emotional harm to the client and the nurses could be charged with slander. This situation also violates the client's right to confidentiality.

*Test-Taking Strategy:* Use the process of elimination and focus on the issue, client's rights and confidentially. This will assist in eliminating options 1 and 4 first. From the remaining options, recall that slander constitutes verbal discussion regarding a client. Review this legal responsibility if you had difficulty with this question.

*Level of Cognitive Ability:* Analysis
*Client Needs:* Safe, Effective Care Environment
*Integrated Concept/Process:* Nursing Process/Analysis
*Content Area:* Fundamental Skills

*Reference*
DeLaune, S., & Ladner, P. (1998). *Fundamentals of nursing: Standards and practice.* Albany, N.Y.: Delmar, p. 233.

---

**160.** A nurse arrives at work and is told that the intensive care unit (ICU) is in need of assistance. The nurse is told by the supervisor that the assignment today is to work in the ICU. The nurse has never worked in the ICU and shares concerns with the supervisor regarding unfamiliarity with the technological equipment used in that unit. The nurse is again told to report to the ICU. The most appropriate action by the nurse is to:

1    Refuse to go to the ICU
2    Go to the ICU, and tell the charge nurse he or she is ill and needs to go home
3    Call the hospital lawyer
4    Go to the ICU and inform the charge nurse of those tasks that cannot be performed

**Answer: 4**

*Rationale:* Legally, a nurse cannot refuse to float unless a union contract guarantees that nurses can only work in a specified area, or the nurse can prove the lack of knowledge for the performance of an assigned task. When encountered with this situation, the nurse should set priorities and identify potential areas of harm to the client. All pertinent facts related to client care problems and safety issues should be documented. The nurse should perform only those tasks in which training has been received. It is the nurse's responsibility to clearly describe these tasks.

*Test-Taking Strategy:* Use the process of elimination. Eliminate option 1 because if a nurse refuses to care for a client, the nurse can be charged with abandonment. Eliminate option 2 next because it is similar to option 1 and because it is ethically unsound. From the remaining options, focusing on the issue, the legalities surrounding floating, will direct you to option 4. Review the issues related to floating and abandonment of the client if you had difficulty with this question.

*Level of Cognitive Ability:* Application
*Client Needs:* Safe, Effective Care Environment
*Integrated Concept/Process:* Nursing Process/Implementation
*Content Area:* Fundamental Skills

*Reference*
Potter, P., & Perry, A. (2001). *Fundamentals of nursing* (5th ed.). St. Louis: Mosby, p. 435.

**161.** A registered nurse (RN) asks a licensed practical nurse (LPN) to change the colostomy bag on a client. The LPN tells the RN that although attendance at the hospital inservice was complete regarding this procedure, the procedure has never been performed on a client. The most appropriate action by the RN is:
1   Request that the LPN review the materials from the inservice before performing the procedure
2   Request that the LPN review the procedure in the hospital manual and to bring the written procedure into the client's room for guidance during the procedure
3   Request that another LPN observe the procedure when it is performed
4   Perform the procedure with the LPN

**Answer: 4**
*Rationale:* The RN must remember that even though a task may be delegated to someone, the nurse who delegates maintains accountability for the overall nursing care of the client. Only the task, not the ultimate accountability may be delegated to another. The RN is responsible for ensuring that competent and accurate care is delivered to the client. Requesting that another LPN observe the procedure does not ensure that the procedure will be done correctly. Since this is a new procedure for this LPN, the RN should accompany the LPN, provide guidance and answer questions following the procedure.

*Test-Taking Strategy:* Use the process of elimination and eliminate options 1 and 2 first. Although it may be important for the LPN to review inservice materials and the hospital procedure manual, these options are not complete. From the remaining options, select option 4 because option 3 does not ensure that the LPN will perform this procedure safely. Additionally, it is the RN's responsibility to educate. Review the principles related to delegating and accountability if you had difficulty with this question.

*Level of Cognitive Ability:* Application
*Client Needs:* Safe, Effective Care Environment
*Integrated Concept/Process:* Nursing Process/Implementation
*Content Area:* Fundamental Skills

*Reference*
DeLaune, S., & Ladner, P. (1998). *Fundamentals of nursing: Standards and practice.* Albany, N.Y.: Delmar, p. 237.

---

**162.** A nurse has applied the patch electrodes of an automatic external defibrillator (AED) to the chest of a client who is pulseless. The defibrillator has interpreted the rhythm to be ventricular fibrillation. The nurse then:
1   Orders any personnel away from the client, charges the machine, and defibrillates through the console
2   Performs cardiopulmonary resuscitation (CPR) for one minute before defibrillating
3   Charges the machine and immediately pushes the "discharge" buttons on the console
4   Administers rescue breathing during the defibrillation

**Answer: 1**
*Rationale:* If the AED advises to defibrillate, the nurse or rescuer orders all persons away from the client, charges the capacitor, and pushes both of the "discharge" buttons on the console at the same time. The charge is delivered through the patch electrodes, and this method is known as "hands off" defibrillation, which is safer for the rescuer. The sequence of charges (up to three consecutive attempts at 200, 300, 360 joules) is similar to that of conventional defibrillation. Option 4 is contraindicated for the safety of any rescuer. Performing CPR delays the defibrillation attempt.

*Test-Taking Strategy:* Use the process of elimination, noting that the question requires prioritizing actions. Recalling the need to avoid contact with the client during this procedure will direct you to option 1. Review this procedure if you had difficulty with this question.

*Level of Cognitive Ability:* Application
*Client Needs:* Safe, Effective Care Environment
*Integrated Concept/Process:* Nursing Process/Implementation
*Content Area:* Adult Health/Cardiovascular

*Reference*
Ignatavicius, D., Workman, M., & Mishler, M. (1999). *Medical-surgical nursing across the health care continuum* (3rd ed.). Philadelphia: W.B. Saunders, p. 798.

**163.** A nurse is planning care for a client diagnosed with deep vein thrombosis (DVT) of the left leg. Which intervention would the nurse avoid in the care of this client?
1 Application of moist heat to the left leg
2 Administration of acetaminophen (Tylenol)
3 Elevation of the left leg
4 Ambulation in the hall once per shift

**Answer:** 4

*Rationale:* Standard management of the client with deep vein thrombosis includes bed rest for 5 to 7 days; limb elevation; relief of discomfort with warm moist heat and analgesics as needed; anticoagulant therapy; and monitoring for signs of pulmonary embolism. Ambulation is contraindicated because it increases the likelihood of dislodgment of the tail of the thrombus, which could travel to the lungs as a pulmonary embolism.

*Test-Taking Strategy:* Use the process of elimination, noting the key word *avoid*. Recalling that pulmonary embolism is a complication of DVT will direct you to option 4. Review care of the client with DVT if you had difficulty with this question.

*Level of Cognitive Ability:* Application
*Client Needs:* Safe, Effective Care Environment
*Integrated Concept/Process:* Nursing Process/Implementation
*Content Area:* Adult Health/Cardiovascular

*Reference*
Ignatavicius, D., Workman, M., & Mishler, M. (1999). *Medical-surgical nursing across the health care continuum* (3rd ed.). Philadelphia: W.B. Saunders, p. 873.

**164.** A nurse is caring for a client with severe toxemia of pregnancy. The client is receiving an intravenous (IV) infusion of magnesium sulfate. Of the following items, which item is considered to be of highest priority to have available?
1 Percussion hammer
2 Tongue blade
3 Potassium chloride injection
4 Calcium gluconate injection

**Answer:** 4

*Rationale:* Toxic effects of magnesium sulfate may cause loss of deep tendon reflexes, heart block, respiratory paralysis, and cardiac arrest. The antidote for magnesium sulfate is calcium gluconate. A percussion hammer may be important to assess reflexes, but is not the highest priority item. An airway rather than a tongue blade is an appropriate item. Potassium chloride is not related to the administration of magnesium sulfate.

*Test-Taking Strategy:* Use the process of elimination. Note the key words *highest priority*. Remember, the percussion hammer would identify the decrease in deep tendon reflexes but the calcium gluconate is required to treat the life-threatening condition that can occur. Review care of the client receiving IV magnesium sulfate if you had difficulty with this question.

*Level of Cognitive Ability:* Application
*Client Needs:* Safe, Effective Care Environment
*Integrated Concept/Process:* Nursing Process/Implementation
*Content Area:* Pharmacology

*Reference*
Hodgson, B., & Kizior, R. (2001). *Saunders Nursing drug handbook 2001.* Philadelphia: W.B. Saunders, p. 618.

**165.** A nurse administers the morning dose of digoxin (Lanoxin) to the client. When the nurse charts the medication, the nurse discovers that a dose of 0.25 mg was administered rather than the prescribed dose of 0.125 mg. Which nursing action is most appropriate?
1  Administer the additional 0.125 mg
2  Tell the client that the dose administered was not the total amount and administer the additional dose
3  Tell the client that too much medication was administered and an error was made
4  Complete an incident report

**Answer: 4**
*Rationale:* In accord with agency's policies, nurses are required to file incident reports when a situation arises that could or did cause client harm. The nurse also contacts the physician. If a dose of 0.125 mg was prescribed, and a dose of 0.25 mg was administered, then the client received too much medication. Additional medication is not required and in fact could be detrimental. The client should be informed when an error has occurred, but in a professional manner so as not to cause great fear and concern. In many situations, the physician will discuss this with the client.

*Test-Taking Strategy:* Use the process of elimination. Simple math calculation will assist in eliminating options 1 and 2. From the remaining options, noting the key words *most appropriate* will direct you to option 4. Remember, the nurse completes an incident report when an error occurs. Review the principles related to incident reports if you had difficulty with this question.

*Level of Cognitive Ability:* Application
*Client Needs:* Safe, Effective Care Environment
*Integrated Concept/Process:* Nursing Process/Implementation
*Content Area:* Fundamental Skills

*Reference*
DeLaune, S., & Ladner, P. (1998). *Fundamentals of nursing: Standards and practice.* Albany, N.Y.: Delmar, p. 237.

**166.** When planning the discharge of a client with chronic anxiety, the nurse directs the goals at promoting a safe environment at home. The most appropriate maintenance goal for the client should focus on which of the following?
1  Maintaining continued contact with a crisis counselor
2  Identifying anxiety-producing situations
3  Ignoring feelings of anxiety
4  Eliminating all anxiety from daily situations

**Answer: 2**
*Rationale:* Recognizing situations that produce anxiety allows the client to prepare to cope with anxiety or avoid specific stimulus. Counselors will not be available for all anxiety producing situations. Additionally, this option does not encourage the development of internal strengths. Ignoring feelings will not resolve anxiety. It is impossible to eliminate all anxiety from life.

*Test-Taking Strategy:* Use the process of elimination. Eliminate option 4 first because of the word *all.* Eliminate option 3 next because feelings should not be ignored. From the remaining options, select option 2 over option 1 because this option is more client-centered and provides the preparation for the client to deal with anxiety should it occur. Review goals of care for the client with anxiety if you had difficulty with this question.

*Level of Cognitive Ability:* Application
*Client Needs:* Safe, Effective Care Environment
*Integrated Concept/Process:* Self-Care
*Content Area:* Mental Health

*Reference*
Stuart, G.W., & Laraia, M.T. (1998). *Principles and practice of psychiatric nursing.* (6th ed.). St. Louis: Mosby, p. 275.

**167.** A nurse is planning to instruct a client with chronic vertigo about safety measures to prevent exacerbation of symptoms or injury. The nurse plans to teach the client that it is important to:
1   Drive at times when the client does not feel dizzy
2   Go to the bedroom and lie down when vertigo is experienced
3   Remove throw rugs and clutter in the home
4   Turn the head slowly when spoken to

**Answer: 3**
*Rationale:* The client with chronic vertigo should avoid driving and using public transportation. The sudden movements involved in each could precipitate an attack. To further prevent vertigo attacks, the client should change position slowly, and should turn the entire body, not just the head, when spoken to. If vertigo does occur, the client should immediately sit down or grasp the nearest piece of furniture. The client should maintain the home in a state that is free of clutter and have throw rugs removed, since the effort of trying to regain balance after slipping could trigger the onset of vertigo.

*Test-Taking Strategy:* Use the process of elimination, focusing on the issue, chronic vertigo and preventing injury. Eliminate options 1 and 2 first, since they put the client at greatest risk of injury secondary to vertigo. From the remaining options, recalling that the client is taught to turn the entire body, not just the head, will direct you to option 3. Review safety measures for the client with chronic vertigo if you had difficulty with this question.

*Level of Cognitive Ability:* Application
*Client Needs:* Safe, Effective Care Environment
*Integrated Concept/Process:* Teaching/Learning
*Content Area:* Adult Health/Ear

*Reference*
Smeltzer, S., & Bare, B. (2000). *Brunner & Suddarth's Textbook of medical-surgical nursing* (9th ed.). Philadelphia: Lippincott Williams & Wilkins, p. 1579.

**168.** A client receiving heparin therapy for acute myocardial infarction has an activated partial thromboplastin time (aPTT) value of 100 seconds. Before reporting the results to the physician, the nurse verifies that which of the following are available for use?
1   Protamine sulfate
2   Vitamin K (AquaMephyton)
3   Vitamin $B_{12}$ (Cyanocobalamin)
4   Methylene blue (Urolene Blue)

**Answer: 1**
*Rationale:* Therapeutic values of the aPTT for clients on heparin ranges between 60 and 70 seconds. A value of 100 seconds indicates that the client has received too much heparin. The antidote for heparin overdosage is protamine sulfate. Vitamin K is the antidote for warfarin sodium (Coumadin) overdosage. Methylene blue is an antidote for cyanide poisoning. Vitamin $B_{12}$ is used to treat clients with pernicious anemia.

*Test-Taking Strategy:* Focus on the issue, heparin therapy and note the key words *available for use*. Recalling that protamine sulfate is the antidote for heparin will direct you to option 1. Review the normal aPTT and the antidote for heparin if you had difficulty with this question.

*Level of Cognitive Ability:* Application
*Client Needs:* Safe, Effective Care Environment
*Integrated Concept/Process:* Nursing Process/Implementation
*Content Area:* Pharmacology

*Reference*
Hodgson, B., & Kizior, R. (2001). *Saunders Nursing drug handbook 2001.* Philadelphia: W.B. Saunders, p. 881.

**169.** A male suicidal client is being discharged home with his family. Which statement by a family member might constitute a criterion for delaying discharge?
1  The client's wife asks, "Does he know that I've already moved out and filed for a divorce?"
2  The client's son states, "One of his friends visited last week to tell us Dad's union is out on strike."
3  The client's daughter states, "I've decided to postpone my wedding until Dad's feeling better."
4  The client's brother asks, "Will my brother be able to continue as executor of our parent's trust ?"

**Answer: 1**
*Rationale:* Single, divorced, and widowed clients have suicide rates that are four to five times greater than those who are married. While the situation of the strike is stressful, the client will probably receive a portion of his wages and can derive hope and a sense of belonging from being a member of the union. While the client might feel responsible for his daughter's postponement of the wedding, if presented as an action to include him, the client will feel loved and cared for. While being suicidal may reduce the ability to concentrate, if the client perceives the executorship positively, taking the role away reinforces the client's low self-esteem and self-worth. This statement by the client's brother indicates a need for the client's brother to be educated about depressive illness.

*Test-Taking Strategy:* Use the process of elimination and focus on the issue, delaying discharge. Recalling the risks associated with a suicide intent will direct you to option 1. Review these risks if you had difficulty with this question.

*Level of Cognitive Ability:* Analysis
*Client Needs:* Safe, Effective Care Environment
*Integrated Concept/Process:* Nursing Process/Analysis
*Content Area:* Mental Health

*Reference*
Stuart, G.W., & Laraia, M.T. (1998). *Principles and practice of psychiatric nursing.* (6th ed.). St. Louis: Mosby, p. 271.

**170.** A nurse is preparing to ambulate a client with Parkinson's disease who has recently been started on L-dopa (levodopa). The nurse assesses which most important item before performing this activity with the client?
1  Assistive devices used by the client
2  The degree of intention tremors exhibited by the client
3  The client's history of falls
4  The client's postural (orthostatic) vital signs

**Answer: 4**
*Rationale:* Clients with Parkinson's disease are at risk for postural (orthostatic) hypotension from the disease. This problem is exacerbated with the introduction of L-dopa, which can also cause postural hypotension and increase the client's risk for falls. Although knowledge of the client's use of assistive devices and history of falls is helpful, it is not the most important piece of assessment data based on the wording of this question. Clients with Parkinson's disease generally have resting not intention tremors.

*Test-Taking Strategy:* Focus on the key words *most important.* Postural hypotension presents the greatest safety risk to the client. Use the ABCs, airway, breathing, and circulation, when prioritizing. Checking postural vital signs is one way to assess circulation. Review the complications associated with Parkinson's disease and the effects of L-dopa if you had difficulty with this question.

*Level of Cognitive Ability:* Application
*Client Needs:* Safe, Effective Care Environment
*Integrated Concept/Process:* Nursing Process/Assessment
*Content Area:* Pharmacology

*Reference*
Salerno, E. (1999). *Pharmacology for health professionals.* St. Louis: Mosby, p. 497.

**171.** A nurse is preparing to transfer an average sized client with right-sided hemiplegia from the bed to the wheelchair. The client is able to support weight on the unaffected side. The nurse plans to use the hemiplegic transfer technique. The client is dangling on the side of the bed. For the safest transfer, the wheelchair should be positioned:

1   Near the client's right leg
2   Next to either leg
3   As space in the room permits
4   Near the client's left leg

**Answer: 4**

*Rationale:* Although space in the room is an important consideration for placement of the wheelchair for a transfer, when the client has an affected lower extremity, movement should always occur toward the client's unaffected (strong) side. For example, if the client's right leg is involved, and the client is sitting on the edge of the bed, position the wheelchair next to the client's left side. This wheelchair position allows the client to use the unaffected leg effectively and safely.

*Test-Taking Strategy:* Use the process of elimination, focusing on the issue, a safe transfer technique. Noting that the client has right-sided hemiplegia and visualizing each of the options will direct you to option 4. Positioning the wheelchair next to the client's unaffected leg allows the client to use the stronger leg more effectively for a safe transfer. Review transfer techniques if you had difficulty with this question.

*Level of Cognitive Ability:* Application
*Client Needs:* Safe, Effective Care Environment
*Integrated Concept/Process:* Nursing Process/Implementation
*Content Area:* Fundamental Skills

*Reference*
Potter, P., & Perry, A. (2001). *Fundamentals of nursing* (5th ed.). St. Louis: Mosby, p. 1539.

**172.** A nurse is caring for a client with a grave clinical condition who is a potential organ donor. Before approaching the family to discuss organ donation, the nurse reviews the client's medical record for contraindications to organ donation, which would include:

1   Allergy to penicillin-type antibiotics
2   Age of 38 years
3   Hepatitis B infection
4   Negative rapid plasma reagin (RPR) laboratory result

**Answer: 3**

*Rationale:* A potential organ donor must meet age eligibility requirements, which vary by organ. For example, age must not exceed 65 years for kidney donation, 55 years for pancreas or liver donation, and 40 years for heart donation. The client should be free of communicable disease, such as human immunodeficiency virus, hepatitis, or syphilis and the involved organ must not be diseased. Another contraindication is malignancy, with the exception of noninvolved skin and cornea.

*Test-Taking Strategy:* Use the process of elimination. Focusing on the issue, contraindications to organ donations, will direct you to option 3. Review these contraindications if you had difficulty with this question.

*Level of Cognitive Ability:* Analysis
*Client Needs:* Safe, Effective Care Environment
*Integrated Concept/Process:* Nursing Process/Assessment
*Content Area:* Fundamental Skills

*Reference*
Smeltzer, S., & Bare, B. (2000). *Brunner & Suddarth's Textbook of medical-surgical nursing* (9th ed.). Philadelphia: Lippincott Williams & Wilkins, p. 1160.

**173.** A nurse is monitoring the ongoing care given to the potential organ donor who has been diagnosed with brain death. The nurse evaluates that the standard of care had been maintained if which of the following data is observed?
1    Urine output 45 mL/hr
2    Capillary refill 5 seconds
3    Serum pH 7.32
4    Blood pressure 90/48 mm Hg

**Answer: 1**
*Rationale:* Adequate perfusion must be maintained to all vital organs in order for the client to remain viable as an organ donor. A urine output of 45 mL/hr indicates adequate renal perfusion. Low blood pressure and delayed capillary refill time are circulatory system indicators of inadequate perfusion. A serum pH of 7.32 is acidotic, which adversely affects all body tissues.

*Test-Taking Strategy:* Use the process of elimination and eliminate options 2, 3, and 4 because they are abnormal values. If this question was difficult, review normal values for physical assessment measurements and the criteria related to organ donation.

*Level of Cognitive Ability:* Analysis
*Client Needs:* Safe, Effective Care Environment
*Integrated Concept/Process:* Nursing Process/Evaluation
*Content Area:* Fundamental Skills

*Reference*
Smeltzer, S., & Bare, B. (2000). *Brunner & Suddarth's Textbook of medical-surgical nursing* (9th ed.). Philadelphia: Lippincott Williams & Wilkins, p. 961.

---

**174.** A client who suffered a severe head injury has had vigorous treatment to control cerebral edema. Brain death has now been determined. The nurse prepares to carry out which of the following that will maintain viability of the kidneys before organ donation?
1    Monitoring temperature
2    Administering IV fluids
3    Assessing lung sounds
4    Performing range of motion exercises to extremities

**Answer: 2**
*Rationale:* Perfusion to the kidney is affected by blood pressure, which is in turn affected by blood vessel tone and fluid volume. Therefore, the client who was previously dehydrated to control intracranial pressure is now in need of rehydration to maintain perfusion to the kidneys. Thus, the nurse prepares to infuse IV fluids as prescribed, and continues to monitor urine output. Options 1, 3, and 4 will not maintain viability of the kidneys.

*Test-Taking Strategy:* Focus on the issue, maintaining viability of the kidneys. Use the process of elimination, noting the relationship between the issue and option 2. Review the concepts related to organ donation of the kidneys if you had difficulty with this question.

*Level of Cognitive Ability:* Application
*Client Needs:* Safe, Effective Care Environment
*Integrated Concept/Process:* Nursing Process/Planning
*Content Area:* Fundamental Skills

*Reference*
Smeltzer, S., & Bare, B. (2000). *Brunner & Suddarth's Textbook of medical-surgical nursing* (9th ed.). Philadelphia: Lippincott Williams & Wilkins, p. 1160.

**175.** A nurse is working in the emergency room of a small local hospital when a client with multiple gunshot wounds arrives by ambulance. Which of the following actions by the nurse is contraindicated in the proper care of handling legal evidence?

**1** Cut clothing along seams, avoiding bullet holes

**2** Initiate a chain of custody log

**3** Place personal belongings in a labeled, sealed paper bag

**4** Give clothing and wallet to the family

**Answer: 4**

*Rationale:* Basic rules for handling evidence include limiting the number of people with access to the evidence; initiating a chain of custody log to track handling and movement of evidence; and careful removal of clothing to avoid destroying evidence. This usually includes cutting clothes along seams, while avoiding areas where there are obvious holes or tears. Potential evidence is never released to the family to take home.

*Test-Taking Strategy:* Focus on the client situation and note the key word *contraindicated*. Use knowledge of basic emergency care principles related to a potential crime to eliminate each of the incorrect options. Remember, giving the client's belongings to the family may be giving up evidence. If this question was difficult, review the legal principles related to care of a client with a gunshot wound.

*Level of Cognitive Ability:* Application
*Client Needs:* Safe, Effective Care Environment
*Integrated Concept/Process:* Nursing Process/Implementation
*Content Area:* Fundamental Skills

**Reference**
Smeltzer, S., & Bare, B. (2000). *Brunner & Suddarth's Textbook of medical-surgical nursing* (9th ed.). Philadelphia: Lippincott Williams & Wilkins, p. 1929.

**176.** A nurse working on a medical nursing unit during an external disaster is called to assist with care for clients coming into the emergency room. Using principles of triage, the nurse initiates immediate care for a client with which of the following injuries?

**1** Bright red bleeding from a neck wound

**2** Penetrating abdominal injury

**3** Fractured tibia

**4** Open massive head injury in deep coma

**Answer: 1**

*Rationale:* The client with arterial bleeding from a neck wound is in *immediate* need of treatment to save the client's life. This client is classified as such and would wear a color tag of red from the triage process. The client with a penetrating abdominal injury would be tagged yellow and classified as "delayed," requiring intervention within 30 to 60 minutes. A green or "minimal" designation would be given to the client with a fractured tibia, who requires intervention but who can provide self-care if needed. A designation of "expectant" would be applied to the client with massive injuries and minimal chance of survival. This client would be color coded "black" in the triage process. The client who is color-coded "black" is given supportive care and pain management, but is given definitive treatment last.

*Test-Taking Strategy:* Use the process of elimination and focus on the key words *initiates immediate care*. Use the principles of triage and prioritize. Noting the words *bright red* in option 1 will direct you to this option. Review disaster planning and the principles of triage if you had difficulty with this question.

*Level of Cognitive Ability:* Application
*Client Needs:* Safe, Effective Care Environment
*Integrated Concept/Process:* Nursing Process/Implementation
*Content Area:* Fundamental Skills

**Reference**
Smeltzer, S., & Bare, B. (2000). *Brunner & Suddarth's Textbook of medical-surgical nursing* (9th ed.). Philadelphia: Lippincott Williams & Wilkins, p. 1902.

**177.** A nurse working on an adult nursing unit is told to review the client census to determine which clients could be discharged if there are a large number of admissions from a newly declared disaster. The nurse interprets that the client with which of the following problems would not be able to be discharged, even if support was available at home?

1   Laparoscopic cholecystectomy (same day)
2   Ongoing ventricular dysrhythmias while on procainamide (Procan)
3   Diabetes mellitus with blood glucose at 180 mg/dL
4   Fractured hip pinned 5 days ago

**Answer: 2**

*Rationale:* The client with ongoing ventricular dysrhythmias requires ongoing medical evaluation and treatment because of potentially lethal complications of the problem. Each of the other problems listed may be managed at home with appropriate agency referrals for home care services, and support from the family at home.

*Test-Taking Strategy:* Use the principles of triage. Severity of illness usually guides the determination of who requires ongoing monitoring and care. Use of the ABCs, airway, breathing, and circulation, will direct you to option 2. Review the principles of triage and prioritizing if you had difficulty with this question.

*Level of Cognitive Ability:* Analysis
*Client Needs:* Safe, Effective Care Environment
*Integrated Concept/Process:* Nursing Process/Analysis
*Content Area:* Fundamental Skills

*Reference*
Smeltzer, S., & Bare, B. (2000). *Brunner & Suddarth's Textbook of medical-surgical nursing* (9th ed.). Philadelphia: Lippincott Williams & Wilkins, p. 1902.

---

**178.** A registered nurse (RN) is orienting a nursing assistant to the clinical nursing unit. The RN would intervene if the nursing assistant did which of the following during a routine handwashing procedure?

1   Kept hands lower than elbows
2   Used 3 to 5 mL of soap from the dispenser
3   Washed continuously for 10 to 15 seconds
4   Dried from forearm down to fingers

**Answer: 4**

*Rationale:* Proper handwashing procedure involves wetting hands and wrists, keeping hands lower than forearms so water flows toward the fingertips. The nurse uses 3 to 5 mL of soap and scrubs for 10 to 15 seconds using rubbing and circular motions. The hands are rinsed and then dried, moving from the fingers to the forearms. The paper towel is then discarded, and a second one is used to turn off the faucet to avoid hand contamination.

*Test-Taking Strategy:* Use the process of elimination. Note that the wording of the question guides you to look for an incorrect option. Use basic principles of medical asepsis and visualize each option to answer this question. If you answered incorrectly, review this fundamental nursing procedure.

*Level of Cognitive Ability:* Application
*Client Needs:* Safe, Effective Care Environment
*Integrated Concept/Process:* Nursing Process/Implementation
*Content Area:* Fundamental Skills

*Reference*
Potter, P., & Perry, A. (2001). *Fundamentals of nursing* (5th ed.). St. Louis: Mosby, p. 852.

**179.** A client who is immunosuppressed is being admitted to the hospital and will be placed on neutropenic precautions. The nurse plans to ensure that which of the following does not occur in the care of the client?

**1** Placing a mask on the client if the client leaves the room

**2** Removing a vase with fresh flowers left by a previous client

**3** Admitting the client to a semi-private room

**4** Placing a precaution sign on the door to the room

**Answer: 3**

*Rationale:* The client who is on neutropenic precautions is immunosuppressed, and is admitted to a single (private) room on the nursing unit. A precaution sign should be placed on the door to the client's room. Removal of standing water and fresh flowers is done to decrease the microorganism count. The client should wear a mask whenever leaving the room to be protected from exposure to microorganisms.

*Test-Taking Strategy:* Use the process of elimination, noting the key words *does not occur.* Recalling that neutropenic precautions are instituted when the client is at risk for infection resulting from impaired immune function will direct you to option 3. If this question was difficult, review this type of infection control precaution.

*Level of Cognitive Ability:* Application
*Client Needs:* Safe, Effective Care Environment
*Integrated Concept/Process:* Nursing Process/Planning
*Content Area:* Adult Health/Oncology

*Reference*
Smeltzer, S., & Bare, B. (2000). *Brunner & Suddarth's Textbook of medical-surgical nursing* (9th ed.). Philadelphia: Lippincott Williams & Wilkins, p. 296.

**180.** A client who received a dose of chemotherapy 12 hours ago is incontinent of urine while in bed. The nurse wears which of the following when cleaning the client?

**1** Mask and gloves

**2** Gown and gloves

**3** Mask, gown, and gloves

**4** Gown, gloves, and eyewear

**Answer: 2**

*Rationale:* The client who has received chemotherapy within the previous 48 hours will have antineoplastic agents or their metabolites in body fluids and excreta. For this reason, the nurse should wear protection for likely sources of contamination. In caring for the incontinent client, the nurse should wear gloves and a gown, to protect the hands and uniform from contamination.

*Test-Taking Strategy:* Use the process of elimination. Note that the potential source of contamination in this situation is the client's urine. Since urine present on the hospital gown and bedclothes is not likely to splash, eliminate options 1, 3, and 4. Review universal precautions if you had difficulty with this question.

*Level of Cognitive Ability:* Application
*Client Needs:* Safe, Effective Care Environment
*Integrated Concept/Process:* Nursing Process/Implementation.
*Content Area:* Adult Health/Oncology

*Reference*
Smeltzer, S., & Bare, B. (2000). *Brunner & Suddarth's Textbook of medical-surgical nursing* (9th ed.). Philadelphia: Lippincott Williams & Wilkins, p. 1352.

**181.** A nurse receives a call that a client is being admitted who will undergo implantation of a sealed internal radiation source. The nurse contacts the admission office clerk to ensure that which of the following rooms is selected for the client?

1   A single room at the distant end of the hall
2   A single room near the nurse's station
3   A semiprivate room between two isolation rooms
4   A semiprivate room near the nurse's station

**Answer: 1**

*Rationale:* The client receiving an implantation of a sealed internal radiation source should be placed in a single room in an area that reduces the risk of exposure to others. For this reason, rooms are often used that are at the end of a hall.

*Test-Taking Strategy:* Use the process of elimination. Use of the principle of shielding related to radiation therapy will assist to eliminate options 2, 3, and 4 since they do not provide distance to protect other clients. Review the protective measures related to the care of a client with a sealed internal radiation source if you had difficulty with this question.

*Level of Cognitive Ability:* Application
*Client Needs:* Safe, Effective Care Environment
*Integrated Concept/Process:* Nursing Process/Planning
*Content Area:* Adult Health/Oncology

*Reference*
Smeltzer, S., & Bare, B. (2000). *Brunner & Suddarth's Textbook of medical-surgical nursing* (9th ed.). Philadelphia: Lippincott Williams & Wilkins, p. 1255.

---

**182.** A nurse is assessing the corneal reflex on an unconscious client. The nurse would use which of the following as the safest stimulus to touch the client's cornea?

1   Wisp of cotton
2   Sterile drop of saline solution
3   Sterile glove
4   Tip of a 1-mL syringe with the needle removed

**Answer: 2**

*Rationale:* The client who is unconscious is at great risk for corneal abrasion. For this reason, the safest way to test the corneal reflex is by using a drop of sterile saline. Use of the items in options 1, 3, and 4 can cause injury to the cornea.

*Test-Taking Strategy:* Use the process of elimination, noting the key word *unconscious*. Remember that options that are similar are not likely to be correct. In this case, each of the incorrect options is a solid substance, while the correct option is a liquid. Review assessment techniques for an unconscious client if you had difficulty with this question.

*Level of Cognitive Ability:* Application
*Client Needs:* Safe, Effective Care Environment
*Integrated Concept/Process:* Nursing Process/Assessment
*Content Area:* Adult Health/Neurological

*Reference*
Smeltzer, S., & Bare, B. (2000). *Brunner & Suddarth's Textbook of medical-surgical nursing* (9th ed.). Philadelphia: Lippincott Williams & Wilkins, p. 1623.

**183.** A nurse is preparing to assist the client from the bed to a chair using a hydraulic lift. The nurse would do which of the following to move the client safely with this device?

1 Have three people available to assist
2 Position the client in the center of the sling
3 Have the client grasp the chains attaching the sling to the lift
4 Lower the client rapidly once positioned over the chair

**Answer: 2**

*Rationale:* When using a hydraulic lift, the client is positioned in the center of the sling, which is then attached to chains or straps that attach the sling to the lift. The client's hands and arms are crossed over the chest, and the client is raised from the bed into a sitting position. The client is also raised off the mattress with the lift, and is lowered slowly once the sling is positioned over the chair.

*Test-Taking Strategy:* Use the process of elimination. Visualize this procedure and each description in the options to direct you to option 2 Review this procedure if you had difficulty with this question.

*Level of Cognitive Ability:* Application
*Client Needs:* Safe, Effective Care Environment
*Integrated Concept/Process:* Nursing Process/Implementation
*Content Area:* Fundamental Skills

*Reference*
Potter, P., & Perry, A. (2001). *Fundamentals of nursing* (5th ed.). St. Louis: Mosby, p. 1534.

**184.** An elderly client in a long-term care facility has a nursing diagnosis of Risk for Injury related to confusion. The client's gait is stable. The nurse uses which of the following methods of restraint to prevent injury to the client?

1 Vest restraint
2 Waist restraint
3 Chair with locking lap tray
4 Alarm-activating bracelet

**Answer: 4**

*Rationale:* If the client is confused and has a stable gait, the least intrusive method of restraint is the use of an alarm activating bracelet, or "wandering bracelet." This allows the client to move about the residence freely while preventing the client from leaving the premises. Options 1, 2, and 3 are restrictive devices and should not be used.

*Test-Taking Strategy:* Use the process of elimination and knowledge of the ethical and legal ramifications related to restraints. Noting the key words *gait is stable* will direct you to option 4. Review the guidelines related to the use of restraints if you had difficulty with this question.

*Level of Cognitive Ability:* Application
*Client Needs:* Safe, Effective Care Environment
*Integrated Concept/Process:* Nursing Process/Implementation
*Content Area:* Fundamental Skills

*Reference*
Potter, P., & Perry, A. (2001). *Fundamentals of nursing* (5th ed.). St. Louis: Mosby, p. 1038.

**185.** Furosemide (Lasix) 40 mg PO has been prescribed for a client. A nurse administers Lasix 80 mg PO to the client at 10:00 A.M. Following discovery of the error, the nurse completes an incident report. Which of the following would the nurse document on this report?

  **1** "Lasix 80 mg was given to the client instead of 40 mg."
  **2** "The wrong dose of medication was given to the client at 10:00 A.M."
  **3** "I meant to give 40 mg of Lasix but I was rushed to get to another client who needed me and I gave the wrong dose."
  **4** "Lasix 80 mg administered at 10:00 A.M."

**Answer: 4**
*Rationale:* When completing an incident report, the nurse should state the fact clearly. The nurse should not record assumptions, opinions, judgments, or conclusions about what occurred. The nurse should not point blame or suggest how to prevent an occurrence of a similar incident.

*Test-Taking Strategy:* Read the occurrence as stated in the question. Use the process of elimination and select the option that clearly and most directly states what has occurred. Options 1 and 2 are similar therefore, eliminate these options. Option 3 provides a judgment. Option 4 clearly and simply states the occurrence. Review the principles associated with incident reports if you had difficulty with this question.

*Level of Cognitive Ability:* Application
*Client Needs:* Safe, Effective Care Environment
*Integrated Concept/Process:* Communication and Documentation
*Content Area:* Fundamental Skills

*Reference*
DeLaune, S., & Ladner, P. (1998). *Fundamentals of nursing: Standards and practice.* Albany, N.Y.: Delmar, pp. 236, 502.

**186.** A registered nurse (RN) on the night shift assists a staff member in completing an incident report for a client who was found sitting on the floor. Following completion of the report, the RN avoids which action?

  **1** Documents in the nurses notes that an incident report was filed
  **2** Forwards the incident report to the Continuous Quality Improvement Department
  **3** Asks the unit secretary to call the physician
  **4** Notifies the nursing supervisor

**Answer: 1**
*Rationale:* Nurses are advised not to document the filing of an incident report in the nurses notes for legal reasons. Incident reports inform the facility's administration of the incident so that risk management personnel can consider changes that might prevent similar occurrences in the future. Incident reports also alert the facility's insurance company to a potential claim and the need for further investigation. Options 2, 3, and 4 are accurate interventions.

*Test-Taking Strategy:* Use the process of elimination. Note the word *avoids* in the stem of the question. Note that options 2, 3, and 4 all relate to notification of key individuals or departments. Option 1 relates to documentation of filing an incident report. Review the concepts that relate to incident reports if you had difficulty with this question.

*Level of Cognitive Ability:* Application
*Client Needs:* Safe, Effective Care Environment
*Integrated Concept/Process:* Nursing Process/Implementation
*Content Area:* Fundamental Skills

*Reference*
DeLaune, S., & Ladner, P. (1998). *Fundamentals of nursing: standards and practice.* Albany, N.Y.: Delmar, p. 502.

**187.** A physician visits a client on the nursing unit. During the visit, the physician is called to another nursing unit to assess a client in extreme pain. The physician states to the nurse, "I'm in a hurry. Can you write the order to decrease the atenolol (Tenormin) to 25 mg daily?" Which of the following is the most appropriate nursing action?
1 Write the order as stated
2 Call the nursing supervisor to write the order
3 Ask the physician to return to the nursing unit to write the order
4 Inform the client of the change of medication

**Answer: 3**
*Rationale:* Nurses are encouraged not to accept verbal orders from the physician because of the risks of error. The only exception to this may be in an emergency situation and then the agency policy and procedure must be adhered to. Although the client will be informed of the change in the treatment plan, this is not the most appropriate action at this time. The physician needs to write the new order. It is inappropriate to ask another individual other than the physician to write the order.

*Test-Taking Strategy:* Use the process of elimination. Recall that verbal orders are not acceptable. Options 1 and 2 are similar, therefore eliminate these options. Option 4 is appropriate, but not at this time. Option 3 clearly identifies the nurse's responsibility in this situation. Review these principles if you had difficulty with this question.

*Level of Cognitive Ability:* Application
*Client Needs:* Safe, Effective Care Environment
*Integrated Concept/Process:* Nursing Process/Implementation
*Content Area:* Fundamental Skills

*Reference*
DeLaune, S., & Ladner, P. (1998). *Fundamentals of nursing: Standards and practice.* Albany, N.Y.: Delmar, p. 237.

**188.** A nurse is caring for a client who has an order for dextroamphetamine (Dexedrine) 25 mg PO daily. The nurse collaborates with the dietician to limit the amount of which of the following items on the client's dietary trays?
1 Starch
2 Caffeine
3 Protein
4 Fat

**Answer: 2**
*Rationale:* Dextroamphetamine is a central nervous system (CNS) stimulant. Caffeine is a stimulant also, and should be limited in the client taking this medication. The client should be taught to limit their caffeine intake as well. Options 1, 3, and 4 are acceptable dietary items.

*Test-Taking Strategy:* Use the process of elimination. Recalling that this medication is a CNS stimulant will direct you to option 2. Review this medication if you had difficulty with this question.

*Level of Cognitive Ability:* Application
*Client Needs:* Safe, Effective Care Environment
*Integrated Concept/Process:* Nursing Process/Implementation
*Content Area:* Pharmacology

*Reference*
Hodgson, B., & Kizior, R. (2001). *Saunders Nursing drug handbook 2001.* Philadelphia: W.B. Saunders, p. 300.

**189.** A nurse is planning preoperative care for a client scheduled for insertion of an inferior vena cava (IVC) filter. The nurse questions the physician about withholding which regularly scheduled medication on the day before surgery?
1 Furosemide (Lasix)
2 Potassium chloride (K-Dur)
3 Docusate (Colace)
4 Warfarin sodium (Coumadin)

**Answer: 4**
*Rationale:* In the preoperative period, the nurse consults with the physician about discontinuing warfarin sodium to avoid the occurrence of hemorrhage. Furosemide is a diuretic, potassium chloride is a supplement, and docusate is a stool softener.

*Test-Taking Strategy:* Note the issue, witholding a medication. Use the process of elimination evaluating each medication in terms of its potential harm to the client. Review these medications if you had difficulty with this question.

*Level of Cognitive Ability:* Application
*Client Needs:* Safe, Effective Care Environment
*Integrated Concept/Process:* Communication and Documentation
*Content Area:* Adult Health/Cardiovascular

*Reference*
Ignatavicius, D., Workman, M., & Mishler, M. (1999). *Medical-surgical nursing across the health care continuum* (3rd ed.). Philadelphia: W.B. Saunders, p. 687.

**190.** A hospitalized client with hypertension has been started on captopril (Capoten). The nurse ensures that the client does which of the following specific to this medication?
1 Eats foods that are high in potassium
2 Takes in sufficient amounts of high-fiber foods
3 Moves from a sitting to a standing position slowly
4 Drinks plenty of water

**Answer: 3**
*Rationale:* Orthostatic hypotension is a concern for clients taking antihypertensive medications. Clients are advised to avoid standing in one position for lengthy amounts of time, to change positions slowly, and avoid extreme warmth (showers, bath, weather). Clients are also taught to recognize the symptoms of orthostatic hypotension, including dizziness, lightheadedness, weakness, and syncope. Options 1, 2, and 4 are not specific to this medication.

*Test-Taking Strategy:* Use the process of elimination. Recalling that captopril is an antihypertensive will direct you to option 3. Remember the risk of orthostatic hypotension is present with all types of antihypertensives. Review the effects of this medication if you had difficulty with this question.

*Level of Cognitive Ability:* Application
*Client Needs:* Safe, Effective Care Environment
*Integrated Concept/Process:* Nursing Process/Evaluation
*Content Area:* Adult Health/Cardiovascular

*Reference*
Hodgson, B., & Kizior, R. (2001). *Saunders Nursing drug handbook 2001.* Philadelphia: W.B. Saunders, p. 142.

**191.** The physician's order reads heparin sodium 25,000 units in 250 mL 5% dextrose in water to run continuously at a rate of 800 units per hour by IV. The nurse sets the intravenous pump to how many mL per hour?

1   8
2   32
3   40
4   80

**Answer: 1**

*Rationale:* Use the formula for calculating milliliters per hour with the use of an infusion pump.

*Desired:* 800 units/hour
*Available:* 25,000 units/250 mL 5% dextrose in water

First, divide the 25,000 units by the 250 mL to yield a concentration of 100 units per mL.
Next, 800 units/hour is divided by 100 units/mL. The nurse would set the pump at 8 mL per hour.

*Test-Taking Strategy:* Think about what the question is asking. Determine units per milliliter and then use the standard "desired over available" formula. Also, note that options 2, 3 and 4 are high doses. Review this formula if you had difficulty with this question.

*Level of Cognitive Ability:* Application
*Client Needs:* Safe, Effective Care Environment
*Integrated Concept/Process:* Nursing Process/Implementation
*Content Area:* Fundamental Skills

**Reference**

Kee, J., & Marshall, S. (2000). *Clinical calculations: With applications to general and specialty areas* (4th ed.). Philadelphia: W.B. Saunders, pp. 240-241.

---

**192.** A client receiving lisinopril (Prinivil) has a white blood cell (WBC) count of 3800/mm$^3$. The nurse plans to do which of the following in the care of this client?

1   Follow aseptic technique diligently
2   Request prophylactic antibiotics from the physician
3   Place the client on respiratory isolation
4   Use antibacterial soap when bathing the client

**Answer: 1**

*Rationale:* The client taking angiotensin-converting enzymes (ACE) inhibitors, such as lisinopril, is at risk of developing neutropenia. These clients require the use of strict aseptic technique by all who care for the client. The client should also be taught to report signs and symptoms of infection, such as sore throat and fever to the physician. The WBC count with differential may be monitored monthly for up to 6 months in clients deemed at risk.

*Test-Taking Strategy:* Use the process of elimination. This question can be correctly answered even without knowing that ACE inhibitors cause neutropenia, as long as you can recognize abnormally low WBC values. Recognizing that a WBC count of 3800/mm$^3$ is a low count and that a low count places the client at risk for infection directs you to option 1. Review this medication if you had difficulty with this question.

*Level of Cognitive Ability:* Application
*Client Needs:* Safe, Effective Care Environment
*Integrated Concept/Process:* Nursing Process/Planning
*Content Area:* Pharmacology

**Reference**

Hodgson, B., & Kizior, R. (2001). *Saunders Nursing drug handbook 2001.* Philadelphia: W.B. Saunders, p. 596.

**193.** A nurse is taking a temperature on a client using a glass thermometer. The nurse shakes down the thermometer and drops the thermometer on the floor. Which of the following actions will the nurse take?

1 Carefully wipe up the spill, avoiding getting cut from the glass
2 Use a mop and dustpan to clean up the spill, avoiding contact with the glass and mercury
3 Notify the Environmental Services Department of the spill
4 Call housekeeping department to clean up the spill and broken glass

**Answer: 3**
*Rationale:* Mercury is a hazardous material. Accidental breakage of a mercury-in-glass thermometer is a health hazard to the client, nurse, and other health care workers. Mercury droplets are not to be touched. If a breakage or spill occurs, the Environmental Services Department is called and a mercury spill kit is used to clean up the spill.

*Test-Taking Strategy:* Use the process of elimination. Remembering that mercury is a hazardous material will direct you to option 3. Review the principles associated with mercury spills if you had difficulty with this question.

*Level of Cognitive Ability:* Application
*Client Needs:* Safe, Effective Care Environment
*Integrated Concept/Process:* Nursing Process/Implementation
*Content Area:* Fundamental Skills

*Reference*
Potter, P., & Perry, A. (2001). *Fundamentals of nursing* (5th ed.). St. Louis: Mosby, p. 685.

**194.** A nurse is called to a client's room by another nurse. When the nurse arrives at the room, the nurse discovers that a fire has occurred in the client's waste basket. The first nurse has removed the client from the room. What is the second nurse's next action?

1 Evacuate the unit
2 Extinguish the fire
3 Confine the fire
4 Activate the fire alarm

**Answer: 4**
*Rationale:* Remember the acronym RACE to set priorities if a fire occurs. "R" stands for rescue. "A" stands for alarm. "C" stands for confine. "E" stands for extinguish. In this situation, the client has been rescued from the immediate vicinity of the fire. The next action is to activate the fire alarm.

*Test-Taking Strategy:* Use the RACE acronym to set priorities and answer the question. If you had difficulty with this question, review fire safety.

*Level of Cognitive Ability:* Application
*Client Needs:* Safe, Effective Care Environment
*Integrated Concept/Process:* Nursing Process/Implementation
*Content Area:* Fundamental Skills

*Reference*
Potter, P., & Perry, A. (2001). *Fundamentals of nursing* (5th ed.). St. Louis: Mosby, p. 1044.

**195.** A nurse is caring for a client with cervical cancer who has an internal radiation implant. Which of the following items would the nurse ensure is kept in the client's room during this treatment?

1 A bedside commode
2 A lead apron
3 Long-handled forceps and a lead container
4 A number 16 Foley catheter

**Answer: 3**
*Rationale:* In the case of dislodgment of an internal radiation implant, the radioactive source is never touched with the bare hands. It is retrieved with long-handled forceps and placed in the lead container kept in the client's room. In many situations, the client has a Foley catheter inserted and is on bed rest during treatment to prevent dislodgment. A lead apron, although one may be in the room, is not the required item. Nurses wear a dosimeter badge while in the client's room to measure the exposure to radiation.

*Test-Taking Strategy:* Use knowledge regarding radioactive materials and care to the client with a radiation implant to answer the question. Note the key word *ensure.* Eliminate option 1 and 4 because they are similar and relate to urinary output. From the remaining options, select option 3 over option 2 keeping in mind that the risk of dislodgment can occur. Review these principles if you had difficulty with this question.

*Level of Cognitive Ability:* Application
*Client Needs:* Safe, Effective Care Environment
*Integrated Concept/Process:* Nursing Process/Implementation
*Content Area:* Fundamental Skills

**Reference**
Smeltzer, S., & Bare, B. (2000). *Brunner & Suddarth's Textbook of medical-surgical nursing* (9th ed.). Philadelphia: Lippincott Williams & Wilkins, p. 1255.

---

**196.** A nurse enters the client's room and finds the client lying on the floor. Following assessment of the client, the nurse calls the nursing supervisor and the physician to inform them of the occurrence. The nursing supervisor instructs the nurse to complete an incident report. The nurse understands that incident reports allow the analysis of adverse client events by:

1    Evaluating quality care and the potential risks for injury to the client
2    Determining the effectiveness of nursing interventions in relation to outcomes
3    Providing a method of reporting injuries to local, state, and federal agencies
4    Providing clients with necessary stabilizing treatments

**Answer: 1**
*Rationale:* Proper documentation of unusual occurrences, incidents, and accidents, and the nursing actions taken as a result of the occurrence, are internal to the institution or agency and allow the nurse and administration to review the quality of care and determine any potential risks present. Incident reports are not routinely filled out for interventions nor are they used to report occurrences to other agencies.

*Test-Taking Strategy:* Use the process of elimination and knowledge regarding the purpose of incident reports. Eliminate option 2, recalling that incident reports are not routinely filled out for interventions. Eliminate option 3 because incident reports are not used to report occurrences to other agencies. Option 4 is unrelated to the purpose of an incident report. If you had difficulty with this question, review the purpose of incident reports.

*Level of Cognitive Ability:* Analysis
*Client Needs:* Safe, Effective Care Environment
*Integrated Concept/Process:* Nursing Process/Analysis
*Content Area:* Fundamental Skills

**Reference**
Kozier, B., Erb, G., Berman, A., & Burke, K. (2000). *Fundamentals of nursing: Concepts, process, and practice* (6th ed.). Upper Saddle River, N.J.: Prentice-Hall, p. 66.

**197.** A nurse observes that the client received pain medication 1 hour ago from another nurse, but that the client still has severe pain. The nurse has previously observed this same occurrence. The nurse practice act requires the observing nurse to do which of the following?

1   Talk with the nurse who gave the medication
2   Report the information to a nursing supervisor
3   Call the impaired nurse organization
4   Report the information to the police

**Answer: 2**

*Rationale:* Nurse practice acts require reporting the suspicion of impaired nurses. The board of nursing has jurisdiction over the practice of nursing and may develop plans for treatment and supervision. This suspicion needs to be reported to the nursing supervisor, who will then report to the board of nursing.

*Test-Taking Strategy:* Use the process of elimination and knowledge regarding the agency channels of communication when reporting an incident. Review nursing responsibilities related to suspicion of an impaired nurse if you had difficulty with this question.

*Level of Cognitive Ability:* Application
*Client Needs:* Safe, Effective Care Environment
*Integrated Concept/Process:* Nursing Process/Implementation
*Content Area:* Fundamental Skills

*Reference*
Brent, N. (1997). *Nurses and the law.* Philadelphia: W.B. Saunders, p. 347.

---

**198.** A nurse lawyer provides an education session to the nursing staff regarding client rights. A staff nurse asks the lawyer to describe an example that might relate to invasion of client privacy. Which of the following indicates a violation of this right?

1   Taking photographs of the client without consent
2   Telling the client that he or she cannot leave the hospital
3   Threatening to place a client in restraints
4   Performing a surgical procedure without consent

**Answer: 1**

*Rationale:* Invasion of privacy takes place when an individual's private affairs are unreasonably intruded into. Telling the client that he or she cannot leave the hospital constitutes false imprisonment. Threatening to place a client in restraints constitutes assault. Performing a surgical procedure without consent is an example of battery.

*Test-Taking Strategy:* Use the process of elimination, noting the key words *invasion of client privacy.* These key words should easily direct you to option 1. If you had difficulty with this question, review those situations that include invasion of privacy.

*Level of Cognitive Ability:* Analysis
*Client Needs:* Safe, Effective Care Environment
*Integrated Concept/Process:* Nursing Process/Analysis
*Content Area:* Fundamental Skills

*Reference*
Harkreader, H. (2000). *Fundamentals of nursing: Caring and clinical judgment.* Philadelphia: W.B. Saunders, p. 24.

**199.** A nurse witnesses an automobile accident and provides care to the open wound of a young child at the scene of the accident. The family is extremely grateful and insists that the nurse accept monetary compensation for the care provided to the child. Because of the family insistence, the nurse accepts the compensation to avoid offending the family. The child develops an infection and sepsis and is hospitalized. The family files suit against the nurse who provided care to the child at the scene of the accident. Which of the following is accurate regarding the nurse's immunity from this suit?

1 The Good Samaritan Law will protect the nurse
2 The Good Samaritan Law will protect the nurse if the care given at the scene was not negligent
3 The Good Samaritan Law will not provide immunity from suit if the nurse accepted compensation for the care provided
4 The Good Samaritan Law protects lay persons and not professional health care providers

**Answer: 3**
*Rationale:* A Good Samaritan Law is passed by a state legislator to encourage nurses and other health care providers to provide care to a person when an accident, emergency, or injury occurs, without fear of being sued for the care provided. Called immunity from suit, this protection usually applies only if all of the conditions of the law are met, such as the health care provider receives no compensation for the care provided, and the care given is not willfully and wantonly negligent.

*Test-Taking Strategy:* If you read the question carefully, you will note the key words *accept monetary compensation*. This will easily direct you to option 3. Additionally, options 1, 2, and 4 are similar. Review the Good Samaritan Law if you had difficulty with this question.

*Level of Cognitive Ability:* Analysis
*Client Needs:* Safe, Effective Care Environment
*Integrated Concept/Process:* Nursing Process/Analysis
*Content Area:* Fundamental Skills

*Reference*
Leahy, J., & Kizilay, P. (1998). *Foundations of nursing practice: A nursing process approach.* Philadelphia: W.B. Saunders, p. 73.

**200.** A client brought to the emergency room after a serious accident is unconscious and bleeding profusely. Surgery is required immediately in order to save the client's life. In regard to informed consent for the surgical procedure, which of the following is the best nursing action?

1 Try to obtain the spouse's telephone number and call the spouse to obtain telephone consent before the surgical procedure
2 Transport the client to the operating room immediately as required by the physician without obtaining an informed consent
3 Ask the friend that accompanied the client to the emergency room to sign the consent form
4 Call the nursing supervisor to initiate a court order for the surgical procedure

**Answer: 2**
*Rationale:* Generally, the informed consent of an adult client is not needed in two instances. One instance is when an emergency is present and delaying treatment for the purpose of obtaining informed consent would result in injury or death to the client. The second instance is when the client waives the right to give informed consent. Option 3 is inappropriate. Options 1 and 4 would delay treatment.

*Test-Taking Strategy:* Use the process of elimination. Option 3 can be easily eliminated first because it is inappropriate. Note the key words *surgery is required immediately*. Eliminate options 1 and 4 because these actions would delay treatment. Review the issues surrounding informed consent if you had difficulty with this question.

*Level of Cognitive Ability:* Application
*Client Needs:* Safe, Effective Care Environment
*Integrated Concept/Process:* Nursing Process/ Implementation
*Content Area:* Fundamental Skills

*Reference*
Craven, R., & Hirnle, C. (2000). *Fundamentals of nursing: Human health and function* (3rd ed.). Philadelphia: Lippincott, p. 99.

**201.** A home health care nurse arrives at the client's home for the scheduled home visit. The client's lawyer is present and the client is preparing a living will. The living will requires that the client's signature be witnessed, and the client asks the nurse to witness the signature. Which of the following is the most appropriate nursing action?

1   Sign the will as a witness to signature only
2   Sign the will, clearly identifying credentials and employment agency
3   Decline to sign the will
4   Call the home health care office and notify the supervisor that the will is being witnessed

**Answer: 3**

*Rationale:* Living wills are required to be in writing and signed by the client. The client's signature either must be witnessed by specified individuals or notarized. Many states prohibit any employee, including a nurse of a facility where the declaring is receiving care, from being a witness. The nurse should decline to sign the will.

*Test-Taking Strategy:* Use the process of elimination and note the key words *most appropriate*. This may indicate that more than one option may be correct. Options 1 and 2 are similar and should be eliminated first. From the remaining options, option 3 is most appropriate. Review legal implications associated with wills if you had difficulty with this question.

*Level of Cognitive Ability:* Application
*Client Needs:* Safe, Effective Care Environment
*Integrated Concept/Process:* Nursing Process/Implementation
*Content Area:* Fundamental Skills

**Reference**
Kozier, B., Erb, G., Berman, A., & Burke, K. (2000). *Fundamentals of nursing: Concepts, process, and practice* (6th ed.). Upper Saddle River, N.J.: Prentice-Hall, p. 58.

**202.** An elderly woman is brought to the emergency room. On physical assessment, the nurse notes old and new ecchymotic areas on both arms and buttocks. The nurse asks the client how the bruises were sustained. The client, although reluctant, tells the nurse in confidence that her daughter frequently hits her if she gets in the way. Which of the following is the most appropriate nursing response?

1   "I promise I will not tell anyone but let's see what we can do about this."
2   "I have a legal obligation to report this type of abuse."
3   "Let's talk about ways that will prevent your daughter from hitting you."
4   "This should not be happening, and if it happens again you must call the emergency department."

**Answer: 2**

*Rationale:* Confidential issues are not to be discussed with nonmedical personnel or the person's family or friends without the person's permission. Clients should be assured that information is kept confidential, unless it places the nurse under a legal obligation. The nurse must report situations related to child or elderly abuse, gunshot wounds, and certain infectious diseases.

*Test-Taking Strategy:* Use the process of elimination. Option 4 can be eliminated first because this action does not protect the client from injury. Options 1 and 3 are similar and should be eliminated. Review the nursing responsibilities related to reporting obligations if you had difficulty with this question.

*Level of Cognitive Ability:* Application
*Client Needs:* Safe, Effective Care Environment
*Integrated Concept/Process:* Nursing Process/Implementation
*Content Area:* Fundamental Skills

**Reference**
Craven, R., & Hirnle, C. (2000). *Fundamentals of nursing: Human health and function* (3rd ed.). Philadelphia: Lippincott, p. 91.

**203.** A client is brought to the emergency room by the ambulance team following collapse at home. Cardiopulmonary resuscitation is attempted but is unsuccessful. The wife of the client tells the nurse that the client is an organ donor and that the eyes are to be donated. Which of the following is the most appropriate nursing action?

1   Elevate the head of the bed of the deceased and place dry sterile dressings over the eyes
2   Call the National Donor Association to confirm that the client is a donor
3   Close the deceased client's eyes and place wet saline gauze pads and an ice pack on the eyes
4   Ask the wife to obtain the legal documents regarding organ donation from the lawyer

**Answer: 3**

*Rationale:* When a corneal donor dies, the eyes are closed and gauze pads wet with saline solution are placed over them with a small ice pack. Within 2 to 4 hours the eyes are enucleated. The cornea is usually transplanted within 24 to 48 hours. The head of the bed should also be elevated.

*Test-Taking Strategy:* Use the process of elimination. Note that the key issue relates to donation of the eyes. This should assist in eliminating options 2 and 4. From the remaining options, knowledge regarding care to the eyes of the deceased who is a donor is required. Review this procedure if you had difficulty with the question.

*Level of Cognitive Ability:* Application
*Client Needs:* Safe, Effective Care Environment
*Integrated Concept/Process:* Nursing Process/Implementation
*Content Area:* Fundamental Skills

*Reference*
Monahan, F., & Neighbors, M. (1998). *Medical-surgical nursing: Foundations for clinical practice* (2nd ed.). Philadelphia: W. B. Saunders. p. 1954.

**204.** A client tells the home health care nurse of the decision to refuse external cardiac massage. Which of the following is the most appropriate initial nursing action?

1   Notify the physician of the client's request
2   Document the client's request in the home health nursing care plan
3   Conduct a client conference with the home health care staff to share the client's request
4   Discuss the client's request with the family

**Answer: 1**

*Rationale:* External cardiac massage is one type of treatment that a client can refuse. The most appropriate nursing action is to notify the physician because a written "Do Not Resuscitate" (DNR) order from the physician must be present. The DNR order must be reviewed or renewed on a regular basis per agency policy. Although options 2, 3, and 4 may be appropriate, remember that first a written physician's order is necessary.

*Test-Taking Strategy:* Use the process of elimination and prioritize the options. Note the key words *most appropriate initial*. These key words may indicate that more than one option may be correct. Although options 2, 3, and 4 may be appropriate, remember that first a written physician's order is necessary. Review DNR procedures if you had difficulty with this question.

*Level of Cognitive Ability:* Application
*Client Needs:* Safe, Effective Care Environment
*Integrated Concept/Process:* Nursing Process/Implementation
*Content Area:* Fundamental Skills

*Reference*
Harkreader, H. (2000). *Fundamentals of nursing: Caring and clinical judgment.* Philadelphia: W.B. Saunders, p. 37.

**205.** A nurse is caring for a client with severe cardiac disease. While caring for the client, the client states to the nurse, "If anything should happen to me, please make sure that the doctors do not try to push on my chest and revive me." The most appropriate nursing action is to:

1    Tell the client that this procedure cannot legally be refused by a client if the doctor feels that it is necessary to save the client's life

2    Tell the client that it is necessary to notify the physician of the client's request

3    Tell the client that the family must agree with the request

4    Plan a client conference with the nursing staff to share the client's request

**Answer: 2**

*Rationale:* External cardiac massage is one type of treatment that a client can refuse. The most appropriate nursing action is to notify the physician because a written "Do Not Resuscitate (DNR)" order from the physician must be present on the client's record. The DNR order must be reviewed or renewed on a regular basis per agency policy. Options 1 and 3 are inaccurate. Option 4 may be appropriate but only after the physician is contacted and notified of the client's request.

*Test-Taking Strategy:* The key words *most appropriate* may indicate that more than one option may be correct. Prioritize the nursing actions. Options 1 and 3 are inaccurate and can be eliminated first. From the remaining options, the priority is to notify the physician. Review DNR procedures if you had difficulty with this question.

*Level of Cognitive Ability:* Application
*Client Needs:* Safe, Effective Care Environment
*Integrated Concept/Process:* Nursing Process/Implementation
*Content Area:* Fundamental Skills

*Reference*
Harkreader, H. (2000). *Fundamentals of nursing: Caring and clinical judgment.* Philadelphia: W.B. Saunders, p. 37.

**206.** A nursing instructor is discussing professional liability insurance to the senior class of nursing students. The instructor most appropriately advises the students who will be graduating in two months:

1    To obtain their own malpractice insurance

2    That malpractice insurance is not required and is expensive

3    To discuss liability insurance with the employment agency

4    That most lawsuits are filed against physicians

**Answer: 1**

*Rationale:* Nurses need their own liability insurance for protection against malpractice law suits. Nurses erroneously assume that they are protected by an agency's professional liability policies. Usually when a nurse is sued, the employer is also sued for the nurse's actions or inaction's. Even though this is the norm, nurses are encouraged to have their own malpractice insurance.

*Test-Taking Strategy:* Note the key words *most appropriately* in the stem of the question. These key words tell you that one or more than one option may correct. Although options 2, 3, and 4 may be accurate, the most appropriate advise is identified in option 1. Review liability related to malpractice insurance if you had difficulty with this question.

*Level of Cognitive Ability:* Application
*Client Needs:* Safe, Effective Care Environment
*Integrated Concept/Process:* Nursing Process/Implementation
*Content Area:* Fundamental Skills

*Reference*
Harkreader, H. (2000). *Fundamentals of nursing: Caring and clinical judgment.* Philadelphia: W.B. Saunders, p. 40.

**207.** A nurse educator at the local community hospital is conducting an orientation session for nurses who are newly employed at the hospital. The nurse educator informs the new nurses that the policy of the hospital requires that nurses "float" to other nursing departments when client census is high on other units. The nurse educator advises the new nurses that if this situation arises, and if the nurse is unfamiliar with the unit in which the nurse must float, to:

1 Refuse to float
2 Call the nurse educator
3 Report to the unit and identify tasks that can be safely performed
4 Call the nursing supervisor

**Answer: 3**
*Rationale:* Floating is an acceptable, legal practice used by hospitals to solve their understaffing problems. Legally, a nurse cannot refuse to float unless union contract guarantees that nurses can only work in a specified area or the nurse can prove the lack of knowledge for the performance of assigned tasks. When encountered with this situation, nurses should set priorities and identify potential areas of harm to the client. The nursing supervisor and the nurse educator may need to become involved in the situation at some point if the nurse requires assistance or education regarding a new skill, but the action that the nurse must take is identified in option 3.

*Test-Taking Strategy:* Use the process of elimination. Option 1 can be easily eliminated. It is premature to call the nursing supervisor or the nurse educator therefore eliminate these options. Review nursing responsibilities related to "floating" if you had difficulty with this question.

*Level of Cognitive Ability:* Application
*Client Needs:* Safe, Effective Care Environment
*Integrated Concept/Process:* Nursing Process/Implementation
*Content Area:* Fundamental Skills

*Reference*
Leahy, J., & Kizilay, P. (1998). *Foundations of nursing practice: A nursing process approach.* Philadelphia: W.B. Saunders, p. 69.

**208.** A nurse has received the client assignment for the day and is organizing the required tasks. Which of the following will not be a component of the plan for time management?

1 Prioritizing client needs and daily tasks
2 Providing time for unexpected tasks
3 Gathering supplies before beginning a task
4 Documenting task completion at the end of the day

**Answer: 4**
*Rationale:* The nurse should document task completion continuously throughout the day. Options 1, 2, and 3 identify accurate components of time management.

*Test-Taking Strategy:* Note the key word *not* in the stem of the question. Use the process of elimination and knowledge regarding the guidelines for time management to answer the question. If you had difficulty with this question, review time management principles and the principles related to documentation.

*Level of Cognitive Ability:* Application
*Client Needs:* Safe, Effective Care Environment
*Integrated Concept/Process:* Nursing Process/Planning
*Content Area:* Fundamental Skills

*Reference*
Harkreader, H. (2000). *Fundamentals of nursing: Caring and clinical judgment.* Philadelphia: W.B. Saunders, p. 242.

**209.** A registered nurse (RN) is a preceptor for a new nursing graduate and is describing critical paths and variance analysis to the new graduate. The RN instructs the new nursing graduate that a variance analysis is performed on all clients:
1    Daily during hospitalization
2    Every other day of hospitalization
3    Every third day of hospitalization
4    Continuously

**Answer:** 4
*Rationale:* Variance analysis occurs continually as the case manager and other caregivers monitor client outcomes against critical paths. The goal of critical paths is to anticipate and recognize negative variance early so that appropriate action can be taken. A negative variance occurs when untoward events preclude a timely discharge and the length of stay is longer than planned for a client on a specific critical path. Options 1, 2, and 3 are incorrect.

*Test-Taking Strategy:* Use the process of elimination and knowledge regarding the characteristics of critical paths and variance analysis. Options 2 and 3 can be easily eliminated first. From the remaining options, remember that it is best to monitor a client continuously rather than on a daily basis. Review the characteristics of critical paths and variance analysis if you had difficulty with this question.

*Level of Cognitive Ability:* Application
*Client Needs:* Safe, Effective Care Environment
*Integrated Concept/Process:* Teaching/Learning
*Content Area:* Fundamental Skills

*Reference*
Rocchiccioli, J., & Tilbury, M. (1998). *Clinical leadership in nursing.* Philadelphia: W.B. Saunders, pp. 38-39.

**210.** A nurse manager employs a leadership style in which decisions regarding the management of the nursing unit are made without input from the staff. The type of leadership style that is implemented by this nurse manager is:
1    Autocratic
2    Situational
3    Democratic
4    Laissez-faire

**Answer:** 1
*Rationale:* The autocratic style of leadership is task oriented and directive. The leader uses his or her power and position in an authoritarian manner to set and implement organizational goals. Decisions are made without input from the staff. Democratic styles best empower staff toward excellence because this style of leadership allows nurses an opportunity to grow professionally. Situational leadership style utilizes a style depending on the situation and events. Laissez-faire allows staff to work without assistance, direction, or supervision.

*Test-Taking Strategy:* Use the process of elimination. Noting the key words *made without input from the staff* will assist in directing you to option 1. If you had difficulty with this question review the various leadership styles.

*Level of Cognitive Ability:* Application
*Client Needs:* Safe, Effective Care Environment
*Integrated Concept/Process:* Nursing Process/Implementation
*Content Area:* Fundamental Skills

*Reference*
Rocchiccioli, J., & Tilbury, M. (1998). *Clinical leadership in nursing.* Philadelphia: W.B. Saunders, pp. 103-104.

**211.** A hospital administration has implemented a change in the method of assignments of nurses to nursing units. Nurses will now be required to work in other nursing departments and will not be specifically assigned to a nursing unit. A group of registered nurses is resistant to the change and it is anticipated by nursing administration that they will not facilitate the process of change. Which of the following would be the best approach on the part of administration in dealing with the resistance?
1 Ignore the resistance
2 Exert coercion with the nurses
3 Manipulate the nurses to participate in the change
4 Confront the nurses to encourage verbalization of feelings regarding the change

**Answer: 4**
*Rationale:* Confrontation is an important strategy to meet resistance head-on. Face-to-face meetings to confront the issue at hand will allow verbalization of feelings, identification of problems and issues, and the development of strategies to solve the problem. Option 1 will not address the problem. Option 2 may produce additional resistance. Option 3 may provide a temporary solution to the resistance, but will not specifically address the concern.

*Test-Taking Strategy:* Use the process of elimination. Options 1 and 2 can be easily eliminated first. From the remaining options, select option 4 over option 3 because this option specifically addresses the issue and would provide problem solving measures. If you had difficulty with this question review the strategies associated with dealing with resistance to change.

*Level of Cognitive Ability:* Application
*Client Needs:* Safe, Effective Care Environment
*Integrated Concept/Process:* Nursing Process/Implementation
*Content Area:* Fundamental Skills

*Reference*
Harkreader, H. (2000). *Fundamentals of nursing: Caring and clinical judgment.* Philadelphia: W.B. Saunders, p. 357.

**212.** A registered nurse (RN) in charge is preparing the assignments for the day. The RN assigns a nursing assistant to make beds and bathe one of the clients on the unit and assigns another nursing assistant to fill the water pitchers and to serve juice to all the clients. Another RN is assigned to administer all medications. Based on the assignments designed by the RN in charge, which type of nursing care is being implemented?
1 Functional nursing
2 Team nursing
3 Exemplary model of nursing
4 Primary nursing

**Answer: 1**
*Rationale:* The functional model of care involves an assembly line approach to client care, with major tasks being delegated by the charge nurse to individual staff members. Team nursing is characterized by a high degree of communication and collaboration between members. The team is generally led by a registered nurse who is responsible for assessing, developing nursing diagnoses, planning, and evaluating each client's plan of care. In an exemplary model of nursing, each staff member works fully within the realm of his or her educational and clinical experience in an effort to provide comprehensive individualized client care. Each staff member is accountable for client care and outcomes of care. In primary nursing, the concern is with keeping the nurse at the bedside actively involved in care, providing goal-directed and individualized client care.

*Test-Taking Strategy:* Knowledge regarding the different models of nursing delivery systems is required to answer this question. Focus on the information provided in the question to assist in directing you to the correct option. If you had difficulty with this question review the various nursing delivery systems.

*Level of Cognitive Ability:* Application
*Client Needs:* Safe, Effective Care Environment
*Integrated Concept/Process:* Nursing Process/Implementation
*Content Area:* Fundamental Skills

*Reference*
Rocchiccioli, J., & Tilbury, M. (1998). *Clinical leadership in nursing.* Philadelphia: W.B. Saunders, pp. 29-32.

**213.** A nurse is receiving a client in transfer from the postanesthesia care unit following a left above-the-knee amputation. The nurse should take which of the following most important actions when positioning the client at this time?

1   Put the bed in reverse Trendelenburg position
2   Keep the stump flat with the client lying on the operative side
3   Position the stump flat on the bed
4   Elevate the foot of the bed

**Answer: 4**
*Rationale:* Edema of the stump is controlled by elevating the foot of the bed for the first 24 hours after surgery. Following the first 24 hours, the stump is placed flat on the bed to prevent hip contracture. Edema is also controlled by stump wrapping techniques.

*Test-Taking Strategy:* Use the process of elimination. A key issue in this question is that the client has just returned from surgery. Using basic principles related to immediate postoperative care will assist in directing you to option 4. If you had difficulty with this question, review postoperative positioning following amputation.

*Level of Cognitive Ability:* Application
*Client Needs:* Safe, Effective Care Environment
*Integrated Concept/Process:* Nursing Process/Implementation
*Content Area:* Fundamental Skills

*Reference*
LeMone, P., & Burke, K. (2000). *Medical-surgical nursing: Critical thinking in client care* (2nd ed.). Upper Saddle River, N.J.: Prentice-Hall, p. 1608.

**214.** A clinic nurse is caring for a pregnant client with herpes genitalis. The nurse provides instructions to the mother regarding treatment modalities that may be necessary for treatment of this condition. Which of the following statements if made by the mother indicates an understanding of these treatment measures?

1   "I need to abstain from sexual intercourse until after delivery."
2   "I need to use vaginal creams after the douche every day."
3   "I need to douche and perform a sitz bath three times a day."
4   "It may be necessary to have a cesarean section for delivery."

**Answer: 4**
*Rationale:* If a woman has an active lesion, either recurrent or primary at the time of labor, delivery should be by cesarean section. Clients are advised to abstain from sexual contact while the lesions are present. If it is an initial infection, the client should continue to abstain from sexual intercourse until the cultures are negative because prolonged viral shedding may occur. Douches are contraindicated and the genital area should be kept clean and dry to promote healing.

*Test-Taking Strategy:* Use the process of elimination and knowledge regarding the physiology and treatment associated with herpes genitalis. Options 2 and 3 can be eliminated first because they are similar. Next eliminate option 1 because of the absolute word *abstain*. If you are unfamiliar with the treatment measures associated with this infection, review this content area.

*Level of Cognitive Ability:* Analysis
*Client Needs:* Safe, Effective Care Environment
*Integrated Concept/Process:* Teaching/Learning
*Content Area:* Maternity

*Reference*
Ladewig, P., London. M., & Olds, S. (1998). *Maternal-newborn nursing care: The nurse, the family, and the community* (4th ed.). Menlo Park, Calif.: Addison Wesley Longman, p. 315.

**215.** A pregnant client tests positive for the hepatitis B virus. The client asks the nurse if she will be able to breastfeed the baby as planned after delivery. Which of the following responses is most appropriate by the nurse?

1 "You will not be able to breast-feed the baby until 6 months after delivery."

2 "Breastfeeding is not a problem and you will be able to breastfeed immediately after delivery."

3 "Breastfeeding is allowed if the baby receives prophylaxis at birth and remains on the scheduled immunization."

4 "Breastfeeding is not advised, and you should seriously consider bottle-feeding the baby."

**Answer: 3**

*Rationale:* The pregnant client who tests positive for hepatitis B virus should be reassured that breastfeeding is not contraindicated if their infant receives prophylaxis at birth and remains on the schedule for immunizations. Options 1, 2, and 4 are incorrect.

*Test-Taking Strategy:* Use the process of elimination. Eliminate options 1, 2, and 4 because of the absolute word *not*. Also use therapeutic communication techniques to direct you to option 3. Review the management of hepatitis B virus if you had difficulty with this question.

*Level of Cognitive Ability:* Application
*Client Needs:* Safe, Effective Care Environment
*Integrated Concept/Process:* Teaching/Learning
*Content Area:* Maternity

*Reference*
Lowdermilk, D., Perry, S., & Bobak, I. (2000). *Maternity & women's health care* (7th ed.). St. Louis: Mosby, p. 163.

---

**216.** A nurse manager is planning to implement a change in the method of the documentation system in the nursing unit. Many problems have occurred as a result of the present documentation system and the nurse manager determines that a change is required. The initial step in the process of change for the nurse manager is which of the following?

1 Plan strategies to implement the change

2 Identify potential solutions and strategies for the change process

3 Set goals and priorities regarding the change process

4 Identify the inefficiency that needs improvement or correction

**Answer: 4**

*Rationale:* When beginning the change process, the nurse should identify and define the problem that needs improvement or correction. This important first step can prevent many future problems, because if the problem is not correctly identified, a plan for change may be aimed at the wrong problem. This is followed by goal setting, prioritizing, and identifying potential solutions and strategies to implement the change.

*Test-Taking Strategy:* Use the steps of the nursing process and knowledge regarding the change process to answer this question. Option 4 is the only option that identifies an assessment step. If you had difficulty with this question, review the steps of the change process.

*Level of Cognitive Ability:* Application
*Client Needs:* Safe, Effective Care Environment
*Integrated Concept/Process:* Nursing Process/Planning
*Content Area:* Fundamental Skills

*Reference*
Rocchiccioli, J., & Tilbury, M. (1998). *Clinical leadership in nursing.* Philadelphia: W.B. Saunders, p. 187.

**217.** A delivery room nurse is preparing a client for a cesarean delivery. The client is placed on the delivery room table and the nurse positions the client:
1   In Trendelenburg position
2   In semi-Fowler's position
3   Supine position with a wedge under the right hip
4   In the prone position

**Answer: 3**
*Rationale:* Vena cava and descending aorta compression by the pregnant uterus impedes blood return from the lower trunk and extremities, therefore decreasing cardiac return, cardiac output, and blood flow to the uterus and subsequently the fetus. The best position to prevent this would be side-lying with the uterus displaced off the abdominal vessels. Positioning for abdominal surgery necessitates a supine position; however a wedge placed under the right hip provides displacement of the uterus. Trendelenburg positioning places pressure from the pregnant uterus on the diaphragm and lungs, decreasing respiratory capacity and oxygenation. A semi-Fowler's or prone position is not practical for this type of abdominal surgery.

*Test-Taking Strategy:* Knowledge regarding the optimal positioning for cesarean section is required to answer this question. Use the process of elimination and visualize each of the positions as you select the correct option. You should easily be directed to option 3. If you had difficulty answering this question, review positioning concepts.

*Level of Cognitive Ability:* Application
*Client Needs:* Safe, Effective Care Environment
*Integrated Concept/Process:* Nursing Process/Implementation
*Content Area:* Maternity

*Reference*
Gorrie, T., McKinney, E., & Murray, S. (1998). *Foundations of maternal-newborn nursing* (2nd ed.) Philadelphia: W.B. Saunders, p. 126.

**218.** A nurse in the day care center is told that a child with autism will be attending the center. The nurse collaborates with the staff of the day care center and plans activities that will meet the child's needs. The priority consideration in planning activities for the child is to ensure:
1   Social interactions with other children in the same age group
2   Safety with activities
3   Familiarity with all activities and providing orientation throughout the activities
4   That activities provide verbal stimulation

**Answer: 2**
*Rationale:* Safety with all activities is a priority in planning activities with the child. The child with autism is unable to anticipate danger, has a tendency for self-mutilation, and has sensory perceptual deficits. Although social interactions, verbal communications, and providing familiarity and orientation are also appropriate interventions, the priority is safety.

*Test-Taking Strategy:* Use Maslow's Hierarchy of Needs theory to answer this question. Physiological needs take priority. When a physiological need does not exist, safety needs are the priority. None of the options address a physiological need. Option 2 addresses the safety need. Options 1, 3, and 4 address psychosocial needs. Review care to the child with autism if you had difficulty with this question.

*Level of Cognitive Ability:* Application
*Client Needs:* Safe, Effective Care Environment
*Integrated Concept/Process:* Nursing Process/Planning
*Content Area:* Child Health

*Reference*
Ball, J., & Bindler, R. (1999). *Pediatric nursing: Caring for children* (2nd ed.). Stamford, Conn.: Appleton & Lange, p. 961.

**219.** A nurse is preparing a plan of care for a child who is being admitted to the pediatric unit with a diagnosis of seizures. Which of the following will not be included in the plan of care for this child?
1    Pad the side rails of the bed with blankets
2    Maintain the bed in a low position
3    Restrain the child if a seizure occurs
4    Place the child in a side lying lateral position if a seizure occurs

**Answer: 3**

*Rationale:* Restraints are not to be applied to a child with a seizure, because they could cause injury to the child. The side rails of the bed are padded with blankets and the bed is maintained in low position to provide safety in the event that the child has a seizure. Positioning the child on his or her side will prevent aspiration as the saliva drains out of the child's mouth during the seizure.

*Test-Taking Strategy:* Use the process of elimination. Note the key word *not* in the stem of the question. Focus on safety as you eliminate the incorrect options recalling that restraints are not to be used. Review safety measures related to the child with seizures if you had difficulty with this question.

*Level of Cognitive Ability:* Application
*Client Needs:* Safe, Effective Care Environment
*Integrated Concept/Process:* Nursing Process/Planning
*Content Area:* Child Health

*Reference*
Wong, D. (1999). *Whaley & Wong's Nursing care of infants and children* (6th ed.). St. Louis: Mosby, p. 1820.

---

**220.** Penicillin V (Pen-Vee K), 250 mg PO every 8 hours, is prescribed for a child with a respiratory infection. The medication label reads: Penicillin V, 125 mg per 5 mL. The nurse has determined that the dosage prescribed is safe for the child. The nurse prepares to administer how many milliliters per dose to the child?
1    2 mL
2    4 mL
3    8 mL
4    10 mL

**Answer: 4**

*Rationale:* Use the following formula for calculating medication dosages:

$$\frac{\text{Desired}}{\text{Available}} \times \text{Volume} = \frac{250 \text{ mg}}{125 \text{ mg}} \times 5 \text{ mL} = 10 \text{ mL per dose}$$

*Test-Taking Strategy:* Identify the key components of the question and what the question is asking. In this case, the question asks for the milliliters per dose. Use the formula to determine the correct dosage. Review medication calculations if you had difficulty with this question.

*Level of Cognitive Ability:* Application
*Client Needs:* Safe, Effective Care Environment
*Integrated Concept/Process:* Nursing Process/Planning
*Content Area:* Child Health

*Reference*
Kee, J., & Marshall, S. (2000). *Clinical calculations: With applications to general and specialty areas* (4th ed). Philadelphia: W.B. Saunders, p. 78.

**221.** A cooling blanket is prescribed for a child with a fever. A nurse caring for the child has never used this type of equipment. The charge nurse provides instructions to the nurse and assists the nurse assigned to the child. Which action by the nurse would indicate the need for further instructions in the use of the cooling blanket?

1 Placing the cooling blanket on the bed and covering it with a sheet
2 Checking the skin condition of the child before, during, and after the use of the cooling blanket
3 Keeping the child uncovered to assist in reducing the fever
4 Keeping the child dry while on the cooling blanket to prevent the risk of frostbite

**Answer: 3**

*Rationale:* While on a cooling blanket, the child should be covered lightly to maintain privacy and reduce shivering. Options 1, 2, and 4 are important interventions to prevent shivering, frostbite, and skin breakdown.

*Test-Taking Strategy:* Use the process of elimination and note the key words *indicate the need for further instructions.* Recalling the physiological response associated with fever will direct you to the correct option. Review the procedure associated with the use of a cooling blanket if you had difficulty with this question.

*Level of Cognitive Ability:* Analysis
*Client Needs:* Safe, Effective Care Environment
*Integrated Concept/Process:* Teaching/Learning
*Content Area:* Child Health

*Reference*
Wong, D. (1999). *Whaley & Wong's Nursing care of infants and children* (6th ed.). St. Louis: Mosby, p. 1241.

---

**222.** A child with respiratory syncytial virus (RSV) who is in an oxygen tent is receiving ribavirin (Virazole). Which precaution will the nurse specifically take while caring for the child?

1 Wear a mask
2 Wear goggles
3 Wear a gown
4 Wear a gown and mask

**Answer: 2**

*Rationale:* Some caregivers experience headaches, burning nasal passages and eyes, and crystallization of soft contact lenses as a result of contact with ribavirin (Virazole). Specific to this medication is the use of goggles. A mask may be worn. A gown is not necessary.

*Test-Taking Strategy:* Use the process of elimination. Note the key words *specifically take* in the question. Eliminate options 1, 3, and 4 because they contain similar components. If you had difficulty with this question, review the concepts related to the administration of this medication.

*Level of Cognitive Ability:* Application
*Client Needs:* Safe, Effective Care Environment
*Integrated Concept/Process:* Nursing Process/Implementation
*Content Area:* Child Health

*Reference*
Clark, J., Queener, S., & Karb, V. (2000). Pharmacologic basis of nursing practice (6th ed.). St. Louis: Mosby, p. 585.

**223.** A nurse receives a telephone call from the emergency room and is told that a child with a diagnosis of tonic-clonic seizures will be admitted to the pediatric unit. The nurse prepares for the admission of the child and instructs the nursing assistant to place which of the following items at the bedside?

1 Suction apparatus and an airway
2 A tracheotomy set and oxygen
3 An emergency cart and padded side rails
4 An endotracheal tube and an airway

**Answer: 1**

*Rationale:* Tonic-clonic seizures cause tightening of all body muscles followed by tremors. Obstructed airway and increased oral secretions are the major complications during and following a seizure. Suction is helpful to prevent choking and cyanosis. Options 2 and 4 are incorrect because inserting an endotracheal tube or a tracheostomy is not done. It is not necessary to have an emergency cart at the bedside but a cart should be available in the treatment room or on the nursing unit.

*Test-Taking Strategy:* Use the process of elimination. Knowing that tonic-clonic seizures produce excessive oral secretions and airway obstruction will assist in selecting the correct option. If you had difficulty with this question, review the plan of care associated with seizure precautions.

*Level of Cognitive Ability:* Application
*Client Needs:* Safe, Effective Care Environment
*Integrated Concept/Process:* Nursing Process/Planning
*Content Area:* Child Health

*Reference*
Ball, J., & Bindler, R. (1999). *Pediatric nursing: Caring for children* (2nd ed.). Stamford, Conn.: Appleton & Lange, p. 764.

---

**224.** The nurse in a well baby clinic is providing safety instructions to a mother of a 1-month-old infant. Which of the following safety instructions is most appropriate at this age?

1 Cover electrical outlets
2 Remove hazardous objects from low places
3 Lock all poisons
4 Never shake the infant's head

**Answer: 4**

*Rationale:* The age-appropriate instruction that is most important is to instruct the mother not to shake or vigorously jiggle the baby's head. Options 1, 2, and 3 are most important instructions to provide to the mother as the child reaches the age of 6 months and begins to explore the environment.

*Test-Taking Strategy:* Focus on the age of the infant to direct you to the correct option. A 1-month-old infant is not at a developmental level to explore the environment, which will assist in eliminating options 1, 2, and 3. Review age-appropriate safety measures if you had difficulty with this question.

*Level of Cognitive Ability:* Application
*Client Needs:* Safe, Effective Care Environment
*Integrated Concept/Process:* Teaching/Learning
*Content Area:* Child Health

*Reference*
Wong, D. (1999). *Whaley & Wong's Nursing care of infants and children* (6th ed.). St. Louis: Mosby, p. 760.

**225.** A nurse is caring for a 9-month-old child following cleft palate repair. The nurse has applied elbow restraints to the child. The mother visits the child and asks the nurse to remove the restraints. Which of the following is the most appropriate nursing action?

1   Remove both restraints
2   Tell the mother that the restraints cannot be removed
3   Remove a restraint from one extremity
4   Loosen the restraints but tell the mother that they cannot be removed

**Answer:  3**

*Rationale:* Elbow restraints are used following cleft palate repair to prevent the child from touching the repair site, which could cause accidental rupture and tearing of the sutures. The restraints can be removed one at a time only if a parent or nurse is in constant attendance. Options 1, 2 and 4 are inaccurate nursing actions.

*Test-Taking Strategy:* Use the process of elimination. Eliminate options 2 and 4 first because they are similar. From the remaining options recall the purpose of the restraints following this surgical procedure. This may assist in directing you to option 3, the safest nursing action. Review postoperative nursing interventions following cleft palate repair if you had difficulty with this question.

*Level of Cognitive Ability:* Application
*Client Needs:* Safe, Effective Care Environment
*Integrated Concept/Process:* Nursing Process/Implementation
*Content Area:* Child Health

*Reference*
Wong, D. (1999). *Whaley & Wong's Nursing care of infants and children* (6th ed.). St. Louis: Mosby, p. 1248.

# CRITICAL THINKING: FREE-TEXT ENTRY

**1.** A nurse has documented an entry regarding client care in the client's medical record. When checking the entry, the nurse realizes that incorrect information was documented. How does the nurse correct the error?

**Answer:** Draws one line to cross out the incorrect entry, then initials the change.

*Rationale:* To correct an error documented in a medical record, the nurse draws one line through the incorrect entry and then initials the error. An error is never erased and "white-out" is never used in a medical record.

*Test-Taking Strategy:* Focus on the issue, correcting an error in a medical record. Recalling the principles related to documentation will assist in answering the question. Review these principles if you are unfamiliar with them.

*Level of Cognitive Ability:* Application
*Client Needs:* Safe, Effective Care Environment
*Integrated Concept/Process:* Communication and Documentation
*Content Area:* Fundamental Skills

*Reference*
Ignatavicius, D., Workman, M., & Mishler, M. (1999). *Medical-surgical nursing across the health care continuum* (3rd ed.). Philadelphia: W.B. Saunders, p. 17.

**2.** A registered nurse (RN) is planning the assignments for the day. The RN has a licensed practical nurse (LPN) and a nursing assistant (NA) working on the team. The clients include a client scheduled for a cardiac catheterization, a client with dementia and the client's roommate who requires enemas in preparation for a sigmoidoscopy, a 1-day postoperative mastectomy client, and a client who requires some assistance with bathing and ambulation. The RN will not be assigned to provide client care. Which clients would the RN assign to the LPN and to the NA?

**Answer:** LPN: Client scheduled for a cardiac catheterization and the 1-day postoperative mastectomy client; NA: Client with dementia, the client's roommate who requires enemas in preparation for a sigmoidoscopy, and the client who requires some assistance with bathing and ambulation.

*Rationale:* Assignment of tasks needs to be implemented based on the job description of the LPN and NA, the level of education and clinical competence, and state law. The client scheduled for a cardiac catheterization and the 1-day postoperative mastectomy client will need care that requires the skill of a licensed nurse. The nursing assistant has the skills to care for a client with dementia, a client who requires enemas, and the client who requires some assistance with bathing and ambulation. Also, two of the clients assigned to the NA are in the same room. Since the LPN will be performing higher level skills than the NA, it is best to assign three clients to the NA, as long as the care required by the clients is within the realm of the NA's job description.

*Test-Taking Strategy:* Focus on the clients described in the question and the job description and level of education of the LPN and NA. Think about the needs of each client to assist in determining the assignment. Remember that the LPN will be performing at a higher skill level than the NA. Review the principles associated with delegating and assignment making if you had difficulty with this question.

*Level of Cognitive Ability:* Application
*Client Needs:* Safe, Effective Care Environment
*Integrated Concept/Process:* Nursing Process/Planning
*Content Area:* Fundamental Skills

*Reference*
Yoder-Wise, P. (1999). *Leading and managing in nursing* (2nd ed.). St. Louis: Mosby, pp. 310-311.

---

**3.** A nurse is told that an assigned client has acquired multidrug-resistant *Staphylococcus aureus* (MRSA). In addition to standard precautions, the nurse places the client on which type of transmission-based precautions?

**Answer:** Contact precautions

*Rationale:* Contact precautions are precautions that include standard precautions and the use of barrier precautions such as gloves and impermeable gowns. Contact precautions are used for clients with diarrhea, draining wounds not contained by a sterile dressing, or clients who have acquired antibiotic-resistant infections. The goal of these precautions is to eliminate disease transmission resulting either from direct contact with the client or indirect contact through an intermediary infected object or surface that has been in contact with the client, such as instruments, linens, or dressing materials.

*Test-Taking Strategy:* Focus on the client's diagnosis and think about the method of transmission of the infection to others. Recalling that MRSA can be transmitted by contact with the infecting organism will assist in answering the question. Review contact precautions if you had difficulty with this question.

*Level of Cognitive Ability:* Application
*Client Needs:* Safe, Effective Care Environment
*Integrated Concept/Process:* Nursing Process/Implementation
*Content Area:* Fundamental Skills

### Reference

Harkreader, H. (2000). *Fundamentals of nursing: Caring and clinical judgment.* Philadelphia: W.B. Saunders, pp. 618-619.

---

**4.** A client is scheduled for a colonoscopy and the physician has provided detailed information to the client regarding the procedure. The nurse brings the informed consent form into the client to obtain the client's signature and discovers that the client cannot write. What is the nurse's next most appropriate action?

**Answer:** Obtain a second nurse to also act as a witness and ask the client to sign the form with an X.

**Rationale:** Clients who cannot write may sign an informed consent with an X. This is witnessed by two nurses. Nurses serve as witnesses to the client's signature, and not to the fact that the client is informed. It is the physician's responsibility to inform the client about a procedure. The nurse clarifies facts presented by the physician.

**Test-Taking Strategy:** Note the key word *next.* Also, note that in this situation the physician has informed the client about the procedure. Keeping this in mind, and recalling the principles related to informed consent, will assist in answering the question. Review the principles related to informed consent if you had difficulty with this question.

*Level of Cognitive Ability:* Application
*Client Needs:* Safe, Effective Care Environment
*Integrated Concept/Process:* Nursing Process/Implementation
*Content Area:* Fundamental Skills

### Reference

Ignatavicius, D., Workman, M., & Mishler, M. (1999). *Medical-surgical nursing across the health care continuum* (3rd ed.). Philadelphia: W.B. Saunders, p. 318.

---

## REFERENCES

Ball, J., & Bindler, R. (1999). *Pediatric nursing: Caring for children* (2nd ed.). Stamford, Conn.: Appleton & Lange.

Brent, N. (1997). *Nurses and the law.* Philadelphia: W.B. Saunders.

Clark, J., Queener, S., & Karb, V. (2000). *Pharmacologic basis of nursing practice* (6th ed.). St. Louis: Mosby.

Craven, R., & Hirnle, C. (2000). *Fundamentals of nursing: Human health and function* (3rd ed.). Philadelphia: Lippincott.

Deglin, J., & Vallerand, A. (2001). *Davis's drug guide for nurses* (7th ed.). Philadelphia: F.A. Davis.

DeLaune, S., & Ladner, P. (1998). *Fundamentals of nursing: Standards and practice.* Albany, N.Y.: Delmar.

Fischbach, F. (2000). *A manual of laboratory & diagnostic tests* (6th ed.). Philadelphia: Lippincott Williams & Wilkins.

Gorrie, T., McKinney, E., & Murray, S. (1998). *Foundations of maternal-newborn nursing* (2nd ed.). Philadelphia: W.B. Saunders.

Harkreader, H. (2000). *Fundamentals of nursing: Caring and clinical judgment.* Philadelphia: W.B. Saunders.

Hodgson, B., & Kizior, R. (2001). *Saunders Nursing drug handbook 2001.* Philadelphia: W.B. Saunders.

Ignatavicius, D., Workman, M., & Mishler, M. (1999). *Medical-surgical nursing across the health care continuum* (3rd ed.). Philadelphia: W.B. Saunders.

Kee, J., & Marshall, S. (2000). *Clinical calculations: With applications to general and specialty areas* (4th ed). Philadelphia: W.B. Saunders.

Kozier, B., Erb, G., Berman, A., & Burke, K. (2000). *Fundamentals of nursing: Concepts, process, and practice* (6th ed.). Upper Saddle River, N.J.: Prentice-Hall.

Ladewig, P., London, M., & Olds, S. (1998). *Maternal-newborn care: The nurse, the family, and the community* (4th ed.). Menlo Park, Calif.: Addison-Wesley.

Leahy, J., & Kizilay, P. (1998). *Foundations of nursing practice: A nursing process approach.* Philadelphia: W.B. Saunders.

LeMone, P., & Burke, K. (2000). *Medical-surgical nursing: Critical thinking in client care* (2nd ed.). Upper Saddle River, N.J.: Prentice-Hall.

Lowdermilk, D., Perry, S., & Bobak, I. (2000). *Maternity & women's health care* (7th ed.). St. Louis: Mosby.

Monahan, F., & Neighbors, M. (1998). *Medical-surgical nursing: Foundations for clinical practice* (2nd ed.). Philadelphia: W.B. Saunders.

Olds, S., London. M., & Ladewig, P. (2000). *Maternal-newborn nursing: A family and community-based approach* (6th ed.). Upper Saddle River, N.J.: Prentice-Hall.

Potter, P., & Perry, A. (2001). *Fundamentals of nursing* (5th ed.). St. Louis: Mosby.

Rocchiccioli, J., & Tilbury, M. (1998). *Clinical leadership in nursing.* Philadelphia: W.B. Saunders.

Salerno, E. (1999). *Pharmacology for health professionals.* St. Louis: Mosby.

Smeltzer, S., & Bare, B. (2000). *Brunner & Suddarth's Textbook of medical-surgical nursing* (9th ed.). Philadelphia: Lippincott Williams & Wilkins.

Stuart, G.W., & Laraia, M.T. (1998). *Principles and practice of psychiatric nursing* (6th ed.). St. Louis: Mosby.

Wong, D. (1999). *Whaley & Wong's Nursing care of infants and children* (6th ed.). St. Louis: Mosby.

Yoder-Wise, P. (1999). *Leading and managing in nursing* (2nd ed.). St. Louis: Mosby.

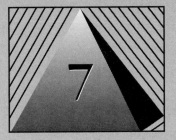

# 7

# Physiological Integrity

1 — 200# ‡♭

1. During an assessment of a perinatal client with a history of left-sided heart failure, a nurse notes that the client is experiencing unusual episodes of a nonproductive cough on minimal exertion. The nurse interprets that this finding may be the first indicator of which important cardiac problem?

1 Orthopnea
2 Decreased blood volume
3 Right-sided heart failure
4 Pulmonary edema

**Answer: 4**
*Rationale:* Pulmonary edema from heart failure may first be manifested as a cough. The cough occurs in response to fluid filling the alveolar spaces. Pulmonary edema develops as a result of left ventricular failure or acute fluid overload. Orthopnea is an assessment finding. Increased rather than decreased blood volume occurs in heart failure. Peripheral edema and organomegaly are signs of right-sided heart failure.

*Test-Taking Strategy:* Use the process of elimination. Note the key words *first indicator*. Focus on the issue: left-sided heart failure. Remember "left" and "lung" to direct you to option 4. Review the complications of left-sided heart failure and the first indicator of pulmonary edema if you had difficulty with this question.

*Level of Cognitive Ability:* Analysis
*Client Needs:* Physiological Integrity
*Integrated Concept/Process:* Nursing Process/Assessment
*Content Area:* Maternity

*Reference*
Lowdermilk, D., Perry, S., & Bobak, I. (2000). *Maternity & women's health care* (7th ed.). St. Louis: Mosby, p. 916.

2. A nurse is performing an assessment on a client with a diagnosis of chronic angina pectoris. The client is receiving sotalol (Betapace) 80 mg PO daily. Which assessment finding indicates to the nurse that the client is experiencing a side effect related to the medication?

1 Difficulty swallowing
2 Diaphoresis
3 Dry mouth
4 Palpitations

**Answer: 4**
*Rationale:* Sotalol (Betapace) is a beta-adrenergic blocking agent. Side effects include bradycardia, palpitations, difficulty breathing, irregular heartbeat, signs of congestive heart failure, and cold hands and feet. Gastrointestinal disturbances, anxiety and nervousness, and unusual tiredness and weakness can also occur.

*Test-Taking Strategy:* Use the process of elimination. Note that the question presents a client with chronic angina pectoris, a cardiac disorder. Remember that medications ending with "lol" (sotalol) are beta-blockers, which are commonly used for cardiac disorders. Note that option 4 is the only option that is directly cardiac related. Review the side effects of sotalol if you had difficulty with this question.

*Level of Cognitive Ability:* Analysis
*Client Needs:* Physiological Integrity
*Integrated Concept/Process:* Nursing Process/Assessment
*Content Area:* Pharmacology

*Reference*
Hodgson, B., & Kizior, R. (2001). *Saunders Nursing drug handbook 2001.* Philadelphia: W.B. Saunders, p. 940.

---

**3.** Before performing a venipuncture to initiate continuous intravenous (IV) therapy, a nurse would:
1  Apply a tourniquet below the chosen vein site
2  Inspect the IV solution for particles or contamination
3  Secure an armboard to the joint located above the IV site
4  Place a cool compress over the vein

**Answer: 2**
*Rationale:* All IV solutions should be free of particles or precipitates. A tourniquet is to be applied above the chosen vein site. Cool compresses will cause vasoconstriction, making the vein less visible. Armboards are applied after the IV is started.

*Test-Taking Strategy:* Note the key word *before*. Use the steps of the nursing process. Option 2 is the only option that reflects assessment, the first step of the nursing process. Review nursing interventions related to initiating an IV if you had difficulty with this question.

*Level of Cognitive Ability:* Application
*Client Needs:* Physiological Integrity
*Integrated Concept/Process:* Nursing Process/Assessment
*Content Area:* Fundamental Skills

*Reference*
Potter, P., & Perry, A. (2001). *Fundamentals of nursing* (5th ed.). St. Louis: Mosby, p. 1220.

---

**4.** A nurse is caring for a client who received an allogenic liver transplant. The client is receiving tacrolimus (Prograf) daily. Which of the following indicates to the nurse that the client is experiencing an adverse reaction to the medication?
1  A decrease in urine output
2  Hypotension
3  Profuse sweating
4  Photophobia

**Answer: 1**
*Rationale:* Tacrolimus (Prograf) is an immunosuppressant medication used in the prophylaxis of organ rejection in clients receiving allogenic liver transplants. Frequent side effects include headache, tremor, insomnia, paresthesia, diarrhea, nausea, constipation, vomiting, abdominal pain, and hypertension. Adverse reactions and toxic effects include nephrotoxicity and pleural effusion. Nephrotoxicity is characterized by an increasing serum creatinine level and a decrease in urine output.

*Test-Taking Strategy:* First, determine the medication classification. Note the client's diagnosis. Look at the medication name Prograf, *Pro* meaning "for" and *graf* indicating "graft," to identify the action of the medication, which is to prevent transplant rejection. This will assist in identifying the classification as an immunosuppressant. Next, recalling the side effects and adverse effects of the medication will direct you to option 1. If you had difficulty with this question, review the adverse effects of this medication.

*Level of Cognitive Ability:* Analysis
*Client Needs:* Physiological Integrity
*Integrated Concept/Process:* Nursing Process/Assessment
*Content Area:* Pharmacology

*Reference*
Hodgson, B., & Kizior, R. (2001). *Saunders Nursing drug handbook 2001.* Philadelphia: W.B. Saunders, pp. 959-960.

---

5. A client was admitted to the hospital 24 hours ago following pulmonary trauma. Which clinical manifestation would first alert the nurse that the client is experiencing adult respiratory distress syndrome (ARDS)?
   1 An increase in respiratory rate
   2 Blood-tinged frothy sputum
   3 Bronchial breath sounds
   4 Diffuse pulmonary infiltrates on the chest x-ray

**Answer: 1**
*Rationale:* Adult respiratory distress syndrome usually develops within 24 to 48 hours after an initiating event. In most cases, tachypnea and dyspnea are the first clinical manifestations. Blood-tinged frothy sputum would present later, after the development of pulmonary edema. Breath sounds in the early stages of ARDS are usually clear but then may progress to bronchial breath sounds when pulmonary edema occurs. Chest x-ray findings may be normal during the early stages but will show infiltrates in the later stages.

*Test-Taking Strategy:* Use the process of elimination. Note the key words *first alert*. It is important to remember with respiratory conditions that tachypnea and dyspnea are often the initial presenting symptoms, along with restlessness, as the hypoxia develops. If you had difficulty with this question, review the early clinical manifestations of ARDS.

*Level of Cognitive Ability:* Analysis
*Client Needs:* Physiological Integrity
*Integrated Concept/Process:* Nursing Process/Assessment
*Content Area:* Adult Health/Respiratory

*Reference*
Smeltzer, S., & Bare, B. (2000). *Brunner & Suddarth's Textbook of medical-surgical nursing* (9th ed.). Philadelphia: Lippincott Williams & Wilkins, p. 467.

---

6. A nurse is caring for a client with Buck's traction. Which assessment finding indicates a complication associated with this type of traction?
   1 Weak pedal pulses
   2 Drainage at the pin sites
   3 Warm toes with brisk capillary refill
   4 Complaints of discomfort

**Answer: 1**
*Rationale:* Weak pedal pulses are a sign of vascular compromise, which can be caused by pressure on the tissues of the leg by the elastic bandage used to secure this type of traction. This type of traction does not use pins; rather, it is secured by elastic bandages or a prefabricated boot. Warm toes with brisk capillary refill is a normal assessment finding. Discomfort is an expected finding.

*Test-Taking Strategy:* Use the ABCs: airway, breathing, and circulation. Option 1 indicates a sign of vascular compromise. If you had difficulty with this question, review care of a client with Buck's traction.

*Level of Cognitive Ability:* Analysis
*Client Needs:* Physiological Integrity
*Integrated Concept/Process:* Nursing Process/Analysis
*Content Area:* Adult Health/Musculoskeletal

**Reference**

Ignatavicius, D., Workman, M., & Mishler, M. (1999). *Medical-surgical nursing across the health care continuum* (3rd ed.). Philadelphia: W.B. Saunders, p. 1289.

**7.** A pregnant client has been diagnosed with a vaginal infection from the organism *Candida albicans.* Which findings would the nurse expect to note on assessment of the client?
1    Absence of any signs and symptoms
2    Pain, itching, and vaginal discharge
3    Proteinuria, hematuria, edema, and hypertension
4    Costovertebral angle pain

**Answer: 2**

*Rationale:* Clinical manifestations of a *Candida* infection include pain, itching, and a thick, white vaginal discharge. Proteinuria, hematuria, edema, hypertension, and costovertebral angle pain are clinical manifestations associated with urinary tract infections.

*Test-Taking Strategy:* Use the process of elimination, focusing on the issue: vaginal infection. Note the relationship between the issue and option 2. Review the signs of a vaginal *Candida* infection if you had difficulty with this question.

*Level of Cognitive Ability:* Analysis
*Client Needs:* Physiological Integrity
*Integrated Concept/Process:* Nursing Process/Assessment
*Content Area:* Maternity

**Reference**

Lowdermilk, D., Perry, S., & Bobak, I. (2000). *Maternity & women's health care* (7th ed.). St. Louis: Mosby, p. 166.

**8.** A pregnant client is suspected of having iron deficiency anemia (IDA). Which of the following would the nurse expect to note regarding the client's status?
1    A low hemoglobin and hematocrit level
2    A high hemoglobin and hematocrit level
3    Fluid volume excess
4    Fluid volume deficit

**Answer: 1**

*Rationale:* When the hemoglobin level is below 11 mg/dL, iron deficiency is suspected. An indirect index of the oxygen-carrying capacity is the packed red blood cell volume or hematocrit level. Pathological anemia of pregnancy is primarily caused by iron deficiency. Options 3 and 4 are nursing diagnoses and not noted in IDA.

*Test-Taking Strategy:* Use the process of elimination. Note the word *deficiency* in the question and the word *low* in option 1. Review the manifestations of IDA if you had difficulty with this question.

*Level of Cognitive Ability:* Analysis
*Client Needs:* Physiological Integrity
*Integrated Concept/Process:* Nursing Process/Assessment
*Content Area:* Maternity

**Reference**

Lowdermilk, D., Perry, S., & Bobak, I. (2000). *Maternity & women's health care* (7th ed.). St. Louis: Mosby, p. 362.

**9.** A nurse is caring for a postpartum client. Which finding would make the nurse suspect endometritis in this client?

1   Fever over 38° Celsius (C), beginning 3 days postpartum
2   Lochia rubra on the second day postpartum
3   Elevated white blood cell count
4   Breast engorgement

**Answer: 1**

*Rationale:* Fever on the third or fourth day postpartum should raise concerns about possible endometritis until proven otherwise. A woman with endometritis normally presents with a temperature higher than 38° C. Lochia rubra on the second day postpartum is a normal finding. The white blood cell count of a postpartum woman is normally increased. Thus this method of detecting infection is not of great value in the puerperium. Breast engorgement is also a normal response and is not associated with endometritis.

*Test-Taking Strategy:* Use the process of elimination, focusing on the issue: endometritis. Recalling the normal findings in the postpartum period will assist in eliminating options 2, 3, and 4. Review the signs of endometritis if you had difficulty with this question.

*Level of Cognitive Ability:* Analysis
*Client Needs:* Physiological Integrity
*Integrated Concept/Process:* Nursing Process/Assessment
*Content Area:* Maternity

*Reference*
Lowdermilk, D., Perry, S., & Bobak, I. (2000). *Maternity & women's health care* (7th ed.). St. Louis: Mosby, p. 208.

**10.** A nurse is performing an assessment on a postmature neonate. Which physical characteristic would the nurse expect to observe?

1   Vernix that covers the body in a thick layer
2   Desquamation over the body
3   Smooth soles without creases
4   Lanugo covering the entire body

**Answer: 2**

*Rationale:* A postmature neonate exhibits dry, peeling, cracked, almost leatherlike skin over the body, which is called *desquamation.* A preterm neonate (24 to 37 weeks) exhibits thick vernix covering the body, smooth soles without creases, and lanugo covering the entire body.

*Test-Taking Strategy:* Use the process of elimination, focusing on the issue: postmature neonate. In options 1, 3, and 4 the physical characteristics are all of a preterm infant. Option 2 is the only option that describes the postmature neonate. If you had difficulty with this question, review the characteristics of preterm and postmature neonates.

*Level of Cognitive Ability:* Analysis
*Client Needs:* Physiological Integrity
*Integrated Concept/Process:* Nursing Process/Assessment
*Content Area:* Maternity

*Reference*
Lowdermilk, D., Perry, S., & Bobak, I. (2000). *Maternity & women's health care* (7th ed.). St. Louis: Mosby, p. 1126.

**11.** A nurse is performing an admission assessment on a small for gestational age (SGA) term infant. The nurse observes tachypnea, grunting, retractions, and nasal flaring. The nurse interprets that these symptoms are most likely the result of:

1 Hypoglycemia
2 Meconium aspiration syndrome
3 Respiratory distress syndrome
4 Transient tachypnea of the newborn

**Answer: 2**

*Rationale:* Tachypnea, grunting, retractions, and nasal flaring are symptoms of respiratory distress related to meconium aspiration syndrome. The SGA infant is most prone to meconium aspiration syndrome. In utero, hypoxia can cause relaxation of the anal sphincter, with passage of meconium into the amniotic fluid. The fetus also gasps in response to hypoxia, which can result in aspiration of meconium in utero or with the first breaths after birth. Transient tachypnea of the newborn is primarily found in infants delivered via cesarean section. Respiratory distress syndrome is a complication of preterm infants. These symptoms are unrelated to hypoglycemia.

*Test-Taking Strategy:* Use the process of elimination, focusing on the symptoms identified in the question. Option 1 is eliminated first because hypoglycemia is not a respiratory condition. From the remaining options, recalling the complications that can occur in an SGA infant will direct you to option 2. If you had difficulty with this question, review these complications.

*Level of Cognitive Ability:* Analysis
*Client Needs:* Physiological Integrity
*Integrated Concept/Process:* Nursing Process/Analysis
*Content Area:* Maternity

*Reference*
Lowdermilk, D., Perry, S., & Bobak, I. (2000). *Maternity & women's health care* (7th ed.). St. Louis: Mosby, p. 1126.

---

**12.** A client had a seizure an hour ago. The family was present during the episode and reported that the client's jaw was moving as though grinding food. In helping to determine the origin of this seizure, the nurse assesses for the evidence of:

1 History of prior trauma
2 Diaphoresis
3 Rotating eye movements
4 Loss of consciousness

**Answer: 1**

*Rationale:* Seizures that originate with specific motor phenomena are considered focal/jacksonian and are indicative of a focal structural lesion in the brain, often caused by trauma, infection, or drug consumption. Options 2, 3, and 4 address signs and symptoms rather than an origin of the seizure.

*Test-Taking Strategy:* Use the process of elimination, focusing on the issue: origin of the seizure. Options 2, 3, and 4 address signs and symptoms. Option 1 is the only option that addresses a possible origin. Review the causes of seizures if you had difficulty with this question.

*Level of Cognitive Ability:* Application
*Client Needs:* Physiological Integrity
*Integrated Concept/Process:* Nursing Process/Assessment
*Content Area:* Adult Health/Neurological

*Reference*
Ignatavicius, D., Workman, M., & Mishler, M. (1999). *Medical-surgical nursing across the health care continuum* (3rd ed.). Philadelphia: W.B. Saunders, p. 1031.

**13.** A nurse is caring for a client with hypertension who is receiving torsemide (Demedex) 5 mg PO daily. Which of the following would indicate to the nurse that the client might be experiencing an adverse reaction related to the medication?
1   A blood urea nitrogen (BUN) level of 15 mg/dL
2   A chloride level of 98 mEq/L
3   A sodium level of 135 mEq/L
4   A potassium level of 3.1 mEq/L

**Answer: 4**
*Rationale:* Torsemide (Demedex) is a loop diuretic. The medication can produce acute, profound water loss, volume and electrolyte depletion, dehydration, decreased blood volume, and circulatory collapse. Option 4 is the only option that indicates an electrolyte depletion since the normal potassium level is 3.5 to 5.1 mEq/L. The normal sodium level is 135 to 145 mEq/L. The normal chloride level is 98 to 107 mEq/L. The normal blood BUN is 5 to 20 mg/dL.

*Test-Taking Strategy:* Use the process of elimination and knowledge of normal laboratory values to assist in selecting option 4, since this is the only abnormal laboratory value presented. If you are unfamiliar with this medication or these normal laboratory values, review this content.

*Level of Cognitive Ability:* Analysis
*Client Needs:* Physiological Integrity
*Integrated Concept/Process:* Nursing Process/Analysis
*Content Area:* Pharmacology

*Reference*
Hodgson, B., & Kizior, R. (2001). *Saunders Nursing drug handbook 2001.* Philadelphia: W.B. Saunders, p. 1008.

---

**14.** A nurse is performing an admission assessment on a client admitted with newly diagnosed Hodgkin's disease. Which of the following would the nurse expect the client to report?
1   Night sweats
2   Severe lymph node pain
3   Weight gain of 2 kg
4   Headache with minor visual changes

**Answer: 1**
*Rationale:* Assessment of a client with Hodgkin's disease most often reveals enlarged, painless lymph nodes, fever, malaise, and night sweats. Weight loss may be present in metastatic disease.

*Test-Taking Strategy:* Use the process of elimination. Eliminate options 2 and 4 first, because they are similar in that they relate to discomfort. Weight gain is rarely the symptom of any cancer diagnosis, so eliminate option 3. If you had difficulty with this question, review content related to Hodgkin's disease.

*Level of Cognitive Ability:* Analysis
*Client Needs:* Physiological Integrity
*Integrated Concept/Process:* Nursing Process/Assessment
*Content Area:* Adult Health/Oncology

*Reference*
Smeltzer, S., & Bare, B. (2000). *Brunner & Suddarth's Textbook of medical-surgical nursing* (9th ed.). Philadelphia: Lippincott Williams & Wilkins, p. 763.

---

**15.** A nurse is assessing a 3-day-old preterm neonate with a diagnosis of respiratory distress syndrome (RDS). Which assessment finding indicates that the neonate's respiratory status is improving?
1   Presence of a systolic murmur
2   Respiratory rate between 60 and 70 breaths/min
3   Edema of the hands and feet
4   Urine output of 1 to 3 mL/kg/hr

**Answer: 4**
*Rationale:* Increased urination is an early sign that the neonate's respiratory condition is improving. Lung fluid, which occurs in RDS, moves from the lungs into the blood stream as the condition improves and the alveoli open. This extra fluid circulates to the kidneys, which results in increased voiding. Systolic murmurs usually indicate the presence of a patent ductus arteriosus, which is a common complication of RDS. Respiratory rates above 60 breaths/min are indicative of tachypnea, which is a sign of respiratory distress. Edema of the hands and feet occurs within the

first 24 hours as a result of low protein concentrations, a decrease in colloidal osmotic pressure, and transudation of fluid from the vascular system to the tissues.

*Test-Taking Strategy:* Use the process of elimination. Note the issue, respiratory status is improving. Option 4 is the only normal finding and indicates a normal urine output, which would indicate resolution of excess lung fluid. Review RDS if you had difficulty answering the question.

*Level of Cognitive Ability:* Analysis
*Client Needs:* Physiological Integrity
*Integrated Concept/Process:* Nursing Process/Evaluation
*Content Area:* Maternity

*Reference*
Lowdermilk, D., Perry, S., & Bobak, I. (2000). *Maternity & women's health care* (7th ed.). St. Louis: Mosby, p. 673.

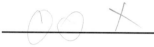

**16.** A nurse is caring for a term newborn. Which assessment finding would alert the nurse to suspect the occurrence of jaundice in this newborn?

1    A negative result to a direct Coombs' test
2    Birth weight of 8 lb 6 oz
3    Presence of a cephalhematoma
4    Infant blood type of O negative

**Answer: 3**

*Rationale:* Enclosed hemorrhage, such as with cephalhematoma, predisposes the newborn to jaundice by producing an increased bilirubin load as the cephalhematoma resolves and is absorbed into the circulatory system. A negative result to a direct Coombs' test indicates that there are no maternal antibodies on fetal erythrocytes. The birth weight in option 2 is within the acceptable ranges for a term newborn and therefore does not contribute to an increased bilirubin level. The classic Rh incompatibility situation involves an Rh-negative mother with an Rh-positive fetus or newborn.

*Test-Taking Strategy:* Use the process of elimination. Recalling the risk factors associated with jaundice and the association between hemorrhage and jaundice will direct you to option 3. Review the risk factors associated with jaundice if you had difficulty with this question.

*Level of Cognitive Ability:* Analysis
*Client Needs:* Physiological Integrity
*Integrated Concept/Process:* Nursing Process/Assessment
*Content Area:* Maternity

*Reference*
Lowdermilk, D., Perry, S., & Bobak, I. (2000). *Maternity & women's health care* (7th ed.). St. Louis: Mosby, p. 1071.

**17.** Which assessment is most important for the nurse to make before advancing a client from liquid to solid food?
1   Food preferences
2   Appetite
3   Presence of bowel sounds
4   Chewing ability

**Answer: 4**
*Rationale:* It may be necessary to modify a client's diet to a soft or mechanically chopped diet if the client has difficulty chewing. Food preferences should be ascertained on admission assessment. Appetite will affect the amount of food eaten, but not the type of diet ordered. Bowel sounds should be present before introducing any diet, including liquids.

*Test-Taking Strategy:* Use the process of elimination, focusing on the issue. Advancing a diet from liquid to solid will direct you to option 4. Review nursing considerations related to dietary measures if you had difficulty with this question.

*Level of Cognitive Ability:* Analysis
*Client Needs:* Physiological Integrity
*Integrated Concept/Process:* Nursing Process/Assessment
*Content Area:* Fundamental Skills

*Reference*
Potter, P., & Perry, A. (2001). *Fundamentals of nursing* (5th ed.). St. Louis: Mosby, p. 1711.

**18.** A nurse is caring for the client who is diagnosed with cystitis. Which assessment finding, if obtained by the nurse, would not be consistent with the typical clinical picture seen in this disorder?
1   Urinary retention
2   Burning on urination
3   Low back pain
4   Hematuria

**Answer: 1**
*Rationale:* Clinical manifestations of cystitis usually include urinary frequency, urgency, dysuria, inability to void, or voiding only small amounts. The urine may be cloudy, with hematuria and bacteriuria. The client may complain of pain that is suprapubic or in the lower back. Nonspecific signs include fever, chills, malaise, and nausea and vomiting. Some clients, particularly the elderly, may be asymptomatic.

*Test-Taking Strategy:* Use the process of elimination. Noting the key word *not* guides you to look for an incorrect option. First, eliminate options 2 and 4, since they are commonly associated with cystitis. Knowing that urgency and frequency, not urinary retention, are signs of cystitis directs you to option 1. Review the signs of cystitis if you had difficulty with this question.

*Level of Cognitive Ability:* Analysis
*Client Needs:* Physiological Integrity
*Integrated Concept/Process:* Nursing Process/Assessment
*Content Area:* Adult Health/Renal

*Reference*
Smeltzer, S., & Bare, B. (2000). *Brunner & Suddarth's Textbook of medical-surgical nursing* (9th ed.). Philadelphia: Lippincott Williams & Wilkins, p. 1136.

**19.** What method would a nurse use to most accurately assess the effectiveness of a weight loss diet for an obese client?

1. Daily weights
2. Serum protein levels
3. Daily calorie counts
4. Daily intake and output

**Answer: 1**

*Rationale:* The most accurate measurement of weight loss is daily weighing of the client at the same time of the day, in the same clothes, and using the same scale. Options 2, 3, and 4 measure nutrition and hydration status.

*Test-Taking Strategy:* Use the process of elimination. Focus on the issue—weight loss—and note the key words *most accurately assess*. Assessing weight will most accurately identify weight changes. Review care of a client on a weight loss program if you had difficulty with this question.

*Level of Cognitive Ability:* Application
*Client Needs:* Physiological Integrity
*Integrated Concept/Process:* Nursing Process/Assessment
*Content Area:* Fundamental Skills

*Reference*
Smeltzer, S., & Bare, B. (2000). *Brunner & Suddarth's Textbook of medical-surgical nursing* (9th ed.). Philadelphia: Lippincott Williams & Wilkins, p. 62.

**20.** A client has fallen and sustained a leg injury. Which question would a nurse ask the client to help determine whether the pain is the result of a fracture?

1. "Does the pain feel like a series of cramps?"
2. "Does the pain feel like pins and needles?"
3. "Is the pain a dull ache?"
4. "Is the pain sharp and piercing?"

**Answer: 4**

*Rationale:* Fracture pain is generally described as sharp and piercing. Bone pain is often described as a boring, dull, deep ache. Pain of muscle origin is often described as an aching or cramping pain, or soreness. Altered sensations, such as paresthesias (pins and needles), indicate that there is pressure on nerves or impairment of circulation.

*Test-Taking Strategy:* Use the process of elimination, focusing on the issue: a fracture. Recalling that a new injury such as a fracture is more likely to be described as sharp will direct you to option 4. If you had difficulty with this question, review assessment of a fracture.

*Level of Cognitive Ability:* Application
*Client Needs:* Physiological Integrity
*Integrated Concept/Process:* Nursing Process/Assessment
*Content Area:* Adult Health/Musculoskeletal

*Reference*
Smeltzer, S., & Bare, B. (2000). *Brunner & Suddarth's Textbook of medical-surgical nursing* (9th ed.). Philadelphia: Lippincott Williams & Wilkins, p. 1835.

**21.** A nurse performs a fingerstick glucose test on a client receiving total parenteral nutrition (TPN). Results show the client's glucose level to be greater than 400 mg/dL. What nursing action is most appropriate at this time?

1. Stop the TPN
2. Decrease the flow rate of the TPN
3. Administer insulin
4. Notify the physician

**Answer: 4**

*Rationale:* Hyperglycemia is a complication of TPN, and the nurse reports abnormalities to the physician. Options 1, 2, and 3 are not done without a physician's order.

*Test-Taking Strategy:* Use the process of elimination. Note that options 1, 2, and 3 are not within the scope of nursing practice and require a physician's order. A blood glucose level greater than 400 mg/dL requires notification of the physician. Review the complications associated with TPN if you had difficulty with this question.

*Level of Cognitive Ability:* Application
*Client Needs:* Physiological Integrity
*Integrated Concept/Process:* Nursing Process/Implementation
*Content Area:* Fundamental Skills

**Reference**
Ignatavicius, D., Workman, M., & Mishler, M. (1999). *Medical-surgical nursing across the health care continuum* (3rd ed.). Philadelphia: W.B. Saunders, p. 1560.

---

**22.** A client with urolithiasis is scheduled for extracorporeal shock wave lithotripsy. The nurse assesses to ensure that which of the following items are in place or maintained before sending the client for the procedure?

1. Signed consent, clear liquid restriction, Foley catheter
2. Signed consent, NPO status, IV line
3. IV line, clear liquid restriction, Foley catheter
4. IV line, NPO status, Foley catheter

**Answer: 2**

*Rationale:* Extracorporeal shock wave lithotripsy is done under epidural or general anesthesia. The client must sign an informed consent form for the procedure and must be NPO for the procedure. The client needs an IV line for the procedure as well. A Foley catheter is not needed.

*Test-Taking Strategy:* Use the process of elimination. Begin to answer by eliminating options 3 and 4, since the client must sign an informed consent for this procedure. From the remaining options, recalling that the client is premedicated before the procedure will direct you to option 2. If you had difficulty with this question, review the preprocedure preparation for extracorporeal shock wave lithotripsy.

*Level of Cognitive Ability:* Application
*Client Needs:* Physiological Integrity
*Integrated Concept/Process:* Nursing Process/Assessment
*Content Area:* Adult Health/Renal

**Reference**
Ignatavicius, D., Workman, M., & Mishler, M. (1999). *Medical-surgical nursing across the health care continuum* (3rd ed.). Philadelphia: W.B. Saunders, p. 1841.

---

**23.** A client has developed atrial fibrillation with a ventricular rate of 150 beats/min. The nurse assesses the client for:

1. Hypotension and dizziness
2. Nausea and vomiting
3. Hypertension and headache
4. Flat neck veins

**Answer: 1**

*Rationale:* The client with uncontrolled atrial fibrillation with a ventricular rate over 100 beats/min is at risk for low cardiac output as a result of loss of atrial kick. The nurse assesses the client for palpitations, chest pain or discomfort, hypotension, pulse deficit, fatigue, weakness, dizziness, syncope, shortness of breath, and distended neck veins.

*Test-Taking Strategy:* Use the process of elimination. Recalling that flat neck veins are normal or indicate hypovolemia will assist in eliminating option 4, and remembering that nausea and vomiting are associated with vagus nerve activity, not a tachycardic state, will assist in eliminating option 2. From the remaining options, thinking of the effects of a falling cardiac output will direct you to option 1. Review the symptoms related to atrial fibrillation if you had difficulty with this question.

*Level of Cognitive Ability:* Application
*Client Needs:* Physiological Integrity
*Integrated Concept/Process:* Nursing Process/Assessment
*Content Area:* Adult Health/Cardiovascular

*Reference*
Ignatavicius, D., Workman, M., & Mishler, M. (1999). *Medical-surgical nursing across the health care continuum* (3rd ed.). Philadelphia: W.B. Saunders, p. 777.

24. A preschooler with a history of cleft palate repair comes to the clinic for a routine well-child checkup. To determine whether this child has a long-term effect associated with cleft palate, a nurse should ask which question?
    1 "Was the child recently treated for pneumonia?"
    2 "Does the child play with an imaginary friend?"
    3 "Is the child unresponsive when given directions?"
    4 "Has the child had any difficulty swallowing food?"

**Answer: 3**
*Rationale:* Unresponsiveness may be an indication that the child has a hearing loss. A child who has a history of cleft palate should be routinely checked for hearing loss. Options 1 and 4 are unrelated to cleft palate after repair. Option 2 is normal behavior for a preschool child. Many preschoolers with vivid imaginations have imaginary friends.

*Test-Taking Strategy:* Use the process of elimination, focusing on the issue: a long-term effect. Recalling that hearing loss can occur in a child with cleft palate will direct you to option 3. If you had difficulty with this question, review content related to cleft palate.

*Level of Cognitive Ability:* Application
*Client Needs:* Physiological Integrity
*Integrated Concept/Process:* Nursing Process/Assessment
*Content Area:* Child Health

*Reference*
Wong, D. (1999). *Whaley & Wong's Nursing care of infants and children* (6th ed.). St. Louis: Mosby, p. 517.

25. A nurse is performing a respiratory assessment on a client with asthma. The nurse is alert to a worsening of the client's respiratory status when which of the following occurs?
    1 Loud wheezing heard throughout the lung fields
    2 The absence of wheezing during inhalation
    3 Wheezing heard only during exhalation
    4 Noticeably diminished breath sounds

**Answer: 4**
*Rationale:* Wheezing is not a reliable manifestation to determine the severity of an asthma attack. Clients with minor attacks may experience loud wheezes, while others with severe attacks may not wheeze. The client with severe asthma attacks may have no audible wheezing because of the decrease of airflow. For wheezing to occur, the client must be able to move sufficient air to produce breath sounds. Wheezing usually occurs first on exhalation. As the asthma attack progresses, the client may wheeze during both inspiration and expiration. Noticeably diminished breath sounds are an indication of severe obstruction and respiratory failure.

*Test-Taking Strategy:* Use the ABCs: airway, breathing, and circulation. Note the key words *worsening of the client's respiratory status*. Remember that diminished breath sounds in a client indicates obstruction and possibly respiratory failure. Review care of a client with asthma if you had difficulty with this question.

*Level of Cognitive Ability:* Analysis
*Client Needs:* Physiological Integrity
*Integrated Concept/Process:* Nursing Process/Assessment
*Content Area:* Adult Health/Respiratory

*Reference*
Smeltzer, S., & Bare, B. (2000). *Brunner & Suddarth's Textbook of medical-surgical nursing* (9th ed.). Philadelphia: Lippincott Williams & Wilkins, p. 461.

---

**26.** A nurse is assessing the casted extremity of a client. The nurse would assess for which of the following signs and symptoms indicative of infection?
1   Coolness and pallor of the extremity
2   Presence of a "hot spot" on the cast
3   Diminished distal pulse
4   Dependent edema

**Answer: 2**
*Rationale:* Signs and symptoms of infection under a casted area include odor or purulent drainage from the cast, or the presence of "hot spots," which are areas on the cast that are warmer than others. The physician should be notified if any of these occur. Signs of impaired circulation in the distal extremity include coolness and pallor of the skin, diminished arterial pulse, and edema.

*Test-Taking Strategy:* Use the process of elimination and focus on the issue: infection. Thinking about the signs of infection (redness, swelling, heat, and drainage) will direct you to option 2. The "hot spot" on the cast could signify infection underneath that area. Review the signs and symptoms of infection if you had difficulty with this question.

*Level of Cognitive Ability:* Application
*Client Needs:* Physiological Integrity
*Integrated Concept/Process:* Nursing Process/Assessment
*Content Area:* Adult Health/Musculoskeletal

*Reference*
Smeltzer, S., & Bare, B. (2000). *Brunner & Suddarth's Textbook of medical-surgical nursing* (9th ed.). Philadelphia: Lippincott Williams & Wilkins, p. 1783.

---

**27.** A home care client with chronic obstructive pulmonary disease (COPD) is complaining of increased dyspnea. The client is on home oxygen via a concentrator at 2 L/min. The respiratory rate is 22 breaths/min. The most appropriate nursing action is to:
1   Determine the need to increase the oxygen
2   Conduct further assessment of the client's respiratory status
3   Call emergency services to come to the home
4   Reassure the client that there is no need to worry

**Answer: 2**
*Rationale:* Obtaining further assessment data is the most appropriate nursing action. Reassuring the client that there is no need to worry is inappropriate. Calling emergency services is a premature action. Oxygen is not increased without the approval of the physician, especially since the client with COPD can retain carbon dioxide.

*Test-Taking Strategy:* Use the process of elimination. Remember, assessment is the first step of the nursing process. Also use the ABCs: airway, breathing, and circulation, to direct you to option 2. Review care of a client with COPD if you had difficulty with this question.

*Level of Cognitive Ability:* Application
*Client Needs:* Physiological Integrity

*Integrated Concept/Process:* Nursing Process/Implementation
*Content Area:* Adult Health/Respiratory

**Reference**

Smeltzer, S., & Bare, B. (2000). *Brunner & Suddarth's Textbook of medical-surgical nursing* (9th ed.). Philadelphia: Lippincott Williams & Wilkins, p. 456.

---

**28.** A client with schizophrenia tells a nurse, "I stopped taking my chlorpromazine (Thorazine) because of the way it made me feel." Which side effect is the nurse likely to note during further assessment of the client's complaint?
  1  Polyuria, thirst, weight gain, mild nausea
  2  Constipation, drowsiness, hypotension, dizziness
  3  Fine hand tremor, hypertension, photophobia
  4  Dry eyes, diarrhea, headache, lip smacking

**Answer: 2**
*Rationale:* Side effects associated with chlorpromazine can include hypotension, dizziness and fainting (especially with parenteral use), drowsiness, blurred vision, dry mouth, lethargy, constipation or diarrhea, nasal congestion, peripheral edema, and urinary retention. Options 1, 3, and 4 are not side effects of chlorpromazine.

*Test-Taking Strategy:* Knowledge of the side effects of chlorpromazine is required to answer this question. If you are unfamiliar with the side effects of this medication, review this information.

*Level of Cognitive Ability:* Analysis
*Client Needs:* Physiological Integrity
*Integrated Concept/Process:* Nursing Process/Assessment
*Content Area:* Pharmacology

**Reference**

Hodgson, B., & Kizior, R. (2001). *Saunders Nursing drug handbook 2001.* Philadelphia: W.B. Saunders, p. 210.

---

**29.** A home health nurse is making follow-up visits to a client following renal transplant. The nurse assesses for signs of acute graft rejection, which include:
  1  Hypotension, graft tenderness, and anemia
  2  Hypertension, oliguria, thirst, and hypothermia
  3  Fever, vomiting, hypotension, and copious amounts of dilute urine
  4  Fever, hypertension, graft tenderness, and malaise

**Answer: 4**
*Rationale:* Acute rejection usually occurs within the first 3 months after transplant, although it can occur for up to 2 years after transplant. The client exhibits fever, hypertension, malaise, and graft tenderness. Treatment is immediately begun with corticosteroids, and possibly also with monoclonal antibodies and antilymphocyte agents.

*Test-Taking Strategy:* Use the process of elimination. Begin to answer this question by eliminating options 1 and 3, since hypotension is not part of the clinical picture with graft rejection. From the remaining options, recalling that fever rather than hypothermia accompanies this complication will direct you to option 4. Review the signs of acute graft rejection if you had difficulty with this question.

*Level of Cognitive Ability:* Application
*Client Needs:* Physiological Integrity
*Integrated Concept/Process:* Nursing Process/Assessment
*Content Area:* Adult Health/Renal

**Reference**

Smeltzer, S., & Bare, B. (2000). *Brunner & Suddarth's Textbook of medical-surgical nursing* (9th ed.). Philadelphia: Lippincott Williams & Wilkins, p. 1160.

**30.** A nurse is caring for a client diagnosed with a skin infection. The client is receiving tobramycin sulfate (Nebcin) intravenously every 8 hours. Which of the following would indicate to the nurse that the client is experiencing an adverse reaction related to the medication?
1 A blood urea nitrogen (BUN) of 30 mg/dL
2 A white blood cell count of 6000/μl
3 A sedimentation rate of 15 mm/hr
4 A total bilirubin of 0.5 mg/dL

**Answer: 1**
*Rationale:* Adverse reactions or toxic effects of tobramycin sulfate include nephrotoxicity as evidenced by an increased BUN and serum creatinine; irreversible ototoxicity as evidenced by tinnitus, dizziness, ringing or roaring in the ears, and reduced hearing; and neurotoxicity as evidenced by headaches, dizziness, lethargy, tremors, and visual disturbances. A normal white blood cell count is 4500 to 11,000/μl. The normal sedimentation rate is 0 to 30 mm/hr. The normal total bilirubin level is less than 1.5 mg/dL. The normal blood urea nitrogen (BUN) is 8 to 25 mg/dL.

*Test-Taking Strategy:* Use the process of elimination and knowledge of normal laboratory values to assist in directing you to option 1, since this is the only abnormal laboratory value presented in the options. If you are unfamiliar with this medication or these laboratory values, review this content.

*Level of Cognitive Ability:* Analysis
*Client Needs:* Physiological Integrity
*Integrated Concept/Process:* Nursing Process/Analysis
*Content Area:* Pharmacology

*Reference*
Hodgson, B., & Kizior, R. (2001). *Saunders Nursing drug handbook 2001.* Philadelphia: W.B. Saunders, p. 998.

---

**31.** A client arrives in the emergency department and carbon monoxide poisoning is suspected. Nursing assessment of the client is primarily directed toward assessment of the:
1 Level of consciousness
2 Cardiac status
3 Respiratory rate
4 Skin color

**Answer: 1**
*Rationale:* The neurological system is primarily affected by carbon monoxide poisoning. With high levels of carbon monoxide, the neurological status progressively deteriorates. Although cardiac status, respiratory rate, and skin color are components of assessment, neurological status is primarily affected.

*Test-Taking Strategy:* Use the process of elimination. Note the key word *primarily*. Recalling that the neurological system is affected in carbon monoxide poisoning will direct you to option 1. If you are unfamiliar with the assessment findings in carbon monoxide poisoning, review this content.

*Level of Cognitive Ability:* Application
*Client Needs:* Physiological Integrity
*Integrated Concept/Process:* Nursing Process/Assessment
*Content Area:* Adult Health/Respiratory

*Reference*
Smeltzer, S., & Bare, B. (2000). *Brunner & Suddarth's Textbook of medical-surgical nursing* (9th ed.). Philadelphia: Lippincott Williams & Wilkins, p. 1921.

**32.** A nurse is assessing a preoperative client. Which of the following questions will help the nurse determine the client's risk for developing malignant hyperthermia postoperatively?

1 "What is your normal body temperature?"

2 "Do you experience frequent infections?"

3 "Do you have a family history of problems with general anesthesia?"

4 "Have you ever suffered from heat exhaustion or heat stroke?"

**Answer: 3**

*Rationale:* Malignant hyperthermia is a genetic disorder in which a combination of anesthetic agents (succinylcholine and inhalation agents such as halothanes) trigger uncontrolled skeletal muscle contractions. This quickly leads to a potentially fatal hyperthermia. Questioning the client about any family history of general anesthesia problems may reveal this as a possibility for the client. Options 1, 2, and 4 are unrelated to this surgical complication.

*Test-Taking Strategy:* Use the process of elimination. Recalling that this disorder is genetic will direct you to option 3. If you had difficulty with this question, review the characteristics of malignant hypertension.

*Level of Cognitive Ability:* Analysis
*Client Needs:* Physiological Integrity
*Integrated Concept/Process:* Nursing Process/Assessment
*Content Area:* Fundamental Skills

**Reference**
Smeltzer, S., & Bare, B. (2000). *Brunner & Suddarth's Textbook of medical-surgical nursing* (9th ed.). Philadelphia: Lippincott Williams & Wilkins, p. 343.

---

**33.** A nursing instructor has taught a student about increased intracranial pressure (ICP). The instructor asks the student about the three types of noncompressible cranial contents. The student responds correctly by stating that these include the:

1 Ventricles, blood volume, and the subarachnoid space

2 Cerebrospinal fluid, brain, and the foramen ovale

3 Semisolid brain, cerebrospinal fluid, and the intravascular blood

4 Gray matter, white matter, and the extrapyramidal tract

**Answer: 3**

*Rationale:* When the volume of any of these three components increases, one or both of the other components must decrease, proportionally, or an increase in ICP will occur.

*Test-Taking Strategy:* Note the key word *noncompressible* and use knowledge regarding the anatomy and physiology of the brain to answer this question. If you had difficulty with this question, review anatomy and physiology of the brain and the pathophysiology associated with ICP.

*Level of Cognitive Ability:* Analysis
*Client Needs:* Physiological Integrity
*Integrated Concept/Process:* Teaching/Learning
*Content Area:* Adult Health/Neurological

**Reference**
Smeltzer, S., & Bare, B. (2000). *Brunner & Suddarth's Textbook of medical-surgical nursing* (9th ed.). Philadelphia: Lippincott Williams & Wilkins, p. 1634.

**34.** A client has been taking methyldopa (Aldomet) for approximately 2 months. A home care nurse monitoring the effects of therapy determines that drug tolerance has developed if which of the following is noted?

1 Decrease in weight
2 Decrease in blood pressure
3 Output greater than intake
4 Gradual rise in blood pressure

**Answer: 4**

*Rationale:* During the second or third month of therapy with methyldopa, drug tolerance can develop, which is evident by rising blood pressure levels. The physician should be notified, who may then increase the medication dosage or add a diuretic to the medication regimen. The client is also at risk of developing fluid retention, which would be manifested as dependent edema, intake greater than output, and an increase in weight. This would also warrant adding a diuretic to the course of therapy.

*Test-Taking Strategy:* Use the process of elimination. First, recall that methyldopa is an antihypertensive. Next, recall the definition of drug tolerance; that is, as one adjusts to a medication, the therapeutic effect diminishes. These concepts will direct you to option 4. If you had difficulty with this question, review the effects of methyldopa and the definition of tolerance.

*Level of Cognitive Ability:* Analysis
*Client Needs:* Physiological Integrity
*Integrated Concept/Process:* Nursing Process/Assessment
*Content Area:* Pharmacology

*Reference*
Hodgson, B., & Kizior, R. (2001). *Saunders Nursing drug handbook 2001.* Philadelphia: W.B. Saunders, p. 662.

**35.** A client with a history of panic disorder comes to the emergency department and tells a nurse, "Please help me. I think I'm having a heart attack." What is the priority nursing action?

1 Identify the client's activity during the pain
2 Assess the signs related to the panic disorder
3 Assess the client's vital signs
4 Determine the client's use of relaxation techniques

**Answer: 3**

*Rationale:* Clients with panic disorders experience acute physical symptoms, such as chest pain and palpitations. The priority is to assess the client's physical condition to rule out a physiological disorder.

*Test-Taking Strategy:* Use Maslow's Hierarchy of Needs theory. Remember that physiological needs are the priority. Review care of a client with a panic disorder if you had difficulty with this question.

*Level of Cognitive Ability:* Application
*Client Needs:* Physiological Integrity
*Integrated Concept/Process:* Nursing Process/Implementation
*Content Area:* Mental Health

*Reference*
Stuart, G.W., & Laraia, M.T. (1998). *Principles and practice of psychiatric nursing* (6th ed.). St. Louis: Mosby, p. 287.

**36.** A nurse is caring for a client with trigeminal neuralgia (tic douloureux). The client asks for a snack and something to drink. The nurse determines that the most appropriate choice for this client to meet nutritional needs is:

1 Hot herbal tea with graham crackers
2 Iced coffee with peanut butter and crackers
3 Vanilla wafers and milk
4 Cocoa with honey and toast

**Answer: 3**

*Rationale:* Because mild tactile stimulation of the face of clients with trigeminal neuralgia can trigger pain, the client needs to eat or drink lukewarm, nutritious foods that are soft and easy to chew. Extremes of temperature will cause trigeminal pain.

*Test-Taking Strategy:* Use the process of elimination. Note the similarity between options 1, 2, and 4. These options contain hot or iced items and foods that are mechanically difficult to chew and swallow. Review care of a client with trigeminal neuralgia if you had difficulty with this question.

*Level of Cognitive Ability:* Application
*Client Needs:* Physiological Integrity
*Integrated Concept/Process:* Nursing Process/Implementation
*Content Area:* Adult Health/Neurological

*Reference*
Smeltzer, S., & Bare, B. (2000). *Brunner & Suddarth's Textbook of medical-surgical nursing* (9th ed.). Philadelphia: Lippincott Williams & Wilkins, p. 1752.

---

**37.** A nurse is preparing to perform an assessment on a client with peptic ulcer disease. The nurse understands that which data are unrelated to the client's disorder?

1 Use of acetaminophen (Tylenol)
2 A history of tarry black stools
3 Complaints of gastric pain 2 to 4 hours after meals
4 History of alcohol abuse

**Answer: 1**

*Rationale:* Unlike aspirin, acetaminophen has little effect on platelet function, does not affect bleeding time, and generally produces no gastric bleeding. Therefore, acetaminophen is not a risk factor for bleeding from peptic ulcers. Options 2 and 3 are signs and symptoms of peptic ulcers and bleeding peptic ulcers. Because alcohol may aggravate the stomach mucosa, a history of alcohol abuse is often seen in clients with peptic ulcer disease.

*Test-Taking Strategy:* Note the key word *unrelated*. Use the process of elimination and focus on the client's diagnosis, peptic ulcer disease. Recall that bleeding is a concern and select the object that is not related to this concern. Review assessment of the client with peptic ulcer disease if you had difficulty with this question.

*Level of Cognitive Ability:* Analysis
*Client Needs:* Physiological Integrity
*Integrated Concept/Process:* Nursing Process/Assessment
*Content Area:* Adult Health/Gastrointestinal

*Reference*
Smeltzer, S., & Bare, B. (2000). *Brunner & Suddarth's Textbook of medical-surgical nursing* (9th ed.). Philadelphia: Lippincott Williams & Wilkins, p. 860.

**38.** A child is admitted to the orthopedic unit after insertion of a Harrington rod for the treatment of scoliosis. Which assessment is most important in the immediate postoperative period?
1 Capillary refill, sensation, and motion in all extremities
2 Pain level
3 Ability to turn using the logroll technique
4 Ability to flex and extend the lower extremities

**Answer: 1**
*Rationale:* When the spinal column is manipulated during surgery, altered neurovascular status is a possible complication; therefore neurovascular checks, including circulation, sensation, and motion, should be performed every 2 hours. Level of pain is an important postoperative assessment, but circulatory status is most important. Assessment of flexion and extension of the lower extremities is a component of option 1, which includes checking motion. Logrolling is performed by nurses.

*Test-Taking Strategy:* Use the ABCs (airway, breathing, and circulation) and the process of elimination. Option 1 addresses circulatory status. Review priority nursing assessments following Harrington rod insertion if you had difficulty with this question.

*Level of Cognitive Ability:* Application
*Client Needs:* Physiological Integrity
*Integrated Concept/Process:* Nursing Process/Assessment
*Content Area:* Child Health

*Reference*
Wong, D. (1999). *Whaley & Wong's Nursing care of infants and children* (6th ed.). St. Louis: Mosby, p. 1946.

**39.** A nurse has just finished assisting a physician in placing a central intravenous (IV) line. Which of the following is a priority nursing intervention?
1 Obtain a temperature to monitor for infection
2 Monitor the blood pressure (BP) to assess for fluid volume overload
3 Label the dressing with the date and time of catheter insertion
4 Prepare the client for a chest x-ray examination

**Answer: 4**
*Rationale:* A major risk associated with central line placement is the possibility of a pneumothorax developing from an accidental puncture of the lung. Assessing the results of a chest x-ray examination is one of the best methods to determine whether this complication has occurred and to verify catheter tip placement before initiating intravenous (IV) therapy. A temperature elevation would not likely occur immediately after placement. Although BP assessment is always important in assessing a client's status after an invasive procedure, fluid volume overload is not a concern until IV fluids are started. Labeling the dressing site is important but is not the priority.

*Test-Taking Strategy:* Use the process of elimination and note the key words *priority nursing intervention* and *has just finished*. Recall that assessment of accurate placement is essential before initiating IV therapy. Review care of a client following central line placement if you had difficulty with this question.

*Level of Cognitive Ability:* Application
*Client Needs:* Physiological Integrity
*Integrated Concept/Process:* Nursing Process/Implementation
*Content Area:* Fundamental Skills

*Reference*
Smeltzer, S., & Bare, B. (2000). *Brunner & Suddarth's Textbook of medical-surgical nursing* (9th ed.). Philadelphia: Lippincott Williams & Wilkins, p. 852.

**40.** A nurse is admitting a client with suspected tuberculosis (TB) to the hospital. The nurse understands that the most accurate method for diagnosing TB is:

1 The client's long history of hemoptysis
2 A positive result to a purified protein derivative (PPD) test
3 A sputum culture positive for *Mycobacterium tuberculosis*
4 A chest x-ray examination that is positive for lung lesions

**Answer: 3**

*Rationale:* The most accurate means of diagnosing TB is by sputum culture. Establishing the presence of tubercle bacilli is essential for a definitive diagnosis. Hemoptysis is not a common finding and is usually associated with more advanced cases of TB. A positive PPD indicates exposure to TB. Other diseases may mimic TB on the chest x-ray film.

*Test-Taking Strategy:* Use the process of elimination. Note the issue, the most accurate method of diagnosing TB. Consider which test or data would be most definitive. The actual presence of *Mycobacterium* in the sputum culture is the most accurate method. Review the diagnostic tests related to TB if you had difficulty with this question.

*Level of Cognitive Ability:* Analysis
*Client Needs:* Physiological Integrity
*Integrated Concept/Process:* Nursing Process/Assessment
*Content Area:* Adult Health/Respiratory

*Reference*
Smeltzer, S., & Bare, B. (2000). *Brunner & Suddarth's Textbook of medical-surgical nursing* (9th ed.). Philadelphia: Lippincott Williams & Wilkins, p. 438.

---

**41.** A child has just returned from surgery and has a hip spica cast. A nursing priority at this time is to:

1 Elevate the head of the bed
2 Abduct the hips using pillows
3 Assess the circulatory status
4 Turn the child on the right side

**Answer: 3**

*Rationale:* During the first few hours after a cast is applied, the chief concern is swelling that may cause the cast to act as tourniquet and obstruct circulation. Therefore circulatory assessment is a high priority. Elevating the head of the bed of a child in a hip spica cast would cause discomfort. Using pillows to abduct the hips is not necessary, because a hip spica cast immobilizes the hip and knee. Turning the child side to side at least every 2 hours is important, because it allows the body cast to dry evenly and prevents complications related to immobility; however, it is not a higher priority than checking circulation.

*Test-Taking Strategy:* Use the process of elimination and the ABCs (airway, breathing, and circulation) to answer this question. Also, use the nursing process to answer this question. Since assessment is the first step in the nursing process, it is likely that the priority is to assess. If you had difficulty with this question, review nursing care following application of a spica cast.

*Level of Cognitive Ability:* Application
*Client Needs:* Physiological Integrity
*Integrated Concept/Process:* Nursing Process/Implementation
*Content Area:* Child Health

*Reference*
Wong, D. (1999). *Whaley & Wong's Nursing care of infants and children* (6th ed.). St. Louis: Mosby, p. 915.

**42.** A nurse is assessing a client with a brainstem injury. In addition to performing the Glasgow Coma Scale, the nurse plans to:
1 Check cranial nerve functioning and respiratory rate and rhythm
2 Perform arterial blood gas measurement
3 Assist with a lumbar puncture
4 Perform a pulmonary wedge pressure measurement

**Answer: 1**
*Rationale:* Assessment should be specific to the area of the brain involved. Assessing the respiratory status and cranial nerve function is a critical component of the assessment process in a client with a brainstem injury. Options 2, 3, and 4 are incorrect.

*Test-Taking Strategy:* Use the process of elimination. Recall the anatomical location of the respiratory center to direct you to option 1. Remember, the respiratory center is located in the brainstem. If you had difficulty with this question, review content and nursing care related to brainstem injuries.

*Level of Cognitive Ability:* Application
*Client Needs:* Physiological Integrity
*Integrated Concept/Process:* Nursing Process/Planning
*Content Area:* Adult Health/Neurological

*Reference*
Smeltzer, S., & Bare, B. (2000). *Brunner & Suddarth's Textbook of medical-surgical nursing* (9th ed.). Philadelphia: Lippincott Williams & Wilkins, p. 1680.

---

**43.** A client has had a Miller-Abbott tube in place for 24 hours. Which assessment finding indicates that the tube is located in the intestine?
1 Aspirate from the tube that has a pH of 7
2 The abdominal x-ray film indicates that the end of the tube is above the pylorus
3 Bowel sounds are absent
4 The client continues to be nauseated

**Answer: 1**
*Rationale:* The Miller-Abbott tube is a nasoenteric tube that is used to decompress the intestine and to correct a bowel obstruction. The end of the tube should be located in the intestine. The pH of the gastric fluid is acidic and the pH of the intestinal fluid is alkaline (7 or higher). Location of the tube can also be determined by x-ray evaluation.

*Test-Taking Strategy:* Use the process of elimination. Focus on the issue: a Miller-Abbott tube and intestinal location. Recalling that intestinal fluid is alkaline will direct you to option 1. Review the purpose and nursing care of a client with a Miller-Abbott tube if you had difficulty with this question.

*Level of Cognitive Ability:* Analysis
*Client Needs:* Physiological Integrity
*Integrated Concept/Process:* Nursing Process/Analysis
*Content Area:* Adult Health/Gastrointestinal

*Reference*
Smeltzer, S., & Bare, B. (2000). *Brunner & Suddarth's Textbook of medical-surgical nursing* (9th ed.). Philadelphia: Lippincott Williams & Wilkins, p. 834.

**44.** While a nurse is admitting a client with myxedema to the hospital, the client reports having a lack of energy, cold intolerance, and puffiness around the eyes and face. The nurse knows that these symptoms are caused by a lack of production of which hormone or hormones?

**1** Luteinizing hormone (LH)
**2** Adrenocorticotropic hormone (ACTH)
**3** Triiodothyronine ($T_3$) and thyroxine ($T_4$)
**4** Prolactin (PRL) and growth hormone (GH)

**Answer: 3**
*Rationale:* While all of these hormones originate from the anterior pituitary, only $T_3$ and $T_4$ are associated with the client's symptoms. Myxedema results from inadequate thyroid hormone levels ($T_3$ and $T_4$). Low levels of thyroid hormone result in an overall decrease in the basal metabolic rate, affecting virtually every body system and leading to weakness and fatigue. Many metabolic processes are affected and the client experiences a decrease in heat production. There is also an accumulation of hydrophilic proteoglycans in the interstitial space, which causes increased interstitial fluid and subsequent edema. A decrease in LH results in the loss of secondary sex characteristics. A decrease in ACTH is seen in Addison's disease along with a decrease in glucocorticoids and mineralocorticoid hormones, resulting in hypoglycemia and orthostatic hypotension. PRL affects mammary glands to stimulate breast milk production, and GH affects bone and soft tissue by promoting growth through protein anabolism and lipolysis.

*Test-Taking Strategy:* Use the process of elimination. Recalling that myxedema is associated with the thyroid gland will assist in making a relationship between what the question is asking and option 3. Review content and laboratory values related to myxedema if you had difficulty with this question.

*Level of Cognitive Ability:* Analysis
*Client Needs:* Physiological Integrity
*Integrated Concept/Process:* Nursing Process/Analysis
*Content Area:* Adult Health/Endocrine

*Reference*
Smeltzer, S., & Bare, B. (2000). *Brunner & Suddarth's Textbook of medical-surgical nursing* (9th ed.). Philadelphia: Lippincott Williams & Wilkins, p. 1038.

**45.** A 33-year-old woman is admitted to the hospital with a tentative diagnosis of Graves' disease. Which symptom related to the client's menstrual cycle would the client most likely report during the initial assessment?

**1** Dysmenorrhea
**2** Metrorrhagia
**3** Amenorrhea
**4** Menorrhagia

**Answer: 3**
*Rationale:* Amenorrhea or a decreased menstrual flow is not uncommon in a client with Graves' disease. Dysmenorrhea, metrorrhagia, and menorrhagia are also disorders related to the female reproductive system; however, they do not manifest themselves in the presence of Graves' disease.

*Test-Taking Strategy:* Use the process of elimination. Thinking about the pathophysiology associated with Graves' disease will direct you to option 3. Review the clinical manifestations of Graves' disease if you had difficulty with this question.

*Level of Cognitive Ability:* Analysis
*Client Needs:* Physiological Integrity
*Integrated Concept/Process:* Nursing Process/Assessment
*Content Area:* Adult Health/Endocrine

*Reference*
Smeltzer, S., & Bare, B. (2000). *Brunner & Suddarth's Textbook of medical-surgical nursing* (9th ed.). Philadelphia: Lippincott Williams & Wilkins, p. 1041.

**46.** A nurse is performing an assessment on a client with pregnancy-induced hypertension (PIH) who is in labor. The nurse most likely expects to note:

1  Decelerations and increased variability of the fetal heart rate
2  Increased blood pressure
3  Decreased brachial reflexes
4  Increased urine output

**Answer: 2**
*Rationale:* The major symptom of PIH is elevated blood pressure. As the disease progresses, it is possible that increased brachial reflexes, decreased fetal heart rate and variability, and decreased urine output will occur, particularly during labor.

*Test-Taking Strategy:* Use the process of elimination. Noting the name of the disorder will easily direct you to option 2. Review the manifestations associated with PIH if you had difficulty with this question.

*Level of Cognitive Ability:* Analysis
*Client Needs:* Physiological Integrity
*Integrated Concept/Process:* Nursing Process/Assessment
*Content Area:* Maternity

*Reference*
Lowdermilk, D., Perry, S., & Bobak, I. (2000). *Maternity & women's health care* (7th ed.). St. Louis: Mosby, p. 816.

---

**47.** A nurse has just administered a purified protein derivative (PPD) skin test to a client. The nurse determines that the test is positive if which of the following occurs?

1  An induration of 10 mm or greater
2  A large area of erythema
3  The presence of a wheal
4  Client complaints of constant itching

**Answer: 1**
*Rationale:* An induration of 10 mm or greater is usually considered a positive result. Erythema is not a positive reaction. The presence of a wheal would indicate that the skin test was administered appropriately. Itching is not an indication of a positive PPD.

*Test-Taking Strategy:* Use the process of elimination. Focusing on the issue, a positive test, will direct you to option 1. Review the interpretation of PPD results if you had difficulty with this question.

*Level of Cognitive Ability:* Analysis
*Client Needs:* Physiological Integrity
*Integrated Concept/Process:* Nursing Process/Assessment
*Content Area:* Adult Health/Respiratory

*Reference*
Smeltzer, S., & Bare, B. (2000). *Brunner & Suddarth's Textbook of medical-surgical nursing* (9th ed.). Philadelphia: Lippincott Williams & Wilkins, p. 438.

---

**48.** A nurse is performing an otoscopic examination on a client with a suspected diagnosis of mastoiditis. The nurse would expect to note which of the following if this disorder was present?

1  An immobile tympanic membrane
2  A pearly colored tympanic membrane
3  A mobile tympanic membrane
4  A transparent tympanic membrane

**Answer: 1**
*Rationale:* Otoscopic examination in a client with mastoiditis reveals a red, dull, thick, and immobile tympanic membrane with or without perforation. Options 2, 3, and 4 indicate normal findings in an otoscopic examination.

*Test-Taking Strategy:* Use the process of elimination and knowledge of normal assessment findings on an ear examination to direct you to option 1, the only abnormal finding. If you had difficulty with this question, review the assessment findings associated with this disorder.

*Level of Cognitive Ability:* Analysis
*Client Needs:* Physiological Integrity
*Integrated Concept/Process:* Nursing Process/Assessment
*Content Area:* Adult Health/Ear

*Reference*
Ignatavicius, D., Workman, M., & Mishler, M. (1999). *Medical-surgical nursing across the health care continuum* (3rd ed.). Philadelphia: W.B. Saunders, p. 1215.

---

**49.** A nurse is reviewing the record of a client with a disorder involving the inner ear. Which of the following would the nurse expect to see documented as an assessment finding in this client?

1    Severe hearing loss
2    Complaints of severe pain in the affected ear
3    Complaints of burning in the ear
4    Complaints of tinnitus

**Answer: 4**
*Rationale:* Tinnitus is the most common complaint of clients with otological disorders, especially disorders involving the inner ear. Symptoms of tinnitus range from mild ringing in the ear, which can go unnoticed during the day, to a loud roaring in the ear, which can interfere with the client's thinking process and attention span. The assessment findings noted in options 1, 2, and 3 are not specifically noted in a client with an inner ear disorder.

*Test-Taking Strategy:* Focus on the issue of the question, inner ear disorder. Recalling the function of the inner ear will direct you to option 4. If you had difficulty with this question or are unfamiliar with the signs and symptoms associated with an inner ear disorder, review this content.

*Level of Cognitive Ability:* Analysis
*Client Needs:* Physiological Integrity
*Integrated Concept/Process:* Nursing Process/Assessment
*Content Area:* Adult Health/Ear

*Reference*
Ignatavicius, D., Workman, M., & Mishler, M. (1999). *Medical-surgical nursing across the health care continuum* (3rd ed.). Philadelphia: W.B. Saunders, p. 1216.

---

**50.** A nurse has an order to administer hydroxyzine (Vistaril) to a client by the intramuscular (IM) route. The nurse explains which of the following to the client before administering the medication?

1    There will be some pain at the injection site
2    There will be relief from nausea within 5 minutes
3    Excessive salivation is a side effect
4    The client will have increased alertness for about 2 hours

**Answer: 1**
*Rationale:* Hydroxyzine is an antiemetic and sedative/hypnotic that may be used in conjunction with narcotic analgesics for added effect. The injection can be extremely painful. Medications administered by the IM route generally take 20 to 30 minutes to be come effective. Hydroxyzine causes dry mouth and drowsiness as side effects.

*Test-Taking Strategy:* Use the process of elimination and read each option carefully. Begin to answer this question by eliminating options 2 and 4, which are the least likely effects. From the remaining options, noting that the medication is administered by the IM route will direct you to option 1. If you had difficulty with this question, review the side effects of this medication.

*Level of Cognitive Ability:* Application
*Client Needs:* Physiological Integrity
*Integrated Concept/Process:* Nursing Process/Implementation
*Content Area:* Pharmacology

*Reference*
Deglin, J., & Vallerand, A. (2001). *Davis's drug guide for nurses* (7th ed.). Philadelphia: F.A. Davis, p. 493.

---

**51.** A client with diabetes mellitus has a blood glucose level of 644 mg/dL. The nurse interprets that this client is most at risk of developing which type of acid-base imbalance?
1   Respiratory acidosis
2   Respiratory alkalosis
3   Metabolic acidosis
4   Metabolic alkalosis

**Answer: 3**
*Rationale:* Diabetes mellitus can lead to metabolic acidosis. When the body does not have sufficient circulating insulin, the blood glucose level rises. At the same time, the cells of the body utilize all available glucose. The body then breaks down glycogen and fat for fuel. The byproducts of fat metabolism are acidotic and can lead to the condition known as diabetic ketoacidosis. Options 1, 2, and 4 are incorrect.

*Test-Taking Strategy:* Use the process of elimination. Noting the client's diagnosis will assist in eliminating options 1 and 2. From the remaining options, remember that the client with diabetes mellitus is at risk for developing metabolic acidosis. Review the causes of metabolic acidosis if you had difficulty with this question.

*Level of Cognitive Ability:* Analysis
*Client Needs:* Physiological Integrity
*Integrated Concept/Process:* Nursing Process/Analysis
*Content Area:* Fundamental Skills

*Reference*
Ignatavicius, D., Workman, M., & Mishler, M. (1999). *Medical-surgical nursing across the health care continuum* (3rd ed.). Philadelphia: W.B. Saunders, p. 299.

---

**52.** A nurse is reviewing the client's most recent blood gas results and the results indicate a pH of 7.42, $P_{CO_2}$ of 31 mm Hg, and $HCO_3$ of 21 mEq/L. The nurse interprets these results as indicative of which acid-base imbalance?
1   Uncompensated metabolic alkalosis
2   Compensated metabolic acidosis
3   Uncompensated respiratory acidosis
4   Compensated respiratory alkalosis

**Answer: 4**
*Rationale:* The normal pH is 7.35 to 7.45. The normal $P_{CO_2}$ is 35 to 45 mm Hg and the normal $HCO_3$ is 22 to 27 mEq/L. The pH is elevated in alkalosis and low in acidosis. In a respiratory condition, an opposite effect will be seen between the pH and the $P_{CO_2}$. In an metabolic condition, the pH and the bicarbonate move in the same direction. Since the pH is within the normal range of 7.35 to 7.45, compensation has occurred.

*Test-Taking Strategy:* Remember that in a respiratory imbalance you will find an opposite response between the pH and the $P_{CO_2}$, as indicated in the question. Therefore, options 1 and 2 are eliminated first. Next remember that the pH is elevated with alkalosis and compensation has occurred as evidenced by a normal pH. Option 4 reflects a respiratory alkalotic condition and compensation, and describes the blood gas values as indicated in the question. Review the steps related to reading blood gas values if you had difficulty with this question.

*Level of Cognitive Ability:* Analysis
*Client Needs:* Physiological Integrity
*Integrated Concept/Process:* Nursing Process/Analysis
*Content Area:* Fundamental Skills

*Reference*
LeMone, P., & Burke, K. (2000). *Medical-surgical nursing: Critical thinking in client care* (2nd ed.). Upper Saddle River, N.J.: Prentice-Hall, p. 153.

---

**53.** A nurse is caring for a client with a nasogastric tube that is attached to low suction. The nurse assesses the client for symptoms of which acid-base disorder?
1    Metabolic acidosis
2    Metabolic alkalosis
3    Respiratory acidosis
4    Respiratory alkalosis

**Answer: 2**
*Rationale:* Loss of gastric fluid via nasogastric suction or vomiting causes metabolic alkalosis. This is because of the loss of hydrochloric acid, which is a potent acid in the body. Thus this situation results in an alkalotic condition. The respiratory system is not involved.

*Test-Taking Strategy:* Eliminate options 1 and 3 first, since the loss of hydrochloric acid would cause an alkalotic condition. Since the question addresses a situation other than a respiratory one, the acid base disorder would be metabolic alkalosis. If you had difficulty with this question, review the causes of metabolic alkalosis.

*Level of Cognitive Ability:* Application
*Client Needs:* Physiological Integrity
*Integrated Concept/Process:* Nursing Process/Assessment
*Content Area:* Fundamental Skills

*Reference*
Ignatavicius, D., Workman, M., & Mishler, M. (1999). *Medical-surgical nursing across the health care continuum* (3rd ed.). Philadelphia: W.B. Saunders, p. 301.

---

**54.** A nurse is caring for a client with late stage salicylate poisoning who is experiencing metabolic acidosis. The client has a chemistry blood profile drawn. The nurse anticipates that which laboratory value is related to the client's acid-base disturbance?
1    Sodium of 145 mEq/L
2    Magnesium 2.0 mEq/L
3    Potassium 5.2 mEq/L
4    Phosphorus 2.3 mEq/L

**Answer: 3**
*Rationale:* The client with late stage salicylate poisoning is at risk for metabolic acidosis because of the effects of acetylsalicylic acid in the body. Clinical manifestations of metabolic acidosis include hyperpnea with Kussmaul's respirations, headache, nausea, vomiting, diarrhea, fruity-smelling breath because of improper fat metabolism, central nervous system depression, twitching, convulsions, and hyperkalemia. The other laboratory values listed are within the normal reference ranges.

*Test-Taking Strategy:* Knowledge about the clinical manifestations of metabolic acidosis along with normal laboratory values will easily direct you to option 3. Use the process of elimination and note that the only abnormal laboratory value is the potassium level. Review normal laboratory values and the clinical manifestations of metabolic acidosis if this question was difficult.

*Level of Cognitive Ability:* Analysis
*Client Needs:* Physiological Integrity
*Integrated Concept/Process:* Nursing Process/Analysis
*Content Area:* Fundamental Skills

*Reference*
Ignatavicius, D., Workman, M., & Mishler, M. (1999). *Medical-surgical nursing across the health care continuum* (3rd ed.). Philadelphia: W.B. Saunders, p. 299.

---

**55.** An emergency department nurse prepares to treat a child with acetaminophen (Tylenol) overdose. The nurse reviews the physician's orders expecting that which of the following will be prescribed?
1  Vitamin K (Aqua-Mephyton)
2  Protamine sulfate
3  Succimer (Chemet)
4  *N*-Acetylcysteine (NAC)

**Answer: 4**
*Rationale:* *N*-Acetylcysteine (NAC) is the antidote for Tylenol overdose. It is administered orally with juice or soda or via a nasogastric tube. Vitamin K is the antidote for warfarin (Coumadin). Protamine sulfate is the antidote for heparin. Succimer (Chemet) is used in the treatment of lead poisoning.

*Test-Taking Strategy:* Use the process of elimination. Knowledge regarding the antidote for Tylenol overdose is required to answer this question. Learn the major antidotes for medication overdose if you are unfamiliar with them.

*Level of Cognitive Ability:* Analysis
*Client Needs:* Physiological Integrity
*Integrated Concept/Process:* Nursing Process/Analysis
*Content Area:* Child Health

*Reference*
Wong, D. (1999). *Whaley & Wong's Nursing care of infants and children* (6th ed.). St. Louis: Mosby, p. 742.

---

**56.** A 1000-mL intravenous (IV) solution of normal saline solution 0.9% is prescribed for the client. The nurse understands that which of the following is not a characteristic of this type of solution?
1  Is isotonic with the plasma and other body fluids
2  Is hypotonic with the plasma and other body fluids
3  Does not affect the plasma osmolarity
4  Is the same solution as sodium chloride 0.9%

**Answer: 2**
*Rationale:* Sodium chloride 0.9% is the same solution as normal saline solution 0.9%. This solution is isotonic, and isotonic solutions are frequently used for IV infusion because they do not affect the plasma osmolarity.

*Test-Taking Strategy:* Use the process of elimination and note the key word *not* in the stem of the question. If you knew that normal saline was the same as sodium chloride, you could eliminate option 4. Noting the words *normal saline solution* will assist in eliminating options 1 and 3. Remember that normal saline solution is isotonic and would not affect plasma osmolarity.

*Level of Cognitive Ability:* Analysis
*Client Needs:* Physiological Integrity
*Integrated Concept/Process:* Nursing Process/Analysis
*Content Area:* Fundamental Skills

*Reference*
LeMone, P., & Burke, K. (2000). *Medical-surgical nursing: Critical thinking in client care* (2nd ed.). Upper Saddle River, N.J.: Prentice Hall, p. 110.

**57.** A client who has fallen from a ladder and fractured three ribs has arterial blood gas results of pH 7.38, $P_{CO_2}$ 38 mm Hg, $P_{O_2}$ 86 mm Hg, $HCO_3$ 23 mEq/L. The nurse interprets that the client's arterial blood gases (ABGs) indicate which of the following?

1 Normal results
2 Metabolic alkalosis
3 Metabolic acidosis
4 Respiratory acidosis

**Answer: 1**

*Rationale:* Normal ABG results include a pH of 7.35 to 7.45, a $P_{CO_2}$ of 35 to 45 mm Hg, a $P_{O_2}$ of 80 to 100, and an $HCO_3$ of 22 to 27 mm Hg. The client's results fall in the normal range.

*Test-Taking Strategy:* Specific knowledge related to arterial blood gas analysis is needed to answer this question correctly. Review the normal ABG levels if you had difficulty with this question.

*Level of Cognitive Ability:* Analysis
*Client Needs:* Physiological Integrity
*Integrated Concept/Process:* Nursing Process/Analysis
*Content Area:* Adult Health/Respiratory

*Reference*
Fischbach, F. (2000). *A manual of laboratory & diagnostic tests* (6th ed.). Philadelphia: Lippincott Williams & Wilkins, p. 989.

---

**58.** An adult client has undergone a lumbar puncture to obtain cerebrospinal fluid (CSF) for analysis. A nurse assesses for which of the following values that should be negative if the CSF is normal?

1 Protein
2 Glucose
3 White blood cells
4 Red blood cells

**Answer: 4**

*Rationale:* An adult with normal cerebrospinal fluid has no red blood cells in the CSF. The client may have small levels of white blood cells (0 to 5 cells). Protein (15 to 45 mg/dL) and glucose (45 to 80 mg/dL) are normally present in CSF.

*Test-Taking Strategy:* Use the process of elimination and note the key word *normal* in the stem of the question. Recalling that the presence of red blood cells would indicate blood vessel rupture or meningeal irritation will direct you to option 4. Review normal CSF values if you had difficulty with this question.

*Level of Cognitive Ability:* Analysis
*Client Needs:* Physiological Integrity
*Integrated Concept/Process:* Nursing Process/Assessment
*Content Area:* Adult Health/Neurological

*Reference*
Fischbach, F. (2000). *A manual of laboratory & diagnostic tests* (6th ed.). Philadelphia: Lippincott Williams & Wilkins, pp. 308-309.

---

**59.** A client with a burn injury is transferred to the nursing unit, and a regular diet has been prescribed. Which dietary items should the nurse encourage the client to eat in order to promote wound healing?

1 Veal, potatoes, Jell-O, orange juice
2 Peanut butter and jelly, cantaloupe, tea
3 Chicken breast, broccoli, strawberries, milk
4 Spaghetti with tomato sauce, garlic bread, ginger ale

**Answer: 3**

*Rationale:* Protein and vitamin C are necessary for wound healing. Poultry and milk are good sources of protein. Broccoli and strawberries are good sources of vitamin C. Peanut butter is a source of niacin. Jell-O and jelly have no nutrient value. Spaghetti is a complex carbohydrate.

*Test-Taking Strategy:* Remember that all components of an option must be correct in order for the option to be correct. Knowledge that protein and vitamin C are necessary for wound healing would assist in selecting the option that contains those nutrients. Eliminate options 1 and 2 first because jelly and Jell-O have no nutrient value related to healing. From the remaining options, select option 3 over option 4 because of the greater nutrient value in these food items. Review foods high in protein and vitamin C if you had difficulty with this question.

*Level of Cognitive Ability:* Application
*Client Needs:* Physiological Integrity
*Integrated Concept/Process:* Nursing Process/Implementation
*Content Area:* Fundamental Skills

*Reference*
Grodner, M., Anderson, S., & DeYoung, S. (2000). *Foundations and clinical applications of nutrition: A nursing approach.* St. Louis: Mosby, p. 189.

---

**60.** A nurse caring for a client with a neurological disorder is planning care to maintain nutritional status. The nurse is concerned about the client's swallowing ability. Which of the following food items would the nurse plan to avoid in this client's diet?

1  Cheese casserole
2  Scrambled eggs
3  Mashed potatoes
4  Spinach

**Answer: 4**
*Rationale:* In general, flavorful, warm, or well-chilled foods with texture stimulate the swallow reflex. Moist pastas, casseroles, egg dishes, and potatoes are usually effective. Raw vegetables, chunky vegetables such as diced beets, and stringy vegetables such as spinach, corn, and peas are foods commonly excluded from the diet of a client with a poor swallow reflex.

*Test-Taking Strategy:* Note the key words *swallowing ability* and *avoid.* Use the process of elimination to select option 4 as the food that is stringy and with the least amount of substance or consistency. If you had difficulty with this question, review feeding measures for a client with altered swallowing ability.

*Level of Cognitive Ability:* Application
*Client Needs:* Physiological Integrity
*Integrated Concept/Process:* Nursing Process/Planning
*Content Area:* Adult Health/Neurological

*Reference*
Grodner, M., Anderson, S., & DeYoung, S. (2000). *Foundations and clinical applications of nutrition: A nursing approach.* St. Louis: Mosby, p. 463.

---

**61.** A nurse reviews the assessment data of a client admitted to the hospital with a diagnosis of anxiety. The nurse assigns priority to which assessment finding?

1  Tearful, withdrawn, oriented times four, isolated
2  Blood pressure 160/100 mm Hg; pulse 120 beats/min; respirations 18 breaths/min
3  Temperature 99.4° F, affect bland
4  Fist clenched, pounding table, fearful

**Answer: 4**
*Rationale:* Tearful, withdrawn, isolated, and elevated vital signs are abnormal findings. These findings are not life threatening, although they should be monitored. Anxiety symptoms may take the form of physical harm, and if these symptoms occur, they are a priority.

*Test-Taking Strategy:* Use the process of elimination and focus on the client's diagnosis. Remembering that safety of the client and others is the priority will direct you to option 4. If you had difficulty with this question, review the interventions for anxiety.

*Level of Cognitive Ability:* Analysis
*Client Needs:* Physiological Integrity
*Integrated Concept/Process:* Nursing Process/Analysis
*Content Area:* Mental Health

*Reference*
Stuart, G.W., & Laraia, M.T. (1998). *Principles and practice of psychiatric nursing.* (6th ed.). St. Louis: Mosby, p. 275.

**62.** A client is resuming a diet after hemigastrectomy. To minimize complications from eating, the nurse would tell the client to avoid doing which of the following?
1 Eating six small meals per day
2 Avoiding concentrated sweets
3 Lying down after eating
4 Drinking liquids with meals

**Answer: 4**
*Rationale:* The client who has had a hemigastrectomy is at risk for dumping syndrome. The client should avoid drinking liquids with meals to prevent this syndrome. This client should be placed on a diet that is high in protein, moderate in fat, and high in calories. Frequent small meals are encouraged and the client should avoid concentrated sweets.

*Test-Taking Strategy:* Note the key word *avoid* in the stem of the question. Use the process of elimination. Focusing on the diagnosis and thinking about the complications of this surgical procedure will direct you to option 4. If you had difficulty with this question, review the complications of hemigastrectomy and the prevention and management of the complications.

*Level of Cognitive Ability:* Application
*Client Needs:* Physiological Integrity
*Integrated Concept/Process:* Teaching/Learning
*Content Area:* Adult Health/Gastrointestinal

*Reference*
Grodner, M., Anderson, S., & DeYoung, S. (2000). *Foundations and clinical applications of nutrition: A nursing approach.* St. Louis: Mosby, p. 501.

**63.** A nurse is preparing to administer diazepam (Valium) by the IV route to a child that is having a seizure. The nurse prepares to administer the medication by:
1 Diluting the prescribed dose in 50 mL of 5% dextrose in water ($D_5W$)
2 Administering the prescribed dose at a rate of 5 mg/min
3 Mixing the prescribed dose into the existing IV of 5% dextrose in normal saline solution
4 Administering the prescribed dose directly into the vein

**Answer: 4**
*Rationale:* IV diazepam must be given directly into the vein (not the tubing, because it interacts with plastic), at a rate no greater that 1 mg/min. It should not be mixed with other medications or solutions and can be diluted only with normal saline solution.

*Test-Taking Strategy:* Knowledge regarding the procedure for IV administration of diazepam is required to answer this question. Eliminate options 1 and 3 first because they are similar. From the remaining options, it is necessary to know that this medication is administered at a rate no greater than 1 mg per min. Review the procedure for the administration of IV diazepam if you had difficulty with this question.

*Level of Cognitive Ability:* Application
*Client Needs:* Physiological Integrity
*Integrated Concept/Process:* Nursing Process/Implementation
*Content Area:* Pharmacology

*Reference*
Wong, D. (1999). *Whaley & Wong's Nursing care of infants and children* (6th ed.). St. Louis: Mosby, p. 1817.

**64.** A nurse is assessing a child with increased intracranial pressure who has been exhibiting decorticate posturing. On assessment the nurse notes that the child is now exhibiting decerebrate posturing. The nurse interprets that this change in the child's condition indicates which of the following?
1 An improvement in condition
2 Decreasing intracranial pressure
3 Deteriorating neurological function
4 An insignificant finding

**Answer: 3**
*Rationale:* The progression from decorticate to decerebrate posturing usually indicates deteriorating neurological function and warrants physician notification. Options 1, 2, and 4 are inaccurate interpretations.

*Test-Taking Strategy:* Use the process of elimination. Eliminate options 1 and 2 first because they are similar. Recalling the significance of decerebrate posturing will assist in eliminating option 4. Review the significance of assessment findings in the child with increased intracranial pressure if you had difficulty with this question.

*Level of Cognitive Ability:* Analysis
*Client Needs:* Physiological Integrity
*Integrated Concept/Process:* Nursing Process/Analysis
*Content Area:* Child Health

*Reference*
Wong, D. (1999). *Whaley & Wong's Nursing care of infants and children* (6th ed.). St. Louis: Mosby, p. 1772.

**65.** A nurse is caring for a hospitalized infant and is monitoring for increased intracranial pressure (ICP). The nurse notes that the anterior fontanel bulges when the infant cries. Based on this assessment finding, which action would the nurse take?
1 Lower the head of the bed
2 Document the findings
3 Place the infant on NPO status
4 Notify the physician immediately

**Answer: 2**
*Rationale:* The anterior fontanel is diamond-shaped and located on the top of the head. It should be soft and flat in a normal infant, and it normally closes by 12 to 18 months of age. The posterior fontanel closes by 2 to 3 months of age. A bulging or tense fontanel may result from crying or increased ICP. Noting a bulging fontanel when the infant cries is a normal finding that should be documented and monitored. It is not necessary to notify the physician for this finding. Options 1 and 3 are inappropriate actions.

*Test-Taking Strategy:* Use the process of elimination and focus on the information provided in the question. Note the key words *bulges when the infant cries.* This should provide you with the clue that this is a normal finding. Remember that a bulging or tense fontanel may result from crying. If you had difficulty with this question, review normal assessment findings in an infant.

*Level of Cognitive Ability:* Application
*Client Needs:* Physiological Integrity
*Integrated Concept/Process:* Nursing Process/Implementation
*Content Area:* Child Health

*References*
Ladewig, P., London, M., & Olds, S. (1998). *Maternal-newborn care: The nurse, the family, and the community* (4th ed.). Menlo Park, Calif.: Addison-Wesley, p. 340.
Wong, D. (1999). *Whaley & Wong's Nursing care of infants and children* (6th ed.). St. Louis: Mosby, p. 321.

**66.** A nurse is assessing the vital signs of a 3-year-old child hospitalized with a diagnosis of croup. The nurse notes that the respiratory rate is 28 breaths/min. Based on this finding, which nursing action is most appropriate?

1 Reassess the respiratory rate in 15 minutes
2 Notify the physician
3 Document the findings
4 Administer oxygen

**Answer: 3**
*Rationale:* The normal respiratory rate for a 3-year-old is 20 to 30 breaths/min. Since the respiratory rate is normal, options 1, 2, and 4 are unnecessary actions. The nurse would document the findings.

*Test-Taking Strategy:* Use the process of elimination. Knowing that the normal respiratory rate for a 3-year-old is 20 to 30 breaths/min will direct you to option 3. If you had difficulty with this question, review the normal vital signs in a 3-year-old.

*Level of Cognitive Ability:* Application
*Client Needs:* Physiological Integrity
*Integrated Concept/Process:* Nursing Process/Implementation
*Content Area:* Child Health

*Reference*
Bindler, R., & Ball, J. (1999). *Quick reference to pediatric clinical skills.* Stamford, Conn.: Appleton & Lange, p. 21.

**67.** A nurse is performing an assessment on a female client who is suspected of having mittelschmerz. Which of the following would the nurse expect to note on assessment of the client?

1 Client complains of pain at the beginning of menstruation
2 Profuse vaginal bleeding
3 Sharp pain located on the right side of the pelvis
4 Pain that occurs during intercourse

**Answer: 3**
*Rationale:* Mittelschmerz (middle pain) refers to pelvic pain that occurs midway between menstrual periods or at the time of ovulation. The pain is caused by growth of the dominant follicle within the ovary, or rupture of the follicle and subsequent spillage of follicular fluid and blood into the peritoneal space. The pain is fairly sharp and is felt on the right or left side of the pelvis. It generally lasts one to three days, and slight vaginal bleeding may accompany the discomfort.

*Test-Taking Strategy:* Use the process of elimination. Knowledge that mittelschmerz is "middle pain" will assist in eliminating option 1. Knowing that this occurs as a result of growth of the follicle or rupture of the follicle will assist in eliminating options 2 and 4. Review this disorder if you are unfamiliar with it.

*Level of Cognitive Ability:* Analysis
*Client Needs:* Physiological Integrity
*Integrated Concept/Process:* Nursing Process/Assessment
*Content Area:* Maternity

*Reference*
Sherwen, L., Scoloveno, M.A., & Weingarten, C. (1999). *Maternity nursing: Care of the childbearing family* (3rd ed.). Stamford, Conn.: Appleton & Lange, p. 126.

**68.** A client has been seen in the health care clinic and has been diagnosed with endometriosis. The client asks the nurse to describe this condition. The nurse tells the client that endometriosis:

1   Is the presence of tissue outside the uterus that resembles the endometrium
2   Is pain the occurs during ovulation
3   Is also known as primary dysmenorrhea
4   Causes the cessation of menstruation

**Answer: 1**

*Rationale:* Endometriosis is defined as the presence of tissue outside the uterus that resembles the endometrium in both structure and function. The response of this tissue to the stimulation of estrogen and progesterone during the menstrual cycle is identical to that of the endometrium. Primary dysmenorrhea refers to menstrual pain without identified pathology. Mittelschmerz refers to pelvic pain that occurs midway between menstrual periods, and amenorrhea is the cessation of menstruation for a period of at least 3 cycles or 6 months in a woman who has established a pattern of menstruation and can result from a variety of causes.

*Test-Taking Strategy:* Use the process of elimination and knowledge regarding the pathophysiology associated with endometriosis to answer this question. Note the relationship between *endometriosis* in the question and *endometrium* in the correct option. Review this disorder if you had difficulty with this question.

*Level of Cognitive Ability:* Application
*Client Needs:* Physiological Integrity
*Integrated Concept/Process:* Nursing Process/Implementation
*Content Area:* Maternity

*Reference*
Lowdermilk, D., Perry, S., & Bobak, I. (2000). *Maternity & women's health care* (7th ed.). St. Louis: Mosby, p. 121.

---

**69.** A client calls the physician's office to schedule an appointment because a home pregnancy test was performed and the results were positive. A nurse determines that the home pregnancy test identified the presence of which of the following in the urine?

1   Estrogen
2   Progesterone
3   Human chorionic gonadotropin (hCG)
4   Follicle stimulating hormone (FSH)

**Answer: 3**

*Rationale:* In early pregnancy, hCG is produced by trophoblastic cells that surround the developing embryo. This hormone is responsible for positive pregnancy tests. Options 1, 2, and 4 are incorrect.

*Test-Taking Strategy:* Use the process of elimination. Knowledge regarding the changes caused by placental hormones in early pregnancy is required to answer this question. Review this pregnancy test if you are unfamiliar with it.

*Level of Cognitive Ability:* Analysis
*Client Needs:* Physiological Integrity
*Integrated Concept/Process:* Nursing Process/Assessment
*Content Area:* Maternity

*Reference*
Sherwen, L., Scoloveno, M.A., & Weingarten, C. (1999). *Maternity nursing: Care of the childbearing family* (3rd ed.). Stamford, Conn.: Appleton & Lange, pp. 417-418.

**70.** A hepatitis B screen is performed on a pregnant client, and the results indicate the presence of antigens in the maternal blood. Which of the following would the nurse anticipate to be prescribed?
  1 Repeat hepatitis screen
  2 Retesting the mother in 1 week
  3 Administration of hepatitis vaccine and hepatitis B immune globulin to the neonate within 12 hours after birth
  4 Administration of antibiotics during pregnancy

**Answer: 3**
*Rationale:* A hepatitis B screen is performed to detect the presence of antigens in maternal blood. If antigens are present, the neonate needs to receive the hepatitis vaccine and hepatitis B immune globulin within 12 hours after birth. Options 1, 2, and 4 are incorrect actions or treatment measures.

*Test-Taking Strategy:* Use the process of elimination. Eliminate options 1 and 2 because they are similar. From the remaining options, recalling that the concern is the effect on the fetus and neonate will assist in directing you to the correct option. Review the purpose and the significance of the hepatitis B screen if you had difficulty with this question.

*Level of Cognitive Ability:* Analysis
*Client Needs:* Physiological Integrity
*Integrated Concept/Process:* Nursing Process/Analysis
*Content Area:* Maternity

*Reference*
Lowdermilk, D., Perry, S., & Bobak, I. (2000). *Maternity & women's health care* (7th ed.). St. Louis: Mosby, p. 742.

**71.** A pregnant client is seen in the health care clinic. During the prenatal visit the client informs the nurse that she is experiencing pain in the calf when she walks. Which of the following would be the most appropriate nursing action?
  1 Tell the client that this is normal during pregnancy
  2 Instruct the client to avoid walking
  3 Assess for the presence of Homans' sign
  4 Instruct the client to elevate the legs consistently throughout the day

**Answer: 3**
*Rationale:* If a woman complains of calf pain during walking, it could be an indication of venous thrombosis of the lower extremities. The most appropriate nursing action would be to assess for Homans' sign, which would assist in determining the presence of venous thrombosis. It is not appropriate to tell the mother that this is normal during pregnancy. Ambulation is a necessary exercise and the woman should be encouraged to ambulate during pregnancy. Although it is important to elevate the legs during pregnancy, elevating the legs consistently is not the appropriate nursing action.

*Test-Taking Strategy:* Note the key words *most appropriate* in the stem of the question. Use the nursing process to assist in answering the question. Option 3 is the only option that addresses assessment. Review normal and abnormal expectations in the prenatal period if you had difficulty with this question.

*Level of Cognitive Ability:* Application
*Client Needs:* Physiological Integrity
*Integrated Concept/Process:* Nursing Process/Implementation
*Content Area:* Maternity

*Reference*
Olds, S., London. M., & Ladewig, P. (2000). *Maternal-newborn nursing: A family and community-based approach* (6th ed.). Upper Saddle River, N.J.: Prentice-Hall Health, p. 925.

**72.** A clinic nurse is performing an assessment on a client seen in the health care clinic for a first prenatal visit. The nurse asks the client when the first day of the last menstrual period (LMP) was and the client reports February 9, 2002. Using Nagele's rule, the nurse determines that the estimated date of confinement is:

**1** October 16, 2002
**2** November 16, 2002
**3** October 7, 2002
**4** November 7, 2002

**Answer: 2**

*Rationale:* Accurate use of Nagele's rule requires that the woman have a regular 28-day menstrual cycle. To calculate the estimated date of confinement, the nurse would add 7 days to the first day of the LMP, subtract 3 months, and then add 1 year. First day of last menstrual period: February 9, 2002, add 7 days: February 16, 2002, subtract three months: November 16, 2001, and add 1 year, November 16, 2002.

*Test-Taking Strategy:* Use the process of elimination and knowledge regarding the use of Nagele's rule to answer this question. Be careful when following the steps to determine the estimated data of confinement using this rule. Avoid taking shortcuts, particularly when math is involved. Read all of the options carefully noting the dates and years before selecting an option. Review Nagele's rule if you had difficulty with this question.

*Level of Cognitive Ability:* Analysis
*Client Needs:* Physiological Integrity
*Integrated Concept/Process:* Nursing Process/Assessment
*Content Area:* Maternity

*Reference*
Lowdermilk, D., Perry, S., & Bobak, I. (2000). *Maternity & women's health care* (7th ed.). St. Louis: Mosby, pp. 381-382.

**73.** A nurse is preparing to access an implanted vascular port to administer chemotherapy. The nurse:

**1** Anchors the port with the dominant hand
**2** Palpates the port to locate the center of the septum
**3** Places a warm pack over the area for several minutes to alleviate possible discomfort
**4** Cleans the area with alcohol working from the outside inward

**Answer: 2**

*Rationale:* Before accessing an implanted port, the nurse must palpate the port to locate the center of the septum. The port should then be anchored with the nondominant hand. Cool compresses over the site can help to alleviate pain upon entry. The site should be cleansed with alcohol working from the inside out to prevent introducing germs into the access site.

*Test-Taking Strategy:* Use the process of elimination. Remembering the principles related to the effects of applying cool applications and the principles of aseptic technique will assist in eliminating options 3 and 4. From the remaining options, select option 2 over option 1 because it does not make sense to anchor the port with the dominant hand. The nurse would need the dominant hand to perform the access. Review the concepts related to implanted vascular ports if you had difficulty answering this question.

*Level of Cognitive Ability:* Application
*Client Needs:* Physiological Integrity
*Integrated Concept/Process:* Nursing Process/Implementation
*Content Area:* Fundamental Skills

*Reference*
Potter, P., & Perry, A. (2001). *Fundamentals of nursing* (5th ed.). St. Louis: Mosby, p. 1219.

**74.** A nurse is measuring the fundal height of a client who is at 36 weeks' gestation. In preparing to perform the procedure the nurse would:

1 Turn the client onto her left side
2 Instruct the client to lie in a prone position
3 Place the client in a prone position with the head of the bed elevated
4 Have the client stand for the procedure

**Answer: 1**

*Rationale:* When measuring fundal height, the nurse has the client lie in a supine position and instructs the women to turn onto her left side, or the nurse can elevate the left buttock by placing a pillow under the area. Options 2, 3, and 4 are incorrect client positions for measuring fundal height.

*Test-Taking Strategy:* Use the process of elimination. Focus on the issue of the question and think about the physiological effects of an enlarged uterus at 36 weeks' gestation. Eliminate options 2 and 3 first because they are similar. Next, recalling the potential for vena cava syndrome or knowing that the standing position is inappropriate for measuring fundal height will assist in directing you to option 1. Review the procedure for measuring fundal height if you had difficulty with this question.

*Level of Cognitive Ability:* Application
*Client Needs:* Physiological Integrity
*Integrated Concept/Process:* Nursing Process/Implementation
*Content Area:* Maternity

*Reference*
Gorrie, T., McKinney, E., & Murray, S. (1998). *Foundations of maternal-newborn nursing* (2nd ed.). Philadelphia: W.B. Saunders, p. 143.

**75.** A nurse is performing a measurement of fundal height on a client who is at 36 weeks' gestation. During the measurement the client begins to feel light-headed. Based on the nurse's knowledge of the physiological occurrences of pregnancy, the nurse determines that this is most likely the result of:

1 Emotional instability
2 Compression of the vena cava
3 A full bladder
4 Insufficient iron intake

**Answer: 2**

*Rationale:* Compression of the inferior vena cava and aorta by the uterus may cause supine hypotension syndrome late in pregnancy. Having the woman turn onto her left side or elevating the left buttock during fundal height measurement will correct or prevent the problem. Options 1, 3, and 4 are unrelated to this syndrome.

*Test-Taking Strategy:* Use the process of elimination. Noting the word *physiological* in the question will assist in eliminating option 1. Recalling that compression of the inferior vena cava and aorta by the uterus may cause supine hypotension syndrome will easily direct you to option 2. Review vena cava syndrome if you had difficulty with this question.

*Level of Cognitive Ability:* Analysis
*Client Needs:* Physiological Integrity
*Integrated Concept/Process:* Nursing Process/Analysis
*Content Area:* Maternity

*Reference*
Gorrie, T., McKinney, E., & Murray, S. (1998). *Foundations of maternal-newborn nursing* (2nd ed.). Philadelphia: W.B. Saunders, p. 126.

**76.** A nurse in the prenatal clinic is monitoring a client who is pregnant with twins. The nurse monitors the client most closely for which complication that is most likely associated with a twin pregnancy?

1   Maternal anemia
2   Postterm labor
3   Hemorrhoids
4   Gestational diabetes

**Answer: 1**

*Rationale:* Maternal anemia often occurs in twin pregnancies because of a greater demand for iron by the fetuses. Option 2 is incorrect because twin pregnancies often end in prematurity. Hemorrhoids occur in pregnancy but are not the most likely occurrence associated with a twin pregnancy. Option 4 is not a complication of a twin pregnancy.

*Test-Taking Strategy:* Use the process of elimination, focusing on the issue of the question, a twin pregnancy. Also note the key words *most likely*. Think about the physiological occurrences in a twin pregnancy to direct you to option 1. Review the risks associated with a twin pregnancy if you had difficulty with this question.

*Level of Cognitive Ability:* Application
*Client Needs:* Physiological Integrity
*Integrated Concept/Process:* Nursing Process/Assessment
*Content Area:* Maternity

*Reference*
Lowdermilk, D., Perry, S., & Bobak, I. (2000). *Maternity & women's health care* (7th ed.). St. Louis: Mosby, p. 426.

**77.** A nurse is conducting a clinic visit with a prenatal client with heart disease. The nurse carefully assesses the client's vital signs, weight, and fluid and nutritional status to detect complications caused by:

1   Hypertrophy and increased contractility of the heart
2   The increase in circulating blood volume
3   Fetal cardiomegaly
4   Rh incompatibility

**Answer: 2**

*Rationale:* Pregnancy taxes the circulating system of every woman because both the blood volume and cardiac output increase. Options 1, 3, and 4 are not directly associated with pregnancy in a client with a cardiac condition.

*Test-Taking Strategy:* Use the process of elimination and focus on the client of the question. Eliminate options 3 and 4 first because they address the fetus, not the prenatal client. Knowledge of the pathophysiology regarding the changes that take place in the woman during pregnancy will direct you to option 2. Also, remember that hypertrophy of the heart may occur in cardiac disease but the outcome would be a decrease in contractility, not an increase. Review the pathophysiology in relation to cardiac disease in the pregnant client if you had difficulty with this question.

*Level of Cognitive Ability:* Application
*Client Needs:* Physiological Integrity
*Integrated Concept/Process:* Nursing Process/Assessment
*Content Area:* Maternity

*Reference*
Sherwen, L., Scoloveno, M.A., & Weingarten, C. (1999). *Maternity nursing: Care of the childbearing family* (3rd ed.). Stamford, Conn.: Appleton & Lange, p. 594.

**78.** A nurse has assisted the physician with a liver biopsy that was done at the bedside. On completion of the procedure, the nurse assists the client into which of the following positions?

1  Left side-lying with a small pillow or towel under the puncture site
2  Right side-lying with a small pillow or towel under the puncture site
3  Left side-lying with the right arm elevated above the head
4  Right side-lying with the left arm elevated above the head

**Answer: 2**

*Rationale:* Following a liver biopsy, the client is assisted to assume a right side-lying position with a small pillow or folded towel under the puncture site for 2 hours. This position compresses the liver against the chest wall at the biopsy site.

*Test-Taking Strategy:* Use the process of elimination and knowledge regarding the anatomy of the body to answer this question. Remember that the liver is on the right side of the body, and that the application of pressure on the right side will minimize the escape of blood or bile through the puncture site. Review care of a client following a liver biopsy if you had difficulty with this question.

*Level of Cognitive Ability:* Application
*Client Needs:* Physiological Integrity
*Integrated Concept/Process:* Nursing Process/Implementation
*Content Area:* Fundamental Skills

*Reference*
Altman, G., Buchsel, P., & Coxon, V. (2000). *Delmar's Fundamental & advanced nursing skills.* Albany, N.Y.: Delmar, p. 1320.

**79.** A client has an order for "enemas until clear" before major bowel surgery. After preparing the equipment and solution, the nurse assists the client into which of the following positions to administer the enema?

1  Left-lateral Sims' position
2  Right-lateral Sims' position
3  Left side-lying with the head of the bed elevated 45 degrees
4  Right side-lying with the head of the bed elevated 45 degrees

**Answer: 1**

*Rationale:* For administration of an enema, the client is placed in a left-lateral Sims' position so that the enema solution can flow by gravity in the natural direction of the colon. The head of the bed is not elevated in the Sims' position.

*Test-Taking Strategy:* Use the process of elimination and knowledge regarding the anatomy of the bowel to answer the question. This will assist in eliminating options 2 and 4. Attempt to visualize the procedure for administering an enema and eliminate option 3 because the head of the bed should be flat during enema administration. Review the procedure for administering an enema if you had difficulty with this question.

*Level of Cognitive Ability:* Application
*Client Needs:* Physiological Integrity
*Integrated Concept/Process:* Nursing Process/Implementation
*Content Area:* Fundamental Skills

*Reference*
Potter, P., & Perry, A. (2001). *Fundamentals of nursing* (5th ed.). St. Louis: Mosby, p. 1463.

**80.** A physician has just inserted a Cantor tube in a client with a bowel obstruction. When the procedure is complete, the nurse assists the client into which of the following positions initially to maximize the effect of the tube?

1 Right side
2 Left side
3 Prone
4 Supine

**Answer: 1**
*Rationale:* The Cantor tube is a single-lumen, mercury-weighted tube. The weight of the mercury carries the tube by gravity. Following insertion, to facilitate movement of the tube, the client is positioned for 2 hours on the right side, 2 hours on the back with the head elevated, and then 2 hours on the left.

*Test-Taking Strategy:* Use the process of elimination. Note the key word *initially*. Knowledge of the anatomy of the gastrointestinal tract and the Cantor tube will easily direct you to option 1. If you had difficulty with this question, review nursing care related to the client with a Cantor tube.

*Level of Cognitive Ability:* Application
*Client Needs:* Physiological Integrity
*Integrated Concept/Process:* Nursing Process/Implementation
*Content Area:* Fundamental Skills

**Reference**
Phipps, W., Sands, J., & Marek, J. *Medical-surgical nursing: Concepts & clinical practice* (6th ed.). St. Louis: Mosby, p. 1346.

---

**81.** A nurse is caring for a client following craniotomy who has a supratentorial incision. The nurse places a sign above the client's bed stating that the client should be maintained in which of the following positions?

1 Semi-Fowler's position
2 Dorsal recumbent
3 Prone
4 Supine

**Answer: 1**
*Rationale:* Following supratentorial surgery (surgery above the brain's tentorium), the client's head is usually elevated 30 degrees to promote venous outflow through the jugular veins. Options 2, 3, and 4 are incorrect positions following this surgery.

*Test-Taking Strategy:* Use the process of elimination and knowledge regarding supratentorial surgery and craniotomy to answer this question. A helpful strategy is to remember *supra*, above the brain's tentorium, head up. If you had difficulty with this question, review positioning following craniotomy surgery.

*Level of Cognitive Ability:* Application
*Client Needs:* Physiological Integrity
*Integrated Concept/Process:* Nursing Process/Implementation
*Content Area:* Fundamental Skills

**Reference**
Ignatavicius, D., Workman, M., & Mishler, M. (1999). *Medical-surgical nursing across the health care continuum* (3rd ed.). Philadelphia: W.B. Saunders, p. 1142.

82. A postpartum nurse is reviewing the records of the new mothers admitted to the postpartum unit. The nurse determines that which of the following mothers would be at least risk for developing a puerperal infection?
    1 A mother with a history of previous infections
    2 A mother who experienced prolonged rupture of the membranes
    3 A mother who had an excessive number of vaginal examinations
    4 A mother who underwent a vaginal delivery of the newborn

**Answer: 4**
*Rationale:* Risk factors associated for puerperal infection include a history of previous infections, cesarean births, trauma, prolonged rupture of the membranes, prolonged labor, excessive number of vaginal examinations, and retained placental fragments.

*Test-Taking Strategy:* Use the process of elimination, noting the key words *at least risk*. Knowledge that cesarean birth rather than vaginal birth presents a risk factor for infection will assist in directing you to option 4. Review the risk factors associated with puerperal infection if you had difficulty with this question.

*Level of Cognitive Ability:* Analysis
*Client Needs:* Physiological Integrity
*Integrated Concept/Process:* Nursing Process/Assessment
*Content Area:* Maternity

*Reference*
Gorrie, T., McKinney, E., & Murray, S. (1998). *Foundations of maternal-newborn nursing* (2nd ed.). Philadelphia: W.B. Saunders, p. 797.

83. A nurse in the delivery room is assisting with the delivery of a newborn infant. Following delivery, the nurse prepares to prevent heat loss in the newborn infant from conduction by:
    1 Wrapping the newborn in a blanket
    2 Closing the doors to the delivery room
    3 Drying the newborn with a warm blanket
    4 Placing a warm pad on the crib before placing the newborn in the crib

**Answer: 4**
*Rationale:* Hypothermia caused by conduction occurs when the newborn infant is on a cold surface, such as a cold pad or mattress. Warming the crib pad will assist in preventing hypothermia by conduction. Evaporation of moisture from a wet body dissipates heat along with the moisture. Keeping the newborn infant dry by drying the wet newborn infant at birth will prevent hypothermia via evaporation. Convection occurs as air moves across the newborn infant's skin from an open door and heat is transferred to the air. Radiation occurs when heat from the newborn infant radiates to a colder surface.

*Test-Taking Strategy:* Use the process of elimination. Note the key word *conduction* in the question to assist in selecting the correct option. Knowledge that conduction occurs when a baby is on a cold surface will assist in directing you to option 4. Review these heat loss concepts if you had difficulty with this question.

*Level of Cognitive Ability:* Application
*Client Needs:* Physiological Integrity
*Integrated Concept/Process:* Nursing Process/Planning
*Content Area:* Maternity

*Reference*
Sherwen, L., Scoloveno, M.A., & Weingarten, C. (1999). *Maternity nursing: Care of the childbearing family* (3rd ed.). Stamford, Conn.: Appleton & Lange, p. 922.

**84.** A nurse provides a class to new mothers on newborn care. In teaching cord care, the nurse tells the mother:

1   If triple dye has been applied to the cord, it is not necessary to do anything else to it
2   To apply alcohol to the cord, ensuring that all areas around the cord are cleaned two or three times a day
3   To apply alcohol thoroughly to the cord, being careful not to move the cord because it will cause the newborn infant pain
4   All that is necessary is to wash the cord with antibacterial soap, allowing it to air dry one time a day

**Answer: 2**

*Rationale:* The umbilical cord and base should be cleaned two or three times per day using alcohol or other agents. The steps are to lift the cord, wipe around the cord starting at the top, clean the base of the cord, and fold the diaper below the cord to allow the cord to air dry and to prevent contamination from urine. Continuation of cord care is necessary until the cord falls off within 7 to 14 days. The cord needs to be cleansed with alcohol thoroughly. The infant does not feel pain in this area. Water and soap are not necessary, and in fact the cord should be kept from getting wet.

*Test-Taking Strategy:* Use the process of elimination. Simply recalling that the cord should be cleansed two to three times a day will direct you to the correct option. Review the principles related to cord care if you had difficulty with this question.

*Level of Cognitive Ability:* Application
*Client Needs:* Physiological Integrity
*Integrated Concept/Process:* Teaching/Learning
*Content Area:* Maternity

*Reference*
Sherwen, L., Scoloveno, M.A., & Weingarten, C. (1999). *Maternity nursing: Care of the childbearing family* (3rd ed.). Stamford, Conn.: Appleton & Lange, p. 922.

---

**85.** A nurse is monitoring a preterm newborn infant for signs of respiratory distress syndrome (RDS). The nurse monitors the infant for:

1   Cyanosis, tachypnea, retractions, grunting respirations, and nasal flaring
2   Acrocyanosis, apnea, pneumothorax, and grunting
3   Barrel-shaped chest, hypotension, and bradycardia
4   Acrocyanosis, emphysema, and interstitial edema

**Answer: 1**

*Rationale:* The newborn infant with respiratory distress syndrome may present with clinical signs of cyanosis, tachypnea or apnea, nasal flaring, chest wall retractions, or audible grunts. Acrocyanosis is the bluish discoloration of the hands and feet, is associated with immature peripheral circulation, and is not uncommon in the first few hours of life. Options 2, 3, and 4 do not indicate clinical signs of RDS.

*Test-Taking Strategy:* Use the process of elimination. Recalling that acrocyanosis may be a normal sign in a newborn infant will assist in eliminating options 2 and 4. From the remaining options, it is necessary to be familiar with the signs of respiratory distress syndrome. Also, note the relationship between the diagnosis and the signs noted in option 1. If you had difficulty with this question, review the signs of RDS.

*Level of Cognitive Ability:* Application
*Client Needs:* Physiological Integrity
*Integrated Concept/Process:* Nursing Process/Assessment
*Content Area:* Maternity

*Reference*
Ladewig, P., London. M., & Olds, S. (1998). *Maternal-newborn nursing care: The nurse, the family, and the community* (4th ed.). Menlo Park, Calif.: Addison Wesley Longman, p. 679.

**86.** A nurse is preparing to assess the apical heart rate of a newborn infant in the newborn nursery. The nurse performs the procedure and notes that the heart rate is normal if which of the following is noted?

1    A heart rate of 90 beats/min
2    A heart rate of 140 beats/min
3    A heart rate of 180 beats/min
4    A heart rate of 190 beats/min

*[handwritten: 3 year-old Respiratory rate 20-30 beat]*

**Answer: 2**

*Rationale:* The normal heart rate in a newborn infant is 100 to 170 beats/min. Options 1, 3, and 4 are incorrect. Option 1 indicates bradycardia and options 3 and 4 indicate tachycardia.

*Test-Taking Strategy:* Use the process of elimination and knowledge regarding the normal heart rate for a newborn infant to answer this question. If you are unfamiliar with this normal finding, review this content.

*Level of Cognitive Ability:* Analysis
*Client Needs:* Physiological Integrity
*Integrated Concept/Process:* Nursing Process/Assessment
*Content Area:* Maternity

*Reference*
Ball, J., & Bindler, R. (1999). *Quick reference to pediatric clinical skills.* Stamford, Conn.: Appleton & Lange, p. 20.

---

**87.** A nurse reviews the electrolyte values of a client with congestive heart failure. The nurse notes that the potassium level is low and notifies the physician. The physician prescribes a dose of intravenous potassium. When administering the potassium solution, the nurse plans to:

1    Inject it as a bolus
2    Dilute it as instructed
3    Use a filter in the IV line
4    Apply cool compresses to the IV site during administration

**Answer: 2**

*Rationale:* Potassium is very irritating to the vein and needs to be diluted to prevent phlebitis. Potassium is never administered as a bolus injection. A filter is not necessary for potassium solutions. Cool compresses would vasoconstrict the IV site, which could possibly be more irritating to the vein.

*Test-Taking Strategy:* Use the process of elimination. Recalling that potassium is always diluted before administration will direct you to option 2. Review the procedure for administering IV potassium if you had difficulty with this question.

*Level of Cognitive Ability:* Application
*Client Needs:* Physiological Integrity
*Integrated Concept/Process:* Nursing Process/Planning
*Content Area:* Pharmacology

*Reference*
Hodgson, B., & Kizior, R. (2001). *Saunders Nursing drug handbook 2001.* Philadelphia: W.B. Saunders, p. 847.

---

**88.** A childbirth educator teaches a class of expectant parents that it is standard routine to instill a medication into the eyes of a newborn infant as a preventive measure against ophthalmia neonatorum. The educator tells the class that the medication currently used for the prophylaxis of ophthalmia neonatorium is:

1    Erythromycin ophthalmic eye ointment
2    Neomycin ophthalmic eye ointment
3    Penicillin ophthalmic eye ointment
4    Vitamin K injection

**Answer: 1**

*Rationale:* Ophthalmic erythromycin 0.5% ointment is a broad-spectrum antibiotic and is used prophylactically to prevent ophthalmia neonatorum, an eye infection acquired from the newborn infant's passage through the birth canal. Infection from these organisms can cause blindness or serious eye damage. Erythromycin is effective against *Neisseria gonorrhoeae* and *Chlamydia trachomatis*. Vitamin K is administered to the newborn infant to prevent abnormal bleeding and to promote liver formation of the clotting factors II, VII, IX, and X. Options 2 and 3 are incorrect.

*Test-Taking Strategy:* Use the process of elimination. It is necessary to know that ophthalmic erythromycin 0.5% ointment is used prophylactically to prevent ophthalmia neonatorum. If you had difficulty with this question, review initial care of the newborn infant.

*Level of Cognitive Ability:* Application
*Client Needs:* Physiological Integrity
*Integrated Concept/Process:* Teaching/Learning
*Content Area:* Maternity

**Reference**
Lowdermilk, D., Perry, S., & Bobak, I. (2000). *Maternity & women's health care* (7th ed.). St. Louis: Mosby, p. 725.

---

**89.** A nurse is developing a teaching plan for the mother of a newborn infant who is human immunodeficiency virus (HIV)-positive. Which specific instruction should be included in the teaching plan?
1 Instruct the mother to provide meticulous skin care of the newborn infant and to change the infant's diaper after each voiding or stool
2 Instruct the mother to feed the newborn infant in an upright position with the head and chest tilted slightly back to avoid aspiration
3 Instruct the mother to feed the newborn infant with a special nipple and bubble the infant frequently to decrease the tendency to swallow air
4 Instruct the mother to check the anterior fontanel for bulging and sutures for widening each day

**Answer: 1**
*Rationale:* Meticulous skin care helps protect the HIV-infected newborn infant from secondary infections. Feeding the newborn in an upright position, using a special nipple, and bulging fontanels are unrelated to the pathology associated with HIV.

*Test-Taking Strategy:* Read the question carefully and use the process of elimination. The question specifically asks for instructions to be given to the mother regarding HIV. Although options 2, 3, and 4 may be correct or partially correct in substance, the content does not specifically relate to care of the newborn infant infected with HIV. Review care of an infant infected with HIV if you had difficulty with this question.

*Level of Cognitive Ability:* Application
*Client Needs:* Physiological Integrity
*Integrated Concept/Process:* Teaching/Learning
*Content Area:* Maternity

**Reference**
Olds, S., London, M., & Ladewig, P. (2000). *Maternal-newborn nursing: A family and community-based approach* (6th ed.). Upper Saddle River, N.J.: Prentice-Hall, pp. 840-841.

---

**90.** Based on assessment and diagnostic evaluation, it has been determined that a client has Lyme disease, stage II. The nurse assesses the client for which of the following that is most indicative of this stage?
1 Erythematous rash
2 Neurological deficits
3 Headache
4 Lethargy

**Answer: 2**
*Rationale:* Stage II of Lyme disease develops within 1 to 6 months in the majority of untreated individuals. The most serious problems in this stage include cardiac conduction defects and neurological disorders such as Bell's palsy and paralysis. These problems are not usually permanent. Flulike symptoms and a rash appear in stage I.

*Test-Taking Strategy:* Use the process of elimination. Recalling that a rash and flulike symptoms occur in stage I will easily direct you to the correct option. If you had difficulty with this question, review the clinical manifestations associated with each stage of Lyme disease.

*Level of Cognitive Ability:* Analysis
*Client Needs:* Physiological Integrity
*Integrated Concept/Process:* Nursing Process/Assessment
*Content Area:* Adult Health/Integumentary

*Reference*
Phipps, W., Sands, J., & Marek, J. (1999). *Medical-surgical nursing: Concepts & clinical practice* (6th ed.). St. Louis: Mosby, p. 1993.

**91.** A nurse is caring for a client with a diagnosis of pemphigus. On assessment of the client, the nurse looks for which hallmark sign characteristic of this condition?

1    Homans' sign
2    Chvostek's sign
3    Trousseau's sign
4    Nikolsky's sign

**Answer: 4**
*Rationale:* A hallmark sign of pemphigus is Nikolsky's sign. Nikolsky's sign is when the epidermis can be rubbed off by slight friction or injury. Other characteristics include flaccid bullae that rupture easily and emit a foul-smelling drainage, leaving crusted, denuded skin. The lesions are common on the face, back, chest, and umbilicus. Even slight pressure on an intact blister may cause spread to adjacent skin. Trousseau's sign is a sign for tetany, in which carpal spasm can be elicited by compressing the upper arm and causing ischemia to the nerves distally. Chvostek's sign, seen in tetany, is a spasm of the facial muscles elicited by tapping the facial nerve in the region of the parotid gland. Homans' sign, a sign of thrombosis in the leg, is discomfort in the calf on forced dorsiflexion of the foot.

*Test-Taking Strategy:* Use the process of elimination. Eliminate options 2 and 3 first because they are both related to tetany. Recalling that Homans' sign is related to thrombophlebitis will direct you to option 4. If you had difficulty with this question, review these various signs.

*Level of Cognitive Ability:* Analysis
*Client Needs:* Physiological Integrity
*Integrated Concept/Process:* Nursing Process/Assessment
*Content Area:* Adult Health/Integumentary

*Reference*
LeMone, P., & Burke, K. (2000). *Medical-surgical nursing: Critical thinking in client care* (2nd ed.). Upper Saddle River, N.J.: Prentice Hall, p. 595.

**92.** Following tonsillectomy, which of the following fluid or food items is most appropriate to offer to the child?

1    Cool cherry Kool-Aid
2    Vanilla pudding
3    Cold ginger ale
4    Jell-O

**Answer: 4**
*Rationale:* Following tonsillectomy, clear, cool liquids should be administered. Citrus, carbonated, and extremely hot or cold liquids should be avoided because they may irritate the throat. Red liquids should be avoided because they give the appearance of blood if the child vomits. Milk and milk products (pudding) are avoided because they coat the throat and cause the child to clear the throat, increasing the risk of bleeding.

*Test-Taking Strategy:* Use the process of elimination. Note the key words *most appropriate*. Avoiding foods and fluids that may irritate or cause bleeding is the concern. This will assist in eliminating options 2 and 3. The word *cherry* in option 1 should be the clue that this is not an appropriate food item. Review dietary measures following tonsillectomy if you had difficulty with this question.

*Level of Cognitive Ability:* Application
*Client Needs:* Physiological Integrity
*Integrated Concept/Process:* Nursing Process/Implementation
*Content Area:* Child Health

**Reference**
Wong, D. (1999). *Whaley & Wong's Nursing care of infants and children* (6th ed.). St. Louis: Mosby, p. 1466.

---

**93.** A nurse is checking postoperative orders and planning care for a 110-lb child after spinal fusion. Morphine sulfate, 8 mg subcutaneously (SC) every 4 hours PRN for pain, is prescribed. The pediatric drug reference states that the safe dose is 0.1 to 0.2 mg/kg/dose every 2 to 4 hours. From this information, the nurse determines that:

1  The dose is too low
2  The dose is too high
3  The dose is within the safe dosage range
4  There is not enough information to determine the safe dose

**Answer: 3**
*Rationale:* Use the following formula to determine the dosage parameters:

Convert pounds to kilograms by dividing by 2.2.
110 lb ÷ 2.2 = 50 kg
Dosage parameters: 0.1 mg/kg/dose × 50 kg = 5 mg
0.2 mg/kg/dose × 50 kg = 10 mg
Dosage is within the safe dosage range.

*Test-Taking Strategy:* Identify the key components of the question and what the question is asking. In this case, the question asks for the safe dosage range for medication. Change pounds to kilograms. Calculate the dosage parameters using the safe dose range identified in the question and the child's weight in kg. Review medication calculations if you had difficulty with this question.

*Level of Cognitive Ability:* Analysis
*Client Needs:* Physiological Integrity
*Integrated Concept/Process:* Nursing Process/Analysis
*Content Area:* Child Health

**Reference**
Kee, J., & Marshall, S. (2000). *Clinical calculations: With applications to general and specialty areas* (4th ed.). Philadelphia: W.B. Saunders, p. 219.

---

**94.** A physician's order reads "acetaminophen (Tylenol) liquid, 450 mg PO every 4 hours PRN for pain." The medication label reads "160 mg/5 mL." The nurse prepares how many milliliters to administer one dose?

1  0.1 mL
2  5 mL
3  10 mL
4  14 mL

**Answer: 4**
*Rationale:* Use the following formula for calculating medication dosages:

$$\frac{\text{Desired}}{\text{Available}} \times \text{Volume} = \text{mL/dose}$$

$$\frac{450 \text{ mg}}{160 \text{ mg}} \times 5 \text{ mL} = 14 \text{ mL}$$

*Test-Taking Strategy:* Identify the key components of the question and what the question is asking. In this case, the question asks for milliliters per one dose. Set up the formula knowing that the desired dose is 450 mg, available as 160 mg/5 mL. Review medication calculations if you had difficulty with this question.

*Level of Cognitive Ability:* Application
*Client Needs:* Physiological Integrity
*Integrated Concept/Process:* Nursing Process/Planning
*Content Area:* Fundamental Skills

**Reference**
Kee, J., & Marshall, S. (2000). *Clinical calculations: With applications to general and specialty areas* (4th ed.). Philadelphia: W.B. Saunders, p. 78.

**95.** A pediatric nurse specialist provides an educational session to the nursing students about childhood communicable diseases. A nursing student asks the pediatric nurse specialist to describe the signs and symptoms associated with the most common complication of mumps. The pediatric nurse specialist responds knowing that which of the following signs or symptoms are indicative of the most common complication of this communicable disease?

1   A red, swollen testicle
2   Nuchal rigidity
3   Pain
4   Deafness

**Answer: 2**
*Rationale:* The most common complication of mumps is aseptic meningitis with the virus being identified in the cerebrospinal fluid. Common signs include nuchal rigidity, lethargy, and vomiting. A red, swollen testicle may be indicative of orchitis. Although this complication appears to cause most concern among parents, it is not the most common complication. Although mumps is one of the leading causes of unilateral nerve deafness, this does not occur frequently. Muscular pain, parotid pain, or testicular pain may occur, but pain is not a sign of a common complication.

*Test-Taking Strategy:* Use the process of elimination. Knowledge that aseptic meningitis is the most common complication of mumps will easily direct you to option 2. If you had difficulty with this question, review the complications associated with mumps.

*Level of Cognitive Ability:* Analysis
*Client Needs:* Physiological Integrity
*Integrated Concept/Process:* Teaching/Learning
*Content Area:* Child Health

**Reference**
Ball, J., & Bindler, R. (1999). *Pediatric nursing: Caring for children* (2nd ed.). Stamford, Conn.: Appleton & Lange, p. 390.

**96.** A 5-year-old child is hospitalized with Rocky Mountain spotted fever (RMSF). The nursing assessment reveals that the child was bitten by a tick 2 weeks ago. The child presents with complaints of headache, fever, and anorexia. The nurse notes a rash on the palms of the hands and soles of the feet. The nurse reviews the physician's orders and anticipates that which of the following medications will be prescribed?

1   Tetracycline (Achromycin)
2   Amphotericin B (Ketoconazole)
3   Ganciclovir (Foscarnet)
4   Amantadine (Rimantadine)

**Answer: 1**
*Rationale:* The nursing care of a child with RMSF will include the administration of tetracycline. An alternative medication is chloramphenicol, a fluoroquinolone. Amphotericin B is used for fungal infections. Ganciclovir is used to treat cytomegalovirus. Amantadine is used to treat influenza A virus.

*Test-Taking Strategy:* Knowledge regarding the treatment plan associated with RMSF is required to answer this question. If you are unfamiliar with this treatment plan or with the medications identified in the options, review this content.

*Level of Cognitive Ability:* Analysis
*Client Needs:* Physiological Integrity
*Integrated Concept/Process:* Nursing Process/Analysis
*Content Area:* Child Health

**Reference**
Wong, D. (1999). *Whaley & Wong's Nursing care of infants and children* (6th ed.). St. Louis: Mosby, p. 847.

**97.** A nursing instructor assigns a student nurse to present a clinical conference to the student group about brain tumors in children. The nursing student prepares for the conference and includes which of the following information in the presentation?

1 Surgery is not normally performed because of the risk of functional deficits occurring as a result of the surgery
2 Head shaving is no longer required before removal of the brain tumor
3 Chemotherapy is the treatment of choice
4 The most significant symptoms are headaches and vomiting

**Answer: 4**
*Rationale:* The hallmark symptoms of children with brain tumors are headache and vomiting. The treatment of choice is total surgical removal of the tumor without residual neurological damage. Before surgery the child's head will be shaved, although every effort is made to shave only as much hair as necessary.

*Test-Taking Strategy:* Use the process of elimination. Knowledge regarding the clinical manifestations and therapeutic interventions associated with a brain tumor is required to eliminate options 1, 2, and 3. If you are unfamiliar with the clinical manifestations and interventions associated with a brain tumor, review this content.

*Level of Cognitive Ability:* Application
*Client Needs:* Physiological Integrity
*Integrated Concept/Process:* Nursing Process/Planning
*Content Area:* Child Health

*Reference*
Wong, D. (1999). *Whaley & Wong's Nursing care of infants and children* (6th ed.). St. Louis: Mosby, p. 1740.

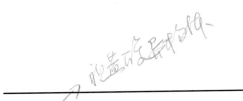

**98.** A brain tumor is suspected in a 9-year-old child, and a magnetic resonance imaging (MRI) and positron emission tomography (PET) scan are ordered. A sedative is prescribed to be administered before these procedures. Which medication does the nurse anticipate will be prescribed for this child?

1 Ondansetron hydrochloride (Zofran)
2 Dexamethasone (Decadron)
3 Chloral hydrate (Noctec)
4 Ofloxacin (Floxin)

**Answer: 3**
*Rationale:* Noctec is a sedative and the medication used most often to sedate young children. Zofran is an antiemetic used during chemotherapy. Decadron is administered to reduce some of the brain tissue swelling that occurs from the manipulation of tissue during surgery. Floxin is an antiinfective medication.

*Test-Taking Strategy:* Use the process of elimination. Noting the key word *sedative* in the question will direct you to option 3. Review these medications if you are unfamiliar with them.

*Level of Cognitive Ability:* Analysis
*Client Needs:* Physiological Integrity
*Integrated Concept/Process:* Nursing Process/Analysis
*Content Area:* Child Health

*Reference*
Hodgson, B., & Kizior, R. (2001). *Saunders Nursing drug handbook 2001.* Philadelphia: W.B. Saunders, pp. 198; 296; 772; 766.

**99.** Tretinoin (Retin-A) is prescribed for a client with acne. The client calls the clinic nurse and says that the skin has become very red and is beginning to peel. Which of the following nursing statements to the client would be most appropriate?

1 "Come to the clinic immediately."
2 "Discontinue the medication."
3 "Notify the physician."
4 "This is a normal occurrence with the use of this medication."

**Answer: 4**
*Rationale:* Tretinoin decreases cohesiveness of the epithelial cells, increasing cell mitosis and turnover. It is potentially irritating, particularly when used correctly. Within 48 hours of use, the skin generally becomes red and begins to peel. Options 1, 2, and 3 are incorrect responses to the client.

*Test-Taking Strategy:* Use the process of elimination. Options 1 and 3 can be eliminated first because they are similar. Eliminate option 2 next because it is not within the scope of nursing practice to advise a client to discontinue a medication. Review the effects of this medication if you had difficulty with this question.

*Level of Cognitive Ability:* Application
*Client Needs:* Physiological Integrity
*Integrated Concept/Process:* Teaching/Learning
*Content Area:* Pharmacology

*Reference*
Kuhn, M. (1998). *Pharmacotherapeutics: A nursing process approach* (4th ed.). Philadelphia: F.A. Davis, p. 997.

---

**100.** A child is hospitalized with a diagnosis of lead poisoning, and chelation therapy is prescribed. The nurse caring for the child would prepare to administer which of the following medications?
1    Activated charcoal
2    Sodium bicarbonate
3    Ipecac syrup
4    Dimercaprol (BAL)

**Answer: 4**
*Rationale:* Dimercaprol (BAL) is a chelating agent that is used to treat lead poisoning. Sodium bicarbonate may be used in salicylate poisoning. Ipecac syrup is used in poisonings to induce vomiting. Activated charcoal is used to decrease absorption in certain poisoning situations.

*Test-Taking Strategy:* Use the process of elimination and knowledge regarding the treatment related to lead poisoning to answer this question. Review this treatment if you are unfamiliar with it.

*Level of Cognitive Ability:* Application
*Client Needs:* Physiological Integrity
*Integrated Concept/Process:* Nursing Process/Planning
*Content Area:* Child Health

*Reference*
Ball, J., & Bindler, R. (1999). *Pediatric nursing: Caring for children* (2nd ed.). Stamford, Conn.: Appleton & Lange, p. 657.

---

**101.** A nurse is performing pin site care on a client in skeletal traction. Which finding would the nurse expect to note when assessing the pin sites?
1    Redness and swelling around the pin sites
2    Loose pin sites
3    Purulent drainage from the pin sites
4    Serosanguineous draining from the pin sites

**Answer: 4**
*Rationale:* A small amount of serosanguineous drainage may be expected after cleaning and removing crusting around the pin sites. Redness and swelling around the pin sites and purulent drainage may be indicative of an infection. Pins should not be loose and if this is noted, the physician should be notified.

*Test-Taking Strategy:* Use the process of elimination. Option 2 is not an expected finding and can be eliminated first because loose pins would not provide a secure hold with the traction. Eliminate options 1 and 3 next because they are similar and indicate signs of infection. Review assessment of pin sites in the client with skeletal traction if you had difficulty with this question.

*Level of Cognitive Ability:* Analysis
*Client Needs:* Physiological Integrity
*Integrated Concept/Process:* Nursing Process/Assessment
*Content Area:* Adult Health/Musculoskeletal

*Reference*
Monahan, F., & Neighbors, M. (1998). *Medical-surgical nursing: Foundations for clinical practice* (2nd ed.). Philadelphia: W.B Saunders, p. 863.

**102.** A nurse is caring for a client who has been placed in Buck's extension traction while awaiting surgical repair of a fractured femur. The nurse prepares to perform a complete neurovascular assessment of the affected extremity and plans to assess:

1 Color, sensation, movement, capillary refill, and pulse of the affected extremity
2 Warmth of the skin and the pedal pulse in the affected extremity
3 Vital signs and bilateral lung sounds
4 Nail thickness and for the presence of edema in the affected extremity

**Answer: 1**

*Rationale:* A complete neurological assessment of an extremity includes color, sensation, movement, capillary refill, and pulse of the affected extremity. Option 2 identifies only some of the components of a neurological assessment. Options 3 and 4 do not identify the components of a neurovascular assessment.

*Test-Taking Strategy:* Focus on the key words *complete neurovascular assessment of the affected extremity.* Use the process of elimination and knowledge regarding neurovascular assessment to assist in directing you to option 1. Review the components of a neurovascular assessment if you had difficulty with this question.

*Level of Cognitive Ability:* Application
*Client Needs:* Physiological Integrity
*Integrated Concept/Process:* Nursing Process/Assessment
*Content Area:* Adult Health/Musculoskeletal

*Reference*
Monahan, F., & Neighbors, M. (1998). *Medical-surgical nursing: Foundations for clinical practice* (2nd ed.). Philadelphia: W.B Saunders, p. 862.

---

**103.** A client in the emergency department has a plaster of Paris spica cast applied. The client arrives to the nursing unit and the nurse prepares to transfer the client into the bed by:

1 Supporting the cast with the fingertips only
2 Using the crossbar on the cast
3 Placing ice on top of the cast to decrease swelling
4 Using the palms of the hands and using soft pillows to support the cast

**Answer: 4**

*Rationale:* The palms or the flat surface of the extended fingers should be used when moving a wet cast to prevent indentations. Pillows are used to support the curves of the cast to prevent cracking or flattening of the cast from the weight of the body. Half-full bags of ice may be placed next to the cast to prevent swelling but this action would be performed after the client is placed in bed. Lifting a cast by the crossbars is never done and could cause breakage of the cast.

*Test-Taking Strategy:* Use the process of elimination. Focusing on the issue of the question, *transfer the client into the bed,* will assist in eliminating option 3. Eliminate option 2 next recalling that this action can cause breakage of the cast. Recalling that a wet plaster cast can easily be molded will direct you to option 4. Review care of a client in a newly applied plaster cast if you had difficulty with this question.

*Level of Cognitive Ability:* Application
*Client Needs:* Physiological Integrity
*Integrated Concept/Process:* Nursing Process/Planning
*Content Area:* Adult Health/Musculoskeletal

*Reference*
Smeltzer, S., & Bare, B. (2000). *Brunner & Suddarth's Textbook of medical-surgical nursing* (9th ed.). Philadelphia: Lippincott Williams & Wilkins, pp. 1782.

**104.** A physician orders the deflation of the esophageal balloon of a Sengstaken-Blakemore tube in a client. The nurse prepares for the procedure knowing that the deflation of the esophageal balloon places the client at risk for:
1 Increased ascites
2 Esophageal necrosis
3 Recurrent hemorrhage from the esophageal varices
4 Gastritis

**Answer: 3**
*Rationale:* A Sengstaken-Blakemore tube is inserted in clients with cirrhosis who have ruptured esophageal varices. It has esophageal and gastric balloons. The esophageal balloon exerts pressure on the ruptured esophageal varices and stops the bleeding. The pressure of the esophageal balloon is released at intervals to decrease the risk of trauma to the esophageal tissues including esophageal rupture or necrosis. When the balloon is deflated, the client may begin to bleed again from the esophageal varices.

*Test-Taking Strategy:* Focus on the issue and recall the purpose of the esophageal balloon of the Sengstaken-Blakemore tube. Remembering that the esophageal balloon exerts pressure on the ruptured esophageal varices and stops the bleeding will assist in directing you to the correct option. Review the complications associated with this type of tube if you are unfamiliar with it.

*Level of Cognitive Ability:* Analysis
*Client Needs:* Physiological Integrity
*Integrated Concept/Process:* Nursing Process/Planning
*Content Area:* Adult Health/Gastrointestinal

*Reference*
Smeltzer, S., & Bare, B. (2000). *Brunner & Suddarth's Textbook of medical-surgical nursing* (9th ed.). Philadelphia: Lippincott Williams & Wilkins, p. 839.

**105.** A physician tells a nurse that a client can be given droperidol (Inapsine) for the relief of postoperative nausea. The nurse anticipates that the physician will order the medication by which of the following routes?
1 Oral
2 Intravenous
3 Subcutaneous
4 Intranasal

**Answer: 2**
*Rationale:* Droperidol may be administered by the intramuscular or intravenous routes. The IV route is the route used when relief of nausea is needed. The IM route may be used when the medication is used as an adjunct to anesthesia. Options 1, 3, and 4 are not routes of administration of this medication.

*Test-Taking Strategy:* Use the process of elimination. Noting that the client is a postoperative client will assist in directing you to option 2. Review this medication if you had difficulty with this question.

*Level of Cognitive Ability:* Analysis
*Client Needs:* Physiological Integrity
*Integrated Concept/Process:* Nursing Process/Analysis
*Content Area:* Pharmacology

*Reference*
Hodgson, B., & Kizior, R. (2001). *Saunders Nursing drug handbook 2001.* Philadelphia: W.B. Saunders, p. 358.

**106.** A nurse is teaching the parents of a child with celiac disease about dietary measures. The nurse tells the parents to:
1. Read all label ingredients carefully to avoid hidden sources of gluten
2. Restrict corn and rice in the diet
3. Restrict fresh starchy vegetables in the diet
4. Substitute grain cereals with pasta products

**Answer: 1**
*Rationale:* Gluten is found primarily in the grains of wheat and rye. Corn and rice become substitute foods. Gluten is added to many foods as hydrolyzed vegetable protein that is derived from cereal grains, therefore labels need to be read. Corn and rice as well as vegetables are acceptable in a gluten-free diet. Many pasta products contain gluten. Grains are frequently added to processed foods for thickness or fillers.

*Test-Taking Strategy:* Use the process of elimination. Remembering that a gluten-free diet is required in celiac disease will assist in directing you to the correct option. If you had difficulty with this question, review the dietary measures in celiac disease.

*Level of Cognitive Ability:* Application
*Client Needs:* Physiological Integrity
*Integrated Concept/Process:* Teaching/Learning
*Content Area:* Child Health

*Reference*
Ball, J., & Bindler, R. (1999). *Pediatric nursing: Caring for children* (2nd ed.). Stamford, Conn.: Appleton & Lange, pp. 642-643.

**107.** A 45-year-old client is admitted to the hospital for evaluation of recurrent runs of ventricular tachycardia noted on Holter monitoring. The client is scheduled for electrophysiology studies (EPS) the following morning. Which statement would the nurse include in a teaching plan for this client?
1. "During the procedure, a special wire is used to increase the heart rate and produce the irregular beats that caused your signs and symptoms."
2. "You will be sedated during the procedure and will not remember what has happened."
3. "This test is a noninvasive method of determining the effectiveness of your medication regimen."
4. "You will continue to take your medications until the morning of the test."

**Answer: 1**
*Rationale:* The purpose of EPS is to study the heart's electrical system. During this invasive procedure, a special wire is introduced into the heart to produce dysrhythmias. To prepare for this procedure, the client should be NPO for 6 to 8 hours before and all antidysrhythmics are held for at least 24 hours before the test in order to study the dysrhythmias without the influence of medications. Since the client's verbal response to the rhythm changes are extremely important, heavy sedation is avoided if possible.

*Test-Taking Strategy:* Specific knowledge regarding the client preparation for EPS studies is needed to answer this question. Review this procedure if you had difficulty with this question.

*Level of Cognitive Ability:* Application
*Client Needs:* Physiological Integrity
*Integrated Concept/Process:* Teaching/Learning
*Content Area:* Adult Health/Cardiovascular

*Reference*
Fischbach, F. (2000). *A manual of laboratory & diagnostic tests* (6th ed.). Philadelphia: Lippincott Williams & Wilkins, p. 1046.

**108.** A nurse is providing diet teaching to a client with congestive heart failure (CHF). The nurse tells the client to avoid:

1    Leafy green vegetables
2    Catsup
3    Cooked cereal
4    Sherbet

**Answer: 2**

*Rationale:* Catsup is high in sodium. Leafy green vegetables, cooked cereal, and sherbet are all low in sodium. Clients with CHF should monitor sodium intake.

*Test-Taking Strategy:* Use the process of elimination, noting that options 1, 3, and 4 are similar in that they are low-sodium foods. Recalling that the client with CHF should limit sodium intake will direct you to option 2. Review dietary measures for the client with CHF if you had difficulty with this question.

*Level of Cognitive Ability:* Application
*Client Needs:* Physiological Integrity
*Integrated Concept/Process:* Teaching/Learning
*Content Area:* Adult Health/Cardiovascular

*Reference*
Smeltzer, S., & Bare, B. (2000). *Brunner & Suddarth's Textbook of medical-surgical nursing* (9th ed.). Philadelphia: Lippincott Williams & Wilkins, p. 668.

---

**109.** A home care nurse is developing a plan of care for an elderly client with diabetes mellitus who has gastroenteritis. In order to maintain food and fluid intake to prevent dehydration, the nurse plans to:

1    Offer water, only, until the client is able to tolerate solid foods
2    Withhold all fluids until vomiting has ceased for at least 4 hours
3    Encourage the client to take 8 to 12 ounces of fluid every hour while awake
4    Maintain a clear liquid diet for at least 5 days before advancing to solids to allow inflammation of the bowel to dissipate

**Answer: 3**

*Rationale:* The client should be offered liquids containing both glucose and electrolytes. Small amounts of fluid may be tolerated even when vomiting is present. The diet should be advanced as tolerated and should include a minimum of 100 to 150 g of carbohydrates daily. Offering water only and maintaining liquids for 5 days will not prevent dehydration but may promote it in this client.

*Test-Taking Strategy:* Eliminate options 1 and 2 because of the words *only* and *all*. From the remaining options, note the words *for at least 5 days* in option 4. Thinking about the issue, a client with diabetes mellitus and preventing dehydration, will direct you to option 3. Review sick day rules for a client with diabetes mellitus if you had difficulty with this question.

*Level of Cognitive Ability:* Application
*Client Needs:* Physiological Integrity
*Integrated Concept/Process:* Nursing Process/Planning
*Content Area:* Adult Health/Endocrine

*Reference*
Smeltzer, S., & Bare, B. (2000). *Brunner & Suddarth's Textbook of medical-surgical nursing* (9th ed.). Philadelphia: Lippincott Williams & Wilkins, p. 1882.

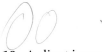

**110.** A client is unable to expectorate to yield a sputum sample and the nurse decides to use the saline inhalation method to obtain the sample. The nurse instructs the client to inhale the warm saline vapor via nebulizer by:

1 Holding the nebulizer under the nose
2 Keeping the lips closed lightly over the mouthpiece
3 Keeping the lips closely tightly over the mouthpiece
4 Alternating one vapor breath with one breath from room air

**Answer: 2**

*Rationale:* The inhalation of heated vapor helps the client to cough productively because the vapor condenses on the tracheo-bronchial mucosa and stimulates the production of secretions and a cough reflex. The client is told to lightly cover the mouthpiece with the lips and not to form a tight seal. The client inhales vaporized saline until coughing results.

*Test-Taking Strategy:* Use the process of elimination. Visualize this procedure, keeping in mind the purpose of the procedure, to direct you to option 2. Review this variation of the procedure for obtaining a sputum sample if you had difficulty with the question.

*Level of Cognitive Ability:* Application
*Client Needs:* Physiological Integrity
*Integrated Concept/Process:* Teaching/Learning
*Content Area:* Fundamental Skills

*Reference*
Monahan, F., & Neighbors, M. (1998). *Medical surgical nursing: Foundations for clinical practice* (2nd ed.). Philadelphia: W.B. Saunders, p. 546.

**111.** A nurse has completed tracheostomy care for a client whose tracheostomy tube has a nondisposable inner cannula. The nurse reinserts the inner cannula into the tracheostomy immediately after:

1 Suctioning the client's airway
2 Rinsing it with sterile water
3 Tapping it against a sterile surface to dry it
4 Drying it thoroughly with a sterile gauze

**Answer: 3**

*Rationale:* After washing and rinsing the inner cannula, the nurse dries it by tapping it against a sterile surface. The nurse then inserts the cannula into the tracheostomy and turns it clockwise to lock it into place. Options 1, 2, and 4 are inaccurate actions.

*Test-Taking Strategy:* Use the process of elimination. Eliminate option 1 first because you would not suction a client without an inner cannula in place. Eliminate option 2 next because a wet cannula should not be inserted. From the remaining options, eliminate option 4 because using a sterile gauze to dry the cannula can cause particles of the gauze to gather on the cannula leading to respiratory problems following insertion. Review the procedure for tracheotomy care if you had difficulty with this question.

*Level of Cognitive Ability:* Application
*Client Needs:* Physiological Integrity
*Integrated Concept/Process:* Nursing Process/Implementation
*Content Area:* Fundamental Skills

*Reference*
DeLaune, S., & Ladner, P. (1998). *Fundamentals of nursing: Standards and practice.* Albany, N.Y.: Delmar, p. 803.

**112.** A nurse suspects that an air embolism has occurred in a client receiving total parenteral nutrition (TPN) through a central venous catheter when the central line disconnects from the IV tubing. The nurse immediately turns the client to the:

1  Left side with the head higher than the feet
2  Right side with the head higher than the feet
3  Left side with the feet higher than the head
4  Right side with the feet higher than the head

**Answer: 3**

*Rationale:* If the client experiences air embolism, the immediate action is to place the client on the left side with the feet higher than the head. This position traps air in the right atrium. If necessary, the air can then be directly removed by intracardiac aspiration. Options 1, 2, and 4 are incorrect positions.

*Test-Taking Strategy:* Use the process of elimination. Recalling that the goal of action is to trap air in the right atrium will direct you to option 3. Review emergency care of a client with an air embolism if you had difficulty with this question.

*Level of Cognitive Ability:* Application
*Client Needs:* Physiological Integrity
*Integrated Concept/Process:* Nursing Process/Implementation
*Content Area:* Fundamental Skills

*Reference*
Monahan, F., & Neighbors, M. (1998). *Medical-surgical nursing: Foundations for clinical practice* (2nd ed.). Philadelphia: W.B. Saunders, p. 988.

---

**113.** An anxious client enters the emergency department seeking treatment for a laceration of the finger that occurred when using a power tool. The client's vital signs are pulse (P) 96 beats/min, blood pressure (BP) 148/88 mm Hg, and respirations (R) 24 breaths/min. After cleansing the injury and reassuring the client, the nurse rechecks the vital signs and notes P 82 beats/min, BP 130/80 mm Hg, and R 20 breaths/min. The nurse determines that the change in vital signs is caused by:

1  Reduced stimulation of the sympathetic nervous system
2  The cooling effects of the cleansing solution
3  The body's physical adaptation to the air conditioning
4  Possible impending cardiovascular collapse

**Answer: 1**

*Rationale:* Physical or emotional stress triggers a sympathetic nervous system response. Responses that are reflected in the vital signs include an increased pulse, increased blood pressure, and increased respiratory rate. Stress reduction, then, returns these parameters to baseline. Options 2, 3, and 4 are unrelated to the changes in vital signs.

*Test-Taking Strategy:* Note the information in the question, that the client is anxious and has an injury. These two elements guide you to think about the body's response to stress. Recalling the relationship of stress to the sympathetic nervous system will direct you to option 1. Review the effects of physical stress on the vital signs if you had difficulty with this question.

*Level of Cognitive Ability:* Analysis
*Client Needs:* Physiological Integrity
*Integrated Concept/Process:* Nursing Process/Analysis
*Content Area:* Fundamental Skills

*Reference*
Smeltzer, S., & Bare, B. (2000). *Brunner & Suddarth's Textbook of medical-surgical nursing* (9th ed.). Philadelphia: Lippincott Williams & Wilkins, p. 75.

**114.** A nurse is scheduling multiple diagnostic procedures for a client with activity intolerance. The procedures ordered include an echocardiogram, chest x-ray examination, and a computed axial tomography (CT) scan. The nurse schedules the procedure in which sequence to best meet the needs of this client?

1 Chest x-ray examination in the morning, echocardiogram in the afternoon, and the CT scan the morning of the following day

2 Chest x-ray examination and echocardiogram together in the morning, and the CT scan in the afternoon of the same day

3 Echocardiogram in the morning, and the chest x-ray examination and CT scan together in the afternoon of the same day

4 CT scan in the morning, and the chest x-ray examination and echocardiogram on the following morning

**Answer: 1**

*Rationale:* Echocardiograms can be done at the bedside. Chest x-ray examinations and CT scans are performed in the radiology department (unless a portable chest x-ray examination is ordered). The best sequence would be to have the client go to a procedure in another department in the morning (when most rested); have a rest period; have another procedure on the unit in the afternoon (when more fatigued); and go off the nursing unit again the next morning (when rested again). A client who has activity intolerance will do best when activities are spaced.

*Test-Taking Strategy:* Use the process of elimination. Focus on the issue: activity intolerance. Recalling that the client will do best if activities are spaced will direct you to option 1. Review interventions for the client with activity tolerance if you had difficulty with this question.

*Level of Cognitive Ability:* Application
*Client Needs:* Physiological Integrity
*Integrated Concept/Process:* Nursing Process/Planning
*Content Area:* Fundamental Skills

*Reference*
Johnson, M., Bulechek, G., Dochterman, J., Maas, M., Moorhead, S. (2001). *Nursing diagnoses, outcomes, and interventions.* St. Louis: Mosby, p. 41.

**115.** A nurse is preparing to initiate an intravenous nitroglycerin drip for a client with acute myocardial infarction. In the absence of an invasive (arterial) monitoring line, the nurse prepares to have which piece of equipment for use at the bedside?

1 Defibrillator
2 Pulse oximeter
3 Central venous pressure (CVP) tray
4 Noninvasive blood pressure monitor

**Answer: 4**

*Rationale:* Nitroglycerin dilates both arteries and veins, causing peripheral blood pooling and thus reducing preload, afterload, and myocardial work. This action accounts for the primary side effect of nitroglycerin, which is hypotension. In the absence of an arterial monitoring line, the nurse should have a noninvasive blood pressure monitor for use at the bedside.

*Test-Taking Strategy:* Use the process of elimination, noting the key words *absence of an invasive (arterial) monitoring line.* Recalling the purpose of this type of monitoring device and recalling the action of nitroglycerin will direct you to option 4. Review nursing responsibilities when administering a nitroglycerin drip if you had difficulty with this question.

*Level of Cognitive Ability:* Application
*Client Needs:* Physiological Integrity
*Integrated Concept/Process:* Nursing Process/Planning
*Content Area:* Adult Health/Cardiovascular

*Reference*
Smeltzer, S., & Bare, B. (2000). *Brunner & Suddarth's Textbook of medical-surgical nursing* (9th ed.). Philadelphia: Lippincott Williams & Wilkins, p. 629.

**116.** A client in labor has a concurrent diagnosis of sickle cell anemia. Because the client is at high risk for sickling crisis, which nursing action is the priority to assist in preventing a crisis from occurring during labor?

1    Reassure the client
2    Administer oxygen as ordered throughout labor
3    Maintain strict asepsis
4    Prevent bearing down

**Answer: 2**

*Rationale:* During the labor process, the client with sickle cell anemia is at high risk for being unable to meet the oxygen demands of labor. Administering oxygen will prevent sickle cell crisis during labor. Options 1 and 3 are appropriate actions but are unrelated to sickle cell crisis. Option 4 is inappropriate.

*Test-Taking Strategy:* Focus on the client's diagnosis and use the ABCs (airway, breathing, and circulation) to direct you to option 2. Review care of a client with sickle cell anemia in labor if you had difficulty with this question.

*Level of Cognitive Ability:* Application
*Client Needs:* Physiological Integrity
*Integrated Concept/Process:* Nursing Process/Implementation
*Content Area:* Maternity

*Reference*
Lowdermilk, D., Perry, S., & Bobak, I. (2000). *Maternity & women's health care* (7th ed.). St. Louis: Mosby, p. 902.

**117.** A client is scheduled for several diagnostic tests to rule out renal disease. As an essential component of the nursing assessment, the nurse plans to ask the client about a history of:

1    Frequent antibiotic use
2    Long-term diuretic therapy
3    Allergy to shellfish or iodine
4    Familial renal disease

**Answer: 3**

*Rationale:* The client undergoing any type of diagnostic testing should be questioned about allergy to shellfish, seafood, or iodine. This is essential to identify the risk for potential allergic reaction to contrast dye, which may be used in some diagnostic tests. The other items are also useful as part of the assessment but are not as critical as the allergy determination.

*Test-Taking Strategy:* Note the key word *essential*. This implies that more than one or all options may be correct. However, one of them is of highest priority. Since the question indicates that diagnostic testing is planned, the items are evaluated against their potential connection to this aspect of care. Recalling that contrast dye is used in many diagnostic tests will direct you to option 3. Review client assessment related to diagnostic testing if you had difficulty with this question.

*Level of Cognitive Ability:* Application
*Client Needs:* Physiological Integrity
*Integrated Concept/Process:* Nursing Process/Assessment
*Content Area:* Adult Health/Renal

*Reference*
Ignatavicius, D., Workman, M., & Mishler, M. (1999). *Medical-surgical nursing across the health care continuum* (3rd ed.). Philadelphia: W.B. Saunders, p. 812.

**118.** A nurse has an order to obtain a 24-hour urine collection on a client with a renal disorder. The nurse avoids which of the following to ensure proper collection of the 24-hour specimen?

1  Have the client void at the start time, and place this specimen in the container

2  Discard the first voiding; save all subsequent voidings during the 24-hour time period

3  Place the container on ice, or in a refrigerator

4  Have the client void at the end time, and place this specimen in the container

**Answer: 1**

*Rationale:*  The nurse asks the client to void at the beginning of the collection period and discards this urine sample. All subsequent voided urine is saved in a container, which is placed on ice or refrigerated. The client is asked to void at the finish time, and this sample is added to the collection. The container is labeled, placed on fresh ice, and sent to the laboratory immediately.

*Test-Taking Strategy:*  Use the process of elimination and note the key word *avoids*. Focusing on the issue: a 24-hour urine collection will assist in eliminating options 2 and 3. From the remaining options, think about the procedure. Having the client void at the finish time makes sense, because this captures the urine that the bladder has stored between the last time of voiding and the finish time for the specimen. On the other hand, if you save the first specimen, you do not know how long that urine has been stored in the bladder. Therefore, you would not be getting a true "24-hour" collection. Review this procedure if you had difficulty with this question.

*Level of Cognitive Ability:*  Application
*Client Needs:*  Physiological Integrity
*Integrated Concept/Process:*  Nursing Process/Implementation
*Content Area:*  Fundamental Skills

*Reference*
Potter, P., & Perry, A. (2001). *Fundamentals of nursing* (5th ed.). St. Louis: Mosby, p. 1398.

---

**119.** A nurse is caring for a client in active labor. The nurse performs which of the following to best prevent fetal heart rate decelerations?

1  Increases the rate of the oxytocin (Pitocin) infusion

2  Encourages upright or side-lying maternal positions

3  Monitors the fetal heart rate every 30 minutes

4  Prepares the client for a Cesarean delivery

**Answer: 2**

*Rationale:*  Side-lying and upright positions like walking, standing, and squatting can improve venous return and encourage effective uterine activity. The nurse should discontinue an oxytocin infusion in the presence of fetal heart rate decelerations, thereby reducing uterine activity and increasing uteroplacental perfusion. Monitoring the fetal heart rate every 30 minutes will not prevent fetal heart rate decelerations. There are many nursing actions to prevent fetal heart rate decelerations, without necessitating surgical intervention.

*Test-Taking Strategy:*  Use the process of elimination and focus on the issue, *best prevent fetal heart rate decelerations*. Options 1, 3, and 4 will not prevent fetal heart rate decelerations. Side-lying and upright positions will encourage effective uterine activity. Review nursing interventions for the client in labor if you had difficulty with this question.

*Level of Cognitive Ability:*  Application
*Client Needs:*  Physiological Integrity
*Integrated Concept/Process:*  Nursing Process/Implementation
*Content Area:*  Maternity

*Reference*
Lowdermilk, D., Perry, S., & Bobak, I. (2000). *Maternity & women's health care* (7th ed.). St. Louis: Mosby, p. 528.

**120.** A client with diabetes mellitus is at 36 weeks' gestation. The client has had weekly nonstress tests for the last 3 weeks, and the results have been reactive. This week the nonstress test was nonreactive after 40 minutes. Based on these results the nurse would anticipate the client will be prepared for:

1    Immediate induction of labor
2    Hospitalization with continuous fetal monitoring
3    A return appointment in 2 to 7 days to repeat the nonstress test
4    A contraction stress test

**Answer: 4**

*Rationale:* A nonreactive test needs further assessment. There is not enough data in the question to indicate that the procedures in options 1 and 2 are necessary at this time. To send the client home for 2 to 7 days may put the fetus in jeopardy. A contraction stress test is the next test needed to further assess the fetal status.

*Test-Taking Strategy:* Use the process of elimination, focusing on the issue: a change in test results from reactive to nonreactive. Options 1 and 2 can be eliminated first because they are unnecessary at this time. Option 3 can be eliminated next because repeating the test at a later time is not a safe intervention, especially considering that previous test results were reactive. Review the meanings of the test results related to a nonstress test if you had difficulty with this question.

*Level of Cognitive Ability:* Analysis
*Client Needs:* Physiological Integrity
*Integrated Concept/Process:* Nursing Process/Planning
*Content Area:* Maternity

*Reference*
Lowdermilk, D., Perry, S., & Bobak, I. (2000). *Maternity & women's health care* (7th ed.). St. Louis: Mosby, p. 811.

---

**121.** A nurse is administering magnesium sulfate to a client for severe preeclampsia. During the administration of the medication, the nurse:

1    Assesses for signs and symptoms of labor, since the client's level of consciousness will be altered
2    Assesses the client's temperature every 2 hours, since the client is at high risk for infection
3    Schedules a nonstress test every 4 hours to assess fetal well-being
4    Schedules daily ultrasonography to assess fetal movement

**Answer: 1**

*Rationale:* Because of the sedative effect of the magnesium sulfate, the client may not perceive labor. This client is not at high risk for infection. A nonstress test may be done, but not every 4 hours. Daily ultrasonography is not necessary for this client.

*Test-Taking Strategy:* Use the nursing process to answer the question. Assessment is the first step, so eliminate options 3 and 4. From the remaining options, knowledge that the client is not at high risk for infection will assist in directing you to option 1. Review nursing responsibilities when administering magnesium sulfate if you had difficulty with this question.

*Level of Cognitive Ability:* Application
*Client Needs:* Physiological Integrity
*Integrated Concept/Process:* Nursing Process/Implementation
*Content Area:* Maternity

*Reference*
Lowdermilk, D., Perry, S., & Bobak, I. (2000). *Maternity & women's health care* (7th ed.). St. Louis: Mosby, p. 829.

**122.** A client's nasogastric (NG) feeding tube has become clogged. The nurse's first action is to:
1  Flush the tube with warm water
2  Aspirate the tube
3  Flush with carbonated liquids, such as cola
4  Replace the tube

**Answer: 2**

*Rationale:* The nurse first attempts to unclog a feeding tube by aspirating the tube. If this is not successful, the nurse then tries to flush the tube with warm water. Carbonated liquids, such as cola, are sometimes used to prevent clogging, but the tube must be rinsed thoroughly to avoid stickiness. Replacement of the tube is the last step if other actions are unsuccessful.

*Test-Taking Strategy:* Use the process of elimination. Focusing on the key words *first action* will assist in eliminating option 4. Next, eliminate options 1 and 3 because they are similar. Review care of a client with an NG tube if you had difficulty with this question.

*Level of Cognitive Ability:* Application
*Client Needs:* Physiological Integrity
*Integrated Concept/Process:* Nursing Process/Implementation
*Content Area:* Fundamental Skills

*Reference*
Monahan, F., & Neighbors, M. (1998). *Medical surgical nursing: Foundations for clinical practice* (2nd ed.). Philadelphia: W.B. Saunders, p. 986.

---

**123.** A nurse is planning to give a tepid tub bath to a child who has hyperthermia. The nurse plans to:
1  Obtain isopropyl alcohol to add to the bath water
2  Warm the water to the same body temperature of the child
3  Have cool water available to add to the bath water
4  Allow 5 minutes for the child to soak in the tub

**Answer: 3**

*Rationale:* Adding cool water to an already warm bath allows the water temperature to drop slowly. The child is able to adjust to the changing water temperature gradually and will not experience chilling. Alcohol is toxic and contraindicated for tepid sponge or tub baths. To achieve the best cooling results, the water temperature should be at least 2° F lower than the child's body temperature. The child should be in a tepid tub bath for 20 to 30 minutes to achieve maximum results.

*Test-Taking Strategy:* Use the process of elimination. Eliminate option 1, recalling that alcohol is toxic. Eliminate option 2, because water that is the same as body temperature will not reduce hyperthermia. Eliminate option 4 because of the 5-minute time frame. Review measures for hyperthermia and the procedure for giving a tepid bath to a child if you had difficulty with this question.

*Level of Cognitive Ability:* Application
*Client Needs:* Physiological Integrity
*Integrated Concept/Process:* Nursing Process/Planning
*Content Area:* Child Health

*Reference*
Wong, D. (1999). *Whaley & Wong's Nursing care of infants and children* (6th ed.). St. Louis: Mosby, p. 1241.

**124.** A nurse is assigned to care for a child who is on postoperative day 1 following surgical repair of a cleft lip. Which nursing intervention is most appropriate when caring for this child's surgical incision?
1 Clean the incision only when serous exudate forms
2 Rub the incision gently with a sterile cotton-tipped swab
3 Rinse the incision with sterile water after feeding
4 Replace the Logan bar carefully after cleaning the incision

**Answer: 3**
*Rationale:* The incision should be rinsed with sterile water after every feeding. Rubbing alters the integrity of the suture line. Rather, the incision should be patted or dabbed. The purpose of the Logan bar is to maintain the integrity of the suture line. Removing the Logan bar on the first postoperative day would increase tension on the surgical incision.

*Test-Taking Strategy:* Use the process of elimination. Eliminate options 1 and 2 first because of the word *only* in option 1 and *rub* in option 2. Focus on the words *postoperative day 1*. This should assist in eliminating option 4. Review care of a child following surgical repair of a cleft lip if you had difficulty with this question.

*Level of Cognitive Ability:* Application
*Client Needs:* Physiological Integrity
*Integrated Concept/Process:* Nursing Process/Implementation
*Content Area:* Child Health

*Reference*
Wong, D. (1999). *Whaley & Wong's Nursing care of infants and children* (6th ed.). St. Louis: Mosby, pp. 519-520.

**125.** A client is in ventricular tachycardia, and the physician orders a STAT dose of lidocaine (Xylocaine) by intravenous (IV) bolus. An IV of 5% dextrose in water ($D_5W$) is infusing. To administer the lidocaine, the nurse:
1 Stops the IV, flushes the IV line, and then gives the lidocaine
2 Stops the IV and gives the lidocaine directly into the IV line
3 Starts another IV site
4 Checks for incompatibility of lidocaine with other IV medications

**Answer: 2**
*Rationale:* A bolus of lidocaine can be given directly into an IV line if 5% dextrose in water ($D_5W$) is infusing, because it is compatible with $D_5W$. If $D_5W$ is the primary solution, the IV line does not need to be flushed. A new IV line is not required for the administration of this medication in this situation. There are no data in this question that other IV medications are being administered; therefore option 4 is unnecessary.

*Test-Taking Strategy:* Use the process of elimination. Eliminate option 4 first because there are no data indicating that other medications are being administered. Eliminate option 3 next, because this action is avoided if possible. From the remaining options, recalling that lidocaine is compatible with $D_5W$ will direct you to option 2. Review the procedure for administering this medication if you had difficulty with this question.

*Level of Cognitive Ability:* Application
*Client Needs:* Physiological Integrity
*Integrated Concept/Process:* Nursing Process/Implementation
*Content Area:* Adult Health/Cardiovascular

*Reference*
Hodgson, B., & Kizior, R. (2001). *Saunders Nursing drug handbook 2001.* Philadelphia: W.B. Saunders, p. 591.

**126.** A client receiving total parenteral nutrition (TPN) via a central intravenous (IV) line is scheduled to receive an antibiotic by the IV route. Which action by the nurse is appropriate before hanging the antibiotic solution?
1   Ensure a separate IV access for the antibiotic
2   Turn off the TPN for 30 minutes before administering the antibiotic
3   Check with the pharmacy to be sure the antibiotic can be hung through the TPN line
4   Flush the central line with 60 mL of normal saline solution before hanging the antibiotic

**Answer: 1**
*Rationale:* The TPN line is used only for the administration of the TPN solution. Any other intravenous medication must be administered though a separate IV access site.

*Test-Taking Strategy:* Use the process of elimination. Eliminate options 2, 3, and 4 because they are similar in that they all involve using the TPN line for the administration of the antibiotic. Review care of a client receiving TPN if you had difficulty with this question.

*Level of Cognitive Ability:* Application
*Client Needs:* Physiological Integrity
*Integrated Concept/Process:* Nursing Process/Implementation
*Content Area:* Fundamental Skills

*Reference*
Potter, P., & Perry, A. (2001). *Fundamentals of nursing* (5th ed.). St. Louis: Mosby, p. 1218.

---

**127.** A nurse is inserting an indwelling urinary catheter into a male client. As the nurse inflates the balloon, the client complains of discomfort. The nurse:
1   Removes the syringe from the balloon because discomfort is normal and temporary
2   Aspirates the fluid, advances the catheter farther, then reinflates the balloon
3   Aspirates the fluid, withdraws the catheter slightly, then reinflates the balloon
4   Aspirates the fluid, removes the catheter, and reinserts a new catheter

**Answer: 2**
*Rationale:* If the balloon is positioned in the urethra, inflating the balloon could produce trauma and cause pain. If pain occurs, the fluid should be aspirated and the catheter inserted a little farther to provide sufficient space to inflate the balloon. The catheter's balloon is behind the opening at the insertion tip. Inserting the catheter the extra distance will ensure that the balloon is inflated inside the bladder and not in the urethra. There is no need to remove the catheter and reinsert a new one. Pain when the balloon is inflated is not normal.

*Test-Taking Strategy:* Note the issue, the client's complaint of discomfort on balloon inflation. Use the process of elimination and attempt to visualize the procedure to direct you to option 2. Review the complications associated with insertion of a urinary catheter if you had difficulty with this question.

*Level of Cognitive Ability:* Application
*Client Needs:* Physiological Integrity
*Integrated Concept/Process:* Nursing Process/Implementation
*Content Area:* Fundamental Skills

*Reference*
Kozier, B., Erb, G., & Blais, K. (1998). *Fundamentals of nursing: concepts, process, and practice* (5th ed.). Menlo Park, Calif.: Addison-Wesley, pp. 1256-1257.

**128.** A client with acquired immunodeficiency syndrome (AIDS) who has cytomegalovirus (CMV) retinitis is receiving ganciclovir sodium (Cytovene). The nurse implements which of the following in the care of this client?

1 Monitors blood glucose levels for elevation
2 Administers the medication on an empty stomach only
3 Tells the client to use a soft toothbrush and an electric razor
4 Applies pressure to venipuncture sites for at least 2 minutes

**Answer: 3**

*Rationale:* Ganciclovir causes neutropenia and thrombocytopenia as the most frequent side effects. For this reason the nurse monitors the client for signs and symptoms of bleeding and implements the same precautions that are used for a client receiving anticoagulant therapy. Thus, venipuncture sites should be held for approximately 10 minutes. The medication does not have to be taken on an empty stomach. The medication may cause hypoglycemia, but not hyperglycemia.

*Test-Taking Strategy:* Use the process of elimination. Recalling that this medication causes thrombocytopenia will direct you to option 3. Review the nursing considerations related to this medication if you had difficulty with this question.

*Level of Cognitive Ability:* Application
*Client Needs:* Physiological Integrity
*Integrated Concept/Process:* Nursing Process/Implementation
*Content Area:* Adult Health/Immune

*Reference*
Hodgson, B., & Kizior, R. (2001). *Saunders Nursing drug handbook 2001.* Philadelphia: W.B. Saunders, p. 457.

**129.** A client without history of respiratory disease has experienced sudden onset of chest pain and dyspnea, and pulmonary embolus is diagnosed. The nurse immediately implements which of the following therapeutic orders prescribed for this client?

1 Semi-Fowler's position, oxygen at 4 L/min, and morphine sulfate (MS) 2 mg intravenously (IV)
2 Semi-Fowler's position, oxygen at 1 L/min, and meperidine hydrochloride (Demerol) 100 mg intramuscularly (IM)
3 High-Fowler's position, oxygen at 4 L/min, and 2 tablets acetaminophen with codeine (Tylenol #3)
4 High-Fowler's position, oxygen at 1 L/min, and MS 10 mg IV

**Answer: 1**

*Rationale:* Standard therapeutic intervention for the client with pulmonary embolus includes proper positioning, oxygen, and intravenous analgesics. The head of the bed is placed in semi-Fowler's position. High-Fowler's is avoided because extreme hip flexure slows venous return from the legs and increases the risk of new thrombi. The client without preexisting respiratory disorders can tolerate oxygen at levels exceeding 2 to 3 L/min. The usual analgesic of choice is MS administered IV. This medication reduces pain, alleviates anxiety, and can diminish congestion of blood in the pulmonary vessels because it causes peripheral venous dilatation.

*Test-Taking Strategy:* Use the process of elimination. Noting the key words *without history of respiratory disease* should indicate that the client can tolerate a high oxygen flow. Thus, eliminate options 2 and 4. From the remaining options, recalling either that semi-Fowler's position is best or that MS is the medication of choice will direct you to option 1. Review care of a client with pulmonary embolus if you had difficulty with this question.

*Level of Cognitive Ability:* Application
*Client Needs:* Physiological Integrity
*Integrated Concept/Process:* Nursing Process/Implementation
*Content Area:* Adult Health/Respiratory

*Reference*
Ignatavicius, D., Workman, M., & Mishler, M. (1999). *Medical-surgical nursing across the health care continuum* (3rd ed.). Philadelphia: W.B. Saunders, p. 683.

**130.** A client who recently experienced myocardial infarction is scheduled to have a percutaneous transluminal coronary angioplasty (PTCA). The nurse plans to teach the client that during this procedure a balloon-tipped catheter will:

1  Cut away the plaque from the coronary vessel wall using a cutting blade
2  Be used to compress the plaque against the coronary blood vessel wall
3  Inflate a meshlike device that will spring open and keep the plaque against the coronary vessel wall
4  Be positioned in a coronary artery to take pressure measurements in the vessel

**Answer: 2**

*Rationale:* Option 1 describes coronary atherectomy. Option 2 describes PTCA. Option 3 describes placement of a coronary stent, and option 4 describes part of the process used in cardiac catheterization.

*Test-Taking Strategy:* Use the process of elimination. Look at the name of the procedure. "Angioplasty" refers to repair of a blood vessel, which should narrow your choices to options 1 and 2. Usually a procedure that cuts something away would have the suffix "-ectomy," which then eliminates option 1. Review this procedure if you had difficulty with this question.

*Level of Cognitive Ability:* Application
*Client Needs:* Physiological Integrity
*Integrated Concept/Process:* Teaching/Learning
*Content Area:* Adult Health/Cardiovascular

*Reference*
Smeltzer, S., & Bare, B. (2000). *Brunner & Suddarth's Textbook of medical-surgical nursing* (9th ed.). Philadelphia: Lippincott Williams & Wilkins, p. 601.

---

**131.** A nurse is caring for a client who has been placed in Buck's extension traction. The nurse provides for countertraction to reduce shear and friction by:

1  Slightly elevating the head of the bed
2  Slightly elevating the foot of the bed
3  Providing an overhead trapeze
4  Using a footboard

**Answer: 2**

*Rationale:* The part of the bed under an area in traction is usually elevated to aid in countertraction. For the client in Buck's extension traction (which is applied to a leg), the foot of the bed is elevated. An overhead trapeze or footboard is not used for the purpose of providing countertraction. Option 2 provides a force that opposes the traction force effectively without harming the client, and is the answer to the question.

*Test-Taking Strategy:* Use the process of elimination. Eliminate option 1 recalling that Buck's extension traction is applied to the leg. From the remaining options, focus on the issue—providing countertraction—to eliminate options 3 and 4. Review Buck's traction if you had difficulty with this question.

*Level of Cognitive Ability:* Application
*Client Needs:* Physiological Integrity
*Integrated Concept/Process:* Nursing Process/Implementation
*Content Area:* Adult Health/Musculoskeletal

*Reference*
Smeltzer, S., & Bare, B. (2000). *Brunner & Suddarth's Textbook of medical-surgical nursing* (9th ed.). Philadelphia: Lippincott Williams & Wilkins, p. 1787.

**132.** A nurse has inserted a nasogastric (NG) tube to the level of the oropharynx and has repositioned the client's head in a flexed-forward position. The client has been asked to begin swallowing. The nurse starts to slowly advance the NG tube with each swallow. The client begins to cough, gag, and choke. Which of the following nursing actions would least likely result in proper tube insertion and promote client relaxation?
1    Continuing to advance the tube to the desired distance
2    Pulling the tube back slightly
3    Checking the back of the pharynx using a tongue blade and flashlight
4    Instructing the client to breathe slowly

**Answer: 1**
*Rationale:*  As the NG tube is passed through the oropharynx, the gag reflex is stimulated, which may cause coughing, gagging, and choking. Instead of passing through to the esophagus, the NG tube may coil around itself in the oropharynx, or it may enter the larynx and obstruct the airway. Since the tube may enter the larynx, advancing the tube may position it in the trachea. Slow breathing helps the client relax to reduce the gag response. The tube may be advanced after the client relaxes.

*Test-Taking Strategy:*  Note the key words *least likely*. Noting that the client is coughing, gagging, and choking will direct you to option 1. Review this procedure if you had difficulty with this question.

*Level of Cognitive Ability:*  Application
*Client Needs:*  Physiological Integrity
*Integrated Concept/Process:*  Nursing Process/Implementation
*Content Area:*  Adult Health/Gastrointestinal

*Reference*
Potter, P., & Perry, A. (2001). *Fundamentals of nursing* (5th ed.). St. Louis: Mosby, p. 1467.

**133.** A nurse is planning care for a client with heart failure. The nurse asks the dietary department to remove which item from all meal trays before delivering them to the client?
1    Salt packets
2    1% milk
3    Margarine
4    Decaffeinated tea

**Answer: 1**
*Rationale:* Sodium restriction reduces water retention and improves cardiac efficiency. A standard dietary modification for the client with heart failure is sodium restriction.

*Test-Taking Strategy:*  Use the process of elimination. Focusing on the client's diagnosis will assist in recalling the need for sodium restriction and direct you to option 2. Review care of a client with heart failure if you had difficulty with this question.

*Level of Cognitive Ability:*  Application
*Client Needs:*  Physiological Integrity
*Integrated Concept/Process:*  Nursing Process/Implementation
*Content Area:*  Adult Health/Cardiovascular

*Reference*
Smeltzer, S., & Bare, B. (2000). *Brunner & Suddarth's Textbook of medical-surgical nursing* (9th ed.). Philadelphia: Lippincott Williams & Wilkins, p. 668.

**134.** A nurse is caring for an infant with spina bifida (meningomyelocele type) who had the gibbus (sac on the back containing cerebrospinal fluid, the meninges, and the spinal cord) surgically removed. The nurse plans which of the following in the postoperative period to maintain the infant's safety?
1   Elevating the head with the infant in the prone position
2   Covering the back dressing with a binder
3   Placing the infant in a head-down position
4   Strapping the infant in a baby seat sitting up

**Answer: 1**
*Rationale:* Elevating the head will decrease the chance of cerebrospinal fluid collecting in the cranial cavity. The fluid amount will take several weeks to decrease in volume after the gibbus reservoir is removed. The infant needs to be prone for several days to decrease the pressure on the surgical site on the back. Binders and a baby seat should not be used because of the pressure they would exert on the surgical site.

*Test-Taking Strategy:* Recall that preventing pressure on the surgical site and preventing intracranial cerebrospinal fluid collection are goals for the postoperative period. Use the process of elimination. Options 2 and 4 would increase pressure on the surgical site, and option 3 would not promote drainage of cerebrospinal fluid from the cranial cavity. Review postoperative nursing care following this procedure if you had difficulty with this question.

*Level of Cognitive Ability:* Application
*Client Needs:* Physiological Integrity
*Integrated Concept/Process:* Nursing Process/Planning
*Content Area:* Child Health

*Reference*
Ball, J., & Bindler, R. (1999). *Pediatric nursing: Caring for children* (2nd ed.). Stamford, Conn.: Appleton & Lange, p. 788.

**135.** A nurse is administering iron dextran (Infed) to a client by the intravenous route. The nurse checks that which of the following medications is available for use if needed as an antidote to the iron?
1   Deferoxamine (Desferal)
2   Dirithromycin (Dynabac)
3   Ferrous fumarate (Feostat)
4   Ferrous sulfate (Slow Fe)

**Answer: 1**
*Rationale:* The antidote to iron dextran is deferoxamine, which is a heavy metal antagonist. This medication chelates unbound iron in the circulation and forms a water-soluble complex that can be eliminated by the kidneys. Dirithromycin is a macrolide antiinfective. Ferrous sulfate and ferrous fumarate are forms of iron supplements.

*Test-Taking Strategy:* Specific knowledge regarding the antidote to iron dextran is needed to answer this question. Memorize the antidote, if this question was difficult.

*Level of Cognitive Ability:* Application
*Client Needs:* Physiological Integrity
*Integrated Concept/Process:* Nursing Process/Planning
*Content Area:* Pharmacology

*Reference*
Hodgson, B., & Kizior, R. (2001). *Saunders Nursing drug handbook 2001.* Philadelphia: W.B. Saunders, p. 302.

**136.** A client with pulmonary edema has oxygen via nasal cannula at 6 liters per minute. Arterial blood gas (ABG) results indicate the following: pH 7.29, $P_{CO_2}$ 49 mm Hg, $P_{O_2}$ 58 mm Hg, $HCO_3$ 18 mEq/L. The nurse anticipates that the physician will order which of the following for respiratory support?

1    Lowering the oxygen to 4 liters per minute via nasal cannula
2    Keeping the oxygen at 6 liters per minute via nasal cannula
3    Adding a partial rebreather mask to the current order
4    Intubation and mechanical ventilation

**Answer: 4**

*Rationale:* If respiratory failure occurs, endotracheal intubation and mechanical ventilation are necessary. The client is exhibiting respiratory acidosis, metabolic acidosis, and persistent hypoxemia. Lowering or keeping the oxygen at the same liter flow will not improve the client's condition. A partial rebreather mask will raise $CO_2$ levels even further.

*Test-Taking Strategy:* Use the process of elimination, noting the ABG values. Noting that the oxygen level is low will eliminate options 1 and 2. Knowing that the $P_{CO_2}$ is high will eliminate option 3, because a partial rebreather mask will raise $CO_2$ levels even further. Review ABG values if you had difficulty with this question.

*Level of Cognitive Ability:* Analysis
*Client Needs:* Physiological Integrity
*Integrated Concept/Process:* Nursing Process/Analysis
*Content Area:* Adult Health/Respiratory

*Reference*
Fischbach, F. (2000). *A manual of laboratory & diagnostic tests* (6th ed.). Philadelphia: Lippincott Williams & Wilkins, p. 986.

---

**137.** A client with an arteriovenous (AV) shunt in place for hemodialysis is at risk for bleeding. The nurse does which of the following as a priority action to prevent this complication?

1    Checks the results of partial thromboplastin time (PTT) tests as they are ordered
2    Checks the shunt once per shift
3    Checks the shunt for the presence of a bruit and thrill
4    Ensures that small clamps are attached to the AV shunt dressing

**Answer: 4**

*Rationale:* An AV shunt is a less common form of access site, but carries a risk for bleeding when it is used. This is because two ends of a cannula are tunneled subcutaneously into an artery and a vein, and the ends of the cannula are joined. If accidental disconnection occurs, the client could lose blood rapidly. For this reason, small clamps are attached to the dressing that covers the insertion site for use if needed. The shunt should be checked at least every 4 hours. Checking the results of the PTT does not prevent bleeding. Checking for the presence of a bruit and thrill assesses the patency.

*Test-Taking Strategy:* Use the process of elimination, focusing on the issue: preventing bleeding. The only option that relates to this issue is option 4. Review care of a client with an AV shunt if you had difficulty with this question.

*Level of Cognitive Ability:* Application
*Client Needs:* Physiological Integrity
*Integrated Concept/Process:* Nursing Process/Implementation
*Content Area:* Adult Health/Renal

*Reference*
Smeltzer, S., & Bare, B. (2000). *Brunner & Suddarth's Textbook of medical-surgical nursing* (9th ed.). Philadelphia: Lippincott Williams & Wilkins, p. 1113.

**138.** A client is due in hydrotherapy for a burn dressing change. To ensure that the procedure is most tolerable for the client, the nurse takes which of the following actions?
1 Sends dressing supplies with the client to hydrotherapy
2 Ensures that the client has a robe and slippers
3 Administers an analgesic 20 minutes before therapy
4 Administers the intravenous antibiotic 30 minutes before therapy

**Answer: 3**
*Rationale:* The client should receive pain medication approximately 20 minutes before a burn dressing change. This will help the client to tolerate an otherwise painful procedure. Antibiotics are timed evenly around the clock, and not necessarily in relation to timing of burn dressing changes. Dressing supplies are generally available in the hydrotherapy area and do not need to be sent with the client. A robe and slippers are beneficial for the client's comfort if traveling by wheelchair, but pain medication is more essential.

*Test-Taking Strategy:* Use Maslow's Hierarchy of Needs theory to answer this question. Also, noting the key words *most tolerable* will direct you to option 3. Review care of a burn client if you had difficulty with this question.

*Level of Cognitive Ability:* Application
*Client Needs:* Physiological Integrity
*Integrated Concept/Process:* Nursing Process/Implementation
*Content Area:* Adult Health/Integumentary

**Reference**
Smeltzer, S., & Bare, B. (2000). *Brunner & Suddarth's Textbook of medical-surgical nursing* (9th ed.). Philadelphia: Lippincott Williams & Wilkins, p. 1520.

**139.** A nurse caring for a client with heart failure receives a telephone call from the laboratory and is told that the client has a magnesium level of 1.5 mg/dL. The nurse plans to:
1 Encourage increased intake of phosphate antacids
2 Monitor the client for dysrhythmias
3 Administer ordered magnesium in normal saline
4 Encourage intake of foods such as ground beef, eggs, or chicken breast

**Answer: 2**
*Rationale:* The normal magnesium is 1.6 to 2.6 mg/dL. Phosphate use should be limited in the presence of hypomagnesemia because it worsens the condition. The client should be monitored for dysrhythmias, since the client is at risk for ventricular dysrhythmias. Magnesium sulfate is not administration in saline solutions. Ground beef, eggs, and chicken breast are examples of foods that are low in magnesium.

*Test-Taking Strategy:* Recalling the normal magnesium level and noting that the client is experiencing hypomagnesemia will direct you to option 2. If this question was difficult, review this electrolyte disorder and its treatment.

*Level of Cognitive Ability:* Application
*Client Needs:* Physiological Integrity
*Integrated Concept/Process:* Nursing Process/Planning
*Content Area:* Fundamental Skills

**Reference**
Fischbach, F. (2000). *A manual of laboratory & diagnostic tests* (6th ed.). Philadelphia: Lippincott Williams & Wilkins, p. 346.

**140.** A nurse is preparing to care for a client who has undergone a parathyroidectomy. The nurse plans care anticipating which postoperative order?
1    Place in a flat position with the head and neck immobilized
2    Take a rectal temperature only until discharge
3    Maintain endotracheal tube for 24 hours
4    Administer a continuous mist of room air or oxygen

**Answer: 4**
*Rationale:* Humidification of air or oxygen helps to liquefy mucous secretions and promotes easier breathing following parathyroidectomy. Pooling of thick mucous secretions in the trachea, bronchi, and lungs will cause respiratory obstruction. Semi-Fowler's position is the position of choice to assist in lung expansion and prevent edema. Rectal temperatures are not required. Tympanic temperatures can be taken. The client will not necessarily have an endotracheal tube.

*Test-Taking Strategy:* Use the ABCs (airway, breathing, and circulation) to direct you to option 4. Review care of a client following parathyroidectomy if you had difficulty with this question.

*Level of Cognitive Ability:* Application
*Client Needs:* Physiological Integrity
*Integrated Concept/Process:* Nursing Process/Planning
*Content Area:* Adult Health/Endocrine

**Reference**
Smeltzer, S., & Bare, B. (2000). *Brunner & Suddarth's Textbook of medical-surgical nursing* (9th ed.). Philadelphia: Lippincott Williams & Wilkins, p. 1051.

---

**141.** A client with carbon monoxide poisoning is to receive hyperbaric oxygen therapy. During the therapy, the nurse implements which priority intervention?
1    Assessing that oxygen is being delivered
2    Maintaining an intravenous access
3    Administering sedation to prevent claustrophobia
4    Providing emotional support to the client's family

**Answer: 1**
*Rationale:* Hyperbaric oxygen therapy is a process by which 100% oxygen is administered at greater than normal pressure. In carbon monoxide poisoning this therapy causes an increase in alveolar oxygen pressure and allows the carbon monoxide that is attached to the hemoglobin to be replaced by oxygen. Since the client is placed in a closed chamber, the administration of oxygen is of primary importance. Although options 2, 3, and 4 may be appropriate interventions, option 1 is the priority.

*Test-Taking Strategy:* Use the ABCs (airway, breathing, and circulation) to direct you to option 1. Review nursing care related to this therapy if you had difficulty with this question.

*Level of Cognitive Ability:* Application
*Client Needs:* Physiological Integrity
*Integrated Concept/Process:* Nursing Process/Implementation
*Content Area:* Adult Health/Respiratory

**Reference**
Smeltzer, S., & Bare, B. (2000). *Brunner & Suddarth's Textbook of medical-surgical nursing* (9th ed.). Philadelphia: Lippincott Williams & Wilkins, p. 1916.

**142.** A nurse is caring for a client with a herniated lumbar intervertebral disc. The nurse plans to place the client in which position to minimize the pain?
1  High-Fowler's position with the foot of the bed flat
2  Semi-Fowler's position with the knee gatch slightly raised
3  Semi-Fowler's position with the foot of the bed flat
4  Flat with the knee gatch raised

**Answer: 2**
*Rationale:* Clients with low back pain are often more comfortable when placed in semi-Fowler's position with the knee gatch raised sufficiently to flex the knees. This relaxes the muscles of the lower back and relieves pressure on the spinal nerve root. Keeping the foot of the bed flat will enhance extension of the spine. Keeping the bed flat with the knee gatch raised would excessively stretch the lower back and would also put the client at risk for thrombophlebitis.

*Test-Taking Strategy:* Use the process of elimination. Focus on the client's diagnosis and the issue, the position that will minimize pain. Visualize each of the positions, noting that option 2 places the least pressure on the spine. Review care of a client with a lumbar disc if you had difficulty with this question.

*Level of Cognitive Ability:* Application
*Client Needs:* Physiological Integrity
*Integrated Concept/Process:* Nursing Process/Planning
*Content Area:* Adult Health/Neurological

**Reference**
Smeltzer, S., & Bare, B. (2000). *Brunner & Suddarth's Textbook of medical-surgical nursing* (9th ed.). Philadelphia: Lippincott Williams & Wilkins, p. 1089.

**143.** A mother arriving at the emergency department with her child states that she just found the child sitting on the floor next to an empty bottle of aspirin. On assessment, the nurse notes that the child is drowsy but conscious. The nurse prepares to administer:
1  Ipecac syrup
2  Activated charcoal
3  Magnesium citrate
4  Magnesium sulfate

**Answer: 1**
*Rationale:* Ipecac is administered to induce vomiting. In this situation the child is conscious and the ingested substance (aspirin) will not damage the esophagus or lungs. Therefore the nurse prepares to administer the ipecac syrup. Activated charcoal may be used as an antidote in some poisoning situations, but its action is to absorb ingested toxic substances. Options 3 and 4 are unrelated to treatment for this occurrence.

*Test-Taking Strategy:* Use the process of elimination. Eliminate options 3 and 4 first because they are unrelated to the issue of poisoning. From the remaining options, note that the child is conscious. Also, think about the effect that the specific poison may have on the esophagus if vomited. Noting that the question states that the child was *just found* and considering that this ingestion will not harm the esophagus will direct you to option 1. Review measures to treat aspirin poisoning if you had difficulty with this question.

*Level of Cognitive Ability:* Application
*Client Needs:* Physiological Integrity
*Integrated Concept/Process:* Nursing Process/Planning
*Content Area:* Child Health

**Reference**
Wong, D. (1999). *Whaley & Wong's Nursing care of infants and children* (6th ed.). St. Louis: Mosby, p. 741.

**144.** A client with myasthenia gravis is admitted to the hospital. The nursing history reveals that the client is taking pyridostigmine (Mestinon). The nurse assesses the client for side effects of the medication and asks the client about the presence of:

1   Muscle cramps
2   Mouth ulcers
3   Feelings of depression
4   Unexplained weight gain

**Answer: 1**

*Rationale:* Mestinon is an acetylcholinesterase inhibitor. Muscle cramps and small muscle contractions are side effects and occur as a result of overstimulation of neuromuscular receptors. Options 2, 3, and 4 are not associated with this medication.

*Test-Taking Strategy:* Recall that myasthenia gravis is a neuromuscular disorder. Select the option that is most closely associated with this disorder. This will direct you to option 1. Review the side effects associated with this medication if you had difficulty with this question.

*Level of Cognitive Ability:* Application
*Client Needs:* Physiological Integrity
*Integrated Concept/Process:* Nursing Process/Assessment
*Content Area:* Pharmacology

*Reference*
Hodgson, B., & Kizior, R. (2001). *Saunders Nursing drug handbook 2001.* Philadelphia: W.B. Saunders, p. 888.

**145.** A client with a fractured right ankle has a short leg plaster cast applied in the emergency department. During discharge teaching, the nurse provides which information to the client to prevent complications?

1   Keep the right ankle elevated with pillows above the heart for 24 to 48 hours
2   Weight-bear on the right leg only after the cast is dry
3   Expect burning and tingling sensations under the cast for 3 to 4 days
4   Trim the rough edges of the cast after it is dry

**Answer: 1**

*Rationale:* Leg elevation is important to increase venous return and decrease edema, which can cause compartment syndrome, a major complication of fractures and casting. Weight-bearing on a fractured extremity is prescribed by the physician during follow-up examination, after an x-ray film is taken. Although the client may feel heat after the cast is applied, burning or tingling sensations indicate nerve damage or ischemia and are not expected. These complaints should be reported immediately. Option 4 is incorrect, because any cast modifications should be done by trained personnel under medical supervision. The client and family may be taught how to "petal" the cast to prevent skin irritation and breakdown, but rough edges, if trimmed, can fall into the cast and cause a break in skin integrity.

*Test-Taking Strategy:* Use the process of elimination and the ABCs (airway, breathing, and circulation). Option 1 is associated with maintenance of circulation. Review client teaching points related to cast care if you had difficulty with this question.

*Level of Cognitive Ability:* Application
*Client Needs:* Physiological Integrity
*Integrated Concept/Process:* Teaching/Learning
*Content Area:* Adult Health/Musculoskeletal

*Reference*
Smeltzer, S., & Bare, B. (2000). *Brunner & Suddarth's Textbook of medical-surgical nursing* (9th ed.). Philadelphia: Lippincott Williams & Wilkins, p. 1782.

**146.** An older adult woman client with a fractured left tibia has a long leg cast and is using crutches to ambulate. In caring for the client, the nurse assesses for which of the following signs and symptoms that indicate a complication associated with crutch walking?
1 Forearm muscle weakness
2 Left leg discomfort
3 Triceps muscle spasms
4 Weak biceps brachii

**Answer: 1**
*Rationale:* Forearm muscle weakness is a sign of radial nerve injury caused by crutch pressure on the axillae. When clients lack upper body strength, especially in the flexor and extensor muscles of the arms, they frequently allow their weight to rest on their axillae instead of their arms while ambulating with crutches. Leg discomfort is expected as a result of the injury. Triceps muscle spasms may occur as a result of increased muscle use but is not a complication of crutch walking. Weak biceps brachii is a common physical assessment finding in older adults and is not a complication of crutch walking.

*Test-Taking Strategy:* Focus on the issue: a complication of crutch walking. When asked about a complication of the use of crutches, think about nerve injury caused by crutch pressure on the axillae. This will direct you to option 1. Review this complication if you had difficulty with this question.

*Level of Cognitive Ability:* Analysis
*Client Needs:* Physiological Integrity
*Integrated Concept/Process:* Nursing Process/Assessment
*Content Area:* Adult Health/Musculoskeletal

*Reference*
Potter, P., & Perry, A. (2001). *Fundamentals of nursing* (5th ed.). St. Louis: Mosby, p. 1008.

**147.** A client with myasthenia gravis is experiencing prolonged periods of weakness. The physician orders an edrophonium (Tensilon) test. A test dose is administered and the client becomes weaker. The nurse interprets this test result as:
1 Normal
2 Positive
3 Myasthenia crisis
4 Cholinergic crisis

**Answer: 4**
*Rationale:* A Tensilon test may be performed to determine whether increasing weakness in a client with previously diagnosed myasthenia is caused by a cholinergic crisis (overmedication with anticholinesterase drugs) or myasthenic crisis (under medication with cholinesterase inhibitors). Worsening of the symptoms after the test dose of medication is administered indicates a cholinergic crisis.

*Test-Taking Strategy:* Use the process of elimination. Focus on the issue: the client becomes weaker after edrophonium is administered. Review this test and the interpretation of results if you had difficulty with this question.

*Level of Cognitive Ability:* Analysis
*Client Needs:* Physiological Integrity
*Integrated Concept/Process:* Nursing Process/Analysis
*Content Area:* Adult Health/Neurological

*Reference*
Smeltzer, S., & Bare, B. (2000). *Brunner & Suddarth's Textbook of medical-surgical nursing* (9th ed.). Philadelphia: Lippincott Williams & Wilkins, p. 1736.

**148.** A nurse notes an isolated premature ventricular contraction (PVC) on the cardiac monitor. The most appropriate nursing action is to:

1    Continue to monitor the rhythm
2    Notify the physician immediately
3    Prepare for defibrillation
4    Administer the ordered lidocaine hydrochloride (LidoPen)

**Answer: 1**

*Rationale:* As an isolated occurrence, the PVC is not life threatening. In this situation the nurse should continue to monitor the client. Frequent PVCs, however, may be precursors of more life-threatening rhythms, such as ventricular tachycardia and ventricular fibrillation. If this occurred, the physician needs to be notified.

*Test-Taking Strategy:* Focus on the information in the question. Note the key word *isolated*. This should direct you to the option that addresses continued monitoring. If you had difficulty with this question, review the implications of PVCs and the associated interventions.

*Level of Cognitive Ability:* Application
*Client Needs:* Physiological Integrity
*Integrated Concept/Process:* Nursing Process/Implementation
*Content Area:* Adult Health/Cardiovascular

**Reference**
Smeltzer, S., & Bare, B. (2000). *Brunner & Suddarth's Textbook of medical-surgical nursing* (9th ed.). Philadelphia: Lippincott Williams & Wilkins, p. 574.

**149.** A nurse is caring for a client admitted with the diagnosis of active tuberculosis (TB). This nurse determines that this diagnosis was confirmed by a:

1    Mantoux test
2    Sputum culture
3    Tine test
4    Chest x-ray evaluation

**Answer: 2**

*Rationale:* A sputum culture showing *Mycobacterium tuberculosis* confirms the diagnosis of TB. Usually three sputum samples are obtained for the acid-fast smear. After the initiation of medication therapy, sputum samples are obtained again to determine the effectiveness of therapy. A positive result to a tine or Mantoux test indicates exposure to TB but does not confirm the presence of *M. tuberculosis*. A positive chest x-ray evaluation may indicate the presence of tuberculosis lesions but again does not confirm active disease.

*Test-Taking Strategy:* Note the key word *confirmed* in the stem of the question. Active TB can be confirmed only by the presence of the bacilli. The sputum culture is the only method of determining the presence of this organism. Review tests associated with TB if you had difficulty with this question.

*Level of Cognitive Ability:* Analysis
*Client Needs:* Physiological Integrity
*Integrated Concept/Process:* Nursing Process/Assessment
*Content Area:* Adult Health/Respiratory

**Reference**
Smeltzer, S., & Bare, B. (2000). *Brunner & Suddarth's Textbook of medical-surgical nursing* (9th ed.). Philadelphia: Lippincott Williams & Wilkins, p. 438.

**150.** A clinic nurse prepares to assess the fundal height in a client in the second trimester of pregnancy. When measuring the fundal height, the nurse will most likely expect the measurement to:
1  Correlate with gestational age
2  Be greater than gestational age
3  Be less than gestational age
4  Have no correlation to gestational age

**Answer: 1**
*Rationale:* Up until the third trimester the measurement of fundal height will, on average, correlate with the gestational age. Options 2, 3, and 4 are incorrect.

*Test-Taking Strategy:* Note the key words *most likely*. Focus on the issue: second trimester and fundal height. Recall the correlation of fundal height and gestational age to direct you to option 1. If you had difficulty with this question, review this prenatal assessment.

*Level of Cognitive Ability:* Analysis
*Client Needs:* Physiological Integrity
*Integrated Concept/Process:* Nursing Process/Assessment
*Content Area:* Maternity

*Reference*
Lowdermilk, D., Perry, S., & Bobak, I. (2000). *Maternity & women's health care* (7th ed.). St. Louis: Mosby, p. 401.

**151.** A pregnant client tells a nurse that she felt wetness on her peri-pad and that she found some clear fluid. The nurse immediately inspects the perineum and notes the presence of the umbilical cord. The nurse's initial action is to:
1  Notify the physician
2  Monitor the fetal heart rate
3  Transfer the client to the delivery room
4  Place the client in Trendelenburg position

**Answer: 4**
*Rationale:* On inspection of the perineum, if the umbilical cord is noted, the nurse immediately places the client into Trendelenburg position while pushing the presenting part upward to relieve the cord compression. This position is maintained and the physician is notified. The nurse monitors the fetal heart rate. The client is transferred to the delivery room when prescribed by the physician.

*Test-Taking Strategy:* Note the key words *notes the presence of the umbilical cord*, which indicates the need for an immediate action on the nurse's part to prevent or relieve cord compression. The only action that will achieve this is option 4. The physician is notified after the client is positioned. Review nursing actions when this complication occurs if you had difficulty with this question.

*Level of Cognitive Ability:* Application
*Client Needs:* Physiological Integrity
*Integrated Concept/Process:* Nursing Process/Implementation
*Content Area:* Maternity

*Reference*
Lowdermilk, D., Perry, S., & Bobak, I. (2000). *Maternity & women's health care* (7th ed.). St. Louis: Mosby, pp. 4014-4015.

**152.** A nurse admits a newborn infant to the nursery. On assessment of the infant, the nurse palpates the anterior fontanel and notes that it feels soft. The nurse determines that this finding indicates:

1  Increased intracranial pressure
2  Dehydration
3  Decreased intracranial pressure
4  A normal finding

**Answer: 4**

*Rationale:* The anterior fontanel is normally 2 to 3 cm in width, 3 to 4 cm in length, and diamond-shaped. It can be described as soft, which is normal, or full and bulging, which could be indicative of increased intracranial pressure. Conversely, a depressed fontanel could mean that the infant is dehydrated.

*Test-Taking Strategy:* Use the process of elimination. Focusing on the key word *soft* will direct you to option 4. Review the normal findings related to the fontanels if you had difficulty with this question.

*Level of Cognitive Ability:* Analysis
*Client Needs:* Physiological Integrity
*Integrated Concept/Process:* Nursing Process/Assessment
*Content Area:* Maternity

**Reference**

Lowdermilk, D., Perry, S., & Bobak, I. (2000). *Maternity & women's health care* (7th ed.). St. Louis: Mosby, p. 698.

**153.** A client with acquired immunodeficiency syndrome (AIDS) is admitted to the hospital for chills, fever, nonproductive cough, and pleuritic chest pain. A diagnosis of *Pneumocystis carinii* pneumonia is made, and the client is started on IV pentamidine (Nebupent). The nurse plans to infuse the medication over:

1  1 hour with the client in a supine position
2  30 minutes with the client in a reclining position
3  1 hour and the client may be ambulatory
4  15 minutes with the client in a supine position

**Answer: 1**

*Rationale:* IV pentamidine is infused over 1 hour with the client supine to minimize severe hypotension and dysrhythmias. Options 2, 3, and 4 are inaccurate in either the length of time pentamidine is administered or the client's position.

*Test-Taking Strategy:* Use the process of elimination. Eliminate option 4 first because this time frame is very short for an IV medication. From the remaining options, recalling that the medication causes hypotension will direct you to option 1, the option that addresses both the supine position and the longest time of administration. Review this medication if you had difficulty with this question.

*Level of Cognitive Ability:* Application
*Client Needs:* Physiological Integrity
*Integrated Concept/Process:* Nursing Process/Planning
*Content Area:* Adult Health/Immune

**Reference**

Hodgson, B., & Kizior, R. (2001). *Saunders Nursing drug handbook 2001.* Philadelphia: W.B. Saunders, p. 801.

*[handwritten notes]*

**154.** A nurse is caring for a client who has returned to a surgical unit from a critical care unit after having a pelvic exenteration. The client complains of pain in the calf area. The nurse would:

1  Administer meperidine hydrochloride (Demerol) PRN as prescribed
2  Check the calf for temperature, color, and size
3  Lightly massage the area to relieve the pain
4  Ask the client to walk, and observe the gait

**Answer: 2**

*Rationale:* The nurse monitors for postoperative complications such as deep vein thrombosis, pulmonary emboli, and wound infection. Pain in the calf could indicate a deep vein thrombosis. Change in color, temperature, or size of the client's calf could also indicate this complication. Options 3 and 4 could result in an embolus if in fact this client had a deep vein thrombosis. Pain medication for this client complaint is not the appropriate nursing action. Further assessment is needed.

*Test-Taking Strategy:* Use the steps of the nursing process. Assessment is the first step. Option 2 is the only option that addresses assessment. Review postoperative complications and appropriate interventions if you had difficulty with this question.

*Level of Cognitive Ability:* Application
*Client Needs:* Physiological Integrity
*Integrated Concept/Process:* Nursing Process/Assessment
*Content Area:* Fundamental Skills

*Reference*
Smeltzer, S., & Bare, B. (2000). *Brunner & Suddarth's Textbook of medical-surgical nursing* (9th ed.). Philadelphia: Lippincott Williams & Wilkins, p. 361.

---

**155.** A nurse is preparing to assess the respirations of a newborn infant just admitted to the newborn nursery. The nurse performs the procedure and determines that the respiratory rate is normal if which of the following are noted?

1  A respiratory rate of 20 breaths/min
2  A respiratory rate of 40 breaths/min
3  A respiratory rate of 90 breaths/min
4  A respiratory rate of 100 breaths/min

**Answer: 2**

*Rationale:* Normal respiratory rate varies from 30 to 80 breaths/min when the infant is not crying. Respirations should be counted for 1 full minute to ensure an accurate measurement because the newborn infant is a periodic breather. Observing and palpating respirations while the infant is quiet promotes accurate assessment. Palpation aids observation in determining the respiratory rate. Option 1 indicates bradypnea, and options 3 and 4 indicate tachypnea.

*Test-Taking Strategy:* Use the process of elimination and knowledge regarding the normal respiratory rate for a newborn infant to answer this question. If you are unfamiliar with this normal finding, review this content.

*Level of Cognitive Ability:* Analysis
*Client Needs:* Physiological Integrity
*Integrated Concept/Process:* Nursing Process/Assessment
*Content Area:* Maternity

*Reference*
Ball, J., & Bindler, R. (1999). *Quick reference to pediatric clinical skills.* Stamford, Conn.: Appleton & Lange, p. 21.

**156.** A client is in her second trimester of pregnancy. During her routine prenatal visit, she states that she frequently has calf pain when she walks. Which of the following should the nurse assess to assist in identifying the origin of the discomfort?
1   Chadwick's sign
2   Leopold's sign
3   Homans' sign
4   Kernig's sign

**Answer: 3**

*Rationale:* Homans' sign tests for venous thrombosis of the lower extremity. Pain in the calf during walking could indicate venous thrombosis. Chadwick's sign is a cervical change and is a probable sign of pregnancy. Leopold's sign is a fictitious term. Leopold's maneuvers are a series of abdominal palpation maneuvers that provide information regarding fetal presentation, position, presenting part, attitude, and descent. Kernig's sign tests for meningeal irritability.

*Test-Taking Strategy:* Use the process of elimination. Focus on the key words *frequently has calf pain when she walks* to assist in directing you to option 3. Review the signs identified in the options if you had difficulty with this question.

*Level of Cognitive Ability:* Analysis
*Client Needs:* Physiological Integrity
*Integrated Concept/Process:* Nursing Process/Assessment
*Content Area:* Maternity

*Reference*
Olds, S., London, M., & Ladewig, P. (2000). *Maternal-newborn nursing: A family and community-based approach* (6th ed.). Upper Saddle River, N.J.: Prentice Hall, p. 925.

**157.** A nurse is evaluating the patency of a peripheral intravenous (IV) site and suspects an infiltration. The nurse does which of the following to determine whether the IV has infiltrated?
1   Gently palpates the surrounding tissue for edema and coolness
2   Strips the tubing quickly while assessing for a rapid blood return
3   Increases the IV flow rate and observes the site for immediate tightening of tissue
4   Checks the area around the IV site for discomfort, redness, and warmth

**Answer: 1**

*Rationale:* In the assessment of an IV for signs and symptoms of infiltration, it is important to assess the site for edema and coolness, signifying leakage of the IV fluid into the surrounding tissues. Stripping the tubing will not cause a blood return but will force IV fluids into the vein or surrounding tissues, which could cause more tissue damage. Increasing the flow rate may be damaging to the tissues if the IV has infiltrated. The IV site will feel cool if the IV fluid has infiltrated into the surrounding tissues.

*Test-Taking Strategy:* Use the process of elimination, focusing on the issue: infiltration. Recalling that the site will feel cool will direct you to option 1. Review the signs of infiltration if you had difficulty with this question.

*Level of Cognitive Ability:* Application
*Client Needs:* Physiological Integrity
*Integrated Concept/Process:* Nursing Process/Implementation
*Content Area:* Fundamental Skills

*Reference*
Potter, P., & Perry, A. (2001). *Fundamentals of nursing* (5th ed.). St. Louis: Mosby, p. 1233.

**158.** A client is brought into the emergency department after being in a car accident. A neck injury is suspected. The client is unresponsive and pulseless. The nurse opens the client's airway by which method?
1   Head tilt–chin lift
2   Lifting the head up, placing the head on two pillows, and attempting to ventilate
3   Jaw-thrust maneuver
4   Keeping the client flat and grasping the tongue

**Answer: 3**
*Rationale:* In suspected neck injuries the most appropriate way to open the airway is the jaw-thrust maneuver. If a neck injury is present, this maneuver will prevent further injury. Options 1, 2, and 4 are incorrect.

*Test-Taking Strategy:* Note the key words *neck injury is suspected.* Knowledge regarding airway management will assist in eliminating options 2 and 4. From the remaining options, eliminate option 1, because this method would cause further damage to a neck injury. Review basic life support measures if you had difficulty with this question.

*Level of Cognitive Ability:* Application
*Client Needs:* Physiological Integrity
*Integrated Concept/Process:* Nursing Process/Implementation
*Content Area:* Fundamental Skills

*Reference*
Potter, P., & Perry, A. (2001). *Fundamentals of nursing* (5th ed.). St. Louis: Mosby, p. 1184.

**159.** A nurse is caring for a child with Reye's syndrome. The nurse monitors for which major symptom associated with this syndrome?
1   Persistent vomiting
2   Protein in the urine
3   A history of a staphylococcal infection
4   Symptoms of hyperglycemia

**Answer: 1**
*Rationale:* Intracranial pressure and encephalopathy are major symptoms of Reye's syndrome. Persistent vomiting is a major symptom associated with intracranial pressure. Protein is not present in the urine. Reye's syndrome is related to a history of viral infections, and hypoglycemia is a symptom of this disease.

*Test-Taking Strategy:* Use the process of elimination, focusing on the issue: a major symptom. Recalling that intracranial pressure is associated with this syndrome and that vomiting is a symptom of intracranial pressure will direct you to option 1. If you had difficulty with this question, review the symptoms of Reye's syndrome and the signs of intracranial pressure.

*Level of Cognitive Ability:* Application
*Client Needs:* Physiological Integrity
*Integrated Concept/Process:* Nursing Process/Assessment
*Content Area:* Child Health

*Reference*
Wong, D. (1999). *Whaley & Wong's Nursing care of infants and children* (6th ed.). St. Louis: Mosby, p. 1806.

**160.** A child is admitted to the hospital with a suspected diagnosis of pneumococcal pneumonia. The nurse prepares to:
1. Have a chest x-ray film taken to determine how much consolidation there is in the lungs
2. Allow the child to go to the playroom to play with other children
3. Monitor the child's respiratory rate and breath sounds
4. Start antibiotic therapy immediately

**Answer:** 3
*Rationale:* A complication of pneumococcal pneumonia is pleural effusion, so the respiratory status of the child should be monitored. Option 1 is medical management, not nursing care. Antibiotic therapy is not started until cultures are obtained. The child should not be allowed in the playroom at this time.

*Test-Taking Strategy:* Use the steps of the nursing process. Assessment is the first step. This option also addresses the ABCs (airway, breathing, and circulation). It is also the option that is directly related to the child's diagnosis. Review care of a client with pneumonia if you had difficulty with this question.

*Level of Cognitive Ability:* Application
*Client Needs:* Physiological Integrity
*Integrated Concept/Process:* Nursing Process/Implementation
*Content Area:* Child Health

*Reference*
Wong, D. (1999). *Whaley & Wong's Nursing care of infants and children* (6th ed.). St. Louis: Mosby, p. 1482.

**161.** A nurse admits a client to the hospital with a suspected diagnosis of bulimia nervosa. When performing the admission assessment, the nurse elicits data knowing that the client with bulimia:
1. Overeats for the enjoyment of food
2. Binge eats, then purges
3. Overeats in response to losing control over a weight loss diet
4. Is accepting of body size

**Answer:** 2
*Rationale:* Individuals with bulimia nervosa develop cycles of binge eating, followed by purging. They seldom attempt to diet and have no sense of loss of control. Options 1, 3, and 4 are true of an obese person who may binge eat.

*Test-Taking Strategy:* Use the process of elimination. Eliminate options 1 and 3 because they are similar. From the remaining options, recalling the definition of bulimia will direct you to option 2. If you had difficulty with this question, review the characteristics associated with this disorder.

*Level of Cognitive Ability:* Analysis
*Client Needs:* Physiological Integrity
*Integrated Concept/Process:* Nursing Process/Assessment
*Content Area:* Mental Health

*Reference*
Stuart, G.W., & Laraia, M.T. (1998). *Principles and practice of psychiatric nursing.* (6th ed.). St. Louis: Mosby, p. 534.

**162.** A nurse is caring for the client who develops compartment syndrome from a severely fractured arm. The client asks the nurse how this can happen. The nurse's response is based on the understanding that:

1   An injured artery causes impaired arterial perfusion through the compartment
2   The fascia expands with injury, causing pressure on underlying nerves and muscles
3   A bone fragment has injured the nerve supply in the area
4   Bleeding and swelling cause increased pressure in an area that cannot expand

**Answer: 4**

*Rationale:* Compartment syndrome is caused by bleeding and swelling within a compartment, which is lined by fascia that does not expand. The bleeding and swelling places pressure on the nerves, muscles, and blood vessels in the compartment, triggering the symptoms.

*Test-Taking Strategy:* Use the process of elimination. Option 1 is eliminated first because this syndrome is not caused by an arterial injury. Knowing that the fascia itself cannot expand eliminates option 2. From the remaining options, it is necessary to know that bleeding and swelling cause the symptoms, not a nerve injury. Review the physiology associated with compartment syndrome if you had difficulty with this question.

*Level of Cognitive Ability:* Analysis
*Client Needs:* Physiological Integrity
*Integrated Concept/Process:* Nursing Process/Analysis
*Content Area:* Adult Health/Musculoskeletal

*Reference*
Smeltzer, S., & Bare, B. (2000). *Brunner & Suddarth's Textbook of medical-surgical nursing* (9th ed.). Philadelphia: Lippincott Williams & Wilkins, p. 1783.

**163.** A client has undergone fasciotomy to treat compartment syndrome of the leg. The nurse prepares to provide which type of wound care of the fasciotomy site?

1   Dry sterile dressings
2   Moist sterile saline dressings
3   Hydrocolloid dressings
4   One-half strength Betadine dressings

**Answer: 2**

*Rationale:* The fasciotomy site is not sutured but is left open to relieve pressure and edema. The site is covered with moist sterile saline dressings. After 3 to 5 days, when perfusion is adequate and edema subsides, the wound is debrided and closed. A hydrocolloid dressing is not indicated for use with clean, open incisions. The incision is clean, not dirty, so there should be no reason to require Betadine. In addition, Betadine can be irritating to normal tissues.

*Test-Taking Strategy:* Use the process of elimination and knowledge of what a fasciotomy involves and the basics of wound care. Recall that the skin is not sutured closed but is left open for pressure relief. Remembering that moist tissue needs to remain moist will direct you to option 2. Review care of a fasciotomy site if you had difficulty with this question.

*Level of Cognitive Ability:* Application
*Client Needs:* Physiological Integrity
*Integrated Concept/Process:* Nursing Process/Planning
*Content Area:* Adult Health/Musculoskeletal

*Reference*
Smeltzer, S., & Bare, B. (2000). *Brunner & Suddarth's Textbook of medical-surgical nursing* (9th ed.). Philadelphia: Lippincott Williams & Wilkins, p. 1528.

**164.** A nurse is caring for a female client who was recently admitted to the hospital with a diagnosis of anorexia nervosa. When the nurse enters the room, the client is engaged in rigorous push-ups. Which nursing action would be best?

1    Allow the client to complete the exercise program
2    Tell the client that she is not allowed to exercise rigorously
3    Interrupt the client and offer to take her for a walk
4    Interrupt the client and weigh her immediately

**Answer: 3**

*Rationale:* Clients with anorexia nervosa are frequently preoccupied with rigorous exercise and push themselves beyond normal limits to work off caloric intake. The nurse must provide for appropriate exercise as well as place limits on rigorous activities.

*Test-Taking Strategy:* Use the process of elimination, noting the key word *best*. Focus on the need for the nurse to set firm limits with clients who have this disorder. Also, recalling that the nurse needs to provide and guide the client to perform appropriate exercise will direct you to option 3. Review interventions for clients with this disorder if you had difficulty with this question.

*Level of Cognitive Ability:* Application
*Client Needs:* Physiological Integrity
*Integrated Concept/Process:* Nursing Process/Implementation
*Content Area:* Mental Health

*Reference*
Stuart, G.W., & Laraia, M.T. (1998). *Principles and practice of psychiatric nursing.* (6th ed.). St. Louis: Mosby, p. 536.

**165.** A nurse assesses the peripheral intravenous (IV) site dressing and notes that it is damp and the tape is loose. The first most appropriate nursing action is to:

1    Stop the infusion immediately and notify the physician
2    Check that the tubing is securely attached to the catheter and redress the site
3    Increase the IV flow rate to assess for further leaking
4    Remove the tape, slow the IV rate, and then discontinue the IV

**Answer: 2**

*Rationale:* If there is leakage at the IV site, the nurse should first locate the source. The nurse should assess the site further to be certain that all connections are secure. The nurse should not increase the flow rate. While it is true that it may leak more, it may also cause more tissue damage if the IV was infiltrating. While the infusion most likely will need to be stopped, the physician would not need to be notified. Slowing and discontinuing the IV is also premature. The IV must first be assessed as to the cause of the leaking.

*Test-Taking Strategy:* Note the key words *first* and *most appropriate*. Remember that the priority is to determine the cause of the leaking. Use the steps of the nursing process. Remember that assessment is the first step. Review care of a client with an IV if you had difficulty with this question.

*Level of Cognitive Ability:* Application
*Client Needs:* Physiological Integrity
*Integrated Concept/Process:* Nursing Process/Implementation
*Content Area:* Fundamental Skills

*Reference*
Potter, P., & Perry, A. (2001). *Fundamentals of nursing* (5th ed.). St. Louis: Mosby, p. 1234.

**166.** A nurse assists the physician with the removal of a chest tube. During removal of the chest tube, the nurse instructs the client to:
1  Breathe out forcefully
2  Breathe in deeply
3  Hold the breath
4  Breathe normally

**Answer: 3**
*Rationale:* The client is instructed in the Valsalva maneuver so that the client can hold the breath and bear down as the physician removes the chest tube. This maneuver will increase intrathoracic pressure, thereby lessening the potential for air to enter the pleural space. Options 1, 2, and 4 are incorrect.

*Test-Taking Strategy:* Use the process of elimination. Eliminate options 2 and 4 because they are similar in that breathing will cause air to enter the pleural space. From the remaining options, eliminate option 1 because of the word *forcefully*. Review the procedure for the removal of chest tubes if you had difficulty with this question.

*Level of Cognitive Ability:* Application
*Client Needs:* Physiological Integrity
*Integrated Concept/Process:* Nursing Process/Implementation
*Content Area:* Adult Health/Respiratory

*Reference*
Smeltzer, S., & Bare, B. (2000). *Brunner & Suddarth's Textbook of medical-surgical nursing* (9th ed.). Philadelphia: Lippincott Williams & Wilkins, p. 518.

**167.** A nurse assesses the water seal chamber of a closed chest drainage system and notes fluctuations in the chamber. The nurse determines that this finding indicates that:
1  An air leak is present
2  The tubing is kinked
3  The lung has reexpanded
4  The system is functioning as expected

**Answer: 4**
*Rationale:* Fluctuations (tidaling) in the water seal chamber are normal during inhalation and exhalation until the lung reexpands and the client no longer requires chest drainage. If fluctuations are absent, it could indicate an air leak, kinking, or that the lung has reexpanded.

*Test-Taking Strategy:* Note the key words *water seal chamber* and *fluctuations*. Recalling the normal expectations related to the functioning of chest tube drainage systems will direct you to option 4. Review the normal expectations and the indications of complications if you had difficulty with this question.

*Level of Cognitive Ability:* Analysis
*Client Needs:* Physiological Integrity
*Integrated Concept/Process:* Nursing Process/Analysis
*Content Area:* Adult Health/Respiratory

*Reference*
Smeltzer, S., & Bare, B. (2000). *Brunner & Suddarth's Textbook of medical-surgical nursing* (9th ed.). Philadelphia: Lippincott Williams & Wilkins, p. 518.

**168.** A nurse is caring for a client with depression who has not responded to antidepressant medication. The nurse anticipates that what treatment modality may be prescribed?
1  Electroconvulsive therapy
2  Psychosurgery
3  Insulin therapy medication
4  Neuroleptic medication

**Answer: 1**
*Rationale:* Electroconvulsive therapy is an effective treatment for depression that has not responded to medication. Psychosurgery is rarely performed and would not treat depression. Insulin therapy is an outmoded form of therapy. Neuroleptics are not effective in the treatment of depression.

*Test-Taking Strategy:* Use the process of elimination. Eliminate option 2 first because it is the most invasive of the options given. From the remaining options, recalling that insulin therapy and neuroleptics are not used will direct you to option 1. Review treatment measures for depression if you had difficulty with this question.

*Level of Cognitive Ability:* Analysis
*Client Needs:* Physiological Integrity
*Integrated Concept/Process:* Nursing Process/Analysis
*Content Area:* Mental Health

*Reference*
Stuart, G.W., & Laraia, M.T. (1998). *Principles and practice of psychiatric nursing.* (6th ed.). St. Louis: Mosby, p. 373.

---

**169.** A client arrives in the emergency department after being in an automobile accident. The client was physically unharmed yet was hyperventilating and complaining of dizziness and nausea. In addition, the client appeared confused and had difficulty focusing on what was going on. The nurse assesses the client's level of anxiety as:

1    Mild
2    Moderate
3    Severe
4    Panic

**Answer: 3**
*Rationale:* The person whose anxiety is assessed as severe is unable to solve problems and has difficulty focusing on what is happening in the environment. Somatic symptoms are usually present. The individual with mild anxiety is only mildly uncomfortable and may even find performance enhanced. The individual with moderate anxiety grasps less information about a situation and has some difficulty problem solving. The individual in panic will demonstrate markedly disturbed behavior and may lose touch with reality.

*Test-Taking Strategy:* Use the process of elimination. Focus on the signs and symptoms presented in the question to eliminate options 1 and 4. Noting the fact that the client had difficulty focusing on what was going on, should direct you to option 3. Review the characteristics related to the levels of anxiety if you had difficulty with this question.

*Level of Cognitive Ability:* Analysis
*Client Needs:* Physiological Integrity
*Integrated Concept/Process:* Nursing Process/Assessment
*Content Area:* Mental Health

*Reference*
Stuart, G.W., & Laraia, M.T. (1998). *Principles and practice of psychiatric nursing.* (6th ed.). St. Louis: Mosby, p. 275.

---

**170.** A child is admitted to the hospital with a diagnosis of acute rheumatic fever (RF). The nurse reviews the blood laboratory findings knowing that which of the following will confirm the likelihood of this disorder?

1    Increased leukocyte count
2    Decreased hemoglobin count
3    Increased antistreptolysin-O (ASO)
4    Decreased erythrocyte sedimentation rate

**Answer: 3**
*Rationale:* Children with suspected RF are tested for streptococcal antibodies. The best and most reliable standardized test to confirm the diagnosis is the ASO titer. An elevated level is indicative of the presence of RF.

*Test-Taking Strategy:* Use the process of elimination. Focusing on the diagnosis will assist in eliminating options 2 and 4. From the remaining options, recall that an increased leukocyte count indicates the presence of infection but is not specific in confirming a particular diagnosis. Review the diagnostic tests for RF if you had difficulty with this question.

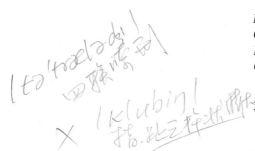

*Level of Cognitive Ability:* Analysis
*Client Needs:* Physiological Integrity
*Integrated Concept/Process:* Nursing Process/Assessment
*Content Area:* Child Health

**Reference**
Wong, D. (1999). *Whaley & Wong's Nursing care of infants and children* (6th ed.). St. Louis: Mosby, pp. 1630-1631.

---

**171.** A 5-year-old child is admitted to the hospital for heart surgery to repair tetralogy of Fallot. The nurse reviews the child's record and notes that the child has clubbed fingers. The nurse understands that the clubbing is most likely caused by:
1   Peripheral hypoxia
2   Delayed physical growth
3   Chronic hypertension
4   Destruction of bone marrow

**Answer: 1**
*Rationale:* Clubbing, a thickening and flattening of the tips of the fingers and toes, is thought to occur because of a chronic tissue hypoxia and polycythemia. Options 2, 3, and 4 do not cause clubbing.

*Test-Taking Strategy:* Use the ABCs (airway, breathing, and circulation). Hypoxia relates to oxygenation, a concern with this disorder. If you had difficulty with this question, review the manifestations associated with tetralogy of Fallot.

*Level of Cognitive Ability:* Analysis
*Client Needs:* Physiological Integrity
*Integrated Concept/Process:* Nursing Process/Analysis
*Content Area:* Child Health

**Reference**
Wong, D. (1999). *Whaley & Wong's Nursing care of infants and children* (6th ed.). St. Louis: Mosby, p. 1615.

---

**172.** An elderly client admitted to the hospital with a hip fractures is placed in Buck's traction. The nurse plans to frequently monitor the client's:
1   Vital signs
2   Mental state
3   Range of motion
4   Neurovascular status

**Answer: 4**
*Rationale:* The neurovascular status of the extremity of the client in Buck's traction must be assessed every 2 hours for the first 24 hours. Elderly clients are especially at risk for neurovascular compromise because many elderly clients already have disorders that affect the peripheral vascular system. The client's physiological status determines the frequency of vital signs, not the presence or absence of Buck's traction. Although clients in some types of traction do become depressed after a few days or weeks, Buck's traction is usually used preoperatively, which typically involves a few hours or 1 to 2 days at the most. Range of motion of the involved leg is contraindicated in hip fractures.

*Test-Taking Strategy:* Use the process of elimination, focusing on the issue: Buck's traction. Recalling the purpose of this traction and visualizing its use will direct you to option 4. Review nursing care of the client in Buck's traction if you had difficulty with this question.

*Level of Cognitive Ability:* Application
*Client Needs:* Physiological Integrity
*Integrated Concept/Process:* Nursing Process/Assessment
*Content Area:* Adult Health/Musculoskeletal

*Reference*

Smeltzer, S., & Bare, B. (2000). *Brunner & Suddarth's Textbook of medical-surgical nursing* (9th ed.). Philadelphia: Lippincott Williams & Wilkins, p. 1787.

---

**173.** A client who has a renal mass asks the nurse why ultrasonography has been scheduled, as opposed to other diagnostic tests that may be ordered. The nurse formulates a response based on the understanding that:

1   Ultrasonography can differentiate a solid mass from a fluid-filled cyst
2   Ultrasonography is much more cost effective than other diagnostic tests
3   All other tests are more invasive than ultrasonography
4   All other tests require more elaborate postprocedure care

**Answer: 1**

*Rationale:* A significant advantage of ultrasonography is that it can differentiate a solid mass from a fluid-filled cyst. It is noninvasive and does not require any special aftercare. There are other diagnostic tests, such as magnetic resonance imaging and computed tomography scanning, that are also noninvasive (unless a contrast agent is used) and that require no special aftercare either. However, it is ultrasonography that can discriminate between solid and fluid masses most optimally.

*Test-Taking Strategy:* Eliminate options 3 and 4 first because of the absolute word *all*. From the remaining options, focus on the client's diagnosis to direct you to option 1. Review the purpose of ultrasonography if you had difficulty with this question.

*Level of Cognitive Ability:* Application
*Client Needs:* Physiological Integrity
*Integrated Concept/Process:* Nursing Process/Planning
*Content Area:* Adult Health/Renal

*Reference*

Smeltzer, S., & Bare, B. (2000). *Brunner & Suddarth's Textbook of medical-surgical nursing* (9th ed.). Philadelphia: Lippincott Williams & Wilkins, p. 1094.

---

**174.** A client has been admitted to the hospital with a diagnosis of acute glomerulonephritis. On assessment, the nurse first asks the client about a recent history of:

1   Bleeding ulcer
2   Hypertension
3   Fungal infection
4   Streptococcal infection

**Answer: 4**

*Rationale:* The predominant cause of acute glomerulonephritis is infection with beta-hemolytic *Streptococcus* 3 weeks before the onset of symptoms. In addition to bacteria, infectious agents that could trigger the disorder include viruses or parasites. Hypertension and bleeding ulcer are not precipitating causes.

*Test-Taking Strategy:* Use the process of elimination. Recalling that infection is a common trigger for glomerulonephritis assists in eliminating options 1 and 2 first. From the remaining options, is necessary to know that streptococcal infections, rather than fungal infections, are a common cause of this problem. Review the causes of acute glomerulonephritis if you had difficulty with this question.

*Level of Cognitive Ability:* Application
*Client Needs:* Physiological Integrity
*Integrated Concept/Process:* Nursing Process/Assessment
*Content Area:* Adult Health/Renal

*Reference*
Smeltzer, S., & Bare, B. (2000). *Brunner & Suddarth's Textbook of medical-surgical nursing* (9th ed.). Philadelphia: Lippincott Williams & Wilkins, p. 1142.

---

**175.** A male client has just been admitted to the emergency department with chest pain. Serum enzyme levels are drawn. Results indicate an elevated creatinine phosphokinase (CPK), elevated CPK-MB, and elevated lactic dehydrogenase (LDH), with the $LDH_2$ exceeding $LDH_1$. The nurse concludes that these results are compatible with:

1   New onset myocardial infarction (MI)
2   Myocardial infarction of at least 3 days' duration
3   Unstable angina
4   Prinzmetal's angina

**Answer: 1**
*Rationale:* CPK and its cardiac isoenzyme, CPK-MB, are sensitive indicators of myocardial damage. Levels begin to rise 3 to 6 hours after the onset of chest pain, peak at approximately 24 hours, and return to normal in about 3 days. Normal values for males are 12 to 70 U/mL or 38 to 174 U/L. LDH begins to rise in 24 hours, peaks at 48 to 72 hours, and returns to normal in 7 to 14 days. $LDH_1$ rises above the level of $LDH_2$ with MI. The elevations identified in the question are consistent with new onset MI.

*Test-Taking Strategy:* Use the process of elimination. Recall that there is no permanent myocardial damage with unstable angina or Prinzmetal's angina, which eliminates options 3 and 4. From the remaining options, focus on the data in the question and note that the client is in the emergency department. These data will assist in directing you to option 1. Review the diagnostic laboratory values related to MI if you had difficulty to this question.

*Level of Cognitive Ability:* Analysis
*Client Needs:* Physiological Integrity
*Integrated Concept/Process:* Nursing Process/Analysis
*Content Area:* Adult Health/Cardiovascular

*Reference*
Smeltzer, S., & Bare, B. (2000). *Brunner & Suddarth's Textbook of medical-surgical nursing* (9th ed.). Philadelphia: Lippincott Williams & Wilkins, p. 626.

---

**176.** A client with heart failure has cardiomegaly noted on a chest x-ray film. As part of cardiac assessment, the nurse auscultates the apical rate and places the stethoscope:

1   At the normal point of maximal impulse (PMI)
2   Slightly upward and medial to the normal PMI
3   Slightly downward and medial to the normal PMI
4   Lateral to the normal PMI

**Answer: 4**
*Rationale:* The point of maximal impulse (PMI), where the apical rate is auscultated, is normally located in the fifth intercostal space, midclavicular line. With heart failure, the heart enlarges, shifting the PMI laterally.

*Test-Taking Strategy:* First it is necessary to recall the thoracic landmarks. Next, visualize the position of the heart in the thoracic cavity and picture the displacement of the heart when enlarged. This will direct you to option 4. Review thoracic landmarks if you had difficulty with this question.

*Level of Cognitive Ability:* Application
*Client Needs:* Physiological Integrity
*Integrated Concept/Process:* Nursing Process/Assessment
*Content Area:* Adult Health/Cardiovascular

*Reference*
Smeltzer, S., & Bare, B. (2000). *Brunner & Suddarth's Textbook of medical-surgical nursing* (9th ed.). Philadelphia: Lippincott Williams & Wilkins, p. 547.

---

**177.** A nurse is caring for a client receiving bolus feedings via a Levin-type nasogastric tube. As the nurse is finishing the feeding, the client asks for the bed to be positioned flat to sleep. The nurse explains to the client that the most appropriate position at this time is which of the following?

1 Head of the bed flat with the client in the supine position for at least 30 minutes
2 Head of the bed elevated 35 to 40 degrees with the client in the right-lateral position for at least 30 minutes
3 Head of the bed elevated 45 to 60 degrees with the client in the supine position for at least 60 minutes
4 Head of the bed in semi-Fowler's position with the client in the left-lateral position for at least 60 minutes

**Answer: 2**

*Rationale:* Aspiration is a possible complication associated with nasogastric tube feeding. The head of the bed is elevated 35 to 40 degrees for at least 30 minutes following bolus tube feeding to prevent vomiting and aspiration. The right-lateral position uses gravity to facilitate gastric retention to prevent vomiting. The flat supine position is avoided for the first 30 minutes after a tube feeding.

*Test-Taking Strategy:* Use the process of elimination. Note that each option includes the level of elevation of the head, the client's position, and the duration. Option 1 is eliminated first because the flat position could result in aspiration. Option 3 is also eliminated because of the supine position and the longer duration. From the remaining options, it is necessary to recall that the right-lateral position facilitates gravity. Review care of a client receiving tube feedings if you had difficulty with this question.

*Level of Cognitive Ability:* Application
*Client Needs:* Physiological Integrity
*Integrated Concept/Process:* Nursing Process/Implementation
*Content Area:* Fundamental Skills

*Reference*
Smeltzer, S., & Bare, B. (2000). *Brunner & Suddarth's Textbook of medical-surgical nursing* (9th ed.). Philadelphia: Lippincott Williams & Wilkins, p. 840.

---

**178.** A nurse is caring for a client with acute pancreatitis who has a history of alcoholism. The nurse closely monitors the client for paralytic ileus knowing that which assessment data indicate this complication of pancreatitis?

1 Firm, nontender mass palpable at the lower right costal margin
2 Severe, constant pain with rapid onset
3 Inability to pass flatus
4 Loss of anal sphincter control

**Answer: 3**

*Rationale:* An inflammatory reaction such as acute pancreatitis can cause paralytic ileus, the most common form of nonmechanical obstruction. Inability to pass flatus is a clinical manifestation of paralytic ileus. Option 1 is the description of the physical finding of liver enlargement. The liver is usually enlarged in the client with cirrhosis or hepatitis. Although this client may have an enlarged liver, an enlarged liver is not a sign of paralytic ileus or intestinal obstruction. Pain is associated with paralytic ileus, but the pain usually presents as a more constant generalized discomfort. Pain that is severe, constant, and rapid in onset is more likely caused by strangulation of the bowel. Loss of sphincter control is not a sign of paralytic ileus.

*Test-Taking Strategy:* Focus on the issue: a sign of paralytic ileus. Recalling the definition of this complication will direct you to option 3. Review the signs of paralytic ileus if you had difficulty with this question.

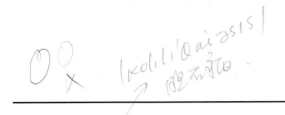

Level of Cognitive Ability: Application
*Client Needs:* Physiological Integrity
*Integrated Concept/Process:* Nursing Process/Assessment
*Content Area:* Adult Health/Gastrointestinal

*Reference*
Smeltzer, S., & Bare, B. (2000). *Brunner & Suddarth's Textbook of medical-surgical nursing* (9th ed.). Philadelphia: Lippincott Williams & Wilkins, p. 368.

**179.** After performing an initial abdominal assessment on a client with a diagnosis of cholelithiasis, the nurse documents that the bowel sounds are normal. Which of the following descriptions best describes this assessment finding?
1   Waves of loud gurgles auscultated in all four quadrants
2   Very high-pitched loud rushes auscultated especially in one or two quadrants
3   Relatively high-pitched clicks or gurgles auscultated in all four quadrants
4   Low-pitched swishing auscultated in one or two quadrants

**Answer: 3**
*Rationale:* Although frequency and intensity of bowel sounds will vary depending on the phase of digestion, normal bowel sounds are relatively high-pitched clicks or gurgles. Loud gurgles (borborygmi) indicate hyperperistalsis. Bowel sounds will be more high pitched and loud (hyperresonance) when the intestines are under tension, such as in intestinal obstruction. A swishing or buzzing sound represents turbulent blood flow associated with a bruit. No aortic bruits should be heard.

*Test-Taking Strategy:* Use the process of elimination. Normally, bowel sounds should be audible in all four quadrants, and therefore options 2 and 4 can be eliminated. From the remaining options, select option 3 because it is more thoroughly descriptive of normal bowel sounds. Review normal abdominal assessment findings if you had difficulty with this question.

*Level of Cognitive Ability:* Analysis
*Client Needs:* Physiological Integrity
*Integrated Concept/Process:* Nursing Process/Assessment
*Content Area:* Adult Health/Gastrointestinal

*Reference*
Potter, P., & Perry, A. (2001). *Fundamentals of nursing* (5th ed.). St. Louis: Mosby, p. 802.

**180.** A nurse is assigned to care for a client with nephrotic syndrome. The nurse assesses which of the following most important parameters on a daily basis?
1   Albumin levels
2   Weight
3   Blood urea nitrogen (BUN) level
4   Activity tolerance

**Answer: 2**
*Rationale:* The client with nephrotic syndrome typically presents with edema, hypoalbuminemia, and proteinuria. The nurse carefully assesses the fluid balance of the client, which includes daily monitoring of weight, intake and output, edema, and girth measurements. Albumin levels are monitored as they are prescribed, as are the BUN and creatinine levels. The client's activity level is adjusted according to the amount of edema and water retention. As edema increases, the client's activity level should be restricted.

*Test-Taking Strategy:* Use the process of elimination noting the key words *daily basis*. Recalling the typical signs of nephrotic syndrome will direct you to option 2. Review these signs if you had difficulty with this question.

*Level of Cognitive Ability:* Application
*Client Needs:* Physiological Integrity
*Integrated Concept/Process:* Nursing Process/Assessment
*Content Area:* Adult Health/Renal

*Reference*
Smeltzer, S., & Bare, B. (2000). *Brunner & Suddarth's Textbook of medical-surgical nursing* (9th ed.). Philadelphia: Lippincott Williams & Wilkins, p. 1142.

---

**181.** A client is being admitted to the hospital with a diagnosis of urolithiasis and ureteral colic. The nurse assesses the client for pain that is:

1　Dull and aching in the costovertebral area
2　Sharp and radiating posteriorly to the spinal column
3　Excruciating, wavelike, and radiating toward the genitalia
4　Aching and cramplike throughout the abdomen

**Answer: 3**

*Rationale:* The pain of ureteral colic is caused by movement of a stone through the ureter and is sharp, excruciating and wavelike, radiating to the genitalia and thigh. The stone causes reduced flow of urine, and the urine also contains blood because of the stone's abrasive action on urinary tract mucosa. Stones in the renal pelvis cause pain that is a deep ache in the costovertebral area. Renal colic is characterized by pain that is acute, with tenderness over the costovertebral area.

*Test-Taking Strategy:* Use the process of elimination, focusing on the diagnosis, urolithiasis and ureteral colic. Recall the anatomical location of the kidneys and the ureters. Since the kidneys are located in the posterior abdomen near the ribcage, pain in the costovertebral area is more likely to be associated with stones in the renal pelvis. On the other hand, sharp wavelike pain that radiates toward the genitalia is more consistent with the location of the ureters in the abdomen. Review the assessment findings in this disorder if you had difficulty with this question.

*Level of Cognitive Ability:* Analysis
*Client Needs:* Physiological Integrity
*Integrated Concept/Process:* Nursing Process/Assessment
*Content Area:* Adult Health/Renal

*Reference*
Smeltzer, S., & Bare, B. (2000). *Brunner & Suddarth's Textbook of medical-surgical nursing* (9th ed.). Philadelphia: Lippincott Williams & Wilkins, p. 1163.

---

**182.** A nurse is assessing a client with left-sided heart failure. The client states that it is necessary to use three pillows under the head and chest at night to be able to breathe comfortably while sleeping. The nurse documents that the client is experiencing:

1　Dyspnea on exertion
2　Dyspnea at rest
3　Orthopnea
4　Paroxysmal nocturnal dyspnea

**Answer: 3**

*Rationale:* Dyspnea is a subjective complaint that can range from an awareness of breathing to physical distress and does not necessarily correlate with the degree of heart failure. Dyspnea can be exertional or at rest. Orthopnea is a more severe form of dyspnea, requiring the client to assume a "three-point" position while upright and to use pillows to support the head and thorax at night. Paroxysmal nocturnal dyspnea is a severe form of dyspnea occurring suddenly at night as a result of rapid fluid reentry into the vasculature from the interstitium during sleep.

*Test-Taking Strategy:* Use the process of elimination and knowledge of the different degrees of dyspnea. Eliminate options 1 and 4 because the question mentions nothing about exertion or a sudden (paroxysmal) event. From the remaining options, select option 3 over 2 because the client is breathing "comfortably" with the use of pillows. Review the various descriptions of dyspnea if you had difficulty with this question.

*Level of Cognitive Ability:* Analysis
*Client Needs:* Physiological Integrity
*Integrated Concept/Process:* Communication and Documentation
*Content Area:* Adult Health/Cardiovascular

*Reference*

Smeltzer, S., & Bare, B. (2000). *Brunner & Suddarth's Textbook of medical-surgical nursing* (9th ed.). Philadelphia: Lippincott Williams & Wilkins, p. 664.

---

**183.** A nurse witnesses a client going into pulmonary edema. The client exhibits respiratory distress, but the blood pressure is stable at this time. As an immediate action before help arrives, the nurse plans to first:

1 Suction the client's airway vigorously
2 Place the client in high-Fowler's position
3 Begin assembling medications that the nurse anticipates will be given
4 Call the respiratory therapy department for a ventilator

**Answer: 2**

*Rationale:* The client in pulmonary edema is placed in high-Fowler's position, if the blood pressure is stable. Vigorous suctioning may deplete the client of vital oxygen at a time when the respiratory system is compromised. Assembling medications is useful, but not critical to the immediate well-being of the client. The client may or may not need mechanical ventilation.

*Test-Taking Strategy:* Use the process of elimination. Note the key words *respiratory distress* and *first* to assist in eliminating options 3 and 4. From the remaining options, note that option 2 is preferable because it will enhance the client's respirations, while option 1 may impair oxygenation, as implied by the word *vigorously* in that option. Review the initial nursing interventions for a client in pulmonary edema if you had difficulty with this question.

*Level of Cognitive Ability:* Application
*Client Needs:* Physiological Integrity
*Integrated Concept/Process:* Nursing Process/Implementation
*Content Area:* Adult Health/Cardiovascular

*Reference*

Smeltzer, S., & Bare, B. (2000). *Brunner & Suddarth's Textbook of medical-surgical nursing* (9th ed.). Philadelphia: Lippincott Williams & Wilkins, p. 657.

**184.** A nurse suspects that cardiogenic shock is developing in a client who had a myocardial infarction. The nurse assesses for which of the following peripheral vascular manifestations of this complication?

1    Flushed, dry skin with bounding pedal pulses
2    Warm, moist skin with irregular pedal pulses
3    Cool, dry skin with alternating weak and strong pedal pulses
4    Cool, clammy skin with weak or thready pedal pulses

**Answer: 4**

*Rationale:* Classic signs of cardiogenic shock include increased pulse (weak and thready), decreased blood pressure, decreasing urinary output, signs of cerebral ischemia (confusion, agitation), and cool, clammy skin.

*Test-Taking Strategy:* Use the process of elimination and recall the signs and symptoms of shock. The word *clammy* in option 4 should direct you to this option. Review the signs of cardiogenic shock if you had difficulty with this question.

*Level of Cognitive Ability:* Analysis
*Client Needs:* Physiological Integrity
*Integrated Concept/Process:* Nursing Process/Assessment
*Content Area:* Adult Health/Cardiovascular

*Reference*
Smeltzer, S., & Bare, B. (2000). *Brunner & Suddarth's Textbook of medical-surgical nursing* (9th ed.). Philadelphia: Lippincott Williams & Wilkins, p. 672.

**185.** A nurse is caring for a client who returns from cardiac surgery with chest tubes in place. The nurse measures the drainage on an hourly basis and assesses that the client is stable as long as drainage does not exceed how many milliliters over the first 24 hours?

1    100
2    200
3    500
4    1000

**Answer: 3**

*Rationale:* Approximately 500 mL of drainage is expected in the first 24 hours after cardiac surgery. Up to 100 mL may be lost in the first hour postoperatively. The nurse measures and records the drainage on an hourly basis. The drainage is initially dark red and becomes more serous over time.

*Test-Taking Strategy:* Focus on the issue: a postoperative client. Eliminate options 1 and 2 because the values are so small. From the remaining options, try converting the drainage to liters, recalling that 1000 mL = 1 L and 500 mL = 0.5 L. Knowing that there is only about 6 L of blood circulating in the body will direct you to option 3. Review the expected postoperative findings following cardiac surgery if you had difficulty with this question.

*Level of Cognitive Ability:* Analysis
*Client Needs:* Physiological Integrity
*Integrated Concept/Process:* Nursing Process/Analysis
*Content Area:* Adult Health/Cardiovascular

*Reference*
Ignatavicius, D., Workman, M., & Mishler, M. (1999). *Medical-surgical nursing across the health care continuum* (3rd ed.). Philadelphia: W.B. Saunders, p. 649.

**186.** A client with renal cancer is being treated preoperatively with radiation therapy. The nurse evaluates that the client has an understanding of proper care of the skin over the treatment field if the client states the need to:
1 Avoid skin exposure to direct sunlight and chlorinated water
2 Use lanolin-based cream on the affected skin on a daily basis
3 Remove the lines or ink marks using a gentle soap after each treatment
4 Use the hottest water possible to wash the treatment site twice daily

**Answer: 1**
*Rationale:* The client undergoing radiation therapy should avoid washing the site until instructed to do so. The client should then wash using mild soap and warm or cool water, and pat the area dry. No lotions, creams, alcohol, or deodorants should be placed on the skin over the treatment site. Lines or ink marks that are placed on the skin to guide the radiation therapy should be left in place. The affected skin should be protected from temperature extremes, direct sunlight, and chlorinated water (as from swimming pools).

*Test-Taking Strategy:* Use the process of elimination, noting the key words *understanding of proper care*. Eliminate options 2 and 4 first because of the words *lanolin-based cream* and *hottest*. From the remaining options, recalling that the lines and ink marks guide therapy will direct you to option 1. Review client teaching related to radiation if you had difficulty with this question.

*Level of Cognitive Ability:* Analysis
*Client Needs:* Physiological Integrity
*Integrated Concept/Process:* Self Care
*Content Area:* Adult Health/Oncology

*Reference*
Smeltzer, S., & Bare, B. (2000). *Brunner & Suddarth's Textbook of medical-surgical nursing* (9th ed.). Philadelphia: Lippincott Williams & Wilkins, p. 276.

**187.** A client with renal failure is receiving epoetin alfa (Epogen) to support erythropoiesis. The nurse questions the client about compliance with taking which of the following medications that supports red blood cell (RBC) production?
1 Calcium supplement
2 Iron supplement
3 Magnesium supplement
4 Zinc supplement

**Answer: 2**
*Rationale:* Iron is needed for RBC production. Otherwise, the body cannot produce sufficient erythrocytes or produce cells that are deficient in iron. In either case, the client is not receiving the full benefit of epoetin alfa therapy if iron is not taken.

*Test-Taking Strategy:* Use the process of elimination. Note the relationship of RBC production in the question and iron in the correct option. Review the concepts related to epoetin alfa and RBC production if you had difficulty with this question.

*Level of Cognitive Ability:* Application
*Client Needs:* Physiological Integrity
*Integrated Concept/Process:* Nursing Process/Assessment
*Content Area:* Adult Health/Renal

*Reference*
Monahan, F., & Neighbors, M. (1998). *Medical-surgical nursing: Foundations for clinical practice* (2nd ed.). Philadelphia: W.B. Saunders, p. 469.

**188.** A home health nurse is performing an initial assessment on a client who has arrived home with a permanent pacemaker following cardiac surgery. The nurse determines the client's ability regarding self-care related to the pacemaker when the nurse:

1 Asks the client to take the pulse in the wrist or neck and checks the accuracy of the client's reading

2 Determines whether the client knows not to operate a microwave oven

3 Determines whether the client knows that he or she can resume sexual activity immediately

4 Asks the client to move the arms and shoulders vigorously to check pacemaker functioning

**Answer: 1**

*Rationale:* Clients with permanent pacemakers must be able to take their pulse in the wrist or neck accurately in order to note any variation in the pulse rate or rhythm that may need to be reported to the physician. Clients can safely operate microwave ovens, VCRs, AM-FM radios, electric blankets, lawn mowers, leaf blowers, and cars. Proper grounding must be ensured if the client is to operate electric typewriters, copying machines, and personal computers. Sexual activity is not resumed until 6 weeks after surgery. The arms and shoulders should not be moved vigorously for 6 weeks after insertion.

*Test-Taking Strategy:* Use the process of elimination. Eliminate option 3 because of the word *immediately* and option 4 because of the word *vigorously*. From the remaining options, select option 1 because a pacemaker assists in controlling cardiac rate and rhythm. Review client teaching points related to a pacemaker if you had difficulty with this question.

*Level of Cognitive Ability:* Analysis
*Client Needs:* Physiological Integrity
*Integrated Concept/Process:* Teaching/Learning
*Content Area:* Adult Health/Cardiovascular

*Reference*
Smeltzer, S., & Bare, B. (2000). *Brunner & Suddarth's Textbook of medical-surgical nursing* (9th ed.). Philadelphia: Lippincott Williams & Wilkins, pp. 588-589.

---

**189.** A client with a severe major depressive episode is unable to address activities of daily living. The most appropriate nursing intervention would be to:

1 Feed, bathe, and dress the client as needed until the client can perform these activities independently

2 Structure the client's day so that adequate time can be devoted to the client's assuming responsibility for the activities of daily living

3 Offer the client choices and describe the consequences of failure to comply with the expectation of maintaining activities of daily living

4 Have the client's peers confront the client about how noncompliance in addressing activities of daily living affects the milieu

**Answer: 1**

*Rationale:* The symptoms of major depression include depressed mood, loss of interest or pleasure, changes in appetite and sleep patterns, psychomotor agitation or retardation, fatigue, feelings of worthlessness or guilt, diminished ability to think or concentrate, and recurrent thoughts of death. Often, the client does not have the energy or interest to complete activities of daily living. Option 2 is incorrect because the client still lacks the energy and motivation to do these independently. Option 3 may lead to increased feelings of worthlessness as the client fails to meet expectations. Option 4 will increase the client's feelings of poor self-esteem and unworthiness.

*Test-Taking Strategy:* Focus on the client's diagnosis and the issue of the question. Use Maslow's Hierarchy of Needs theory. Remember, physiological needs are the priority. Review care of a client with depression if you had difficulty with this question.

*Level of Cognitive Ability:* Application
*Client Needs:* Physiological Integrity
*Integrated Concept/Process:* Nursing Process/Implementation
*Content Area:* Mental Health

*Reference*
Stuart, G.W., & Laraia, M.T. (1998). *Principles and practice of psychiatric nursing.* (6th ed.). St. Louis: Mosby, p. 352.

**190.** A pregnant woman who is at 32 weeks' gestation is admitted to the obstetric unit for observation after an automobile accident. The client is experiencing slight vaginal bleeding and mild cramps. The nurse does which of the following to determine the viability of the fetus?

1   Inserts an intravenous line and begins an infusion at 125 mL/hr
2   Administers oxygen to the woman via a face mask at 7 to 10 L/min
3   Positions and connects the ultrasound transducer and the tocotransducer to the external fetal monitor
4   Positions and connects a spiral electrode to the fetal monitor for internal fetal monitoring

**Answer: 3**

*Rationale:* External fetal monitoring will allow the nurse to determine any change in the fetal heart rate and rhythm that would indicate that the fetus is in jeopardy. Internal monitoring is contraindicated when there is vaginal bleeding of an unstated cause, especially in preterm labor. Since fetal distress has not been determined at this time, oxygen administration is premature. The amount of bleeding described is insufficient to require intravenous fluid replacement.

*Test-Taking Strategy:* Focus on the client of the question, the fetus. Next, use the steps of the nursing process, and note that option 3 is the noninvasive measure. Review fetal assessment techniques if you had difficulty with this question.

*Level of Cognitive Ability:* Application
*Client Needs:* Physiological Integrity
*Integrated Concept/Process:* Nursing Process/Implementation
*Content Area:* Maternity

**Reference**
Lowdermilk, D., Perry, S., & Bobak, I. (2000). *Maternity & women's health care* (7th ed.). St. Louis: Mosby, p. 491.

---

**191.** A nurse is reviewing the results of a sweat test performed on a child with cystic fibrosis (CF). The nurse would expect to note which finding?

1   A sweat sodium concentration less than 40 mEq/L
2   A sweat potassium concentration less than 40 mEq/L
3   A sweat potassium concentration greater than 40 mEq/L
4   A sweat chloride concentration greater than 60 mEq/L

**Answer: 4**

*Rationale:* A consistent finding of an abnormally high sodium and chloride concentrations in the sweat is a unique characteristic of CF. Normally, the sweat chloride concentration is less than 40 mEq/L. A chloride concentration greater than 60 mEq/L is diagnostic of CF. Potassium concentration is unrelated to the sweat test.

*Test-Taking Strategy:* Use the process of elimination. Eliminate options 2 and 3 first because the potassium level is unrelated to the sweat test. From the remaining options, note that option 4 indicates a "greater" value. Review this test if you had difficulty with this question.

*Level of Cognitive Ability:* Analysis
*Client Needs:* Physiological Integrity
*Integrated Concept/Process:* Nursing Process/Analysis
*Content Area:* Child Health

**Reference**
Wong, D. (1999). *Whaley & Wong's Nursing care of infants and children* (6th ed.). St. Louis: Mosby, p. 1521.

**192.** A nurse is assessing a client with a Miller-Abbott tube. Which finding indicates correct placement of the tube?

  1   A pH of aspirate of 7.0 or greater
  2   A pH of aspirate less than 7.0
  3   The presence of gastric contents when checking residuals
  4   The auscultation of air when the tube is inserted into the abdomen

**Answer: 1**
*Rationale:* The Miller-Abbott tube is an intestinal tube. The nurse ensures intestinal placement by checking the pH of aspirate. A pH reading greater than 7 indicates intestinal contents; one less than 7 indicates gastric contents.

*Test-Taking Strategy:* Use the process of elimination. Recalling that the Miller-Abbott tube is an intestinal tube will assist in eliminating options 3 and 4. From the remaining options, recalling that intestinal fluid is alkaline will assist in directing you to option 1. Review the principles associated with the care of a client with a Miller-Abbott tube if you had difficulty with this question.

*Level of Cognitive Ability:* Analysis
*Client Needs:* Physiological Integrity
*Integrated Concept/Process:* Nursing Process/Analysis
*Content Area:* Adult Health/Gastrointestinal

*Reference*
Smeltzer, S., & Bare, B. (2000). *Brunner & Suddarth's Textbook of medical-surgical nursing* (9th ed.). Philadelphia: Lippincott Williams & Wilkins, p. 838.

**193.** A nurse performs a neurovascular assessment on a client with a newly applied cast. Close observation and further evaluation would be required if the nurse notes:

  1   Capillary refill less than 6 seconds
  2   Palpable pulses distal to the cast
  3   Sensation when the area distal to the cast is pinched
  4   Blanching of the nail bed when depressed

**Answer: 1**
*Rationale:* To assess for adequate circulation, the nail bed of each finger or toe is depressed until it blanches, and then the pressure is released. Optimally, the color will change from white to pink rapidly (less than 3 seconds). If this does not occur, the toes or fingers will require close observation and further evaluation. Palpable pulses and sensations distal to the cast are expected. However, if pulses could not be palpated or if the client complained of numbness or tingling, the physician should be notified.

*Test-Taking Strategy:* Use the process of elimination. Note the key words *close observation and further evaluation.* Eliminate options 2, 3, and 4 because these options identify normal expected findings. Option 1 identifies an abnormal or unexpected finding. Review assessment of capillary refill if you had difficulty with this question.

*Level of Cognitive Ability:* Analysis
*Client Needs:* Physiological Integrity
*Integrated Concept/Process:* Nursing Process/Assessment
*Content Area:* Adult Health/Neurological

*Reference*
Smeltzer, S., & Bare, B. (2000). *Brunner & Suddarth's Textbook of medical-surgical nursing* (9th ed.). Philadelphia: Lippincott Williams & Wilkins, p. 1783.

**194.** A nurse is preparing to care for a client arriving from the operating room following a wedge resection of the right lower lobe. In planning for the client's safety, the nurse:

1   Removes obstructions to the transport stretcher
2   Notifies the pharmacy of the client's location
3   Places rubber-shod clamps at the bedside
4   Ensures that the wall suction unit is operational

**Answer: 3**

*Rationale:* Following wedge resection, the client will have a chest tube. Clamps should always be available at the bedside of a client with a closed drainage system so that they can be applied in the event of an accidental disconnection of the drainage tubing. It is also important to remember that chest tubes are never clamped without specific orders of the physician, except in emergencies. While operational wall suction is desirable, it does not directly affect the safety of the client. Option 1 relates to safety but is less directly related to the client. Option 2 is unrelated to the issue of the question.

*Test-Taking Strategy:* Focus on the issue of safety and note that the client had a wedge resection. Recalling that the client will have a chest tube will direct you to option 3. Review postoperative expectations following wedge resection if you had difficulty with this question.

*Level of Cognitive Ability:* Application
*Client Needs:* Physiological Integrity
*Integrated Concept/Process:* Nursing Process/Planning
*Content Area:* Adult Health/Respiratory

*Reference*
Smeltzer, S., & Bare, B. (2000). *Brunner & Suddarth's Textbook of medical-surgical nursing* (9th ed.). Philadelphia: Lippincott Williams & Wilkins, p. 518.

**195.** A nurse is caring for a client admitted to the surgical nursing unit following right modified radical mastectomy. The nurse includes which of the following in the nursing plan of care for this client?

1   Position the client supine with the right arm elevated on a pillow
2   Take blood pressures in the right arm only
3   Draw serum laboratory samples from the right arm only
4   Check the right posterior axilla area when assessing the surgical dressing

**Answer: 4**

*Rationale:* If there is drainage or bleeding from the surgical site after mastectomy, gravity will cause the drainage to seep down and soak the posterior axillary portion of the dressing first. The nurse checks this area to detect early bleeding. The client should be positioned with the head in semi-Fowler's position and the arm elevated on pillows to decrease edema. Edema is likely to occur because lymph drainage channels have been resected during the surgical procedure. Blood pressure, venipunctures, and IV sites should not involve use of the operative arm.

*Test-Taking Strategy:* Use the process of elimination. Eliminate options 2 and 3 first because of the words *right arm only*. From the remaining options, use knowledge of the effects of gravity to direct you to option 4. Review care of a client following mastectomy if you had difficulty with this question.

*Level of Cognitive Ability:* Application
*Client Needs:* Physiological Integrity
*Integrated Concept/Process:* Nursing Process/Planning
*Content Area:* Adult Health/Oncology

*Reference*
Smeltzer, S., & Bare, B. (2000). *Brunner & Suddarth's Textbook of medical-surgical nursing* (9th ed.). Philadelphia: Lippincott Williams & Wilkins, p. 1273.

**196.** A nurse is assisting the client with hepatic encephalopathy to fill out the dietary menu. The nurse advises the client to avoid which of the following entree items that could aggravate the client's condition?

1 Fresh fruit plate
2 Tomato soup
3 Vegetable lasagna
4 Ground beef patty

**Answer: 4**

*Rationale:* Clients with hepatic encephalopathy have impaired ability to convert ammonia to urea and must limit dietary intake of protein- and ammonia-containing foods. The client should avoid foods such as chicken, beef, ham, cheese, buttermilk, Idaho potatoes, onions, peanut butter, and gelatin.

*Test-Taking Strategy:* Use the process of elimination, focusing on the client's diagnosis. Note that options 1, 2, and 3 are similar in that they address food items of a fruit and vegetable nature. Review dietary measures for the client with hepatic encephalopathy if you had difficulty with this question.

*Level of Cognitive Ability:* Application
*Client Needs:* Physiological Integrity
*Integrated Concept/Process:* Teaching/Learning
*Content Area:* Adult Health/Gastrointestinal

*Reference*
Smeltzer, S., & Bare, B. (2000). *Brunner & Suddarth's Textbook of medical-surgical nursing* (9th ed.). Philadelphia: Lippincott Williams & Wilkins, p. 938.

**197.** A client with a colostomy is complaining of gas building up in the colostomy bag. The nurse instructs the client that which of the following food items will not aggravate this problem?

1 Beans
2 Cauliflower
3 Potatoes
4 Corn

**Answer: 3**

*Rationale:* Gas-forming foods include corn, cauliflower, onions, beans, and cabbage. These should be avoided by the client with a colostomy until tolerance to them is determined.

*Test-Taking Strategy:* Focus on the issue: gas-forming foods. Note the similarity between options 1, 2, and 4 in terms of their food substance. Review those food items that are gas-forming if you had difficulty with this question.

*Level of Cognitive Ability:* Application
*Client Needs:* Physiological Integrity
*Integrated Concept/Process:* Teaching/Learning
*Content Area:* Adult Health/Gastrointestinal

*Reference*
Monahan, F., & Neighbors, M. (1998). *Medical-surgical nursing: Foundations for clinical practice* (2nd ed.). Philadelphia: W.B. Saunders, p. 961

**198.** A client receiving total parenteral nutrition (TPN) complains of nausea, excessive thirst, and increased frequency of voiding. A nurse initially assesses which of the following client data?

1 Serum blood urea nitrogen and creatinine
2 Capillary blood glucose
3 Last serum potassium
4 Rectal temperature

**Answer: 2**

*Rationale:* The symptoms exhibited by the client are consistent with hyperglycemia. The nurse would need to assess the client's blood glucose level to verify these data. Clients receiving TPN are at risk for hyperglycemia related to the increased glucose load of the solution. The other options would not provide any information that would correlate with the client symptoms.

*Test-Taking Strategy:* Focus on the client's symptoms and think about the complications of TPN. Recalling that hyperglycemia is a complication will direct you to option 2. Review the complications associated with TPN if you had difficulty with this question.

*Level of Cognitive Ability:* Analysis
*Client Needs:* Physiological Integrity
*Integrated Concept/Process:* Nursing Process/Assessment
*Content Area:* Adult Health/Gastrointestinal

*Reference*
Monahan, F., & Neighbors, M. (1998). *Medical-surgical nursing: Foundations for clinical practice* (2nd ed.). Philadelphia: W.B. Saunders, p. 987.

**199.** A client admitted to the hospital with a diagnosis of cirrhosis has massive ascites and has difficulty breathing. A nurse performs which intervention as a priority measure to assist the client with breathing?
1 Auscultates the lung fields every 4 hours
2 Repositions side to side every 2 hours
3 Encourages deep breathing exercises every 2 hours
4 Elevates the head of the bed 60 degrees

**Answer: 4**
*Rationale:* The client is having difficulty breathing because of upward pressure on the diaphragm from the ascitic fluid. Elevating the head of the bed enlists the aid of gravity in relieving pressure on the diaphragm. The other options are general measures to promote lung expansion in the client with ascites, but the priority measure is the one that relieves diaphragmatic pressure.

*Test-Taking Strategy:* Note the key words *priority measure* and the issue: assisting with breathing. Recalling that elevating the head will provide immediate relief of symptoms will direct you to option 4. Review care of a client with ascites who is having difficulty breathing if you had difficulty with this question.

*Level of Cognitive Ability:* Application
*Client Needs:* Physiological Integrity
*Integrated Concept/Process:* Nursing Process/Implementation
*Content Area:* Adult Health/Gastrointestinal

*Reference*
Monahan, F., & Neighbors, M. (1998). *Medical-surgical nursing: Foundations for clinical practice* (2nd ed.). Philadelphia: W.B. Saunders, p. 1190.

**200.** A client with diverticulitis has just been advanced from a liquid diet to solids. The nurse encourages the client to eat foods that are:
1 Low residue
2 High residue
3 Moderate in fat
4 High roughage

**Answer: 1**
*Rationale:* The purpose of a low-residue diet for a client with diverticulitis is to allow the bowel to rest while the inflammation subsides. The client should avoid foods such as nuts, corn, popcorn, and raw celery, which are high in roughage.

*Test-Taking Strategy:* Use the process of elimination. Eliminate options 2 and 4 first because they are similar. From the remaining options, recalling that diverticulitis indicates inflammation will direct you to option 1. If this question was difficult, review the diet prescribed for this disorder.

*Level of Cognitive Ability:* Application
*Client Needs:* Physiological Integrity
*Integrated Concept/Process:* Nursing Process/Implementation
*Content Area:* Adult Health/Gastrointestinal

*Reference*
Monahan, F., & Neighbors, M. (1998). *Medical-surgical nursing: Foundations for clinical practice* (2nd ed.). Philadelphia: W.B. Saunders, pp. 1083-1084.

**201.** A client with Cushing's syndrome is being admitted to the hospital after a stab wound to the abdomen. The nurse places highest priority on which of the following nursing diagnoses developed for this client?
1    Risk for Fluid Volume Deficit
2    Risk for Infection
3    Body Image Disturbance
4    Altered Health Maintenance

**Answer: 2**
*Rationale:* The client with a stab wound has a break in the body's first line of defense against infection. The client with Cushing's syndrome is at great risk for infection as a result of excess cortisol secretion, subsequent impaired antibody function, and decreased proliferation of lymphocytes. The client may also have an Altered Health Maintenance and Body Image Disturbance, but these are not the highest priority at this time. The client would be at risk for Fluid Volume Excess, not Fluid Volume Deficit, with Cushing's syndrome.

*Test-Taking Strategy:* Note the key words *highest priority*. Use Maslow's Hierarchy of Needs theory to eliminate options 3 and 4. From the remaining options, focus on the client's diagnosis. Eliminate option 1 because it is the opposite of what is expected with this disorder. Review the needs of a client with Cushing's syndrome if you had difficulty with this question.

*Level of Cognitive Ability:* Analysis
*Client Needs:* Physiological Integrity
*Integrated Concept/Process:* Nursing Process/Analysis
*Content Area:* Adult Health/Endocrine

*Reference*
Monahan, F., & Neighbors, M. (1998). *Medical-surgical nursing: Foundations for clinical practice* (2nd ed.). Philadelphia: W.B. Saunders, pp. 1286-1289.

**202.** A female adolescent client is admitted to the mental health unit after medical stabilization for an overdose of acetaminophen (Tylenol). The client's boyfriend broke up with her 2 weeks ago. The client stopped eating at that time and has lost 15 pounds. The nurse avoids which of the following when caring for the client?
1    Offer frequent, nutritious snacks
2    Provide meals on a tray that contains no glass or metal utensils
3    Stand the client in front of a mirror to show her how thin she is
4    Offer bland, easy to digest foods

**Answer: 3**
*Rationale:* The client has been denying herself food as a means of self-harm. Reinforcing her success at this is not therapeutic. Meeting her nutritional needs is the nursing care priority. Options 1 and 4 meet the client's nutritional needs. Option 2 is a necessary safety measure.

*Test-Taking Strategy:* Note the key word *avoids*. Use Maslow's Hierarchy of Needs theory. Options 1 and 4 address a physiological need. Option 2 addresses both a physiological and safety need. Option 3 addresses a psychosocial need. Review care of a client at risk for self-harm if you had difficulty with this question.

*Level of Cognitive Ability:* Application
*Client Needs:* Physiological Integrity
*Integrated Concept/Process:* Nursing Process/Implementation
*Content Area:* Mental Health

*Reference*
Stuart, G.W., & Laraia, M.T. (1998). *Principles and practice of psychiatric nursing.* (6th ed.). St. Louis: Mosby, p. 538.

1 kari baksi'himəglobin !
- ⅔ ⅞ 을 ⅞ ₱12 ℓ.

**203.** A nurse evaluates a client following treatment for carbon monoxide poisoning. The nurse would document that the treatment was effective when the:
1   Client is awake and talking
2   Carboxyhemoglobin levels are less than 5%
3   Heart monitor shows sinus tachycardia
4   Client is sleeping soundly

**Answer: 2**
*Rationale:* Normal carboxyhemoglobin levels are less than 5%. Clients can be awake and talking with abnormally high levels. The symptoms of carbon monoxide poisoning are tachycardia, tachypnea, and central nervous system depression.

*Test-Taking Strategy:* Note the relationship between carbon monoxide poisoning and option 2. Option 2 is the only option that specifically addresses this issue. Review the normal carboxyhemoglobin levels if you had difficulty with this question.

*Level of Cognitive Ability:* Analysis
*Client Needs:* Physiological Integrity
*Integrated Concept/Process:* Nursing Process/Evaluation
*Content Area:* Adult Health/Respiratory

*Reference*
Smeltzer, S., & Bare, B. (2000). *Brunner & Suddarth's Textbook of medical-surgical nursing* (9th ed.). Philadelphia: Lippincott Williams & Wilkins, p. 1921.

---

**204.** A nurse instructs a preoperative client in the proper use of an incentive spirometer. Postoperative assessment of the effectiveness of its use is determined if the client exhibits:
1   Coughing
2   Shallow breaths
3   Wheezing in one lung field
4   Unilateral chest expansion

**Answer: 1**
*Rationale:* Incentive devices have many desired and positive effects. Incentive devices provide the stimulus for a spontaneous deep breath. Spontaneous deep breathing, using the sustained maximal inspiration concept, reduces atelectasis, opens airways, stimulates coughing, and actively encourages individual participation in recovery. Shallow breaths, wheezing, and unilateral chest expansion would indicate that the incentive spirometry was not effective. Wheezing indicates narrowing or obstruction of the airway, and unilateral chest expansion could indicate atelectasis.

*Test-Taking Strategy:* Focus on the issue: the effectiveness of an incentive spirometer. Options 2, 3, and 4 indicate abnormal findings. Review the purpose of an incentive spirometer if you had difficulty with this question.

*Level of Cognitive Ability:* Analysis
*Client Needs:* Physiological Integrity
*Integrated Concept/Process:* Nursing Process/Evaluation
*Content Area:* Fundamental Skills

*Reference*
Potter, P., & Perry, A. (2001). *Fundamentals of nursing* (5th ed.). St. Louis: Mosby, p. 1172.

**205.** A client is to be started on prazosin hydrochloride (Minipress). The client asks the nurse why the first three doses must be taken at bedtime. The nurse's response is based on the understanding that during early use, prazosin:

1   Can cause dizziness, lightheadedness, or possible syncope
2   Results in extreme drowsiness
3   Should be taken when the stomach is empty
4   Can cause significant dependent edema

**Answer: 1**

*Rationale:* Prazosin is an alpha-adrenergic blocking agent. During early therapy the client may have a "first-dose hypotensive reaction," which is characterized by dizziness, lightheadedness, and possible loss of consciousness. This can also occur when the dosage is increased. This effect usually disappears with continued use or when the dosage is decreased.

*Test-Taking Strategy:* Note the name of the medication, Minipress. This will assist in determining that the medication is an antihypertensive agent. Recalling that orthostatic hypotension occurs with the use of antihypertensives will direct you to option 1. Review the effects of this medication if you had difficulty with this question.

*Level of Cognitive Ability:* Application
*Client Needs:* Physiological Integrity
*Integrated Concept/Process:* Teaching/Learning
*Content Area:* Pharmacology

*Reference*
Hodgson, B., & Kizior, R. (2001). *Saunders Nursing drug handbook 2001.* Philadelphia: W.B. Saunders, p. 851.

---

**206.** A nurse has applied the prescribed dressing to the leg of a client with an ischemic arterial leg ulcer. The nurse would use which of the following methods to cover the dressing?

1   Apply a large, soft pad, and tape it to the skin
2   Apply a Kerlix roll, and tape it to the skin
3   Apply small Montgomery straps, and tie the edges together
4   Apply a Kling roll, and tape the edge of the roll onto the bandage

**Answer: 4**

*Rationale:* With an arterial ulcer, the nurse applies tape only to the bandage itself. Tape is never used directly on the skin because it could cause further tissue damage. For the same reason, Montgomery straps could not be applied to the skin (although these are generally intended for use on abdominal wounds, anyway). Standard dressing technique includes the use of Kling rolls on circumferential dressings.

*Test-Taking Strategy:* Use the process of elimination, noting that options 1, 2, and 3 are similar. Recalling that tape is not applied to the skin, eliminate options 1 and 2. For the same reason, eliminate option 3, because the Montgomery straps would need to be adhered to the skin as well. Review care of a client with an arterial leg ulcer if you had difficulty with this question.

*Level of Cognitive Ability:* Application
*Client Needs:* Physiological Integrity
*Integrated Concept/Process:* Nursing Process/Implementation
*Content Area:* Adult Health/Cardiovascular

*Reference*
Smeltzer, S., & Bare, B. (2000). *Brunner & Suddarth's Textbook of medical-surgical nursing* (9th ed.). Philadelphia: Lippincott Williams & Wilkins, p. 711.

**207.** A child is admitted to the pediatric unit with a diagnosis of celiac disease. Based on this diagnosis, the nurse expects that the child's stools will be:
1   Dark in color
2   Abnormally small in amount
3   Unusually hard
4   Malodorous

**Answer: 4**
*Rationale:* The stools of a child with celiac disease are characteristically malodorous, pale, large (bulky), and soft (loose). Excessive flatus is common, and bouts of diarrhea may occur.

*Test-Taking Strategy:* Use the process of elimination, thinking about the pathophysiology that occurs in celiac disease. Review these manifestations if you had difficulty with this question.

*Level of Cognitive Ability:* Analysis
*Client Needs:* Physiological Integrity
*Integrated Concept/Process:* Nursing Process/Assessment
*Content Area:* Child Health

*Reference*
Wong, D. (1999). *Whaley & Wong's Nursing care of infants and children* (6th ed.). St. Louis: Mosby, p. 1567.

**208.** A clinic nurse is caring for a client suspected of a diagnosis of pregnancy-induced hypertension (PIH). The nurse assesses the client expecting to note which of the following if PIH is present?
1   Glycosuria, hypertension, and obesity
2   Edema, ketonuria, and obesity
3   Edema, tachycardia, and ketonuria
4   Hypertension, edema, and proteinuria

**Answer: 4**
*Rationale:* PIH is the most common hypertensive disorder in pregnancy. It is characterized by the development of hypertension, proteinuria, and edema. Glycosuria and ketonuria occur in diabetes mellitus. Tachycardia and obesity are not specifically related to diagnosing PIH.

*Test-Taking Strategy:* Use the process of elimination. Eliminate options 2 and 3 because they do not address hypertension. From the remaining options, recalling that glycosuria is an indication of diabetes mellitus will assist in directing you to option 4. Review the clinical manifestations associated with PIH if you had difficulty with this question.

*Level of Cognitive Ability:* Application
*Client Needs:* Physiological Integrity
*Integrated Concept/Process:* Nursing Process/Assessment
*Content Area:* Maternity

*Reference*
Lowdermilk, D., Perry, S., & Bobak, I. (2000). *Maternity & women's health care* (7th ed.). St. Louis: Mosby, pp. 817-818.

**209.** A client who undergoes a gastric resection is at risk for developing dumping syndrome. The nurse monitors the client for:
1   Extreme thirst
2   Bradycardia
3   Dizziness
4   Constipation

**Answer: 3**
*Rationale:* Early manifestations of dumping syndrome occur 5 to 30 minutes after eating. Symptoms include vasomotor disturbances such as dizziness, tachycardia, syncope, sweating, pallor, palpitations, and the desire to lie down.

*Test-Taking Strategy:* Use the process of elimination. Recalling that the symptoms of this disorder are vasomotor in nature will direct you to option 3. Review this disorder and the appropriate treatment measures if you had difficulty with this question.

*Level of Cognitive Ability:* Application
*Client Needs:* Physiological Integrity
*Integrated Concept/Process:* Nursing Process/Assessment
*Content Area:* Adult Health/Gastrointestinal

*Reference*
Ignatavicius, D., Workman, M., & Mishler, M. (1999). *Medical-surgical nursing across the health care continuum* (3rd ed.). Philadelphia: W.B. Saunders, p. 1396.

---

**210.** A nurse is caring for a client who had a craniotomy. When assessing the client for the major postoperative complication, the nurse monitors for:

1. Restlessness
2. Bleeding
3. Hypotension
4. Bradycardia

**Answer: 1**

*Rationale:* The major postoperative complication is increased intracranial pressure (ICP) from cerebral edema, hemorrhage, or obstruction of the normal flow of cerebrospinal fluid (CSF). Symptoms of increased ICP include severe headache, deteriorating level of consciousness, restlessness, irritability, and dilated or pinpoint pupils that are slow to react or nonreactive to light. Without prompt recognition and treatment, herniation syndromes develop and death can occur.

*Test-Taking Strategy:* Note the client's diagnosis. Always monitor the neurological client for increased ICP. Remember that changes in the level of consciousness (LOC) are the first key indicator of increased ICP. Option 1 is the only option that addresses LOC. Review the signs of increased ICP and postoperative complications following craniotomy if you had difficulty with this question.

*Level of Cognitive Ability:* Analysis
*Client Needs:* Physiological Integrity
*Integrated Concept/Process:* Nursing Process/Assessment
*Content Area:* Adult Health/Neurological

*Reference*
Ignatavicius, D., Workman, M., & Mishler, M. (1999). *Medical-surgical nursing across the health care continuum* (3rd ed.). Philadelphia: W.B. Saunders, p. 1144.

---

**211.** Buck's traction is applied to an elderly client following a hip fracture. The client asks the nurse about the traction. The nurse tells the client that this type of traction is:

1. Skin traction involving the use of elastic bandages applied to the skin and soft tissues
2. Skeletal traction involving the use of surgically inserted pins
3. Circumferential traction involving the use of a belt around the body
4. Plaster traction involving the use of a cast

**Answer: 1**

*Rationale:* Buck's traction is a form of skin traction and involves the use of elastic bandages applied to the skin and soft tissues. The purpose of this type of traction is to decrease painful muscle spasms that accompany fractures. The weight that is used as a pulling force is limited (5 to 10 lb), to prevent injury to the skin. Options 2, 3, and 4 are incorrect descriptions.

*Test-Taking Strategy:* Recalling that Buck's traction is a skin traction will assist in eliminating options 2, 3, and 4. Review the purpose and principles related to this type of traction if you had difficulty with this question.

*Level of Cognitive Ability:* Application
*Client Needs:* Physiological Integrity

*Integrated Concept/Process:* Teaching/Learning
*Content Area:* Adult Health/Musculoskeletal

*Reference*
Ignatavicius, D., Workman, M., & Mishler, M. (1999). *Medical-surgical nursing across the health care continuum* (3rd ed.). Philadelphia: W.B. Saunders, p. 1289.

---

**212.** An adult client arrives in the emergency unit with burns to both legs and perineal areas. Using the Rule of Nines, the nurse would determine that approximately what percentage of the client's body surface has been burned?
1 19%
2 46%
3 37%
4 65%

**Answer: 3**
*Rationale:* The most rapid method used to calculate the size of a burn injury in adult clients whose weights are in normal proportion to their heights is the Rule of Nines. This method divides the body into areas that are in multiples of 9%. Each leg is 18%, each arm is 9%, and the head is 9%. The trunk is 36% and the perineal area is 1%. Both legs and the perineal area equal 37%.

*Test-Taking Strategy:* Knowledge regarding the percentages associated with this method of calculating burn injuries is required to answer this question. Memorize these percentages if you had difficulty with this question.

*Level of Cognitive Ability:* Analysis
*Client Needs:* Physiological Integrity
*Integrated Concept/Process:* Nursing Process/Assessment
*Content Area:* Adult Health/Integumentary

*Reference*
Ignatavicius, D., Workman, M., & Mishler, M. (1999). *Medical-surgical nursing across the health care continuum* (3rd ed.). Philadelphia: W.B. Saunders, p. 1766.

---

**213.** Skin closure with heterograft is performed on the burn client. The client asks the nurse about the meaning of a heterograft. The nurse tells the client that a heterograft is skin from:
1 Another species
2 A cadaver
3 The burned client
4 A skin bank

**Answer: 1**
*Rationale:* Biological dressings are usually heterograft or homograft material. Heterograft is skin from another species. The most commonly used type of heterograft is pigskin because of its availability and its relative compatibility with human skin. Homograft is skin from another human, which is usually obtained from a cadaver and is provided through a skin bank. Autograft is skin from the client.

*Test-Taking Strategy:* Focus on the key word *heterograft.* Options 2, 3, and 4 are similar, and all relate to grafts from human skin. Review the various types of skin closure grafts if you had difficulty with this question.

*Level of Cognitive Ability:* Application
*Client Needs:* Physiological Integrity
*Integrated Concept/Process:* Nursing Process/Implementation
*Content Area:* Adult Health/Integumentary

*Reference*
Ignatavicius, D., Workman, M., & Mishler, M. (1999). *Medical-surgical nursing across the health care continuum* (3rd ed.). Philadelphia: W.B. Saunders, p. 1776.

**214.** A nurse is caring for a client admitted to the hospital after sustaining a head injury. The nurse most appropriately positions the client:

1   With the head elevated on pillow
2   In left Sims' position
3   In reverse Trendelenburg position
4   With the head of the bed elevated 30 to 45 degrees

**Answer: 4**

*Rationale:* The client with a head injury is positioned to avoid extreme flexion or extension of the neck and to maintain the head in the midline, neutral position. The client is logrolled when turned to avoid extreme hip flexion. The head of the bed is elevated 30 to 45 degrees. All of these measures are used to enhance venous drainage, which helps prevent increased intracranial pressure (ICP).

*Test-Taking Strategy:* Use the process of elimination, recalling that the client with a head injury is at risk for increased ICP. Bearing this in mind, and considering the principles of gravity, will direct you to option 4. Review care of a client following a head injury if you had difficulty with this question.

*Level of Cognitive Ability:* Application
*Client Needs:* Physiological Integrity
*Integrated Concept/Process:* Nursing Process/Implementation
*Content Area:* Adult Health/Neurological

*Reference*
Ignatavicius, D., Workman, M., & Mishler, M. (1999). *Medical-surgical nursing across the health care continuum* (3rd ed.). Philadelphia: W.B. Saunders, p. 1130.

**215.** An infant is admitted to the pediatric unit with a diagnosis of tracheoesophageal fistula (TEF). The nurse assesses the infant, knowing that a typical finding in an infant with TEF is:

1   Continuous drooling
2   Diaphragmatic breathing
3   Slowed reflexes
4   Passage of large amounts of frothy stool

**Answer: 1**

*Rationale:* Esophageal atresia prevents the passage of swallowed mucus and saliva into the stomach. After fluid has accumulated in the pouch, it flows from the mouth and the infant then drools continuously. The inability to swallow amniotic fluid prevents the accumulation of normal meconium, and a lack of stools results. Responsiveness of the infant to stimulus would depend on the overall condition of the infant and is not considered a classic sign of tracheoesophageal fistula (TEF). Diaphragmatic breathing is not associated with TEF.

*Test-Taking Strategy:* Use the process of elimination. Eliminate options 3 and 4 by considering the anatomical location of the disorder. From the remaining options, recalling that diaphragmatic breathing is not associated with TEF will direct you to option 1. Review the manifestations associated with this disorder if you had difficulty with this question.

*Level of Cognitive Ability:* Analysis
*Client Needs:* Physiological Integrity
*Integrated Concept/Process:* Nursing Process/Assessment
*Content Area:* Child Health

*Reference*
Wong, D. (1999). *Whaley & Wong's Nursing care of infants and children* (6th ed.). St. Louis: Mosby, p. 520.

**216.** A nurse is determining the need for suctioning in a client with an endotracheal (ET) tube attached to a mechanical ventilator. Which observation by the nurse is not consistent with the need for suctioning?

1   Low peak inspiratory pressure on the ventilator
2   Gurgling sound with respiration
3   Restlessness
4   Presence of rhonchi

**Answer: 1**

*Rationale:* Indications for suctioning include moist, wet respirations, restlessness, rhonchi on auscultation of the lungs, visible mucus bubbling in the ET tube, increased pulse and respiratory rates, and increased peak inspiratory pressures on the ventilator. A low peak inspiratory pressure would indicate a leak in the mechanical ventilation system.

*Test-Taking Strategy:* Note the key word *not* and focus on the issue: the need for suctioning. Rhonchi and gurgling sounds are obvious indications for suctioning and are eliminated first. Recalling that restlessness is a sign of hypoxia (which could result from the need for suctioning) helps to eliminate option 3. Review assessment of the client being mechanically ventilated if you had difficulty with this question.

*Level of Cognitive Ability:* Analysis
*Client Needs:* Physiological Integrity
*Integrated Concept/Process:* Nursing Process/Assessment
*Content Area:* Adult Health/Respiratory

*Reference*
Smeltzer, S., & Bare, B. (2000). *Brunner & Suddarth's Textbook of medical-surgical nursing* (9th ed.). Philadelphia: Lippincott Williams & Wilkins, p. 499.

---

**217.** A client is intubated and receiving mechanical ventilation. The physician has added 5 cm of positive end expiratory pressure (PEEP) to the ventilator settings of the client. The nurse assesses for which of the following expected but adverse effects of PEEP?

1   Systolic blood pressure decrease from 122 to 98 mm Hg
2   Decreased heart rate from 78 to 64 beats/min
3   Decreased peak pressure on the ventilator
4   Increased temperature from 98° to 100° F rectally

**Answer: 1**

*Rationale:* PEEP leads to increased intrathoracic pressure, which in turn leads to decreased cardiac output. This is manifested in the client by decreased blood pressure and increased pulse (compensatory). Peak pressures on the ventilator should not be affected, although the pressure at the end of expiration remains positive at the level set for the PEEP. Fever would indicate respiratory infection, or infection from another source.

*Test-Taking Strategy:* Note the key words *expected but adverse.* Knowing that PEEP increases intrathoracic pressure leads you to look for the option that reflects a consequence of this event. Fever is irrelevant, so option 4 is eliminated first. From the remaining options, think about the effects of PEEP to direct you to option 1. Review the effects of PEEP if you had difficulty with this question.

*Level of Cognitive Ability:* Analysis
*Client Needs:* Physiological Integrity
*Integrated Concept/Process:* Nursing Process/Assessment
*Content Area:* Adult Health/Respiratory

*Reference*
Smeltzer, S., & Bare, B. (2000). *Brunner & Suddarth's Textbook of medical-surgical nursing* (9th ed.). Philadelphia: Lippincott Williams & Wilkins, p. 506.

**218.** A nurse is assessing the respiratory status of the client following thoracentesis. The nurse would become most concerned with which of the following assessment findings?

1    Respiratory rate of 22 breaths/min
2    Equal bilateral chest expansion
3    Few scattered wheezes, unchanged from baseline
4    Diminished breath sounds on the affected side

**Answer: 4**

*Rationale:* Following thoracentesis, the nurse assesses vital signs and breath sounds. The nurse especially notes increased respiratory rates, dyspnea, retractions, diminished breath sounds, or cyanosis, which could indicate pneumothorax. Any of these signs should be reported to the physician.

*Test-Taking Strategy:* Use the process of elimination noting the key words *most concerned*. Eliminate options 1 and 2 first, because they are normal findings. Option 3 is an abnormality, but note that the wheezes are unchanged from the client's baseline. Option 4 is the abnormal finding. Review the signs of complications following a thoracentesis if you had difficulty with this question.

*Level of Cognitive Ability:* Analysis
*Client Needs:* Physiological Integrity
*Integrated Concept/Process:* Nursing Process/Analysis
*Content Area:* Adult Health/Respiratory

*Reference*
Smeltzer, S., & Bare, B. (2000). *Brunner & Suddarth's Textbook of medical-surgical nursing* (9th ed.). Philadelphia: Lippincott Williams & Wilkins, p. 399.

---

**219.** A nurse is preparing to administer a Mantoux skin test to a client. The nurse determines that which area is most appropriate for injection of the medication?

1    Inner aspect of the forearm that is not heavily pigmented
2    Inner aspect of the forearm that is close to a burn scar
3    Dorsal aspect of the upper arm near a mole
4    Dorsal aspect of the upper arm that has a small amount of hair

**Answer: 1**

*Rationale:* Intradermal injections are most commonly given in the inner surface of the forearm. Other sites include the dorsal area of the upper arm or the upper back beneath the scapulae. The nurse finds an area that is not heavily pigmented and is clear of hairy areas or lesions that could interfere with reading the results.

*Test-Taking Strategy:* Use the process of elimination. Note that options 2, 3, and 4 are similar in that they indicate areas that are not clear of lesions or hair. If this question was difficult, review the basics of intradermal injection techniques.

*Level of Cognitive Ability:* Application
*Client Needs:* Physiological Integrity
*Integrated Concept/Process:* Nursing Process/Assessment
*Content Area:* Adult Health/Respiratory

*Reference*
Smeltzer, S., & Bare, B. (2000). *Brunner & Suddarth's Textbook of medical-surgical nursing* (9th ed.). Philadelphia: Lippincott Williams & Wilkins, p. 438.

---

**220.** A home care nurse is planning therapeutic measures for the client who experienced a rib fracture 2 days earlier. The nurse avoids including which of the following items in the nursing care plan?

1    Rest
2    Local heat
3    Ice
4    Analgesics

**Answer: 3**

*Rationale:* Common therapies for fractured ribs include rest, analgesics, and the local application of heat. Heat has an analgesic effect and speeds resolution of inflammation.

*Test-Taking Strategy:* Use the process of elimination, focusing on the client's injury and noting the key word *avoids*. Recalling that ice is used only in the first 24 hours after an injury will direct you to option 3. Review client teaching points related to measures in treating a rib fracture if you had difficulty with this question.

*Level of Cognitive Ability:* Application
*Client Needs:* Physiological Integrity
*Integrated Concept/Process:* Nursing Process/Planning
*Content Area:* Adult Health/Respiratory

*Reference*
Smeltzer, S., & Bare, B. (2000). *Brunner & Suddarth's Textbook of medical-surgical nursing* (9th ed.). Philadelphia: Lippincott Williams & Wilkins, p. 482.

---

**221.** A hospitalized client is dyspneic, and left pneumothorax has been diagnosed on the basis of chest x-ray evaluation. Which of the following signs or symptoms observed by the nurse most clearly indicates that the pneumothorax is rapidly worsening?
1 Pain with respiration
2 Hypertension
3 Tracheal deviation to the right
4 Tracheal deviation to the left

**Answer: 3**
*Rationale:* A pneumothorax is characterized by distended neck veins, displaced point of maximal impulse (PMI), subcutaneous emphysema, tracheal deviation to the unaffected side, decreased fremitus, and worsening cyanosis. The client could have pain with respiration even with milder pneumothorax. The increased intrathoracic pressure would cause the blood pressure to fall, not to rise.

*Test-Taking Strategy:* Focus on the client's diagnosis and the key words *rapidly worsening*. Pain and hypertension are the least specific indicators and are eliminated first. From the remaining options, remember that a large pneumothorax causes the trachea to be pushed in the opposite direction, to the unaffected side. Review the complications of pneumothorax if you had difficulty with this question.

*Level of Cognitive Ability:* Analysis
*Client Needs:* Physiological Integrity
*Integrated Concept/Process:* Nursing Process/Assessment
*Content Area:* Adult Health/Respiratory

*Reference*
Smeltzer, S., & Bare, B. (2000). *Brunner & Suddarth's Textbook of medical-surgical nursing* (9th ed.). Philadelphia: Lippincott Williams & Wilkins, p. 392.

---

**222.** A client is admitted to the hospital with a diagnosis of right lower lobe pneumonia. The nurse auscultates the right lower lobe, expecting to note which of the following types of breath sounds?
1 Bronchial
2 Bronchovesicular
3 Vesicular
4 Absent

**Answer: 1**
*Rationale:* A client with pneumonia will have bronchial breath sounds over area(s) of consolidation, because the consolidated tissue carries bronchial sounds to the peripheral lung fields. The client may also have crackles in the affected area as a result of fluid in the interstitium and alveoli. Absence of breath sounds is not likely to occur unless a serious complication of the pneumonia occurs. Options 2 and 3 are not noted in pneumonia.

*Test-Taking Strategy:* Use the process of elimination. Recalling that vesicular breath sounds are normal in the lung periphery helps to eliminate option 3. From the remaining options, recall that the pneumonia transmits the bronchial breath sounds, so they are heard over the area of consolidation. Review assessment findings in pneumonia if you had difficulty with this question.

*Level of Cognitive Ability:* Analysis
*Client Needs:* Physiological Integrity
*Integrated Concept/Process:* Nursing Process/Assessment
*Content Area:* Adult Health/Respiratory

*Reference*
Smeltzer, S., & Bare, B. (2000). *Brunner & Suddarth's Textbook of medical-surgical nursing* (9th ed.). Philadelphia: Lippincott Williams & Wilkins, p. 426.

---

**223.** A nurse assesses the client with acquired immunodeficiency syndrome (AIDS) for early signs of Kaposi's sarcoma. The nurse observes the client for lesion(s) that are:

1  Unilateral, raised, and bluish purple
2  Bilateral, flat, and pink, turning to dark violet or black
3  Unilateral, red, raised, and resembling a blister
4  Bilateral, flat, and brownish and scaly in appearance

**Answer: 2**
*Rationale:* Kaposi's sarcoma generally starts with an area that is flat and pink and then changes to a dark violet or black color. The lesions are usually present bilaterally. They may appear in many areas of the body and are treated with radiation, chemotherapy, and cryotherapy.

*Test-Taking Strategy:* Use the process of elimination. Recalling that Kaposi's sarcoma occurs in a bilateral pattern eliminates options 1 and 3. From the remaining options, recalling the character of the lesions will direct you to option 2. Review the characteristics of this disorder if you had difficulty with this question.

*Level of Cognitive Ability:* Analysis
*Client Needs:* Physiological Integrity
*Integrated Concept/Process:* Nursing Process/Assessment
*Content Area:* Adult Health/Immune

*Reference*
Smeltzer, S., & Bare, B. (2000). *Brunner & Suddarth's Textbook of medical-surgical nursing* (9th ed.). Philadelphia: Lippincott Williams & Wilkins, p. 1491.

---

**224.** A client has a suspected pleural effusion. The nurse assesses the client for which typical manifestations of this respiratory problem?

1  Dyspnea at rest and moist, productive cough
2  Dyspnea on exertion and moist, productive cough
3  Dyspnea at rest and dry, nonproductive cough
4  Dyspnea on exertion and dry, nonproductive cough

**Answer: 4**
*Rationale:* Typical assessment findings in the client with a pleural effusion include dyspnea, which usually occurs with exertion, and a dry, nonproductive cough. The cough is caused by bronchial irritation and possible mediastinal shift.

*Test-Taking Strategy:* Use the process of elimination. Recalling that a pleural effusion is in the pleural space and not the airways helps to eliminate options 1 and 2. Knowing that dyspnea occurs on exertion before it occurs at rest will direct you to option 4 from the remaining options. Review the manifestations of plural effusion if you had difficulty with this question.

*Level of Cognitive Ability:* Application
*Client Needs:* Physiological Integrity
*Integrated Concept/Process:* Nursing Process/Assessment
*Content Area:* Adult Health/Respiratory

*Reference*
Smeltzer, S., & Bare, B. (2000). *Brunner & Suddarth's Textbook of medical-surgical nursing* (9th ed.). Philadelphia: Lippincott Williams & Wilkins, p. 444.

**225.** A client with pleural effusion had a thoracentesis and a sample of fluid was sent to the laboratory. Analysis of the fluid reveals a high red blood cell count. The nurse interprets that this result is most consistent with:

1　Trauma
2　Infection
3　Congestive heart failure (CHF)
4　Liver failure

**Answer: 1**

*Rationale:* Pleural effusion that has a high red blood cell count may result from trauma and may be treated with placement of a chest tube for drainage. Other causes of pleural effusion include infection, CHF, liver or renal failure, malignancy, or inflammatory processes. Infection would be accompanied by increased white blood cells. The fluid portion of the serum would accumulate with liver failure and heart failure.

*Test-Taking Strategy:* Use the process of elimination. Noting the key words *red blood cell count* will direct you to option 1. Review the causes of pleural effusion if you had difficulty with this question.

*Level of Cognitive Ability:* Analysis
*Client Needs:* Physiological Integrity
*Integrated Concept/Process:* Nursing Process/Analysis
*Content Area:* Adult Health/Respiratory

*Reference*
Smeltzer, S., & Bare, B. (2000). *Brunner & Suddarth's Textbook of medical-surgical nursing* (9th ed.). Philadelphia: Lippincott Williams & Wilkins, p. 444.

**226.** A nurse is scheduling a client for diagnostic studies of the gastrointestinal (GI) system. Which of the following studies, if ordered, should the nurse schedule last?

1　Abdominal scan
2　Ultrasonography
3　Colonoscopy
4　Barium enema

**Answer: 4**

*Rationale:* Barium is instilled into the lower GI tract during a barium enema and may take up to 72 hours to clear the GI tract. The presence of barium could cause interference with obtaining clear visualization and accurate results of the other tests listed, if they are performed before the client has fully excreted the barium. For this reason, diagnostic studies that involve barium contrast are scheduled at the conclusion of other diagnostic studies.

*Test-Taking Strategy:* Use the process of elimination. Note the key word *last*. Recall that barium shows up on x-ray as opaque and that this substance would impair visualization during other tests. Review the procedure for the diagnostic tests listed in the options if you had difficulty with this question.

*Level of Cognitive Ability:* Application
*Client Needs:* Physiological Integrity
*Integrated Concept/Process:* Nursing Process/Planning
*Content Area:* Adult Health/Gastrointestinal

*Reference*
Smeltzer, S., & Bare, B. (2000). *Brunner & Suddarth's Textbook of medical-surgical nursing* (9th ed.). Philadelphia: Lippincott Williams & Wilkins, p. 798.

**227.** A nurse is caring for a client who is scheduled to have a liver biopsy. Before this procedure, it is most important for the nurse to assess the client's:

1. History of nausea and vomiting
2. Tolerance for pain
3. Allergy to iodine or shellfish
4. Ability to lie still and hold the breath

**Answer: 4**

*Rationale:* It is most important for the nurse to assess the client's ability to lie still and hold the breath for the procedure. This helps the physician to avoid complications, such as puncturing the lung or other organs. Assessment of allergy to iodine or shellfish is unnecessary for this procedure, because no contrast dye is used. Knowledge of the history related to nausea and vomiting is generally a part of assessment of the gastrointestinal system but has no relationship to the procedure. The client's tolerance for pain is a useful item to know. However, the area will receive a local anesthetic.

*Test-Taking Strategy:* Use the process of elimination. Visualizing this procedure and thinking about its complications will direct you to option 4. Review this procedure if you had difficulty with this question.

*Level of Cognitive Ability:* Application
*Client Needs:* Physiological Integrity
*Integrated Concept/Process:* Nursing Process/Assessment
*Content Area:* Adult Health/Gastrointestinal

*Reference*
Smeltzer, S., & Bare, B. (2000). *Brunner & Suddarth's Textbook of medical-surgical nursing* (9th ed.). Philadelphia: Lippincott Williams & Wilkins, p. 924.

**228.** A nurse is caring for a client who has a diagnosis of pneumonia. The nurse plans which of the following as the best time to take the client for a short walk?

1. After the client uses the metered-dose inhaler
2. After oxygen saturation is recorded on the bedside flow sheet
3. After the client eats lunch
4. After the client has a brief nap

**Answer: 1**

*Rationale:* The nurse should schedule activities for the client with pneumonia after the client has received respiratory treatments or medications. After the administration of bronchodilators (often administered by metered-dose inhaler), the client has the best oxygen exchange possible and would tolerate the activity best. Still, the nurse implements activity cautiously so as not to increase the client's dyspnea.

*Test-Taking Strategy:* Use the process of elimination, noting the key word *best*. Use the ABCs (airway, breathing, and circulation). The use of bronchodilator medication would widen the air passages, allowing more air to enter the client's lungs. Review care of a client with pneumonia if you had difficulty with this question.

*Level of Cognitive Ability:* Application
*Client Needs:* Physiological Integrity
*Integrated Concept/Process:* Nursing Process/Planning
*Content Area:* Adult Health/Respiratory

*Reference*
Smeltzer, S., & Bare, B. (2000). *Brunner & Suddarth's Textbook of medical-surgical nursing* (9th ed.). Philadelphia: Lippincott Williams & Wilkins, p. 429.

**229.** A nurse has just inserted an indwelling Foley catheter into the bladder of a postoperative client who has not voided for 6 hours and has a distended bladder. After the tubing is secured and the collection bag is hung on the bed frame, the nurse notices that 750 mL of urine has drained into the collection bag. The most appropriate nursing action for the safety of the client is to:

1 Clamp the tubing for 30 minutes and then release
2 Provide suprapubic pressure to maintain a steady flow of urine
3 Check the specific gravity of the urine
4 Raise the collection bag high enough to slow the rate of drainage

**Answer: 1**
*Rationale:* Rapid emptying of a large volume of urine may cause engorgement of pelvic blood vessels and hypovolemic shock. Clamping the tubing for 30 minutes allows equilibration to prevent complications. Option 2 would increase the flow of urine, which would lead to hypovolemic shock. Option 3 is an assessment and would not affect the flow of urine or prevent the possible hypovolemic shock. Option 4 could cause backflow of urine. Infection is likely to develop if urine is allowed to flow back into the bladder.

*Test-Taking Strategy:* Use the process of elimination. Note the key words *750 mL*. Recall the physiology of the hemodynamic changes following the rapid collapse of an overdistended bladder. Eliminate option 2 because slowing the rate of urine drainage is the issue. Note that option 3 is an assessment action rather than an action that affects the amount of urine drainage. Option 4 is an inappropriate action. Review the complications associated with inserting a Foley catheter in a client with a distended bladder if you had difficulty with this question.

*Level of Cognitive Ability:* Application
*Client Needs:* Physiological Integrity
*Integrated Concept/Process:* Nursing Process/Implementation
*Content Area:* Fundamental Skills

**Reference**
Smeltzer, S., & Bare, B. (2000). *Brunner & Suddarth's Textbook of medical-surgical nursing* (9th ed.). Philadelphia: Lippincott Williams & Wilkins, p. 1120.

**230.** A nurse has an order to administer amphotericin B (Fungizone) intravenously to a client with histoplasmosis. The nurse plans to do which of the following during administration of the medication?

1 Monitor for hypothermia
2 Administer a concurrent fluid challenge
3 Assess the intravenous infusion site
4 Monitor for an excessive urine output

**Answer: 3**
*Rationale:* Amphotericin B is a toxic medication that can produce symptoms during administration such as chills, fever, headache, vomiting, and impaired renal function. The medication is also very irritating to the IV site, commonly causing thrombophlebitis. The nurse administering this medication monitors for these complications.

*Test-Taking Strategy:* Use the process of elimination, recalling the toxic effects of this medication. Knowing that fever and chills can occur eliminates option 1. Recalling that the medication can be toxic to the kidneys eliminates option 4. From the remaining options, knowing that there is no rationale for giving concurrent fluids will direct you to option 3. Review nursing care related to the administration of this medication if you had difficulty with this question.

*Level of Cognitive Ability:* Application
*Client Needs:* Physiological Integrity
*Integrated Concept/Process:* Nursing Process/Planning
*Content Area:* Adult Health/Immune

**Reference**
Hodgson, B., & Kizior, R. (2001). *Saunders Nursing drug handbook 2001.* Philadelphia: W.B. Saunders, p. 57.

**231.** A client with repeated pleural effusions from inoperable lung cancer is to undergo pleurodesis. The nurse plans to do which of the following after the physician injects the sclerosing agent through the chest tube?

1  Clamp the chest tube
2  Ambulate the client
3  Ask the client to cough and deep breathe
4  Ask the client to remain in one position only

**Answer: 1**

*Rationale:* After injection of the sclerosing agent, the nurse clamps the chest tube to prevent the agent from draining back out of the pleural space. A repositioning schedule is used by some physicians, but its usefulness in dispersing the agent is controversial. Ambulation, coughing, and deep breathing have no specific purpose in the immediate period after injection.

*Test-Taking Strategy:* Note that the client is having a pleurodesis. This will assist in eliminating option 2. Eliminate option 4 because of the word *only*. From the remaining options, recall the purpose of the procedure. It is most reasonable to clamp the chest tube so that the sclerosing agent cannot flow back out of the tube. Coughing and deep breathing have no specific purpose in this situation. Review this procedure if you had difficulty with this question.

*Level of Cognitive Ability:* Application
*Client Needs:* Physiological Integrity
*Integrated Concept/Process:* Nursing Process/Planning
*Content Area:* Adult Health/Respiratory

*Reference*
Ignatavicius, D., Workman, M., & Mishler, M. (1999). *Medical-surgical nursing across the health care continuum* (3rd ed.). Philadelphia: W.B. Saunders, p. 649.

**232.** A client with a bladder injury has had surgical repair of the injured area and placement of a suprapubic catheter. The nurse plans to do which of the following to prevent complications of this procedure?

1  Monitor urine output every shift
2  Encourage a high intake of oral fluids
3  Prevent kinking of the catheter tubing
4  Measure specific gravity once a shift

**Answer: 3**

*Rationale:* A complication after surgical repair of the bladder is disruption of sutures caused by tension on them from urine buildup. The nurse prevents this from happening by ensuring that the catheter is able to drain freely. This involves basic catheter care, including keeping the tubing free from kinks, keeping the tubing below the level of the bladder, and monitoring the flow of urine frequently. A high oral fluid intake and measurement of urine specific gravity do not prevent complications of a suprapubic catheter. Monitoring of urine output every shift is insufficient to detect decreased flow from catheter kinking.

*Test-Taking Strategy:* Use the process of elimination. Eliminate option 4 first because specific gravity measurement is not a preventive action. Eliminate option 1 next, because measurement once a shift is not a preventive action and is also insufficient in frequency. From the remaining options, knowing that a high oral fluid intake will not prevent complications of a suprapubic catheter directs you to option 3. Review care of a client with a suprapubic catheter if you had difficulty with this question.

*Level of Cognitive Ability:* Application
*Client Needs:* Physiological Integrity
*Integrated Concept/Process:* Nursing Process/Planning
*Content Area:* Adult Health/Renal

*Reference*
Ignatavicius, D., Workman, M., & Mishler, M. (1999). *Medical-surgical nursing across the health care continuum* (3rd ed.). Philadelphia: W.B. Saunders, p. 2029.

**233.** A client with benign prostatic hyperplasia undergoes transurethral resection of the prostate (TURP). The nurse orders which of the following solutions from the pharmacy so that it is available postoperatively for continuous bladder irrigation (CBI)?
1    Sterile water
2    Sterile normal saline solution
3    Sterile Dakin's solution
4    Sterile water with 5% dextrose

**Answer: 2**

*Rationale:* Continuous bladder irrigation is done following TURP using sterile normal saline, which is isotonic. Sterile water is not used because the solution could be absorbed systemically, precipitating hemolysis and possibly renal failure. Dakin's solution contains hypochlorite and is used only for wound irrigation in selected circumstances. Solutions containing dextrose are not introduced into the bladder.

*Test-Taking Strategy:* Use the process of elimination, noting the issue, a continuous bladder irrigation. Recalling that normal saline is isotonic will direct you to option 2. Review the procedure for CBI if you had difficulty with this question.

*Level of Cognitive Ability:* Application
*Client Needs:* Physiological Integrity
*Integrated Concept/Process:* Nursing Process/Implementation
*Content Area:* Adult Health/Renal

*Reference*
Ignatavicius, D., Workman, M., & Mishler, M. (1999). *Medical-surgical nursing across the health care continuum* (3rd ed.). Philadelphia: W.B. Saunders, p. 2024.

**234.** A client with acquired immunodeficiency syndrome (AIDS) is being admitted for treatment of *Pneumocystis carinii* infection. Which of the following activities that assists in maintaining comfort does the nurse plan to include in the care of this client?
1    Assess respiratory rate, rhythm, depth, and breath sounds every 8 hours
2    Evaluate arterial blood gas results
3    Keep the head of the bed elevated
4    Monitor vital signs every hour

**Answer: 3**

*Rationale:* Clients with respiratory difficulties are often more comfortable with the head of the bed elevated. Options 1, 2, and 4 are appropriate measures to evaluate respiratory function and to avoid complications. Option 3 is the only option that addresses planning for client comfort.

*Test-Taking Strategy:* Use the process of elimination. Focusing on the issue—maintaining comfort—will direct you to option 3. Also, note that options 1, 2, and 4 are similar and are all measures to evaluate respiratory function. Review measures to promote comfort in a client with a respiratory infection if you had difficulty with this question.

*Level of Cognitive Ability:* Application
*Client Needs:* Physiological Integrity
*Integrated Concept/Process:* Nursing Process/Planning
*Content Area:* Adult Health/Immune

*Reference*
Ignatavicius, D., Workman, M., & Mishler, M. (1999): *Medical-surgical nursing across the health care continuum* (3rd ed.). Philadelphia: W.B. Saunders, p. 673.

**235.** A client with significant flail chest has arterial blood gas (ABG) results that reveal a $Pao_2$ of 68 and a $Paco_2$ of 51. Two hours ago the $Pao_2$ was 82 and the $Paco_2$ was 44. Based on these changes, the nurse obtains which of the following items?

1 Injectable lidocaine (Xylocaine)
2 Portable chest x-ray machine
3 Intubation tray
4 Chest tube insertion set

**Answer: 3**

*Rationale:* The client with flail chest has painful, rapid, shallow respirations while experiencing severe dyspnea. The effort of breathing and the paradoxical chest movement have the net effect of producing hypoxia and hypercapnia. Respiratory failure develops, and the client requires intubation and mechanical ventilation, usually with positive end expiratory pressure (PEEP). Therefore, an intubation tray is necessary.

*Test-Taking Strategy:* Use the process of elimination, noting the changes in the ABG values. Recall that a falling arterial oxygen level and a rising carbon dioxide level indicate respiratory failure. The usual treatment for respiratory failure is intubation, which makes option 3 the correct option. Review the complications of flail chest and the signs of respiratory failure if you had difficulty with this question.

*Level of Cognitive Ability:* Application
*Client Needs:* Physiological Integrity
*Integrated Concept/Process:* Nursing Process/Implementation
*Content Area:* Adult Health/Respiratory

*Reference*
Ignatavicius, D., Workman, M., & Mishler, M. (1999). *Medical-surgical nursing across the health care continuum* (3rd ed.). Philadelphia: W.B. Saunders, p. 709.

**236.** A client with empyema is to have a thoracentesis performed at the bedside. The nurse plans to have which of the following available in the event that the procedure is not effective?

1 Code cart
2 Chest tube and drainage system
3 Extra large drainage bottle
4 A small-bore needle

**Answer: 2**

*Rationale:* If the exudate is too thick for drainage via thoracentesis, the client may require placement of a chest tube to adequately drain the purulent effusion. A small-bore needle would not effectively allow exudate to drain. Options 1 and 3 are also unnecessary.

*Test-Taking Strategy:* Note the client's diagnosis. In this condition many times the exudate is very thick. Recalling that the purpose of thoracentesis is to provide drainage of the pleura will direct you to option 2. Review care of a client undergoing a thoracentesis if you had difficulty with this question.

*Level of Cognitive Ability:* Application
*Client Needs:* Physiological Integrity
*Integrated Concept/Process:* Nursing Process/Planning
*Content Area:* Adult Health/Respiratory

*Reference*
Smeltzer, S., & Bare, B. (2000). *Brunner & Suddarth's Textbook of medical-surgical nursing* (9th ed.). Philadelphia: Lippincott Williams & Wilkins, p. 397.

**237.** A nurse is administering a dose of fentanyl (Sublimaze) to the client via an epidural catheter after nephrectomy. Before administering the medication, the nurse plans to:

1  Aspirate to ensure that there is a cerebrospinal fluid (CSF) return
2  Ensure that naloxone (Narcan) is readily available
3  Place the head of the bed flat
4  Flush the catheter with 6 mL of sterile water

**Answer: 2**

*Rationale:* Epidural analgesia is used for clients with high levels of expected postoperative pain. The nurse carefully checks the medication, notes the client's level of sedation, and makes sure that the head of the bed is elevated 30 degrees unless contraindicated. The nurse aspirates to make sure there is no CSF return. If CSF returns with aspiration, the catheter has migrated from the epidural space into the subarachnoid space. The catheter is not flushed with 6 mL of sterile water. Narcan should be readily available for use if respiratory depression should occur.

*Test-Taking Strategy:* Use the process of elimination, focusing on the key word *epidural.* Eliminate option 4 first because flushing 6 mL of sterile water through an epidural catheter is dangerous. Option 1 is eliminated next, since CSF aspiration should not occur with an epidural catheter. From the remaining options, either recalling that the antidote to fentanyl is naloxone or that the head of the bed should be elevated at least 30 degrees will direct you to option 2. Review the procedure for administrating medication through an epidural catheter if you had difficulty with this question.

*Level of Cognitive Ability:* Application
*Client Needs:* Physiological Integrity
*Integrated Concept/Process:* Nursing Process/Planning
*Content Area:* Pharmacology

*Reference*
Smeltzer, S., & Bare, B. (2000). *Brunner & Suddarth's Textbook of medical-surgical nursing* (9th ed.). Philadelphia: Lippincott Williams & Wilkins, p. 357.

---

**238.** A nurse is planning care for a client with a chest tube attached to a Pleur-Evac drainage system. The nurse avoids which of the following activities to prevent a tension pneumothorax?

1  Adding water to the suction chamber as it evaporates
2  Taping the connection between the chest tube and the drainage system
3  Maintaining the collection chamber below the client's waist
4  Clamping the chest tube

**Answer: 4**

*Rationale:* To prevent a tension pneumothorax, the nurse avoids clamping the chest tube, unless specifically ordered. In many facilities, clamping of the chest tube is contraindicated by agency policy. Adding water to the suction control chamber is an appropriate nursing action and is done as needed to maintain the full suction level ordered. Taping the connection between the chest tube and system is also indicated to prevent accidental disconnection. Maintaining the system below waist level is indicated to prevent fluid from reentering the pleural space.

*Test-Taking Strategy:* Use the process of elimination, noting the key word *avoids.* Recall that tension pneumothorax occurs when air is trapped in the pleural space and has no exit. Therefore, it is necessary to evaluate each of the options in terms of relative risk for air trapping in the pleural space. Clamping the chest tube could trap air in the pleural space and is avoided by the nurse. Review the causes of tension pneumothorax and care of the client with a chest tube if you had difficulty with this question.

*Level of Cognitive Ability:* Application
*Client Needs:* Physiological Integrity
*Integrated Concept/Process:* Nursing Process/Implementation
*Content Area:* Adult Health/Respiratory

*Reference*
Smeltzer, S., & Bare, B. (2000). *Brunner & Suddarth's Textbook of medical-surgical nursing* (9th ed.). Philadelphia: Lippincott Williams & Wilkins, p. 515.

---

**239.** A nurse is assisting a client with a chest tube to get out of bed. The tubing accidentally gets caught in the bed rail and disconnects. During the attempt to reestablish the connection, the Pleur-Evac drainage system falls over and cracks. The nurse should first:

1  Call the physician
2  Immerse the chest tube in a bottle of sterile normal saline
3  Apply a petrolatum gauze over the end of the chest tube
4  Clamp the chest tube

**Answer: 2**
*Rationale:* If a chest tube accidentally disconnects from the tubing of the drainage apparatus, the nurse should first reestablish underwater seal to prevent tension pneumothorax and mediastinal shift. This can be accomplished by reconnecting the chest tube, or in this case, immersing the chest tube in a bottle of sterile normal saline or water. The physician should be notified after corrective action is taken. If the physician is called first, tension pneumothorax has time to develop. Clamping the chest tube could also cause tension pneumothorax. A petrolatum gauze would be applied to the skin over the chest tube insertion site if the entire chest tube was accidentally removed from the chest.

*Test-Taking Strategy:* Use the process of elimination, noting the key word *first*. Eliminate option 1 as too time consuming to be the first action. Option 4 would create a tension pneumothorax, since this action does not reestablish an underwater seal. From the remaining options, noting that an underwater seal must be established will direct you to option 2. Review care of a client with a chest tube if you had difficulty with this question.

*Level of Cognitive Ability:* Application
*Client Needs:* Physiological Integrity
*Integrated Concept/Process:* Nursing Process/Implementation
*Content Area:* Adult Health/Respiratory

*Reference*
Ignatavicius, D., Workman, M., & Mishler, M. (1999). *Medical-surgical nursing across the health care continuum* (3rd ed.). Philadelphia: W.B. Saunders, p. 654.

---

**240.** A nurse is caring for a client with a diagnosis of Cushing's syndrome. The nurse plans which of these measures to prevent complications from this medical condition?

1  Monitoring glucose levels
2  Monitoring epinephrine levels
3  Encouraging daily jogging
4  Encouraging visits from friends

**Answer: 1**
*Rationale:* In the client with Cushing's syndrome, increased levels of glucocorticoids can result in hyperglycemia and signs and symptoms of diabetes mellitus. Epinephrine levels are not affected. Clients experience activity intolerance related to muscle weakness and fatigue, so option 3 is incorrect. Visitors should be limited because of the client's impaired immune response.

*Test-Taking Strategy:* Focus on the clinical manifestations and complications of Cushing's syndrome. Remember that hyperglycemia can occur to direct you to option 1. Review the clinical manifestations associated with Cushing's syndrome if you had difficulty with this question.

*Level of Cognitive Ability:* Analysis
*Client Needs:* Physiological Integrity
*Integrated Concept/Process:* Nursing Process/Planning
*Content Area:* Adult Health/Endocrine

*Reference*

Ignatavicius, D., Workman, M., & Mishler, M. (1999). *Medical-surgical nursing across the health care continuum* (3rd ed.). Philadelphia: W.B. Saunders, p. 1605.

---

**241.** A client receiving hemodialysis suddenly becomes short of breath and complains of chest pain. The client is tachycardic, pale, and anxious. The nurse, suspecting an air embolism, should:

1. Continue dialysis at a slower rate after checking the lines for air
2. Discontinue dialysis and notify the physician
3. Monitor vital signs every 15 minutes for the next hour
4. Administer a 500-mL bolus of normal saline to break up the air embolus

**Answer: 2**

*Rationale:* If the client experiences air embolus during hemodialysis, the nurse should terminate dialysis immediately, notify the physician, and administer oxygen as needed. The other options are incorrect.

*Test-Taking Strategy:* Focus on the signs and symptoms in the question and think about the actions to take if an air embolism is suspected. The physician needs to be notified if a life-threatening condition exists. This will direct you to option 2. Review the interventions for an air embolism if you had difficulty with this question.

*Level of Cognitive Ability:* Application
*Client Needs:* Physiological Integrity
*Integrated Concept/Process:* Nursing Process/Implementation
*Content Area:* Adult Health/Renal

*Reference*

Ignatavicius, D., Workman, M., & Mishler, M. (1999). *Medical-surgical nursing across the health care continuum* (3rd ed.). Philadelphia: W.B. Saunders, p. 1902.

---

**242.** A nurse notes on the cardiac monitor that a client with aldosteronism is experiencing a dysrhythmia. The nurse immediately assesses the client's:

1. Plasma potassium level
2. Intake and output
3. Peripheral pulses
4. Superficial reflexes

**Answer: 1**

*Rationale:* Aldosteronism can lead to hypokalemia, which in turn can cause life-threatening dysrhythmias. Options 2, 3, and 4 are not immediate priorities for this client.

*Test-Taking Strategy:* Note the key word *immediately*. Recalling the complications associated with this disorder and that altered potassium levels can cause dysrhythmias will direct you to option 1. Review the complications of aldosteronism if you had difficulty with this question.

*Level of Cognitive Ability:* Application
*Client Needs:* Physiological Integrity
*Integrated Concept/Process:* Nursing Process/Implementation
*Content Area:* Adult Health/Endocrine

*Reference*

Smeltzer, S., & Bare, B. (2000). *Brunner & Suddarth's Textbook of medical-surgical nursing* (9th ed.). Philadelphia: Lippincott Williams & Wilkins, p. 218.

**243.** A nurse is monitoring the results of serial arterial blood gases for a client in whom carbon monoxide poisoning has been diagnosed. The client does not want to keep the oxygen in place. The nurse evaluates that the oxygen may be safely removed once the carboxyhemoglobin level decreases to less than:
1  5%
2  10%
3  15%
4  25%

**Answer: 1**
*Rationale:* Oxygen may be removed safely from the client with carbon monoxide poisoning once carboxyhemoglobin levels are less than 5%. Options 2, 3, and 4 are elevated levels.

*Test-Taking Strategy:* Focus on the issue: safely removing the oxygen. If you are unsure, it would be best to select the lowest level as identified in option 1. Review the normal carboxyhemoglobin levels if you had difficulty with this question.

*Level of Cognitive Ability:* Analysis
*Client Needs:* Physiological Integrity
*Integrated Concept/Process:* Teaching/Learning
*Content Area:* Adult Health/Respiratory

*Reference*
Smeltzer, S., & Bare, B. (2000). *Brunner & Suddarth's Textbook of medical-surgical nursing* (9th ed.). Philadelphia: Lippincott Williams & Wilkins, p. 1921.

**244.** A nurse is teaching a pregnant client about nutrition. The nurse includes which information in the client's teaching plan?
1  The nutritional status of the mother significantly influences fetal growth and development
2  All mothers are at high risk for nutritional deficiencies
3  Calcium is not important until the third trimester
4  Iron supplements are not necessary unless the mother has iron-deficiency anemia

**Answer: 1**
*Rationale:* Poor nutrition during pregnancy can negatively influence fetal growth and development. Although pregnancy poses some nutritional risk for the mother, not all clients are at high risk. Calcium is critical during the third trimester but must be increased from the onset of pregnancy. Intake of dietary iron is insufficient for the majority of pregnant women, and iron supplements are routinely prescribed.

*Test-Taking Strategy:* Use the process of elimination. Option 2 uses the absolute word *all;* therefore, eliminate this option. Options 3 and 4 offer specific time frames or conditions for interventions; therefore, eliminate these options. Option 1 is a general or global option that is true for any stage of pregnancy. Review the importance of nutrition during pregnancy if you had difficulty with this question.

*Level of Cognitive Ability:* Application
*Client Needs:* Physiological Integrity
*Integrated Concept/Process:* Nursing Process/Implementation
*Content Area:* Maternity

*Reference*
Lowdermilk, D., Perry, S., & Bobak, I. (2000). *Maternity & women's health care* (7th ed.). St. Louis: Mosby, p. 362.

**245.** A nurse is formulating a plan of care for a client receiving enteral feedings. The nurse identifies which nursing diagnosis as the highest priority for this client?
1  Altered nutrition, less than body requirements
2  High risk for aspiration
3  High risk for fluid volume deficit
4  Diarrhea

**Answer: 2**
*Rationale:* Any condition in which gastrointestinal motility is slowed or esophageal reflux is possible places a client at risk for aspiration. Although options 1, 3, and 4 may be a concern, these are not the priority.

*Test-Taking Strategy:* Use the ABCs (airway, breathing, circulation). Option 2 addresses airway maintenance. Options 1, 3, and 4 are possible problems, but not as high a priority as airway

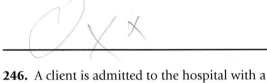

maintenance. Review care of a client receiving enteral feedings if you had difficulty with this question.

*Level of Cognitive Ability:* Analysis
*Client Needs:* Physiological Integrity
*Integrated Concept/Process:* Nursing Process/Analysis
*Content Area:* Fundamental Skills

*Reference*
Potter, P., & Perry, A. (2001). *Fundamentals of nursing* (5th ed.). St. Louis: Mosby, p. 1365.

---

**246.** A client is admitted to the hospital with a diagnosis of Cushing's syndrome. The nurse monitors the client for which of the following that is most likely to occur in this client?

1    Fluid volume deficit
2    Hypoglycemia
3    Hypovolemia
4    Mental status changes

**Answer: 4**

*Rationale:* When Cushing's syndrome develops, the normal function of the glucocorticoids becomes exaggerated and the classic picture of the syndrome emerges. This exaggerated physiological action can cause mental status changes, including memory loss, poor concentration and cognition, euphoria, and depression. It can also cause persistent hyperglycemia along with sodium and water retention, producing edema and hypertension.

*Test-Taking Strategy:* Use the process of elimination. Eliminate options 1 and 3 first because they are similar. Recalling that hyperglycemia rather than hypoglycemia occurs in this condition will direct you to option 4. Review the manifestations of Cushing's syndrome if you had difficulty with this question.

*Level of Cognitive Ability:* Application
*Client Needs:* Physiological Integrity
*Integrated Concept/Process:* Nursing Process/Assessment
*Content Area:* Adult Health/Endocrine

*Reference*
Smeltzer, S., & Bare, B. (2000). *Brunner & Suddarth's Textbook of medical-surgical nursing* (9th ed.). Philadelphia: Lippincott Williams & Wilkins, p. 1060.

---

**247.** A physician is performing direct visualization of the larynx on a client to rule out laryngeal cancer. The nurse tells the client to do which of the following to decrease the sensation of gagging during the procedure?

1    Try to swallow
2    Hold the breath
3    Breathe in and out normally
4    Roll the tongue to the back of the mouth

**Answer: 3**

*Rationale:* The client is instructed to breathe in and out normally, to decrease the sensation of gagging during the procedure. The tongue cannot be moved back because it would occlude the airway. Swallowing cannot be done with the instrument in place. The procedure takes longer than the time the client would be able to hold the breath, and this action is ineffective anyway.

*Test-Taking Strategy:* Use the process of elimination. Option 4 is eliminated first because it is not possible to move the tongue back with the instrument in place. It would also cause the airway to become occluded. Given the length of time needed to perform the procedure, the client could not realistically hold the breath, so option 2 is eliminated next. Trying to swallow would actually cause the larynx to move against the instrument and could cause gagging. Review care of a client during laryngoscopy if you had difficulty with this question.

*Level of Cognitive Ability:* Application
*Client Needs:* Physiological Integrity
*Integrated Concept/Process:* Nursing Process/Implementation
*Content Area:* Adult Health/Oncology

*Reference*
Ignatavicius, D., Workman, M., & Mishler, M. (1999). *Medical-surgical nursing across the health care continuum* (3rd ed.). Philadelphia: W.B. Saunders, p. 561.

---

**248.** A nurse is caring for a client scheduled for a bilateral adrenalectomy for treatment of an adrenal tumor that is producing excessive aldosterone. The nurse most appropriately tells the client which of the following?
1. "You will most likely need to undergo chemotherapy after surgery."
2. "You will need to take hormone replacements for the rest of your life."
3. "You will need to wear an abdominal binder after surgery."
4. "You will not require any special long-term treatment after surgery."

**Answer: 2**
*Rationale:* The major cause of primary hyperaldosteronism is an aldosterone-secreting tumor called an aldosteronoma. Surgery is the treatment of choice. Clients undergoing a bilateral adrenalectomy will need permanent replacement of adrenal hormones. Options 1, 3, and 4 are inaccurate.

*Test-Taking Strategy:* Note the key word *bilateral*. Recalling the function of the adrenal glands and that glucocorticoids and mineralocorticoids are essential to sustain life will direct you to option 2. Review care following bilateral adrenalectomy if you had difficulty with this question.

*Level of Cognitive Ability:* Application
*Client Needs:* Physiological Integrity
*Integrated Concept/Process:* Teaching/Learning
*Content Area:* Adult Health/Endocrine

*Reference*
Smeltzer, S., & Bare, B. (2000). *Brunner & Suddarth's Textbook of medical-surgical nursing* (9th ed.). Philadelphia: Lippincott Williams & Wilkins, p. 1061.

---

**249.** A nurse is caring for a client who is scheduled for an adrenalectomy. The nurse plans to administer which medication in the preoperative period to prevent Addison's crisis?
1. Spironolactone (Aldactone) intramuscularly
2. Methylprednisolone sodium succinate (Solu-Medrol) intravenously
3. Prednisone (Deltasone) orally
4. Fludrocortisone (Florinef) subcutaneously

**Answer: 2**
*Rationale:* A glucocorticoid preparation will be administered intravenously or intramuscularly in the immediate preoperative period to a client scheduled for an adrenalectomy. Methylprednisolone sodium succinate protects the client from acute adrenal insufficiency (Addison's crisis), which occurs as a result of the adrenalectomy. Aldactone is a potassium-sparing diuretic. Prednisone is an oral corticosteroid. Fludrocortisone is a mineralocorticoid.

*Test-Taking Strategy:* Focus on the issue: preventing Addison's crisis in a client scheduled for adrenalectomy. Recalling the function of the adrenal glands will assist in eliminating options 1 and 4. From the remaining options, select option 2 because the client is preoperative and should receive medications via routes other than orally. Review preoperative care for the client scheduled for adrenalectomy if you had difficulty with this question.

*Level of Cognitive Ability:* Application
*Client Needs:* Physiological Integrity
*Integrated Concept/Process:* Nursing Process/Planning
*Content Area:* Adult Health/Endocrine

*Reference*
Smeltzer, S., & Bare, B. (2000). *Brunner & Suddarth's Textbook of medical-surgical nursing* (9th ed.). Philadelphia: Lippincott Williams & Wilkins, p. 1062.

---

**250.** A nurse prepares a nursing care plan for a client with Graves' disease who is to receive radioactive iodine therapy. Which of the following statements would be most appropriate for the nurse to include in the teaching plan for this client?

1. The radioactive iodine is designed to destroy the entire thyroid gland with just one dose
2. It takes 6 to 8 weeks after treatment to experience relief from the symptoms of the disease
3. The high levels of radioactivity prohibit contact with family for 4 weeks after initial treatment
4. Following the initial dose, subsequent treatments must continue lifelong

**Answer: 2**
*Rationale:* Following treatment with radioactive iodine therapy, a decrease in thyroid hormone level should be noted, which would help to alleviate symptoms. Relief of symptoms does not occur until 6 to 8 weeks after initial treatment. This form of therapy is not designed to destroy the entire gland; rather, some of the cells that synthesize thyroid hormone will be destroyed by the local radiation. The nurse needs to reassure the client and family that unless the dosage is extremely high, clients are not required to observe radiation precautions. The rationale for this is that the radioactivity dissipates quickly. Occasionally, a client may require a second or third dose, but treatments are never lifelong.

*Test-Taking Strategy:* Use the process of elimination and knowledge regarding this treatment. Note the absolute words *entire*, *prohibit*, and *must* in the incorrect options. Review this treatment if you had difficulty with this question.

*Level of Cognitive Ability:* Application
*Client Needs:* Physiological Integrity
*Integrated Concept/Process:* Nursing Process/Planning
*Content Area:* Adult Health/Endocrine

*Reference*
Ignatavicius, D., Workman, M., & Mishler, M. (1999). *Medical-surgical nursing across the health care continuum* (3rd ed.). Philadelphia: W.B. Saunders, p. 1617.

---

**251.** A client arrives at the emergency department with upper gastrointestinal (GI) bleeding and is in moderate distress. The priority nursing action is to:

1. Ask the client about the precipitating events
2. Insert a nasogastric (NG) tube and perform a Hematest on the emesis
3. Complete an abdominal physical examination
4. Obtain vital signs

**Answer: 4**
*Rationale:* The priority action is to obtain vital signs to determine whether the client is in shock from blood loss and to obtain a baseline by which to monitor the progress of treatment. The client may not be able to provide subjective data until the immediate physical needs are met. Insertion of an NG tube may be prescribed but is not the priority action. A complete abdominal physical examination needs to be performed but is not the priority.

*Test-Taking Strategy:* Use the process of elimination, noting the key word *priority*. Recall that the client with a GI bleed is at risk for shock. Also option 4 addresses the ABCs (airway, breathing, and circulation). Review care of a client with a GI bleed if you had difficulty with this question

*Level of Cognitive Ability:* Application
*Client Needs:* Physiological Integrity
*Integrated Concept/Process:* Nursing Process/Implementation
*Content Area:* Adult Health/Gastrointestinal

*Reference*
Ignatavicius, D., Workman, M., & Mishler, M. (1999). *Medical-surgical nursing across the health care continuum* (3rd ed.). Philadelphia: W.B. Saunders, p. 1387.

---

**252.** A fluid restriction of 1500 mL per day is ordered for a client with acute renal failure. The nurse best plans to assist the client with maintaining the restriction by:

1 Prohibiting beverages with sugar to minimize thirst
2 Using mouthwash with alcohol for mouth care
3 Asking the client to calculate the IV fluids into the total daily allotment
4 Removing the water pitcher from the bedside

**Answer: 4**
*Rationale:* The nurse can help the client maintain fluid restriction through a variety of means. One way is to provide frequent mouth care; however, alcohol-based products should be avoided because they are drying to mucous membranes. The use of ice chips and lip ointments are other interventions that may be helpful to the client on a fluid restriction. Beverages that the client enjoys are provided and are not restricted based on sugar content. The client is not asked to keep track of IV fluid intake; this is the responsibility of the nurse. The water pitcher should be removed from the bedside to aid in compliance.

*Test-Taking Strategy:* Use the process of elimination. Eliminate option 3 because this is a nursing responsibility. Eliminate option 2 next, since alcohol-based products are drying to oral mucous membranes and could exacerbate thirst. From the remaining options, focus on the key word *best* to direct you to option 4. Review measures to promote compliance with fluid restrictions if you had difficulty with this question.

*Level of Cognitive Ability:* Application
*Client Needs:* Physiological Integrity
*Integrated Concept/Process:* Nursing Process/Implementation
*Content Area:* Adult Health/Renal

*Reference*
Smeltzer, S., & Bare, B. (2000). *Brunner & Suddarth's Textbook of medical-surgical nursing* (9th ed.). Philadelphia: Lippincott Williams & Wilkins, p. 1149.

---

**253.** A nurse has administered approximately half of a high cleansing enema when the client complains of pain and cramping. Which nursing action is the most appropriate?

1 Raising the enema bag so that the solution can be completed quickly
2 Clamping the tubing for 30 seconds and restarting the flow at a slower rate
3 Reassuring the client and continuing the flow
4 Discontinuing the enema and notifying the physician

**Answer: 2**
*Rationale:* The enema fluid should be administered slowly. If the client complains of pain or cramping, the flow is stopped for 30 seconds and restarted at a slower rate. Slow enema administration and stopping the flow temporarily, if necessary, will decrease the likelihood of intestinal spasm and premature ejection of the solution. The higher the solution container is held above the rectum, the faster the flow and the greater the force in the rectum. There is no need to discontinue the enema and notify the physician at this time.

*Test-Taking Strategy:* Use the process of elimination, focusing on the issue: alleviating pain and cramping. Eliminate options 1 and 3 first because they are similar. From the remaining options, noting that there is no need to notify the physician will direct you to option 2. Review the procedure for enema administration if you had difficulty with this question.

*Level of Cognitive Ability:* Application
*Client Needs:* Physiological Integrity
*Integrated Concept/Process:* Nursing Process/Implementation
*Content Area:* Fundamental Skills

*Reference*
Potter, P., & Perry, A. (2001). *Fundamentals of nursing* (5th ed.). St. Louis: Mosby, p. 1460.

---

**254.** A client with chronic renal failure who is scheduled for hemodialysis this morning is due to receive a daily dose of enalapril (Vasotec). The nurse plans to administer this medication:
1  Just before dialysis
2  During dialysis
3  Upon return from dialysis
4  The day after dialysis

**Answer: 3**
*Rationale:* Antihypertensive medications, such as enalapril, are administered to the client following hemodialysis. This prevents the client from becoming hypotensive during dialysis and also from having the medication removed from the bloodstream by dialysis. There is no rationale for waiting a full day to resume the medication. This would lead to ineffective control of the blood pressure.

*Test-Taking Strategy:* Use the process of elimination. Think about the effects of an antihypertensive medication on the blood pressure when fluid is being removed from the body. Since hypotension is much more likely to occur in this circumstance, eliminate options 1 and 2. Since most clients are hemodialyzed three times a week, if the medication was held for dialysis until the following day, the client would miss three of the seven doses that would usually be given in a week. This would lead to ineffective blood pressure control. Therefore, eliminate option 4. Review the procedure for preparing a client for dialysis if you had difficulty with this question.

*Level of Cognitive Ability:* Application
*Client Needs:* Physiological Integrity
*Integrated Concept/Process:* Nursing Process/Planning
*Content Area:* Pharmacology

*Reference*
Smeltzer, S., & Bare, B. (2000). *Brunner & Suddarth's Textbook of medical-surgical nursing* (9th ed.). Philadelphia: Lippincott Williams & Wilkins, p. 1115.

---

**255.** A nurse is preparing to administer a high cleansing enema. The nurse positions the client in the:
1  Left-lateral position with the right leg acutely flexed
2  Supine position with the legs elevated
3  Dorsal recumbent position
4  Right-lateral position with the left leg acutely flexed

**Answer: 1**
*Rationale:* The sigmoid and descending colon are located on the left side. Therefore, the left-lateral position uses gravity to facilitate the flow of solution into the sigmoid and descending colon. Acute flexion of the right leg allows for adequate exposure of the anus. Options 2, 3, and 4 are incorrect positions.

*Test-Taking Strategy:* Use the process of elimination. Visualize this procedure and think about the anatomy of the colon to direct you to option 1. Review this procedure if you had difficulty with this question.

*Level of Cognitive Ability:* Application
*Client Needs:* Physiological Integrity
*Integrated Concept/Process:* Nursing Process/Implementation
*Content Area:* Fundamental Skills

*Reference*
Potter, P., & Perry, A. (2001). *Fundamentals of nursing* (5th ed.). St. Louis: Mosby, p. 1460.

---

**256.** A nurse is preparing to care for a client returning from the operating room following a subtotal thyroidectomy. The nurse anticipates the need for which of the following items to be placed at the bedside?

1. Emergency tracheostomy kit
2. Ampule of saturated solution of potassium iodide (SSKI)
3. Hypothermia blanket
4. Magnesium sulfate in a ready-to-inject vial

**Answer: 1**
*Rationale:* Respiratory distress can occur following thyroidectomy as a result of swelling in the tracheal area. The nurse would ensure that an emergency tracheostomy kit is available. SSKI is typically administered preoperatively to block thyroid hormone synthesis and release, as well as place the client in an euthyroid state. Iodine makes the thyroid gland less vascular before surgery. Surgery on the thyroid does not alter the heat control mechanism of the body. Magnesium sulfate would not be indicated, since the incidence of hypomagnesemia is not a common problem after thyroidectomy.

*Test-Taking Strategy:* Recall the anatomical location of the thyroid gland to direct you to option 1. Also, use the ABCs (airway, breathing, and circulation). Maintaining a patent airway is critical. Review care of a client following thyroidectomy if you had difficulty with this question.

*Level of Cognitive Ability:* Application
*Client Needs:* Physiological Integrity
*Integrated Concept/Process:* Nursing Process/Planning
*Content Area:* Adult Health/Endocrine

*Reference*
Smeltzer, S., & Bare, B. (2000). *Brunner & Suddarth's Textbook of medical-surgical nursing* (9th ed.). Philadelphia: Lippincott Williams & Wilkins, p. 1051.

---

**257.** Sodium nitroprusside (Nipride) is prescribed for a client with a diagnosis of cardiogenic shock. The nurse plans to do which of the following when preparing to administer this medication?

1. Protect the solution from light
2. Add potassium to the infusion
3. Administer only through a central line
4. Obtain a baseline thiocyanate level

**Answer: 1**
*Rationale:* Sodium nitroprusside becomes unstable when exposed to light and must be protected. No other medications are added to the infusion. It can be given through a peripheral line. The level of thiocyanate (a nitroprusside metabolite similar to cyanide) is usually drawn if the client is maintained on this therapy for several days.

*Test-Taking Strategy:* Use the process of elimination and knowledge of the principles related to administering IV medications. Options 2 and 3 can be eliminated even without knowledge of this medication using these basic principles. Usually, levels of any medication or its byproducts are measured after administration has been ongoing, so eliminate option 4. Review this medication if you had difficulty with this question.

*Level of Cognitive Ability:* Application
*Client Needs:* Physiological Integrity
*Integrated Concept/Process:* Nursing Process/Planning
*Content Area:* Pharmacology

*Reference*
Hodgson, B., & Kizior, R. (2001). *Saunders Nursing drug handbook 2001.* Philadelphia: W.B. Saunders, p. 754.

---

**258.** A nurse is encouraging the client to cough and deep breathe after cardiac surgery. The nurse ensures that which of the following items is available to maximize the effectiveness of this procedure?
1   Ambu bag
2   Incisional splinting device
3   Suction equipment
4   Nebulizer

**Answer: 2**
*Rationale:* The use of an incisional splint such as a "cough pillow" can ease discomfort during coughing and deep breathing. The client who is comfortable will do more effective deep breathing and coughing exercises. Use of an incentive spirometer is also indicated. Options 1, 3, and 4 will not encourage the client to cough and deep breathe.

*Test-Taking Strategy:* Use the process of elimination. Focus on the issue: an item that will maximize effectiveness. This issue eliminates options 1 and 3, which are items used by the nurse. A nebulizer (option 4) is used to deliver medication. Review measures that will assist the postoperative client to cough and deep breathe if you had difficulty with this question.

*Level of Cognitive Ability:* Application
*Client Needs:* Physiological Integrity
*Integrated Concept/Process:* Nursing Process/Implementation
*Content Area:* Adult Health/Respiratory

*Reference*
Smeltzer, S., & Bare, B. (2000). *Brunner & Suddarth's Textbook of medical-surgical nursing* (9th ed.). Philadelphia: Lippincott Williams & Wilkins, p. 323.

---

**259.** A nurse is preparing to administer an intermittent tube feeding through a nasogastric tube. The nurse assesses gastric residual before administering the tube feeding to:
1   Confirm proper nasogastric tube placement
2   Determine patency of the tube
3   Assess fluid and electrolyte status
4   Evaluate absorption of the last feeding

**Answer: 4**
*Rationale:* All stomach contents are aspirated and measured before administering a tube feeding. This procedure measures the gastric residual. The gastric residual is determined in order to evaluate whether undigested formula from a previous feeding remains. It is important to assess gastric residual because administration of a tube feeding to a full stomach could result in overdistention, thus predisposing the client to regurgitation and possible aspiration. Assessing residual does not confirm placement, determine patency, or assess fluid and electrolyte status.

*Test-Taking Strategy:* Focus on the issue: the purpose for assessing the residual. Note the relationship between the issue and option 4. Review the purpose of assessing residual if you had difficulty with this question.

*Level of Cognitive Ability:* Application
*Client Needs:* Physiological Integrity
*Integrated Concept/Process:* Nursing Process/Assessment
*Content Area:* Fundamental Skills

*Reference*
Smeltzer, S., & Bare, B. (2000). *Brunner & Suddarth's Textbook of medical-surgical nursing* (9th ed.). Philadelphia: Lippincott Williams & Wilkins, p. 840.

---

**260.** A nurse is caring for a client scheduled to undergo a renal biopsy. To minimize the risk of postprocedure complications, the nurse reports which of the following laboratory results before the procedure?
1   Blood urea nitrogen (BUN) 20 mg/dL
2   Serum creatinine 1.2 mg/dL
3   Bleeding time 13 minutes
4   Potassium 3.8 mEq/L

**Answer: 3**
*Rationale:* Postprocedure hemorrhage is a significant complication after renal biopsy. Because of this, bleeding times are assessed before the procedure. The normal bleeding time is 1 to 6 minutes depending on the type of test performed by the laboratory. The nurse assures that these results are available, and reports abnormalities promptly. Options 1, 2, and 4 identify normal values. The normal BUN is 8 to 25 mg/dL. The normal serum creatinine is 0.6 to 1.3 mg/dL and the normal potassium is 3.5 to 5.1 mEq/L.

*Test-Taking Strategy:* When a client is to have a biopsy, remember that bleeding is a concern. This will direct you to option 3. Also note that options 1, 2, and 4 identify normal values. Review the complications of renal biopsy and normal laboratory values if you had difficulty with this question.

*Level of Cognitive Ability:* Analysis
*Client Needs:* Physiological Integrity
*Integrated Concept/Process:* Nursing Process/Implementation
*Content Area:* Adult Health/Renal

*Reference*
Smeltzer, S., & Bare, B. (2000). *Brunner & Suddarth's Textbook of medical-surgical nursing* (9th ed.). Philadelphia: Lippincott Williams & Wilkins, p. 1096.

---

**261.** A client involved in a house fire is experiencing respiratory distress and an inhalation injury is suspected. The nurse monitors which of the following for the presence of carbon monoxide poisoning?
1   Pulse oximetry
2   Urine myoglobin
3   Sputum carbon levels
4   Serum carboxyhemoglobin levels

**Answer: 4**
*Rationale:* Serum carboxyhemoglobin levels are the most direct measure of carbon monoxide poisoning, provide the level of poisoning, and thus determine the appropriate treatment measures. The carbon monoxide molecule has a 200 times greater affinity for binding with hemoglobin than an oxygen molecule, causing decreased availability of oxygen to the cells. Clients are treated with 100% oxygen. Options 1, 2, and 3 would not identify carbon monoxide poisoning.

*Test-Taking Strategy:* Use the process of elimination. Note the relationship between *carbon monoxide* and option 4. Review carbon monoxide poisoning if you had difficulty with this question.

*Level of Cognitive Ability:* Application
*Client Needs:* Physiological Integrity
*Integrated Concept/Process:* Nursing Process/Assessment
*Content Area:* Adult Health/Respiratory

*Reference*
Smeltzer, S., & Bare, B. (2000). *Brunner & Suddarth's Textbook of medical-surgical nursing* (9th ed.). Philadelphia: Lippincott Williams & Wilkins, p. 1506.

---

**262.** A nurse is assigned to care for a client with hypertonic labor contractions. The nurse plans to conserve the client's energy and promote rest by:

1  Avoiding uncomfortable procedures such as intravenous infusions or epidural anesthesia

2  Assisting the client with breathing and relaxation techniques

3  Keeping the room brightly lit so the client can watch her monitor

4  Keeping the television (TV) or radio on to provide distraction

**Answer: 2**
*Rationale:* Breathing and relaxation techniques aid the client in coping with the discomfort of labor and in conserving energy. The use of intravenous or epidural pain relief can be useful. Intravenous hydration can increase perfusion and oxygenation of maternal and fetal tissues and provide glucose for energy needs. Noise from a TV or radio and light stimulation does not promote rest. A quiet, dim environment would be more advantageous.

*Test-Taking Strategy:* Focus on the issue: conserving energy and promoting rest for the client. Noting the key word *assisting* in option 2 will direct you to this option. Review care of a client with hypertonic labor contractions if you had difficulty with this question.

*Level of Cognitive Ability:* Application
*Client Needs:* Physiological Integrity
*Integrated Concept/Process:* Nursing Process/Planning
*Content Area:* Maternity

*Reference*
Lowdermilk, D., Perry, S., & Bobak, I. (2000). *Maternity & women's health care* (7th ed.). St. Louis: Mosby, p. 994.

---

**263.** A client with acute pyelonephritis has nausea and is vomiting. The client is scheduled for an intravenous pyelogram. The nurse places highest priority on which action?

1  Place the client on hourly intake and output measurements

2  Request an order for an IV infusion from the physician

3  Ask the client to sign the informed consent

4  Explain the procedure thoroughly to the client

**Answer: 2**
*Rationale:* The highest priority of the nurse would be to obtain an order for intravenous therapy. This is needed to replace fluid lost with vomiting, will be necessary for dye injection for the procedure, and will assist with the elimination of the dye following the procedure. The intake and output should be measured, but this will not assist in preventing dehydration. The procedure is explained and the signed consent is obtained once the client's physiological needs are met.

*Test-Taking Strategy:* Using Maslow's Hierarchy of Needs theory will assist in eliminating options 3 and 4. From the remaining options, noting that the client is vomiting will direct you to option 2. Review care of a client who is vomiting if you had difficulty with this question.

*Level of Cognitive Ability:* Application
*Client Needs:* Physiological Integrity
*Integrated Concept/Process:* Nursing Process/Implementation
*Content Area:* Adult Health/Renal

*Reference*
Smeltzer, S., & Bare, B. (2000). *Brunner & Suddarth's Textbook of medical-surgical nursing* (9th ed.). Philadelphia: Lippincott Williams & Wilkins, p. 1095.

---

**264.** A nurse is planning care for a client with a T3 spinal cord injury. The nurse includes which intervention in the plan to prevent autonomic dysreflexia (hyperreflexia)?

1  Assess vital signs, and observe for hypotension, tachycardia, and tachypnea
2  Teach the client that this condition is relatively minor with few symptoms
3  Assist the client to develop a daily bowel routine to prevent constipation
4  Administer dexamethasone (Decadron) as per the physician's order

**Answer: 3**
*Rationale:* Autonomic dysreflexia (hyperreflexia) may be triggered by bowel distention. A daily bowel program eliminates this trigger. A client with autonomic dysreflexia would be hypertensive and bradycardic. Autonomic dysreflexia is potentially life threatening if intervention does not occur. Removal of the stimuli results in prompt resolution of the signs and symptoms. Option 4 is unrelated to this specific condition.

*Test-Taking Strategy:* Focus on the key word *prevent* to eliminate options 1 and 2. From the remaining options, remembering that this condition may be triggered by bowel distention will direct you to option 3. If you are unfamiliar with this syndrome, review its causes.

*Level of Cognitive Ability:* Application
*Client Needs:* Physiological Integrity
*Integrated Concept/Process:* Nursing Process/Planning
*Content Area:* Adult Health/Neurological

*Reference*
Smeltzer, S., & Bare, B. (2000). *Brunner & Suddarth's Textbook of medical-surgical nursing* (9th ed.). Philadelphia: Lippincott Williams & Wilkins, p. 1693.

---

**265.** A client in cardiogenic shock has an order for an intravenous (IV) nitroglycerin (Nitrostat) drip for control of chest pain and to increase myocardial tissue perfusion. The nurse understands that the nitroglycerin must be prepared by mixing the medication:

1  In a solution that is in a plastic bag
2  In a solution that is in a glass bottle
3  Every hour because of its unstable chemical structure
4  Under a laminar flow hood

**Answer: 2**
*Rationale:* IV nitroglycerin is prepared only in glass bottles, using the administration sets provided. Standard plastic (polyvinyl chloride) tubing will adsorb the nitroglycerin, reducing the potency and reliability of the medication. It should also be protected from extremes of light and temperature. It should be remixed every 4 hours. It does not require mixture under a laminar flow hood.

*Test-Taking Strategy:* Use the process of elimination. Eliminate option 3, because "every hour" is much too frequent. From the remaining options, note that options 1 and 2 provide two opposite methods of administration. This should provide a clue that one of these methods may be accurate. Remember, standard plastic will adsorb the nitroglycerin. Review the procedure for preparing IV nitroglycerin if you had difficulty with this question.

*Level of Cognitive Ability:* Analysis
*Client Needs:* Physiological Integrity
*Integrated Concept/Process:* Nursing Process/Implementation
*Content Area:* Pharmacology

**Reference**
Hodgson, B., & Kizior, R. (2001). *Saunders Nursing drug handbook 2001.* Philadelphia: W.B. Saunders, p. 750.

---

**266.** A client has a left pleural effusion that has not yet been treated. The nurse plans to have which of the following items available for immediate use?
1  Thoracentesis tray
2  Paracentesis tray
3  Intubation tray
4  Central line insertion tray

**Answer: 1**
*Rationale:* The client with a significant pleural effusion is usually treated by thoracentesis. This procedure allows drainage of the fluid, which may then be analyzed to determine the precise cause of the effusion. The nurse ensures that a thoracentesis tray is readily available, in case the client's symptoms should rapidly become more severe. A paracentesis tray is needed for the removal of abdominal effusion. Options 3 and 4 are not specifically indicated for this procedure.

*Test-Taking Strategy:* Use the process of elimination and knowledge regarding the usual treatment for pleural effusion. Note the relationship between the words *pleural* in the question and *thoracentesis* in the correct option. If this question was difficult, review the treatment for pleural effusion.

*Level of Cognitive Ability:* Application
*Client Needs:* Physiological Integrity
*Integrated Concept/Process:* Nursing Process/Planning
*Content Area:* Adult Health/Respiratory

**Reference**
Smeltzer, S., & Bare, B. (2000). *Brunner & Suddarth's Textbook of medical-surgical nursing* (9th ed.). Philadelphia: Lippincott Williams & Wilkins, p. 444.

---

**267.** A client has been taking procainamide (Pronestyl) 750 mg PO BID. The nurse prepares to administer the medication and implements which of the following before giving the medication?
1  Nothing, because this is a nontoxic medication
2  Assesses the client for the side effects of the medication
3  Schedules the client for a drug level 1 hour after the first dose
4  Monitors the vital signs and the ECG continuously

**Answer: 2**
*Rationale:* This medication may cause side effects such as diarrhea, nausea and vomiting, and heart failure; therefore, the client should be assessed before the administration of the medication. Although vital signs need to be monitored, continuous monitoring is not necessary. Option 1 is incorrect, and option 3 is not an action taken before administration of the medication.

*Test-Taking Strategy:* Use the process of elimination. Focus on the key words *before* in the question and use the steps of the nursing process. This will direct you to option 2. Review this medication if you had difficulty with this question.

*Level of Cognitive Ability:* Application
*Client Needs:* Physiological Integrity

*Integrated Concept/Process:* Nursing Process/Implementation
*Content Area:* Pharmacology

*Reference*
Hodgson, B., & Kizior, R. (2001). *Saunders Nursing drug handbook 2001.* Philadelphia: W.B. Saunders, p. 861.

---

**268.** A client with urolithiasis is being evaluated to determine the type of stone that is being formed. The nurse plans to keep which of the following items available in the client's room to assist in this process?
1   A calorie count sheet
2   A strainer
3   An intake and output record
4   A vital signs graphic sheet

**Answer: 2**
*Rationale:* The urine is strained until the stone is passed and obtained for analysis. Straining the urine will catch small stones that may be sent to the laboratory for analysis. Once the type of stone is determined, an individualized plan of care for prevention and treatment is developed. Options 1, 3, and 4 are unrelated to the question.

*Test-Taking Strategy:* Focus on the issue: an item that will help to determine the type of stone. Eliminate options 1, 3, and 4, since these items give information about food intake, vital signs, and fluid balance but will not provide data that will help determine the type of stone. Review care of a client with urolithiasis if you had difficulty with this question.

*Level of Cognitive Ability:* Application
*Client Needs:* Physiological Integrity
*Integrated Concept/Process:* Nursing Process/Planning
*Content Area:* Adult Health/Renal

*Reference*
Smeltzer, S., & Bare, B. (2000). *Brunner & Suddarth's Textbook of medical-surgical nursing* (9th ed.). Philadelphia: Lippincott Williams & Wilkins, p. 1163.

---

**269.** A client develops bilateral wheezes, orthopnea, and tachypnea, and the nurse notes the presence of 2+ pitting edema. The nurse suspects pulmonary edema and notifies the physician. While awaiting the physician's arrival, the nurse avoids which action?
1   Preparing to administer IV morphine sulfate
2   Placing the client in the high-Fowler's position
3   Elevating the client's legs
4   Preparing to administer IV furosemide (Lasix)

**Answer: 3**
*Rationale:* Elevating the client's legs would rapidly increase venous return to the right side of the heart and worsen the client's condition. The feet should be in the horizontal position, or the client could dangle at the bedside if the client's condition permits. Morphine sulfate reduces anxiety and is likely to be prescribed. Anxiety causes an increase in the oxygen demands on the heart. A high-Fowler's position increases the thoracic capacity, which improves ventilation. Furosemide will be prescribed because of its diuretic action.

*Test-Taking Strategy:* Use the process of elimination and note the key word *avoids*. Recalling that the pulmonary system is congested will direct you to option 3 because this action would cause further congestion of the pulmonary system. Review care of a client with pulmonary edema if you had difficulty with this question.

*Level of Cognitive Ability:* Application
*Client Needs:* Physiological Integrity
*Integrated Concept/Process:* Nursing Process/Implementation
*Content Area:* Adult Health/Cardiovascular

*Reference*
Smeltzer, S., & Bare, B. (2000). *Brunner & Suddarth's Textbook of medical-surgical nursing* (9th ed.). Philadelphia: Lippincott Williams & Wilkins, p. 657.

---

**270.** A nurse is caring for a client following a ureterolithotomy. The client has a ureteral tube. On review of the physician's orders, the nurse notes that the client has a PRN order to irrigate the tube. The nurse plans to avoid which of the following in the management of this tube?

1  Irrigating using gentle force
2  Irrigating using gravity
3  Clamping the tube
4  Using a separate drainage bag for the ureteral catheter

**Answer: 3**

*Rationale:* A ureteral tube is never clamped, because the renal pelvis can hold only about 5 mL at a time. The nurse who has an order to irrigate the tube may do so using gravity or gentle force only. A drainage bag attached to the ureteral catheter is used so that accurate measurement of urine flow can be done.

*Test-Taking Strategy:* Use the process of elimination, noting the key word *avoid*. Focus on the issue—a ureteral tube—and think about the anatomy of the kidney to direct you to option 3. Remember, ureteral tubes are never clamped. Review care of a client with a ureteral tube if you had difficulty with this question.

*Level of Cognitive Ability:* Application
*Client Needs:* Physiological Integrity
*Integrated Concept/Process:* Nursing Process/Planning
*Content Area:* Adult Health/Renal

*Reference*
Potter, P., & Perry, A. (2001). *Fundamentals of nursing* (5th ed.). St. Louis: Mosby, p. 1424.

---

**271.** Before administering a tube feeding, a nurse aspirates 40 mL of undigested formula from a client's nasogastric tube. The nurse understands that before administering the tube feeding, the 40 mL of gastric aspirate should be:

1  Discarded properly and recorded as output on the client's I&O record
2  Poured into the nasogastric tube through a syringe with the plunger removed
3  Mixed with the formula and poured into the nasogastric tube through a syringe without a plunger
4  Diluted with water and injected into the nasogastric tube by putting pressure on the plunger

**Answer: 2**

*Rationale:* After checking residual feeding contents, the nurse reinstills the gastric contents into the stomach by removing the syringe bulb or plunger and pouring the gastric contents via the syringe into the nasogastric tube. Gastric contents should be reinstilled to maintain the client's electrolyte balance. It does not need to be mixed with water, nor should it be discarded or mixed with formula.

*Test-Taking Strategy:* Use the process of elimination. Remembering that the removal of the gastric contents could disturb the client's electrolyte balance will assist in eliminating option 1. Eliminate option 4 because of the word *pressure*. From the remaining options, recalling that gastric contents aspirated should be immediately replaced will assist in directing you to the correct option. Review this procedure if you had difficulty with this question.

*Level of Cognitive Ability:* Application
*Client Needs:* Physiological Integrity
*Integrated Concept/Process:* Nursing Process/Implementation
*Content Area:* Fundamental Skills

*Reference*
Smeltzer, S., & Bare, B. (2000). *Brunner & Suddarth's Textbook of medical-surgical nursing* (9th ed.). Philadelphia: Lippincott Williams & Wilkins, p. 842.

---

**272.** A nurse is caring for a client with suspected carbon monoxide poisoning. Of the following interventions that the nurse assists in implementing, which is of highest priority?
1   Requesting a building inspection at the site of the incident from the local health department
2   Drawing blood for carboxyhemoglobin levels
3   Frequently observing the client
4   Administering 100% oxygen

**Answer: 4**
*Rationale:* 100% oxygen is administered at atmospheric pressure or hyperbaric pressure to speed up the elimination of carbon monoxide from the hemoglobin and to reverse hypoxia. The next most important action is constant observation of the client. The client may exhibit a variety of symptoms caused by central nervous system damage, which include ataxia, spastic paralysis, visual disturbances, personality changes, and psychoses. Blood is drawn serially to monitor carboxyhemoglobin levels; once they drop under 5%, oxygen may be removed. If the episode was unintentional and precipitated by conditions in a dwelling, the health department is notified.

*Test-Taking Strategy:* Use the process of elimination, noting the key words *highest priority*. Use the ABCs (airway, breathing, and circulation) to direct you to option 4. Review care of a client with carbon monoxide poisoning if you had difficulty with this question.

*Level of Cognitive Ability:* Application
*Client Needs:* Physiological Integrity
*Integrated Concept/Process:* Nursing Process/Implementation
*Content Area:* Adult Health/Respiratory

*Reference*
Smeltzer, S., & Bare, B. (2000). *Brunner & Suddarth's Textbook of medical-surgical nursing* (9th ed.). Philadelphia: Lippincott Williams & Wilkins, p. 1921.

---

**273.** A client with adult respiratory distress syndrome has an order to be placed on a continuous positive airway pressure (CPAP) face mask. The nurse ensures that which of the following is implemented, for this procedure to be most effective?
1   Apply the mask to the face with a snug fit
2   Obtain baseline arterial blood gases
3   Obtain baseline arterial oxygen saturation levels
4   Allow the client to remove the mask frequently for coughing

**Answer: 1**
*Rationale:* The face mask must be applied over the nose and mouth with a snug fit, which is necessary to maintain positive pressure in the client's airways. The nurse obtains baseline respiratory assessments and arterial blood gases to evaluate the effectiveness of therapy, but these are not done to increase the effectiveness of the procedure. A disadvantage of the CPAP face mask is that the client must remove it for coughing, eating, or drinking. This removes benefit of positive pressure in the airway each time the mask is removed.

*Test-Taking Strategy:* Focus on the issue: a nursing action that will make the procedure most effective. Options 2 and 3 do not make the therapy more effective and are eliminated. From the remaining options, knowing that positive pressure must be maintained to be effective will direct you to option 1. Review care of a client with a CPAP face mask if you had difficulty with this question.

*Level of Cognitive Ability:* Application
*Client Needs:* Physiological Integrity
*Integrated Concept/Process:* Nursing Process/Implementation
*Content Area:* Adult Health/Respiratory

**Reference**
Smeltzer, S., & Bare, B. (2000). *Brunner & Suddarth's Textbook of medical-surgical nursing* (9th ed.). Philadelphia: Lippincott Williams & Wilkins, p. 493.

---

**274.** A nurse is caring for a client scheduled to undergo a cardiac catheterization for the first time. The nurse tells the client that:

1  The procedure is performed in the operating room (OR), with the personnel wearing scrub gowns and masks
2  The client may feel fatigue and have various aches, because it is necessary to lie quietly on a hard x-ray table for about 4 hours
3  The client may feel certain sensations at various points during the procedure, such as a fluttery feeling, a flushed warm feeling, a desire to cough, or palpitations
4  Initial catheter insertion is quite painful; after that, there is little or no pain

**Answer: 3**

*Rationale:* Preprocedure teaching points include that the procedure is done in a darkened cardiac catheterization room and that ECG leads are attached to the client. A local anesthetic is used, so there is little to no pain with catheter insertion. The x-ray table is hard and may be tilted periodically. The procedure may take up to 2 hours, and the client may feel various sensations with catheter passage and dye injection.

*Test-Taking Strategy:* Use the process of elimination. The location (operating room) eliminates option 1. The duration of the procedure, 4 hours, eliminates option 2. From the remaining options, noting the words *quite painful* in option 4 will direct you to option 3. If you had difficulty with this question, review the client preparation for this procedure.

*Level of Cognitive Ability:* Application
*Client Needs:* Physiological Integrity
*Integrated Concept/Process:* Teaching/Learning
*Content Area:* Adult Health/Cardiovascular

**Reference**
Smeltzer, S., & Bare, B. (2000). *Brunner & Suddarth's Textbook of medical-surgical nursing* (9th ed.). Philadelphia: Lippincott Williams & Wilkins, p. 557.

---

**275.** A client with acquired immunodeficiency syndrome will be receiving aerosolized pentamidine isethionate (NebuPent) prophylactically once every 4 weeks. The home health nurse visits and instructs the client about the medication. Which statement by the client indicates a need for further teaching?

1  "If you develop a cough or shortness of breath after receiving the inhalation therapy, I need to let a doctor or nurse know."
2  "If I have any visual disturbances, I need to let the doctor know."
3  "There are no known side effects of this therapy."
4  "I may experience some nausea with the inhalation therapy."

**Answer: 3**

*Rationale:* Side effects associated with this therapy include nausea, visual disturbances, or shortness of breath. The client needs to inform the health care provider if cough, shortness of breath, or visual disturbances occur.

*Test-Taking Strategy:* Use the process of elimination. Note the key words *indicates a need for further teaching*. Noting the words *no known side effects* will direct you to this option. Review this medication if you had difficulty with this question.

*Level of Cognitive Ability:* Analysis
*Client Needs:* Physiological Integrity
*Integrated Concept/Process:* Self Care
*Content Area:* Adult Health/Immune

**Reference**
Hodgson, B., & Kizior, R. (2001). *Saunders Nursing drug handbook 2001.* Philadelphia: W.B. Saunders, p. 801.

**276.** A nurse admits a client with myocardial infarction (MI) to the coronary care unit (CCU). The nurse plans to do which of the following in delivering care to this client?

1. Administer oxygen at a rate of 6 liters/minute by nasal cannula
2. Infuse intravenous (IV) fluid at a rate of 150 mL/hr
3. Begin a continuous heparin infusion at a rate of 2000 U/hr
4. Place the client on continuous cardiac monitoring

**Answer: 4**

*Rationale:* Standard interventions upon admittance to the CCU as they relate to this question include continuous cardiac monitoring, oxygen at a rate of 2 L/min unless otherwise ordered, and an IV line insertion or intermittent lock. If an IV infusion is administered, it is maintained at a keep vein open rate to prevent fluid overload and heart failure. A heparin drip may be instituted according to protocol, but a rate of 2000 units per hour is excessive.

*Test-Taking Strategy:* Use the process of elimination. Note the relationship between the client's diagnosis and option 4. Also, note that the values in options 1, 2, and 3 related to the rates of oxygen, IV fluid, and heparin infusion are high. Review care of a client following MI if you had difficulty with this question.

*Level of Cognitive Ability:* Application
*Client Needs:* Physiological Integrity
*Integrated Concept/Process:* Nursing Process/Planning
*Content Area:* Adult Health/Cardiovascular

*Reference*
Smeltzer, S., & Bare, B. (2000). *Brunner & Suddarth's Textbook of medical-surgical nursing* (9th ed.). Philadelphia: Lippincott Williams & Wilkins, pp. 629-630.

---

**277.** A nurse is trying to analyze an ECG rhythm strip on an assigned client and asks another nurse how much time each small box on the ECG paper represents. The second nurse responds that each small box measures:

1. 0.02 second
2. 0.04 second
3. 0.20 second
4. 0.40 second

**Answer: 2**

*Rationale:* Standard ECG graph paper measurements are 0.04 second for each small box on the horizontal axis (measuring time) and 1 mm (measuring voltage) for each small box on the vertical axis.

*Test-Taking Strategy:* Knowledge regarding ECG basics is necessary to answer this question. Review these basics because they will be helpful in answering questions related to dysrhythmias.

*Level of Cognitive Ability:* Comprehension
*Client Needs:* Physiological Integrity
*Integrated Concept/Process:* Teaching/Learning
*Content Area:* Adult Health/Cardiovascular

*Reference*
Ignatavicius, D., Workman, M., & Mishler, M. (1999). *Medical-surgical nursing across the health care continuum* (3rd ed.). Philadelphia: W.B. Saunders, p. 761.

**278.** A nurse is applying ECG electrodes to a diaphoretic client. The nurse does which of the following to keep the electrodes from coming loose?

1  Secures the electrodes with adhesive tape
2  Places clear, transparent dressings over the electrodes
3  Applies lanolin to the skin before applying the electrodes
4  Applies a little benzoin to the skin before applying the electrodes

**Answer: 4**

*Rationale:* Tincture of benzoin is commonly used on a diaphoretic client to help the electrodes adhere to the skin. Placing adhesive tape or a clear dressing over the electrodes will not help the adhesive gel of the actual electrode to make better contact with the diaphoretic skin. Lanolin or any other lotion makes the skin slippery and prevents good initial adherence.

*Test-Taking Strategy:* Use the process of elimination. Note that options 1 and 2 are similar in that they both provide an external form of providing security of the electrodes. From the remaining options, note that option 4 addresses direct contact with the skin. Review the procedure for attaching ECG electrodes if you had difficulty with this question.

*Level of Cognitive Ability:* Application
*Client Needs:* Physiological Integrity
*Integrated Concept/Process:* Nursing Process/Implementation
*Content Area:* Adult Health/Cardiovascular

*Reference*
Smeltzer, S., & Bare, B. (2000). *Brunner & Suddarth's Textbook of medical-surgical nursing* (9th ed.). Philadelphia: Lippincott Williams & Wilkins, p. 567.

---

**279.** A nurse has developed a plan of care for a client with a diagnosis of anterior cord syndrome. Which intervention would the nurse include in the plan of care?

1  Assess the client for pain before physical therapy
2  Remind the client to change positions slowly
3  Assess the sensation of touch and vibration above the level of injury
4  Teach the client about loss of motor function and temperature sensation

**Answer: 4**

*Rationale:* Clinical findings related to anterior cord syndrome include loss of motor function and temperature sensation below the level of injury. The syndrome is not painful and does not affect sensations of touch, motion, position, and vibration.

*Test-Taking Strategy:* Specific knowledge of anterior cord syndrome is necessary to answer this question. If you are unfamiliar with this syndrome, review the nursing interventions related to the disorder.

*Level of Cognitive Ability:* Application
*Client Needs:* Physiological Integrity
*Integrated Concept/Process:* Nursing Process/Planning
*Content Area:* Adult Health/Neurological

*Reference*
Smeltzer, S., & Bare, B. (2000). *Brunner & Suddarth's Textbook of medical-surgical nursing* (9th ed.). Philadelphia: Lippincott Williams & Wilkins, p. 1688.

**280.** A nurse is caring for a client with a thoracic spinal cord injury. As part of the nursing care plan, the nurse monitors for spinal shock. In the event that spinal shock occurs, the nurse anticipates that the most likely intravenous (IV) fluid to be prescribed would be:

1. 5% dextrose in water ($D_5W$)
2. Dextran
3. 5% dextrose in normal saline solution ($D_5NS$)
4. Normal saline solution (NS)

**Answer: 4**

*Rationale:* NS is an isotonic solution that primarily remains in the intravascular space, increasing intravascular volume. This IV fluid would increase the client's blood pressure. Dextran is rarely used in spinal shock because isotonic fluid administration is usually sufficient. Additionally, Dextran has potentially serious side effects. $D_5W$ is a hypotonic solution that pulls fluid out of the intravascular space and is not indicated for shock. $D_5NS$ is hypertonic and indicated for shock resulting from hemorrhage or burns.

*Test-Taking Strategy:* Focus on the issue: spinal shock. Knowledge of the treatment for spinal shock and the purpose of the various IV fluids will direct you to option 4. Review the IV therapy associated with this disorder if you had difficulty with this question.

*Level of Cognitive Ability:* Application
*Client Needs:* Physiological Integrity
*Integrated Concept/Process:* Nursing Process/Planning
*Content Area:* Adult Health/Neurological

*Reference*
Smeltzer, S., & Bare, B. (2000). *Brunner & Suddarth's Textbook of medical-surgical nursing* (9th ed.). Philadelphia: Lippincott Williams & Wilkins, p. 259.

**281.** A client with myocardial infarction begins to experience multiform premature ventricular contractions (PVCs). The nurse plans to have which of the following medications available for immediate use?

1. Digoxin (Lanoxin)
2. Metoprolol (Lopressor)
3. Verapamil (Isoptin) — Calcium-channel-blocking agent
4. Lidocaine hydrochloride (Xylocaine)

**Answer: 4**

*Rationale:* Lidocaine hydrochloride is a Class 1 antidysrhythmic that is the medication of choice to treat ventricular dysrhythmias associated with acute myocardial ischemia or infarction. Digoxin is a cardiac glycoside; metoprolol is a beta-adrenergic blocking agent; verapamil is a calcium channel–blocking agent.

*Test-Taking Strategy:* Use the process of elimination, focusing on the issue: PVCs. Recalling the classification of each medication listed in the options will direct you to option 4. Review the treatment for PVCs if you had difficulty with this question.

*Level of Cognitive Ability:* Application
*Client Needs:* Physiological Integrity
*Integrated Concept/Process:* Nursing Process/Planning
*Content Area:* Pharmacology

*Reference*
Smeltzer, S., & Bare, B. (2000). *Brunner & Suddarth's Textbook of medical-surgical nursing* (9th ed.). Philadelphia: Lippincott Williams & Wilkins, p. 581.

**282.** A client has Buck's extension traction applied to the right leg. The nurse plans which of the following interventions to prevent complications of the device?
1 Massage the skin of the right leg with lotion every 8 hours
2 Provide pin care once a shift
3 Inspect the skin on the right leg at least once every 8 hours
4 Release the weights on the right leg for range of motion exercises daily

**Answer: 3**
*Rationale:* Buck's extension traction is a type of skin traction. The nurse inspects the skin of the limb in traction at least once every 8 hours for irritation or inflammation. Massaging the skin with lotion is not indicated. The nurse never releases the weights of traction unless specifically ordered by the physician. There are no pins to care for with skin traction.

*Test-Taking Strategy:* Focus on the issue: Buck's extension traction. Recalling that there are no pins in Buck's traction and that the nurse never removes weights without a specific order to do so eliminates options 2 and 4. From the remaining options, noting that the device would have to be removed to apply lotion will direct you to option 3. Review care of a client in Buck's traction if you had difficulty with this question.

*Level of Cognitive Ability:* Application
*Client Needs:* Physiological Integrity
*Integrated Concept/Process:* Nursing Process/Planning
*Content Area:* Adult Health/Musculoskeletal

*Reference*
Ignatavicius, D., Workman, M., & Mishler, M. (1999). *Medical-surgical nursing across the health care continuum* (3rd ed.). Philadelphia: W.B. Saunders, p. 1289.

**283.** A nurse is in the room of a client on a cardiac monitor whose cardiac rhythm changes to ventricular fibrillation (VF). The nurse calls for help, knowing that which of the following items will be needed immediately?
1 Pacemaker insertion tray
2 Ventilator
3 Defibrillator
4 Lidocaine hydrochloride (Xylocaine)

**Answer: 3**
*Rationale:* A defibrillator is needed to correct VF. Options 1 and 2 will do nothing to correct this rhythm. Lidocaine is given for ventricular tachycardia (an organized, although potentially deadly rhythm).

*Test-Taking Strategy:* Use the process of elimination. Note the relationship between *fibrillation* in the question and *defibrillator* in the correct option. Review treatment for VF if you had difficulty with this question.

*Level of Cognitive Ability:* Application
*Client Needs:* Physiological Integrity
*Integrated Concept/Process:* Nursing Process/Implementation
*Content Area:* Adult Health/Cardiovascular

*Reference*
Ignatavicius, D., Workman, M., & Mishler, M. (1999). *Medical-surgical nursing across the health care continuum* (3rd ed.). Philadelphia: W.B. Saunders, p. 767.

**284.** A nurse is caring for a client with a newly applied plaster leg cast. The nurse prevents the development of compartment syndrome by:
1    Elevating the limb and applying ice to the affected leg
2    Elevating the limb and covering the limb with bath blankets
3    Placing the leg in a slightly dependent position and applying ice
4    Keeping the leg horizontal and applying ice to the affected leg

**Answer: 1**
*Rationale:* Compartment syndrome is prevented by controlling edema. This is achieved most optimally with the use of elevation and the application of ice. The use of bath blankets or a dependent or horizontal leg position will not prevent this syndrome.

*Test-Taking Strategy:* Use the process of elimination. Recalling that edema is controlled or prevented with limb elevation helps to eliminate options 3 and 4. From the remaining options, think about the effects of ice versus bath blankets. Ice will further control edema, while bath blankets will produce heat and prevent air circulation needed for the cast to dry. Review interventions to prevent complications following cast application if you had difficulty with this question.

*Level of Cognitive Ability:* Application
*Client Needs:* Physiological Integrity
*Integrated Concept/Process:* Nursing Process/Implementation
*Content Area:* Adult Health/Musculoskeletal

*Reference*
Smeltzer, S., & Bare, B. (2000). *Brunner & Suddarth's Textbook of medical-surgical nursing* (9th ed.). Philadelphia: Lippincott Williams & Wilkins, p. 1783.

---

**285.** A client undergoing hemodialysis becomes hypotensive. The nurse avoids taking which of the following contraindicated actions?
1    Administering albumin
2    Administering a bolus of 250 mL normal saline (NS) solution
3    Increasing the blood flow into the dialyzer
4    Raising the client's legs and feet

**Answer: 3**
*Rationale:* To treat hypotension during hemodialysis, the nurse raises the client's feet and legs to enhance cardiac return. An NS bolus of up to 500 mL may be given to increase circulating volume. Albumin may be given as per protocol to increase colloid oncotic pressure. Finally, the transmembrane hydrostatic pressure or the blood flow rate into the dialyzer may be decreased. All of these measures should improve the circulating volume and blood pressure (BP).

*Test-Taking Strategy:* Focus on the issue—hypotension—and note that the client is being dialyzed. Thinking about each action in the options and how it may affect the BP will direct you to option 3. Review the treatment for this complication of dialysis if you had difficulty with this question.

*Level of Cognitive Ability:* Application
*Client Needs:* Physiological Integrity
*Integrated Concept/Process:* Nursing Process/Implementation
*Content Area:* Adult Health/Renal

*Reference*
Smeltzer, S., & Bare, B. (2000). *Brunner & Suddarth's Textbook of medical-surgical nursing* (9th ed.). Philadelphia: Lippincott Williams & Wilkins, p. 1114.

**286.** A nurse is preparing a client for cardioversion using anterolateral paddle placement. The nurse places the conductive gel pads at which areas on the client's chest in preparation for this procedure?
1. Right second intercostal space, and left fifth intercostal space at anterior axillary line
2. Left second intercostal space, and left fifth intercostal space at midaxillary line
3. Right fourth intercostal space, and left fifth intercostal space at anterior axillary line
4. Left fourth intercostal space, and left fifth intercostal space at midaxillary line

**Answer: 1**
*Rationale:* Anterolateral paddle placement for external counter-shock involves placing one paddle at the right second intercostal space and the other at the fifth intercostal space at the anterior axillary line.

*Test-Taking Strategy:* Use the process of elimination. Remember that the paddles are positioned so the electric shock travels through as much myocardium as possible. Visualize each of the placements as described, and use knowledge of cardiothoracic landmarks, remembering the position of the heart in the chest. This will direct you to option 1. Review the procedure for cardioversion if you had difficulty with this question.

*Level of Cognitive Ability:* Application
*Client Needs:* Physiological Integrity
*Integrated Concept/Process:* Nursing Process/Implementation
*Content Area:* Adult Health/Cardiovascular

*Reference*
Smeltzer, S., & Bare, B. (2000). *Brunner & Suddarth's Textbook of medical-surgical nursing* (9th ed.). Philadelphia: Lippincott Williams & Wilkins, p. 580.

**287.** A nurse is planning care for a client scheduled for venography. The nurse plans care knowing that which action does not have to be implemented before this procedure?
1. Asking the client about allergies to iodine or shellfish
2. Obtaining a signed informed consent
3. Determining the location and strength of peripheral pulses
4. Placing the client on an NPO after midnight status

**Answer: 4**
*Rationale:* Venography is similar to arteriography, except it evaluates the venous system. A radiopaque dye is injected into selected veins to evaluate patency and blood flow characteristics. The client signs an informed consent because venography is an invasive procedure. Allergies to shellfish or iodine must be noted. Peripheral pulses are assessed so that comparisons can be made after the procedure. The client is usually given clear liquids for 3 to 4 hours before the procedure to help with dye excretion afterward.

*Test-Taking Strategy:* Use the process of elimination, noting the key word *not*. Since venography is an invasive procedure using a contrast agent, options 1 and 2 are eliminated first, because they must be done. From the remaining options, recall that an NPO status will promote dehydration rather than dye clearance and that assessing peripheral pulses is necessary to identify potential complications. Review preprocedure care for venography if you had difficulty with this question.

*Level of Cognitive Ability:* Application
*Client Needs:* Physiological Integrity
*Integrated Concept/Process:* Nursing Process/Planning
*Content Area:* Adult Health/Cardiovascular

*Reference*
Fischbach, F. (2000). *A manual of laboratory & diagnostic tests* (6th ed.). Philadelphia: Lippincott Williams & Wilkins, p. 800.

**288.** A physician writes an order to obtain a 12-lead ECG on a client. The nurse informs the client of the procedure. Which client statement indicates that the client understands the procedure?
1   "I cannot breathe while the ECG is running."
2   "When the ECG begins, I must take a deep breath."
3   "I need to lie still while the ECG is being done."
4   "If I move when the ECG begins, I will be shocked."

**Answer: 3**
*Rationale:* Good contact between the skin and electrodes are necessary to obtain a clear 12-lead ECG printout. Therefore, the electrodes are placed on the flat surfaces of the skin just above the ankles and wrists. Movement may cause a disruption in that contact. The client does not need to hold the breath or take a deep breath during the procedure. The client needs to be reassured that a shock will not be received. Options 1, 2, and 4 are inappropriate statements.

*Test-Taking Strategy:* Use the process of elimination, focusing on the issue: performing an ECG. Recalling that good contact is required to obtain a clear ECG will direct you to option 3. Review this procedure if you had difficulty with this question.

*Level of Cognitive Ability:* Analysis
*Client Needs:* Physiological Integrity
*Integrated Concept/Process:* Teaching/Learning
*Content Area:* Adult Health/Cardiovascular

*Reference*
Ignatavicius, D., Workman, M., & Mishler, M. (1999). *Medical-surgical nursing across the health care continuum* (3rd ed.). Philadelphia: W.B. Saunders, p. 742.

**289.** A nurse is giving a bed bath to a client who is on strict bed rest. To increase venous return, the nurse bathes the client's extremities by using:
1   Long, firm strokes from distal to proximal areas
2   Firm circular strokes from proximal to distal areas
3   Short, patting strokes from distal to proximal areas
4   Smooth, light strokes back and forth from proximal to distal areas

**Answer: 1**
*Rationale:* Long, firm strokes in the direction of venous flow promote venous return when bathing the extremities. Circular strokes are used on the face. Short, patting strokes and light strokes are not as comfortable for the client, and they do not promote venous return.

*Test-Taking Strategy:* Use the process of elimination, focusing on the issue: increase venous return. Eliminate options 2 and 4 first because a stroke from proximal to distal will not promote venous return. From the remaining options, focusing on the issue will direct you to option 1. Review the principles related to a bed bath if you had difficulty with this question.

*Level of Cognitive Ability:* Application
*Client Needs:* Physiological Integrity
*Integrated Concept/Process:* Nursing Process/Implementation
*Content Area:* Fundamental Skills

*Reference*
Potter, P., & Perry, A. (2001). *Fundamentals of nursing* (5th ed.). St. Louis: Mosby, p. 1078.

**290.** A nurse is preparing to give an intramuscular injection that is irritating to the subcutaneous tissues. The drug reference recommends that it be given using the Z-track technique. The nurse avoids which of the following with this administration technique?

1. Prepare a 0.2-mL air lock in the syringe after drawing up the medication
2. Massage the site after injecting the medication
3. Attach a new sterile needle to the syringe after drawing up the medication
4. Retract the skin to the side before piercing the skin with the needle

**Answer: 2**

*Rationale:* The Z-track variation of the standard intramuscular technique is used to administer intramuscular medications that are highly irritating to subcutaneous and skin tissues. Attaching a new sterile needle is done because the new needle will not have any medication adhering to the outside that could be irritating to the tissues. Preparing an air lock keeps the needle clean of medication on insertion, and as the air is injected behind the medication, it will provide a seal at the point of insertion to prevent tracking of the medication. Retracting the skin provides a seal over the injected medication to prevent tracking through the subcutaneous tissues. The site should not be massaged because this can lead to tissue irritation.

*Test-Taking Strategy:* Focus on the issue: Z-track injection. Recalling the purpose of using the Z-track technique will direct you to option 2. Review this procedure for administering medications if you had difficulty with this question.

*Level of Cognitive Ability:* Application
*Client Needs:* Physiological Integrity
*Integrated Concept/Process:* Nursing Process/Implementation
*Content Area:* Fundamental Skills

*Reference*
Potter, P., & Perry, A. (2001). *Fundamentals of nursing* (5th ed.). St. Louis: Mosby, p. 947.

---

**291.** A nurse is preparing to suction a client's tracheostomy. To promote deep breathing and coughing, the client should be positioned in the:

1. Supine position
2. Lateral position
3. High-Fowler's position
4. Semi-Fowler's position

**Answer: 4**

*Rationale:* If not contraindicated, before a tracheostomy is suctioned, the client is placed in semi-Fowler's position to promote deep breathing, maximum lung expansion, and productive coughing. In this position, gravity pulls downward on the diaphragm, which allows greater chest expansion and lung volume. High-Fowler's position, the supine position, or the lateral position would not allow easy visualization of the tracheostomy or easy access of the suction catheter.

*Test-Taking Strategy:* Use the process of elimination and focus on the issue: the position that will promote deep breathing and coughing during suctioning. Visualize each position as you focus on this issue. The semi-Fowler's position promotes deep breathing, maximum lung expansion, and productive coughing. Review this procedure if you had difficulty with this question.

*Level of Cognitive Ability:* Application
*Client Needs:* Physiological Integrity
*Integrated Concept/Process:* Nursing Process/Implementation
*Content Area:* Fundamental Skills

*Reference*
Potter, P., & Perry, A. (2001). *Fundamentals of nursing* (5th ed.). St. Louis: Mosby, p. 1164.

**292.** A client is at term pregnancy. The fetal heart rate (FHR) is being monitored for a baseline rate. The nurse is satisfied with the results and tells the client that the baby's heart rate is within normal limits. The nurse then documents which FHR finding?

1   90 beats/min
2   140 beats/min
3   180 beats/min
4   200 beats/min

**Answer: 2**
*Rationale:* The normal FHR range is 110 to 160 beats/min; therefore, option 2 is the only correct option.

*Test-Taking Strategy:* Knowledge of the normal fetal heart rate is required to answer this question. Review this content if you are unfamiliar with it.

*Level of Cognitive Ability:* Application
*Client Needs:* Physiological Integrity
*Integrated Concept/Process:* Communication and Documentation
*Content Area:* Maternity

*Reference*
Lowdermilk, D., Perry, S., & Bobak, I. (2000). *Maternity & women's health care* (7th ed.). St. Louis: Mosby, p. 493.

**293.** A client receiving chemotherapy has an infiltrated intravenous line and extravasation at the site. The nurse avoids doing which of the following in the management of this situation?

1   Stopping the administration of the medication
2   Leaving the needle in place and aspirating any residual medication
3   Administering an available antidote as prescribed
4   Applying direct manual pressure to the site

**Answer: 4**
*Rationale:* General recommendations for managing extravasation of a chemotherapeutic agent include stopping the infusion, leaving the needle in place and attempting to aspirate any residual medication from the site, administering an antidote if available, and assessing the site for complications. Direct pressure is not applied to the site because it could further injure tissues exposed to the chemotherapeutic agent.

*Test-Taking Strategy:* Use the process of elimination, noting the key word *avoids*. Noting that the client was receiving chemotherapy and that "extravasation" occurred will direct you to option 4. Review treatment measures for extravasation if you had difficulty with this question.

*Level of Cognitive Ability:* Application
*Client Needs:* Physiological Integrity
*Integrated Concept/Process:* Nursing Process/Implementation
*Content Area:* Adult Health/Oncology

*Reference*
Smeltzer, S., & Bare, B. (2000). *Brunner & Suddarth's Textbook of medical-surgical nursing* (9th ed.). Philadelphia: Lippincott Williams & Wilkins, p. 277.

**294.** A nurse is suctioning the airway of a client with a tracheostomy. To properly perform the procedure, the nurse:

1   Turns on the wall suction to 180 mm Hg
2   Inserts the catheter until coughing or resistance is felt
3   Withdraws the catheter while suctioning continuously
4   Reenters the tracheostomy after suctioning the mouth

**Answer: 2**
*Rationale:* The wall suction unit is usually set to 80 to 120 mm Hg pressure. This allows adequate removal of secretions while protecting the airway from trauma. The nurse inserts the catheter until resistance is felt, and then withdraws it 1 cm to move away from mucosa. The nurse suctions intermittently and does not reenter the tracheostomy after suctioning the client's mouth.

*Test-Taking Strategy:* Use the process of elimination. Eliminate option 3 because of the word *continuously* and option 4 because the trachea is not reentered. From the remaining options, it is necessary to know that 180 mm Hg pressure would cause trauma to the mucosa. If you had difficulty with this question, review this procedure.

*Level of Cognitive Ability:* Application
*Client Needs:* Physiological Integrity
*Integrated Concept/Process:* Nursing Process/Implementation
*Content Area:* Adult Health/Respiratory

*Reference*
Smeltzer, S., & Bare, B. (2000). *Brunner & Suddarth's Textbook of medical-surgical nursing* (9th ed.). Philadelphia: Lippincott Williams & Wilkins, p. 502.

---

**295.** A nurse has prepared a client for an intravenous pyelogram. The nurse evaluates that the client is knowledgeable about the procedure if the client states the need to report which of the following sensations immediately?

1 Nausea
2 Difficulty breathing
3 Warm flushed feeling in the body
4 Salty taste in the mouth

**Answer: 2**

*Rationale:* Intravenous pyelography is a contrast study of the kidneys to determine a variety of disorders of the kidneys, ureters, and bladder. Normal sensations during injection of the iodine-based radiopaque dye include a warm flushed feeling, salty taste in the mouth, and transient nausea. Difficulty breathing, wheezing, hives, or itching signals an allergic response and should be reported immediately. This complication is prevented by inquiring about allergies to iodine or shellfish before the procedure.

*Test-Taking Strategy:* Use the process of elimination, and recall that this diagnostic test involves injection of an iodine-based radiopaque dye. Use of the ABCs (airway, breathing, and circulation) will direct you to option 2. Review this diagnostic procedure if you had difficulty with this question.

*Level of Cognitive Ability:* Analysis
*Client Needs:* Physiological Integrity
*Integrated Concept/Process:* Teaching/Learning
*Content Area:* Adult Health/Renal

*Reference*
Fischbach, F. (2000). *A manual of laboratory & diagnostic tests* (6th ed.). Philadelphia: Lippincott Williams & Wilkins, p. 789.

---

**296.** A client who is 15 years old is pregnant and is being treated by a dermatologist for acne. The clinic nurse asks the client about the treatment prescribed for the acne knowing that which treatment will be avoided?

1 Topical erythromycin
2 Exfoliation
3 Cleansing with antibacterial soap
4 Oral tetracycline

**Answer: 4**

*Rationale:* Tetracycline use during pregnancy may lead to discoloration of the child's teeth when they erupt. This treatment for acne will be avoided during pregnancy. Options 1, 2, and 3 are appropriate treatments.

*Test-Taking Strategy:* Use the process of elimination. Focus on the safety factor for the unseen client (fetus), and note the key word *avoided*. Eliminate options 1, 2, and 3 because they are similar and are all topical treatments. Review the concepts related to medications and safety during pregnancy if you had difficulty with this question.

*Level of Cognitive Ability:* Analysis
*Client Needs:* Physiological Integrity
*Integrated Concept/Process:* Nursing Process/Assessment
*Content Area:* Maternity

*Reference*
Hodgson, B., & Kizior, R. (2001). *Saunders Nursing drug handbook 2001.* Philadelphia: W.B. Saunders, p. 977.

---

**297.** A client with a bone infection is to have indium imaging done. The client asks a nurse to explain how the procedure is done. The nurse's response is based on the understanding that:

1. Indium is injected into the bloodstream and collects in normal bone, but not in infected areas
2. Indium is injected into the bloodstream and highlights the vascular supply to the bone
3. A sample of the client's leukocytes is tagged with indium and will subsequently accumulate in infected bone
4. A sample of the client's red blood cells is tagged with indium and will subsequently accumulate in normal bone.

**Answer: 3**
*Rationale:* A sample of the client's blood is collected, and the leukocytes are tagged with indium. The leukocytes are then reinjected into the client. They accumulate in infected areas of bone and can be detected with scanning. No special preparation or aftercare is necessary. Options 1, 2, and 4 are incorrect descriptions.

*Test-Taking Strategy:* Use the process of elimination, focusing on the information in the question. Note that the client has a bone infection. Recall that with any type of infection, leukocytes migrate to the area (and bone is not a highly vascular area). This will direct you to option 3. Review this test if you had difficulty with this question.

*Level of Cognitive Ability:* Application
*Client Needs:* Physiological Integrity
*Integrated Concept/Process:* Teaching/Learning
*Content Area:* Fundamental Skills

*Reference*
Fischbach, F. (2000). *A manual of laboratory & diagnostic tests* (6th ed.). Philadelphia: Lippincott Williams & Wilkins, p. 722.

---

**298.** A client with repeated episodes of pulmonary emboli from thromboembolism is scheduled for insertion of an inferior vena cava filter. A nurse determines that the client has an adequate understanding of the procedure if the client makes which of the following statements?

1. "The filter will keep new blood clots from forming in my legs."
2. "I don't mind having a filter in my artery if it means I don't have any more trouble."
3. "The filter will be like a catcher's mitt and keep the clots from going to my lungs."
4. "It's too bad I have to continue anticoagulant therapy after the surgery."

**Answer: 3**
*Rationale:* Insertion of an inferior vena cava filter is indicated for clients with recurrent deep vein thrombosis or pulmonary emboli who do not respond to medical therapy and cannot tolerate anticoagulant therapy. The filter device or "umbrella" is inserted percutaneously in the inferior vena cava, where it springs open and attaches itself to the vena caval wall. The device has holes to allow blood flow but traps larger clots, thus preventing pulmonary emboli. The filter does not prevent blood clots from forming and is not placed in an artery.

*Test-Taking Strategy:* Specific knowledge regarding this filter is required to answer this question. Thinking about the purpose and the action of a filter will direct you to option 3. Review this content if you had difficulty with this question.

*Level of Cognitive Ability:* Analysis
*Client Needs:* Physiological Integrity

*Integrated Concept/Process:* Teaching/Learning
*Content Area:* Adult Health/Cardiovascular

*Reference*
Ignatavicius, D., Workman, M., & Mishler, M. (1999). *Medical-surgical nursing across the health care continuum* (3rd ed.). Philadelphia: W.B. Saunders, p. 687.

---

**299.** A client is admitted to the hospital with a diagnosis of infective endocarditis from *Streptococcus viridans*. The client asks the nurse about the antibiotic therapy that will be given. Knowing that the client has no medication allergies, the nurse prepares the client to receive:

1  Penicillin G benzathine (Bicillin) intravenously (IV) for 10 days, followed by oral doses for 2 weeks

2  Penicillin G benzathine (Bicillin) IV for 4 to 6 weeks, continuing at home after hospital discharge

3  Amphotericin B (Fungizone) IV for 10 days, followed by oral doses for 3 weeks

4  Amphotericin B (Fungizone) IV for 4 to 6 weeks, continuing at home after hospital discharge

**Answer: 2**
*Rationale:* Penicillin is frequently the medication of choice for treating endocarditis of bacterial origin. The standard duration of therapy is 4 to 6 weeks, with home care support after hospital discharge, which is usually for 7 to 10 days. Amphotericin B is an antifungal agent and would not be effective with this type of infection.

*Test-Taking Strategy:* Use the process of elimination. Recalling that amphotericin B is an antifungal agent eliminates options 3 and 4. From the remaining options, note that the severity and nature of the infection makes continued IV therapy necessary; therefore, option 2 is the best option. Review the treatment for this disorder if you had difficulty with this question.

*Level of Cognitive Ability:* Analysis
*Client Needs:* Physiological Integrity
*Integrated Concept/Process:* Nursing Process/Planning
*Content Area:* Adult Health/Cardiovascular

*Reference*
Ignatavicius, D., Workman, M., & Mishler, M. (1999). *Medical-surgical nursing across the health care continuum* (3rd ed.). Philadelphia: W.B. Saunders, p. 827.

---

**300.** A nurse is doing a dressing change on a venous stasis ulcer that is clean and has a growing bed of granulation tissue. The nurse avoids using which of the following dressing materials on this wound?
1  Wet-to-dry saline dressing
2  Wet-to-wet saline dressing
3  Hydrocolloid dressing
4  Vaseline gauze dressing

**Answer: 1**
*Rationale:* The use of wet-to-dry saline dressings provides a nonselective mechanical debridement, whereby both devitalized and viable tissue are removed. This method should never be used on a clean, granulating wound. Granulation tissue in a venous stasis ulcer is protected through the use of wet-to-wet saline dressings, Vaseline gauze, or moist occlusive dressings, such as hydrocolloid dressings.

*Test-Taking Strategy:* Use the process of elimination. Note that the question specifically tells you that the wound is clean with granulation tissue (which needs protection). Next, look at the options and note that options 2, 3, and 4 are similar and have one thing in common, that is, continuous moisture. The wet-to-dry saline dressing could disrupt this healing tissue. Review care of a venous stasis ulcer if you had difficulty with this question.

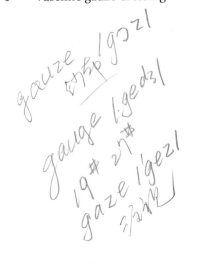

*Level of Cognitive Ability:* Application
*Client Needs:* Physiological Integrity
*Integrated Concept/Process:* Nursing Process/Implementation
*Content Area:* Fundamental Skills

*Reference*
Smeltzer, S., & Bare, B. (2000). *Brunner & Suddarth's Textbook of medical-surgical nursing* (9th ed.). Philadelphia: Lippincott Williams & Wilkins, p. 1453.

---

**301.** A nurse is preparing to admit an elderly client to the hospital who has severe digoxin toxicity from accidental ingestion of a week's supply of the medication. The nurse calls the hospital pharmacy and requests that which medication be brought to the nursing unit?

1. Digoxin immune FAB (Digibind)
2. Potassium chloride (K-Dur)
3. Protamine sulfate (Protamine)
4. Furosemide (Lasix)

**Answer: 1**
*Rationale:* Digibind is an antidote for severe digoxin toxicity. It uses an antibody produced in sheep, which antigenically binds any unbound digoxin in the serum and removes it. As more digoxin reenters the bloodstream from the tissues, it binds that also for excretion by the kidneys.

*Test-Taking Strategy:* Note the client's diagnosis and note the names of the medications in the options. Noting the relationship between the diagnosis and option 1 will direct you to this option. Review the treatment for digoxin toxicity if you had difficulty with this question.

*Level of Cognitive Ability:* Application
*Client Needs:* Physiological Integrity
*Integrated Concept/Process:* Nursing Process/Implementation
*Content Area:* Pharmacology

*Reference*
Hodgson, B., & Kizior, R. (2001). *Saunders Nursing drug handbook 2001.* Philadelphia: W.B. Saunders, p. 324.

---

**302.** The parents of a 6-month-old male report that the infant has been screaming and drawing the knees up to the chest and has passed stools mixed with blood and mucus that are jellylike. A nurse recognizes these signs and symptoms as indicative of:

1. Hirschsprung's disease
2. Peritonitis
3. Intussusception
4. Appendicitis

**Answer: 3**
*Rationale:* The classic signs and symptoms of intussusception are acute, colicky abdominal pain with currant jelly–like stools. Clinical manifestations of Hirschsprung's disease include constipation, abdominal distention, and ribbonlike, foul-smelling stools. Peritonitis is a serious complication that may follow intestinal obstructions and perforation. The most common symptom of appendicitis is colicky, periumbilical or lower abdominal pain in the right quadrant.

*Test-Taking Strategy:* Use the process of elimination. Eliminate options 2 and 4 because they are similar. Recalling that in Hirschsprung's disease the stools are ribbonlike will assist in eliminating option 1. If you had difficulty with this question, review the clinical manifestations of intussusception.

*Level of Cognitive Ability:* Analysis
*Client Needs:* Physiological Integrity
*Integrated Concept/Process:* Nursing Process/Assessment
*Content Area:* Child Health

### Reference

Wong, D. (1999). *Whaley & Wong's Nursing care of infants and children* (6th ed.). St. Louis: Mosby, p. 1565.

---

**303.** A nurse is caring for a client who has been placed in seclusion. The nurse is documenting care provided to the client and addresses which items in the client's record?

1  Vital signs, toileting, and checking the client based on protocol time frame, such as every 15 minutes

2  Ambulating, toileting, and checking the client based on protocol time frame, such as every 15 minutes

3  Vital signs, toileting, feeding and fluid intake, and checking the client based on protocol time frame, such as every 15 minutes

4  Vital signs, reason for the procedure, date and time

**Answer: 3**

*Rationale:* The client in seclusion is assessed continuously or at least every 15 minutes, or according to agency protocol. Vital signs, food and fluid intake, and toileting needs are assessed. Options 1 and 2 are not complete in terms of identification of physiological needs. Option 4 contains client documentation that would precede seclusion.

*Test-Taking Strategy:* Use Maslow's Hierarchy of Needs theory and the process of elimination. Note that option 3 is the most complete in terms of the client's basic needs. If you had difficulty with this question, review care of a client in seclusion.

*Level of Cognitive Ability:* Application
*Client Needs:* Physiological Integrity
*Integrated Concept/Process:* Communication and Documentation
*Content Area:* Mental Health

### Reference

Stuart, G.W., & Laraia, M.T. (1998). *Principles and practice of psychiatric nursing.* (6th ed.). St. Louis: Mosby, p. 634.

---

**304.** During the admission assessment, the nurse asks the client to run the heel of one foot down the lower anterior surface of the other leg. The nurse notices rhythmic tremors of the leg being tested and concludes that the client has an alteration in the area of:

1  Muscle strength and flexibility

2  Balance and coordination

3  Sensation and reflexes

4  Bowel and bladder function

**Answer: 2**

*Rationale:* In this situation, the nurse is performing one test of cerebellar function and is testing for ataxia. Alterations in the cerebellar function are noted by alterations in balance and coordination.

*Test-Taking Strategy:* Use the process of elimination. Note the relationship between the words *tremors* in the question and *coordination* in option 2. If you had difficulty with this question, review assessment for cerebellar function and coordination.

*Level of Cognitive Ability:* Analysis
*Client Needs:* Physiological Integrity
*Integrated Concept/Process:* Nursing Process/Assessment
*Content Area:* Adult Health/Neurological

### Reference

Smeltzer, S., & Bare, B. (2000). *Brunner & Suddarth's Textbook of medical-surgical nursing* (9th ed.). Philadelphia: Lippincott Williams & Wilkins, p. 1622.

**305.** A nurse is monitoring the intracranial pressure (ICP) of a client with a head injury. The cerebrospinal fluid pressure (CSF) is averaging 25 mm Hg. The nurse analyzes these results as:

1 Normal
2 Compensation, indicating adequate brain adaptation
3 Borderline in elevation, indicating the initial stage of compensation
4 Increased, indicating a serious compromise in cerebral perfusion

**Answer: 4**
*Rationale:* The normal CSF pressure is 5 to 15 mm Hg. A pressure of 25 mm Hg is increased.

*Test-Taking Strategy:* Use the process of elimination. Eliminate options 2 and 3 because they are similar. From the remaining options, knowledge of normal CSF pressure will direct you to option 4. Review intracranial pressure and the normal CSF pressure if you had difficulty with this question.

*Level of Cognitive Ability:* Analysis
*Client Needs:* Physiological Integrity
*Integrated Concept/Process:* Nursing Process/Analysis
*Content Area:* Adult Health/Neurological

*Reference*
Smeltzer, S., & Bare, B. (2000). *Brunner & Suddarth's Textbook of medical-surgical nursing* (9th ed.). Philadelphia: Lippincott Williams & Wilkins, p. 1636.

**306.** A woman at 32 weeks' gestation is brought into the emergency department after an automobile accident. The client is bleeding vaginally, and fetal assessment indicates moderate fetal distress. Which of the following will the nurse do first in an attempt to reduce the stress on the fetus?

1 Start intravenous (IV) fluids at a keep open rate
2 Administer oxygen via a facemask at 7 to 10 liters per minute
3 Elevate the head of the bed to a semi-Fowler's position
4 Set up for an immediate cesarean section delivery

**Answer: 2**
*Rationale:* Administering oxygen will increase the amount of oxygen for transport to the fetus, partially compensating for the loss of circulating blood volume. This action is essential regardless of the cause or amount of bleeding. IV fluids may be initiated. The client will be positioned per physician's order. There are no data that indicate an "immediate" cesarean delivery is necessary.

*Test-Taking Strategy:* Note the key word *first* in the stem of the question. Using the ABCs (airway, breathing, circulation) will direct you to option 2. Review care of the obstetric client when fetal distress occurs if you had difficulty with this question.

*Level of Cognitive Ability:* Application
*Client Needs:* Physiological Integrity
*Integrated Concept/Process:* Nursing Process/Implementation
*Content Area:* Maternity

*Reference*
Olds, S., London. M., & Ladewig, P. (2000). *Maternal-newborn nursing: A family and community-based approach* (6th ed.). Upper Saddle River, N.J.: Prentice Hall Health, p. 630.

**307.** A client with a Sengstaken-Blakemore tube in place is admitted to the nursing unit from the emergency department. The nurse plans care knowing that the purpose of this tube is to:

1 Control bleeding from gastritis
2 Apply pressure to esophageal varices
3 Control ascites
4 Remove ammonia-forming bacteria from the gastrointestinal tract

**Answer: 2**
*Rationale:* A Sengstaken-Blakemore tube is inserted in clients with cirrhosis who have ruptured esophageal varices. It has esophageal and gastric balloons. The esophageal balloon exerts pressure on the ruptured esophageal varices and stops the bleeding. The gastric balloon holds the tube in correct position and prevents migration of the esophageal balloon. Options 1, 3, and 4 are not the purpose of this tube.

*Test-Taking Strategy:* Focus on the issue: the purpose of a Sengstaken-Blakemore tube. Recalling the relationship between this tube and ruptured esophageal varices will direct you to option

2. Review the concepts related to this type of tube, if you are unfamiliar with them.

*Level of Cognitive Ability:* Application
*Client Needs:* Physiological Integrity
*Integrated Concept/Process:* Nursing Process/Planning
*Content Area:* Adult Health/Gastrointestinal

*Reference*
Smeltzer, S., & Bare, B. (2000). *Brunner & Suddarth's Textbook of medical-surgical nursing* (9th ed.). Philadelphia: Lippincott Williams & Wilkins, p. 834.

---

**308.** A home health care nurse is instructing a client with chronic obstructive pulmonary disease (COPD) how to perform breathing techniques that will assist in exhaling carbon dioxide and open the airways. The nurse teaches the client which technique?
1   Pursed-lip breathing
2   Intercostal chest expansion
3   Abdominal breathing
4   Chest physical therapy

**Answer: 1**
*Rationale:* Pursed-lip breathing allows the client to slowly exhale carbon dioxide while keeping the airways open. Intercostal chest expansion is not a technique. Abdominal breathing is recommended for clients with dyspnea. Chest physical therapy is not a breathing technique.

*Test-Taking Strategy:* Use the process of elimination and focus on the issue: breathing techniques for the client with COPD. Eliminate options 2 and 4 first because these are not breathing techniques. From the remaining options, remembering that pursed lip breathing is associated with the COPD client will assist in directing you to the correct option. Review pursed-lip breathing and abdominal breathing if you are unfamiliar with the purposes and techniques.

*Level of Cognitive Ability:* Application
*Client Needs:* Physiological Integrity
*Integrated Concept/Process:* Teaching/Learning
*Content Area:* Adult Health/Respiratory

*Reference*
Smeltzer, S., & Bare, B. (2000). *Brunner & Suddarth's Textbook of medical-surgical nursing* (9th ed.). Philadelphia: Lippincott Williams & Wilkins, p. 448.

---

**309.** A physician has ordered a partial re-breather facemask for a client who has terminal lung cancer. The nurse prepares to implement the order knowing that the mask:

1 Delivers accurate fraction of inspired oxygen ($FIO_2$) to the client
2 Conserves oxygen by having the client rebreathe his or her own exhaled air
3 Requires that the reservoir bag deflate during inspiration to work effectively
4 Requires a low liter flow to prevent rebreathing of carbon dioxide

**Answer: 2**

*Rationale:* Rebreathing masks have a reservoir bag that conserves oxygen and requires a high liter flow to achieve concentrations of 40% to 60%. It does not deliver accurate $FIO_2$ to the client. The bag should not deflate during inspiration. Rebreathing bags conserve oxygen by having the client rebreathe their own exhaled air.

*Test-Taking Strategy:* Use the process of elimination. Note the relationship between *partial rebreather* in the question and *rebreathe his or her own exhaled air* in the correct option. Review oxygen delivery system, if you have difficulty with this question.

*Level of Cognitive Ability:* Application
*Client Needs:* Physiological Integrity
*Integrated Concept/Process:* Nursing Process/Planning
*Content Area:* Adult Health/Respiratory

*Reference*
Smeltzer, S., & Bare, B. (2000). *Brunner & Suddarth's Textbook of medical-surgical nursing* (9th ed.). Philadelphia: Lippincott Williams & Wilkins, p. 493.

---

**310.** A client has a slow, regular pulse. On the monitor, the nurse notes regular QRS complexes with no associated P waves and with a ventricular rate of 50 beats/min. The nurse suspects that there is a problem at which part of the cardiac conduction system?
1 The sinoatrial (SA) node
2 The atrioventricular (AV) node
3 The bundle of His
4 The left ventricle

**Answer: 1**

*Rationale:* A normal P wave indicates that the impulse that depolarized the atrium was initiated in the SA node. A change in the form or the absence of a P wave can indicate a problem at this part of the conduction system, with the resulting impulse originating from an alternate site lower in the conduction pathway. Options 2, 3, and 4 are incorrect.

*Test-Taking Strategy:* Use the process of elimination. Option 4 can be eliminated first because it does not identify a mechanism of the conduction system. The question also identifies a regular QRS complex and a ventricular rate of 50 beats/min, indicating an intact AV node; thus the problem lies higher in the conduction system. Correlate a P wave with the SA node. If you had difficulty with this question, review the conduction system of the heart.

*Level of Cognitive Ability:* Analysis
*Client Needs:* Physiological Integrity
*Integrated Concept/Process:* Nursing Process/Analysis
*Content Area:* Adult Health/Cardiovascular

*Reference*
Sole, M.L., Lamborn, M., & Hartshorn, J. (2001). *Introduction to critical care nursing* (3rd ed.). Philadelphia: W.B. Saunders, p. 42.

**311.** A client is hospitalized with a diagnosis of thrombophlebitis and is being treated with heparin infusion therapy. About 24 hours after the infusion has begun, the nurse notes that the client's partial thromboplastin time (PTT) is 100 seconds with a control of 60 seconds. What is the most appropriate initial nursing action?

1 Discontinue the heparin infusion
2 Do nothing; the client is receiving adequate anticoagulation therapy
3 Notify the physician of the laboratory results
4 Prepare to administer protamine sulfate

**Answer: 2**

*Rationale:* The effectiveness of heparin therapy is monitored by the results of the partial thromboplastin time (PTT). Desired ranges for therapeutic anticoagulation are $1\frac{1}{2}$ to $2\frac{1}{2}$ times the control. A PTT of 100 seconds is within the therapeutic range.

*Test-Taking Strategy:* Use the process of elimination. Remember that the desired range for therapeutic anticoagulation is $1\frac{1}{2}$ to $2\frac{1}{2}$ times the control. Noting that the control is 60 and that $1\frac{1}{2}$ to $2\frac{1}{2}$ times the control is a range of 90 to 150 will direct you to option 2. Review care of a client receiving a heparin infusion if you had difficulty with this question.

*Level of Cognitive Ability:* Application
*Client Needs:* Physiological Integrity
*Integrated Concept/Process:* Nursing Process/Implementation
*Content Area:* Pharmacology

*Reference*
Fischbach, F. (2000). *A manual of laboratory & diagnostic tests* (6th ed.). Philadelphia: Lippincott Williams & Wilkins, p. 1207.

**312.** A 48-year-old man is brought to the emergency department and is complaining of chest pain. His vital signs are blood pressure (BP) 150/90 mm Hg, pulse (P) 88 beats/min (beats/min), and respirations (R) 20 breaths/min. The nurse administers nitroglycerin 0.4 mg sublingually. To evaluate the effectiveness of this medication, the nurse should expect which of the following changes in the vital signs?

1 BP 160/100 mm Hg, P 120 beats/min, R 16 breaths/min
2 BP 150/90 mm Hg, P 70 beats/min, R 24 breaths/min
3 BP 100/60 mm Hg, P 96 beats/min, R 20 breaths/min
4 BP 100/60 mm Hg, P 70 beats/min, R 24 breaths/min

**Answer: 3**

*Rationale:* Nitroglycerin dilates both arteries and veins, causing blood to pool in the periphery. This causes a reduced preload and therefore a drop in cardiac output. This vasodilation causes the blood pressure to fall. The drop in cardiac output causes the sympathetic nervous system to respond and attempt to maintain cardiac output by increasing the pulse. Beta blockers, such as propranolol (Inderal), are often used in conjunction with nitroglycerin to prevent this rise in heart rate.

*Test-Taking Strategy:* Use the process of elimination. Knowing that nitroglycerin is a vasodilator and that it causes the BP to drop will assist in eliminating options 1 and 2. Also, if chest pain is reduced and cardiac workload is reduced, the client will be more comfortable; therefore, a rise in respirations should not be seen. This assists in eliminating option 4. If you had difficulty with this question, review the effects of nitroglycerin.

*Level of Cognitive Ability:* Analysis
*Client Needs:* Physiological Integrity
*Integrated Concept/Process:* Nursing Process/Evaluation
*Content Area:* Pharmacology

*Reference*
Hodgson, B., & Kizior, R. (2001). *Saunders Nursing drug handbook 2001.* Philadelphia: W.B. Saunders, pp. 750-753.

**313.** A client who has had an abdominal aortic aneurysm repair is on postoperative day 1. The nurse performs an abdominal assessment and notes the absence of bowel sounds. The nurse's best action is to:

1 Call the physician immediately
2 Remove the nasogastric (NG) tube
3 Feed the client
4 Continue to assess for bowel sounds

**Answer: 4**

*Rationale:* Bowel sounds may be absent for 3 to 4 days after surgery because of bowel manipulation during the procedure. The nurse should continue to monitor the client, the nasogastric tube should stay in place if present, and the client is kept NPO until after the onset of bowel sounds. There is no need to call the physician immediately at this time.

*Test-Taking Strategy:* Use the process of elimination. Note the key words *postoperative day 1.* Eliminate option 2 because there are no data in the question regarding the presence of an NG tube. Additionally, an NG tube would not be removed and the client would not be fed (option 3) if bowel sounds are absent. Recalling that bowel sounds may not return for 3 to 4 days postoperatively will direct you to option 4 from the remaining options. If you had difficulty with this question, review normal postoperative assessment findings.

*Level of Cognitive Ability:* Application
*Client Needs:* Physiological Integrity
*Integrated Concept/Process:* Nursing Process/Implementation
*Content Area:* Adult Health/Gastrointestinal

*Reference*
Smeltzer, S., & Bare, B. (2000). *Brunner & Suddarth's Textbook of medical-surgical nursing* (9th ed.). Philadelphia: Lippincott Williams & Wilkins, p. 367.

---

**314.** A nurse is caring for a client with pregnancy-induced hypertension (PIH) who is in labor. The nurse monitors the client closely for which complication of PIH?

1 Seizures
2 Placenta previa
3 Hallucinations
4 Altered respiratory status

**Answer: 1**

*Rationale:* The major complication of pregnancy-induced hypertension is seizures. Placenta previa, hallucinations, and altered respiratory status are not directly associated with PIH.

*Test-Taking Strategy:* Use the process of elimination. Remembering that seizures are a concern with PIH will direct you to option 1. If you had difficulty with this question, review the complications associated with PIH.

*Level of Cognitive Ability:* Analysis
*Client Needs:* Physiological Integrity
*Integrated Concept/Process:* Nursing Process/Assessment
*Content Area:* Maternity

*Reference*
Lowdermilk, D., Perry, S., & Bobak, I. (2000). *Maternity & women's health care* (7th ed.). St. Louis: Mosby, p. 832.

**315.** A nurse is evaluating the outcomes of care for a client who experienced an acute myocardial infarction. Which of the following findings indicate that an expected outcome for the nursing diagnosis of decreased cardiac output has been met?

**1** Cardiac output of 3 L/min when measured with a pulmonary artery catheter

**2** Cardiac monitor shows a heart rate of 50 beats/min after the client has eaten dinner

**3** The client complains of symptoms that require immediate action following client teaching

**4** The client reports absence of dyspnea and anginal pain with activity

**Answer: 4**

*Rationale:* Dyspnea and angina are signs of altered cardiac output. The absence of these with activity indicates that cardiac output is adequate. Normal adult cardiac output is 4 to 8 L/min. Option 1 identifies a low reading. A low heart rate affects cardiac output. The client's heart rate should be between 60 to 100 beats/min. Complaints of symptoms that require immediate action is not an expected outcome.

*Test-Taking Strategy:* Focus on the issue: an expected outcome. Use the ABCs (airway, breathing, and circulation). Note the key words *absence of dyspnea and anginal pain* in the correct option. If you had difficulty with this question, review normal cardiac output and heart rate.

*Level of Cognitive Ability:* Analysis
*Client Needs:* Physiological Integrity
*Integrated Concept/Process:* Nursing Process/Evaluation
*Content Area:* Adult Health/Cardiovascular

*Reference*
Smeltzer, S., & Bare, B. (2000). *Brunner & Suddarth's Textbook of medical-surgical nursing* (9th ed.). Philadelphia: Lippincott Williams & Wilkins, p. 569.

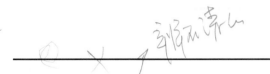

**316.** A nurse analyzed a 6-second ECG strip for a client with left-sided heart failure, as follows; atrial rate: no identifiable P waves; baseline irregular ventricular rate: 160 beats/min; rhythm: irregular PR interval and indiscernible, QRS at 0.08. The nurse interprets the rhythm strip as:

**1** Sinus dysrhythmia
**2** Atrial fibrillation
**3** Ventricular fibrillation
**4** Third-degree heart block

**Answer: 2**

*Rationale:* Atrial fibrillation is characterized by rapid, chaotic atrial depolarization, with ventricular rates ranging from 160 to 180 beats/min. The ECG reveals no identifiable P waves and a baseline that is irregular. The PR interval is irregular. A sinus dysrhythmia has a normal P wave, PR interval, and QRS complex. In ventricular fibrillation, there are no identifiable P waves, QRS complexes, or T waves. In third-degree heart block, the atria and ventricles beat independently.

*Test-Taking Strategy:* Recall that in atrial fibrillation the P wave is erratic or not identifiable. This will direct you to option 2. If you are unfamiliar with the cardiac dysrhythmias identified in the options, review this content.

*Level of Cognitive Ability:* Analysis
*Client Needs:* Physiological Integrity
*Integrated Concept/Process:* Nursing Process/Analysis
*Content Area:* Adult Health/Cardiovascular

*Reference*
Smeltzer, S., & Bare, B. (2000). *Brunner & Suddarth's Textbook of medical-surgical nursing* (9th ed.). Philadelphia: Lippincott Williams & Wilkins, p. 578.

**317.** A nurse is caring for a client with multiple myeloma. The client is receiving intravenous hydration at 100 mL/hr. Which of the following assessment findings would indicate a positive response to the treatment plan?

1    Weight increase of 1 kg
2    White blood cell count of 6000/mm$^3$
3    Respirations of 18 breaths/min
4    Creatinine level of 1 mg/dL

**Answer:  4**
*Rationale:*  Renal failure is a concern in the client with multiple myeloma. In multiple myeloma, hydration is essential to prevent renal damage resulting from precipitation of protein in the renal tubules and from excessive calcium and uric acid in the blood. Creatinine is the most accurate measure of renal status. Options 2 and 3 are unrelated to the issue of hydration. Weight gain is not a positive sign when concerned with renal status.

*Test-Taking Strategy:*  Use the process of elimination. Recalling that renal failure is a concern in multiple myeloma will direct you to option 4. If you had difficulty with this question, review care of a client with multiple myeloma.

*Level of Cognitive Ability:*  Analysis
*Client Needs:*  Physiological Integrity
*Integrated Concept/Process:*  Nursing Process/Evaluation
*Content Area:*  Adult Health/Oncology

*Reference*
Smeltzer, S., & Bare, B. (2000). *Brunner & Suddarth's Textbook of medical-surgical nursing* (9th ed.). Philadelphia: Lippincott Williams & Wilkins, p. 766.

---

**318.** A nurse provides discharge instructions to a client with testicular cancer who had testicular surgery. The nurse tells the client:

1    To report any elevation in temperature to the physician
2    Not to drive for 6 weeks
3    Not to be fitted for a prosthesis for 6 months
4    To refrain from sitting for long periods

**Answer:  1**
*Rationale:*  For the client who has had testicular surgery, the nurse should emphasize the importance of notifying the physician if chills, fever, drainage, redness, or discharge occurs. These symptoms may indicate the presence of an infection. One week after testicular surgery, the client may drive. Often, a prosthesis is inserted during surgery. Sitting needs to be avoided with prostrate surgery because of hemorrhage, but the risk is not as high with testicular surgery.

*Test-Taking Strategy:*  Use Maslow's Hierarchy of Needs theory and principles related to prioritizing. Infection is the priority. After any surgical procedure, elevation of temperature could signal an infection and should be reported. Review posttesticular surgical teaching points if you had difficulty with this question.

*Level of Cognitive Ability:*  Application
*Client Needs:*  Physiological Integrity
*Integrated Concept/Process:*  Teaching/Learning
*Content Area:*  Adult Health/Oncology

*Reference*
Ignatavicius, D., Workman, M., & Mishler, M. (1999). *Medical-surgical nursing across the health care continuum* (3rd ed.). Philadelphia: W.B. Saunders, p. 2042.

**319.** A multidisciplinary team has been working with the spouse of a home care client who has end-stage liver failure and has been teaching the spouse interventions for the management of pain. Which statement by the spouse indicates the need for further teaching?

1 "If the pain increases, I must let the nurse know immediately."
2 "I should have my husband try the breathing exercises to control pain."
3 "This narcotic will cause very deep sleep, which is what my husband needs."
4 "If constipation is a problem, increased fluids will help."

**Answer: 3**

*Rationale:* Changes in level of consciousness are a potential indicator of narcotic overdose, as well as an indicator of fluid, electrolyte, and oxygenation deficits. It is important to teach the spouse the differences between sleep related to relief of pain and changes in neurological status related to a deficit. Options 1, 2, and 4 all are indicative of an understanding of appropriate steps to be taken in the management of pain.

*Test-Taking Strategy:* Use the process of elimination, and note the key words *need for further teaching.* Noting that the client has end-stage liver disease and focusing on the issue—pain management—will direct you to option 3. Review pain management if you had difficulty with this question.

*Level of Cognitive Ability:* Analysis
*Client Needs:* Physiological Integrity
*Integrated Concept/Process:* Teaching/Learning
*Content Area:* Fundamental Skills

*Reference*
Smeltzer, S., & Bare, B. (2000). *Brunner & Suddarth's Textbook of medical-surgical nursing* (9th ed.). Philadelphia: Lippincott Williams & Wilkins, p. 300.

---

**320.** A nurse is reviewing the antenatal history of a client in early labor. The nurse recognizes which of the following factors documented in the history as having the greatest potential for causing neonatal sepsis following delivery?

1 Adequate prenatal care
2 Appropriate maternal nutrition and weight gain
3 Spontaneous rupture of membranes 2 hours ago
4 History of substance abuse during pregnancy

**Answer: 4**

*Rationale:* Risk factors for neonatal sepsis can arise from maternal, intrapartal, or neonatal conditions. Maternal risk factors before delivery include low socioeconomic status, poor prenatal care and nutrition, and a history of substance abuse during pregnancy. Premature rupture of the membranes or prolonged rupture of membranes greater than 18 hours before birth is also a risk factor for neonatal acquisition of infection.

*Test-Taking Strategy:* Use the process of elimination. Options 1 and 2 are optimal findings and can be eliminated. From the remaining options, note the key words *2 hours ago* to assist in eliminating option 3. If you had difficulty with this question, review potential maternal physiological and psychosocial risk factors that may cause neonatal infections.

*Level of Cognitive Ability:* Analysis
*Clients Needs:* Physiological Integrity
*Integrated Concept/Process:* Nursing Process/Assessment
*Content Area:* Maternity

*Reference*
Lowdermilk, D., Perry, S., & Bobak, I. (2000). *Maternity & women's health care* (7th ed.). St. Louis: Mosby, p. 1047.

**321.** A nurse performs a prenatal assessment on a client in the first trimester of pregnancy. The nurse discovers that the client frequently consumes alcohol beverages. The nurse initiates interventions to assist the client to avoid alcohol consumption in order to:

1 Promote the normal psychosocial adaptation of the mother to pregnancy

2 Reduce the potential for fetal growth restriction in utero

3 Minimize the potential for placental abruptions during the intrapartum period

4 Reduce the risk of teratogenic effects to developing fetal organs, tissues, and structures

**Answer: 4**

*Rationale:* The first trimester, or *organogenesis*, is characterized by the differentiation and development of fetal organs, systems, and structures. The effects of alcohol on the developing fetus during this critical period depend not only on the amount of alcohol consumed, but on the interaction of quantity, frequency, type of alcohol, and other drugs that may be abused during this period by the pregnant woman. Eliminating consumption of alcohol during this time may promote normal fetal organ development.

*Test-Taking Strategy:* Use the process of elimination. Focus on the key words *first trimester.* Recall that during this trimester development of fetal organs, tissues, and structures take place. If you had difficulty with this question, review the effects of alcohol on the fetus in the first trimester of pregnancy.

*Level of Cognitive Ability:* Application
*Client Needs:* Physiological Integrity
*Integrated Concept/Process:* Teaching/Learning
*Content Area:* Maternity

*Reference*
Lowdermilk, D., Perry, S., & Bobak, I. (2000). *Maternity & women's health care* (7th ed.). St. Louis: Mosby, p. 412.

**322.** A nurse is admitting a client with a diagnosis of myxedema. The nurse performs which physical assessment technique that will provide data related to this diagnosis?

1 Inspection of facial features

2 Palpation of the adrenal glands

3 Percussion of the thyroid gland

4 Auscultation of lung sounds

**Answer: 1**

*Rationale:* Inspection of facial features will reveal the characteristic coarse features, presence of edema around the eyes and face, and blank expression that are characteristic of myxedema. The assessment techniques in options 2, 3, and 4 will not reveal information related to the diagnosis of myxedema.

*Test-Taking Strategy:* Use the process of elimination. Eliminate options 2 and 4 because they do not relate to the thyroid gland. From the remaining options, recall that palpation, rather than percussion of the thyroid, is the assessment technique used to evaluate the thyroid gland. If you had difficulty with this question, review the clinical manifestations associated with myxedema.

*Level of Cognitive Ability:* Application
*Client Needs:* Physiological Integrity
*Integrated Concept/Process:* Nursing Process/Assessment
*Content Area:* Adult Health/Endocrine

*Reference*
Smeltzer, S., & Bare, B. (2000). *Brunner & Suddarth's Textbook of medical-surgical nursing* (9th ed.). Philadelphia: Lippincott Williams & Wilkins, p. 1038.

**323.** A nurse is teaching a client with chronic obstructive pulmonary disease (COPD) how to purse lip breathe. The nurse tells the client:
1 That inhalation should be twice as long as exhalation
2 To loosen the abdominal muscles while breathing out
3 That exhalation should be twice as long as inhalation
4 To inhale with pursed lips and exhale with the mouth open wide

**Answer: 3**
*Rationale:* Prolonging exhalation time reduces the air trapping caused by airway narrowing that occurs in COPD. Tightening (not loosening) the abdominal muscles aids in expelling air. Exhaling through pursed lips (not with the mouth wide open) increases the intraluminal pressure and prevents the airways from collapsing.

*Test-Taking Strategy:* Use the process of elimination. Knowing that a major purpose of pursed lip breathing is to prevent air trapping during exhalation will direct you to the correct option. Review the principles of pursed lip breathing if you are unfamiliar with this technique.

*Level of Cognitive Ability:* Application
*Client Needs:* Physiological Integrity
*Integrated Concept/Process:* Teaching/Learning
*Content Area:* Adult Health/Respiratory

*Reference*
Smeltzer, S., & Bare, B. (2000). *Brunner & Suddarth's Textbook of medical-surgical nursing* (9th ed.). Philadelphia: Lippincott Williams & Wilkins, p. 448.

**324.** A nurse is caring for a pregnant client with a history of human immunodeficiency virus (HIV). Which nursing diagnosis, if formulated by the nurse, has the highest priority for this client?
1 Self Care Deficit
2 Risk for Infection
3 Nutrition Deficit
4 Activity Intolerance

**Answer: 2**
*Rationale:* Clients with HIV often show some evidence of immune dysfunction and may have increased vulnerability to common infections. HIV infection impairs cellular and humoral immune function. Individuals with HIV are vulnerable to common bacterial infections. Not every client with HIV will have problems with activity, self-care, or nutrition. Although nutritional deficit is a concern, infection is specifically related to HIV and is a priority.

*Test-Taking Strategy:* Use the process of elimination, noting the key words *highest priority*. Focus on the physiology related to HIV to direct you to option 2. Also, recall that infection is a life-threatening condition in the client with HIV. If you had difficulty with this question, review the risks associated with HIV infection.

*Level of Cognitive Ability:* Analysis
*Client Needs:* Physiological Integrity
*Integrated Concept/Process:* Nursing Process/Analysis
*Content Area:* Adult Health/Immune

*Reference*
Lowdermilk, D., Perry, S., & Bobak, I. (2000). *Maternity & women's health care* (7th ed.). St. Louis: Mosby, p. 163.

**325.** A 44-year-old client is taking lithium carbonate (Lithium) for the treatment of bipolar disorder. Which assessment question would the nurse ask the client to determine signs of early lithium toxicity?
1   "Have you been experiencing seizures over the past few days?"
2   "Do you have frequent headaches?"
3   "Have you been experiencing any nausea, vomiting, or diarrhea?"
4   "Have you noted excessive urination?"

**Answer: 3**
*Rationale:* One of the most common early signs of lithium toxicity is gastrointestinal (GI) disturbances such as nausea, vomiting, or diarrhea. The assessment questions in options 1, 2, and 4 are unrelated to the findings in lithium toxicity.

*Test-Taking Strategy:* Use the process of elimination and knowledge regarding the "early" signs of toxicity. Recalling that GI disturbances are early manifestations will direct you to option 3. Review these signs if you had difficulty with this question.

*Level of Cognitive Ability:* Analysis
*Client Needs:* Physiological Integrity
*Integrated Concept/Process:* Nursing Process/Assessment
*Content Area:* Pharmacology

*Reference*
Hodgson, B., & Kizior, R. (2001). *Saunders Nursing drug handbook 2001.* Philadelphia: W.B. Saunders, p. 598.

**326.** A physician's order reads "haloperidol decanoate (Haldol) 175 mg IM." The medication is available in 100 mg per mL. How many milliliters of the medication would a nurse draw into the syringe for injection?
1   1.5 mL
2   1.8 mL
3   1.75 mL
4   1.25 mL

**Answer: 3**
*Rationale:* Use the following formula for calculating medication dosages:

$$Desired = 175 \text{ mg}; Available = 1 \text{ mL} = 100 \text{ mg}$$
$$\text{Ratio: } 175 \text{ mg} : x \text{ mL} :: 100 \text{ mg} : 1 \text{ mL}$$
$$175 = 100x$$
$$x = 1.75 \text{ mL}$$

*Test-Taking Strategy:* When reading math calculation questions, identify the dosage or concentration on hand and the dosage or concentration needed. Once these are identified, set up the mathematical problem and solve for x. Make sure that the answer makes sense. Review the formula for calculating medication dosages if you had difficulty with this question.

*Level of Cognitive Ability:* Application
*Client Needs:* Physiological Integrity
*Integrated Concept/Process:* Nursing Process/Implementation
*Content Area:* Pharmacology

*Reference*
Kee, J., & Marshall, S. (2000). *Clinical calculations: With applications to general and specialty areas* (4th ed.). Philadelphia: W.B. Saunders, p. 78.

**327.** A nurse is performing a prenatal examination on a client in the third trimester. The nurse begins an abdominal examination and performs Leopold's maneuvers. The nurse determines which of the following after performing the first maneuver?
1   Fetal lie and presentation
2   Fetal descent
3   Strength of uterine contractions
4   Placenta previa

**Answer: 1**
*Rationale:* The first maneuver determines the contents of the fundus (either the fetal head or breech) and thereby the fetal lie. Leopold maneuvers should not be performed during a contraction. Placenta previa is diagnosed by ultrasound and not by palpation. Fetal descent is determined with the fourth maneuver.

*Test-Taking Strategy:* Use the process of elimination. Recalling the purpose and procedure of Leopold's maneuvers will assist in eliminating options 3 and 4. From the remaining options, it is necessary to know what the first maneuver determines. Review Leopold's maneuvers if you had difficulty with this question.

*Level of Cognitive Ability:* Analysis
*Client Needs:* Physiological Integrity
*Integrated Concept/Process:* Nursing Process/Assessment
*Content Area:* Maternity

*Reference*
Lowdermilk, D., Perry, S., & Bobak, I. (2000). *Maternity & women's health care* (7th ed.). St. Louis: Mosby, p. 529.

**328.** A nurse is caring for a client with a spinal cord injury who has spinal shock. The nurse performs an assessment on the client knowing that which assessment will provide the best information about recovery from spinal shock?
1   Blood pressure
2   Pulse rate
3   Reflexes
4   Temperature

**Answer: 3**
*Rationale:* Areflexia characterizes spinal shock. Therefore, reflexes would provide the best information about recovery. Vital sign changes (options 1, 2, and 4) are not consistently affected by spinal shock. Because vital signs are affected by many factors, they do not give reliable information about spinal shock recovery. Blood pressure would provide good information about recovery from other types of shock, but not spinal shock.

*Test-Taking Strategy:* Use the process of elimination. Note that options 1, 2, and 4 are similar and are all vital signs. Option 3 is the different option. Review spinal shock, if you are unfamiliar with this content.

*Level of Cognitive Ability:* Analysis
*Client Needs:* Physiological Integrity
*Integrated Concept/Process:* Nursing Process/Assessment
*Content Area:* Adult Health/Neurological

*Reference*
Smeltzer, S., & Bare, B. (2000). *Brunner & Suddarth's Textbook of medical-surgical nursing* (9th ed.). Philadelphia: Lippincott Williams & Wilkins, p. 259.

**329.** A client is admitted to the hospital for repair of an unruptured cerebral aneurysm. Before surgery, the nurse performs frequent assessments on the client. Which assessment finding would be noted first if the aneurysm ruptures?
1   Widened pulse pressure
2   Unilateral slowing of pupil response
3   Unilateral motor weakness
4   A decline in the level of consciousness

**Answer: 4**
*Rationale:* Rupture of a cerebral aneurysm usually results in increased intracranial pressure (ICP). The first sign of pressure in the brain on the brainstem is a change in the level of consciousness. This change in consciousness can be as subtle as drowsiness or restlessness. Because centers that control blood pressure are located lower in the brainstem than those that control consciousness, pulse pressure alteration is a later sign. Slowing of pupil response and motor weakness are also late signs.

*Test-Taking Strategy:* Note the key word *first*. Remember that changes in level of consciousness are the first indication of increased intracranial pressure. Review the clinical manifestations associated with a cerebral aneurysm and ICP if you had difficulty with this question.

*Level of Cognitive Ability:* Analysis
*Client Needs:* Physiological Integrity
*Integrated Concept/Process:* Nursing Process/Assessment
*Content Area:* Adult Health/Neurological

*Reference*
Smeltzer, S., & Bare, B. (2000). *Brunner & Suddarth's Textbook of medical-surgical nursing* (9th ed.). Philadelphia: Lippincott Williams & Wilkins, p. 1714.

---

**330.** An emergency department staff member calls the mental health unit and tells the nurse that a severely depressed client is being transported to the unit. The nurse expects to note which of the following on assessment of this client?

1. Weight gain, hypersomnia, blunted affect
2. Increased crying spells, normal weight, and normal sleep patterns
3. Hesitancy to participate in the activities, but no change in affect
4. Weight loss, insomnia, decreased crying spells

**Answer: 4**
*Rationale:* In a severely depressed client, loss of weight is typical, whereas a mildly depressed client may experience a gain in weight. Sleep is generally affected in a similar way, with hypersomnia in the mildly depressed client and insomnia in the severely depressed client. The severely depressed client may report that no tears are left for crying.

*Test-Taking Strategy:* Use the process of elimination. Note the key words *severely depressed*. Options 2 and 3 identify some degree of normalcy and can be eliminated. Option 1 indicates some degree of normalcy with the term *blunted affect;* therefore eliminate this option. Review assessment findings associated with the severely depressed client if you had difficulty with this question.

*Level of Cognitive Ability:* Analysis
*Client Needs:* Physiological Integrity
*Integrated Concept/Process:* Nursing Process/Assessment
*Content Area:* Mental Health

*Reference*
Stuart, G.W., & Laraia, M.T. (1998). *Principles and practice of psychiatric nursing.* (6th ed.). St. Louis: Mosby, p. 357.

---

**331.** A client with a prior history of suicide attempts is admitted with a diagnosis of depression. The client's therapist reports to the nurse that the client had called earlier and was having severe suicidal thoughts. With this information in mind, the nurse's priority is to assess for:

1. The presence of suicidal thoughts
2. Interaction with peers
3. The amount of food intake for the past 24 hours
4. Information regarding the past treatment regimen

**Answer: 1**
*Rationale:* The critical information from the therapist is that the client is having thoughts of self-harm; therefore, the nurse needs further information about present thoughts of suicide so that the treatment plan may be as appropriate as possible. The nurse must make sure the client is safe. The items in options 2, 3, and 4 should be assessed; however, assessment of suicide potential is most important.

*Test-Taking Strategy:* Use the process of elimination and note the key word *priority*. Note the relationship between *severe suicidal thoughts* in the question and in the correct option. Review assessment of the client at risk for self-harm if you had difficulty with this question.

*Level of Cognitive Ability:* Analysis
*Client Needs:* Physiological Integrity
*Integrated Concept/Process:* Nursing Process/Assessment
*Content Area:* Mental Health

**Reference**
Stuart, G.W., & Laraia, M.T. (1998). *Principles and practice of psychiatric nursing.* (6th ed.). St. Louis: Mosby, p. 389.

---

**332.** A home care nurse finds a client in the bedroom, unconscious, with pill bottle in hand. The pill bottle contained the selective serotonin reuptake inhibitor (SSRI) sertraline (Zoloft). The nurse immediately assesses the client's:
1   Blood pressure
2   Respirations
3   Pulse
4   Urinary output

**Answer: 2**
*Rationale:* In an emergency situation, the nurse should determine breathlessness first, then pulselessness. Blood pressure would be assessed after these assessments were determined. Urinary output is also important, but not the priority at this time.

*Test-Taking Strategy:* Use the ABCs (airway, breathing, and circulation) as the guide for answering this question. Respirations specifically relate to breathing and airway. Review priority assessments in an unconscious client with a suspected overdose of sertraline if you had difficulty with this question.

*Level of Cognitive Ability:* Analysis
*Client Needs:* Physiological Integrity
*Integrated Concept/Process:* Nursing Process/Assessment
*Content Area:* Fundamental Skills

**Reference**
Hodgson, B., & Kizior, R. (2001). *Saunders Nursing drug handbook 2001.* Philadelphia: W.B. Saunders, pp. 926-927.

---

**333.** A nurse is checking a unit of blood received from the blood bank and notes the presence of gas bubbles in the bag. The nurse should take which of the following actions?
1   Add 10 mL of normal saline solution to the bag
2   Agitate the bag gently to mix contents
3   Add 100 units of heparin to the bag
4   Return the bag to the blood bank

**Answer: 4**
*Rationale:* The nurse should return the unit of blood to the blood bank. The presence of gas bubbles in the bag indicates possible bacterial growth, and the unit is considered contaminated. Options 1, 2, and 3 are incorrect actions.

*Test-Taking Strategy:* Use the process of elimination. Recalling that the presence of gas bubbles indicates bacterial growth will direct you to option 4. Remember: when in doubt, consult with the blood bank. Review concepts related to transfusion of blood, if this question was difficult.

*Level of Cognitive Ability:* Application
*Client Needs:* Physiological Integrity
*Integrated Concept/Process:* Nursing Process/Implementation
*Content Area:* Fundamental Skills

**Reference**
Monahan, F., & Neighbors, M. (1998). *Medical surgical nursing: Foundations for clinical practice* (2nd ed.). Philadelphia: W.B. Saunders, p. 457.

**334.** A nurse has an order to infuse a unit of blood. The nurse checks the client's intravenous line to make sure that the gauge of the intravenous catheter is at least:

1. 14 gauge
2. 19 gauge
3. 22 gauge
4. 24 gauge

**Answer: 2**

*Rationale:* An intravenous line used to infuse blood should be 19-gauge or larger. This allows infusion of the blood elements without clogging the line or the IV access site.

*Test-Taking Strategy:* Focus on the issue: infusion of blood. This focus will assist in eliminating options 3 and 4. From the remaining options, think about the gauge of IV catheters to direct you to option 2. Review IV lines and blood transfusions if you had difficulty with this question.

*Level of Cognitive Ability:* Application
*Client Needs:* Physiological Integrity
*Integrated Concept/Process:* Nursing Process/Implementation
*Content Area:* Fundamental Skills

**Reference**
Monahan, F., & Neighbors, M. (1998). *Medical surgical nursing: Foundations for clinical practice* (2nd ed.). Philadelphia: W.B. Saunders, p. 457.

---

**335.** A client began receiving a unit of blood 30 minutes ago. The client rings the call bell and complains of breathing difficulty, itching, and a tight sensation in the chest. Which of the following is the first action of the nurse?

1. Recheck the unit of blood for compatibility
2. Check the client's temperature
3. Stop the transfusion
4. Call the physician

**Answer: 3**

*Rationale:* The symptoms reported by the client are compatible with transfusion reaction. The first action of the nurse when a transfusion reaction is suspected is to discontinue the transfusion. The IV line is kept open with normal saline. The physician is notified. Depending on agency protocol, the nurse may then obtain a urine specimen for urinalysis, draw a sample of blood, and return the unit of blood and tubing to the blood bank. The nurse also institutes supportive care for the client, which may include administration of antihistamines, crystalloids, epinephrine, or vasopressors as prescribed.

*Test-Taking Strategy:* Noting that the question asks for the "first action" will direct you to option 3. Review the nursing actions when a transfusion reaction occurs if you had difficulty with this question.

*Level of Cognitive Ability:* Application
*Client Needs:* Physiological Integrity
*Integrated Concept/Process:* Nursing Process/Implementation
*Content Area:* Fundamental Skills

**Reference**
Monahan, F., & Neighbors, M. (1998). *Medical surgical nursing: Foundations for clinical practice* (2nd ed.). Philadelphia: W.B. Saunders, pp. 460-461.

**336.** A client has not eaten or had anything to drink for 4 hours following two episodes of nausea and vomiting. Which of the following items would be best to offer the client who is ready to try resuming oral intake?

1   Ginger ale
2   Gelatin
3   Toast
4   Dry cereal

**Answer: 1**

*Rationale:* Clear liquids are best tolerated first after episodes of nausea and vomiting. If the client tolerates sips (20 to 30 mL at a time) of clear liquids, such as water or ginger ale, the amounts may be increased and gelatin, tea, and broth may be added. Once these are tolerated, easily digested solid foods such as toast, cereal, and chicken may be tried.

*Test-Taking Strategy:* Use the process of elimination. Begin to answer this question by eliminating options 3 and 4, which identify solid foods and are less well tolerated than liquids. Choose ginger ale over gelatin because it is a liquid at all temperatures.

*Level of Cognitive Ability:* Application
*Client Needs:* Physiological Integrity
*Integrated Concept/Process:* Nursing Process/Implementation
*Content Area:* Adult Health/Gastrointestinal

*Reference*
Monahan, F., & Neighbors, M. (1998). *Medical surgical nursing: Foundations for clinical practice* (2nd ed.). Philadelphia: W.B. Saunders, p. 960.

**337.** A client has just undergone an upper gastrointestinal (GI) series. The nurse provides which of the following upon the client's return to the unit as an important part of routine postprocedure care?

1   Increased fluids
2   Bland diet
3   NPO status
4   Laxative

**Answer: 4**

*Rationale:* Barium sulfate, which is used as a contrast material during an upper GI series, is constipating. If it is not eliminated from the GI tract, it can cause obstruction. Therefore, laxatives or cathartics are administered as part of routine postprocedure care. Fluids are also helpful but do not act in the same way as a laxative to eliminate the barium. Options 2 and 3 are not routine postprocedure measures.

*Test-Taking Strategy:* Use the process of elimination. Focus on the diagnostic test and the key words *routine postprocedure*. Recalling that barium is used will direct you to option 4. Review postprocedure care following an upper GI series if you had difficulty with this question.

*Level of Cognitive Ability:* Application
*Client Needs:* Physiological Integrity
*Integrated Concept/Process:* Nursing Process/Implementation
*Content Area:* Adult Health/Gastrointestinal

*Reference*
Monahan, F., & Neighbors, M. (1998). *Medical surgical nursing: Foundations for clinical practice* (2nd ed.). Philadelphia: W.B. Saunders, p. 970.

**338.** A nurse has an order to discontinue the nasogastric tube of an assigned client. After explaining the procedure to the client, the nurse raises the bed to a semi-Fowler's position, places a towel across the chest, clears the tube with normal saline, clamps the tube, and removes the tube:

1   During inspiration
2   During expiration
3   After inspiration, but before expiration
4   After expiration, but before inspiration

**Answer: 2**
*Rationale:* A nasogastric tube is removed during expiration, so that air and the tube are moving in the same direction. Options 1, 3, and 4 are incorrect.

*Test-Taking Strategy:* Use the process of elimination. Visualize this procedure. Thinking about the action that occurs during this procedure will direct you to option 2. If this question was difficult, review this procedure.

*Level of Cognitive Ability:* Application
*Client Needs:* Physiological Integrity
*Integrated Concept/Process:* Nursing Process/Implementation
*Content Area:* Fundamental Skills

*Reference*
Monahan, F., & Neighbors, M. (1998). *Medical surgical nursing: Foundations for clinical practice* (2nd ed.). Philadelphia: W.B. Saunders, p. 980.

---

**339.** A nurse is caring for a client who has an order to receive an intravenous intralipid infusion. Which of the following actions does the nurse take as part of proper procedure before hanging the infusion?

1   Add 100 mL of normal saline solution to the bottle
2   Attach an in-line filter
3   Remove the bottle from the refrigerator
4   Check the solution for separation or an oily appearance

**Answer: 4**
*Rationale:* Intralipid solutions should not be refrigerated. There should be no additives placed in the bottle because this could affect the stability of the solution. The solution should be checked for separation or an oily appearance. If found, it should not be used. An in-line filter is not used because it could disturb the flow of solution or become clogged.

*Test-Taking Strategy:* Use the process of elimination. Think about the consistency of this solution to direct you to option 4. If you are unfamiliar with the procedure for infusing intralipid solutions, review this content.

*Level of Cognitive Ability:* Application
*Client Needs:* Physiological Integrity
*Integrated Concept/Process:* Nursing Process/Implementation
*Content Area:* Fundamental Skills

*Reference*
Monahan, F., & Neighbors, M. (1998). *Medical surgical nursing: Foundations for clinical practice* (2nd ed.). Philadelphia: W.B. Saunders, p. 990.

---

**340.** A nurse is administering continuous tube feedings to a client. The nurse takes which of the following actions as part of routine care for this client?

1   Checks the residual every 4 hours
2   Changes the feeding bag and tubing every 12 hours
3   Pours additional feeding into the bag when 25 mL are left
4   Holds the feeding if greater than 200 mL are aspirated.

**Answer: 1**
*Rationale:* The nasogastric feeding tube is checked at least every 4 hours for residual when administering continuous tube feedings. It is checked before each bolus with intermittent feedings. The feeding should be withheld for 30 to 60 minutes if the residual is greater than 30 mL, or per agency policy. The bag and tubing are completely changed every 24 hours. The bag should be rinsed before adding new formula to the bag that is hanging.

*Test-Taking Strategy:* Note the key words *continuous tube feedings*. Use the steps of the nursing process to answer the question. Option 1 is the only option that addresses assessment. If you had difficulty with this question, review the nursing care associated with this procedure.

*Level of Cognitive Ability:* Application
*Client Needs:* Physiological Integrity
*Integrated Concept/Process:* Nursing Process/Implementation
*Content Area:* Fundamental Skills

### Reference
Monahan, F., & Neighbors, M. (1998). *Medical surgical nursing: Foundations for clinical practice* (2nd ed.). Philadelphia: W.B. Saunders, p. 985.

---

**341.** A physician is inserting a chest tube. The nurse selects which of the following materials to be used as the first layer of the dressing at the chest tube insertion site?
1  Sterile 4 × 4 gauze pad
2  Absorbent Kerlix dressing
3  Gauze impregnated with povidone-iodine
4  Petrolatum jelly gauze

**Answer: 4**
*Rationale:* The first layer of the chest tube dressing is petrolatum gauze, which allows for an occlusive seal at the chest tube insertion site. Additional layers of gauze cover this layer, and the dressing is secured with a strong adhesive tape or Elastoplast tape.

*Test-Taking Strategy:* Use the process of elimination, noting the key words *first layer*. Recall that an occlusive seal at the site is needed and think about which dressing material will help achieve this seal. Review care of a client requiring chest tube insertion if you had difficulty with this question.

*Level of Cognitive Ability:* Application
*Client Needs:* Physiological Integrity
*Integrated Concept/Process:* Nursing Process/Implementation
*Content Area:* Adult Health/Respiratory

### Reference
Monahan, F., & Neighbors, M. (1998). *Medical surgical nursing: Foundations for clinical practice* (2nd ed.). Philadelphia: W.B. Saunders, p. 577.

---

**342.** A client being seen in the physician's office for follow-up 2 weeks after pneumonectomy complains of numbness and tenderness at the surgical site. The nurse tells the client that this is:
1  A severe problem, and the client will probably be rehospitalized
2  Often the first sign of wound infection, and checks the client's temperature
3  Probably caused by permanent nerve damage as a result of surgery
4  Not likely to be permanent, but may last for some months

**Answer: 4**
*Rationale:* Clients who undergo pneumonectomy may experience numbness, altered sensation, or tenderness in the area that surrounds the incision. These sensations may last for months. It is not considered to be a severe problem and is not indicative of wound infection.

*Test-Taking Strategy:* Use the process of elimination. Eliminate option 1 because of the word *severe*. Eliminate option 2 because numbness and tenderness are not signs of infection. Eliminate option 3 because of the word *permanent*. Review this surgical procedure if you are not familiar with it.

*Level of Cognitive Ability:* Application
*Client Needs:* Physiological Integrity
*Integrated Concept/Process:* Nursing Process/Implementation
*Content Area:* Adult Health/Respiratory

### Reference
Monahan, F., & Neighbors, M. (1998). *Medical surgical nursing: Foundations for clinical practice* (2nd ed.). Philadelphia: W.B. Saunders, pp. 581-582.

**343.** A client scheduled for pneumonectomy asks the nurse how long the chest tubes will be in place. The nurse responds that:
1. They will be in place for 24 to 48 hours
2. They will be removed after 3 to 4 days
3. They usually function for a full week after surgery
4. Most likely, there will be no chest tubes in place after surgery

**Answer: 4**
*Rationale:* Pneumonectomy involves removal of the entire lung, usually because of extensive disease such as bronchogenic carcinoma, unilateral tuberculosis, or lung abscess. Chest tubes are not inserted because the cavity is left to fill with serosanguineous fluid, which later solidifies. The phrenic nerve is severed or crushed to elevate the diaphragm, further decreasing the size of the chest cavity on the operative side.

*Test-Taking Strategy:* Focus on the surgical procedure. Recall that the entire lung is removed with this procedure. This would guide you to reason that chest tubes are unnecessary, since there is no lung remaining to reinflate to fill the pleural space. Review care of a client following pneumonectomy if you had difficulty with this question.

*Level of Cognitive Ability:* Application
*Client Needs:* Physiological Integrity
*Integrated Concept/Process:* Nursing Process/Implementation
*Content Area:* Adult Health/Respiratory

*Reference*
Monahan, F., & Neighbors, M. (1998). *Medical surgical nursing: Foundations for clinical practice* (2nd ed.). Philadelphia: W.B. Saunders, p. 581.

**344.** A nurse is caring for a client with a dissecting abdominal aortic aneurysm. The nurse avoids which of the following while caring for the client?
1. Turning the client to the side to look for ecchymoses on the lower back
2. Auscultating the arteries for bruits
3. Performing deep palpation of the abdomen
4. Telling the client to report back, shoulder, or neck pain

**Answer: 3**
*Rationale:* The nurse avoids deep palpation in the client in which a dissecting aneurysm is known or suspected. Doing so could place the client at risk for rupture. The nurse looks for ecchymoses on the lower back to determine whether the aneurysm is leaking, and tells the client to report back, neck, shoulder, or extremity pain. The nurse may auscultate the arteries for bruits.

*Test-Taking Strategy:* Use the process of elimination. Note the key word *avoids* in the stem of the question. This tells you that the correct option will be an incorrect nursing action, or one that is contraindicated. With the diagnosis presented, the only option that could cause harm is the option related to deep palpation. Review care of a client with a dissecting abdominal aortic aneurysm if you had difficulty with this question.

*Level of Cognitive Ability:* Application
*Client Needs:* Physiological Integrity
*Integrated Concept/Process:* Nursing Process/Implementation
*Content Area:* Adult Health/Cardiovascular

*Reference*
Monahan, F., & Neighbors, M. (1998). *Medical-surgical nursing: Foundations for clinical practice* (2nd ed.). Philadelphia: W.B. Saunders, p. 372.

**345.** A client has undergone angioplasty of the iliac artery. The nurse best detects bleeding from the angioplasty in the region of the iliac artery by:

1. Measuring abdominal girth
2. Auscultating over the area with a doppler
3. Periodically asking the client about mild pain in the area
4. Palpating the pedal pulses

**Answer: 1**

*Rationale:* Bleeding after iliac artery angioplasty causes blood to accumulate in the retroperitoneal area. This can most directly be detected by measuring abdominal girth. Palpation and auscultation of pulses determine patency. Assessment of pain is routinely done, and mild regional discomfort is expected.

*Test-Taking Strategy:* Use the process of elimination. Focus on the key words *bleeding* and *iliac artery*. Select the option that addresses an abdominal assessment, since the iliac arteries are located in the peritoneal cavity. This will direct you to option 1. Review this procedure if you had difficulty with this question.

*Level of Cognitive Ability:* Analysis
*Client Needs:* Physiological Integrity
*Integrated Concept/Process:* Nursing Process/Assessment
*Content Area:* Adult Health/Cardiovascular

*Reference*
Monahan, F., & Neighbors, M. (1998). *Medical-surgical nursing: Foundations for clinical practice* (2nd ed.). Philadelphia: W.B. Saunders, p. 344.

---

**346.** A client is scheduled for a right femoral-popliteal bypass graft. The client has a nursing diagnosis of Altered Peripheral Tissue Perfusion. The nurse takes which of the following actions before surgery to address this nursing diagnosis?

1. Completes a preoperative checklist
2. Marks the location of pedal pulses on the right leg
3. Has the client void before surgery
4. Checks the results of any baseline coagulation studies

**Answer: 2**

*Rationale:* A nursing diagnosis of Altered Peripheral Tissue Perfusion in the client scheduled for femoral-popliteal bypass grafting indicates that the client is likely to have diminished peripheral pulses. It is important to mark the location of any pulses that are palpated or auscultated. This provides a baseline for comparison in the postoperative period. The other options are part of routine preoperative care.

*Test-Taking Strategy:* Note the key words *to address this nursing diagnosis*. In this case, each of the incorrect options is an action that is part of routine preoperative care and are not specific to this nursing diagnosis. Review care of a client with altered tissue perfusion if you had difficulty with this question.

*Level of Cognitive Ability:* Application
*Client Needs:* Physiological Integrity
*Integrated Concept/Process:* Nursing Process/Implementation
*Content Area:* Adult Health/Cardiovascular

*Reference*
Monahan, F., & Neighbors, M. (1998). *Medical-surgical nursing: Foundations for clinical practice* (2nd ed.). Philadelphia: W.B. Saunders, p. 347.

**347.** A client who underwent peripheral arterial bypass surgery 16 hours ago complains of increasing pain in the leg at rest, which worsens with movement and is accompanied by paresthesias. The nurse should take which of the following actions?

1   Administer a narcotic analgesic
2   Apply warm moist heat for comfort
3   Apply ice to minimize any developing swelling
4   Call the physician

**Answer: 4**

*Rationale:* The classic signs of compartment syndrome are pain at rest that intensifies with movement, and the development of paresthesias. Compartment syndrome is characterized by increased pressure within a muscle compartment that results from bleeding or excessive edema. It compresses the nerves in the area and can cause vascular compromise. The physician is notified immediately because the client could require an emergency fasciotomy. Options 1, 2, and 3 are incorrect actions.

*Test-Taking Strategy:* Use the process of elimination. Note the key words *increasing pain.* Note that the surgery was 16 hours ago. The signs and symptoms described indicate a new problem. These factors should indicate that the physician needs to be notified. Review the complications of this type of surgery if you had difficulty with this question.

*Level of Cognitive Ability:* Application
*Client Needs:* Physiological Integrity
*Integrated Concept/Process:* Nursing Process/Implementation
*Content Area:* Adult Health/Cardiovascular

*Reference*
Monahan, F., & Neighbors, M. (1998). *Medical-surgical nursing: Foundations for clinical practice* (2nd ed.). Philadelphia: W.B. Saunders, p. 347.

**348.** A nurse in an ambulatory care clinic takes a client's blood pressure (BP). The nurse measures the client's BP in the left arm as 200/118 mm Hg. The first action of the nurse is to:

1   Notify the physician
2   Inquire about the presence of kidney disorders
3   Check the blood pressure in the right arm
4   Recheck the pressure in the same arm within 30 seconds

**Answer: 3**

*Rationale:* When a high BP reading is noted, the nurse takes the pressure in the opposite arm to see if the blood pressure is elevated in one extremity only. The nurse would also recheck the blood pressure in the same arm, but would wait at least 2 minutes between readings. The nurse would inquire about the presence of kidney disorders that could contribute to the elevated blood pressure. The nurse would notify the physician because immediate treatment may be required, but this would not be done without obtaining verification of the elevation.

*Test-Taking Strategy:* Use the process of elimination. Note the key word *first.* This tells you that more than one or all of the options may be partially or totally correct. In this situation, eliminate option 4 first because of the time frame, 30 seconds. From the remaining options, select option 3 because it provides verification of the initial reading. Review the procedures for BP measurement if you had difficulty with this question.

*Level of Cognitive Ability:* Application
*Client Needs:* Physiological Integrity
*Integrated Concept/Process:* Nursing Process/Implementation
*Content Area:* Adult Health/Cardiovascular

*Reference*
Monahan, F., & Neighbors, M. (1998). *Medical-surgical nursing: Foundations for clinical practice* (2nd ed.). Philadelphia: W.B. Saunders, p. 375.

**349.** Thrombophlebitis has been diagnosed in a hospitalized client. A nurse would avoid doing which of the following during the care of this client?

1    Maintaining the client on bed rest
2    Applying moist heat to the leg
3    Elevating the feet above heart level
4    Placing a pillow under the client's knees

**Answer: 4**

*Rationale:* The nurse avoids placing a pillow under the knees of a client with thrombophlebitis because it obstructs venous return to the heart and exacerbates impairment of blood flow. The client is maintained on bed rest for 3 to 7 days after a diagnosis of thrombophlebitis is made to prevent occurrence of pulmonary embolus. The feet are elevated above heart level to aid in venous return, and warm moist heat may be used to aid in comfort and reduce venospasm.

*Test-Taking Strategy:* Use the process of elimination. Note the key word *avoid*. This tells you that the correct option will be an incorrect nursing action. Use principles related to gravity and relief of inflammation to direct you to option 4. Review care of a client with thrombophlebitis if you had difficulty with this question.

*Level of Cognitive Ability:* Application
*Client Needs:* Physiological Integrity
*Integrated Concept/Process:* Nursing Process/Implementation
*Content Area:* Adult Health/Cardiovascular

*Reference*
Monahan, F., & Neighbors, M. (1998). *Medical-surgical nursing: Foundations for clinical practice* (2nd ed.). Philadelphia: W.B. Saunders, p. 387.

**350.** A new prenatal client is 6 months pregnant. On the first prenatal visit, the nurse notes that the client is gravida 4, para 0, aborta 3. The client is 5'6" tall, weighs 130 lb, and is 25 years old. The client states, "I get really tired after working all day, and I can't keep up with my housework." Which factor in the above data would lead the nurse to suspect gestational diabetes?

1    Fatigue
2    Obesity
3    Maternal age
4    Previous fetal demise

**Answer: 4**

*Rationale:* Fatigue is a normal occurrence during pregnancy. A client 5'6" tall and 130 lb does not meet the criteria of 20% over ideal weight. Therefore the client is not obese. To be at high risk for gestational diabetes, the maternal age should be greater than 30 years. A previous history of unexplained stillbirths or miscarriages puts the client at high risk for gestational diabetes.

*Test-Taking Strategy:* Use the process of elimination. Option 1 can be eliminated because fatigue is a normal occurrence during pregnancy. Recalling the risk factors associated with gestational diabetes will indicate that options 2 and 3 do not apply to this client. If you had difficulty with this question, review the risk factors associated with gestational diabetes.

*Level of Cognitive Ability:* Analysis
*Client Needs:* Physiological Integrity
*Integrated Concept/Process:* Nursing Process/Analysis
*Content Area:* Maternity

*Reference*
Lowdermilk, D., Perry, S., & Bobak, I. (2000). *Maternity & women's health care* (7th ed.). St. Louis: Mosby, p. 876.

**351.** A nurse is caring for a client with preeclampsia. The nurse develops a plan of care knowing that if the client progresses from preeclampsia to eclampsia, the nurse's first action is to:

1    Administer IV magnesium sulfate
2    Assess the blood pressure and fetal heart tones
3    Clear and maintain an open airway
4    Administer oxygen by face mask

**Answer: 3**

*Rationale:* It is important as a first action to keep an open airway and prevent injuries to the client. Options 1, 2, and 4 are all procedures that should be done but are not the first action.

*Test-Taking Strategy:* Note the key words *first action.* Use the ABCs (airway, breathing, and circulation) to direct you to option 3. Review care of a client with preeclampsia or eclampsia if you had difficulty with this question.

*Level of Cognitive Ability:* Application
*Client Needs:* Physiological Integrity
*Integrated Concept/Process:* Nursing Process/Implementation
*Content Area:* Maternity

*Reference*
Lowdermilk, D., Perry, S., & Bobak, I. (2000). *Maternity & women's health care* (7th ed.). St. Louis: Mosby, p. 834.

**352.** A nurse in the emergency department admits a client who is bleeding freely from a scalp laceration obtained during a fall from a stepladder when the client was doing outdoor home repair. The nurse takes which of the following actions first in the care of this wound?

1    Asks the client about timing of the last tetanus vaccination
2    Cleanses the wound with sterile normal saline
3    Prepares for suturing the area
4    Administers a prophylactic antibiotic

**Answer: 2**

*Rationale:* The initial nursing action is to cleanse the wound thoroughly with sterile normal saline. This removes dirt or foreign matter from the wound and allows visualization of the size of the wound. Direct pressure is applied as needed to control bleeding. If suturing is necessary, the surrounding hair may be shaved. Prophylactic antibiotics are often ordered. The date of the client's last tetanus shot is determined, and prophylaxis is given if needed.

*Test-Taking Strategy:* Use the process of elimination. Note the key words *first* and *care of this wound.* The key word *first* implies that more than one or all of the options may be partially or totally correct. Focusing on the issue, care of the wound, will direct you to option 2. Review care of a client with a laceration if you had difficulty with this question.

*Level of Cognitive Ability:* Application
*Client Needs:* Physiological Integrity
*Integrated Concept/Process:* Nursing Process/Implementation
*Content Area:* Adult Health/Integumentary

*Reference*
Monahan, F., & Neighbors, M. (1998). *Medical-surgical nursing: Foundations for clinical practice* (2nd ed.). Philadelphia: W.B. Saunders, p. 817.

**353.** A client was admitted to the nursing unit with a closed head injury 6 hours ago. After report, the nurse finds that the client has vomited, is confused, and complains of dizziness and headache. Which of the following is the most important nursing action?

1 Administer an antiemetic
2 Change the client's gown and bed linens
3 Reorient the client to surroundings
4 Notify the physician

**Answer: 4**

*Rationale:* The client with a closed head injury is at risk for increased intracranial pressure (ICP). This is evidenced by such symptoms as headache, dizziness, confusion, weakness, and vomiting. Because of the implications of the symptoms, the most important nursing action is to notify the physician. Other nursing actions that are appropriate include physical care of the client and reorientation to surroundings.

*Test-Taking Strategy:* Use the process of elimination. Note the key words *most important.* This directs you to prioritize the possible nursing actions. Considering the client's diagnosis, a closed head injury, and the signs and symptoms, the nurse should suspect increased ICP. The physician needs to be notified. Review care of a client with increased ICP if you had difficulty with this question.

*Level of Cognitive Ability:* Application
*Client Needs:* Physiological Integrity
*Integrated Concept/Process:* Nursing Process/Implementation
*Content Area:* Adult Health/Neurological

*Reference*
Monahan, F., & Neighbors, M. (1998). *Medical-surgical nursing: Foundations for clinical practice* (2nd ed.). Philadelphia: W.B. Saunders, p. 819.

**354.** A client is being brought into the emergency department after suffering a head injury. The first action by the nurse is to determine the client's:

1 Respiratory rate and depth
2 Pulse and blood pressure
3 Level of consciousness
4 Ability to move extremities

**Answer: 1**

*Rationale:* The first action of the nurse is to ensure that the client has an adequate airway and respiratory status. In rapid sequence, the client's circulatory status is evaluated (option 2), followed by evaluation of the neurological status (options 3 and 4).

*Test-Taking Strategy:* In emergency situations, use the ABCs (airway, breathing, and circulation). The correct option will most often be the option that deals with the client's airway. Respiratory rate and depth support this action. Review initial care of the client who sustains a head injury if you had difficulty with this question.

*Level of Cognitive Ability:* Application
*Client Needs:* Physiological Integrity
*Integrated Concept/Process:* Nursing Process/Implementation
*Content Area:* Adult Health/Neurological

*Reference*
Monahan, F., & Neighbors, M. (1998). *Medical-surgical nursing: Foundations for clinical practice* (2nd ed.). Philadelphia: W.B. Saunders, p. 821.

**355.** A client with a spinal cord injury is at risk for foot drop. The nurse uses which of the following as the most effective preventive measure?

  1  Heel protectors
  2  Posterior splints
  3  Pneumatic boots
  4  Foot board

**Answer: 2**

*Rationale:* The most effective means of preventing foot drop is the use of posterior splints or high-top sneakers. A foot board prevents plantar flexion but also places the client at greater risk for pressure ulcers of the feet. Pneumatic boots prevent deep vein thrombosis but not foot drop. Heel protectors protect the skin but do not prevent foot drop.

*Test-Taking Strategy:* Note that the issue of the question is "prevention" of foot drop. This guides you to select the option that immobilizes the foot in a functional position while protecting the skin of the extremities. This will direct you to option 2. Review the purposes of the devices identified in the options if you had difficulty with this question.

*Level of Cognitive Ability:* Application
*Client Needs:* Physiological Integrity
*Integrated Concept/Process:* Nursing Process/Implementation
*Content Area:* Adult Health/Neurological

*Reference*
Monahan, F., & Neighbors, M. (1998). *Medical-surgical nursing: Foundations for clinical practice* (2nd ed.). Philadelphia: W.B. Saunders, p. 826.

---

**356.** A client is ambulatory and wearing a halo vest after a cervical spine fracture. The nurse tells the client to avoid which of the following, since the client has a risk for injury?

  1  Bending at the waist
  2  Using a walker
  3  Wearing rubber-soled shoes
  4  Scanning the environment

**Answer: 1**

*Rationale:* The client with a halo vest should avoid bending at the waist, since the halo vest is heavy and the client's trunk is limited in flexibility. It is helpful for the client to scan the environment visually because the client's peripheral vision is diminished from keeping the neck in a stationary position. Use of a walker and rubber-soled shoes may help prevent falls and injury and is therefore also helpful.

*Test-Taking Strategy:* Use the process of elimination. Note the key word *avoid*. This guides you to look for an action that could place the client at risk for injury. Visualize each of the items or actions in the options to assist in identifying how injury could be prevented. Review teaching points for a client with a halo vest if you had difficulty with this question.

*Level of Cognitive Ability:* Application
*Client Needs:* Physiological Integrity
*Integrated Concept/Process:* Self Care
*Content Area:* Adult Health/Neurological

*Reference*
Monahan, F., & Neighbors, M. (1998). *Medical-surgical nursing: Foundations for clinical practice* (2nd ed.). Philadelphia: W.B. Saunders, p. 826.

**357.** A nurse is caring for a client who has undergone transsphenoidal resection of a pituitary adenoma. The nurse measures which of the following to detect occurrence of the most common complication of this surgery?

1. Pulse rate
2. Temperature
3. Urine output
4. Oxygen saturation

**Answer: 3**

*Rationale:* The most common complication of surgery on the pituitary gland is temporary diabetes insipidus. This results from a deficiency in antidiuretic hormone (ADH) secretion as a result of surgical trauma. The nurse measures the client's urine output to determine whether this complication is occurring. Options 1, 2, and 4 are not specifically related to the most common complication following this surgery.

*Test-Taking Strategy:* Use the process of elimination. Recalling that the pituitary gland is responsible for the production of ADH will direct you to option 3. Review the complications of this surgical procedure if you had difficulty with this question.

*Level of Cognitive Ability:* Analysis
*Client Needs:* Physiological Integrity
*Integrated Concept/Process:* Nursing Process/Assessment
*Content Area:* Adult Health/Neurological

*Reference*
Monahan, F., & Neighbors, M. (1998). *Medical-surgical nursing: Foundations for clinical practice* (2nd ed.). Philadelphia: W.B. Saunders, pp. 1267, 1275.

---

**358.** A nurse is sending an arterial blood gas (ABG) specimen to the laboratory for analysis. The nurse does not need to write which of the following pieces of information on the laboratory requisition?

1. The date and time the specimen was drawn
2. A list of client allergies
3. Any supplemental oxygen the client is receiving
4. The client's temperature

**Answer: 2**

*Rationale:* An ABG requisition usually contains information about the date and time the specimen was drawn, the client's temperature, whether the specimen was drawn on room air or using supplemental oxygen, and the ventilator settings if the client is receiving mechanical ventilation. The client's allergies do not have a direct bearing on the laboratory results.

*Test-Taking Strategy:* Use the process of elimination. Note the key word *not*. Review the options from the viewpoint of the relevance of the item to the client's airway status or oxygen utilization. This will direct you to option 2. Review the procedure related to drawing ABGs if you had difficulty with this question.

*Level of Cognitive Ability:* Application
*Client Needs:* Physiological Integrity
*Integrated Concept/Process:* Communication and Documentation
*Content Area:* Adult Health/Respiratory

*Reference*
Monahan, F., & Neighbors, M. (1998). *Medical-surgical nursing: Foundations for clinical practice* (2nd ed.). Philadelphia: W.B. Saunders, p. 543.

**359.** A nurse is preparing postoperative discharge instructions for a client who had one adrenal gland removed. The nurse includes which of the following in the instructions?

1 The need for lifelong replacement of all adrenal hormones
2 Instructions about early signs of a wound infection
3 The reason for maintaining a diabetic diet
4 Teaching proper application of an ostomy pouch

**Answer: 2**

*Rationale:* A client who had a unilateral adrenalectomy will be placed on corticosteroids temporarily to avoid a cortisol deficiency. The client will be gradually weaned from these medications in the postoperative period until they are discontinued. Also, because of the antiinflammatory properties of corticosteroids produced by the adrenal glands, clients who undergo an adrenalectomy are at increased risk for wound infections. Because of this increased risk of infection, it is important for the client to know measures to prevent infection, early signs of infection, and what to do if an infection seems to be present.

*Test-Taking Strategy:* Use the process of elimination. Note the key words *one adrenal gland removed*. Recalling that the hormones from the adrenal glands are needed for proper immune system function will eliminate options 3 and 4. From the remaining options, recalling that one gland can take over the function of two adrenal glands will direct you to option 2. Review care of a client following a unilateral adrenalectomy if you had difficulty with this question.

*Level of Cognitive Ability:* Application
*Client Needs:* Physiological Integrity
*Integrated Concept/Process:* Teaching/Learning
*Content Area:* Adult Health/Endocrine

**Reference**

Smeltzer, S., & Bare, B. (2000). *Brunner & Suddarth's Textbook of medical-surgical nursing* (9th ed.). Philadelphia: Lippincott Williams & Wilkins, p. 1061.

**360.** A nurse is caring for a client who has undergone transsphenoidal surgery for a pituitary adenoma. In the postoperative period, the nurse teaches the client to:

1 Remove the nasal packing after 48 hours
2 Cough and deep breathe hourly
3 Take acetaminophen (Tylenol) for severe headache
4 Report frequent swallowing or postnasal drip

**Answer: 4**

*Rationale:* The client should report frequent swallowing or postnasal drip after transsphenoidal surgery because it could indicate a cerebrospinal fluid (CSF) leakage. The surgeon removes the nasal packing, usually after 24 hours. The client should deep breathe, but coughing is contraindicated because it could cause increased intracranial pressure. The client should also report severe headache because it could indicate increased intracranial pressure.

*Test-Taking Strategy:* Think about the anatomical location of this surgical procedure. Recalling that the concern is increased intracranial pressure and CSF leakage will direct you to option 4. Review care of a client following transsphenoidal surgery if you had difficulty with this question.

*Level of Cognitive Ability:* Application
*Client Needs:* Physiological Integrity
*Integrated Concept/Process:* Teaching/Learning
*Content Area:* Adult Health/Neurological

**Reference**

Monahan, F., & Neighbors, M. (1998). *Medical surgical nursing: Foundations for clinical practice* (2nd ed.). Philadelphia: W.B. Saunders, p. 1269.

**361.** A client is receiving desmopressin (DDAVP) intranasally. The nurse assesses the client knowing that which of the following measurements would not assist in determining the effectiveness of this medication?

1  Urine output
2  Pupillary response
3  Presence of edema
4  Daily weight

**Answer: 2**
*Rationale:* Desmopressin (DDAVP) is an analog of vasopressin (antidiuretic hormone). It is used in the management of diabetes insipidus. The nurse monitors the client's fluid balance to determine the effectiveness of the medication. Fluid status can be evaluated by noting intake and urine output, daily weight, and the presence of edema.

*Test-Taking Strategy:* Use the process of elimination noting the key word *not*. Eliminate options 1, 3, and 4 because they are similar and relate to fluid balance. Review this medication if you had difficulty with this question.

*Level of Cognitive Ability:* Analysis
*Client Needs:* Physiological Integrity
*Integrated Concept/Process:* Nursing Process/Assessment
*Content Area:* Pharmacology

*Reference*
Hodgson, B., & Kizior, R. (2001). *Saunders Nursing drug handbook 2001.* Philadelphia: W.B. Saunders, pp. 293-295.

**362.** As the nurse brings the 10 AM doses of furosemide (Lasix) and nifedipine (Procardia) into the room of an assigned client, the client asks the nurse for a dose of aluminum hydroxide (Amphojel), which is ordered on a PRN basis for dyspepsia. Which of the following actions by the nurse would be best?

1  Administer all three medications at the same time
2  Ask the client if it is possible to wait 1 hour for the aluminum hydroxide
3  Administer the nifedipine and aluminum hydroxide, and the furosemide in 1 hour
4  Administer the furosemide and aluminum hydroxide, and the nifedipine in 1 hour

**Answer: 2**
*Rationale:* Antacids such as aluminum hydroxide often interfere with the absorption of other medications. For this reason, antacids should be separated from other medications by at least 1 hour. Because of the diuretic action of the furosemide and the antihypertensive action of the nifedipine, it is more important to administer them on time if the client can tolerate waiting for the aluminum hydroxide.

*Test-Taking Strategy:* Use the process of elimination. Recalling that antacids interfere with absorption of other medications will assist in eliminating option 1. From the remaining options, knowledge that the diuretic and antihypertensive medication should be administered on time will assist in directing you to option 2. Review these medications if you had difficulty with this question.

*Level of Cognitive Ability:* Application
*Client Needs:* Physiological Integrity
*Integrated Concept/Process:* Nursing Process/Implementation
*Content Area:* Pharmacology

*Reference*
Hodgson, B., & Kizior, R. (2001). *Saunders Nursing drug handbook 2001.* Philadelphia: W.B. Saunders, p. 34.

**363.** A client has been placed on medication therapy with amitriptyline (Elavil). The nurse monitors the client for which common side effect of this medication?

  1   Drowsiness and fatigue
  2   Diarrhea
  3   Hypertension
  4   Polyuria

**Answer: 1**

*Rationale:* Common side effects of amitriptyline (a tricyclic antidepressant) include the central nervous system effects of drowsiness, fatigue, lethargy, and sedation. Other common side effects include dry mouth or eyes, blurred vision, hypotension, and constipation. The nurse monitors the client for these side effects.

*Test-Taking Strategy:* Use the process of elimination. Recalling that this medication is an antidepressant will direct you to option 1. Review this medication if you had difficulty with this question.

*Level of Cognitive Ability:* Application
*Client Needs:* Physiological Integrity
*Integrated Concept/Process:* Nursing Process/Assessment
*Content Area:* Pharmacology

*Reference*
Hodgson, B., & Kizior, R. (2001). *Saunders Nursing drug handbook 2001.* Philadelphia: W.B. Saunders, pp. 49-51.

**364.** A client has been admitted to the mental health unit on a voluntary basis. The client has reported a history of depression over the past 5 years. Which of the following questions by the nurse would elicit the most thorough assessment data regarding the recent sleeping patterns of the client?

  1   "Have you been having trouble sleeping at home?"
  2   "How did you sleep last night?"
  3   "Tell me about your sleeping patterns."
  4   "You look as if you could use some sleep."

**Answer: 3**

*Rationale:* Option 3 is an open-ended question and provides the client the opportunity to express thoughts and feelings. Option 1 could lead to a one-word answer that would not provide thorough assessment data. One night of sleep may not tell the nurse how the pattern has been over time. Anyone may or may not sleep well for one night, and that sleep or loss of sleep does not indicate a problem. Option 4 could be interpreted by the depressed person as a negative statement and could block communication needed for a thorough assessment.

*Test-Taking Strategy:* Use therapeutic communication techniques. Select the option that allows the client to take the lead in the conversation. This will direct you to option 3. Review therapeutic communication techniques if you had difficulty with this question.

*Level of Cognitive Ability:* Application
*Client Needs:* Physiological Integrity
*Integrated Concept/Process:* Nursing Process/Assessment
*Content Area:* Mental Health

*Reference*
Stuart, G.W., & Laraia, M.T. (1998). *Principles and practice of psychiatric nursing.* (6th ed.). St. Louis: Mosby, p. 34.

**365.** A client is admitted to the emergency department with drug-induced anxiety related to overingestion of a prescribed antipsychotic medication. The most important piece of information the nurse should obtain initially is the:

1 The name of the nearest relative and his or her phone number
2 The reason for the suicide attempt and if the client will attempt suicide again
3 The length of time on the medication
4 The name of the ingested medication and the amount ingested

**Answer: 4**

*Rationale:* In an emergency, lifesaving facts are obtained first. The name of and the amount of medication ingested are of utmost importance in treating this potentially life-threatening situation. The relatives and the reason for the suicide attempt are not the most important initial assessment. The length of time on the medication is also not the priority in this situation.

*Test-Taking Strategy:* Use the process of elimination. Note the key words *initially* and *overingestion*. Lifesaving treatment cannot begin until the medication and amount are identified. Review care of a client with a drug overdose if you had difficulty with this question.

*Level of Cognitive Ability:* Application
*Client Needs:* Physiological Integrity
*Integrated Concept/Process:* Nursing Process/Assessment
*Content Area:* Mental Health

*Reference*
Stuart, G.W., & Laraia, M.T. (1998). *Principles and practice of psychiatric nursing.* (6th ed.). St. Louis: Mosby, p. 389.

**366.** A nurse explains to the mother of a newborn the purpose of giving a vitamin K injection to her newborn. The nurse determines that the mother understands if the mother states that vitamin K is administered because the newborn:

1 Has low hemoglobin blood levels
2 Can't produce vitamin K in the liver
3 Lacks vitamins
4 Lacks intestinal bacteria

**Answer: 4**

*Rationale:* The absence of normal flora needed to synthesize vitamin K in the normal newborn gut results in low levels of vitamin K and creates a transient blood coagulation deficiency between the second and fifth day of life. From a low point at about 2 to 3 days after birth, these coagulation factors rise slowly, but do not approach normal adult levels until 9 months of age or later. Increasing levels of these vitamin K–dependent factors indicate a response to dietary intake and bacterial colonization in the intestines. An injection of vitamin K (Aqua-Mephyton) is administered prophylactically on the day of birth to combat the deficiency. Options 1, 2, and 3 are incorrect.

*Test-Taking Strategy:* Recalling the physiology associated with the synthesis of vitamin K in the newborn will direct you to option 4. Review the purpose of administering vitamin K to the newborn if you had difficulty with this question.

*Level of Cognitive Ability:* Analysis
*Client Needs:* Physiological Integrity
*Integrated Concept/Process:* Teaching/Learning
*Content Area:* Maternity

*Reference*
Lowdermilk, D., Perry, S., & Bobak, I. (2000). *Maternity & women's health care* (7th ed.). St. Louis: Mosby, p. 725.

**367.** A nurse is assigned to give a child a tepid tub bath to treat hyperthermia. Following the bath, the nurse plans to:
1. Place the child in bed and cover the child with a blanket
2. Leave the child uncovered for 15 minutes
3. Assist the child to put on a cotton sleep shirt
4. Take the child's axillary temperature in 2 hours

**Answer: 3**
*Rationale:* Cotton is a lightweight material that will protect the child from becoming chilled after the bath. Option 1 is incorrect because a blanket is heavy and may increase the child's body temperature and further increase metabolism. Option 2 is incorrect because the child should not be left uncovered. Option 4 is incorrect because the child's temperature should be reassessed in ½ hour after the bath.

*Test-Taking Strategy:* Use the process of elimination, focusing on the issue: to treat hyperthermia. Eliminate option 1 because of the word *blanket.* Eliminate option 2 because of the word *uncovered.* Eliminate option 4 because of the time frame. If you had difficulty with this question, review care of a child with hyperthermia.

*Level of Cognitive Ability:* Application
*Client Needs:* Physiological Integrity
*Integrated Concept/Process:* Nursing Process/Planning
*Content Area:* Child Health

*Reference*
Wong, D. (1999). *Whaley & Wong's Nursing care of infants and children* (6th ed.). St. Louis: Mosby, p. 1241.

**368.** A nurse is caring for an infant who has diarrhea. The nurse monitors the infant for which early signs of dehydration?
1. Apical pulse rate of 200 beats/min
2. Capillary refill of 4 seconds
3. Gray, mottled skin
4. Cool extremities

**Answer: 1**
*Rationale:* Dehydration causes interstitial fluid to shift to the vascular compartment in an attempt to maintain fluid volume. When the body is unable to compensate for fluid lost, circulatory failure occurs. The blood pressure will decrease, and the pulse rate will increase. This will be followed by peripheral symptoms. Options 2, 3, and 4 are incorrect, and these assessment findings reflect diminished peripheral circulation.

*Test-Taking Strategy:* Use the process of elimination, thinking about the physiology that occurs in dehydration. Also, note that options 2, 3, and 4 are similar and relate directly to circulatory status. If you had difficulty with this question, review the signs of dehydration.

*Level of Cognitive Ability:* Analysis
*Client Needs:* Physiological Integrity
*Integrated Concept/Process:* Nursing Process/Assessment
*Content Area:* Child Health

*Reference*
Wong, D. (1999). *Whaley & Wong's Nursing care of infants and children* (6th ed.). St. Louis: Mosby, p. 1286.

**369.** Acetylsalicylic acid (aspirin) is prescribed for a client with coronary artery disease before a percutaneous transluminal coronary angioplasty (PTCA). The nurse administers the medication knowing that it is prescribed to:
1 Prevent postprocedure hyperthermia
2 Relieve postprocedure pain
3 Prevent thrombus formation
4 Prevent inflammation of the puncture site

**Answer: 3**
*Rationale:* Before PTCA, the client is usually given an anticoagulant, commonly aspirin, to help reduce the risk of occlusion of the artery during the procedure. Options 1, 2, and 4 are unrelated to the purpose of administering aspirin to this client.

*Test-Taking Strategy:* Use the process of elimination. Think about the potential complications of a PTCA and the action and properties of aspirin to direct you to option 3. If you had difficulty with this question, review the action and uses of aspirin and the complications associated with PTCA.

*Level of Cognitive Ability:* Application
*Client Needs:* Physiological Integrity
*Integrated Concept/Process:* Nursing Process/Implementation
*Content Area:* Adult Health/Cardiovascular

*Reference*
Hodgson, B., & Kizior, R. (2001). *Saunders Nursing drug handbook 2001.* Philadelphia: W.B. Saunders, pp. 75-77.

**370.** A nurse reviews a physician's orders and notes that a topical nitrate is prescribed. The nurse notes that acetaminophen (Tylenol) is also prescribed to be administered before the nitrate. The nurse plans to implement the order knowing that the acetaminophen is prescribed because:
1 Headache is a common side effect of nitrates
2 It potentiates the therapeutic effects of nitrates
3 It does not interfere with platelet action as acetylsalicylic acid (aspirin) does
4 Fever usually accompanies myocardial infarction

**Answer: 1**
*Rationale:* Headache occurs as a side effect of nitrates in many clients. Tylenol may be administered before nitrates to prevent headaches or minimize the discomfort from the headaches. Options 2, 3, and 4 are incorrect.

*Test-Taking Strategy:* Use the process of elimination and focus on the issue. Recall that headache is a common side effect of nitrates. Eliminate option 2 first because this is an incorrect statement. Whereas options 3 and 4 are true statements, they do not address the issue of the question. If you had difficulty with this question, review the side effects of nitrates and the purpose of administering acetaminophen before these medications.

*Level of Cognitive Ability:* Application
*Client Needs:* Physiological Integrity
*Integrated Concept/Process:* Nursing Process/Planning
*Content Area:* Pharmacology

*Reference*
Smeltzer, S., & Bare, B. (2000). *Brunner & Suddarth's Textbook of medical-surgical nursing* (9th ed.). Philadelphia: Lippincott Williams & Wilkins, p. 599.

**371.** A nurse develops a plan of care for a client admitted to the hospital with a diagnosis of an acute myocardial infarction (MI). The priority nursing diagnosis in the acute phase would be:
1 Anxiety
2 Altered family processes
3 Altered comfort
4 Impaired tissue integrity

**Answer: 3**
*Rationale:* Pain is the prevailing symptom of acute MI. Relief of pain is a priority. Pain stimulates the autonomic nervous system, increasing myocardial oxygen demand. Although options 1, 2, and 4 are also appropriate nursing diagnoses, the presence of pain has an impact on these additional nursing diagnoses.

*Test-Taking Strategy:* Use Maslow's Hierarchy of Needs theory. Physiological needs are the priority; therefore, options 1 and 2 can be eliminated. From the remaining options, focus on the diagnosis and note the key words *acute phase*. Comfort is the priority over tissue integrity. Review care of a client with an MI if you had difficulty with this question.

*Level of Cognitive Ability:* Analysis
*Client Needs:* Physiological Integrity
*Integrated Concept/Process:* Nursing Process/Analysis
*Content Area:* Adult Health/Cardiovascular

**Reference**
Smeltzer, S., & Bare, B. (2000). *Brunner & Suddarth's Textbook of medical-surgical nursing* (9th ed.). Philadelphia: Lippincott Williams & Wilkins, p. 619.

---

**372.** A nurse is caring for a male client with a diagnosis of urolithiasis. The nurse instructs the client that it is most important to:

1 Turn, cough and deep breathe every 2 hours
2 Restrict physical activities
3 Strain all urine from each voiding
4 Record weight every day

**Answer: 3**
*Rationale:* Obstruction of the urinary tract is the primary problem associated with urolithiasis. Stones recovered from straining urine can be analyzed and can provide direction for prevention of further stone formation. Activities should not be restricted. Option 1 and 4 are not specifically related to the client's diagnosis.

*Test-Taking Strategy:* Focus on the client's diagnosis. Recalling that urolithiasis relates to urinary tract stones will direct you to option 3. Review care of a client with urolithiasis if you had difficulty with this question.

*Level of Cognitive Ability:* Application
*Client Needs:* Physiological Integrity
*Integrated Concept/Process:* Teaching/Learning
*Content Area:* Adult Health/Renal

**Reference**
Smeltzer, S., & Bare, B. (2000). *Brunner & Suddarth's Textbook of medical-surgical nursing* (9th ed.). Philadelphia: Lippincott Williams & Wilkins, p. 1163.

---

**373.** A nurse is caring for a newly delivered breastfeeding infant. Which intervention performed by the nurse would best prevent jaundice in this infant?

1 Encouraging the mother to offer a formula supplement after each breastfeeding session
2 Keeping the infant NPO until the second period of reactivity
3 Placing the infant under phototherapy
4 Encouraging the mother to breastfeed the infant every 2 to 3 hours

**Answer: 4**
*Rationale:* To help prevent jaundice, the mother should feed the infant frequently in the immediate birth period because colostrum is a natural laxative and helps promote the passage of meconium. Offering the infant a formula supplement will cause nipple confusion and decrease the amount of milk produced by the mother. Breastfeeding should begin as soon as possible after birth while the infant is in the first period of reactivity. Delaying breastfeeding decreases the production of prolactin, which decreases the mother's milk production. Phototherapy requires a physician's order and is not implemented until bilirubin levels are 12 mg/dL or higher in the healthy term infant.

*Test-Taking Strategy:* Use the process of elimination. Recalling the physiology associated with jaundice and noting the key words *best prevent* will assist in eliminating options 2 and 3. From the remaining options, select option 4 because option 1 will cause nipple confusion. Review the interventions to prevent jaundice if you had difficulty with this question.

*Level of Cognitive Ability:* Application
*Client Needs:* Physiological Integrity
*Integrated Concept/Process:* Nursing Process/Implementation
*Content Area:* Maternity

**Reference**
Lowdermilk, D., Perry, S., & Bobak, I. (2000). *Maternity & women's health care* (7th ed.). St. Louis: Mosby, p. 773.

---

**374.** A nurse is caring for a client scheduled for an arthroscopy. The nurse develops a postoperative plan of care and includes which priority nursing action in the plan?
1    Monitor intake and output
2    Monitor the area for numbness or tingling
3    Assess the complete blood cell count results
4    Assess the tissue at the surgical site

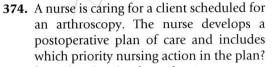
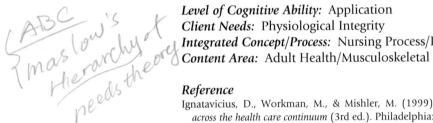

**Answer: 2**
*Rationale:* The priority nursing action is to monitor the affected area for numbness or tingling. Options 1, 3, and 4 are also a component of postoperative care but, from the options presented, are not the priority.

*Test-Taking Strategy:* Use the ABCs (airway, breathing, and circulation) to answer the question. Option 2 relates to circulation. If you had difficulty with this question, review nursing care following arthroscopy.

*Level of Cognitive Ability:* Application
*Client Needs:* Physiological Integrity
*Integrated Concept/Process:* Nursing Process/Planning
*Content Area:* Adult Health/Musculoskeletal

**Reference**
Ignatavicius, D., Workman, M., & Mishler, M. (1999). *Medical-surgical nursing across the health care continuum* (3rd ed.). Philadelphia: W.B. Saunders, p. 1240.

---

**375.** A nurse is caring for a client with active tuberculosis who has started medication therapy that includes rifampin (Rifadin). The nurse instructs the client to expect which side effect of this medication?
1    Orange secretions
2    Bilious urine
3    Yellow sclera
4    Clay-colored stools

**Answer: 1**
*Rationale:* Secretions will become orange as a result of the rifampin. The client should be instructed that this side effect will be likely to occur and should be told that soft contact lenses, if used by the client, will become permanently discolored. Options 2, 3, and 4 are not expected effects.

*Test-Taking Strategy:* Use the process of elimination and knowledge of the side effects of rifampin to answer this question. Eliminate options 2, 3, and 4 because they are similar in that they are all symptoms of intrahepatic obstruction as seen in viral hepatitis. If you had difficulty with this question, review the side effects of this medication.

*Level of Cognitive Ability:* Application
*Client Needs:* Physiological Integrity
*Integrated Concept/Process:* Teaching/Learning
*Content Area:* Adult Health/Respiratory

**Reference**
Hodgson, B., & Kizior, R. (2001). *Saunders Nursing drug handbook 2001.* Philadelphia: W.B. Saunders, pp. 904-905.

**376.** A nurse sends a sputum specimen to the laboratory for culture from a client with suspected active tuberculosis (TB). The results report that *Mycobacterium tuberculosis* is cultured. The nurse analyzes these results as:

1   Positive for active tuberculosis
2   Inconclusive until a repeat sputum is sent
3   Not reliable unless the client has also had a positive Mantoux test result
4   Positive for a less virulent strain of tuberculosis

**Answer: 1**
*Rationale:* Culture of *Mycobacterium tuberculosis* from sputum or other body secretions or tissue is the only method of confirming the diagnosis. Options 2 and 4 are incorrect statements. The Mantoux test is performed to assist in diagnosing TB but does not confirm active disease.

*Test-Taking Strategy:* Use the process of elimination. Recall that culture of the bacteria from sputum confirms the diagnosis. Since tuberculosis affects the respiratory system, it would make sense that the bacteria would be found in the sputum if the client had active disease, therefore confirming the diagnosis. If you had difficulty with this question, review the diagnostic tests associated with active TB.

*Level of Cognitive Ability:* Analysis
*Client Needs:* Physiological Integrity
*Integrated Concept/Process:* Nursing Process/Analysis
*Content Area:* Adult Health/Respiratory

*Reference*
Ignatavicius, D., Workman, M., & Mishler, M. (1999). *Medical-surgical nursing across the health care continuum* (3rd ed.). Philadelphia: W.B. Saunders, p. 676.

**377.** A coronary care unit (CCU) nurse is caring for a client admitted with acute myocardial infarction (MI). The nurse monitors for which most common complication of MI?

1   Cardiogenic shock
2   Cardiac dysrhythmias
3   Congestive heart failure (CHF)
4   Recurrent myocardial infarction

**Answer: 2**
*Rationale:* Dysrhythmias are the most common complication and cause of death after an MI. Cardiogenic shock, CHF, and recurrent MI are also complications but occur less frequently.

*Test-Taking Strategy:* Use the process of elimination. Noting the key words *most common* and knowledge of the complications of MI will direct you to option 2. Review these complications if you had difficulty with this question.

*Level of Cognitive Ability:* Application
*Client Needs:* Physiological Integrity
*Integrated Concept/Process:* Nursing Process/Implementation
*Content Area:* Adult Health/Cardiovascular

*Reference*
Ignatavicius, D., Workman, M., & Mishler, M. (1999). *Medical-surgical nursing across the health care continuum* (3rd ed.). Philadelphia: W.B. Saunders, p. 910.

**378.** A nurse in the newborn nursery is planning for the admission of a large for gestational age (LGA) infant. In preparing to care for this infant, the nurse obtains equipment to perform which diagnostic test?

1   Indirect and direct bilirubin levels
2   Rh and ABO blood typing
3   Heelstick blood glucose
4   Serum insulin level

**Answer: 3**
*Rationale:* After birth, the most common problem in an LGA infant is hypoglycemia, especially if the mother is diabetic. At delivery, when the umbilical cord is clamped and cut, the maternal blood glucose supply is lost. The newborn continues to produce large amounts of insulin, which depletes the infant's blood glucose within the first hours after birth. If immediate identification and treatment of hypoglycemia are not performed, the newborn may suffer central nervous system damage as a result of inadequate circulation of glucose to the brain. Indirect and direct bilirubin levels are usually ordered after the first 24 hours, since jaundice is usually seen at 48 to 72 hours after birth. There is

no rationale for ordering an Rh and ABO blood type, unless the maternal blood is Rh negative. Serum insulin levels are not helpful, since there is no intervention to decrease these levels to prevent hypoglycemia.

*Test-Taking Strategy:* Focus on the issue: an LGA infant. Recalling that hypoglycemia is the concern will direct you to option 3. Review care of the LGA infant if you had difficulty with this question.

*Level of Cognitive Ability:* Application
*Client Needs:* Physiological Integrity
*Integrated Concept/Process:* Nursing Process/Planning
*Content Area:* Maternity

*Reference*
Lowdermilk, D., Perry, S., & Bobak, I. (2000). *Maternity & women's health care* (7th ed.). St. Louis: Mosby, p. 1127.

---

**379.** A nurse is caring for a 30 weeks' gestation client in preterm labor. The physician orders betamethasone (Celestone) intramuscularly. The client asks the nurse why she is receiving corticosteroids. The nurse tells the client that the betamethasone will:
1   Help the baby's lungs mature faster
2   Prevent the membranes from rupturing
3   Decrease the incidence of fetal infection
4   Help stop the labor contractions

**Answer: 1**
*Rationale:* Respiratory distress syndrome (RDS) is the most common cause of morbidity and mortality in preterm infants. Betamethasone, a corticosteroid, is administered to enhance fetal lung maturity in 24- to 34-week gestations. The medication's optimal benefits begin 24 hours after initial therapy. Betamethasone does not prevent rupture of the membranes. Betamethasone does not decrease the incidence of fetal infection and can mask signs of infection when the client has premature rupture of the membranes with preterm labor. Even though betamethasone may be given during the time that tocolytic agents are administered, it does not inhibit preterm labor.

*Test-Taking Strategy:* Use the process of elimination, recalling that betamethasone is a corticosteroid. Noting the key word *preterm* may assist you in recalling that this medication is administered to enhance fetal lung maturity. Review the action of this medication if you had difficulty with this question.

*Level of Cognitive Ability:* Application
*Client Needs:* Physiological Integrity
*Integrated Concept/Process:* Nursing Process/Implementation
*Content Area:* Maternity

*Reference*
Lowdermilk, D., Perry, S., & Bobak, I. (2000). *Maternity & women's health care* (7th ed.). St. Louis: Mosby, p. 975.

**380.** In a client receiving total parenteral nutrition (TPN), chest pain, dyspnea, tachycardia, cyanosis, and decreased level of consciousness suddenly develop. The nurse suspects which complication of TPN?
1    Hyperglycemia
2    Catheter-related sepsis
3    Allergic reaction to the TPN catheter
4    Air embolism

**Answer: 4**
*Rationale:* Symptoms of air embolism include decreased level of consciousness, tachycardia, dyspnea, anxiety, feelings of impending doom, chest pain, cyanosis, and hypotension. Options 1, 2, and 3 are unrelated to the symptoms identified in the question.

*Test-Taking Strategy:* Use the process of elimination. Focus on the symptoms in the question to direct you to option 4. Review the signs of air embolism if you had difficulty with this question.

*Level of Cognitive Ability:* Analysis
*Client Needs:* Physiological Integrity
*Integrated Concept/Process:* Nursing Process/Analysis
*Content Area:* Fundamental Skills

*Reference*
Smeltzer, S., & Bare, B. (2000). *Brunner & Suddarth's Textbook of medical-surgical nursing* (9th ed.). Philadelphia: Lippincott Williams & Wilkins, p. 849.

---

**381.** A client has a nursing diagnosis of Fluid Volume Excess. After assessing the client, the nurse records which assessment data in the medical record that support continued use of this nursing diagnosis?
1    Bibasilar crackles
2    Weak pulse
3    Decreased blood pressure
4    Flat neck veins with the head of the bed at 45 degrees

**Answer: 1**
*Rationale:* Signs of fluid volume excess include bounding pulse, elevated blood pressure, crackles or other adventitious breath sounds, edema of the sacrum or lower extremities, and neck vein distention with the head of the bed positioned at a 45-degree angle. Other signs may include peripheral veins that do not flatten when raised above the head for 3 to 5 seconds and changes in level of consciousness if fluid shifts are occurring.

*Test-Taking Strategy:* Focus on the issue: fluid volume excess. Note the key words in the question, *support continued use.* This tells you that the correct option will be consistent with fluid volume excess. Use basic nursing knowledge of the effects of volume on the cardiovascular and respiratory systems to eliminate options 2, 3, and 4. Review the signs of fluid volume excess if you had difficulty with this question.

*Level of Cognitive Ability:* Application
*Client Needs:* Physiological Integrity
*Integrated Concept/Process:* Communication and Documentation
*Content Area:* Adult Health/Cardiovascular

*Reference*
Smeltzer, S., & Bare, B. (2000). *Brunner & Suddarth's Textbook of medical-surgical nursing* (9th ed.). Philadelphia: Lippincott Williams & Wilkins, p. 210.

**382.** A client is experiencing acute cardiac and cerebral symptoms related to fluid volume excess. The nurse implements which of the following measures to increase the client's comfort until specific therapy is ordered by the physician?

1   Administers oxygen at 4 liters per minute by nasal cannula
2   Elevates the client's head to at least 45 degrees
3   Measures urine output on an hourly basis
4   Measures intravenous and oral fluid intake

**Answer: 2**

*Rationale:* Elevating the head of the bed to 45 degrees decreases venous return to the heart from the lower body, thus reducing the volume of blood that has to be pumped. It also promotes venous drainage from the brain, reducing cerebral symptoms. Oxygen is a medication and is not administered without an order. Intake and output should be monitored and recorded to provide current information about the client's volume status. Options 1, 3, and 4 are important measures, although they do not improve the client's comfort.

*Test-Taking Strategy:* Use the process of elimination, focusing on the issue "increase the client's comfort." This tells you that the correct option is one that directly involves care delivery to the client. With this in mind, eliminate options 3 and 4, since they are assessment measures and will not improve the condition of the client. From the remaining options, note that option 2 identifies the nursing measure. Review care of a client with fluid volume excess if you had difficulty with this question.

*Level of Cognitive Ability:* Application
*Client Needs:* Physiological Integrity
*Integrated Concept/Process:* Nursing Process/Implementation
*Content Area:* Adult Health/Cardiovascular

*Reference*
Smeltzer, S., & Bare, B. (2000). *Brunner & Suddarth's Textbook of medical-surgical nursing* (9th ed.). Philadelphia: Lippincott Williams & Wilkins, p. 210.

---

**383.** A nurse notes that a client's urinalysis report contains a notation of positive red blood cells (RBCs). The nurse interprets that this finding is unrelated to which of the following items that is part of the client's clinical picture?

1   Diabetes mellitus
2   Concurrent anticoagulant therapy
3   History of kidney stones
4   History of recent blow to the right flank

**Answer: 1**

*Rationale:* Hematuria can be caused by trauma to the kidney, such as with blunt trauma to the lower posterior trunk or flank. Kidney stones can cause hematuria as they scrape the endothelial lining of the urinary system. Anticoagulant therapy can cause hematuria as a side effect. Diabetes mellitus does not cause hematuria, although it can lead to renal failure from prerenal causes.

*Test-Taking Strategy:* Use the process of elimination, noting the key word *unrelated*. Eliminate options 2 and 4, which are most likely to cause RBCs in the urine. From the remaining options, recalling that the scraping of the stones against mucosa could cause minor trauma and bleeding will assist to eliminate this option as well. Thus, diabetes mellitus is the item unrelated to positive RBCs in the urine. Review these causes if you had difficulty with this question.

*Level of Cognitive Ability:* Analysis
*Client Needs:* Physiological Integrity
*Integrated Concept/Process:* Nursing Process/Analysis
*Content Area:* Adult Health/Renal

*Reference*
Smeltzer, S., & Bare, B. (2000). *Brunner & Suddarth's Textbook of medical-surgical nursing* (9th ed.). Philadelphia: Lippincott Williams & Wilkins, p. 1022.

**384.** A nurse has an order to ambulate a client with a nephrostomy tube in the hall four times a day. The nurse determines that the safest way to accomplish this while maintaining the integrity of the nephrostomy tube is to:
1 Tie the drainage bag to the client's waist while ambulating
2 Hang the drainage bag from a walker while the client is ambulating
3 Tell the client to hold the drainage bag higher than the level of the bladder
4 Change the drainage bag to a leg collection bag

**Answer: 4**
*Rationale:* The safest approach to protect the integrity and safety of the nephrostomy tube with a mobile client is to attach the tube to a leg collection bag. This allows for greater freedom of movement, while preventing accidental disconnection or dislodgment. The drainage bag is kept below the level of the bladder. Option 2 presents the risk of tension or pulling on the nephrostomy tube by the client during ambulation.

*Test-Taking Strategy:* Use the process of elimination. Note that options 1, 2, and 3 are similar because they all indicate placing the drainage bag above the level of the bladder. Review care of a client with a nephrostomy tube if you had difficulty with this question.

*Level of Cognitive Ability:* Analysis
*Client Needs:* Physiological Integrity
*Integrated Concept/Process:* Nursing Process/Analysis
*Content Area:* Adult Health/Renal

*Reference*
Smeltzer, S., & Bare, B. (2000). *Brunner & Suddarth's Textbook of medical-surgical nursing* (9th ed.). Philadelphia: Lippincott Williams & Wilkins, p. 1126.

---

**385.** A client with newly diagnosed polycystic kidney disease has just finished speaking with the physician about the disorder. The client asks the nurse to explain again what the most serious complication of the disorder might be. In formulating a response, the nurse incorporates the understanding that the most serious complication is:
1 Diabetes insipidus
2 Syndrome of inappropriate antidiuretic hormone (ADH) secretion
3 End stage renal disease (ESRD)
4 Chronic urinary tract infection (UTI)

**Answer: 3**
*Rationale:* The most serious complication of polycystic kidney disease is ESRD, which would be managed with dialysis or transplant. There is no reliable way to predict who will ultimately progress to ESRD. Chronic UTIs are the most common complication because of the altered anatomy of the kidney and from development of resistant strains of bacteria. Diabetes insipidus and syndrome of inappropriate ADH secretion are unrelated disorders.

*Test-Taking Strategy:* Use the process of elimination, noting the key words *most serious*. Eliminate options 1 and 2 because these imbalances are usually temporary and are amenable to treatment. From the remaining options, focusing on the key words will direct you to option 3. Also recalling that ESRD is life threatening and requires dialysis for treatment will direct you to the correct option. Review the complications of polycystic kidney disease if you had difficulty with this question.

*Level of Cognitive Ability:* Application
*Client Needs:* Physiological Integrity
*Integrated Concept/Process:* Nursing Process/Implementation
*Content Area:* Adult Health/Renal

*Reference*
Ignatavicius, D., Workman, M., & Mishler, M. (1999). *Medical-surgical nursing across the health care continuum* (3rd ed.). Philadelphia: W.B. Saunders, p. 1857.

**386.** A nurse is assigned to care for a client who has returned to the nursing unit following left nephrectomy. The nurse places highest priority on obtaining which of the following assessments?
1  Tolerance for sips of clear liquids
2  Temperature
3  Hourly urine output
4  Ability to turn side to side

**Answer: 3**
*Rationale:* Following nephrectomy, it is imperative to measure the urine output on an hourly basis. This is done to monitor the effectiveness of the remaining kidney and to detect renal failure early, if it should occur. The client may also experience significant pain after this surgery, which could affect the client's ability to reposition, cough, and deep breathe. Therefore the next most important measurements are vital signs (including temperature), pain level, and bed mobility. Clear liquids are not given until the client has bowel sounds.

*Test-Taking Strategy:* Use the process of elimination, noting the key words *highest priority*. Note the relationship between *nephrectomy* in the question and *urine output* in the correct option. Review care of a client following nephrectomy if you had difficulty with this question.

*Level of Cognitive Ability:* Application
*Client Needs:* Physiological Integrity
*Integrated Concept/Process:* Nursing Process/Assessment
*Content Area:* Adult Health/Renal

*Reference*
Ignatavicius, D., Workman, M., & Mishler, M. (1999). *Medical-surgical nursing across the health care continuum* (3rd ed.). Philadelphia: W.B. Saunders, p. 1873.

**387.** A client with a history of respiratory disease is ambulating with the nurse to the doorway of the hospital room. The client becomes pale and dyspneic. The nurse has the client sit down and takes the client's vital signs. The respiratory rate is 32 breaths/min, oxygen saturation is 90%, and the heart rate has increased from 76 to 98 beats/min. The nurse interprets that this client is experiencing:
1  Impaired Physical Mobility
2  Activity Intolerance
3  Ineffective Breathing Pattern
4  Ineffective Airway Clearance

**Answer: 2**
*Rationale:* Activity Intolerance is characterized by exertional dyspnea, adverse changes in blood pressure or heart rate with activity, and fatigue. Ineffective Breathing Pattern occurs when the rate, timing, depth, or rhythm of breathing is insufficient to maintain optimal ventilation. Ineffective Airway Clearance occurs when the client is unable to clear own secretions from the airway. Impaired Physical Mobility occurs when the client is limited in physical movement and has limited muscle strength, range of motion, or coordination.

*Test-Taking Strategy:* Use the process of elimination and focus on the data in the question. The question does not mention information about the pattern of breathing or secretions, so eliminate options 3 and 4 first. From the remaining options, noting that the item triggering the dyspnea is ambulation guides you to select Activity Intolerance over Impaired Physical Mobility. Review the characteristics of Activity Intolerance if you had difficulty with this question.

*Level of Cognitive Ability:* Analysis
*Client Needs:* Physiological Integrity
*Integrated Concept/Process:* Nursing Process/Analysis
*Content Area:* Adult Health/Respiratory

*Reference*
Johnson, M., Bulechek, G., Dochterman, J., Maas, M., Moorhead, S. (2001). *Nursing diagnoses, outcomes, and interventions.* St. Louis: Mosby, p. 41.

**388.** A client with cancer is receiving cisplatin (Platinol). On assessment of the client, which of the following findings indicates that the client is having an adverse reaction to the medication?
1 Excessive urination
2 Tinnitus
3 Increased appetite
4 Yellow halos in front of the eyes

**Answer: 2**
*Rationale:* An adverse reaction related to the administration of cisplatin, an antineoplastic medication, is ototoxicity with hearing loss. The nurse should assess for this adverse reaction when administering this medication. Options 1, 3, and 4 are not adverse reactions to this medication.

*Test-Taking Strategy:* Use the process of elimination. Recalling that ototoxicity is an adverse effect will direct you to option 2. Review the effects of this medication and the nursing responsibilities during its administration if you had difficulty with this question.

*Level of Cognitive Ability:* Analysis
*Client Needs:* Physiological Integrity
*Integrated Concept/Process:* Nursing Process/Assessment
*Content Area:* Pharmacology

*Reference*
Hodgson, B., & Kizior, R. (2001). *Saunders Nursing drug handbook 2001.* Philadelphia: W.B. Saunders, p. 226.

**389.** A nurse is caring for a client in whom psychomotor retarded depression has been diagnosed. In this condition the nurse would expect to note which of the following behaviors in the client?
1 Standing without moving, as if a statue, for long periods of time
2 Slowed walking and talking
3 Verbalization of increasingly angry feelings
4 Rapid pacing back and forth

**Answer: 2**
*Rationale:* Slowness in walking and talking is a characteristic behavior of a psychomotor retarded depression. The physical symptoms may be explained by the person's pessimistic view of the future, leading to the psychomotor inhibition or vegetative signs typically seen with depressed clients. Options 3 and 4 may occur in any agitated state. Option 1 is behavior more likely seen in schizophrenia.

*Test-Taking Strategy:* Use the process of elimination. The words *psychomotor retarded depression* should assist in eliminating options 3 and 4. From the remaining options, recalling that option 1 is most likely seen in the client with schizophrenia will direct you to option 2. Review the characteristics of this disorder if you had difficulty with this question.

*Level of Cognitive Ability:* Analysis
*Client Needs:* Physiological Integrity
*Integrated Concept/Process:* Nursing Process/Assessment
*Content Area:* Mental Health

*Reference*
Varcarolis, E. (1998). *Foundations of psychiatric mental health nursing* (3rd ed.). Philadelphia: W.B. Saunders, p. 558.

**390.** It has been 12 hours since a client's delivery of a newborn. A nurse assesses the mother for the process of involution and documents that it is progressing normally when palpation of the client's fundus is noted:

1 At the level of the umbilicus
2 Midway between the umbilicus and the symphysis pubis
3 1 fingerbreadth below the umbilicus
4 2 fingerbreadths below the umbilicus

**Answer: 1**

*Rationale:* The term "involution" is used to describe the rapid reduction in size and the return of the uterus to a normal condition similar to its prepregnant state. Immediately following the delivery of the placenta, the uterus contracts to the size of a large grapefruit. The fundus is situated in the midline between the symphysis pubis and the umbilicus. Within 6 to 12 hours after birth, the fundus of the uterus rises to the level of the umbilicus. The top of the fundus remains at the level of the umbilicus for about a day and then descends into the pelvis approximately 1 fingerbreadth on each succeeding day.

*Test-Taking Strategy:* Use the process of elimination. Note the key words *12 hours since the client's delivery*. Attempt to visualize the process of assessment of involution and the expected finding at this time to answer the question. Review this process if you had difficulty with this question.

*Level of Cognitive Ability:* Application
*Client Needs:* Physiological Integrity
*Integrated Concept/Process:* Communication and Documentation
*Content Area:* Maternity

*Reference*
Sherwen, L., Scoloveno, M.A., & Weingarten, C. (1999). *Maternity nursing: Care of the childbearing family* (3rd ed.). Stamford, Conn.: Appleton & Lange, p. 834.

**391.** A client with a gastric tumor is scheduled for a subtotal gastrectomy (Billroth II procedure). The nurse explains the procedure to the client and tells the client that the:

1 Proximal end of the distal stomach is anastomosed to the duodenum
2 Antrum of the stomach is removed with the remaining portion anastomosed to the duodenum
3 Entire stomach is removed and the esophagus is anastomosed to the duodenum
4 Lower portion of the stomach is removed and the remainder is anastomosed to the jejunum

**Answer: 4**

*Rationale:* In the Billroth II procedure, the lower portion of the stomach is removed and the remainder is anastomosed to the jejunum. The duodenal stump is preserved to permit bile flow to the jejunum. Options 1, 2, and 3 are incorrect descriptions.

*Test-Taking Strategy:* Use the process of elimination. The word *gastrectomy* indicates removal of the stomach. This should assist in eliminating option 1. From the remaining options note the word *subtotal*, which indicates "lower and a part of." This should easily direct you to option 4. If you had difficulty with this question, review this surgical procedure.

*Level of Cognitive Ability:* Application
*Client Needs:* Physiological Integrity
*Integrated Concept/Process:* Nursing Process/Implementation
*Content Area:* Adult Health/Gastrointestinal

*Reference*
Smeltzer, S., & Bare, B. (2000). *Brunner & Suddarth's Textbook of medical-surgical nursing* (9th ed.). Philadelphia: Lippincott Williams & Wilkins, p. 864.

**392.** A client with diabetes mellitus receives Humulin Regular insulin 8 units SC at 7:30 AM. The nurse would be most alert to signs of hypoglycemia at what time during the day?

1. 9:30 AM to 11:30 AM
2. 11:30 AM to 1:30 PM
3. 1:30 PM to 3:30 PM
4. 3:30 PM to 5:30 PM

**Answer: 1**

*Rationale:* Humulin Regular insulin is a short-acting insulin. Its onset of action occurs in ½ hour, and the effect peaks in 2 to 4 hours. Its duration of action is 4 to 6 hours. A hypoglycemic reaction will most likely occur at peak time, which in this situation is between 9:30 AM and 11:30 AM.

*Test-Taking Strategy:* Use the process of elimination and knowledge regarding the onset, peak, and duration of action of Regular insulin to answer this question. Recalling that Regular insulin is a short-acting insulin will direct you to option 1. Review both NPH and Regular insulin if you had difficulty with this question.

*Level of Cognitive Ability:* Analysis
*Client Needs:* Physiological Integrity
*Integrated Concept/Process:* Nursing Process/Assessment
*Content Area:* Pharmacology

*Reference*
Hodgson, B., & Kizior, R. (2001). *Saunders Nursing drug handbook 2001.* Philadelphia: W.B. Saunders, p. 530.

**393.** A nurse prepares a postoperative plan of care for a client scheduled for hypophysectomy. The nurse avoids including which of the following in the plan?

1. Mouth care
2. Coughing and deep breathing
3. Monitoring intake and output
4. Daily weights

**Answer: 2**

*Rationale:* Toothbrushing, sneezing, coughing, nose blowing, and bending are activities that should be avoided postoperatively in the client that underwent a hypophysectomy. These activities interfere with the healing of the incision and can disrupt the graft. Options 1, 3, and 4 are appropriate postoperative interventions.

*Test-Taking Strategy:* Note the key word *avoids.* Consider the anatomical location of the surgical procedure. Although coughing and deep breathing are usually a normal component of postoperative care, in this situation coughing is contraindicated. Review care following a hypophysectomy if you had difficulty with this question.

*Level of Cognitive Ability:* Application
*Client Needs:* Physiological Integrity
*Integrated Concept/Process:* Nursing Process/Planning
*Content Area:* Adult Health/Endocrine

*Reference*
Ignatavicius, D., Workman, M., & Mishler, M. (1999). *Medical-surgical nursing across the health care continuum* (3rd ed.). Philadelphia: W.B. Saunders, p. 1594.

**394.** A client undergoes a thyroidectomy. The nurse monitors the client for signs of damage to the parathyroid glands postoperatively. Which of the following findings would indicate damage to the parathyroid glands?
1 Hoarseness
2 Tingling around the mouth
3 Respiratory distress
4 Neck pain

**Answer: 2**
*Rationale:* The parathyroid glands can be damaged or their blood supply impaired during thyroid surgery. Hypocalcemia and tetany result when parathyroid (PTH) levels decrease. The nurse monitors for complaints of tingling around the mouth or of the toes or fingers, and muscular twitching because these are signs of calcium deficiency. Additional later signs of hypocalcemia are positive Chvostek's and Trousseau's signs.

*Test-Taking Strategy:* Use the process of elimination. Recalling that hypocalcemia results when PTH levels decrease will assist in directing you to the correct option. Review postoperative care following thyroidectomy and the signs of parathyroid damage if you had difficulty with this question.

*Level of Cognitive Ability:* Analysis
*Client Needs:* Physiological Integrity
*Integrated Concept/Process:* Nursing Process/Assessment
*Content Area:* Adult Health/Endocrine

*Reference*
Ignatavicius, D., Workman, M., & Mishler, M. (1999). *Medical-surgical nursing across the health care continuum* (3rd ed.). Philadelphia: W.B. Saunders, p. 1619.

**395.** A nurse is caring for a client who is comatose. The nurse notes in the chart that the client is exhibiting decerebrate posturing. Based on this documented finding, the nurse expects to note which of the following?
1 Extension of the extremities after a stimulus
2 Flexion of the extremities after a stimulus
3 Upper extremity flexion with lower extremity extension
4 Upper extremity extension with lower extremity flexion

**Answer: 1**
*Rationale:* Decerebrate posturing, which can occur with upper brainstem injury, is the extension of the extremities after a stimulus. Options 2, 3, and 4 are incorrect descriptions of this type of posturing.

*Test-Taking Strategy:* Use the process of elimination. Remember that decerebrate may also be known as extension. Recalling this concept will direct you to option 1. Review posturing and its relationship to neurological disorders if you had difficulty with this question.

*Level of Cognitive Ability:* Analysis
*Client Needs:* Physiological Integrity
*Integrated Concept/Process:* Nursing Process/Assessment
*Content Area:* Adult Health/Neurological

*Reference*
Ignatavicius, D., Workman, M., & Mishler, M. (1999). *Medical-surgical nursing across the health care continuum* (3rd ed.). Philadelphia: W.B. Saunders, p. 1014.

**396.** A nurse teaches a postpartum client about observation of lochia. The nurse determines the client's understanding when the client says that on the second day postpartum, the lochia should be:
1 Yellow
2 White
3 Pink
4 Red

**Answer: 4**
*Rationale:* The uterus rids itself of the debris that remains after birth through a discharge called lochia, which is classified according to its appearance and contents. Lochia rubra is dark red. It occurs from delivery to 3 days postpartum and contains epithelial cells, erythrocytes, leukocytes, shreds of decidua, and occasionally fetal meconium, lanugo, and vernix caseosa. Lochia serosa is a brownish pink discharge that occurs from days 4 to 10. Lochia alba is a white discharge that occurs from days 10 to 14. Lochia should not be yellow or contain large clots; if it does, the cause should be investigated without delay.

*Test-Taking Strategy:* Use knowledge regarding the characteristics of lochia. Noting the words *second day postpartum* will direct you to option 4. If you had difficulty with this question, review the normal postpartum assessment findings.

*Level of Cognitive Ability:* Analysis
*Client Needs:* Physiological Integrity
*Integrated Concept/Process:* Teaching/Learning
*Content Area:* Maternity

*Reference*
Lowdermilk, D., Perry, S., & Bobak, I. (2000). *Maternity & women's health care* (7th ed.). St. Louis: Mosby, p. 582.

**397.** A nurse is caring for a client with depression who is being treated with a monoamine oxidase inhibitor (MAOI). The nurse who is monitoring the client for hypertensive crisis ensures that which medication is available for administration if a crisis occurs?
1 Metoprolol tartrate (Lopressor)
2 Prazosin hydrochloride (Minipress)
3 Furosemide (Lasix)
4 Phentolamine mesylate (Regitine)

**Answer: 4**
*Rationale:* While all of the medications identified in the options decrease blood pressure, phentolamine acts quickly and is administered intravenously to treat a hypertensive crisis.

*Test-Taking Strategy:* Use the process of elimination and knowledge of the action and use of these medications. Recalling that phentolamine is rapid-acting will direct you to option 4. Review MAOIs and hypertensive crisis if you had difficulty with this question.

*Level of Cognitive Ability:* Application
*Client Needs:* Physiological Integrity
*Integrated Concept/Process:* Nursing Process/Planning
*Content Area:* Pharmacology

*Reference*
Hodgson, B., & Kizior, R. (2001). *Saunders Nursing drug handbook 2001.* Philadelphia: W.B. Saunders, p. 819.

**398.** An infant with a dislocated hip is placed in Bryant's traction. The nurse plans to assess which of the following while the infant is in traction?
1   Skin integrity over the scapulae
2   Pin sites at the tibia
3   Security of the pelvic belt
4   Pressure over the hip joint

**Answer: 1**
*Rationale:* The infant in Bryant's traction is supine with both legs elevated at a 90-degree angle. The buttocks should just clear the mattress. The scapulas, fibulas, shoulders, and Achilles' tendons are pressure points as a result of positioning and skin traction application. There are no pin sites with Bryant's traction. Pelvic traction is the only traction that uses a pelvic belt. No constructive devices are placed over or near the hip joint with Bryant's traction.

*Test-Taking Strategy:* Remembering that Bryant's traction is a continuous skin traction will assist in eliminating options 2 and 3. Visualizing the alignment and infant positioning in this traction will direct you to option 1. Review the purpose and positioning used in Bryant's traction if you had difficulty with this question.

*Level of Cognitive Ability:* Application
*Client Needs:* Physiological Integrity
*Integrated Concept/Process:* Nursing Process/Assessment
*Content Area:* Child Health

**Reference**
Wong, D. (1999). *Whaley & Wong's Nursing care of infants and children* (6th ed.). St. Louis: Mosby, p. 1921.

**399.** A nurse is caring for a client who had a total knee replacement. Postoperatively, which of the following nursing assessments is of highest priority?
1   Bladder distention
2   Homans' sign
3   Extremity shortening
4   Heel breakdown

**Answer: 2**
*Rationale:* Deep vein thrombosis is a potentially serious complication of lower extremity surgery. Checking for a positive Homans' sign assesses for this complication. Although bladder distention, extremity lengthening or shortening, or heel breakdown can occur, these complications are not potentially serious complications.

*Test-Taking Strategy:* Use the ABCs (airway, breathing, and circulation) to answer the question. Assessment for deep vein thrombosis involves circulation. Review postoperative assessment following total knee replacement if you had difficulty with this question.

*Level of Cognitive Ability:* Analysis
*Client Needs:* Physiological Integrity
*Integrated Concept/Process:* Nursing Process/Assessment
*Content Area:* Adult Health/Musculoskeletal

**Reference**
Smeltzer, S., & Bare, B. (2000). *Brunner & Suddarth's Textbook of medical-surgical nursing* (9th ed.). Philadelphia: Lippincott Williams & Wilkins, p. 1793.

**400.** A nurse is assessing a client's cigarette smoking habit. The client admits to smoking ¾ pack per day for the last 10 years. The nurse calculates that the client has a smoking history of how many pack-years?

1 0.75 pack-years

2 7.5 pack-years

3 15 pack-years

4 30 pack-years

**Answer: 2**

*Rationale:* The standard method for quantifying smoking history is to multiply the number of packs smoked per day by the number of years of smoking. The number is recorded as the number of pack-years. The calculation for the number of pack-years for the client who has smoked ¾ pack a day for 10 years is:

0.75 (¾) packs × 10 years = 7.5 pack-years.

*Test-Taking Strategy:* This question tests a fundamental concept related to history taking and smoking. Knowledge regarding how to calculate pack-years is needed to answer this question. Review this calculation if you had difficulty with this question.

*Level of Cognitive Ability:* Application
*Client Needs:* Physiological Integrity
*Integrated Concept/Process:* Nursing Process/Assessment
*Content Area:* Adult Health/Respiratory

*Reference*
Ignatavicius, D., Workman, M., & Mishler, M. (1999). *Medical-surgical nursing across the health care continuum* (3rd ed.). Philadelphia: W.B. Saunders, pp. 594, 644.

---

**401.** A nurse is conducting a health history on a client with hyperparathyroidism. Which of the following questions made to the client would elicit information about this condition?

1 "Have you had problems with diarrhea lately?"

2 "Do you have tremors in your hands?"

3 "Are you experiencing pain in your joints?"

4 "Do you notice swelling in your legs at night?"

**Answer: 3**

*Rationale:* Hyperparathyroidism causes an oversecretion of parathyroid hormone (PTH), which causes excessive osteoblast growth and activity within the bones. When bone reabsorption is increased, calcium is released from the bones into the blood, causing hypercalcemia. The bones suffer demineralization as a result of calcium loss, leading to bone and joint pain and pathological fractures. Options 1 and 2 relate to assessment of hypoparathyroidism. Option 4 is unrelated to hyperparathyroidism.

*Test-Taking Strategy:* Knowledge regarding the pathophysiology associated with hyperparathyroidism is required to answer the question. Eliminate options 1 and 2 first because these options provide information about hypoparathyroidism. From the remaining options, it is necessary to know the relationship between hyperparathyroidism, PTH, and joint pain to direct you to option 3. Review this disorder if you had difficulty with this question.

*Level of Cognitive Ability:* Analysis
*Client Needs:* Physiological Integrity
*Integrated Concept/Process:* Nursing Process/Assessment
*Content Area:* Adult Health/Endocrine

*Reference*
Smeltzer, S., & Bare, B. (2000) *Brunner & Suddarth's Textbook of medical-surgical nursing* (9th ed.). Philadelphia: Lippincott Williams & Wilkins, p. 1052.

**402.** An 18-year-old client seeks medical attention for intermittent episodes in which the fingers of both hands become cold, pale, and numb, followed by redness and swelling and throbbing, achy pain. Raynaud's disease is suspected. The nurse further assesses the client to see if these episodes occur with:

1 Exposure to heat
2 Being in a relaxed environment
3 Prolonged episodes of inactivity
4 Ingestion of coffee or chocolate

**Answer: 4**

*Rationale:* Raynaud's disease is a bilateral form of intermittent arteriolar spasm, which can be classified as obstructive or vasospastic. Episodes are characterized by pallor, cold, numbness, and possible cyanosis of the fingers, followed by erythema, tingling, and aching pain. Attacks are triggered by exposure to cold, nicotine, caffeine, trauma to the fingertips, and stress. Prolonged episodes of inactivity is unrelated to these episodes.

*Test-Taking Strategy:* Use the process of elimination, focusing on the symptoms identified in the question. Recalling that symptoms occur with vasoconstriction will assist in eliminating options 1, 2, and 3 because these events are unlikely to cause vasoconstriction. Review the characteristics associated with Raynaud's disease if you had difficulty with this question.

*Level of Cognitive Ability:* Analysis
*Client Needs:* Physiological Integrity
*Integrated Concept/Process:* Nursing Process/Assessment
*Content Area:* Adult Health/Cardiovascular

*Reference*
Smeltzer, S., & Bare, B. (2000) *Brunner & Suddarth's Textbook of medical-surgical nursing* (9th ed.). Philadelphia: Lippincott Williams & Wilkins, p. 704.

**403.** A client is admitted to the hospital with a diagnosis of pericarditis. A nurse assesses the client for which manifestation that differentiates pericarditis from other cardiopulmonary problems?

1 Chest pain that worsens on inspiration
2 Pericardial friction rub
3 Anterior chest pain
4 Weakness and irritability

**Answer: 2**

*Rationale:* A pericardial friction rub is heard when there is inflammation of the pericardial sac, during the inflammatory phase of pericarditis. Chest pain that worsens on inspiration is characteristic of both pericarditis and pleurisy. Anterior chest pain may be experienced with angina pectoris and myocardial infarction. Weakness and irritability are nonspecific complaints and could accompany a wide variety of disorders.

*Test-Taking Strategy:* Note the key word *differentiates.* This tells you that the correct option will be one that is unique to this health problem and should assist in eliminating options 3 and 4. From the remaining options, note the relationship between pericarditis and pericardial. Review the characteristics associated with pericarditis if you had difficulty with this question.

*Level of Cognitive Ability:* Analysis
*Client Needs:* Physiological Integrity
*Integrated Concept/Process:* Nursing Process/Assessment
*Content Area:* Adult Health/Cardiovascular

*Reference*
Monahan, F., & Neighbors, M. (1998). *Medical-surgical nursing: Foundations for clinical practice* (2nd ed.). Philadelphia: W.B. Saunders, p. 238.

**404.** An ambulatory care nurse is assessing a client with chronic sinusitis. The nurse interprets that which of the following client manifestations is unrelated to this problem?

1. Purulent nasal discharge
2. Chronic cough
3. Headache more pronounced in the evening
4. Anosmia

**Answer: 3**

*Rationale:* Chronic sinusitis is characterized by persistent purulent nasal discharge, a chronic cough caused by nasal discharge, anosmia (loss of smell), nasal stuffiness, and headache that is worse upon arising after sleep.

*Test-Taking Strategy:* Use the process of elimination. Noting the key word *unrelated* and knowledge of the signs and symptoms of sinusitis will direct you to option 3. Review these signs and symptoms if you had difficulty with this question.

*Level of Cognitive Ability:* Analysis
*Client Needs:* Physiological Integrity
*Integrated Concept/Process:* Nursing Process/Assessment
*Content Area:* Adult Health/Respiratory

*Reference*
Monahan, F., & Neighbors, M. (1998). *Medical-surgical nursing: Foundations for clinical practice* (2nd ed.). Philadelphia: W.B. Saunders, p. 603.

**405.** A client who just underwent a tonsillectomy is becoming slightly restless, has an increased pulse rate, and exhibits slight pallor. The nurse notes that the client is swallowing frequently. Which of the following interpretations most appropriately describes the cause of the complaints?

1. The client needs pain medication
2. The client may have postoperative bleeding or hemorrhage
3. This is an expected postoperative finding
4. The client has some mild postoperative edema

**Answer: 2**

*Rationale:* Signs of postoperative hemorrhage include pallor, restlessness, frequent swallowing, large amounts of bloody drainage or vomitus, increasing pulse rate, and falling blood pressure. These signs should be reported to the surgeon. While restlessness and an increased pulse could be due to the presence of pain, those signs along with others identified in the question indicate postoperative bleeding.

*Test-Taking Strategy:* Focus on the signs and symptoms identified in the question and use the process of elimination. Noting the key words *swallowing frequently* will direct you to option 2. Review postoperative complications following tonsillectomy if you had difficulty with this question.

*Level of Cognitive Ability:* Analysis
*Client Needs:* Physiological Integrity
*Integrated Concept/Process:* Nursing Process/Assessment
*Content Area:* Adult Health/Respiratory

*Reference*
Monahan, F., & Neighbors, M. (1998). *Medical-surgical nursing: Foundations for clinical practice* (2nd ed.). Philadelphia: W.B. Saunders, p. 607.

**406.** A client has Impaired Verbal Communication as a result of a temporary tracheostomy following a laryngectomy. In planning for communication with this client, a nurse would avoid which of the following methods because it would be least helpful for this particular client?
1. Use of hand or finger signals
2. Nodding and shaking the head for yes and no
3. Use of a picture board
4. Use of a pencil and paper

**Answer: 2**
*Rationale:* Following laryngectomy, the client should not be asked to nod or shake the head because it is painful for the client. The use of eye blink or hand or finger signals is acceptable. Other helpful methods include the use of a pencil and paper, word or picture board, flash cards, or a magic slate.

*Test-Taking Strategy:* Use the process of elimination and note the key words *avoid* and *least helpful*. Remember that options that are similar are not likely to be correct. In this question, each of the incorrect options involves use of the hands. Also focusing on the diagnosis and surgical procedure will direct you to option 2. Review care of a client following laryngectomy if you had difficulty with this question.

*Level of Cognitive Ability:* Application
*Client Needs:* Physiological Integrity
*Integrated Concept/Process:* Communication and Documentation
*Content Area:* Adult Health/Respiratory

*Reference*
Monahan, F., & Neighbors, M. (1998). *Medical-surgical nursing: Foundations for clinical practice* (2nd ed.). Philadelphia: W.B. Saunders, pp. 621-622.

**407.** A client with pneumonia has anorexia because of the effort required for eating while dyspneic and decreased taste sensation. Which of the following actions by the nurse would be most helpful in increasing the client's appetite?
1. Push fluids to 3 L/day
2. Keep water at the bedside
3. Provide three large meals daily
4. Provide mouth care before meals

**Answer: 4**
*Rationale:* The client with pneumonia may experience decreased taste sensation as a result of sputum expectoration. To minimize this adverse effect, the nurse should provide oral hygiene before meals. The client should also have small, frequent meals because of dyspnea. Increased oral fluids and keeping water at the bedside are good measures to prevent fluid deficit associated with pneumonia, but they do nothing to alleviate anorexia.

*Test-Taking Strategy:* Use the process of elimination, focusing on the issue: increasing the client's appetite. Eliminate options 1 and 2 because they are similar. From the remaining options, focusing on the issue will direct you to option 4. Review measures that will increase appetite if you had difficulty with this question.

*Level of Cognitive Ability:* Application
*Client Needs:* Physiological Integrity
*Integrated Concept/Process:* Nursing Process/Implementation
*Content Area:* Adult Health/Respiratory

*Reference*
Monahan, F., & Neighbors, M. (1998). *Medical-surgical nursing: Foundations for clinical practice* (2nd ed.). Philadelphia: W.B. Saunders, p. 646.

**408.** A clinic nurse notes that a large number of clients whose chief complaint is the presence of flulike symptoms are being seen in the clinic. Which of the following recommendations by the nurse is least helpful for these clients?

1    Increase intake of liquids
2    Take antipyretics for fever
3    Get a flu shot immediately
4    Get plenty of rest

**Answer: 3**

*Rationale:* Immunization against influenza is a prophylactic measure and is not used to treat flu symptoms. Treatment for the flu includes getting rest, drinking fluids, and taking in nutritious foods and beverages. Medications such as antipyretics and analgesics may also be used for symptom management.

*Test-Taking Strategy:* Use the process of elimination, noting the key words *least helpful*. Recalling that a flu shot is a prophylactic measure will assist in directing you to the correct option. Review measures for the client with flulike symptoms if you had difficulty with this question.

*Level of Cognitive Ability:* Application
*Client Needs:* Physiological Integrity
*Integrated Concept/Process:* Self Care
*Content Area:* Adult Health/Respiratory

*Reference*
Monahan, F., & Neighbors, M. (1998). *Medical-surgical nursing: Foundations for clinical practice* (2nd ed.). Philadelphia: W.B. Saunders, pp. 649-650.

---

**409.** A nurse is beginning to ambulate a client with a nursing diagnosis of Activity Intolerance who was admitted to the hospital for bacterial endocarditis. The nurse evaluates that the client is best tolerating the exercise if which of the following parameters is noted by the nurse?

1    Pulse rate that increases from 68 to 94 beats/min
2    Blood pressure that increases from 114/82 to 118/86 mm Hg
3    Minimal chest pain rated 1 on the pain scale
4    Mild dyspnea after walking 10 feet

**Answer: 2**

*Rationale:* General indicators that a client is tolerating exercise include an absence of chest pain or dyspnea, a pulse rate increase of less than 20 beats/min, and a blood pressure change of less than 10 mm Hg.

*Test-Taking Strategy:* Use the process of elimination, noting the key words *best tolerating the exercise*. Eliminate options 3 and 4 first, since they represent abnormal data. From the remaining options, note that option 2 reflects the least physiological change as a result of the exercise. Review the defining characteristics of Activity Intolerance if you had difficulty with this question.

*Level of Cognitive Ability:* Analysis
*Client Needs:* Physiological Integrity
*Integrated Concept/Process:* Nursing Process/Evaluation
*Content Area:* Adult Health/Cardiovascular

*Reference*
Monahan, F., & Neighbors, M. (1998). *Medical-surgical nursing: Foundations for clinical practice* (2nd ed.). Philadelphia: W.B. Saunders, p. 235.

**410.** Cardiac monitoring leads are placed on a client who is at risk for premature ventricular contractions (PVCs). The nurse assesses the client's rhythm to detect PVCs by looking for:

1   Premature beats followed by a compensatory pause
2   QRS complexes that are short and narrow
3   Inverted P waves before the QRS complexes
4   A P wave preceding every QRS complex

**Answer: 1**

*Rationale:* PVCs are abnormal ectopic beats originating in the ventricles. They are characterized by an absence of P waves, wide and bizarre QRS complexes, and a compensatory pause that follows the ectopy.

*Test-Taking Strategy:* Use the process of elimination. Note the relationship of *premature ventricular contractions* in the question and *premature beats* in the correct option. If this question was difficult, review the characteristics of a PVC.

*Level of Cognitive Ability:* Analysis
*Client Needs:* Physiological Integrity
*Integrated Concept/Process:* Nursing Process/Assessment
*Content Area:* Adult Health/Cardiovascular

*Reference*
Monahan, F., & Neighbors, M. (1998). *Medical-surgical nursing: Foundations for clinical practice* (2nd ed.). Philadelphia: W.B. Saunders, p. 248.

---

**411.** A client with angina pectoris was given nitroglycerin tablets to take sublingually for chest pain. The client states a dislike for the medication because it causes a headache. The nurse makes which of the following interpretations about the client's statement?

1   This is a common but unhealthy response to the medication
2   This is a common response that will diminish as tolerance to nitroglycerin increases
3   This response is caused by cerebral hypoxia induced by the medication
4   This is an extremely adverse reaction and should be reported to the physician

**Answer: 2**

*Rationale:* Headache is a common side effect of the use of nitroglycerin because of its vasodilator properties. The incidence of headache diminishes over time as the client develops tolerance to the medication. The client should be encouraged to continue its use as needed and to take acetaminophen (Tylenol) or aspirin for headache, according to the preference of the prescribing physician.

*Test-Taking Strategy:* Use the process of elimination. Eliminate options 3 and 4 first because of the words *hypoxia* and *extremely*. Remember, nitroglycerin will dilate vessels and relieve hypoxia to the cardiac tissue. Eliminate option 1 because of the word *unhealthy*. If you had difficulty with this question, review the side effects related to nitroglycerin.

*Level of Cognitive Ability:* Analysis
*Client Needs:* Physiological Integrity
*Integrated Concept/Process:* Nursing Process/Analysis
*Content Area:* Adult Health/Cardiovascular

*Reference*
Monahan, F., & Neighbors, M. (1998). *Medical-surgical nursing: Foundations for clinical practice* (2nd ed.). Philadelphia: W.B. Saunders, p. 266.

**412.** A client is experiencing pulmonary edema as an exacerbation of chronic left-sided heart failure. The nurse assesses this client for which of the following manifestations?

1    Distended neck veins
2    Peripheral pitting edema
3    Weight loss
4    Bilateral crackles

**Answer: 4**

*Rationale:* The client with pulmonary edema presents primarily with symptoms that are respiratory in nature, since the blood flow is stagnant in the lungs, which lie behind the left side of the heart from a circulatory standpoint. The client would experience weight gain from fluid retention, not weight loss. Distended neck veins and peripheral pitting edema are classic signs of right-sided heart failure.

*Test-Taking Strategy:* Use knowledge of circulatory dynamics to answer this question. Knowing that blood flow is stagnant behind the area of failure allows you to eliminate each of the incorrect options. With heart failure, to remember the signs and symptoms, remember "left, lungs" and "right, systemic." Option 4 relates to the lungs. Review the signs of left- and right-sided heart failure if you had difficulty with this question.

*Level of Cognitive Ability:* Application
*Client Needs:* Physiological Integrity
*Integrated Concept/Process:* Nursing Process/Assessment
*Content Area:* Adult Health/Cardiovascular

*Reference*
Monahan, F., & Neighbors, M. (1998). *Medical-surgical nursing: Foundations for clinical practice* (2nd ed.). Philadelphia: W.B. Saunders, p. 270.

**413.** The nurse suspects the occurrence of an air embolism in a client with a triple-lumen catheter. If an air embolism is present, the nurse would most likely note which of the following?

1    Hypertension
2    Diminished breath sounds
3    A "churning" sound heard over the right ventricle on auscultation
4    Rales heard in the lung bases on auscultation

**Answer: 3**

*Rationale:* All clients with IV lines are at risk for air embolism. Because an air embolism can be fatal, it is essential that the nurse monitor for the presence of chest pain, coughing, hypotension, cyanosis, and hypoxia. In addition, if the client does have an air embolism, auscultation over the right ventricle may reveal a churning, windmill type of sound. Options 2 and 4 are not characteristics of an air embolism.

*Test-Taking Strategy:* Use the process of elimination. Note that the issue of the question is air embolism. Remembering that fluid (not air) will produce rales heard in the lung bases will assist in eliminating option 4. From the remaining options, think about the signs of an embolism to direct you to option 3. Review the signs of an air embolism if you had difficulty with this question.

*Level of Cognitive Ability:* Analysis
*Client Needs:* Physiological Integrity
*Integrated Concept/Process:* Nursing Process/Assessment
*Content Area:* Fundamental Skills

*Reference*
Smeltzer, S., & Bare, B. (2000) *Brunner & Suddarth's Textbook of medical-surgical nursing* (9th ed.). Philadelphia: Lippincott Williams & Wilkins, p. 240.

**414.** When administering an intramuscular injection in the gluteal muscle, the nurse places the client in which best position to relax the muscle?
  1  On their side with the knee of the uppermost leg flexed
  2  On their side with the knee of the lowermost leg flexed
  3  Prone with a toe-in position
  4  Sims' with a toe-in position

**Answer: 3**
*Rationale:* A prone toe-in position will promote internal rotation of the hips, which will relax the muscle and make the injection less painful. Options 1, 2, and 4 will not relax the muscle.

*Test-Taking Strategy:* Note the key words *relax the muscle.* Visualize each position described in the options to direct you to option 3. If you are unfamiliar with the position for administering IM medications, review this procedure.

*Level of Cognitive Ability:* Application
*Client Needs:* Physiological Integrity
*Integrated Concept/Process:* Nursing Process/Implementation
*Content Area:* Fundamental Skills

*Reference*
Potter, P., & Perry, A. (2001). *Fundamentals of nursing* (5th ed.). St. Louis: Mosby, p. 944.

**415.** A nurse plans to administer a medication by IV bolus through the IV primary line. The nurse notes that the medication is incompatible with the primary IV solution. The most appropriate nursing action to safely administer the medication is to:
  1  Call the physician for an order to change the route of the medication
  2  Start a new IV line for the medication
  3  Flush the tubing before and after the medication with normal saline
  4  Flush the tubing before and after the medication with sterile water

**Answer: 3**
*Rationale:* When giving a medication by IV bolus, if the medication is incompatible with the IV solution, the tubing is flushed before and after the bolus with infusions of normal saline solution. Option 1 is inappropriate. Option 2 is premature and not necessary. Sterile water is not used for an IV flush.

*Test-Taking Strategy:* Use the process of elimination. Option 1 can be easily eliminated because in this situation, it is not an appropriate action. Option 2 is not necessary and may only cause discomfort for the client. From the remaining options, remember that normal saline is physiologically similar to body fluid and is the best choice. Review the procedures for administering IV bolus medications if you had difficulty with this question.

*Level of Cognitive Ability:* Application
*Client Needs:* Physiological Integrity
*Integrated Concept/Process:* Nursing Process/Implementation
*Content Area:* Fundamental Skills

*Reference*
Harkreader, H. (2000). *Fundamentals of nursing: Caring and clinical judgment.* Philadelphia: W.B. Saunders, p. 579.

**416.** A nurse is preparing to administer ear drops to an infant. The nurse plans to:
1    Pull up and back on the auricle and direct the solution toward the wall of the ear canal
2    Pull down and back on the auricle and direct the solution onto the eardrum
3    Pull down and back on the pinna and direct the solution toward the wall of the canal
4    Pull up and back on the ear lobe and direct the solution toward the wall of the canal

**Answer: 3**
*Rationale:* The infant should be turned on the side with the affected ear uppermost. With the nondominant hand, the nurse pulls down and back on the pinna. The wrist of the dominant hand is rested on the infant's head. The medication is administered by aiming it at the wall of the canal rather than directly onto the eardrum. The infant should be held or positioned with the affected ear uppermost for 10 to 15 minutes to retain the solution. In the adult, the auricle is pulled up and back to straighten the auditory canal.

*Test-Taking Strategy:* Use the process of elimination. Basic safety principles related to the administration of ear medications should assist in eliminating option 2. Option 1 is eliminated because it is the adult procedure. It would be difficult to pull up and back on an earlobe, therefore eliminate option 4. Review the procedure for administering ear medications in an infant and adult if you had difficulty with this question.

*Level of Cognitive Ability:* Application
*Client Needs:* Physiological Integrity
*Integrated Concept/Process:* Nursing Process/Implementation
*Content Area:* Pharmacology

*Reference*
Wong, D. (1999). *Whaley & Wong's Nursing care of infants and children* (6th ed.). St. Louis: Mosby, p. 1270.

**417.** A client seeks treatment in an ambulatory clinic for a complaint of hoarseness that has lasted for 6 weeks. Based on the symptom, the nurse interprets that the client is at risk of having:
1    Laryngeal cancer
2    Acute laryngitis
3    Bronchogenic cancer
4    Thyroid cancer

**Answer: 1**
*Rationale:* Hoarseness is a common early sign of laryngeal cancer, but not of bronchogenic or thyroid cancer. Hoarseness that lasts for 6 weeks is not associated with an acute problem, such as laryngitis.

*Test-Taking Strategy:* Use the process of elimination. Begin to answer this question by eliminating option 2, since an acute problem would not generally last for 6 weeks. From the remaining options, recalling that the vocal cords are in the larynx makes option 1 preferable to any of the others. Review the signs of laryngeal cancer if you had difficulty with this question.

*Level of Cognitive Ability:* Analysis
*Client Needs:* Physiological Integrity
*Integrated Concept/Process:* Nursing Process/Analysis
*Content Area:* Adult Health/Respiratory

*Reference*
Smeltzer, S., & Bare, B. (2000) *Brunner & Suddarth's Textbook of medical-surgical nursing* (9th ed.). Philadelphia: Lippincott Williams & Wilkins, p. 414.

**418.** A client is admitted to the nursing unit following lobectomy. The nurse notes that in the first hour after admission the chest tube drainage was 75 mL. During the second hour, the drainage has dropped to 5 mL. The nurse interprets that:

1   The lung has fully reexpanded
2   This is normal
3   The client needs to cough and deep breathe
4   The tube may be occluded

**Answer: 4**

*Rationale:* Chest tube drainage in the first 24 hours after thoracic surgery may total 500 to 1000 mL. The sudden drop in drainage between the first and second hour indicates that the tube is possibly occluded and requires further assessment by the nurse. Options 1, 2, and 3 are incorrect interpretations.

*Test-Taking Strategy:* Use the process of elimination. Option 1 is the least plausible and is eliminated first. Needing to cough and deep breathe is a response that is unrelated to the client's problem and is eliminated next. From the remaining options, knowing that the drainage should not drop so radically in 1 hour directs you to option 4. Review the concepts related to chest tube drainage systems in the postoperative lobectomy client if you had difficulty with this question.

*Level of Cognitive Ability:* Analysis
*Client Needs:* Physiological Integrity
*Integrated Concept/Process:* Nursing Process/Analysis
*Content Area:* Adult Health/Respiratory

*Reference*
Smeltzer, S., & Bare, B. (2000) *Brunner & Suddarth's Textbook of medical-surgical nursing* (9th ed.). Philadelphia: Lippincott Williams & Wilkins, p. 518.

---

**419.** A nurse is auscultating the chest of a client with new onset of pleurisy. The client does not have a pleural friction rub, which was auscultated the previous day. The nurse interprets that this is most likely due to:

1   Decreased inflammatory reaction at the site
2   The deep breaths that the client is taking
3   Accumulation of pleural fluid in the inflamed area
4   Effectiveness of medication therapy

**Answer: 3**

*Rationale:* Pleural friction rub is auscultated early in the course of pleurisy, before pleural fluid accumulates. Once fluid accumulates in the inflamed area, there is less friction between the visceral and parietal lung surfaces, and the pleural friction rub disappears. Options 1, 2, and 4 are incorrect interpretations.

*Test-Taking Strategy:* Use the process of elimination. Eliminate option 2 first, which would intensify the pain. Options 1 and 4 are similar, and since the question states that the problem is new in onset, these should be eliminated next. Remember, fluid accumulation in the area provides a buffer between the lung and chest wall surfaces, which eliminates the friction rub. Review assessment findings in the client with pleurisy if you had difficulty with this question.

*Level of Cognitive Ability:* Analysis
*Client Needs:* Physiological Integrity
*Integrated Concept/Process:* Nursing Process/Analysis
*Content Area:* Adult Health/Respiratory

*Reference*
Smeltzer, S., & Bare, B. (2000) *Brunner & Suddarth's Textbook of medical-surgical nursing* (9th ed.). Philadelphia: Lippincott Williams & Wilkins, p. 444.

**420.** A client is admitted to the nursing unit with a diagnosis of pleurisy. The nurse assesses the client for which of the following characteristic symptoms of this disorder?

1 Early morning fatigue
2 Dyspnea that is relieved by lying flat
3 Pain that worsens when the breath is held
4 Knifelike pain that worsens on inspiration

**Answer: 4**

*Rationale:* A typical symptom of pleurisy is a knifelike pain that worsens on inspiration. This is due to the friction caused by the rubbing together of inflamed pleural surfaces. This pain usually disappears when the breath is held, because these surfaces stop moving. The client does not experience early morning fatigue or dyspnea relieved by lying flat.

*Test-Taking Strategy:* Use the process of elimination. Option 2 is eliminated first because dyspnea is not relieved by lying flat. Option 1 is eliminated next because fatigue, if it were to occur, would not be present in the morning when the client is most well rested. From the remaining options, keep in mind that pleurisy results from inflammation of the pleura. Since the visceral and parietal lung pleura glide over one another with respiration, it is expected that chest movement precipitates or intensifies the pain. Review the symptoms associated with pleurisy if you had difficulty with this question.

*Level of Cognitive Ability:* Application
*Client Needs:* Physiological Integrity
*Integrated Concept/Process:* Nursing Process/Assessment
*Content Area:* Adult Health/Respiratory

**Reference**
Smeltzer, S., & Bare, B. (2000) *Brunner & Suddarth's Textbook of medical-surgical nursing* (9th ed.). Philadelphia: Lippincott Williams & Wilkins, p. 444.

**421.** A nurse is caring for a client with a cerebral aneurysm. Isoproterenol (Isuprel) and aminophylline IV are administered to the client. Which of the following would indicate a positive client response to the treatment?

1 Nausea, vomiting, diarrhea
2 No change in client assessment
3 Tachycardia, premature ventricular contractions (PVCs), hypotension
4 Increased level of consciousness

**Answer: 4**

*Rationale:* Isoproterenol (Isuprel) and aminophylline are administered to prevent vasospasms and reverse ischemia. Isoproterenol produces vasodilation. Aminophylline reduces cell contractility. These actions should result in improved neurological findings. Nausea, vomiting, diarrhea, tachycardia, PVCs, hypotension, and no change are not positive client responses. Tachycardia, PVCs, and hypotension are side effects for which the nurse should monitor.

*Test-Taking Strategy:* Note the key words *indicate a positive client response*. Options 1, 2, and 3 identify signs that do not indicate a positive response. Option 4 indicates not only a positive response but also a relationship to the diagnosis of the client, that being a neurological condition. If you are unfamiliar with these medications and their relationship to the treatment of cerebral aneurysm, review this content.

*Level of Cognitive Ability:* Analysis
*Client Needs:* Physiological Integrity
*Integrated Concept/Process:* Nursing Process/Evaluation
*Content Area:* Pharmacology

**Reference**
Smeltzer, S., & Bare, B. (2000) *Brunner & Suddarth's Textbook of medical-surgical nursing* (9th ed.). Philadelphia: Lippincott Williams & Wilkins, p. 1716.

**422.** A nurse is performing an assessment on a client with the diagnosis of Brown-Séquard syndrome. Which of the following assessment findings should the nurse expect to note?
1 Ipsilateral paralysis and loss of touch and vibration
2 Bilateral loss of pain and temperature sensation
3 Contralateral paralysis and loss of touch sensation and vibration
4 Complete paraplegia or quadriplegia, depending on the level of injury

**Answer: 1**
*Rationale:* Brown-Séquard syndrome results from hemisection of the spinal cord, resulting in ipsilateral paralysis and loss of touch, pressure, vibration, and proprioception. Contralaterally, pain and temperature sensation is lost because these fibers decussate after entering the cord. Options 2, 3, and 4 are not assessment findings in this syndrome.

*Test-Taking Strategy:* Recalling that Brown-Séquard syndrome results from hemisection of the spinal cord will direct you to option 1. If you are unfamiliar with this syndrome, review the assessment findings and the nursing care.

*Level of Cognitive Ability:* Analysis
*Client Needs:* Physiological Integrity
*Integrated Concept/Process:* Nursing Process/Assessment
*Content Area:* Adult Health/Neurological

*Reference*
Ignatavicius, D., Workman, M., & Mishler, M. (1999). *Medical-surgical nursing across the health care continuum* (3rd ed.). Philadelphia: W.B. Saunders, p. 1066.

---

**423.** A nurse is performing an assessment on a client who has a suspected spinal cord injury. Which of the following is the priority nursing assessment?
1 Pupillary response
2 Respiratory status
3 Mobility level
4 Pain level

**Answer: 2**
*Rationale:* All of the above assessments would be performed on a client with a suspected spinal cord injury. Respiratory status is the priority.

*Test-Taking Strategy:* Use the ABCs (airway, breathing, and circulation) to answer the question. Option 2 addresses airway. Review care of a client with a suspected spinal cord injury if you had difficulty with this question.

*Level of Cognitive Ability:* Application
*Client Needs:* Physiological Integrity
*Integrated Concept/Process:* Nursing Process/Assessment
*Content Area:* Adult Health/Neurological

*Reference*
Ignatavicius, D., Workman, M., & Mishler, M. (1999). *Medical-surgical nursing across the health care continuum* (3rd ed.). Philadelphia: W.B. Saunders, p. 1066.

---

**424.** A nurse is caring for a client who is newly diagnosed with a spinal cord injury. The nurse would anticipate that the most likely medication to be prescribed would be:
1 Propranolol (Inderal)
2 Dexamethasone (Decadron)
3 Furosemide (Lasix)
4 Morphine (Astramorph)

**Answer: 2**
*Rationale:* The most likely medication to be prescribed for a newly diagnosed spinal cord injury is dexamethasone (Decadron). This medication is a short-acting glucocorticoid and would be administered to reduce traumatic edema. The use of propranolol, a beta blocker, furosemide, a diuretic, or morphine (Astramorph), an opioid analgesic, would not be indicated based on the information in this question.

*Test-Taking Strategy:* Use the process of elimination. Note the key words *newly diagnosed* and the diagnosis *spinal cord injury*. Knowledge regarding the association between injury and edema will assist in answering the question. If you are unfamiliar with these medications or the treatment for spinal cord injury, review this content.

*Level of Cognitive Ability:* Analysis
*Client Needs:* Physiological Integrity
*Integrated Concept/Process:* Nursing Process/Analysis
*Content Area:* Adult Health/Neurological

*Reference*
Ignatavicius, D., Workman, M., & Mishler, M. (1999). *Medical-surgical nursing across the health care continuum* (3rd ed.). Philadelphia: W.B. Saunders, p. 1070.

---

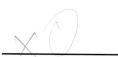

**425.** A nurse is admitting a client with a diagnosis of acquired immunodeficiency syndrome (AIDS) to the medical-surgical unit. The nurse most importantly assesses for which of the following findings?

1. Jaundiced skin
2. White patches in the oral cavity
3. Bradypnea
4. Urine specific gravity of 1.010

**Answer: 2**
*Rationale:* Clients with AIDS frequently have opportunistic infections. *Candida albicans,* the causative organism of thrush, is a common opportunistic infection. Thrush presents as white patches in the oral cavity. Hairy leukoplakia also presents as white patches in the oral cavity. Jaundice is a symptom of hepatic disease. Clients with AIDS frequently acquire pneumonia and may present with tachypnea, not bradypnea. Clients with AIDS frequently have inadequate nutrition and hydration and may present with dehydration, resulting in a high specific gravity rather than a low specific gravity.

*Test-Taking Strategy:* Use the process of elimination. Recalling that the client with AIDS is at risk for developing an infection will direct you to option 2. Review the manifestations associated with AIDS, if you had difficulty with this question.

*Level of Cognitive Ability:* Analysis
*Client Needs:* Physiological Integrity
*Integrated Concept/Process:* Nursing Process/Assessment
*Content Area:* Adult Health/Immune

*Reference*
Ignatavicius, D., Workman, M., & Mishler, M. (1999). *Medical-surgical nursing across the health care continuum* (3rd ed.). Philadelphia: W.B. Saunders, p. 446.

---

**426.** A nurse assesses a client who was involved a motor vehicle accident. The nurse determines the need to prepare for chest tube insertion if the client exhibits:

1. Shortness of breath and tracheal deviation
2. Chest pain and shortness of breath
3. Decreasing oxygen saturation and bradypnea
4. Peripheral cyanosis and hypotension

**Answer: 1**
*Rationale:* Shortness of breath and tracheal deviation result when lung tissue and alveoli have collapsed. The trachea deviates to the unaffected side in the presence of a tension pneumothorax. Air entering the pleural cavity causes the lung to lose its normal negative pressure. The increasing pressure in the affected side displaces contents to the unaffected side. Shortness of breath results from a decreased area available for diffusion of gases. Chest pain and shortness of breath are more commonly associated with myocardial ischemia or infarction. Clients requiring chest tubes exhibit decreasing oxygen saturation but will more likely experience tachypnea related to the hypoxia. Peripheral cyanosis is caused by circulatory disorders. Hypotension may be a result of tracheal shift and impedance of venous return to the heart. However, it may also be the result of other problems such as a failing heart.

*Test-Taking Strategy:* Focus on the issue: preparation for chest tube insertion. Recalling the signs of a tension pneumothorax will direct you to option 1. Review the signs associated with tension pneumothorax and the conditions that require chest tube drainage if you had difficulty with this question.

*Level of Cognitive Ability:* Analysis
*Client Needs:* Physiological Integrity
*Integrated Concept/Process:* Nursing Process/Analysis
*Content Area:* Adult Health/Respiratory

*Reference*
Ignatavicius, D., Workman, M., & Mishler, M. (1999). *Medical-surgical nursing across the health care continuum* (3rd ed.). Philadelphia: W.B. Saunders, p. 710.

---

**427.** A nurse is admitting a client to the mental health unit who has a diagnosis of bipolar disorder, manic phase. In assessing the client regarding sleep patterns and the need for rest, the nurse knows that the most reliable information may be obtained by:

1. Asking the client how many hours of sleep were obtained last night
2. Observing the facial appearance of the client
3. Asking the significant other about the sleep patterns
4. Asking the night shift to record hours of sleep tonight

**Answer: 3**
*Rationale:* Option 3 would provide the most reliable information, since the client may not be able to report sleep patterns accurately. The client may report that sleep has not been a problem when in fact only 3 hours of sleep has been obtained for the last several days. Rest needs are very important, since the manic client may be at the point of exhaustion by the time hospitalization occurs. Facial expressions may be an indicator of fatigue, but they are not quantifiable. Asking the night shift for assessment data is not in the best interest of the client because it delays obtaining needed data.

*Test-Taking Strategy:* Use the process of elimination, focusing on the words *most reliable.* In this situation the significant other is the only one who can provide accurate information. Review assessment of the client with bipolar disorder if you had difficulty with this question.

*Level of Cognitive Ability:* Analysis
*Client Needs:* Physiological Integrity
*Integrated Concept/Process:* Nursing Process/Assessment
*Content Area:* Mental Health

*Reference*
Stuart, G.W., & Laraia, M.T. (1998). *Principles and practice of psychiatric nursing.* (6th ed.). St. Louis: Mosby, p. 352.

**428.** The parents of a male newborn who is not circumcised request information on how to clean the newborn's penis. The best nursing response is:

1   "Retract the foreskin and cleanse the glans when bathing the newborn."
2   "Do not retract the foreskin to cleanse because this may cause adhesions."
3   "Retract the foreskin no farther than it will go and replace it over the glans after cleaning."
4   "Retract the foreskin and cleanse it with every diaper change."

**Answer: 2**

*Rationale:* In newborn males, prepuce is continuous with the epidermis of the glans and is nonretractable. Forced retraction may cause adhesions to develop. It is best to allow separation to occur naturally, which will take place between 3 years and puberty. Most foreskins are retractable by 3 years of age and should be pushed back gently for cleaning once a week.

*Test-Taking Strategy:* Use the process of elimination. Eliminate options 1, 3, and 4 because they are similar and are incorrect because retracting the foreskin is not recommended in an uncircumcised newborn male. Option 2 is the only different option stating that the foreskin should not be retracted. Review parent teaching points related to the care of an uncircumcised newborn if you had difficulty with this question.

*Level of Cognitive Ability:* Application
*Client Needs:* Physiological Integrity
*Integrated Concept/Process:* Teaching/Learning
*Content Area:* Child Health

*Reference*
Lowdermilk, D., Perry, S., & Bobak, I. (2000). *Maternity & women's health care* (7th ed.). St. Louis: Mosby, p. 685.

**429.** The client who has been receiving intravenous aminophylline (Theophylline) has been prescribed an immediate-release oral form of the medication. The IV medication is to be discontinued. The nurse should administer the first dose of the oral medication:

1   Immediately on discontinuing the IV form
2   In 4 to 6 hours after discontinuing the IV form
3   Just before the next meal
4   Just after the next meal

**Answer: 2**

*Rationale:* With an immediate-release preparation, the oral aminophylline should be administered in 4 to 6 hours after discontinuing the IV form of the medication. If the sustained-release form is used, the first oral dose should be administered immediately upon discontinuation of the IV infusion.

*Test-Taking Strategy:* Use the process of elimination. Note the key words *immediate-release*. It then makes sense to wait 4 to 6 hours before administration of the oral form. If this question was difficult, review this medication and its methods of administration.

*Level of Cognitive Ability:* Application
*Client Needs:* Physiological Integrity
*Integrated Concept/Process:* Nursing Process/Implementation
*Content Area:* Pharmacology

*Reference*
Hodgson, B., & Kizior, R. (2001). *Saunders Nursing drug handbook 2001.* Philadelphia: W.B. Saunders, p. 44.

**430.** A client has a serum sodium level of 129 mEq/L as a result of hypervolemia. The nurse consults with the physician to determine whether which of the following most appropriate measures should be instituted?

1  Providing a 2-g sodium diet
2  Providing a 4-g sodium diet
3  Fluid restriction
4  Administering intravenous hypertonic saline

**Answer: 3**

*Rationale:* Hyponatremia is defined as a serum sodium level of less than 135 mEq/L. When it is caused by hypervolemia, it may be treated with fluid restriction. The low serum sodium value is due to hemodilution. Intravenous hypertonic saline is reserved for hyponatremia when the serum sodium level is lower than 125 mEq/L. A 4-gram sodium diet is a no-added-salt diet. A 2-gram sodium restriction would not raise the serum sodium level.

*Test-Taking Strategy:* Use the process of elimination. Note that the serum sodium level is low. With this in mind, you would eliminate option 1. Next, note the key word *hypervolemia.* Knowing that hypervolemia causes hemodilution of the serum sodium would guide you to choose option 3 over options 2 and 4. Review treatment measures for hyponatremia if you had difficulty with this question.

*Level of Cognitive Ability:* Application
*Client Needs:* Physiological Integrity
*Integrated Concept/Process:* Nursing Process/Implementation
*Content Area:* Fundamental Skills

*Reference*
Smeltzer, S., & Bare, B. (2000) *Brunner & Suddarth's Textbook of medical-surgical nursing* (9th ed.). Philadelphia: Lippincott Williams & Wilkins, p. 213.

---

**431.** A nurse is planning care for a client whose oxygenation is being monitored by a pulse oximeter. Which of the following nursing actions would be most important to include in the plan in order to ensure accurate monitoring of the client's oxygenation status?

1  Notify the physician immediately of an oxygen saturation less than 90%
2  Instruct the client not to move the sensor
3  Tape the sensor tightly to the client's finger
4  Place the sensor on a finger below the blood pressure cuff

**Answer: 2**

*Rationale:* The pulse oximeter passes a beam of light through the tissue, and a sensor attached to the fingertip, toe, or ear lobe measures the amount of light absorbed by the oxygen-saturated hemoglobin. The oximeter then gives a reading of the percentage of hemoglobin that is saturated with oxygen ($Sao_2$). Motion at the sensor site changes light absorption. The motion mimics the pulsatile motion of blood, and because the detector cannot distinguish between movement of blood and movement of the finger, results can be inaccurate. The sensor should not be placed distal to blood pressure cuffs, pressure dressings, arterial lines, or any invasive catheters. The sensor should not be taped to the client's finger. If values fall below preset norms (usually 90%), the client should be instructed to deep breathe if this is appropriate.

*Test-Taking Strategy:* Focus on the issue: to ensure accurate monitoring. Eliminate option 1 because although reporting a low oxygen saturation to the physician is important, it is unrelated to ensuring accurate monitoring with a pulse oximeter. Option 4 is inappropriate; therefore eliminate this option. From the remaining options, recalling that motion at the sensor site changes light absorption and noting the word *tightly* in option 3 will direct you to the correct option. Review the principles associated with pulse oximetry if you had difficulty with this question.

*Level of Cognitive Ability:* Application
*Client Needs:* Physiological Integrity
*Integrated Concept/Process:* Nursing Process/Planning
*Content Area:* Adult Health/Respiratory

### Reference

Smeltzer, S., & Bare, B. (2000) *Brunner & Suddarth's Textbook of medical-surgical nursing* (9th ed.). Philadelphia: Lippincott Williams & Wilkins, p. 394.

---

**432.** A nurse is teaching a client with thromboangiitis obliterans (Buerger's disease) about interventions to control the disease process. The nurse avoids telling the client to:
1   Stop smoking immediately
2   Take nifedipine (Procardia) as directed
3   Keep the extremities cool
4   Assess for signs and symptoms of ulceration

**Answer: 3**

*Rationale:* Interventions are directed at preventing the progression of Buerger's disease and include conveying the need for immediate smoking cessation and providing medications prescribed for vasodilation, such as the calcium channel blocker nifedipine (Procardia) or the alpha-adrenergic blocker prazosin (Minipress). The client should maintain warmth to the extremities, especially by avoiding exposure to cold. The client should inspect the extremities and report signs of infection or ulceration.

*Test-Taking Strategy:* Use the process of elimination, noting the key word *avoids*. Since the goals of care for thromboangiitis obliterans are the same as for peripheral arterial disease, the answer to this question is the one that does not promote vasodilatation, option 3. Review home care measures for the client with thromboangiitis obliterans if you had difficulty with this question.

*Level of Cognitive Ability:* Application
*Client Needs:* Physiological Integrity
*Integrated Concept/Process:* Self-Care
*Content Area:* Adult Health/Cardiovascular

### Reference

Smeltzer, S., & Bare, B. (2000) *Brunner & Suddarth's Textbook of medical-surgical nursing* (9th ed.). Philadelphia: Lippincott Williams & Wilkins, p. 699.

---

**433.** A client has been admitted to the mental health unit with a diagnosis of social phobia disorder. Which of the following behaviors would the nurse expect to note on assessment of the client?
1   Panic attack when leaving their house
2   Shortness of breath and palpitations when riding the elevator
3   Persistent hand washing before eating
4   Fear of being humiliated in public and embarrassing self in front of others

**Answer: 4**

*Rationale:* A social phobia is characterized by a fear of appearing incompetent or inept in the presence of others and of doing something embarrassing. Thus these clients becomes anxious when the attention is on them. Option 1 identifies agoraphobia. Option 2 identifies claustrophobia. Option 3 identifies obsessive-compulsive behavior.

*Test-Taking Strategy:* Use the process of elimination. Focus on the key words *social phobia*. This should assist in directing you to option 4. Review the characteristics of the various phobias if you had difficulty with this question.

*Level of Cognitive Ability:* Analysis
*Client Needs:* Physiological Integrity

*Integrated Concept/Process:* Nursing Process/Assessment
*Content Area:* Mental Health

### Reference
Stuart, G.W., & Laraia, M.T. (1998). *Principles and practice of psychiatric nursing.* (6th ed.). St. Louis: Mosby, p. 286.

---

**434.** A nurse is caring for a client with Parkinson's disease. The client is taking benztropine mesylate (Cogentin) PO daily. The priority nursing action when caring for the client on this medication is to monitor the:
1 Pupil response
2 Partial thromboplastin time (PTT)
3 Intake and output
4 Prothrombin time (PT)

**Answer: 3**
*Rationale:* Urinary retention is a side effect of benztropine mesylate. The nurse needs to observe for dysuria, distended abdomen, infrequent voiding of small amounts, and overflow incontinence. Options 1, 2, and 4 are unrelated to the side effects of this medication.

*Test-Taking Strategy:* Use the process of elimination. Eliminate options 2 and 4 first because they are similar. From the remaining options, it is necessary to know that urinary retention is a concern with this medication. Review this medication and its side effects if you had difficulty with this question.

*Level of Cognitive Ability:* Application
*Client Needs:* Physiological Integrity
*Integrated Concept/Process:* Nursing Process/Assessment
*Content Area:* Pharmacology

### Reference
Hodgson, B., & Kizior, R. (2001). *Saunders Nursing drug handbook 2001.* Philadelphia: W.B. Saunders, p. 102.

---

**435.** A home health nurse is assessing a client who has begun using peritoneal dialysis. The nurse would determine that which of the following manifestations noted in the client would most likely indicate the onset of peritonitis?
1 Temperature of 99° F oral
2 History of gastrointestinal (GI) upset 1 week ago
3 Cloudy dialysate output
4 Presence of crystals in dialysate output

**Answer: 3**
*Rationale:* Typical symptoms of peritonitis include fever, nausea, malaise, rebound abdominal tenderness, and cloudy dialysate output. The very slight temperature elevation in option 1 is not the clearest indicator of infection. The complaint of GI upset is too vague to indicate peritonitis. Peritonitis would cause cloudy dialysate, but would not cause crystals to appear in the dialysate.

*Test-Taking Strategy:* Note the key words *most likely* and the issue: indicator of peritonitis. Begin to answer this question by eliminating options 1 and 2 first, since both of these manifestations are nonspecific. From the remaining options, recall that infection would cause white blood cells to be present in the dialysate, which would yield cloudiness, not crystals, in the dialysate output. Review the signs of peritonitis in the client receiving peritoneal dialysis if you had difficulty with this question.

*Level of Cognitive Ability:* Analysis
*Client Needs:* Physiological Integrity
*Integrated Concept/Process:* Nursing Process/Assessment
*Content Area:* Adult Health/Renal

*Reference*
Smeltzer, S., & Bare, B. (2000) *Brunner & Suddarth's Textbook of medical-surgical nursing* (9th ed.). Philadelphia: Lippincott Williams & Wilkins, p. 1121.

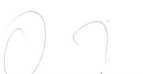

**436.** A nurse is working on a medical surgical nursing unit and is caring for several clients with renal failure. The nurse interprets that which of the following clients is best suited for peritoneal dialysis as a treatment option?

1   A client with severe congestive heart failure
2   A client with a history of ruptured diverticula
3   A client with a history of herniated lumbar disk
4   A client with a history of three previous abdominal surgeries

**Answer: 1**
*Rationale:* Peritoneal dialysis may be the treatment option of choice for clients with severe cardiovascular disease. Severe cardiac disease can be worsened by the rapid shifts in fluid, electrolytes, urea, and glucose that occurs with hemodialysis. For the same reason peritoneal dialysis may be indicated for the client with diabetes mellitus. Contraindications to peritoneal dialysis include diseases of the abdomen such as ruptured diverticula or malignancies; extensive abdominal surgeries; history of peritonitis; obesity; and those with a history of back problems, which could be aggravated by the fluid weight of the dialysate. Severe disease of the vascular system may also be a relative contraindication.

*Test-Taking Strategy:* Note the issue: which of the clients presented would be the best candidate for peritoneal dialysis. Eliminate options 2 and 4 first because they are similar and indicate clients with an abdominal condition. From the remaining options, recall the concepts related to fluid shifts in the body to direct you to option 1. Review the indications for peritoneal dialysis if you had difficulty with this question.

*Level of Cognitive Ability:* Analysis
*Client Needs:* Physiological Integrity
*Integrated Concept/Process:* Nursing Process/Analysis
*Content Area:* Adult Health/Renal

*Reference*
Smeltzer, S., & Bare, B. (2000) *Brunner & Suddarth's Textbook of medical-surgical nursing* (9th ed.). Philadelphia: Lippincott Williams & Wilkins, p. 1119.

**437.** A client undergoing long-term peritoneal dialysis is currently experiencing a problem with reduced outflow from the dialysis catheter. The home health nurse inquires whether the client has had a recent problem with:

1   Vomiting
2   Diarrhea
3   Constipation
4   Flatulence

**Answer: 3**
*Rationale:* Reduced outflow may be due to catheter position and adherence to the omentum, infection, or constipation. Constipation may contribute to reduced outflow in part because peristalsis seems to aid in drainage. For this reason, bisacodyl suppositories are sometimes used prophylactically, even without a history of constipation. The other options are unrelated to impaired catheter drainage.

*Test-Taking Strategy:* Use the process of elimination and focus on the issue: reduced outflow. Evaluate each option in terms of their effect on gut motility, which affects catheter outflow. Each of the incorrect options involves hypermotility of the gastrointestinal tract, which should theoretically facilitate outflow. Constipation is related to decreased gut motility, which could then impair fluid drainage. Review the causes of reduced outflow in peritoneal dialysis if you had difficulty with this question.

*Level of Cognitive Ability:* Analysis
*Client Needs:* Physiological Integrity
*Integrated Concept/Process:* Nursing Process/Assessment
*Content Area:* Adult Health/Renal

*Reference*
Smeltzer, S., & Bare, B. (2000) *Brunner & Suddarth's Textbook of medical-surgical nursing* (9th ed.). Philadelphia: Lippincott Williams & Wilkins, p. 1121.

---

**438.** A client with a history of heart failure who is undergoing peritoneal dialysis has developed crackles in the lower lung fields. The nurse interprets that this finding is most likely related to:
1  Compliance with dietary sodium restriction
2  Adherence to digoxin (Lanoxin) therapy schedule
3  Natural progression of the renal failure
4  Intake greater than output as indicated on the dialysis record

**Answer: 4**
*Rationale:* Crackles in the lung fields of the peritoneal dialysis client result from overhydration or from insufficient fluid removal during dialysis. An intake that is greater than the output of peritoneal dialysis fluid would overhydrate the client, resulting in lung crackles. Adherence to medication and diet therapy should control this sign, not exacerbate it. If dialysis is effective, there is no connection between the progression of renal failure and the development of signs of overhydration.

*Test-Taking Strategy:* Note the key words *developed crackles.* Begin to answer this question by eliminating options 1 and 2. Since adherence to standard therapy should control the signs of heart failure, not exacerbate them, these options are incorrect. From the remaining options, recalling that crackles are due to excess fluid in the body directs you to option 4. Review complications of peritoneal dialysis if you had difficulty with this question.

*Level of Cognitive Ability:* Analysis
*Client Needs:* Physiological Integrity
*Integrated Concept/Process:* Nursing Process/Analysis
*Content Area:* Adult Health/Renal

*Reference*
Smeltzer, S., & Bare, B. (2000). *Brunner & Suddarth's Textbook of medical-surgical nursing* (9th ed.). Philadelphia: Lippincott Williams & Wilkins, p. 1121.

---

**439.** A nurse is teaching the client with asthma how to use a peak flow meter. The nurse tells the client to:
1  Inhale an average size breath
2  Form a loose seal with the mouth around the mouthpiece
3  Blow out as slowly as possible
4  Record the final position of the indicator

**Answer: 4**
*Rationale:* A peak flow meter is used to provide an objective measure of the client's peak expiratory flow. The client is instructed to take the deepest possible breath, form a tight seal around the mouthpiece with the lips, and exhale forcefully and rapidly. The final position of the indicator on the meter is recorded.

*Test-Taking Strategy:* Use the process of elimination and knowledge regarding this piece of equipment and its use. If this question was difficult, review this commonly used device, which may be used to determine when medication adjustments are needed.

*Level of Cognitive Ability:* Application
*Client Needs:* Physiological Integrity
*Integrated Concept/Process:* Teaching/Learning
*Content Area:* Adult Health/Respiratory

*Reference*
Monahan, F., & Neighbors, M. (1998). *Medical-surgical nursing: Foundations for clinical practice* (2nd ed.). Philadelphia: W.B. Saunders, p. 663.

---

**440.** A nurse is teaching the client taking medications by inhalation about the advantages of a newly prescribed spacer. The nurse determines the need for further education if the client states that the spacer:

1. Reduces the frequency of medication to only once per day
2. Reduces the chance of yeast infection because large drops aren't deposited on the oral tissues
3. Disperses medication more deeply and uniformly
4. Reduces the need to coordinate timing between pressing the inhaler and inspiration

**Answer: 1**

*Rationale:* There are key advantages to the use of a spacer for medications administered by inhalation. One is that it reduces the incidence of yeast infections, since large medication droplets are not deposited on oral tissues. The medication is also dispersed more deeply and uniformly than without a spacer. There is less need to coordinate the effort of inhalation with pressing on the canister of the inhaler. Finally, the use of a spacer may decrease either the number or the volume of the puffs taken. Option 1 is too absolute and limiting by description.

*Test-Taking Strategy:* Use the process of elimination and focus on the issue: the need for further education. Note the word *only* in option 1. The use of absolute words such as "only" are likely to make the option incorrect. Review the advantages of the use of the spacer with inhaled medications if you had difficulty with this question.

*Level of Cognitive Ability:* Analysis
*Client Needs:* Physiological Integrity
*Integrated Concept/Process:* Teaching/Learning
*Content Area:* Adult Health/Respiratory

*Reference*
Monahan, F., & Neighbors, M. (1998). *Medical-surgical nursing: Foundations for clinical practice* (2nd ed.). Philadelphia: W.B. Saunders, pp. 661, 663.

---

**441.** A nurse is assessing a client with a tentative diagnosis of pulmonary emphysema. The nurse assesses the client for which of the following signs that distinguishes emphysema from chronic bronchitis?

1. Copious sputum production
2. Marked dyspnea
3. Minimal weight loss
4. Cough that began before the onset of dyspnea

**Answer: 2**

*Rationale:* Key features of pulmonary emphysema include dyspnea that is often marked, late cough (after the onset of dyspnea), scant mucus production, and marked weight loss. By contrast, chronic bronchitis is characterized by early onset of cough (before dyspnea), copious purulent sputum production, minimal weight loss, and milder severity of dyspnea.

*Test-Taking Strategy:* Focus on the issue: the differences between these two respiratory disorders and their associated manifestations. Recalling that marked dyspnea is associated with emphysema will direct you to option 2. Review the manifestations of emphysema and chronic bronchitis if you had difficulty with this question.

*Level of Cognitive Ability:* Analysis
*Client Needs:* Physiological Integrity
*Integrated Concept/Process:* Nursing Process/Assessment
*Content Area:* Adult Health/Respiratory

*Reference*
Monahan, F., & Neighbors, M. (1998). *Medical-surgical nursing: Foundations for clinical practice* (2nd ed.). Philadelphia: W.B. Saunders, p. 669.

---

**442.** A client with late stage emphysema complains of an occipital headache, drowsiness, and difficulty concentrating. The nurse interprets that these symptoms are indicative of which complication of emphysema?

1 Encephalopathy
2 Carbon dioxide narcosis
3 Carbon monoxide poisoning
4 Cerebral embolism

**Answer: 2**

*Rationale:* With late stage emphysema, the retention of carbon dioxide can lead to carbon dioxide narcosis. This is manifested by occipital headache, drowsiness, and inability to concentrate. Other signs are bounding pulse, arterial carbon dioxide level greater than 75 mm Hg, confusion, coma, and asterixis (flap tremor).

*Test-Taking Strategy:* Focus on the issue: a complication of emphysema and on the client's complaints. Recalling that emphysema is characterized by high carbon dioxide levels will direct you to option 2. Review the manifestations and complications associated with emphysema if you had difficulty with this question.

*Level of Cognitive Ability:* Analysis
*Client Needs:* Physiological Integrity
*Integrated Concept/Process:* Nursing Process/Analysis
*Content Area:* Adult Health/Respiratory

*Reference*
Monahan, F., & Neighbors, M. (1998). *Medical-surgical nursing: Foundations for clinical practice* (2nd ed.). Philadelphia: W.B. Saunders, pp. 670-671.

---

**443.** A nurse witnesses an accident in which a pedestrian is hit by an automobile. The nurse stops at the scene and assesses the victim. The nurse notes that the client is responsive and has suffered a flail chest involving at least three ribs. The nurse does which of the following to assist the client's respiratory status until help arrives?

1 Assists the victim to sit up
2 Turns the client onto the side with the flail chest
3 Removes the victim's shirt
4 Applies firm but gentle pressure with the hands to the flail segment

**Answer: 4**

*Rationale:* If significant flail chest is present, the nurse applies firm yet gentle pressure to the flail segments of the ribs to stabilize the chest wall, which will ultimately help the client's respiratory status. The nurse does not move an injured person for fear of worsening an undetected spinal injury. Removing the victim's shirt is of no value in this situation, and could in fact chill the victim, which is counterproductive. Injured persons should be kept warm until help arrives at the scene.

*Test-Taking Strategy:* Use knowledge of the principles of respiration and emergency nursing to answer this question. Eliminate options 1 and 2 because the client should not be moved. From the remaining options, recalling that the client should be kept warm will direct you to option 4. Review emergency care of the client with flail chest if you had difficulty with this question.

*Level of Cognitive Ability:* Application
*Client Needs:* Physiological Integrity
*Integrated Concept/Process:* Nursing Process/Implementation
*Content Area:* Adult Health/Respiratory

*Reference*
Monahan, F., & Neighbors, M. (1998). *Medical-surgical nursing: Foundations for clinical practice* (2nd ed.). Philadelphia: W.B. Saunders, p. 691.

---

**444.** A mental health nurse is assigned to care for a manic client. The nurse reviews the activity schedule for the day and determines that the best activity that this client could participate in is:

1. A brown-bag luncheon and a book review
2. Tetherball
3. Paint by number activity
4. Deep breathing and a progressive relaxation group

**Answer: 2**
*Rationale:* A person who is experiencing mania is overactive, full of energy, lacks concentration, and has poor impulse control. The client needs an activity that will allow him or her to utilize excess energy, yet not endanger others during the process. Options 1, 3 and 4 are relatively sedate activities that require concentration, a quality that is lacking in the manic state. Such activities may lead to increased frustration and anxiety for the client. Tetherball is an exercise that uses the large muscle groups of the body and is a great way to expend the increased energy this client is experiencing.

*Test-Taking Strategy:* Use the process of elimination and focus on the diagnosis of the client. Eliminate options 1, 3, and 4 because they are similar and are sedate activities. Review care of a client with mania if you had difficulty with this question.

*Level of Cognitive Ability:* Analysis
*Client Needs:* Physiological Integrity
*Integrated Concept/Process:* Nursing Process/Planning
*Content Area:* Mental Health

*Reference*
Stuart, G.W., & Laraia, M.T. (1998). *Principles and practice of psychiatric nursing.* (6th ed.). St. Louis: Mosby, p. 354.

---

**445.** A client who has seriously lacerated both wrists is brought to the emergency room by the police. The initial action that the nurse will take is to:

1. Assess and treat the wound sites
2. Secure and record a detailed history
3. Encourage and assist the client to ventilate feelings
4. Administer an antianxiety agent

**Answer: 1**
*Rationale:* The initial action when a client has attempted suicide is to assess and treat any injuries. Although options 2, 3, and 4 may be appropriate at some point, the initial action would be to treat the wounds.

*Test-Taking Strategy:* Use Maslow's Hierarchy of Needs theory to prioritize. Physiological needs come first. Option 1 is the only option that addresses a physiological need. Review initial care of the client who has attempted suicide if you had difficulty with this question.

*Level of Cognitive Ability:* Application
*Client Needs:* Physiological Integrity
*Integrated Concept/Process:* Nursing Process/Implementation
*Content Area:* Mental Health

*Reference*
Stuart, G.W., & Laraia, M.T. (1998). *Principles and practice of psychiatric nursing.* (6th ed.). St. Louis: Mosby, p. 389.

---

**446.** A nurse notes bilateral 2+ edema in the lower extremities of a client with known coronary artery disease who was admitted to the hospital 2 days ago. The nurse plans to do which of the following next after noting this finding?

1   Review the intake and output records for the last 2 days
2   Change the time of diuretic administration from morning to evening
3   Request a sodium restriction of 1 g/day from the physician
4   Order daily weights starting on the following morning

**Answer: 1**
*Rationale:* Edema is the accumulation of excess fluid in the interstitial spaces, which can be measured by intake greater than output, and by a sudden increase in weight (2.2 lb = 1 kg). Diuretics should be administered in the morning whenever possible to avoid nocturia. Strict sodium restrictions are reserved for clients with severe symptoms.

*Test-Taking Strategy:* Note the key word *next*. Use the steps of the nursing process. Option 1 can give the nurse immediate information about fluid balance. Review the manifestations associated with the complications of coronary artery disease if you had difficulty with this question.

*Level of Cognitive Ability:* Application
*Client Needs:* Physiological Integrity
*Integrated Concept/Process:* Nursing Process/Planning
*Content Area:* Adult Health/Cardiovascular

*Reference*
Smeltzer, S., & Bare, B. (2000). *Brunner & Suddarth's Textbook of medical-surgical nursing* (9th ed.). Philadelphia: Lippincott Williams & Wilkins, p. 542.

---

**447.** A nurse in the emergency room is assessing a client with chest pain. Which of the following observations by the nurse helps to determine that this pain is due to myocardial infarction (MI)?

1   The pain, unrelieved by nitroglycerin, was relieved with morphine sulfate
2   The pain was described as substernal and radiating to the left arm
3   The client experienced no nausea or vomiting
4   The client reports that the pain began while the client was pushing a lawnmower

**Answer: 1**
*Rationale:* The pain of angina may radiate to the left arm, is often precipitated by exertion or stress, has few associated symptoms, and is relieved by rest and nitroglycerin. The pain of MI may radiate to the left arm, shoulder, jaw, or neck. It typically begins spontaneously, lasts longer than 30 minutes, is frequently accompanied by associated symptoms (nausea, vomiting, dyspnea, diaphoresis, anxiety), and requires opioid analgesics for relief.

*Test-Taking Strategy:* Note the issue: pain caused by an MI. Recall that a classic hallmark of the pain from MI is that it is unrelieved by rest and nitroglycerin. Review the differences between angina and MI if you had difficulty with this question.

*Level of Cognitive Ability:* Analysis
*Client Needs:* Physiological Integrity

*Integrated Concept/Process:* Nursing Process/Analysis
*Content Area:* Adult Health/Cardiovascular

*Reference*
Ignatavicius, D., Workman, M., & Mishler, M. (1999). *Medical-surgical nursing across the health care continuum* (3rd ed.). Philadelphia: W.B. Saunders, p. 726.

**448.** A nurse is assessing a client hospitalized with acute pericarditis. The nurse monitors the client for cardiac tamponade knowing that which of the following is not associated with this complication of pericarditis?

1. Pulsus paradoxus
2. Distant heart sounds
3. Distended jugular veins
4. Bradycardia

**Answer: 4**

*Rationale:* Assessment findings with cardiac tamponade include tachycardia, distant or muffled heart sounds, jugular vein distention, and a falling blood pressure (BP), accompanied by pulsus paradoxus (a drop in inspiratory BP by greater than 10 mm Hg).

*Test-Taking Strategy:* Note the key word *not*. Think of the consequences of the pressure dynamics in the chest when the pericardial sac is rapidly filling with blood or fluid. The compensatory response would be tachycardia, not bradycardia. Review the signs of cardiac tamponade if you had difficulty with this question.

*Level of Cognitive Ability:* Analysis
*Client Needs:* Physiological Integrity
*Integrated Concept/Process:* Nursing Process/Assessment
*Content Area:* Adult Health/Cardiovascular

*Reference*
Smeltzer, S., & Bare, B. (2000) *Brunner & Suddarth's Textbook of medical-surgical nursing* (9th ed.). Philadelphia: Lippincott Williams & Wilkins, p. 485.

**449.** A nurse is assisting to position the client for pericardiocentesis to treat cardiac tamponade. The nurse positions the client:

1. Lying on left side with a pillow under the chest wall
2. Lying on right side with a pillow under the head
3. Supine with the head of bed elevated at a 45- to 60-degree angle
4. Supine with slight Trendelenburg position

**Answer: 3**

*Rationale:* The client undergoing pericardiocentesis is positioned supine with the head of bed raised to a 45- to 60-degree angle. This places the heart in close proximity to the chest wall for easier insertion of the needle into the pericardial sac. Options 1, 2, and 4 are incorrect positions.

*Test-Taking Strategy:* If you are uncertain how to proceed with this question, visualize each of the positions described. Evaluate how the heart is sitting in the chest with each position, and how easily the pericardial sac could be accessed with a needle. This will direct you to option 3. Review this procedure if you had difficulty with this question.

*Level of Cognitive Ability:* Application
*Client Needs:* Physiological Integrity
*Integrated Concept/Process:* Nursing Process/Implementation
*Content Area:* Adult Health/Cardiovascular

*Reference*
Smeltzer, S., & Bare, B. (2000) *Brunner & Suddarth's Textbook of medical-surgical nursing* (9th ed.). Philadelphia: Lippincott Williams & Wilkins, p. 675.

**450.** A client with multiple sclerosis is treated with diazepam (Valium) for painful muscle spasms. The nurse assesses the client for side effects of the medication and monitors the client for:

1. Urinary frequency
2. Headache
3. Increased salivation
4. Incoordination

**Answer: 4**
*Rationale:* Valium is a centrally acting skeletal muscle relaxant. Incoordination and drowsiness are common side effects resulting from the large doses of the medication that must be used to achieve desired effects. Options 1, 2, and 3 are not side effects.

*Test-Taking Strategy:* Use the process of elimination. Recalling that diazepam is used for muscle spasms will direct you to think that this medication relaxes muscles. The only option that directly relates to this medication action is option 4. Review the action and side effects of this medication if you had difficulty with this question.

*Level of Cognitive Ability:* Analysis
*Client Needs:* Physiological Integrity
*Integrated Concept/Process:* Nursing Process/Assessment
*Content Area:* Pharmacology

*Reference*
Hodgson, B., & Kizior, R. (2001). *Saunders Nursing drug handbook 2001.* Philadelphia: W.B. Saunders, p. 307.

**451.** A client with epilepsy is taking the prescribed dose of phenytoin (Dilantin) to control seizures. A dilantin blood level is drawn and the results reveal a level of 35 μg/mL. Which of the following effects would be expected as a result of this laboratory result?

1. No effects because this is a normal therapeutic dilantin level
2. Slurred speech
3. Tachycardia
4. Nystagmus

**Answer: 2**
*Rationale:* The therapeutic Dilantin level is 10 to 20 μg/mL. Blood levels of dilantin above 30 μg/mL produce slurred speech. Options 1, 3, and 4 are incorrect.

*Test-Taking Strategy:* Knowledge regarding the normal dilantin level and the signs that occur in the client when the level rises is required to answer this question. Review the signs associated with an elevated dilantin level if you had difficulty with this question.

*Level of Cognitive Ability:* Analysis
*Client Needs:* Physiological Integrity
*Integrated Concept/Process:* Nursing Process/Assessment
*Content Area:* Pharmacology

*Reference*
Hodgson, B., & Kizior, R. (2001). *Saunders Nursing drug handbook 2001.* Philadelphia: W.B. Saunders, p. 823.

**452.** A nurse is caring for a child following cleft palate repair. To reduce the risk of aspiration after feeding the child, the nurse places the child in which best position?

1. Right side
2. Left side
3. Supine
4. Prone

**Answer: 1**
*Rationale:* The child with cleft palate repair is placed on the right side after feeding to reduce the chance of aspirating regurgitated formula. Options 2, 3, and 4 are positions that would place the child at risk for aspiration.

*Test-Taking Strategy:* Visualize the anatomical location of the stomach in answering this question. This will assist in eliminating options 3 and 4. From the remaining options, remember that positioning on the right side will aid in absorption and reduce the risk of aspiration. Review care of a child following cleft palate repair if you had difficulty with this question.

*Level of Cognitive Ability:* Application
*Client Needs:* Physiological Integrity
*Integrated Concept/Process:* Nursing Process/Implementation
*Content Area:* Child Health

*Reference*
Wong, D. (1999). *Whaley & Wong's Nursing care of infants and children* (6th ed.). St. Louis: Mosby, p. 518.

**453.** A nurse is monitoring drainage from a nasogastric (NG) tube in a client who had a gastric resection. No drainage has been noted during the past 4 hours, and the client complains of severe nausea. The most appropriate nursing action would be to:
1  Reposition the tube
2  Irrigate the tube
3  Notify the physician
4  Medicate for nausea

**Answer: 3**
*Rationale:* Nausea and vomiting should not occur if the NG tube is patent. The NG tube should not be repositioned or irrigated after gastric surgery because it is placed directly over the suture line. The NG tube is irrigated gently with normal saline only with a physician's order. The client may need medication for the nausea, but in this situation the physician should be notified.

*Test-Taking Strategy:* Note that the client had a surgical procedure that involved the gastric area and that a nasogastric tube is placed in this surgical area. This will assist in eliminating options 1 and 2. From the remaining options, noting the key words *severe nausea* should alert you that the physician needs to be notified. Review postoperative nursing care following gastric surgery if you had difficulty with this question.

*Level of Cognitive Ability:* Application
*Client Needs:* Physiological Integrity
*Integrated Concept/Process:* Nursing Process/Implementation
*Content Area:* Adult Health/Gastrointestinal

*Reference*
Smeltzer, S., & Bare, B. (2000) *Brunner & Suddarth's Textbook of medical-surgical nursing* (9th ed.). Philadelphia: Lippincott Williams & Wilkins, p. 839.

**454.** A nurse explains to a mother that her newborn is being admitted to the neonatal intensive care unit with a probable diagnosis of fetal alcohol syndrome (FAS). The nurse explains the expected effects of FAS to the mother. The nurse evaluates the effectiveness of the explanation when the mother states:
1  "Withdrawal symptoms will occur after 3 days."
2  "Mental retardation is unlikely to happen."
3  "Withdrawal symptoms are tremors, crying, seizures, and reflexes that aren't normal."
4  "The reason the child is so large is because of the fetal alcohol syndrome."

**Answer: 3**
*Rationale:* The long-term prognosis for newborns with FAS is poor. Symptoms of withdrawal include tremors, sleeplessness, seizures, abdominal distention, hyperactivity, and uncontrollable crying. Central nervous system (CNS) disorders are the most common problems associated with FAS. Because of the CNS disorders, children born with FAS are often hyperactive and have a high incidence of speech and language disorders. Symptoms of withdrawal often occur within 6 to 12 hours after birth or at the latest, within the first 3 days of life. Most neonates with FAS are mildly to severely mentally retarded. The newborn is usually growth deficient at birth.

*Test-Taking Strategy:* Use the process of elimination and note the key words *effectiveness of the explanation.* Focus on the diagnosis FAS to eliminate options 2 and 4. From the remaining options, it is necessary to know that withdrawal symptoms can appear within 6 to 12 hours after birth or at the latest, within the first 3 days of life. Review the manifestations associated with FAS if you had difficulty with this question.

*Level of Cognitive Ability:* Analysis
*Client Needs:* Physiological Integrity
*Integrated Concept/Process:* Teaching/Learning
*Content Area:* Maternity

*Reference*
Lowdermilk, D., Perry, S., & Bobak, I. (2000). *Maternity & women's health care* (7th ed.). St. Louis: Mosby, p. 1059.

---

**455.** A client at 10 weeks' gestation is receiving prenatal care at a high-risk clinic. She is an insulin-dependent diabetic. The nurse teaches the client about the early signs of hyperglycemia. The nurse evaluates the teaching as effective when the client states that an early sign of hyperglycemia is:
1   Polyuria
2   Nervousness
3   Shakiness
4   Hunger

**Answer: 1**
*Rationale:* Polyuria is an early sign of hyperglycemia. Other signs can include polydipsia, dry mouth, increased appetite, fatigue, nausea, hot flushed skin, rapid deep breathing, abdominal cramps, acetone breath, headache, drowsiness, depressed reflexes, oliguria or anuria, stupor, and coma.

*Test-Taking Strategy:* Use the process of elimination. Options 2 and 3 are similar and are eliminated first. From the remaining options, recalling that hunger is a sign of hypoglycemia will assist in eliminating option 4. Review the signs of both hypoglycemia and hyperglycemia if you had difficulty with this question.

*Level of Cognitive Ability:* Analysis
*Client Needs:* Physiological Integrity
*Integrated Concept/Process:* Teaching/Learning
*Content Area:* Maternity

*Reference*
Lowdermilk, D., Perry, S., & Bobak, I. (2000). *Maternity & women's health care* (7th ed.). St. Louis: Mosby, p. 862.

---

**456.** A client recovering from a craniotomy complains of a "runny nose." The most important nursing action in this situation is to:
1   Provide the client with tissues
2   Tell the client to use the tissues for the drainage
3   Monitor the client for signs of a cold
4   Notify the physician

**Answer: 4**
*Rationale:* If the client has sustained a craniocerebral injury or is recovering from a craniotomy, careful observation of any drainage from the eyes, ears, nose, or traumatic area is critical. Cerebrospinal fluid is colorless and generally nonpurulent, and its presence is indicative of a serious breach of cranial integrity. Any suspicious drainage should be reported immediately.

*Test-Taking Strategy:* Note the key words *most important*. This should provide you with the clue that the situation presented is serious in nature. Eliminate options 1 and 2 because they are similar. From the remaining options, recalling the signs of complications associated with craniotomy should direct you to option 4. Review postoperative nursing care following craniotomy if you had difficulty with this question.

*Level of Cognitive Ability:* Application
*Client Needs:* Physiological Integrity
*Integrated Concept/Process:* Nursing Process/Implementation
*Content Area:* Adult Health/Neurological

*Reference*
Smeltzer, S., & Bare, B. (2000) *Brunner & Suddarth's Textbook of medical-surgical nursing* (9th ed.). Philadelphia: Lippincott Williams & Wilkins, p. 1662.

---

**457.** A nurse is caring for a client who has returned from the postanesthesia care unit following prostatectomy. The client has a three-way Foley catheter with infusion of continuous bladder irrigation. The nurse assesses that the flow rate is adequate if the color of the urinary drainage is:

1  Dark cherry colored
2  Concentrated yellow with small clots
3  Clear as water
4  Pale yellow or slightly pink

**Answer: 4**
*Rationale:* The infusion of bladder irrigant is not at a preset rate, but rather it is increased or decreased to maintain urine that is a clear, pale yellow color or that has just a slight pink tinge. The infusion rate should be increased if the drainage is cherry colored or if clots are seen. Correspondingly, the rate can be slowed down slightly if the returns are as clear as water.

*Test-Taking Strategy:* Use the process of elimination. Eliminate option 2 as the least realistic of all the urine characteristics described. Next, eliminate options 1 and 3 as reflecting inadequate and excessive flow, respectively. With proper flow rate of bladder irrigant, the urine should be pale yellow or pale pink. Review care of a client following prostatectomy if you had difficulty with this question.

*Level of Cognitive Ability:* Analysis
*Client Needs:* Physiological Integrity
*Integrated Concept/Process:* Nursing Process/Assessment
*Content Area:* Adult Health /Renal

*Reference*
Smeltzer, S., & Bare, B. (2000) *Brunner & Suddarth's Textbook of medical-surgical nursing* (9th ed.). Philadelphia: Lippincott Williams & Wilkins, p. 1316.

---

**458.** A nurse is assessing a client who is at risk of developing acute renal failure (ARF). The nurse would become most concerned if which of the following assessments was made?

1  Urine output 30 mL/hr for the last 3 hours, blood urea nitrogen (BUN) 10 mg/dL, creatinine 1.2 mg/dL
2  Urine output 40 mL/hr for the last 3 hours, BUN 15 mg/dL, creatinine 0.8 mg/dL
3  Urine output 20 mL/hr for the last 3 hours, BUN 35 mg/dL, creatinine 2.1 mg/dL
4  Urine output 60 mL/hr for the last 3 hours, BUN 40 mg/dL, creatinine 1.1 mg/dL

**Answer: 3**
*Rationale:* With acute renal failure, the client is often oliguric or anuric, although the client may have nonoliguric renal failure. The BUN and serum creatinine levels also rise, indicating defective kidney function. Normal serum BUN levels are usually 5 to 20 mg/dL. Normal creatinine levels range from 0.6 to 1.3 mg/dL. The client who has the greatest abnormality in urine output and laboratory values is the client in option 3. This is the client who is most at risk for the development of renal failure.

*Test-Taking Strategy:* Focus on the issue: development of renal failure. Recalling the normal BUN and creatinine levels and that the minimum required hourly urine output is 30 mL will direct you to option 3. Review these normal values and the signs of renal failure if you had difficulty with this question.

*Level of Cognitive Ability:* Analysis
*Client Needs:* Physiological Integrity

*Integrated Concept/Process:* Nursing Process/Assessment
*Content Area:* Adult Health/Renal

*Reference*
Smeltzer, S., & Bare, B. (2000) *Brunner & Suddarth's Textbook of medical-surgical nursing* (9th ed.). Philadelphia: Lippincott Williams & Wilkins, p. 1147.

---

**459.** A client with acute renal failure has been treated with sodium polystyrene sulfonate (Kayexalate) by mouth. The nurse would evaluate this therapy as effective if which of the following values was noted on follow-up laboratory testing?
1   Potassium 4.9 mEq/L
2   Sodium 142 mEq/L
3   Phosphorus 3.9 mg/dL
4   Calcium 9.8 mg/dL

**Answer: 1**
*Rationale:* Of all the electrolyte imbalances that accompany renal failure, hyperkalemia is the most dangerous because it can lead to cardiac dysrhythmias and death. If the potassium level rises too high, Kayexalate may be administered to cause excretion of potassium through the gastrointestinal tract. Each of the electrolyte levels noted in the options falls within the normal reference range for that electrolyte. The potassium level, however, is measured following administration of this medication to note the extent of its effectiveness.

*Test-Taking Strategy:* Use the process of elimination and knowledge regarding the purpose of this medication. Note the name of the medication (Kayexalate) and its relationship to option 1. If you had difficulty with this question, review this medication.

*Level of Cognitive Ability:* Analysis
*Client Needs:* Physiological Integrity
*Integrated Concept/Process:* Nursing Process/Evaluation
*Content Area:* Adult Health/Renal

*Reference*
Smeltzer, S., & Bare, B. (2000) *Brunner & Suddarth's Textbook of medical-surgical nursing* (9th ed.). Philadelphia: Lippincott Williams & Wilkins, p. 1147.

---

**460.** A nurse is admitting a client with chronic renal failure (CRF) to the nursing unit. The nurse assesses for which of the following most frequent cardiovascular signs that occurs in the client with CRF?
1   Hypertension
2   Hypotension
3   Tachycardia
4   Bradycardia

**Answer: 1**
*Rationale:* Hypertension is the most common cardiovascular finding in the client with CRF. It is due to a number of mechanisms, including volume overload, renin-angiotensin system stimulation, vasoconstriction from sympathetic stimulation, and the absence of prostaglandins. Hypertension may also be the cause of the renal failure. It is an important item to assess because hypertension can lead to heart failure in the CRF client because of increased cardiac workload in conjunction with fluid overload.

*Test-Taking Strategy:* Use the process of elimination. Recalling that the blood pressure is the key item to assess helps you to eliminate options 3 and 4. From the remaining options, recall the functions of the renal system and the kidneys to direct you to option 1. Review manifestations of CRF if you had difficulty with this question.

*Level of Cognitive Ability:* Analysis
*Client Needs:* Physiological Integrity
*Integrated Concept/Process:* Nursing Process/Assessment
*Content Area:* Adult Health/Renal

*Reference*
Smeltzer, S., & Bare, B. (2000). *Brunner & Suddarth's Textbook of medical-surgical nursing* (9th ed.). Philadelphia: Lippincott Williams & Wilkins, p. 1151.

---

**461.** A client has sustained a closed fracture and has just had a cast applied to the affected arm. The client is complaining of intense pain. The nurse has elevated the limb, applied an ice bag, and administered an analgesic, which has provided very little relief. The nurse interprets that this pain may be due to:

1    Impaired tissue perfusion
2    The newness of the fracture
3    The anxiety of the client
4    Infection under the cast

**Answer: 1**
*Rationale:* Most pain associated with fractures can be minimized with rest, elevation, application of cold, and the administration of analgesics. Pain that is not relieved from these measures should be reported to the physician, because it may be due to impaired tissue perfusion, tissue breakdown, or necrosis. Since this is a new closed fracture and cast, infection would not have had time to set in.

*Test-Taking Strategy:* Use the process of elimination. Focus on the information in the question to eliminate options 2 and 3. Since the fracture and cast are so new, it is extremely unlikely that infection could have set in. Therefore eliminate option 4. Review the complications associated with a casted extremity if you had difficulty with this question.

*Level of Cognitive Ability:* Analysis
*Client Needs:* Physiological Integrity
*Integrated Concept/Process:* Nursing Process/Analysis
*Content Area:* Adult Health/Musculoskeletal

*Reference*
Smeltzer, S., & Bare, B. (2000) *Brunner & Suddarth's Textbook of medical-surgical nursing* (9th ed.). Philadelphia: Lippincott Williams & Wilkins, p. 1780.

---

**462.** The client with a fractured femur experiences sudden dyspnea. A set of arterial blood gases reveal the following: pH 7.32, $Paco_2$ 43, $Pao_2$ 58, $HCO_3$ 20. The nurse interprets that the client probably has experienced fat embolus because of the:

1    $Paco_2$
2    $Pao_2$
3    $HCO_3$
4    pH

**Answer: 2**
*Rationale:* A key feature of fat embolism is a significant degree of hypoxemia, with a $Pao_2$ often less than 60 mm Hg. Other features that distinguish fat embolism from pulmonary embolism are an elevated temperature and the presence of fat in the blood with fat embolus.

*Test-Taking Strategy:* Use the process of elimination. Recalling that fat embolus causes significant hypoxemia will direct you to option 2. Review the manifestations associated with this disorder if you had difficulty with this question.

*Level of Cognitive Ability:* Analysis
*Client Needs:* Physiological Integrity
*Integrated Concept/Process:* Nursing Process/Analysis
*Content Area:* Adult Health/Musculoskeletal

*Reference*
Smeltzer, S., & Bare, B. (2000) *Brunner & Suddarth's Textbook of medical-surgical nursing* (9th ed.). Philadelphia: Lippincott Williams & Wilkins, p. 1837.

**463.** Mannitol (Osmitrol) is administered intravenously to a client admitted to the hospital with loss of consciousness and a closed head injury. The nurse would evaluate the medication was most effective if which of the following outcomes was noted?

1  Diuresis of 500 mL in 2 hours and a blood urea nitrogen (BUN) level of 15 mg/dL
2  Improved level of consciousness and normal intracranial pressure
3  Weight loss of 1 kg and a serum creatinine level of 0.8 mg/dL
4  Serum creatinine level of 1.2 mg/dL and normal intracranial pressure

**Answer: 2**

*Rationale:* Mannitol (Osmitrol) is an osmotic diuretic that can be administered parenterally to treat cerebral edema. Lowering of intracranial pressure occurs within 15 minutes of administration, and diuresis occurs within 1 to 3 hours. Expected effects of the medication include rapid diuresis and fluid loss. For the client with cerebral edema (as in closed head injury), effectiveness is measured by assessing neurological status and intracranial pressure readings.

*Test-Taking Strategy:* Note the key words *most effective* in the stem of the question. This tells you that more than one option is partially or totally correct. Note the relationship between "loss of consciousness" in the question and the correct option. Review this medication if you had difficulty with this question.

*Level of Cognitive Ability:* Analysis
*Client Needs:* Physiological Integrity
*Integrated Concept/Process:* Nursing Process/Evaluation
*Content Area:* Pharmacology

*Reference*
Hodgson, B., & Kizior, R. (2001). *Saunders Nursing drug handbook 2001.* Philadelphia: W.B. Saunders, p. 1141.

**464.** A nurse is caring for a client with a history of renal insufficiency who is having captopril (Capoten) added to the medication regimen. Before administering the first dose, the nurse reviews the medical record for the results of urinalysis, especially noting for the presence of:

1  Casts
2  Red blood cells (RBCs)
3  Protein
4  White blood cells (WBCs)

**Answer: 3**

*Rationale:* Captopril is an angiotensin converting enzyme (ACE) inhibitor that is used for clients who do not respond to the first-line antihypertensive agents. ACE inhibitors are used cautiously in clients with renal impairment. Before treatment begins, baseline assessment of blood pressure, complete white cell count, and urine protein is performed. Nephrotic syndrome may develop in clients with renal insufficiency, so the client may be monitored for proteinuria on a monthly basis for 9 months, and periodically afterward.

*Test-Taking Strategy:* Note the information in the question. The question tells you that the client has renal impairment and directs you to look at urinalysis results. RBCs and WBCs could be indications of trauma or infection, so these options should be eliminated first. Eliminate option 1 because casts are mineral deposits that form along the renal tubules and occasionally appear in the urine. Normally the kidneys conserve large protein molecules, which makes the presence of proteinuria abnormal. Review this medication if you had difficulty with this question.

*Level of Cognitive Ability:* Analysis
*Client Needs:* Physiological Integrity
*Integrated Concept/Process:* Nursing Process/Assessment
*Content Area:* Pharmacology

*Reference*
Hodgson, B., & Kizior, R. (2001). *Saunders Nursing drug handbook 2001.* Philadelphia: W.B. Saunders, p. 142.

**465.** A nurse assesses a client with chronic arterial insufficiency. After walking three blocks the client complains of leg pain and cramping, which are relieved when the client stops and rests. The nurse documents that the client is experiencing:

1    Arterial-venous shunting
2    Deep vein thrombosis
3    Intermittent claudication
4    Venous insufficiency

**Answer: 3**

*Rationale:* Intermittent claudication is a classic symptom of peripheral vascular disease, also known by other names, including peripheral arterial disease and chronic arterial insufficiency. It is described as a cramplike pain that occurs with exercise and is relieved by rest. Intermittent claudication is due to ischemia and is very reproducible; that is, a predictable amount of exercise causes the pain each time. Options 1, 2, and 4 are incorrect.

*Test-Taking Strategy:* Use the process of elimination. Note that the question indicates that the client has an arterial disorder. This eliminates option 2 and 4. From the remaining options, noting the relationship between the timing in the question and the word *intermittent* in option 3 will direct you to this option. Review intermittent claudication if you had difficulty with this question.

*Level of Cognitive Ability:* Application
*Client Needs:* Physiological Integrity
*Integrated Concept/Process:* Communication and Documentation
*Content Area:* Adult Health/Cardiovascular

*Reference*
Smeltzer, S., & Bare, B. (2000) *Brunner & Suddarth's Textbook of medical-surgical nursing* (9th ed.). Philadelphia: Lippincott Williams & Wilkins, p. 683.

**466.** A nurse is caring for a client with cancer who is receiving daunorubicin (Cerubidine) intravenously. The nurse monitors the client for:

1    Hypertension
2    Polycythemia
3    Nausea and vomiting
4    Hypovolemia

**Answer: 3**

*Rationale:* Daunorubicin is an antineoplastic medication. The major gastrointestinal (GI) side effects include nausea, vomiting, stomatitis, and esophagitis. Cardiovascular side effects include congestive heart failure and dysrhythmias. Other frequently occurring side effects are alopecia and bone marrow depression.

*Test-Taking Strategy:* Focusing on the client's diagnosis will assist in determining that the medication is an antineoplastic. Recalling that antineoplastics commonly cause GI side effects will direct you to option 3. Review the side effects of this medication if you had difficulty with this question.

*Level of Cognitive Ability:* Application
*Client Needs:* Physiological Integrity
*Integrated Concept/Process:* Nursing Process/Assessment
*Content Area:* Pharmacology

*Reference*
Hodgson, B., & Kizior, R. (2001). *Saunders Nursing drug handbook 2001.* Philadelphia: W.B. Saunders, pp. 286-289.

**467.** A home health nurse is visiting a client who was discharged to home with orders for continued administration of enoxaparin (Lovenox) 30 mg BID subcutaneously. On assessment, the nurse questions the client about which of the following highest priority items?
1  Fear of needles
2  Bleeding gums or bruising
3  Constipation
4  Nausea or vomiting

**Answer: 2**
*Rationale:* Enoxaparin is an anticoagulant. A common side effect of anticoagulant therapy is bleeding. Because of this, the nurse questions the client about symptoms that could indicate bleeding, such as bleeding gums, bruising, hematuria, or dark tarry stools.

*Test-Taking Strategy:* Use the process of elimination. Recalling that this medication is an anticoagulant will assist in eliminating options 3 and 4 first. From the remaining options, noting the key words *highest priority* will direct you to option 2. Review this medication if you had difficulty with this question.

*Level of Cognitive Ability:* Application
*Client Needs:* Physiological Integrity
*Integrated Concept/Process:* Nursing Process/Assessment
*Content Area:* Pharmacology

*Reference*
Hodgson, B., & Kizior, R. (2001). *Saunders Nursing drug handbook 2001.* Philadelphia: W.B. Saunders, pp. 265-366.

---

**468.** A client has been given a prescription for sulfasalazine (Azulfidine) for the treatment of ulcerative colitis. Before teaching the client about the medication, the nurse asks the client about a history of allergy to:
1  Salicylates or acetaminophen
2  Sulfonamides or salicylates
3  Shellfish or calcium channel blockers
4  Histamine receptor antagonists or beta blockers

**Answer: 2**
*Rationale:* The client who has been prescribed sulfasalazine should be checked for history of allergy to either sulfonamides or salicylates because the chemical compositions of sulfasalazine and these medications are similar. The other options are incorrect.

*Test-Taking Strategy:* Focus on the issue: history of allergy. Note the relationship of *sulfasalazine* in the question and *sulfonamides* in the correct option. Review information about this medication if you had difficulty with this question.

*Level of Cognitive Ability:* Application
*Client Needs:* Physiological Integrity
*Integrated Concept/Process:* Nursing Process/Assessment
*Content Area:* Pharmacology

*Reference*
Hodgson, B., & Kizior, R. (2001). *Saunders Nursing drug handbook 2001.* Philadelphia: W.B. Saunders, pp. 953-955.

---

**469.** A nurse is caring for a client with a nursing diagnosis of Altered Oral Mucous Membranes. The nurse would avoid using which of the following items when giving mouth care of this client?
1  Nonalcoholic mouthwash
2  Soft toothbrush
3  Lip moistener
4  Lemon-glycerin swabs

**Answer: 4**
*Rationale:* The nurse avoids using lemon-glycerin swabs for the client with altered oral mucous membranes because they dry the membranes further and could cause pain. Items that are helpful include a soft toothbrush to prevent trauma, lip moistener to prevent lip cracking, and soothing cleansing rinses, such as nonalcoholic mouthwash and 1:1 saline and hydrogen peroxide mixture.

*Test-Taking Strategy:* Note the key word *avoid.* Use the process of elimination focusing on the client's diagnosis. Evaluate each of the options in terms of the likelihood of causing trauma to at-risk tissue. This approach will direct you to option 4. Review care of a client with altered oral mucous membranes if you had difficulty with this question.

*Level of Cognitive Ability:* Application
*Client Needs:* Physiological Integrity
*Integrated Concept/Process:* Nursing Process/Implementation
*Content Area:* Fundamental Skills

*Reference*
Ignatavicius, D., Workman, M., & Mishler, M. (1999). *Medical-surgical nursing across the health care continuum* (3rd ed.). Philadelphia: W.B. Saunders, p. 506.

---

**470.** A nurse has an order to administer 20 mEq of potassium to a client with a potassium level of 3 mEq/L. The nurse draws up this medication knowing that it will be administered:
1　After dilution in an intravenous solution
2　Directly by IV push
3　Intramuscularly
4　Subcutaneously

**Answer: 1**
*Rationale:* Potassium chloride may be administered by the intravenous route when the client has moderate to severe hypokalemia. It is always diluted in intravenous solution; administration by IV push could cause death by cardiac arrest. It is not administered intramuscularly or subcutaneously. Intravenous potassium should be administered through an infusion pump. A cardiac monitor should also be in use when administering intravenous potassium.

*Test-Taking Strategy:* Use basic knowledge of electrolyte replacement and medication administration to answer this question. Recalling the physiology of the cardiac conduction system and the effects of potassium on the heart will direct you to the correct option. If this question was difficult, review the procedure for administering potassium.

*Level of Cognitive Ability:* Application
*Client Needs:* Physiological Integrity
*Integrated Concept/Process:* Nursing Process/Implementation
*Content Area:* Pharmacology

*Reference*
Hodgson, B., & Kizior, R. (2001). *Saunders Nursing drug handbook 2001.* Philadelphia: W.B. Saunders, p. 846.

---

**471.** A nurse has an order to administer two ophthalmic medications to the client who has undergone eye surgery. The nurse waits how many minutes after the first medication before giving the second?
1　It is not necessary to wait; the second medication can be administered immediately
2　1 to 2
3　3 to 5
4　8 to 10

**Answer: 3**
*Rationale:* The nurse waits 3 to 5 minutes between administration of the two separate ophthalmic medications. This allows for adequate ocular absorption of the medication and prevents the second medication from flushing out the first.

*Test-Taking Strategy:* Use the process of elimination. Eliminate option 1 because it does not address the issue of the question. Next, eliminate option 4 because of the lengthy time frame. From the remaining options, recalling that time is needed for ocular absorption will direct you to option 3. If needed, review the principles of ocular medication administration.

*Level of Cognitive Ability:* Application
*Client Needs:* Physiological Integrity
*Integrated Concept/Process:* Nursing Process/Implementation
*Content Area:* Adult Health/Eye

### Reference

Smeltzer, S., & Bare, B. (2000). *Brunner & Suddarth's Textbook of medical-surgical nursing* (9th ed.). Philadelphia: Lippincott Williams & Wilkins, p. 1574.

---

**472.** A client has a pH of 7.51 with a bicarbonate level of 29 mEq/L. The nurse prepares to administer which of the following medications that would be ordered to treat this acid-base disorder?

1  Sodium bicarbonate
2  Furosemide (Lasix)
3  Acetazolamide (Diamox)
4  Spironolactone (Aldactone)

**Answer: 3**

*Rationale:* Acetazolamide is a diuretic used in the treatment of metabolic alkalosis. This medication causes excretion of sodium, potassium, bicarbonate, and water by inhibiting the action of carbonic anhydrase. Administration of sodium bicarbonate would aggravate the already existing condition and is contraindicated. Furosemide and spironolactone are loop and potassium-sparing diuretics, respectively. These have no value when excretion of bicarbonate is needed.

*Test-Taking Strategy:* Begin to answer this question by interpreting that the acid-base disorder is metabolic alkalosis. Eliminate option 1 first based on this interpretation. From the remaining options, it is necessary to know which diuretic is used to treat metabolic alkalosis. Review the treatment for this acid-base disorder if you had difficulty with this question.

*Level of Cognitive Ability:* Application
*Client Needs:* Physiological Integrity
*Integrated Concept/Process:* Nursing Process/Planning
*Content Area:* Fundamental Skills

### Reference

Hodgson, B., & Kizior, R. (2001). *Saunders Nursing drug handbook 2001.* Philadelphia: W.B. Saunders, p. 8.

---

**473.** A client is admitted to the hospital in metabolic acidosis caused by diabetic ketoacidosis (DKA). The nurse prepares to administer which of the following medications as a primary initial treatment for this problem?

1  Sodium bicarbonate
2  Calcium gluconate
3  Potassium
4  Insulin

**Answer: 4**

*Rationale:* The primary treatment for any acid-base imbalance is treatment of the underlying disorder that caused the problem. In this case the underlying cause of the metabolic acidosis is anaerobic metabolism resulting from lack of ability to use circulating glucose. Administration of insulin corrects this problem. Potassium may be added to the treatment regimen if serum potassium levels indicate its need. Options 1 and 2 would not be used to treat this disorder.

*Test-Taking Strategy:* Focus on the client's diagnosis, diabetic ketoacidosis. Noting the diagnosis and the key words *primary initial treatment* will direct you to option 4. Review the treatment for DKA if you had difficulty with this question.

*Level of Cognitive Ability:* Application
*Client Needs:* Physiological Integrity
*Integrated Concept/Process:* Nursing Process/Planning
*Content Area:* Fundamental Skills

*Reference*
Smeltzer, S., & Bare, B. (2000) *Brunner & Suddarth's Textbook of medical-surgical nursing* (9th ed.). Philadelphia: Lippincott Williams & Wilkins, p. 1004.

---

**474.** A client is diagnosed with respiratory alkalosis induced by gram-negative sepsis. The nurse carries out which of the following prescribed measures as the most effective means to treat the problem?
1  Administers prescribed antibiotics
2  Administers PRN antipyretics
3  Has the client breathe into a paper bag
4  Requests an order for a partial rebreather oxygen mask

**Answer: 1**
*Rationale:* The most effective way to treat an acid-base disorder is to treat the underlying cause of the disorder. In this case the problem is sepsis, which is most effectively treated with antibiotic therapy. Antipyretics will control fever secondary to sepsis but do nothing to treat the acid-base balance. The paper bag and partial rebreather mask will assist the client to rebreathe exhaled carbon dioxide, but again, these do not treat the primary cause of the imbalance.

*Test-Taking Strategy:* Note the key words *sepsis* and *most effective.* Recalling that the most effective treatment of acid-base imbalances involves treatment of the primary cause will direct you to option 1. Remember, sepsis is a systemic infection and is treated with antibiotics. Review the treatment for respiratory alkalosis and sepsis if you had difficulty with this question.

*Level of Cognitive Ability:* Application
*Client Needs:* Physiological Integrity
*Integrated Concept/Process:* Nursing Process/Planning
*Content Area:* Fundamental Skills

*Reference*
Ignatavicius, D., Workman, M., & Mishler, M. (1999). *Medical-surgical nursing across the health care continuum* (3rd ed.). Philadelphia: W.B. Saunders, p. 673.

---

**475.** A client receiving lithium therapy is noted to be drowsy, has slurred speech, and is experiencing muscle twitching and impaired coordination. Which of the following actions should be taken by the nurse?
1  Double the next lithium dose
2  Increase fluids to 2000 mL/day
3  Hold one dose of lithium
4  Call the physician

**Answer: 4**
*Rationale:* Signs and symptoms of lithium toxicity include vomiting, diarrhea, and nervous system changes such as slurred speech, incoordination, drowsiness, muscle weakness, and twitching. Before any further doses are administered, the physician should be notified. As long as no contraindications exist, the client should routinely take in between 2000 to 3000 mL of fluid per day while taking this medication.

*Test-Taking Strategy:* Use the process of elimination. Eliminate options 1 and 3 first because it is not common practice to either hold one dose or double a medication dose without a specific order. From the remaining options, focusing on the client's symptoms will direct you to option 4. Review the signs of toxicity of this medication if you had difficulty with this question.

*Level of Cognitive Ability:* Application
*Client Needs:* Physiological Integrity
*Integrated Concept/Process:* Nursing Process/Implementation
*Content Area:* Pharmacology

*Reference*
Hodgson, B., & Kizior, R. (2001). *Saunders Nursing drug handbook 2001.* Philadelphia: W.B. Saunders, p. 598.

**476.** A client has been started on medication therapy with metoclopramide (Reglan). The nurse monitors which of the following items to determine effectiveness of therapy?
1 Urine output
2 Breath sounds
3 Complaints of headache
4 Episodes of vomiting

**Answer: 4**
*Rationale:* Metoclopramide is an antiemetic. The nurse would monitor to see whether the client has experienced a decrease or absence of vomiting to determine the effectiveness of therapy. Options 1, 2, and 3 are unrelated to the action of this medication.

*Test-Taking Strategy:* Use the process of elimination. Recalling that metoclopramide is an antiemetic will direct you to option 4. Review the action of this medication if you had difficulty with this question.

*Level of Cognitive Ability:* Application
*Client Needs:* Physiological Integrity
*Integrated Concept/Process:* Nursing Process/Evaluation
*Content Area:* Pharmacology

*Reference*
Hodgson, B., & Kizior, R. (2001). *Saunders Nursing drug handbook 2001.* Philadelphia: W.B. Saunders, p. 671.

**477.** A nurse is preparing to administer an intramuscular injection to a 2-year-old child. The best site to select for the injection is the:
1 Ventral gluteal muscle
2 Dorsal gluteal muscle
3 Deltoid muscle
4 Vastus lateralis muscle

**Answer: 4**
*Rationale:* The vastus lateralis muscle is well developed at birth. It is the best choice for all age groups but should always be used in children younger than 3 years of age. This muscle is able to tolerate larger volumes and is not located near vital structures such as nerves and blood vessels.

*Test-Taking Strategy:* Use the process of elimination. Eliminate options 1 and 2 because they are similar. From the remaining options, recall that the deltoid is a smaller muscle close to important nerves and is generally not a preferred site for intramuscular injection. If you had difficulty with this question, review the procedure for administering intramuscular injections to a 2-year-old.

*Level of Cognitive Ability:* Application
*Client Needs:* Physiological Integrity
*Integrated Concept/Process:* Nursing Process/Implementation
*Content Area:* Fundamental Skills

*Reference*
Wong, D. (1999). *Whaley & Wong's Nursing care of infants and children* (6th ed.). St. Louis: Mosby, p. 1263.

**478.** A nurse is developing a plan of care for a school-aged child with a knowledge deficit related to use of inhalers and peak flow meters. An appropriate expected outcome is that the child will:

1. Express feelings of mastery and competence with the breathing devices
2. Have regular respirations at a rate of 18 to 22 breaths/min
3. Deny shortness of breath or difficulty breathing
4. Be encouraged to watch the educational video and read the printed information provided

**Answer: 1**

*Rationale:* School-aged children strive for mastery and competence to achieve the developmental task of industry and accomplishment. Options 2 and 3 do not relate to the knowledge deficit. Option 4 is an intervention rather than an outcome.

*Test-Taking Strategy:* Focus on the issue: an expected outcome. Eliminate options 2 and 3 because they are similar. From the remaining options, eliminate option 4 because it is an intervention rather than an outcome. Also noting that the child is school-aged will direct you to option 1. If you had difficulty with this question, review development tasks of the school-aged child.

*Level of Cognitive Ability:* Analysis
*Client Needs:* Physiological Integrity
*Integrated Concept/Process:* Nursing Process/Planning
*Content Area:* Child Health

*Reference*
Wong, D. (1999). *Whaley & Wong's Nursing care of infants and children* (6th ed.). St. Louis: Mosby, p. 777.

---

**479.** A nurse is caring for a client who is receiving lithium carbonate (Lithium). The measured lithium level is 1.8 mEq/L. The nurse analyzes this result as:

1. Within normal limits
2. Higher than normal limits, indicating toxicity
3. Lower than normal limits
4. Insignificant

**Answer: 2**

*Rationale:* The therapeutic level for lithium is 0.8 to 1.2 mEq/L. A level of 1.8 mEq/L indicates toxicity and necessitates that the medication be withheld and the blood work repeated. The physician should be notified.

*Test-Taking Strategy:* Knowledge regarding the therapeutic lithium level is required to answer this question. If you are unfamiliar with this level, review this content.

*Level of Cognitive Ability:* Analysis
*Client Needs:* Physiological Integrity
*Integrated Concept/Process:* Nursing Process/Analysis
*Content Area:* Pharmacology

*Reference*
Hodgson, B., & Kizior, R. (2001). *Saunders Nursing drug handbook 2001.* Philadelphia: W.B. Saunders, pp. 598-600.

CHAPTER 7 Physiological Integrity 381

**480.** A client calls the ambulatory care clinic and tells a nurse that she found an area that looks like the peel of an orange when performing breast self-examination (BSE) but found no other changes. The nurse should:
1  Tell the client there is nothing to worry about
2  Arrange for the client to be seen at the clinic as soon as possible
3  Tell the client to take her temperature and call back if she has a fever
4  Tell the client to point out the area to the physician at her next regularly scheduled appointment

**Answer: 2**
*Rationale:* Peau d'orange, an orange-peel appearance of the skin over the breast, is associated with late breast cancer. Therefore the nurse would arrange for the client to come to the clinic at the earliest time possible. Peau d'orange is not indicative of an infection.

*Test-Taking Strategy:* Use the process of elimination. Eliminate options 1 and 4 because they are similar. From the remaining options, focus on the client's description to direct you to option 2. If you had difficulty with this question, review the signs of breast cancer.

*Level of Cognitive Ability:* Application
*Client Needs:* Physiological Integrity
*Integrated Concept/Process:* Nursing Process/Implementation
*Content Area:* Adult Health/Oncology

*Reference*
Smeltzer, S., & Bare, B. (2000) *Brunner & Suddarth's Textbook of medical-surgical nursing* (9th ed.). Philadelphia: Lippincott Williams & Wilkins, p. 1272.

---

**481.** A nurse instructs a client about the procedure to perform the Breast Self-Examination (BSE). Which client statement indicates a need for further instructions?
1  "I don't need to do that, I'm too old for that."
2  "I do BSE 7 days after I get my period."
3  "I examine my breasts in the shower."
4  "I lie on my back to examine my breasts."

**Answer: 1**
*Rationale:* BSE should still be done even after menopause. No one is "too old" to get breast cancer. Options 2, 3, and 4 identify correct components of performing BSE.

*Test-Taking Strategy:* Use the process of elimination, noting the key words *need for further instructions*. Recalling that BSE should be performed even after menopause will direct you to option 1. If you had difficulty with this question or are unfamiliar with this procedure, review this content.

*Level of Cognitive Ability:* Analysis
*Client Needs:* Physiological Integrity
*Integrated Concept/Process:* Teaching/Learning
*Content Area:* Fundamental Skills

*Reference*
Smeltzer, S., & Bare, B. (2000) *Brunner & Suddarth's Textbook of medical-surgical nursing* (9th ed.). Philadelphia: Lippincott Williams & Wilkins, p. 1263.

---

**482.** A client with Cushing's syndrome is being instructed by the nurse on follow-up care. Which of these statements, if made by the client, would indicate a need for further instructions?
1  "I should avoid contact sports."
2  "I need to avoid foods high in potassium."
3  "I should check my ankles for swelling."
4  "I need to check my blood glucose regularly."

**Answer: 2**
*Rationale:* Hypokalemia is a common characteristic of Cushing's syndrome and the client is instructed to consume foods high in potassium. Clients experience activity intolerance, osteoporosis, and frequent bruising. Fluid volume excess results from water and sodium retention. Hyperglycemia is caused by an increased cortisol secretion.

*Test-Taking Strategy:* Note the key words *need for further instructions*. Recalling that hypokalemia is a concern will direct you to option 2. If you had difficulty with this question, review this disorder.

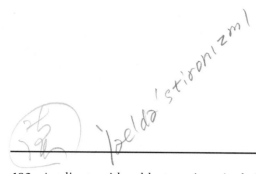

*Level of Cognitive Ability:* Analysis
*Client Needs:* Physiological Integrity
*Integrated Concept/Process:* Teaching/Learning
*Content Area:* Adult Health/Endocrine

**Reference**
Smeltzer, S., & Bare, B. (2000) *Brunner & Suddarth's Textbook of medical-surgical nursing* (9th ed.). Philadelphia: Lippincott Williams & Wilkins, p. 1060.

**483.** A client with aldosteronism is being treated with spironolactone (Aldactone). Which of the following indicates to the nurse that the medication is effective?
1   A decrease in blood pressure
2   A decrease in sodium excretion
3   A decrease in plasma potassium
4   A decrease in body metabolism

**Answer: 1**
*Rationale:* Aldactone antagonizes the effect of aldosterone and decreases circulating volume by inhibiting tubular reabsorption of sodium and water. Thus it produces a decrease in blood pressure. It increases potassium retention and promotes sodium and water excretion. It has no effect on body metabolism.

*Test-Taking Strategy:* Note the key words *medication is effective.* Think about the action of this medication. Recalling that this medication is also used in hypertensive conditions will direct you to option 1. If you had difficulty with this question, review the effects of this medication.

*Level of Cognitive Ability:* Analysis
*Client Needs:* Physiological Integrity
*Integrated Concept/Process:* Nursing Process/Evaluation
*Content Area:* Adult Health/Endocrine

**Reference**
Hodgson, B., & Kizior, R. (2001). *Saunders Nursing drug handbook 2001.* Philadelphia: W.B. Saunders, p. 942.

**484.** A nurse is caring for a postoperative adrenalectomy client. The nurse monitors the client for which of the following?
1   Signs and symptoms of hypocalcemia
2   Peripheral edema
3   Signs and symptoms of hypovolemia
4   Bilateral exophthalmos

**Answer: 3**
*Rationale:* Aldosterone, secreted by the adrenal cortex, plays a major role in fluid volume balance by retaining sodium and water. Thus a deficiency can cause hypovolemia. A deficiency of adrenocortical hormones (adrenalectomy) does not cause the clinical manifestations noted in options 1, 2, and 4.

*Test-Taking Strategy:* Focus on the surgical procedure, adrenalectomy. Recalling the functions of the adrenal glands and the adrenocortical hormones will direct you to option 3. Review care of a client following adrenalectomy if you had difficulty with this question.

*Level of Cognitive Ability:* Application
*Client Needs:* Physiological Integrity
*Integrated Concept/Process:* Nursing Process/Assessment
*Content Area:* Adult Health/Endocrine

**Reference**
Smeltzer, S., & Bare, B. (2000). *Brunner & Suddarth's Textbook of medical-surgical nursing* (9th ed.). Philadelphia: Lippincott Williams & Wilkins, p. 1064.

**485.** A client with cancer who is receiving chemotherapy tells the nurse that the food on the meal tray tastes "funny." Which intervention by the nurse is appropriate?
  1 Keep the client NPO
  2 Administer an antiemetic as ordered
  3 Provide oral hygiene care
  4 Obtain an order for total parenteral nutrition (TPN)

**Answer: 3**
*Rationale:* Cancer treatments may cause distortion of taste. Frequent oral hygiene aids in preserving taste function. Keeping a client NPO increases nutritional risks. Antiemetics are used when nausea and vomiting are a problem. TPN is used when oral intake is not possible.

*Test-Taking Strategy:* Focus on the issue: taste sensation. Only option 3 addresses this issue. Note the relationship between *tastes* and *oral hygiene care*. If you had difficulty with this question, review the effects of cancer treatments and the appropriate nursing interventions.

*Level of Cognitive Ability:* Application
*Client Needs:* Physiological Integrity
*Integrated Concept/Process:* Nursing Process/Implementation
*Content Area:* Adult Health/Oncology

*Reference*
Potter, P., & Perry, A. (2001). *Fundamentals of nursing* (5th ed.). St. Louis: Mosby, p. 1063.

**486.** A nurse notes redness, warmth, and a purulent drainage at the insertion site of a central venous catheter in a client receiving total parenteral nutrition (TPN). The nurse notifies the physician of this finding because:
  1 Infections of a central catheter site can lead to septicemia
  2 The client is experiencing an allergy to the TPN solution
  3 The TPN solution has infiltrated and must be stopped
  4 The client is allergic to the dressing material covering the site

**Answer: 1**
*Rationale:* Redness, warmth, and purulent drainage are signs of an infection, not allergic reaction. Infiltration causes the surrounding tissue to become cool and pale.

*Test-Taking Strategy:* Focus on the issue—signs of infection—noting the key words *redness, warmth,* and *drainage.* Eliminate options 2 and 4 because they are similar and address an allergy. From the remaining options, note that option 1 addresses septicemia, which can be life threatening to the client. If you had difficulty with this question, review nursing interventions related to monitoring for complications of TPN.

*Level of Cognitive Ability:* Application
*Client Needs:* Physiological Integrity
*Integrated Concept/Process:* Nursing Process/Implementation
*Content Area:* Fundamental Skills

*Reference*
Smeltzer, S., & Bare, B. (2000) *Brunner & Suddarth's Textbook of medical-surgical nursing* (9th ed.). Philadelphia: Lippincott Williams & Wilkins, p. 852.

**487.** A nurse is performing a health history on a client with chronic pancreatitis. The nurse expects to most likely note which of the following when obtaining information regarding the client's health history?
  1 Abdominal pain relieved with food or antacids
  2 Exposure to occupational chemicals
  3 Weight gain
  4 Use of alcohol

**Answer: 4**
*Rationale:* Chronic pancreatitis occurs most often in alcoholics. Abstinence from alcohol is important to prevent the client from developing chronic pancreatitis. Clients usually experience malabsorption with weight loss. Pain will not be relieved with food or antacids. Chemical exposure is associated with cancer of the pancreas.

*Test-Taking Strategy:* Focus on the issue: the cause of pancreatitis. Recalling the relationship between alcohol use and pancreatitis will direct you to option 4. If you had difficulty with this question, review the causes of pancreatitis.

*Level of Cognitive Ability:* Analysis
*Client Needs:* Physiological Integrity
*Integrated Concept/Process:* Nursing Process/Assessment
*Content Area:* Adult Health/Gastrointestinal

*Reference*
Ignatavicius, D., Workman, M., & Mishler, M. (1999). *Medical-surgical nursing across the health care continuum* (3rd ed.). Philadelphia: W.B. Saunders, p. 1507.

---

**488.** A client has been taking glucocorticoids to control rheumatoid arthritis. For which abnormal laboratory value is the client at risk as a result of taking this medication?
1. Elevated serum potassium
2. Decreased serum sodium
3. Increased serum glucose
4. Increased white blood cells

**Answer: 3**

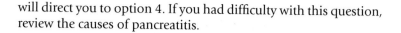

*Rationale:* Glucocorticoids have three primary uses: replacement therapy for adrenal insufficiency, immunosuppressive therapy, and antiinflammatory therapy. Exogenous glucocorticoids cause the same effects on cellular activity as the naturally produced glucocorticoids, but exogenous glucocorticoids may produced undesired effects. The glucocorticoids stimulate appetite and increase caloric intake. They also increase the availability of glucose for energy. These combined effects cause the blood glucose level to rise, making the client prone to hyperglycemia. Options 1, 2, and 4 are not expected effects of the use of glucocorticoids.

*Test-Taking Strategy:* Use the process of elimination. First, eliminate options 1 and 2 because they are similar in that they both relate to electrolytes. From the remaining options, recalling that glucocorticoids increase the availability of glucose for energy will direct you to option 3. If you are unfamiliar with these medications, including their uses, side effects, and contraindications, review this content.

*Level of Cognitive Ability:* Analysis
*Client Needs:* Physiological Integrity
*Integrated Concept/Process:* Nursing Process/Analysis
*Content Area:* Pharmacology

*Reference*
Salerno, E. (1999). *Pharmacology for health professionals.* St. Louis: Mosby, pp. 852-853.

**489.** A client with a diagnosis of Cushing's syndrome is undergoing a dexamethasone suppression test. The nurse plans to implement which steps during this test?

1 Administer 1 mg of dexamethasone orally at night and obtain serum cortisol levels the next morning and evening

2 Administer an injection of dexamethasone, and then collect a 24-hour urine specimen to measure serum cortisol levels

3 Draw blood samples before and after exercise to evaluate the effect of exercise on serum cortisol levels

4 Administer an injection of adrenocorticotropic hormone (ACTH) 30 minutes before drawing blood to measure serum cortisol levels

**Answer: 1**

*Rationale:* The dexamethasone suppression test is performed to evaluate the function of the adrenal cortex. The procedure for this test is to administer 1 mg of dexamethasone at 11 PM to suppress ACTH formation and then obtain 8 AM and 8 PM serum cortisol levels on the following day.

*Test-Taking Strategy:* Recall that Cushing's syndrome is a disorder caused by excessive amounts of cortisol. Since the test is a dexamethasone suppression test, you would expect that dexamethasone would be given to suppress cortisol production. Keeping this in mind, options 3 and 4 can be eliminated. From the remaining options, eliminate option 2 because serum cortisol levels cannot be measured via the urine. If you had difficulty with this question, review this test.

*Level of Cognitive Ability:* Application
*Client Needs:* Physiological Integrity
*Integrated Concept/Process:* Nursing Process/Planning
*Content Area:* Adult Health/Endocrine

*Reference*
Fischbach, F. (2000). *A manual of laboratory & diagnostic tests* (6th ed.). Philadelphia: Lippincott Williams & Wilkins, p. 407.

---

**490.** A nurse is performing an abdominal assessment on a client. The nurse determines that which of the following findings should be reported to the physician?

1 Concave, midline umbilicus

2 Pulsation between the umbilicus and pubis

3 Bowel sound frequency of 15 sounds per minute

4 Absence of a bruit

**Answer: 2**

*Rationale:* The umbilicus should be in the midline, with a concave appearance. The presence of pulsation between the umbilicus and the pubis could indicate an abdominal aortic aneurysm and should be reported to the physician. Bowel sounds vary according to the timing of the last meal and usually range in frequency from 5 to 35 per minute. Bruits are not normally present.

*Test-Taking Strategy:* Use basic nursing knowledge related to physical assessment to answer this question. Note that the wording of the question guides you to look for an abnormal finding. Review abdominal assessment if you had difficulty with this question.

*Level of Cognitive Ability:* Analysis
*Client Needs:* Physiological Integrity
*Integrated Concept/Process:* Nursing Process/Assessment
*Content Area:* Adult Health/Gastrointestinal

*Reference*
Smeltzer, S., & Bare, B. (2000) *Brunner & Suddarth's Textbook of medical-surgical nursing* (9th ed.). Philadelphia: Lippincott Williams & Wilkins, p. 797.

**491.** A nurse is performing a cardiovascular assessment on a client. Which of the following items would the nurse assess to gain the best information about the client's left-sided heart function?

1 Breath sounds
2 Peripheral edema
3 Jugular vein distention
4 Hepatojugular reflux

**Answer: 1**

*Rationale:* The client with heart failure may present with different symptoms depending on whether the right or the left side of the heart is failing. Peripheral edema, jugular vein distention, and hepatojugular reflux are all indicators of right-sided heart function. Breath sounds are an accurate indicator of left-sided heart function.

*Test-Taking Strategy:* Focus on the issue: left-sided heart function. Remember, "left and lungs." Left-sided heart failure leads to respiratory signs and symptoms. Review the signs of the right- and left-sided heart failure if you had difficulty with this question.

*Level of Cognitive Ability:* Application
*Client Needs:* Physiological Integrity
*Integrated Concept/Process:* Nursing Process/Assessment
*Content Area:* Adult Health/Respiratory

*Reference*
Smeltzer, S., & Bare, B. (2000). *Brunner & Suddarth's Textbook of medical-surgical nursing* (9th ed.). Philadelphia: Lippincott Williams & Wilkins, p. 664.

**492.** A nurse is caring for the following group of clients on the clinical nursing unit. The nurse interprets that which of these clients is at most risk for the development of pulmonary embolism?

1 A 65-year-old man out of bed 1 day after prostate resection
2 A 73-year-old woman who has just had a pinning of a hip fracture
3 A 25-year-old woman with diabetic ketoacidosis
4 A 38-year-old man with a pulmonary contusion after an automobile accident

**Answer: 2**

*Rationale:* Clients frequently at risk for pulmonary embolism include clients who are immobilized. This is especially true in immobilized postoperative clients. Other clients at risk include those of advanced age, with endothelial disease, or with conditions characterized by hypercoagulability.

*Test-Taking Strategy:* The options can best be compared by evaluating the degree of immobility of each client and also the age of the client, which is provided in each option. The clients in options 1 and 3 have the least long-term anticipated immobility and therefore should be eliminated first. From the remaining options, the younger client with the pulmonary contusion would be expected to be less immobile than the elderly woman with hip fracture. Review the causes of pulmonary embolism if you had difficulty with this question.

*Level of Cognitive Ability:* Analysis
*Client Needs:* Physiological Integrity
*Integrated Concept/Process:* Nursing Process/Assessment
*Content Area:* Adult Health/Respiratory

*Reference*
Smeltzer, S., & Bare, B. (2000). *Brunner & Suddarth's Textbook of medical-surgical nursing* (9th ed.). Philadelphia: Lippincott Williams & Wilkins, p. 472.

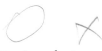

**493.** A graduate nurse is assigned to admit a client with a diagnosis of anorexia nervosa to the nursing unit. The nurse preceptor would remind the graduate nurse that assessment findings may indicate:

1. Elevated potassium levels
2. Low blood urea nitrogen
3. Weight loss of at least 4% of original weight over a short period
4. That the client has extensive knowledge of nutrition

**Answer: 4**
*Rationale:* The potassium level is usually low and the blood urea nitrogen is usually high in clients with anorexia nervosa. These clients lose at least 15% of their original body weight in a short period of time. They are very knowledgeable about nutrition and the caloric value of food.

*Test-Taking Strategy:* Use the process of elimination, focusing on the client's diagnosis. Option 3 is eliminated because this small amount of weight loss may not be a cause for concern of many people. Eliminate options 1 and 2 because these findings do not occur in starvation or in the fluid or electrolyte deficiency typical of anorexia nervosa. Review the typical assessment findings in the client with anorexia nervosa if you had difficulty with this question.

*Level of Cognitive Ability:* Analysis
*Client Needs:* Physiological Integrity
*Integrated Concept/Process:* Nursing Process/Assessment
*Content Area:* Mental Health

*Reference*
Stuart, G.W., & Laraia, M.T. (1998). *Principles and practice of psychiatric nursing.* (6th ed.). St. Louis: Mosby, p. 534.

---

**494.** A physician has inserted a nasoenteric tube into a client for the treatment of intestinal obstruction. Following insertion, the nurse tells the client to lie in which position to help the tube advance into the duodenum, past the pyloric sphincter?

1. Supine with the head of the bed flat
2. Supine with the head elevated 30 degrees
3. On the right side
4. On the left side

**Answer: 3**
*Rationale:* Following insertion of a nasoenteric tube, the client is instructed to lie on the right side to aid the passage of the tube from the stomach into the duodenum, past the pyloric sphincter. Options 1, 2, and 4 are incorrect positions.

*Test-Taking Strategy:* Use knowledge of basic anatomy and the position of the stomach in the abdomen to help eliminate options 1, 2, and 4. Knowledge of this position can be applied to the management of a client with any type of nasoenteric tube. Review care of a client with a nasoenteric tube if you had difficulty with this question.

*Level of Cognitive Ability:* Application
*Client Needs:* Physiological Integrity
*Integrated Concept/Process:* Nursing Process/Implementation
*Content Area:* Adult Health/Gastrointestinal

*Reference*
Smeltzer, S., & Bare, B. (2000). *Brunner & Suddarth's Textbook of medical-surgical nursing* (9th ed.). Philadelphia: Lippincott Williams & Wilkins, p. 838.

**495.** A client with coronary artery disease suddenly complains of palpitations and an irregular heartbeat. The nurse would assess for which of the following to determine an inadequacy of stroke volume?

  1   Pulse pressure
  2   Pulse deficit
  3   Pulsus alternans
  4   Water-hammer pulse

**Answer: 2**

*Rationale:* Palpitations are often a subjective complaint that accompanies dysrhythmias. Irregular rhythms produce varying strengths of stroke volume because of irregular ventricular filling times, and therefore arterial pulsations may become weakened or intermittently absent. The nurse determines this by assessing an apical-radial pulse. An apical rate that is greater than the radial rate is called a pulse deficit. The pulse pressure is an indirect indicator of overall cardiac output. A water-hammer pulse may accompany events that produce an increased cardiac output. Pulsus alternans has a regular rhythm accompanied by a pulse volume that alternates strong with weak.

*Test-Taking Strategy:* Use the process of elimination. Remember that "stroke volume × heart rate = cardiac output." Measures that give a general indication of cardiac output are not specific enough to answer this question, so eliminate options 1 and 4. Pulsus alternans (option 3) occurs with a regular rhythm. Review the definition of pulse deficit if you had difficulty with this question.

*Level of Cognitive Ability:* Analysis
*Client Needs:* Physiological Integrity
*Integrated Concept/Process:* Nursing Process/Assessment
*Content Area:* Adult Health/Cardiovascular

*Reference*
Smeltzer, S., & Bare, B. (2000). *Brunner & Suddarth's Textbook of medical-surgical nursing* (9th ed.). Philadelphia: Lippincott Williams & Wilkins, p. 542.

---

**496.** A nurse is listening to the client's breath sounds and hears a creaking, grating sound on inspiration and expiration over the posterior right lower lobe. The nurse documents that this client has:

  1   Crackles
  2   Wheezes
  3   Rhonchi
  4   Pleural friction rub

**Answer: 4**

*Rationale:* The nurse is hearing a pleural friction rub, which is characterized by sounds that are described as creaking, groaning, or grating in quality. The sounds are localized over an area of inflammation of the pleura and may be heard in both the inspiratory and expiratory phases of the respiratory cycle. Crackles have the sound that is heard when a few strands of hair are rubbed together near the ear; they indicate fluid in the alveoli. Wheezes are musical noises heard on inspiration, expiration, or both. They are the result of narrowed air passages. Rhonchi are usually heard on expiration when there is excessive production of mucus, which accumulates in the air passages.

*Test-Taking Strategy:* Note the key words *creaking, grating sound.* The image called to mind by these sounds is most compatible with the words *friction rub,* and that may be sufficient to help you answer the question correctly. In addition, knowing that these sounds are not the classic descriptors for crackles, wheezes, or rhonchi helps you to eliminate each of the other options. Review the characteristics of a pleural friction rub if you had difficulty with this question.

*Level of Cognitive Ability:* Analysis
*Client Needs:* Physiological Integrity
*Integrated Concept/Process:* Communication and Documentation
*Content Area:* Adult Health/Respiratory

*Reference*
Smeltzer, S., & Bare, B. (2000). *Brunner & Suddarth's Textbook of medical-surgical nursing* (9th ed.). Philadelphia: Lippincott Williams & Wilkins, p. 392.

---

**497.** A nurse is assessing the renal function of a client. After directly noting urine volume and characteristics, the nurse assesses which of the following items as the best indirect indicator of renal function?

1  Bladder distention
2  Level of consciousness
3  Pulse rate
4  Blood pressure

**Answer: 4**
*Rationale:* The kidneys normally receive 20% to 25% of the cardiac output, even under conditions of rest. For kidney function to be optimal, adequate renal perfusion is necessary. Perfusion can best be estimated by the blood pressure, which is an indirect reflection of the adequacy of cardiac output. The pulse rate affects the cardiac output but can be altered by factors unrelated to kidney function. Bladder distention reflects a problem or obstruction that is most often distal to the kidneys. Level of consciousness is an unrelated item.

*Test-Taking Strategy:* Focus on the issue: renal function. Eliminate option 2 first as the item most unrelated to kidney function. Since bladder distention can be affected by a number of other factors besides renal function, this is eliminated next. From the remaining options, remember that the cardiac output = heart rate × stroke volume. The cardiac output overall helps determine the blood pressure and renal perfusion. Thus blood pressure is the more global option and is the one more directly related to kidney perfusion. Review assessment of renal function if you had difficulty with this question.

*Level of Cognitive Ability:* Application
*Client Needs:* Physiological Integrity
*Integrated Concept/Process:* Nursing Process/Assessment
*Content Area:* Adult Health/Renal

*Reference*
Smeltzer, S., & Bare, B. (2000). *Brunner & Suddarth's Textbook of medical-surgical nursing* (9th ed.). Philadelphia: Lippincott Williams & Wilkins, p. 246.

---

**498.** A nurse notes that the infusion bag of a client receiving total parenteral nutrition (TPN) has become empty. The nurse calls the pharmacy, but the next bag will not be delivered for another 30 minutes. The nurse hangs which of the following solutions until the TPN arrives?

1  5% dextrose in water ($D_5W$)
2  10% dextrose in water ($D_{10}W$)
3  50% dextrose in saline solution ($D_{50}NS$)
4  5% dextrose in 0.45% saline solution ($D_5 \frac{1}{2}NS$)

**Answer: 2**
*Rationale:* If a TPN solution bag stops running or becomes empty, the nurse should hang an infusion of 10% dextrose in water until another TPN solution arrives or the problem is fixed. This minimizes the chance that hypoglycemia will develop, since the body produces more insulin in the presence of the high TPN glucose load.

*Test-Taking Strategy:* Use the process of elimination, recalling that the glucose concentration of TPN is high. Eliminate option 3 because there is no such solution of this type. Remember that options that are similar are not likely to be correct. This guides you to eliminate options 1 and 4, since the percentage of dextrose is the same. Review care of a client receiving TPN if you had difficulty with this question.

*Level of Cognitive Ability:* Application
*Client Needs:* Physiological Integrity
*Integrated Concept/Process:* Nursing Process/Implementation
*Content Area:* Adult Health/Gastrointestinal

*Reference*
Smeltzer, S., & Bare, B. (2000). *Brunner & Suddarth's Textbook of medical-surgical nursing* (9th ed.). Philadelphia: Lippincott Williams & Wilkins, p. 854.

---

**499.** A client seen in the ambulatory care clinic has ascites and slight jaundice. The nurse assesses the client for a history of chronic use of which of the following medications?

1 Acetaminophen (Tylenol)
2 Acetylsalicylic acid (Aspirin)
3 Ibuprofen (Advil)
4 Ranitidine (Zantac)

**Answer: 1**

*Rationale:* Acetaminophen is a potentially hepatotoxic medication. Use of this medication and other hepatotoxic agents should be investigated whenever a client presents with symptoms compatible with liver disease (such as ascites and jaundice). Hepatotoxicity is not an adverse effect of the medications identified in options 2, 3, and 4.

*Test-Taking Strategy:* Focus on the signs noted in the question, and recall that these symptoms are compatible with liver disease. With this in mind, evaluate each of the options in relation to their relative ability to be toxic to the liver. Recalling that acetaminophen is hepatotoxic will direct you to option 1. Review these medications if you are unfamiliar with them.

*Level of Cognitive Ability:* Analysis
*Client Needs:* Physiological Integrity
*Integrated Concept/Process:* Nursing Process/Assessment
*Content Area:* Adult Health/Gastrointestinal

*Reference*
Smeltzer, S., & Bare, B. (2000). *Brunner & Suddarth's Textbook of medical-surgical nursing* (9th ed.). Philadelphia: Lippincott Williams & Wilkins, p. 1925.

---

**500.** A nurse is assigned to care for a client who has just undergone eye surgery. The nurse plans to instruct the client that which of the following activities is permitted in the postoperative period?

1 Reading
2 Watching television
3 Bending over
4 Lifting objects

**Answer: 2**

*Rationale:* The client is taught to avoid activities that raise intraocular pressure and could cause complications in the postoperative period. The client is also taught to avoid activities that cause rapid eye movements, which are irritating in the presence of postoperative inflammation. For these reasons the client is taught to avoid bending over, lifting heavy objects, straining, sneezing, making sudden movements, or reading. Watching television is permissible, since the eye does not need to move rapidly with this activity and it does not increase the intraocular pressure.

*Test-Taking Strategy:* Focus on the issue of intraocular pressure when answering this question. Eliminate options 3 and 4 first, since they increase intraocular pressure. From the remaining options, select option 2 because it is less taxing to the eyes. Review postoperative client instructions following eye surgery if you had difficulty with this question.

*Level of Cognitive Ability:* Application
*Client Needs:* Physiological Integrity
*Integrated Concept/Process:* Teaching/Learning
*Content Area:* Adult Health/Eye

*Reference*
Smeltzer, S., & Bare, B. (2000). *Brunner & Suddarth's Textbook of medical-surgical nursing* (9th ed.). Philadelphia: Lippincott Williams & Wilkins, p. 1557.

---

**501.** A nurse is listening to the lungs of a client who has left lower lobe pneumonia. The nurse interprets that the pneumonia is resolving if which of the following is heard over the affected lung area?

1   Bronchophony
2   Egophony
3   Vesicular breath sounds
4   Whispered pectoriloquy

**Answer: 3**
*Rationale:* Vesicular breath sounds are normal sounds that are heard over peripheral lung fields where the air enters the alveoli. A return of breath sounds to normal is consistent with a resolving pneumonia. Bronchophony is an abnormal finding indicative of lung consolidation and is identified if the nurse can clearly hear the client say "ninety-nine" through the stethoscope. (Normally the client's words are unintelligible if heard through a stethoscope). Egophony, which occurs when the sound of the letter "e" is heard as an "a" with auscultation, also indicates lung consolidation. Finally, whispered pectoriloquy is present if the nurse hears the client when "one-two-three" is whispered. This is an abnormal finding, again heard over an area of consolidation. Consolidation typically occurs with pneumonia.

*Test-Taking Strategy:* Use knowledge regarding physical assessment techniques and findings to answer the question. Knowing the areas where bronchial, vesicular, and bronchovesicular breath sounds are heard will direct you to option 3. Review these types of breath sounds if you had difficulty with this question.

*Level of Cognitive Ability:* Analysis
*Client Needs:* Physiological Integrity
*Integrated Concept/Process:* Nursing Process/Evaluation
*Content Area:* Adult Health/Respiratory

*Reference*
Smeltzer, S., & Bare, B. (2000). *Brunner & Suddarth's Textbook of medical-surgical nursing* (9th ed.). Philadelphia: Lippincott Williams & Wilkins, pp. 390, 432.

---

**502.** A female client with a history of chronic infection of the urinary system complains of burning and urinary frequency. To determine whether the current problem is of renal origin, the nurse would assess whether the client has pain or discomfort in the:

1   Suprapubic area
2   Right or left costovertebral angle
3   Urinary meatus
4   Labium

**Answer: 2**
*Rationale:* Pain or discomfort from a problem that originates in the kidney is felt at the costovertebral angle on the affected side. Ureteral pain is felt in the ipsilateral labium in the female client, or the ipsilateral scrotum in the male client. Bladder infection is often accompanied by suprapubic pain and by pain or burning at the urinary meatus when voiding.

*Test-Taking Strategy:* Focus on the issue: a renal problem. Note the similarity between options 1, 3, and 4 in that they relate to the lower urinary tract. Knowing that the kidneys sit higher than the level of the bladder and retroperitoneally will also direct you to option 2. Review the signs of both renal and bladder infections if you had difficulty with this question.

*Level of Cognitive Ability:* Analysis
*Client Needs:* Physiological Integrity
*Integrated Concept/Process:* Nursing Process/Assessment
*Content Area:* Adult Health/Renal

*Reference*
Smeltzer, S., & Bare, B. (2000). *Brunner & Suddarth's Textbook of medical-surgical nursing* (9th ed.). Philadelphia: Lippincott Williams & Wilkins, p. 1091.

---

**503.** During a routine visit to the physician's office for monitoring of diabetic control, an elderly client complains to the nurse of vision changes. The client describes blurring of the vision, with difficulty in reading and with driving at night. Given the client's history, the nurse interprets that which of the following conditions is probably developing?

1  Detached retina
2  Papilledema
3  Glaucoma
4  Cataracts

**Answer: 4**
*Rationale:* Although the incidence of cataracts increases with age, the elderly client with diabetes mellitus is at greater risk for cataracts. The most frequent complaint is of blurred vision that is not accompanied by pain. The client may also experience difficulty with reading, night driving, and glare. Options 1, 2, and 3 are not directly associated with this client's history or complaints.

*Test-Taking Strategy:* Note that the client has diabetes mellitus. Use knowledge related to the risks for and signs and symptoms of common eye disorders to answer this question. If this question was difficult, review the signs and symptoms of cataracts and the associated risk factors.

*Level of Cognitive Ability:* Analysis
*Client Needs:* Physiological Integrity
*Integrated Concept/Process:* Nursing Process/Analysis
*Content Area:* Adult Health/Eye

*Reference*
Ignatavicius, D., Workman, M., & Mishler, M. (1999). *Medical-surgical nursing across the health care continuum* (3rd ed.). Philadelphia: W.B. Saunders, p. 1176.

---

**504.** A nurse inquires about smoking history while conducting a hospital admission assessment with a client with coronary artery disease (CAD). The most important item for the nurse to assess is the:

1  Number of pack-years
2  Brand of cigarettes used
3  Desire to quit smoking
4  Number of past attempts to quit smoking

**Answer: 1**
*Rationale:* The number of cigarettes smoked daily and the duration of the habit are used to calculate the number of pack-years, which is the standard method of documenting smoking history. The brand of cigarettes may give a general indication of tar and nicotine levels, but the information has no immediate clinical use. Desire to quit and number of past attempts to quit smoking may be useful when the nurse develops a smoking cessation plan with the client.

*Test-Taking Strategy:* Note the key words *most important item*. The option that would most closely predict the degree of added risk of CAD is the number of pack-years. Review the technique to assess smoking history if you had difficulty with this question.

*Level of Cognitive Ability:* Analysis
*Client Needs:* Physiological Integrity
*Integrated Concept/Process:* Nursing Process/Assessment
*Content Area:* Adult Health/Cardiovascular

**Reference**

Ignatavicius, D., Workman, M., & Mishler, M. (1999). *Medical-surgical nursing across the health care continuum* (3rd ed.). Philadelphia: W.B. Saunders, p. 594.

---

**505.** A client with primary open angle glaucoma has been prescribed timolol acetate (Timoptic) ophthalmic drops. The client asks the nurse how this medication works. The nurse tells the client that the medication lowers intraocular pressure by:

1   Reducing intracranial pressure
2   Increasing contractions of the ciliary muscle
3   Constricting the pupil
4   Decreasing the production of aqueous humor

**Answer: 4**
*Rationale:* Beta-adrenergic blocking agents such as timolol acetate reduces intraocular pressure by decreasing the production of aqueous humor. Miotic agents (such as pilocarpine) increase contractions of the ciliary muscle and constrict the pupil, thereby increasing the outflow of aqueous humor. This medication does not affect intracranial pressure

*Test-Taking Strategy:* Specific knowledge about the action of this medication is needed to answer this question. Review the action of this medication if you are unfamiliar with it.

*Level of Cognitive Ability:* Application
*Client Needs:* Physiological Integrity
*Integrated Concept/Process:* Teaching/Learning
*Content Area:* Pharmacology

**Reference**

Hodgson, B., & Kizior, R. (2001). *Saunders Nursing drug handbook 2001.* Philadelphia: W.B. Saunders, p. 994.

---

**506.** A client is complaining of knee pain. The knee is swollen, reddened, and warm to the touch. The nurse interprets that the client's signs and symptoms are not compatible with:

1   Inflammation
2   Degenerative disease
3   Infection
4   Recent injury

**Answer: 2**
*Rationale:* Redness, heat, and swelling are associated with musculoskeletal inflammation, infection, or a recent injury. Degenerative disease is accompanied by pain, but there is no redness. Swelling may or may not occur.

*Test-Taking Strategy:* Focus on the signs and symptoms in the question and note the key word *not*. Swelling, redness, and warmth are signs of inflammation. This should direct you to option 2. Review the signs of infection and the signs of degenerative disease if you had difficulty with this question.

*Level of Cognitive Ability:* Analysis
*Client Needs:* Physiological Integrity
*Integrated Concept/Process:* Nursing Process/Analysis
*Content Area:* Adult Health/Musculoskeletal

**Reference**

Ignatavicius, D., Workman, M., & Mishler, M. (1999). *Medical-surgical nursing across the health care continuum* (3rd ed.). Philadelphia: W.B. Saunders, p. 405.

**507.** A client seeks treatment in the emergency room for a lower leg injury. There is visible deformity to the lower aspect of the leg, and the injured leg appears shorter than the other. The area is painful, swollen, and beginning to become ecchymotic. The nurse interprets that this client has experienced a:

1 Contusion
2 Fracture
3 Sprain
4 Strain

**Answer:** 2

**Rationale:** Typical signs and symptoms of a fracture include pain, loss of function in the area, deformity, shortening of the extremity, crepitus, swelling, and ecchymosis. Not all fractures lead to the development of every sign. A contusion results from a blow to soft tissue and causes pain, swelling, and ecchymosis. A sprain is an injury to a ligament caused by a wrenching or twisting motion. Symptoms include pain, swelling, and inability to use the joint or bear weight normally. A strain results from a pulling force on the muscle. Symptoms include soreness and pain with muscle use.

**Test-Taking Strategy:** Use the process of elimination and focus on the signs and symptoms in the question. Within the list of signs and symptoms, note the one that states one leg is shorter than another. Only a fractured bone (which shortens with displacement) could cause this sign. This makes it easy to eliminate each of the other incorrect options. Review the signs and symptoms of a fracture if you had difficulty with this question.

**Level of Cognitive Ability:** Analysis
**Client Needs:** Physiological Integrity
**Integrated Concept/Process:** Nursing Process/Assessment
**Content Area:** Adult Health/Musculoskeletal

**Reference**
Ignatavicius, D., Workman, M., & Mishler, M. (1999). *Medical-surgical nursing across the health care continuum* (3rd ed.). Philadelphia: W.B. Saunders, p. 1277.

**508.** A client arrives at the emergency room with a chemical burn of the left eye. The first action of the nurse is to immediately:

1 Flush the eye continuously with a sterile solution
2 Apply a cold compress to the injured eye
3 Apply a light bandage to the eye
4 Perform an assessment on the client

**Answer:** 1

**Rationale:** When the client has suffered a chemical burn of the eye, the nurse immediately flushes the site with a sterile solution continuously for 15 minutes. If a sterile eye irrigation solution is not available, running water may be used. Performing an assessment may be helpful, but is not the priority action. Applying compresses or bandages are incorrect, because they do not rid the eye of the damaging chemical. Cold compresses are used for blows to the eye, while light bandages may be placed over cuts of the eye or eyelid.

**Test-Taking Strategy:** Focus on the injury described in the question, a chemical burn. Next, note the key words *first* and *immediately*. This focus will direct you to option 1. Review emergency care related to chemical burns to the eye, if you had difficulty with this question.

**Level of Cognitive Ability:** Application
**Client Needs:** Physiological Integrity
**Integrated Concept/Process:** Nursing Process/Implementation
**Content Area:** Adult Health/Eye

**Reference**
Smeltzer, S., & Bare, B. (2000). *Brunner & Suddarth's Textbook of medical-surgical nursing* (9th ed.). Philadelphia: Lippincott Williams & Wilkins, p. 1563.

**509.** A client tells the nurse about a pattern of getting a strong urge to void, which is followed by incontinence before the client can get to the bathroom. The nurse formulates which of the following nursing diagnoses for this client?

1. Reflex Incontinence
2. Stress Incontinence
3. Urge Incontinence
4. Total Incontinence

**Answer: 3**

*Rationale:* Urge incontinence occurs when the client has urinary incontinence soon after experiencing urgency. Reflex incontinence occurs when incontinence occurs at rather predictable times that correspond to when a certain bladder volume is attained. Stress incontinence occurs when the client voids in increments that are less than 50 mL, and has increased abdominal pressure. Total incontinence occurs when there is an unpredictable and continuous loss of urine.

*Test-Taking Strategy:* Use the process of elimination. Eliminate option 4 first as having the least degree of relationship with the information in the question. Note that the question includes the word *urge*. This will direct you to option 3 from the remaining options. Review nursing diagnoses related to incontinence if you had difficulty with this question.

*Level of Cognitive Ability:* Analysis
*Client Needs:* Physiological Integrity
*Integrated Concept/Process:* Nursing Process/Analysis
*Content Area:* Adult Health/Renal

*Reference*
Smeltzer, S., & Bare, B. (2000). *Brunner & Suddarth's Textbook of medical-surgical nursing* (9th ed.). Philadelphia: Lippincott Williams & Wilkins, p. 141.

**510.** A 52-year-old male client is seen in the physician's office for a physical examination after experiencing unusual fatigue over the last several weeks. The client's height is 5 feet, 8 inches and weight is 220 lb. Vital signs are: temperature 98.6° F orally, pulse is 86 beats/min, and the respirations are 18 breaths/min. The blood pressure (BP) is 184/100 mm Hg. Random blood glucose is 122 mg/dL. Which of the following questions should the nurse ask the client next?

1. "Do you exercise regularly?"
2. "Are you considering trying to lose weight?"
3. "Is there a history of diabetes mellitus in your family?"
4. "When was the last time you had your blood pressure checked?"

**Answer: 4**

*Rationale:* The client is hypertensive, which is a known major modifiable risk factor for coronary artery disease (CAD). The other major modifiable risk factors not exhibited by this client include smoking and hypercholesterolemia. The client is overweight, which is a contributing risk factor. The client's nonmodifiable risk factors are age and gender. Since the client presents with several risk factors, the nurse places priority of attention on the client's major modifiable risk factors.

*Test-Taking Strategy:* Use the process of elimination, noting the key word *next*. Eliminate options 1 and 2 first because they are similar. From the remaining options, note the client's BP and its relationship to option 4. Review the major risk factors for CAD if you had difficulty with this question.

*Level of Cognitive Ability:* Analysis
*Client Needs:* Physiological Integrity
*Integrated Concept/Process:* Nursing Process/Assessment
*Content Area:* Adult Health/Cardiovascular

*Reference*
Smeltzer, S., & Bare, B. (2000). *Brunner & Suddarth's Textbook of medical-surgical nursing* (9th ed.). Philadelphia: Lippincott Williams & Wilkins, p. 716.

**511.** A nurse is instilling an otic solution into an adult client's left ear. The nurse avoids doing which of the following as part of this procedure?

1   Warming the solution to room temperature
2   Placing the client in a side-lying position with the ear facing up
3   Pulling the auricle backward and upward
4   Placing the tip of the dropper on the edge of the ear canal

**Answer:** 4

*Rationale:* The dropper is not allowed to touch any object or any part of the client's skin. The solution is warmed before use. The client is placed on the side with the affected ear upward. The nurse pulls the auricle backward and upward, and instills the medication by holding the dropper about 1 cm above the ear canal.

*Test-Taking Strategy:* Note the key word *avoids*. Basic knowledge of proper procedure for administering otic solutions and the principles related to aseptic technique will direct you to option 4. If this question was difficult, review this basic nursing procedure.

*Level of Cognitive Ability:* Application
*Client Needs:* Physiological Integrity
*Integrated Concept/Process:* Nursing Process/Implementation
*Content Area:* Adult Health/Ear

*Reference*
Potter, P., & Perry, A. (2001). *Fundamentals of nursing* (5th ed.). St. Louis: Mosby, p. 923.

**512.** Levothyroxine sodium (Synthroid) is administered to a hospitalized child with congenital hypothyroidism. The child vomits 20 minutes after administration of the dose. The most appropriate nursing action is to:

1   Repeat the prescribed dose
2   Give two doses of the prescribed medicine on the next day
3   Contact the physician immediately
4   Hold the dose for today

**Answer:** 1

*Rationale:* Levothyroxine sodium (Synthroid) is the medication of choice for hypothyroidism. The most significant factor adversely affecting the eventual intelligence of children born with congenital hypothyroidism is inadequate treatment. Therefore compliance with the medication regimen is essential. If the infant or child vomits within 1 hour of taking medication, the dose should be administered again.

*Test-Taking Strategy:* Use the process of elimination. General principles related to medication administration will assist in eliminating option 2. Eliminate option 3 because it is not necessary. From the remaining options, recalling the importance of the medication to treat this disorder will direct you to option 1. If you had difficulty with this question review the administration of this medication in congenital hypothyroidism.

*Level of Cognitive Ability:* Application
*Client Needs:* Physiological Integrity
*Integrated Concept/Process:* Nursing Process/Implementation
*Content Area:* Child Health

*Reference*
Hodgson, B., & Kizior, R. (2001). *Saunders Nursing drug handbook 2001.* Philadelphia: W.B. Saunders, p. 589.

**513.** A client diagnosed as having catatonic excitement has been pacing rapidly nonstop for several hours and is not eating or drinking. The nurse recognizes that in this situation:
1 There is an urgent need for physical and medical control
2 There is an urgent need for restraint
3 There is a need to encourage verbalization of feelings
4 The client will soon become catatonic stuporous

**Answer: 1**
*Rationale:* Catatonic excitement is manifested by a state of extreme psychomotor agitation. Clients urgently require physical and medical control because they are often destructive and violent to others and their excitement can cause them to injure themselves or to collapse from complete exhaustion. Options 2, 3, and 4 are incorrect.

*Test-Taking Strategy:* Use Maslow's Hierarchy of Needs theory to answer the question. Physiological needs are the priority. Noting the client's behavior described in the question will direct you to option 1. Review care of a client with catatonic excitement if you had difficulty with this question.

*Level of Cognitive Ability:* Analysis
*Client Needs:* Physiological Integrity
*Integrated Concept/Process:* Nursing Process/Analysis
*Content Area:* Mental Health

*Reference*
Varcarolis, E. (1998). *Foundations of psychiatric mental health nursing* (3rd ed.). Philadelphia: W.B. Saunders, p. 669.

---

**514.** A nurse is caring for a client with type 1 diabetes mellitus. Which of the following laboratory results would indicate a potential complication associated with this disorder?
1 Blood glucose 112 mg/dL
2 Ketonuria
3 Blood urea nitrogen (BUN) 18 mg/dL
4 Potassium 4.2 mEq

**Answer: 2**
*Rationale:* Ketonuria is an abnormal finding in the client with diabetes mellitus indicating ketosis. Ketosis is a metabolic effect from the lack of insulin and incomplete fat metabolism and occurs in type 1 diabetes mellitus. It is associated with the severe complication of diabetic ketoacidosis (hyperglycemia, ketosis, and acidosis). Option 1, 3, and 4 are all normal laboratory findings.

*Test-Taking Strategy:* Use the process of elimination and knowledge of the normal range of laboratory values. Options 1, 3, and 4 are all normal values. If you had difficulty with this question review the complications of type 1 diabetes mellitus and normal laboratory values.

*Level of Cognitive Ability:* Analysis
*Client Needs:* Physiological Integrity
*Integrated Concept/Process:* Nursing Process/Analysis
*Content Area:* Adult Health/Endocrine

*Reference*
Smeltzer, S., & Bare, B. (2000). *Brunner & Suddarth's Textbook of medical-surgical nursing* (9th ed.). Philadelphia: Lippincott Williams & Wilkins, p. 977.

**515.** A nurse employed in a diabetes clinic is caring for a client on insulin pump therapy. Which statement, if made by the client, indicates that a knowledge deficit exists regarding insulin pump therapy?

1. "If my blood glucose is elevated, I can bolus myself with additional insulin as ordered."
2. "I'll need to check my blood glucose before meals in case I need a premeal insulin bolus."
3. "Now that I have this pump, I don't have to worry about insulin reactions or ketoacidosis ever happening again."
4. "I still need to follow a diet and exercise plan even though I don't inject myself daily anymore."

**Answer: 3**

*Rationale:* Hypoglycemic reactions can occur if there is an error in calculating the insulin dose or if the pump malfunctions. Ketoacidosis can occur if too little insulin is used or if there is an increase in metabolic need. The pump does not have a built-in blood glucose monitoring feedback system, so the client is subject to the usual complications associated with insulin administration without the use of a pump. Options 1, 2, and 4 are accurate regarding the use of the insulin pump.

*Test-Taking Strategy:* Knowledge of the basics of insulin therapy is helpful to answer this question even if you know little about insulin pump therapy. Options 1, 2, and 4 are logical statements regarding the use of endogenous insulin. Option 3 however, presumes a guarantee from a complication of insulin therapy. No biomedical equipment is capable of being 100% safe. Review the principles related to an insulin pump if you had difficulty with this question.

*Level of Cognitive Ability:* Analysis
*Client Needs:* Physiological Integrity
*Integrated Concept/Process:* Nursing Process/Evaluation
*Content Area:* Adult Health/Endocrine

**Reference**
Smeltzer, S., & Bare, B. (2000). *Brunner & Suddarth's Textbook of medical-surgical nursing* (9th ed.). Philadelphia: Lippincott Williams & Wilkins, p. 990.

**516.** A client with Graves' disease has exophthalmos and is experiencing photophobia. Which of the following interventions would best assist the client with this problem?

1. Administer methimazole (Tapazole) every 8 hours around the clock
2. Lubricate the eyes with tap water every 2 to 4 hours
3. Instruct the client to avoid straining or heavy lifting since this can increase eye pressure
4. Obtain dark glasses for the client

**Answer: 4**

*Rationale:* Medical therapy for Graves' disease does not help to alleviate the clinical manifestation of exophthalmos. Since photophobia (light intolerance) accompanies this disorder, dark glasses are helpful in alleviating the problem. Tap water, which is hypotonic, could actually cause more swelling to the eye since it could pull fluid into the interstitial space. In addition, the client is at risk for developing an eye infection since the solution is not sterile. There is no need to avoid straining with exophthalmos.

*Test-Taking Strategy:* Focus on the issue: photophobia. Recalling the definition of photophobia will direct you to option 4. Review the measures to treat this problem if you had difficulty with this question.

*Level of Cognitive Ability:* Application
*Client Needs:* Physiological Integrity
*Integrated Concept/Process:* Nursing Process/Implementation
*Content Area:* Adult Health/Endocrine

**Reference**
Smeltzer, S., & Bare, B. (2000). *Brunner & Suddarth's Textbook of medical-surgical nursing* (9th ed.). Philadelphia: Lippincott Williams & Wilkins, p. 1041.

**517.** A nurse is caring for a client with pneumonia who suddenly becomes restless and has a $Pao_2$ of 60 mm Hg. Which of the following nursing diagnoses would be most appropriate for this client?

1. Fatigue related to a debilitated state
2. Impaired gas exchange related to increased pulmonary secretions
3. Ineffective airway clearance related to dilated bronchioles
4. Impaired gas exchange related to pneumonia

**Answer: 2**

*Rationale:* Restlessness and a low $Pao_2$ are hallmark signs of impaired gas exchange. Although many clients with pneumonia experience fatigue, this nursing diagnosis is not the most appropriate in light of the $Pao_2$ level. Dilated bronchioles would be a goal for treatment and not part of the nursing diagnosis. Pneumonia is a medical diagnosis.

*Test-Taking Strategy:* Use the process of elimination. Eliminate option 4 because it is a medical diagnosis. Focus on the data in the question. Eliminate option 1 next because it is unrelated to this data. From the remaining options, recalling that the bronchioles are not dilated in pneumonia, will direct you to option 2. Review care of a client with pneumonia if you had difficulty with this question.

*Level of Cognitive Ability:* Analysis
*Client Needs:* Physiological Integrity
*Integrated Concept/Process:* Nursing Process/Analysis
*Content Area:* Adult Health/Respiratory

*Reference*
Ignatavicius, D., Workman, M., & Mishler, M. (1999). *Medical-surgical nursing across the health care continuum* (3rd ed.). Philadelphia: W.B. Saunders, p. 673.

---

**518.** A client with tuberculosis (TB) is to be started on rifampin (Rifadin). The nurse provides instructions to the client and tells the client:

1. That yellow-colored skin is common
2. To wear glasses instead of soft contact lens
3. To always take the medication on an empty stomach
4. That as soon as the cultures come back negative, the medication may be stopped

**Answer: 2**

*Rationale:* Soft contacts may be permanently damaged by the orange discoloration that rifampin causes in body fluids. Any sign of jaundice (yellow-colored skin) should always be reported. If rifampin is not tolerated on an empty stomach, it may be taken with food. The client may be on the medication for twelve months even if cultures are negative.

*Test-Taking Strategy:* Use the process of elimination. Eliminate option 3 because of the word *always*. Eliminate option 1 because it is an indication of jaundice. From the remaining options, recalling the side effects of rifampin will direct you to option 2. Review this medication if you are unfamiliar with it.

*Level of Cognitive Ability:* Application
*Client Needs:* Physiological Integrity
*Integrated Concept/Process:* Teaching/Learning
*Content Area:* Pharmacology

*Reference*
Hodgson, B., & Kizior, R. (2001). *Saunders Nursing drug handbook 2001.* Philadelphia: W.B. Saunders, p. 906.

**519.** A nurse reviews the physician's orders for a client with Guillain-Barré syndrome. Which order written by the physician should the nurse question?

1 Assess vital signs every 2 to 4 hours
2 Clear liquid diet
3 Passive range of motion exercises TID
4 Bilateral calf measurements TID

**Answer: 2**

*Rationale:* Clients with Guillain-Barré syndrome have dysphagia. Clients with dysphagia are more likely to aspirate clear liquids than thick or semi-solid foods. Since clients with Guillain-Barré syndrome are at risk for hypotension or hypertension, bradycardia, and respiratory depression, frequent monitoring of vital signs is required. Passive range of motion exercises can help prevent contractures, and assessing calf measurements can help detect deep vein thrombosis, for which they are at risk.

*Test-Taking Strategy:* Use the process of elimination, recalling that the client with Guillain-Barré syndrome is at risk for dysphagia. Even if you are unaware that dysphagia is a problem, note that options 1, 3, and 4 are generally part of routine nursing care. Review the manifestations associated with this disorder, if you had difficulty with this question.

*Level of Cognitive Ability:* Analysis
*Client Needs:* Physiological Integrity
*Integrated Concept/Process:* Nursing Process/Implementation
*Content Area:* Adult Health/Neurological

*Reference*
Smeltzer, S., & Bare, B. (2000). *Brunner & Suddarth's Textbook of medical-surgical nursing* (9th ed.). Philadelphia: Lippincott Williams & Wilkins, p. 1755.

**520.** A client with myasthenia gravis arrives to the emergency room and crisis is suspected. The physician plans to administer edrophonium (Tensilon) to differentiate between myasthenic and cholinergic crisis. The nurse prepares to administer which medication if the client is in cholinergic crisis?

1 Atropine sulfate
2 Morphine sulfate
3 Pyridostigmine bromide (Mestinon)
4 Isoproterenol (Isuprel)

**Answer: 1**

*Rationale:* Clients with cholinergic crisis have experienced overdosage of medication. Tensilon will exacerbate symptoms in cholinergic crisis to the point where the client may need intubation and mechanical ventilation. Intravenous atropine sulfate is used to reverse the effects of these anticholinesterase medications. Morphine sulfate and pyridostigmine bromide would worsen the symptoms of cholinergic crisis. Isuprel is not indicated for cholinergic crisis.

*Test-Taking Strategy:* Focus on the issue: cholinergic crisis. Recalling the antidote for anticholinesterase medications will direct you to option 1. Memorize this antidote, if you had difficulty with this question.

*Level of Cognitive Ability:* Application
*Client Needs:* Physiological Integrity
*Integrated Concept/Process:* Nursing Process/Planning
*Content Area:* Adult Health/Neurological

*Reference*
Smeltzer, S., & Bare, B. (2000). *Brunner & Suddarth's Textbook of medical-surgical nursing* (9th ed.). Philadelphia: Lippincott Williams & Wilkins, p. 1736.

**521.** A nurse is completing a health history on a client with diabetes mellitus who has been taking insulin for many years. At present, the client describes experiencing periods of hypoglycemia followed by periods of hyperglycemia. The most likely cause for this occurrence is which of the following?
1 Injecting insulin at a site of lipodystrophy
2 Adjusting insulin according to blood glucose levels
3 Eating snacks between meals
4 Initiating the use of the insulin pump

**Answer: 1**
*Rationale:* Tissue hypertrophy (lipodystrophy) involves thickening of the subcutaneous tissue at the injection sites. This can interfere with the absorption of insulin, resulting in erratic blood glucose levels. Since the client has been on insulin for many years, this is the most likely cause of poor control.

*Test-Taking Strategy:* Note the key words *taking insulin for many years.* This indicates that you must consider a long-term complication of insulin administration as the answer to the question. Options 2, 3, and 4 are eliminated because they are actually appropriate techniques to use in order to regulate blood glucose levels. Review lipodystrophy if you had difficulty with this question.

*Level of Cognitive Ability:* Analysis
*Client Needs:* Physiological Integrity
*Integrated Concept/Process:* Nursing Process/Analysis
*Content Area:* Adult Health/Endocrine

*Reference*
Potter, P., & Perry, A. (2001). *Fundamentals of nursing* (5th ed.). St. Louis: Mosby, p. 939.

**522.** A nurse receives report at the beginning of the shift regarding a client with an intrauterine fetal demise. On assessment of the client, the nurse expects to note which of the following?
1 Elevated blood pressure, proteinuria, and edema
2 Regression of pregnancy symptoms and absence of fetal heart tones
3 Uterine size greater than expected for gestational age
4 Intractable vomiting and dehydration

**Answer: 2**
*Rationale:* Symptoms of a fetal demise include a decrease in fetal movement, no change or a decrease in fundal height, and absent fetal heart tones. Additionally many symptoms of the pregnancy may diminish, such as breast size and tenderness. Option 1 is associated with preeclampsia. Option 4 is associated with hyperemesis gravidarum.

*Test-Taking Strategy:* Focus on the issue: intrauterine fetal demise. Recalling that fetal demise means fetal death will direct you to option 2. Review the signs associated with fetal demise, if you had difficulty with this question.

*Level of Cognitive Ability:* Analysis
*Client Needs:* Physiological Integrity
*Integrated Concept/Process:* Nursing Process/Assessment
*Content Area:* Maternity

*Reference*
Lowdermilk, D., Perry, S., & Bobak, I. (2000). *Maternity & women's health care* (7th ed.). St. Louis: Mosby, p. 1148.

**523.** A client admitted to the nursing unit from the emergency department has a C4 spinal cord injury. Which of the following assessments should the nurse perform first when admitting the client to the nursing unit?

1. Take the temperature
2. Assess extremity muscle strength
3. Observe for dyskinesias
4. Listen to breath sounds

**Answer: 4**

*Rationale:* Because compromise of respiration is a leading cause of death in cervical cord injury, respiratory assessment is the highest priority. Assessment of temperature and strength can be done after adequate oxygenation is assured. Dyskinesias occur in cerebellar disorders, so are not as important in cord-injured clients, unless head injury is suspected.

*Test-Taking Strategy:* Remembering that a cord injury, particularly at the level of C4, can affect respiratory status will direct you to the correct option. Also, use of the ABCs, airway, breathing, and circulation, can guide assessment priorities in this situation. Breath sounds will be diminished if respiratory muscles are weakened or paralyzed. Review priority care of the client with a C4 spinal cord injury if you had difficulty with this question.

*Level of Cognitive Ability:* Application
*Client Needs:* Physiological Integrity
*Integrated Concept/Process:* Nursing Process/Assessment
*Content Area:* Adult Health/Neurological

*Reference*
Smeltzer, S., & Bare, B. (2000). *Brunner & Suddarth's Textbook of medical-surgical nursing* (9th ed.). Philadelphia: Lippincott Williams & Wilkins, p. 1690.

**524.** A nurse is assisting in positioning a client for a surgical procedure. The nurse knows that the respiratory system is most vulnerable to which of the following positions?

1. Lithotomy
2. Supine
3. Lateral
4. Sims'

**Answer: 1**

*Rationale:* The thoracic cage normally expands in all directions except posteriorly. In the lithotomy position, the expansion of the lungs is restricted at the ribs or sternum, and there is a reduction in the ability of the diaphragm to push down against the abdominal muscles. Respiratory function is impaired because of this interference with normal movements. The volume of air that can be inspired is reduced.

*Test-Taking Strategy:* Use the process of elimination. Options 3 and 4 are similar and are eliminated first. From the remaining options, visualize each of these positions and their effect on the process of respiration. The supine position would not interfere with the expansion of the lungs, as the lithotomy position would. Review these positions, if you had difficulty with this question.

*Level of Cognitive Ability:* Analysis
*Client Needs:* Physiological Integrity
*Integrated Concept/Process:* Nursing Process/Analysis
*Content Area:* Fundamental Skills

*Reference*
Potter, P., & Perry, A. (2001). *Fundamentals of nursing* (5th ed.). St. Louis: Mosby, p. 1524.

**525.** A client has frequent runs of ventricular tachycardia. The physician has prescribed flecainide (Tambocor), a very potent anti-dysrhythmic medication. Because of the effects of the medications, the nurse implements which of the following?

1. Assesses the client for neurological problems
2. Monitors the client's vital signs and ECG frequently
3. Tells the client that the bed rails have to stay up
4. Monitors the client's urinary output

**Answer: 2**

*Rationale:* Flecainide (Tambocor) is an antidysrhythmic medication that slows conduction and decreases excitability, conduction velocity, and automaticity. The nurse needs to monitor for the development of a new or a worsening dysrhythmia. Options 1, 3, and 4 are components of standard care.

*Test-Taking Strategy:* Use the process of elimination. Recall that this medication can cause further cardiac problems. Also, note the relationship of antidysrhythmic medication in the question and the nursing action in the correct option. Option 2 is the only option that relates to cardiac status monitoring. Review this medication, if you had difficulty with this question.

*Level of Cognitive Ability:* Analysis
*Client Needs:* Physiological Integrity
*Integrated Concept/Process:* Nursing Process/Implementation
*Content Area:* Pharmacology

*Reference*
Hodgson, B., & Kizior, R. (2001). *Saunders Nursing drug handbook 2001.* Philadelphia: W.B. Saunders, p. 414.

---

**526.** A nurse is monitoring a client with frequent premature ventricular contractions (PVCs) of more than six per minute. The nurse is preparing to administer a bolus of lidocaine (Xylocaine). The nurse monitors the client for which of the following after administering the medication?

1. Skin temperature and neurological status
2. Vital signs, ECG, and neurological status
3. Kidney and liver function, and neurological status
4. Visual changes, and kidney and liver function

**Answer: 2**

*Rationale:* Lidocaine can cause atrioventricular block with conduction defects. It also can cause paresthesia, numbness, disorientation, and agitation. Monitoring the vital signs, ECG, and neurological status is the priority.

*Test-Taking Strategy:* Use the process of elimination, reading each option thoroughly. Note that option 2 is the only option that addresses direct cardiac monitoring. Review this medication if you had difficulty with this question.

*Level of Cognitive Ability:* Application
*Client Needs:* Physiological Integrity
*Integrated Concept/Process:* Nursing Process/Implementation
*Content Area:* Pharmacology

*Reference*
Sole, M.L., Lamborn, M., & Hartshorn, J. (2001). *Introduction to critical care nursing* (3rd ed.). Philadelphia: W.B. Saunders, p. 186.

**527.** A nurse is caring for a client with acute pulmonary edema. The physician tells the nurse that medication will be prescribed to help reduce preload and afterload. The nurse anticipates that the physician will prescribe which medication?

1. Digoxin (Lanoxin)
2. Nitroprusside sodium (Nipride)
3. Morphine sulfate
4. Furosemide (Lasix)

**Answer: 2**
*Rationale:* IV nitroprusside (Nipride) is a potent vasodilator that reduces preload and afterload. It is the medication of choice for the client with pulmonary edema. Digoxin (Lanoxin) is a cardiac glycoside that increases cardiac contractility. Morphine sulfate is a narcotic analgesic. Furosemide (Lasix) is a loop diuretic and can reduce preload by enhancing the renal excretion of sodium and water, which reduces circulating blood volume.

*Test-Taking Strategy:* Focus on the issue: reducing preload and afterload. Use the process of elimination and knowledge of these medications, selecting the one that reduces both preload and afterload. Review these medications, if you had difficulty with this question.

*Level of Cognitive Ability:* Analysis
*Client Needs:* Physiological Integrity
*Integrated Concept/Process:* Nursing Process/Analysis
*Content Area:* Pharmacology

*Reference*
Smeltzer, S., & Bare, B. (2000). *Brunner & Suddarth's Textbook of medical-surgical nursing* (9th ed.). Philadelphia: Lippincott Williams & Wilkins, pp. 658, 661.

**528.** Streptokinase (Streptase) is being administered to a client following an acute inferior myocardial infarction. The nurse understands that the primary purpose of this medication is to:

1. Inhibit further clot formation
2. Reduce myocardial oxygen demand
3. Prevent platelet aggregation
4. Dissolve the thrombus

**Answer: 4**
*Rationale:* Streptokinase is a thrombolytic medication that causes lysis of blood clots. Anticoagulants prevent further clot formation. Beta-blockers, nitrates, and calcium channel blockers are used to reduce myocardial oxygen demand. Streptokinase does not prevent platelet aggregation.

*Test-Taking Strategy:* Recalling that streptokinase is a thrombolytic medication and that these medications dissolve clots will direct you to option 4. Review this medication, if you had difficulty with this question.

*Level of Cognitive Ability:* Analysis
*Client Needs:* Physiological Integrity
*Integrated Concept/Process:* Nursing Process/Analysis
*Content Area:* Pharmacology

*Reference*
Hodgson, B., & Kizior, R. (2001). *Saunders Nursing drug handbook 2001.* Philadelphia: W.B. Saunders, p. 946.

**529.** A nurse is planning to care for a client with pulmonary edema. The nurse establishes a goal to have the client participate in activities that reduce cardiac workload. The nurse identifies which client action as contributing to this goal?

1　Elevating the legs when in bed
2　Sleeping in the supine position
3　Using seasonings to improve the taste of food
4　Using a bedside commode for urinary and bowel elimination

**Answer: 4**
*Rationale:* Using a bedside commode decreases the work of getting to the bathroom or struggling to use the bedpan. Elevating the client's legs increases venous return to the heart, increasing cardiac workload. The supine position increases respiratory effort and decreases oxygenation. This increases cardiac workload. Seasonings are high in sodium.

*Test-Taking Strategy:* Use the process of elimination, focusing on the issue: reducing cardiac overload. Keeping this issue in mind will direct you to option 4. Review measures that will reduce cardiac workload if you had difficulty with this question.

*Level of Cognitive Ability:* Analysis
*Client Needs:* Physiological Integrity
*Integrated Concept/Process:* Nursing Process/Analysis
*Content Area:* Adult Health/Cardiovascular

*Reference*
Smeltzer, S., & Bare, B. (2000). *Brunner & Suddarth's Textbook of medical-surgical nursing* (9th ed.). Philadelphia: Lippincott Williams & Wilkins, p. 662.

**530.** A child is sent to the school nurse by the teacher. As the nurse is assessing the child, the nurse notes that the child has a rash. The nurse suspects that the child has erythema infectiosum (fifth disease) because the skin assessment revealed a rash that is:

1　A discrete rose-pink maculopapular rash on the trunk
2　A highly pruritic, profuse macule to papule rash on the trunk
3　A discrete pinkish red maculopapular rash that is spreading to the trunk
4　An erythema on the face that has a "slapped face" appearance

**Answer: 4**
*Rationale:* The classic rash of erythema infectiosum or fifth disease is the erythema on the face. The discrete rose-pink maculopapular rash is the rash of exanthema subitum (roseola). The highly pruritic, profuse macule to papule rash is the rash of varicella (chickenpox). The discrete pinkish red maculopapular rash is the rash of rubella (German measles).

*Test-Taking Strategy:* Knowledge regarding the characteristics associated with erythema infectiosum is required to answer the question. If you are unfamiliar with this disorder, note that in options 1, 2, and 3, a similarity exists in that the rash is on the trunk. Option 4 addresses a rash on the face. Review this disorder, if you had difficulty with this question.

*Level of Cognitive Ability:* Analysis
*Client Needs:* Physiological Integrity
*Integrated Concept/Process:* Nursing Process/Assessment
*Content Area:* Child Health

*Reference*
Wong, D. (1999). *Whaley & Wong's Nursing care of infants and children* (6th ed.). St. Louis: Mosby, p. 724.

**531.** A client is taking a monoamine oxidase inhibitor (MAOI). The nurse assesses the client closely because:

1. These medications increase the amount of MAO in the liver
2. Hypotensive crisis may be precipitated by foods rich in tyramine and tryptophan
3. Headache, hypertension, and nausea and vomiting may indicate toxicity
4. Hypotension may indicate toxicity

**Answer: 3**

*Rationale:* Headache, hypertension, tachycardia, nausea and vomiting are precursors to hypertensive crisis brought about by the ingestion of foods rich in tyramine and tryptophan while the client is taking MAO inhibitors. These medications act by decreasing the amount of MAO in the liver, which is necessary for the breakdown and utilization of tyramine and tryptophan. Hypertensive crisis may lead to circulatory collapse, intracranial hemorrhage, and death.

*Test-Taking Strategy:* Use the process of elimination. Eliminate 2 and 4 first because they are similar. From the remaining options, recalling the relationship between MAOIs and toxicity will direct you to option 3. Review the actions and side effects of the MAOIs, if you had difficulty with this question.

*Level of Cognitive Ability:* Application
*Client Needs:* Physiological Integrity
*Integrated Concept/Process:* Nursing Process/Assessment
*Content Area:* Pharmacology

*Reference*
Stuart, G.W., & Laraia, M.T. (1998). *Principles and practice of psychiatric nursing.* (6th ed.). St. Louis: Mosby, p. 586.

**532.** A client has returned to the nursing unit following an abdominal hysterectomy. The client is lying supine. To completely assess the client for postoperative bleeding, the nurse should do which of the following?

1. Check the abdominal dressing
2. Check the perineal pad
3. Ask the client about a sensation of moistness
4. Roll the client to one side after checking the perineal pad and the abdominal dressing

**Answer: 4**

*Rationale:* The nurse should roll the client to one side after checking the perineal pad and the abdominal dressing. This allows the nurse to check the rectal area, where blood may pool by gravity if the client is lying supine. Asking the client about a sensation of moistness is not a complete assessment.

*Test-Taking Strategy:* Use the process of elimination. Eliminate option 3 first because it relies on the client. From the remaining options, note that option 4 addresses rolling the client. It is also the most global option. Review care of a client following hysterectomy if you had difficulty with this question.

*Level of Cognitive Ability:* Application
*Client Needs:* Physiological Integrity
*Integrated Concept/Process:* Nursing Process/Implementation
*Content Area:* Fundamental Skills

*Reference*
Smeltzer, S., & Bare, B. (2000). *Brunner & Suddarth's Textbook of medical-surgical nursing* (9th ed.). Philadelphia: Lippincott Williams & Wilkins, pp. 1252-1253.

**533.** A nurse is caring for the client who returned to the nursing unit following suprapubic prostatectomy. The nurse monitors the continuous bladder irrigation to detect which of the following signs of catheter blockage?

1  Drainage that is pale pink
2  Drainage that is bright red
3  Urine leakage around the three-way catheter at the meatus
4  True urine output of 50 mL/hr

**Answer: 3**

*Rationale:* Catheter blockage or occlusion by clots following prostatectomy can result in urine back-up and leakage around the urethral meatus. This would be accompanied by a stoppage of outflow through the catheter into the drainage bag. Drainage that is bright red indicates that the irrigant is running too slowly; drainage that is pale pink indicates sufficient flow. A true urine output of 50 mL/hr indicates catheter patency.

*Test-Taking Strategy:* Use the process of elimination, focusing on the issue: catheter blockage. Eliminate options 1 and 2 first because of the word *drainage*. This implies catheter patency. From the remaining options, apply basic principles related to Foley catheter management. A leakage around the catheter at the meatus indicates blockage. Review care of a client following prostatectomy if you had difficulty with this question.

*Level of Cognitive Ability:* Analysis
*Client Needs:* Physiological Integrity
*Integrated Concept/Process:* Nursing Process/Assessment
*Content Area:* Adult Health/Renal

*Reference*
Smeltzer, S., & Bare, B. (2000). *Brunner & Suddarth's Textbook of medical-surgical nursing* (9th ed.). Philadelphia: Lippincott Williams & Wilkins, p. 1316.

---

**534.** A nurse is assigned to a client returning from the postanesthesia care unit following transurethral prostatectomy. The nurse avoids doing which of the following after this procedure?

1  Reporting signs of confusion
2  Administering a belladonna and opium (B&O) suppository at room temperature
3  Removing the traction tape on the three-way catheter
4  Monitoring hourly urine output

**Answer: 3**

*Rationale:* The nurse would avoid removing the traction tape applied by the surgeon in the operating room. The purpose of this tape is to place pressure on the prostate and reduce hemorrhage. B&O suppositories, ordered on a PRN basis for bladder spasm, should be warmed to room temperature before administration. The nurse routinely monitors hourly urine output since the client has a three-way bladder irrigation running. The nurse also assesses for confusion, which could result from hyponatremia secondary to the hypotonic irrigant used during the surgical procedure.

*Test-Taking Strategy:* Use the process of elimination, noting the key word *avoids*. Eliminate options 1 and 4 first because they are part of routine nursing care, and would not be contraindicated in the care of this client. From the remaining options, recalling the need to reduce hemorrhage will direct you to option 3. Review care of a client following prostatectomy if you had difficulty with this question.

*Level of Cognitive Ability:* Application
*Client Needs:* Physiological Integrity
*Integrated Concept/Process:* Nursing Process/Implementation
*Content Area:* Adult Health/Renal

*Reference*
Ignatavicius, D., Workman, M., & Mishler, M. (1999). *Medical-surgical nursing across the health care continuum* (3rd ed.). Philadelphia: W.B. Saunders. p. 2028.

**535.** A client is due for a dose of bumetanide (Bumex). The nurse would temporarily withhold the dose and notify the physician if which of the following laboratory results was noted?
1   Sodium 137 mEq/L
2   Potassium 2.9 mEq/L
3   Magnesium 2.6 mg/dL
4   Chloride 106 mEq/L

**Answer: 2**
*Rationale:* Bumetanide is a loop diuretic, that is not potassium-sparing. The value given for potassium is below the therapeutic range of 3.5 to 5.1 mEq/L for this electrolyte. The nurse should notify the physician before giving the dose so that potassium may be ordered. Option 1, 3, and 4 identify normal values.

*Test-Taking Strategy:* Note the key words *notify the physician*. Use the process of elimination and knowledge of the normal laboratory values. Option 2 is the only abnormal value. Review this medication, if you had difficulty with this question.

*Level of Cognitive Ability:* Application
*Client Needs:* Physiological Integrity
*Integrated Concept/Process:* Nursing Process/Implementation
*Content Area:* Pharmacology

*Reference*
Hodgson, B., & Kizior, R. (2001). *Saunders Nursing drug handbook 2001.* Philadelphia: W.B. Saunders, p. 127.

**536.** A client with heart failure is receiving furosemide (Lasix) and digoxin (Lanoxin) daily. When the nurse enters the room to administer the morning doses, the client complains of anorexia, nausea, and yellow vision. The nurse should do which of the following first?
1   Administer the medications
2   Give the digoxin only
3   Check the morning serum potassium level
4   Check the morning serum digoxin level

**Answer: 4**
*Rationale:* The nurse should check for the result of the digoxin level that was drawn, since the symptoms are compatible with digoxin toxicity. Knowing that a low potassium level may contribute to digoxin toxicity, checking the serum potassium level may give useful additive information, but the digoxin level is checked first. The digoxin should be withheld until the level is known, making options 1 and 2 incorrect.

*Test-Taking Strategy:* Note the key word *first*. Eliminate options 1 and 2 first, since it is not appropriate to administer the medication without doing further investigation. From the remaining options, recalling the signs of digoxin toxicity will direct you to option 4. Review the signs of digoxin toxicity, if you had difficulty with this question.

*Level of Cognitive Ability:* Application
*Client Needs:* Physiological Integrity
*Integrated Concept/Process:* Nursing Process/Implementation
*Content Area:* Pharmacology

*Reference*
Hodgson, B., & Kizior, R. (2001). *Saunders Nursing drug handbook 2001.* Philadelphia: W.B. Saunders, p. 452.

inaekrolaid / [handwritten characters]

**537.** A nurse is administering an oral dose of erythromycin (E-Mycin) to an assigned client. The nurse administers this medication with a:

1   Full glass of milk
2   Full glass of water
3   Sip of orange juice
4   Any citrus beverage

**Answer: 2**

*Rationale:* Erythromycin is a macrolide antibiotic that should be taken with a full glass of water. Sufficient volume is needed to obtain the maximal effect of the medication. Depending on the specific type of erythromycin, it may need to be administered on an empty stomach, with meals, or regardless of timing of meals. The nurse should verify the best method of administration for the type of erythromycin ordered.

*Test-Taking Strategy:* Use the process of elimination. Eliminate options 3 and 4 first because they are similar. From the remaining options, recalling that medication administered with milk affects absorption will direct you to option 2. Review this medication, if you had difficulty with this question.

*Level of Cognitive Ability:* Application
*Client Needs:* Physiological Integrity
*Integrated Concept/Process:* Nursing Process/Implementation
*Content Area:* Pharmacology

*Reference*
Hodgson, B., & Kizior, R. (2001). *Saunders Nursing drug handbook 2001.* Philadelphia: W.B. Saunders, p. 377.

**538.** A nurse has given the client a dose of intravenous hydralazine (Apresoline). The nurse evaluates the effectiveness of the medication by monitoring which of the following client parameters?

1   Blood pressure
2   Cardiac rhythm
3   Urine output
4   Blood glucose level

**Answer: 1** /hai'drælazin/

*Rationale:* Hydralazine is an antihypertensive medication used in the management of moderate to severe hypertension. It is a vasodilator medication that decreases afterload. The blood pressure needs to be monitored.

*Test-Taking Strategy:* Use the process of elimination. Note the name of the medication, Apresoline, to assist in determining that the medication is an antihypertensive. This will direct you to option 1. Review this medication if it is unfamiliar to you.

*Level of Cognitive Ability:* Analysis
*Client Needs:* Physiological Integrity
*Integrated Concept/Process:* Nursing Process/Evaluation
*Content Area:* Pharmacology

*Reference*
Hodgson, B., & Kizior, R. (2001). *Saunders Nursing drug handbook 2001.* Philadelphia: W.B. Saunders, p. 493.

**539.** A client with a fractured femur who has had an open reduction-internal fixation is receiving ketorolac (Toradol). The nurse evaluates the effectiveness of the medication by monitoring the client's:

1   Serum calcium level
2   White blood cell count
3   Temperature
4   Pain rating

**Answer: 4**

*Rationale:* Ketorolac is a nonopioid analgesic and nonsteroidal antiinflammatory agent (NSAID). It acts by inhibiting prostaglandin synthesis and produces analgesia that is peripherally mediated. The nurse evaluates the effectiveness of this medication by using the pain rating scale with the client.

*Test-Taking Strategy:* Use the process of elimination. Noting the diagnosis of the client, fractured femur, may provide you with the clue that this medication is an analgesic. Review this medication if you had difficulty with this question.

*Level of Cognitive Ability:* Analysis
*Client Needs:* Physiological Integrity
*Integrated Concept/Process:* Nursing Process/Evaluation
*Content Area:* Pharmacology

*Reference*
Hodgson, B., & Kizior, R. (2001). *Saunders Nursing drug handbook 2001.* Philadelphia: W.B. Saunders, p. 568.

---

**540.** A client receiving a dose of intravenous vancomycin (Vancocin) develops chills, tachycardia, syncope, and flushing of the face and trunk. The nurse interprets that:
1 The client is allergic to the medication
2 The medication has interacted with another medication the client is receiving
3 The medication is infusing too rapidly
4 The client is experiencing upper airway obstruction

**Answer: 3**
*Rationale:* The client is experiencing signs and symptoms of what is called "red man" or "red neck" syndrome. This is a response due to histamine release that occurs with rapid or bolus injection. The client may experience chills, fever, flushing of the face and/or trunk, tachycardia, syncope, tingling, and an unpleasant taste in the mouth. The corrective action is to administer the medication more slowly. An antihistamine such as diphenhydramine (Benadryl) may be administered as well.

*Test-Taking Strategy:* This question may be difficult and you may want to quickly select option 1. Remember that options that are similar are not likely to be correct. For this reason, begin to answer this question by eliminating options 1 and 4 first. From the remaining options, recalling the adverse effect of "red neck" syndrome associated with the use of this medication will direct you to option 3. Review the adverse effects of this medication if you had difficulty with this question.

*Level of Cognitive Ability:* Analysis
*Client Needs:* Physiological Integrity
*Integrated Concept/Process:* Nursing Process/Analysis
*Content Area:* Pharmacology

*Reference*
McKenry, L., & Salerno, E. (1998). *Mosby's pharmacology in nursing (20th ed.).* St. Louis: Mosby-Year Book, p. 914.

---

**541.** A client has an order to be given beclomethasone (Beclovent) by the intranasal route. The client also has an order for a nasal decongestant. The nurse plans to:
1 Administer the beclomethasone 15 minutes before the decongestant
2 Administer the decongestant 15 minutes before the beclomethasone
3 Administer the beclomethasone immediately before the decongestant
4 Administer the decongestant immediately before the beclomethasone

**Answer: 2**
*Rationale:* The nasal decongestant should be administered 15 minutes before the beclomethasone (a glucocorticoid) to clear the nasal passages and enhance absorption of the glucocorticoid. Options 1, 3, and 4 are incorrect methods of administration.

*Test-Taking Strategy:* Use the same principles in answering this question that you would when administering bronchodilators and corticosteroids together. Remember, the glucocorticoid is administered last. Review the procedure for administering intranasal medications if you had difficulty with this question.

*Level of Cognitive Ability:* Application
*Client Needs:* Physiological Integrity

*Integrated Concept/Process:* Nursing Process/Planning
*Content Area:* Pharmacology

*Reference*
Hodgson, B., & Kizior, R. (2001). *Saunders Nursing drug handbook 2001.* Philadelphia: W.B. Saunders, p. 98.

**542.** A client has received atropine sulfate intravenously during a surgical procedure. The nurse monitors the client for which of the following effects of the medication in the immediate postoperative period?
1   Bradycardia
2   Excessive salivation
3   Diarrhea
4   Urinary retention

**Answer: 4**
*Rationale:* Atropine sulfate is an anticholinergic medication that causes tachycardia, drowsiness, blurred vision, dry mouth, constipation, and urinary retention. The nurse monitors the client for any of these effects in the immediate postoperative period.

*Test-Taking Strategy:* Use the process of elimination. Recalling that atropine sulfate is an anticholinergic will direct you to option 4. Review the side effects of this medication, if you had difficulty with this question.

*Level of Cognitive Ability:* Application
*Client Needs:* Physiological Integrity
*Integrated Concept/Process:* Nursing Process/Implementation
*Content Area:* Pharmacology

*Reference*
Hodgson, B., & Kizior, R. (2001). *Saunders Nursing drug handbook 2001.* Philadelphia: W.B. Saunders, p. 82.

**543.** A client is receiving tobramycin (Tobrex). The nurse evaluates that the client is responding well to the medication therapy if which of the following laboratory results is noted?
1   White blood cell (WBC) count of 8,000/mm³ and creatinine level of 0.9 mg/dL
2   WBC count of 15,000/mm³ and a blood urea nitrogen (BUN) of 38 mg/dL
3   Sodium of 140 mEq/L and potassium of 3.9 mEq/L
4   Sodium of 145 mEq/L and chloride of 106 mEq/L

**Answer: 1**
*Rationale:* Tobramycin is an antibiotic (aminoglycoside) that causes nephrotoxicity and ototoxicity. The medication is working if the WBC count drops back into the normal range and the kidney function remains normal. Option 2 indicates an abnormal WBC count and BUN level, and options 3 and 4 are unrelated to the use of this medication.

*Test-Taking Strategy:* Use the process of elimination. Begin to answer this question by eliminating options 3 and 4 first knowing that tobramycin is an antibiotic. Recalling that aminoglycosides cause nephrotoxicity, select option 1 using laboratory values as your guide. Review this medication and normal laboratory values, if you had difficulty with this question.

*Level of Cognitive Ability:* Analysis
*Client Needs:* Physiological Integrity
*Integrated Concept/Process:* Nursing Process/Evaluation
*Content Area:* Pharmacology

*Reference*
Hodgson, B., & Kizior, R. (2001). *Saunders Nursing drug handbook 2001.* Philadelphia: W.B. Saunders, pp. 998-1000.

**544.** A nurse is caring for a client who is taking a maintenance dosage of lithium carbonate (Eskalith). The nurse plans to:

1. Monitoring daily serum lithium levels
2. Perform a weekly ECG
3. Observe for remission of depressive states
4. Monitor intake and output

**Answer: 4**

*Rationale:* Lithium is used to treat manic disorders, not depression. Side effects of lithium are nausea, tremors, polyuria, and polydipsia. Serum lithium concentration is assessed approximately every 2 to 4 days during initial therapy, and at longer intervals, thereafter. Toxic levels of lithium may induce electrocardiogram changes, however, there is no need to perform weekly ECGs if maintenance levels are maintained.

*Test-Taking Strategy:* Use the process of elimination. Eliminate options 1 and 2 first because of the words *daily* and *weekly*. From the remaining options, recalling that this medication is used to treat manic disorders will direct you to option 4. If you had difficulty with this question, review the nursing interventions associated with administering this medication.

*Level of Cognitive Ability:* Application
*Client Needs:* Physiological Integrity
*Integrated Concept/Process:* Nursing Process/Planning
*Content Area:* Pharmacology

*Reference*

Hodgson, B., & Kizior, R. (2001). *Saunders Nursing drug handbook 2001.* Philadelphia: W.B. Saunders, p. 598.

**545.** A nurse is caring for a client with neuroleptic malignant syndrome (NMS) that resulted from the use of antipsychotic medications. On assessment, the nurse would expect to note:

1. Bradycardia
2. Dysphagia
3. Hypotension
4. Hyperpyrexia

**Answer: 4**

*Rationale:* Hyperpyrexia up to 107° F may be present in NMS. Symptoms develop suddenly and may include respiratory distress and muscle rigidity. As the condition progresses, there is evidence of tachycardia, hypertension, increasing respiratory distress, confusion, and delirium. The presence and severity of symptoms is compounded when two or more antipsychotics are taken concomitantly.

*Test-Taking Strategy:* Consider the physiological responses that occur in NMS to answer this question. Options 1 and 3 normally occur in conjunction with each other, therefore eliminate these options. From the remaining options it is necessary to know that hyperpyrexia occurs in this disorder. Review the physiological manifestations that occur in NMS, if you had difficulty with this question.

*Level of Cognitive Ability:* Analysis
*Client Needs:* Physiological Integrity
*Integrated Concept/Process:* Nursing Process/Assessment
*Content Area:* Pharmacology

*Reference*

Stuart, G.W., & Laraia, M.T. (1998). *Principles and practice of psychiatric nursing.* (6th ed.). St. Louis: Mosby, p. 591.

**546.** A nurse is performing an admission assessment on a newborn infant admitted with the diagnosis of subdural hematoma following a difficult vaginal delivery. The nurse assesses for major symptoms associated with subdural hematoma when the nurse:

1. Tests for contractures of the extremities
2. Tests for equality of extremities when stimulating reflexes
3. Monitors the urinary output pattern
4. Monitors the urine for blood

**Answer: 2**

*Rationale:* A subdural hematoma can cause pressure on a specific area of the cerebral tissue. This can, especially if the infant is actively bleeding, cause changes in the stimuli responses in the extremities on the opposite side of the body. Option 1 is incorrect because contractures would not occur this soon after delivery. Options 3 and 4 are incorrect. An infant, after delivery, would normally be incontinent of urine. Blood in the urine would indicate abdominal trauma and not be a result of the hematoma.

*Test-Taking Strategy:* Note the key words *major symptoms*. Eliminate options 3 and 4 because they are similar assessments. Remember, the method of assessing for complications and active bleeding into the cranial cavity would be a neurological assessment. Checking newborn reflexes is a neurological assessment. Although, contractures of extremities could occur as residual effects, this would not occur immediately. Review the signs of subdural hematoma in the newborn infant if you had difficulty with this question.

*Level of Cognitive Ability:* Analysis
*Client Needs:* Physiological Integrity
*Integrated Concept/Process:* Nursing Process/Assessment
*Content Area:* Child Health

*Reference*
Lowdermilk, D., Perry, S., & Bobak, I. (2000). *Maternity & women's health care* (7th ed.). St. Louis: Mosby, p. 1023.

---

**547.** A nurse is performing an admission assessment on a client admitted with a diagnosis of Raynaud's disease. The nurse assesses for the symptoms associated with Raynaud's disease by:

1. Observing for softening of the nails or nail beds
2. Palpating for diminished or absent peripheral pulses
3. Checking for a rash on the digits
4. Palpating for a rapid or irregular peripheral pulse

**Answer: 2**

*Rationale:* Raynaud's disease produces closure of the small arteries in the distal extremities in response to cold, vibration, or external stimuli. Palpation for diminished or absent peripheral pulses checks for interruption of circulation. The nails grow slowly, become brittle or deformed and heal poorly around the nail beds when infected. Skin changes include hair loss, thinning or tightening of the skin, and delayed healing of cuts or injuries. Although palpation of peripheral pulses is correct, a rapid or irregular pulse would not be noted. Peripheral pulses may be normal, absent, or diminished.

*Test-Taking Strategy:* Recall the physiological occurrences in Raynaud's disease. Use the ABCs: airway, breathing, and circulation. Review the manifestations associated with this disorder if you had difficulty with this question.

*Level of Cognitive Ability:* Application
*Client Needs:* Physiological Integrity
*Integrated Concept/Process:* Nursing Process/Assessment
*Content Area:* Adult Health/Cardiovascular

*Reference*
Smeltzer, S., & Bare, B. (2000). *Brunner & Suddarth's Textbook of medical-surgical nursing* (9th ed.). Philadelphia: Lippincott Williams & Wilkins, p. 704.

**548.** A depressed client is found unconscious on the floor in the room. The nurse sees several empty bottles of a prescribed tricyclic antidepressant lying near the client. The immediate action of the nurse is to:

1 Call a "Code," because this incident presents a medical emergency
2 Induce vomiting and notify the physician for further orders
3 Call the Poison Control Center
4 Try to figure out the number of pills taken

**Answer: 1**

*Rationale:* Tricyclic antidepressants can be fatal when taken as an overdose regardless of the amount ingested. Serious, life-threatening symptoms can develop after an overdose. Immediate emergency medical attention and cardiac monitoring is necessitated with an overdose of tricyclics. Options 2, 3, and 4 are not the immediate actions.

*Test-Taking Strategy:* Use the process of elimination and note the key word *immediate*. Eliminate options 3 and 4 because these measures would delay immediate treatment. The client is unconscious, therefore the nurse would not induce vomiting because of the risk of aspiration. Review immediate nursing actions when an overdose for a tricyclic antidepressant occurs in a client.

*Level of Cognitive Ability:* Application
*Client Needs:* Physiological Integrity
*Integrated Concept/Process:* Nursing Process/Implementation
*Content Area:* Mental Health

*Reference*
Stuart, G.W., & Laraia, M.T. (1998). *Principles and practice of psychiatric nursing.* (6th ed.). St. Louis: Mosby, p. 582.

**549.** A client is admitted with acute exacerbation of chronic obstructive pulmonary disease (COPD). Which of the following blood gas results would the nurse most likely expect to note?

1 $Po_2$ of 68 and $Pco_2$ of 40
2 $Po_2$ of 55 and $Pco_2$ of 40
3 $Po_2$ of 70 and $Pco_2$ of 50
4 $Po_2$ of 60 and $Pco_2$ of 50

**Answer: 4**

*Rationale:* During an acute exacerbation, the arterial blood gases deteriorate with a decreasing $Po_2$ and an increasing $Pco_2$. In early stages of COPD, arterial blood gases demonstrate mild to moderate hypoxemia with the $Po_2$ in the high 60s to high 70s and a normal arterial $Pco_2$. As the condition advances, hypoxemia increases and hypercapnia may result.

*Test-Taking Strategy:* Note the key words *acute exacerbation*. Recall the physiological manifestations that occur in COPD. Remembering that in COPD, a low $Po_2$ and an elevated $Pco_2$ is the likely occurrence, will direct you to the correct option. Review the clinical manifestations that are likely to occur in an acute exacerbation if you had difficulty with this question.

*Level of Cognitive Ability:* Analysis
*Client Needs:* Physiological Integrity
*Integrated Concept/Process:* Nursing Process/Analysis
*Content Area:* Adult Health/Respiratory

*Reference*
Smeltzer, S., & Bare, B. (2000). *Brunner & Suddarth's Textbook of medical-surgical nursing* (9th ed.). Philadelphia: Lippincott Williams & Wilkins, p. 448.

**550.** A nurse monitors the respiratory status of the client being treated for acute exacerbation of chronic obstructive pulmonary disease (COPD). Which of the following assessment findings would indicate a deterioration in ventilation?
1. Cyanosis
2. Rapid, shallow respirations
3. Hyperinflated chest
4. Coarse crackles bilaterally

**Answer: 2**

*Rationale:*  An increase in the rate of respirations and a decrease in the depth of respirations indicates a deterioration in ventilation. Cyanosis is not a good indicator of oxygenation in the client with COPD. Cyanosis may be present with some clients but not all clients. A hyperinflated chest (barrel-chest) and hypertrophy of the accessory muscles of the upper chest and neck may normally be found in clients with severe COPD. During an exacerbation, coarse crackles are expected to be heard bilateral throughout the lungs but do not indicate deterioration in ventilation.

*Test-Taking Strategy:*  Note the key words *deterioration in ventilation*. Recalling the normal clinical signs seen in COPD and the signs of exacerbation, eliminate options 3 and 4. Since cyanosis is not a good indicator of oxygenation in the client with COPD, eliminate option 1. Review the clinical manifestations associated with COPD and a deterioration in ventilation, if you had difficulty with this question.

*Level of Cognitive Ability:*  Analysis
*Client Needs:*  Physiological Integrity
*Integrated Concept/Process:*  Nursing Process/Assessment
*Content Area:*  Adult Health/Respiratory

*Reference*
Smeltzer, S., & Bare, B. (2000). *Brunner & Suddarth's Textbook of medical-surgical nursing* (9th ed.). Philadelphia: Lippincott Williams & Wilkins, p. 456.

# CRITICAL THINKING: FREE-TEXT ENTRY

**1.** A nurse is caring for a client with chronic obstructive pulmonary disease (COPD) who is receiving aminophylline (Theophylline) intravenously. A theophylline blood serum level is drawn on the client. The nurse monitors the results of this blood test and expects the findings to be within therapeutic range. What is the therapeutic serum level range of theophylline?

**Answer:** The therapeutic serum level range of theophylline is 10 to 20 µg/mL.

*Rationale:*  Aminophylline (Theophylline) is a bronchodilator. The therapeutic serum level range of theophylline is 10 to 20 µg/mL. It is critical that the nurse monitor theophylline blood serum levels daily when a client is on this medication to ensure that a therapeutic range is present and to monitor for the potential for toxicity.

*Test-Taking Strategy:*  Specific knowledge of this medication and the therapeutic serum level range is required to answer this question. Remember that this therapeutic serum level range is the same as the therapeutic serum level range for phenytoin (Dilantin). Review this medication if you had difficulty with this question.

*Level of Cognitive Ability:* Analysis
*Client Needs:* Physiological Integrity
*Integrated Concept/Process:* Nursing Process/Assessment
*Content Area:* Pharmacology

*Reference*

Hodgson, B., & Kizior, R. (2001). *Saunders Nursing drug handbook 2001.* Philadelphia: W.B. Saunders, pp. 44-47.

---

**2.** A nurse is caring for a client with a closed chest drainage system. On assessment of the client, the nurse notes a rise and fall (fluctuation) of fluid in the water seal chamber. Based on this finding, what action will the nurse take?

**Answer:** The nurse would document that the system is functioning accurately.

*Rationale:* Fluid in the water seal compartment should rise with inspiration and fall with expiration (fluctuations). When fluctuations occur, the drainage tubes are patent and the apparatus is functioning properly. Fluctuations stop when the lung has reexpanded or if the chest drainage tubes are kinked or obstructed.

*Test-Taking Strategy:* Focus on the nurse's assessment finding, a rise and fall (fluctuation) of fluid in the water seal chamber. Visualize the chest tube drainage system and think about the function of each chamber to assist in determining the nurse's action. If you had difficulty with this question, review the functioning of chest tube drainage systems.

*Level of Cognitive Ability:* Analysis
*Client Needs:* Physiological Integrity
*Integrated Concept/Process:* Nursing Process/Implementation
*Content Area:* Adult Health/Respiratory

*Reference*

Black, J., Hawks, J., & Keene, A. (2001). *Medical-surgical nursing: Clinical management for positive outcomes* (6th ed.). Philadelphia: W.B. Saunders, p. 1731.

---

**3.** A nurse is measuring the vital signs of a client with increased intracranial pressure (ICP). The respirations have a variable rate. The cycle of respirations begins shallowly with an increasing depth to hyperventilation, and then decreases in depth to apnea. The cycle then repeats itself. The nurse documents that the client is exhibiting what type of respirations?

**Answer:** Cheyne-Stokes respirations

*Rationale:* The client with increased intracranial pressure may exhibit Cheyne-Stokes respirations. This type of respirations has a variable rate. The cycle of respirations begins shallowly and then increases in depth to hyperventilation, followed by a decrease in depth to apnea. The cycle then repeats itself.

*Test-Taking Strategy:* Focus on the description of the respiratory pattern in the question. This description and noting that the client has a diagnosis of increased ICP will assist in identifying the respiratory pattern. Review this type of respiratory pattern if you had difficulty with this question.

*Level of Cognitive Ability:* Analysis
*Client Needs:* Physiological Integrity
*Integrated Concept/Process:* Communication and Documentation
*Content Area:* Adult Health/Neurological

*Reference*
Black, J., Hawks, J., & Keene, A. (2001). *Medical-surgical nursing: Clinical management for positive outcomes* (6th ed.). Philadelphia: W.B. Saunders, p. 184.

---

**4.** A client received a thermal burn caused by the inhalation of steam. The client's mouth is edematous and the nurse notes blisters in the client's mouth. The nurse next assesses which priority item?

**Answer:** Respiratory status and lung sounds

*Rationale:* Thermal burns to the lower airways can occur with the inhalation of steam or explosive gases or with the aspiration of scalding liquids. Thermal burns to the upper airways are more common and generally appear erythematous and edematous with mucosal blisters or ulcerations. The mucosal edema can lead to upper airway obstruction particularly during the first 24 to 48 hours after a burn injury. Assessment of respiratory status is the priority.

*Test-Taking Strategy:* Focus on the type of burn injury described in the question and note the key words *mouth is edematous.* Use the ABCs: airway, breathing, and circulation, to assist in answering this question. Review care of a client with a burn injury if you had difficulty with this question.

*Level of Cognitive Ability:* Analysis
*Client Needs:* Physiological Integrity
*Integrated Concept/Process:* Nursing Process/Assessment
*Content Area:* Adult Health/Respiratory

*Reference*
Black, J., Hawks, J., & Keene, A. (2001). *Medical-surgical nursing: Clinical management for positive outcomes* (6th ed.). Philadelphia: W.B. Saunders, p. 1337.

---

**5.** A nurse hears the alarm sound on the telemetry monitor. The nurse quickly looks at the monitor and notes that a client is in ventricular tachycardia. The nurse rushes to the client's room. Upon reaching the client's bedside, the nurse would initially assess the client for which finding?

**Answer:** Unresponsiveness

*Rationale:* Determining unresponsiveness is the first assessment action to take. When a client is in ventricular tachycardia, there is a significant decrease in cardiac output. However, assessing for unresponsiveness ensures whether the client is affected by the decreased cardiac output.

*Test-Taking Strategy:* Note the key word *initially.* Use the steps of basic life support to answer the question. Remember, determining unresponsiveness is the first action. Review the initial nursing actions when a client experiences ventricular tachycardia if you had difficulty with this question.

*Level of Cognitive Ability:* Application
*Client Needs:* Physiological Integrity
*Integrated Concept/Process:* Nursing Process/Implementation
*Content Area:* Adult Health/Cardiovascular

*Reference*

Black, J., Hawks, J., & Keene, A. (2001). *Medical-surgical nursing: Clinical management for positive outcomes* (6th ed.). Philadelphia: W.B. Saunders, p. 1560.

---

**6.** A nurse is performing a physical assessment on a client and is testing the client's reflexes. What action would the nurse take to assess the pharyngeal reflex?

**Answer:** Stimulate the back of the throat with a tongue depressor

*Rationale:* The pharyngeal (gag) reflex is tested by touching the back of the throat with an object, such as a tongue depressor. A positive response to this reflex is considered normal.

*Test-Taking Strategy:* Focus on the type of reflex addressed in the question. Recalling that *pharyngeal* refers to the pharynx, or back of the throat, will assist in determining how this reflex is tested. Review assessment of reflexes if you had difficulty with this question.

*Level of Cognitive Ability:* Application
*Client Needs:* Physiological Integrity
*Integrated Concept/Process:* Nursing Process/Assessment
*Content Area:* Adult Health/Neurological

*Reference*

Black, J., Hawks, J., & Keene, A. (2001). *Medical-surgical nursing: Clinical management for positive outcomes* (6th ed.). Philadelphia: W.B. Saunders, p. 1886.

---

**7.** A nurse is performing an admission assessment on a client admitted to the hospital with a diagnosis of pheochromocytoma. The nurse prepares to implement what action to assess for the major symptom associated with this disorder?

**Answer:** Take the client's blood pressure

*Rationale:* Hypertension is the major symptom associated with pheochromocytoma. The blood pressure status would be assessed by taking the client's blood pressure.

*Test-Taking Strategy:* Note the key words *major symptom*. Recalling that pheochromocytoma is a tumor of the adrenal gland and recalling the function of the adrenal gland will assist in determining the assessment technique to be implemented. If you had difficulty with this question, review the major clinical manifestations of pheochromocytoma.

*Level of Cognitive Ability:* Application
*Client Needs:* Physiological Integrity
*Integrated Concept/Process:* Nursing Process/Assessment
*Content Area:* Adult Health/Endocrine

*Reference*

Black, J., Hawks, J., & Keene, A. (2001). *Medical-surgical nursing: Clinical management for positive outcomes* (6th ed.). Philadelphia: W.B. Saunders, p. 1135.

**8.** During the administration of a blood transfusion to a client, the nurse notes the presence of crackles (rales) in the client's lung bases. On further assessment, the nurse notes that the client has distended neck veins and an increase in central venous pressure. The nurse suspects that the client is experiencing what complication of the blood transfusion?

**Answer:** Circulatory overload

**Rationale:** Chest or lumbar pain, cyanosis, dyspnea, moist productive cough, crackle (rales) in the lung bases, distended neck veins, and an increase in central venous pressure are clinical indications of circulatory overload caused from excessive infusion amounts or too rapid an infusion rate. The blood should be discontinued.

**Test-Taking Strategy:** Focusing on the signs and symptoms identified in the question will assist in determining that the client is experiencing circulatory overload. Review the signs of circulatory overload if you had difficulty with this question.

**Level of Cognitive Ability:** Analysis
**Client Needs:** Physiological Integrity
**Integrated Concept/Process:** Nursing Process/Assessment
**Content Area:** Fundamental Skills

**Reference**
Smeltzer, S., & Bare, B. (2000). *Brunner & Suddarth's Textbook of medical-surgical nursing* (9th ed.). Philadelphia: Lippincott Williams & Wilkins, p. 782.

## REFERENCES

Altman, G., Buchsel, P., & Coxon, V. (2000). *Delmar's Fundamental & advanced nursing skills.* Albany, N.Y.: Delmar.

Ball, J., & Bindler, R. (1999). *Pediatric nursing: Caring for children* (2nd ed.). Stamford, Conn.: Appleton & Lange.

Ball, J., & Bindler, R. (1999). *Quick reference to pediatric clinical skills.* Stamford, Conn.: Appleton & Lange.

Black, J., Hawks, J., & Keene, A. (2001). *Medical-surgical nursing: Clinical management for positive outcomes* (6th ed.). Philadelphia: W.B. Saunders.

Deglin, J., & Vallerand, A. (2001). *Davis's drug guide for nurses* (7th ed.). Philadelphia: F.A. Davis.

DeLaune, S., & Ladner, P. (1998). *Fundamentals of nursing: Standards and practice.* Albany, N.Y.: Delmar.

Fischbach, F. (2000). *A manual of laboratory & diagnostic tests* (6th ed.). Philadelphia: Lippincott Williams & Wilkins.

Gorrie, T., McKinney, E., & Murray, S. (1998). *Foundations of maternal-newborn nursing* (2 nd ed.). Philadelphia: W.B. Saunders.

Grodner, M., Anderson, S., & DeYoung, S. (2000). *Foundations and clinical applications of nutrition: A nursing approach.* St. Louis: Mosby.

Gutierrez, K. (1999). *Pharmacotherapeutics: Clinical decision-making in nursing.* Philadelphia: W.B. Saunders.

Harkreader, H. (2000). *Fundamentals of nursing: Caring and clinical judgment.* Philadelphia: W.B. Saunders.

Hodgson, B., & Kizior, R. (2001). *Saunders Nursing drug handbook 2001.* Philadelphia: W.B. Saunders.

Ignatavicius, D., Workman, M., & Mishler, M. (1999). *Medical-surgical nursing across the health care continuum* (3rd ed.). Philadelphia: W.B. Saunders.

Johnson, M., Bulechek, G., Dochterman, J., Maas, M., & Moorhead, S. (2001). *Nursing diagnoses, outcomes, and interventions.* St. Louis: Mosby.

Kee, J., & Marshall, S. (2000). *Clinical calculations: With applications to general and specialty areas* (4th ed.). Philadelphia: W.B. Saunders.

Kozier, B., Erb, G., Berman, A., & Burke, K. (2000). *Fundamentals of nursing: Concepts, process, and practice* (6th ed.). Upper Saddle River, N.J.: Prentice-Hall.

Kuhn, M. (1998). *Pharmacotherapeutics: A nursing process approach* (4th ed.). Philadelphia: F.A. Davis.

Ladewig, P., London, M., & Olds, S. (1998). *Maternal-newborn care: The nurse, the family, and the community* (4th ed.). Menlo Park, Calif.: Addison-Wesley.

LeMone, P., & Burke, K. (2000). *Medical-surgical nursing: Critical thinking in client care* (2nd ed.). Upper Saddle River, N.J.: Prentice-Hall.

Lowdermilk, D., Perry, S., & Bobak, I. (2000). *Maternity & women's health care* (7th ed.). St. Louis: Mosby.

McKenry, L., & Salerno, E. (1998). *Mosby's Pharmacology in nursing* (20th ed.). St. Louis: Mosby.

Monahan, F., & Neighbors, M. (1998). *Medical-surgical nursing: Foundations for clinical practice* (2nd ed.). Philadelphia: W.B. Saunders.

Olds, S., London, M., & Ladewig, P. (2000). *Maternal-newborn nursing: A family and community-based approach* (6th ed.). Upper Saddle River, N.J.: Prentice-Hall Health.

Phipps, W., Sands, J., & Marek, J. (1999). *Medical-surgical nursing: Concepts & clinical practice* (6th ed.). St. Louis: Mosby.

Potter, P., & Perry, A. (2001). *Fundamentals of nursing* (5th ed.). St. Louis: Mosby.

Salerno, E. (1999). *Pharmacology for health professionals.* St. Louis: Mosby.

Sherwen, L., Scoloveno, M.A., & Weingarten, C. (1999). *Maternity nursing: Care of the childbearing family* (3rd ed.). Stamford, Conn.: Appleton & Lange.

Smeltzer, S., & Bare, B. (2000). *Brunner & Suddarth's Textbook of medical-surgical nursing* (9th ed.). Philadelphia: Lippincott Williams & Wilkins.

Sole, M.L., Lamborn, M., & Hartshorn, J. (2001). *Introduction to critical care nursing* (3rd ed.). Philadelphia: W.B. Saunders.

Stuart, G.W., & Laraia, M.T. (1998). *Principles and practice of psychiatric nursing.* (6th ed.). St. Louis: Mosby.

Varcarolis, E. (1998). *Foundations of psychiatric mental health nursing* (3rd ed.). Philadelphia: W.B. Saunders.

Wong, D. (1999). *Whaley & Wong's Nursing care of infants and children* (6th ed.). St. Louis: Mosby.

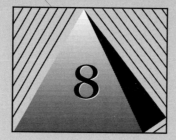

# Psychosocial Integrity

---

**1.** A mother comes to the pediatric clinic because her previously continent 6-year-old son has resumed bedwetting. After learning that there is a new baby in the home, the nurse explains to the mother that the son is most likely using the defense mechanism of:
1  Identification
2  Regression
3  Rationalization
4  Repression

**Answer: 2**
*Rationale:* The defense mechanism of regression is characterized by returning to an earlier form of expressing an impulse. Option 1 occurs when a person models behavior after someone else. Option 3 occurs when a person unconsciously falsifies an experience by giving a "rational" explanation. Option 4 is characterized by blocking a wish or desire from conscious expression.

*Test-Taking Strategy:* Use the process of elimination. Noting the key words *resumed bedwetting* will direct you to option 2. Review defense mechanisms if you had difficulty with this question.

*Level of Cognitive Ability:* Application
*Client Needs:* Psychosocial Integrity
*Integrated Concept/Process:* Nursing Process/Implementation
*Content Area:* Child Health

*Reference*
Wong, D. (1999). *Whaley & Wong's Nursing care of infants and children* (6th ed.). St. Louis: Mosby, p. 679.

---

**2.** A nurse is obtaining a health history for an adolescent. Which statement by the adolescent indicates a need for follow-up assessment and intervention?
1  "I find myself very moody—happy one minute and crying the next."
2  "I can't seem to wake up in the morning. I would sleep until noon if I could."
3  "I don't eat anything with fat in it, and I've lost 8 pounds in 2 weeks."
4  "When I get stressed out about school, I just like to be alone."

**Answer: 3**
*Rationale:* During the adolescent period there is a heightened awareness of body image and peer pressure to go on excessively restrictive diets. The extreme limitation of omitting all fat in the diet and weight loss during a time of growth suggests inadequate nutrition and a possible eating disorder.

*Test-Taking Strategy:* Note the key words *need for follow-up*. Options 1, 2, and 4 are common and normal behaviors or feelings during adolescence. Option 3 indicates a problem or abnormality. If you had difficulty with this question, review the developmental stage of adolescence.

*Level of Cognitive Ability:* Analysis
*Client Needs:* Psychosocial Integrity
*Integrated Concept/Process:* Nursing Process/Analysis
*Content Area:* Child Health

*Reference*
Wong, D. (1999). *Whaley & Wong's Nursing care of infants and children* (6th ed.).
    St. Louis: Mosby, pp. 914-915.

---

**3.** A nurse is caring for a client who has bipolar disorder and is in a manic state. The most appropriate menu choice for this client would be which of the following?
1  Scrambled eggs, orange juice, coffee with cream and sugar
2  Cheeseburger, banana, milk
3  Beef stew, fruit salad, tea
4  Macaroni and cheese, apple, milk

**Answer: 2**
*Rationale:* The client in a manic state often has inadequate food and fluid intake as a result of physical agitation. Foods that the client can eat "on the run" are most appropriate, since the client is too active to sit at meals and use utensils. Additionally, clients in a manic state should not have caffeine-containing products.

*Test-Taking Strategy:* Use the process of elimination, focusing on the key words *manic state*. Note the similarity among options 1, 3, and 4. Remember the concept of finger foods with the client with mania. Review care of a client with mania if you had difficulty with this question.

*Level of Cognitive Ability:* Application
*Client Needs:* Psychosocial Integrity
*Integrated Concept/Process:* Nursing Process/Planning
*Content Area:* Mental Health

*Reference*
Stuart, G.W., & Laraia, M.T. (1998). *Principles and practice of psychiatric nursing* (6th ed.). St. Louis: Mosby, p. 355.

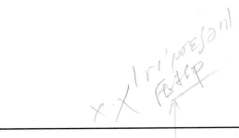

---

**4.** A nurse is caring for a child who is a victim of child abuse. The nurse has determined that the child uses repression to cope with past life experiences. The nurse implements an appropriate plan of care that includes:
1  Placing the child on medications that will help forget the incidents
2  Having the child talk about the abuse in detail during the first therapy session
3  Encouraging the child to use play therapy to act out past experiences
4  Telling the child to let the past go and concentrate on the present and future

**Answer: 3**
*Rationale:* Play therapy is a nonthreatening avenue through which the child can use artwork, dolls, or puppets to act out frightening life experiences. Options 1 and 4 devalue the child and force the child to further repress harmful past experiences rather than face them and move on. Option 2 would be extremely threatening to the child and nontherapeutic.

*Test-Taking Strategy:* Use therapeutic communication techniques to eliminate options 2 and 4. From the remaining options, note the relationship of *past life experiences* in the question and *past experiences* in the correct option. Review care of a child who is a victim of abuse if you had difficulty with this question.

*Level of Cognitive Ability:* Application
*Client Needs:* Psychosocial Integrity
*Integrated Concept/Process:* Nursing Process/Implementation
*Content Area:* Child Health

*Reference*
Wong, D. (1999). *Whaley & Wong's Nursing care of infants and children* (6th ed.).
    St. Louis: Mosby, p. 1173.

**5.** An elderly woman is brought to the emergency department by a family member with whom she lives. A nurse notes that the client has poor hygiene, contractures, and decubitus ulcers on the sacrum, scapula, and heels. The client is suspected of which form of victimization?
1    Emotional abuse
2    Physical abuse
3    Psychological abuse
4    Sexual abuse

**Answer: 2**

*Rationale:* Victimization in a family can take many forms. When analyzing a specific client situation, it is important to understand which form of abuse is being considered. Physical abuse can take the form of battering (hitting, slapping, striking), or can be more subtle, such as neglect (failure to meet basic needs).

*Test-Taking Strategy:* Focus on the data provided in the question. This question identifies only physical signs of victimization. Option 2 is the only option that fits the description in the question. Review the signs of physical abuse in the elderly client if you had difficulty with this question.

*Level of Cognitive Ability:* Analysis
*Client Needs:* Psychosocial Integrity
*Integrated Concept/Process:* Nursing Process/Analysis
*Content Area:* Mental Health

*Reference*
Stuart, G.W., & Laraia, M.T. (1998). *Principles and practice of psychiatric nursing* (6th ed.). St. Louis: Mosby, p. 863.

---

**6.** A female client is admitted to the inpatient mental health unit. When asked her name, she responds, "I am Elizabeth, the Queen of England." The nurse recognizes this response as a(n):
1    Visual illusion
2    Auditory hallucination
3    Grandiose delusion
4    Loose association

**Answer: 3**

*Rationale:* A delusion is an important personal belief that is almost certainly not true and resists modification. An illusion is a misperception or misinterpretation of externally real stimuli. A hallucination is a false perception. Loose association is thinking characterized by speech in which ideas that are unrelated shift from one subject to another.

*Test-Taking Strategy:* Use the process of elimination and focus on the information in the question. Eliminate options 1 and 2, because the client is not having any visual or auditory disturbances. Option 4 is eliminated next, because there is no indication that the client is shifting from one subject to another. Making a reference to being a queen is a grandiose assumption. Review the description of grandiose delusions if you had difficulty with this question.

*Level of Cognitive Ability:* Analysis
*Client Needs:* Psychosocial Integrity
*Integrated Concept/Process:* Nursing Process/Assessment
*Content Area:* Mental Health

*Reference*
Stuart, G.W., & Laraia, M.T. (1998). *Principles and practice of psychiatric nursing* (6th ed.). St. Louis: Mosby, p. 117.

**7.** A newly admitted client with a diagnosis of bipolar disorder is trying to organize a dance with the other clients on the unit and is planning an on-unit supper. To decrease stimulation, the nurse should encourage the client to:

1 Engage the help of other clients on the unit to accomplish the task

2 Seek assistance from other staff members

3 Postpone the dance and engage in a writing activity

4 Firmly tell the client that this task is inappropriate

**Answer: 3**

*Rationale:* Because a client with bipolar disorder is easily stimulated by the environment, sedentary activities are the best outlets for energy release. Since most bipolar clients enjoy writing, the writing task is appropriate. An activity such as planning a dance or supper might be appropriate at some point, but not for a newly admitted client who is likely to have impaired judgment and a short attention span.

*Test-Taking Strategy:* Use the process of elimination. Note the key words *to decrease stimulation.* Options 1 and 2 encourage activity and should be eliminated. Option 4 tells the client that the activity is inappropriate, and this could result in an angry outburst by the client. Option 3 is the only option that limits activity. If you had difficulty with this question, review the appropriate activities for the bipolar client.

*Level of Cognitive Ability:* Application
*Client Needs:* Psychosocial Integrity
*Integrated Concept/Process:* Nursing Process/Implementation
*Content Area:* Mental Health

*Reference*
Stuart, G.W., & Laraia, M.T. (1998). *Principles and practice of psychiatric nursing* (6th ed.). St. Louis: Mosby, p. 352.

---

**8.** A male client with obsessive-compulsive disorder spends many hours during the day and night washing his hands. When initially planning for a safe environment, the nurse allows the client to continue this behavior because it:

1 Relieves the client's anxiety

2 Decreases the chance of infection

3 Gives the client a feeling of self-control

4 Increases self-esteem

**Answer: 1**

*Rationale:* The compulsive act provides immediate relief from anxiety and is used to cope with stress, conflict, or pain. Although the client may feel the need to increase self-esteem, that is not the primary goal of this behavior. Options 2 and 3 are also incorrect.

*Test-Taking Strategy:* Use the process of elimination. Focusing on the key word *initially* and recalling the effect of compulsive acts will direct you to option 1. If you are unfamiliar with this content, review this important disorder.

*Level of Cognitive Ability:* Application
*Client Needs:* Psychosocial Integrity
*Integrated Concept/Process:* Nursing Process/Planning
*Content Area:* Mental Health

*Reference*
Stuart, G.W., & Laraia, M.T. (1998). *Principles and practice of psychiatric nursing* (6th ed.). St. Louis: Mosby, p. 452.

**9.** An adolescent is returning home after psychiatric hospitalization because of a suicide attempt. Which of the following would be least effective in preparing the client to return home?
  1  Identify the family's strengths and weaknesses
  2  Suggest that the mother's boyfriend move out of the home
  3  Provide and offer the family options and resources
  4  Encourage sharing of feelings among the family

**Answer: 2**
*Rationale:* Option 2 is clearly the least effective option because there is no information in the question that indicates that the boyfriend's involvement has anything to do with the suicide attempt. Options 1, 3, and 4 offer helpful ways to enhance the family processes.

*Test-Taking Strategy:* Note the key words *least effective* and focus on the data in the question. Options 1, 3, and 4 identify positive measures. Review the psychosocial issues related to preparing a client for discharge if you had difficulty with this question.

*Level of Cognitive Ability:* Application
*Client Needs:* Psychosocial Integrity
*Integrated Concept/Process:* Nursing Process/Implementation
*Content Area:* Mental Health

*Reference*
Stuart, G.W., & Laraia, M.T. (1998). *Principles and practice of psychiatric nursing* (6th ed.). St. Louis: Mosby, p. 399.

---

**10.** An 11-year-old child scheduled for a diagnostic procedure will have an intravenous (IV) line inserted and will receive an intramuscular (IM) injection. The nurse most appropriately prepares the child for the procedure by:
  1  Teaching the parents so they can explain everything to their child
  2  Using pictures, concrete words, and demonstrations to describe what will happen
  3  Telling the child not to worry because the doctors take care of everything
  4  Reassuring the child that he or she will not feel any pain

**Answer: 2**
*Rationale:* The school-aged child understands best with visual aids and concrete language. Option 1 inappropriately delegates the responsibility for teaching to the parents. Option 3 is not therapeutic. Option 4 is inaccurate information.

*Test-Taking Strategy:* Use the process of elimination and therapeutic communication techniques. In option 1, a nursing responsibility is inappropriately delegated to parents. Options 3 and 4 are nontherapeutic. Review care of a school-aged child if you had difficulty with this question.

*Level of Cognitive Ability:* Application
*Client Needs:* Psychosocial Integrity
*Integrated Concept/Process:* Nursing Process/Implementation
*Content Area:* Child Health

*Reference*
Ball, J., & Bindler, R. (1999). *Pediatric nursing: Caring for children* (2nd ed.). Stamford, Conn.: Appleton & Lange, p. 181.

**11.** A nurse observes an anxious client blocking the hallway, walking three steps forward and then two steps backward. Other clients are agitated, trying to get past. The nurse intervenes by:

1   Standing beside the client and saying, "You're very anxious today."
2   Stopping the behavior and saying, "You're going to get exhausted."
3   Taking the client to the TV lounge and saying, "Relax and watch television now."
4   Walking beside the client and saying, "You're not going anywhere very fast doing this."

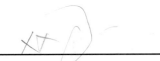

**Answer: 1**

*Rationale:* An important consideration in alleviating the anxiety is to assist the client to recognize their behavior. Options 2 and 3 do not address the increased anxiety and need to control the underlying the behavior and may even escalate the behavior. Option 4 does not raise the client to a functioning level.

*Test-Taking Strategy:* Use the process of elimination. Note the relationship between the word *anxious* in the question and in the correct option. Remember, it is important to assist the client in recognizing his or her behavior. Review measures related to the care of an anxious client if you had difficulty with this question.

*Level of Cognitive Ability:* Application
*Client Needs:* Psychosocial Integrity
*Integrated Concept/Process:* Nursing Process/Implementation
*Content Area:* Mental Health

*Reference*
Stuart, G.W., & Laraia, M.T. (1998). *Principles and practice of psychiatric nursing* (6th ed.). St. Louis: Mosby, p. 355.

---

**12.** A nurse is assisting in providing a form of psychotherapy in which the client enacts situations that are of emotional significance. The nurse understands that this form of therapy is known as:

1   Reality therapy
2   Short-term dynamic psychotherapy
3   Psychoanalytic therapy
4   Psychodrama

**Answer: 4**

*Rationale:* Psychodrama involves enactment of emotionally charged situations. Reality therapy is used for individuals with cognitive impairment. Both short-term dynamic psychotherapy and psychoanalytic therapy depend on techniques drawn from psychoanalysis.

*Test-Taking Strategy:* Note the key words *the client enacts situations.* This will assist in providing you with the definition of psychodrama. If you had difficulty with this question, review these types of therapy.

*Level of Cognitive Ability:* Analysis
*Client Needs:* Psychosocial Integrity
*Integrated Concept/Process:* Nursing Process/Analysis
*Content Area:* Mental Health

*Reference*
Stuart, G.W., & Laraia, M.T. (1998). *Principles and practice of psychiatric nursing* (6th ed.). St. Louis: Mosby, p. 55.

**13.** A female manic client is placed in a seclusion room after an outburst of violent behavior that involved a physical assault on another client. As the client is secluded, the nurse:

1    Remains silent because verbal interaction would be too stimulating
2    Tells the client that she will be allowed to rejoin the others when she can behave
3    Asks the client if she understands why the seclusion is necessary
4    Informs the client that she is being secluded to help regain self-control

**Answer: 4**

*Rationale:* The client is removed to a nonstimulating environment because of behavior. Options 1, 2, and 3 are nontherapeutic actions. Additionally, option 2 implies punishment. It is best to directly inform the client of the purpose of the seclusion.

*Test-Taking Strategy:* Use therapeutic communication techniques. Select the option that presents reality most clearly to the client. Option 4 is the only option that provides a clear and direct purpose for the seclusion. Review care of a client requiring seclusion if you had difficulty with this question.

*Level of Cognitive Ability:* Application
*Client Needs:* Psychosocial Integrity
*Integrated Concept/Process:* Nursing Process/Implementation
*Content Area:* Mental Health

*Reference*
Stuart, G.W., & Laraia, M.T. (1998). *Principles and practice of psychiatric nursing* (6th ed.). St. Louis: Mosby, p. 634.

---

**14.** A client with angina pectoris is extremely anxious after being hospitalized for the first time. The nurse plans to do which of the following to minimize the client's anxiety?

1    Admit the client to a room as far as possible from the nursing station
2    Provide care choices to the client
3    Encourage the client to limit visitors to as few as possible
4    Keep the door open and hallway lights on at night

**Answer: 2**

*Rationale:* General interventions to minimize anxiety in a hospitalized client include providing information, social support, and control over choices related to care, as well as acknowledging the client's feelings. Being far from the nursing station is likely to increase anxiety for this client. Limiting visitors reduces social support, and leaving the door open with hallway lights on may keep the client oriented, but may interfere with sleep and increase anxiety.

*Test-Taking Strategy:* Use the process of elimination, focusing on the issue: minimizing anxiety. Thinking about each option and how it may either increase or minimize anxiety will direct you to option 2. Review interventions to minimize anxiety in the hospitalized client if you had difficulty with this question.

*Level of Cognitive Ability:* Application
*Client Needs:* Psychosocial Integrity
*Integrated Concept/Process:* Nursing Process/Planning
*Content Area:* Adult Health/Cardiovascular

*Reference*
Smeltzer, S., & Bare, B. (2000). *Brunner & Suddarth's Textbook of medical-surgical nursing* (9th ed.). Philadelphia: Lippincott Williams & Wilkins, p. 597.

**15.** A male client diagnosed with catatonic stupor demonstrates severe withdrawal by lying on the bed with his body pulled into a fetal position. The nurse plans to:

1 Leave the client alone and intermittently check on him
2 Take the client into the dayroom with other clients so they can help watch him
3 Sit beside the client in silence and occasionally ask open-ended questions
4 Ask direct questions to encourage talking

**Answer: 3**

*Rationale:* Clients who are withdrawn may be immobile and mute and require consistent, repeated approaches. Intervention includes establishing interpersonal contact. The nurse facilitates communication with the client by sitting in silence, asking open-ended questions, and pausing to provide opportunities for the client to respond. The client is not left alone. Asking direct questions of this client is not therapeutic.

*Test-Taking Strategy:* Use the process of elimination. Eliminate option 1, because the nurse does not leave the client alone. Option 2, which relies on other clients to care for this client, is inappropriate and is eliminated next. From the remaining options, recall that asking direct questions of this client would not be therapeutic. Review care of a client with catatonic stupor if you had difficulty with this question.

*Level of Cognitive Ability:* Application
*Client Needs:* Psychosocial Integrity
*Integrated Concept/Process:* Nursing Process/Planning
*Content Area:* Mental Health

*Reference*
Stuart, G.W., & Laraia, M.T. (1998). *Principles and practice of psychiatric nursing* (6th ed.). St. Louis: Mosby, p. 282.

**16.** A nurse is interviewing a client on admission to the mental health inpatient unit. The client was involved in a fire 2 months ago. The client is complaining of insomnia, difficulty concentrating, nervousness, and hypervigilance and is frequently thinking about fires. The nurse assesses these symptoms to be indicative of:

1 Obsessive-compulsive disorder (OCD)
2 Phobia
3 Posttraumatic stress disorder (PTSD)
4 Dissociative disorder

**Answer: 3**

*Rationale:* PTSD is precipitated by events that are overwhelming, unpredictable, and sometimes life threatening. Typical symptoms of PTSD include difficulty concentrating, sleep disturbances, intrusive recollections of the traumatic event, hypervigilance, and anxiety.

*Test-Taking Strategy:* Focus on the data provided in the question regarding the client's complaints. Recall that having flashbacks of traumatic events is a common symptom of PTSD; this will direct you to option 3. If you are unfamiliar with this disorder, review the clinical manifestations.

*Level of Cognitive Ability:* Analysis
*Client Needs:* Psychosocial Integrity
*Integrated Concept/Process:* Nursing Process/Assessment
*Content Area:* Mental Health

*Reference*
Stuart, G.W., & Laraia, M.T. (1998). *Principles and practice of psychiatric nursing* (6th ed.). St. Louis: Mosby, p. 286.

**17.** A 16-year-old client is hospitalized with pneumonia. Which statement by the client would alert the nurse to a potential developmental problem?

1 "Is it okay if I have a couple of friends in to visit me this evening?"

2 "When my friends get here, I would like to play some computer games with them."

3 "Please tell my friends not to visit, since I'll see them back at school next week."

4 "I'd like my hair washed before my friends get here."

**Answer: 3**

*Rationale:* Adolescents who withdraw from peers into isolation struggle with developing identity, so option 3 should cause the nurse to be concerned. Option 1 shows that the client is eager for companionship. Adolescents often develop special interests within their groups that may help to maximize certain skills, such as with computers. It is appropriate for the client to ask for hygiene measures to be attended to before the client's peers arrive.

*Test-Taking Strategy:* Use the process of elimination. Options 1, 2, and 4 indicate that the client is anticipating the arrival of a peer group, which is appropriate. Option 3 indicates that the client may be withdrawing from appropriate relationships. Review the concepts of growth and development related to an adolescent if you had difficulty answering this question.

*Level of Cognitive Ability:* Analysis
*Client Needs:* Psychosocial Integrity
*Integrated Concept/Process:* Nursing Process/Assessment
*Content Area:* Child Health

*Reference*
Wong, D. (1999). *Whaley & Wong's Nursing care of infants and children* (6th ed.). St. Louis: Mosby, p. 898.

---

**18.** A nurse reviews the client's electrocardiogram (ECG) rhythm strip. The ECG shows that the rate is 90 beats/min. The nurse most appropriately tells the client that:

1 The rate is normal

2 There is no need to worry

3 Medication specific to the problem will be prescribed

4 A slower heart rate is preferred

**Answer: 1**

*Rationale:* A normal adult resting pulse rate ranges between 60 and 100 beats/min.

*Test-Taking Strategy:* Use the process of elimination and knowledge of the basic range of pulse rates for an adult. Telling the client not to worry is an inappropriate action. Options 3 and 4 are similar and indicate that a problem exists. Review normal adult vital signs if you had difficulty with this question.

*Level of Cognitive Ability:* Application
*Client Needs:* Psychosocial Integrity
*Integrated Concept/Process:* Nursing Process/Implementation
*Content Area:* Adult Health/Cardiovascular

*Reference*
Potter, P., & Perry, A. (2001). *Fundamentals of nursing* (5th ed.). St. Louis: Mosby, p. 697.

**19.** A nurse determines that a client recovering from a myocardial infarction is exhibiting signs of depression when the client:
1 Reports insomnia at night
2 Consumes 25% of meals and shows little interest during client teaching
3 Ignores activity restrictions and does not report the experience of chest pain with activity
4 Expresses apprehension about leaving the hospital and requests that someone stay at night

**Answer: 2**
*Rationale:* Signs of depression include withdrawal, lack of interest, crying, anorexia, and apathy. Insomnia may be a sign of anxiety or fear. Ignoring symptoms and activity restrictions is a sign of denial. Apprehension is a sign of anxiety.

*Test-Taking Strategy:* Use the process of elimination, focusing on the issue: signs of depression. Recalling that anorexia and a lack of interest are associated with depression will direct you to option 2. Review the signs of depression if you had difficulty with this question.

*Level of Cognitive Ability:* Analysis
*Client Needs:* Psychosocial Integrity
*Integrated Concept/Process:* Nursing Process/Analysis
*Content Area:* Adult Health/Cardiovascular

*Reference*
Ignatavicius, D., Workman, M., & Mishler, M. (1999). *Medical-surgical nursing across the health care continuum* (3rd ed.). Philadelphia: W.B. Saunders, p. 914.

**20.** A client who recently had a gastrostomy feeding tube inserted refuses to participate in the plan of care, will not make eye contact, and does not speak to the family or visitors. The nurse assesses that the client is using which type of coping mechanism?
1 Self-control
2 Problem solving
3 Accepting responsibility
4 Distancing

**Answer: 4**
*Rationale:* Self-control is demonstrated by stoicism and hiding feelings. Problem solving involves making plans and verbalizing what will be done. Accepting responsibility places the responsibility for a situation on one's self. Distancing is an unwillingness or inability to discuss events.

*Test-Taking Strategy:* Use the process of elimination. Focusing on the client's behavior will direct you to option 4. If you had difficulty with this question, review coping mechanisms.

*Level of Cognitive Ability:* Analysis
*Client Needs:* Psychosocial Integrity
*Integrated Concept/Process:* Nursing Process/Assessment
*Content Area:* Adult Health/Gastrointestinal

*Reference*
Ignatavicius, D., Workman, M., & Mishler, M. (1999). *Medical-surgical nursing across the health care continuum* (3rd ed.). Philadelphia: W.B. Saunders, p. 102.

**21.** A nurse reviews the preoperative teaching plan for a client scheduled for a radical neck dissection. When the nurse is implementing the plan, the nurse's initial assessment should focus on:
1 Postoperative communication techniques
2 The financial status of the client
3 The client's support systems and coping behaviors
4 Information given to the client by the surgeon

**Answer: 4**
*Rationale:* The first step in client teaching is establishing what the client already knows. This allows the nurse not only to correct any misinformation but also to determine the starting point for teaching and to implement the education at the client's level.

*Test-Taking Strategy:* Use the process of elimination. Note the key word *initial.* Remember, determining what the client already knows provides a starting point for teaching. Review the teaching/learning process if you had difficulty with this question.

*Level of Cognitive Ability:* Application
*Client Needs:* Psychosocial Integrity

*Integrated Concept/Process:* Teaching/Learning
*Content Area:* Adult Health/Respiratory

*Reference*
Smeltzer, S., & Bare, B. (2000). *Brunner & Suddarth's Textbook of medical-surgical nursing* (9th ed.). Philadelphia: Lippincott Williams & Wilkins, p. 818.

---

**22.** A nurse is monitoring a client for signs of alcohol withdrawal. Which of the following assessment data would indicate early signs of withdrawal?
1 Anxiety, tremor, insomnia, tachycardia
2 Disorientation, diaphoresis, insomnia
3 Delusions, fever, vomiting, agitation
4 Clouding of consciousness, tachycardia

**Answer: 1**
*Rationale:* The signs of alcohol withdrawal develop within a few hours after cessation or reduction of alcohol intake and peak after 24 to 48 hours. Early signs include anxiety, anorexia, insomnia, tremor, irritability, an elevation in pulse and blood pressure, nausea, vomiting, and poorly formed hallucinations or illusions.

*Test-Taking Strategy:* Use the process of elimination and focus on the key word *early.* Knowledge of the early signs of alcohol withdrawal will direct you to option 1. If you are unfamiliar with the signs and symptoms of alcohol withdrawal, review this content.

*Level of Cognitive Ability:* Analysis
*Client Needs:* Psychosocial Integrity
*Integrated Concept/Process:* Nursing Process/Assessment
*Content Area:* Mental Health

*Reference*
Stuart, G.W., & Laraia, M.T. (1998). *Principles and practice of psychiatric nursing* (6th ed.). St. Louis: Mosby, p. 492.

---

**23.** A preschool child is placed in traction for treatment of a femur fracture. The child, who has reportedly been toilet-trained for at least 1 year, begins bedwetting. The nurse recognizes this as:
1 Attention-seeking behavior requiring intervention by the child psychologist
2 Loss of developmental milestones as a result of prolonged immobilization
3 Regressing to earlier developmental behavior, which is a normal psychological effect of immobilization
4 A body image disturbance

**Answer: 3**
*Rationale:* The monotony of immobilization can lead to sluggish intellectual and psychomotor responses. Regressive behaviors are not uncommon in immobilized children and usually do not require professional intervention. Although *loss of developmental milestones* may seem like an appropriate option, *regressing to earlier developmental behavior* is a more accurate description of the psychological effects of immobilization. Body image may or may not be affected by long-term immobilization and does not relate to the information in the question.

*Test-Taking Strategy:* Use the process of elimination. Eliminate option 4 first because it is unrelated to the question. Eliminate option 1, because bedwetting by an immobilized child is not unusual and a child psychologist is not needed. From the remaining options, recall that regression is a normal psychological response to immobilization to direct you to option 3. Review the psychological effects of immobilization if you had difficulty with this question.

*Level of Cognitive Ability:* Analysis
*Client Needs:* Psychosocial Integrity
*Integrated Concept/Process:* Nursing Process/Analysis
*Content Area:* Child Health

*Reference*
Wong, D. (1999). *Whaley & Wong's Nursing care of infants and children* (6th ed.).
St. Louis: Mosby, p. 1171.

---

**24.** A nurse is assessing a client to determine adjustment to presbycusis. Which of the following noted by the nurse indicates successful adaptation to this problem?
1   Denial of a hearing impairment
2   Proper use of a hearing aid
3   Withdrawal from social activities
4   Reluctance to answer the telephone

**Answer: 2**
*Rationale:* Presbycusis occurs as part of the aging process and is a progressive sensorineural hearing loss. Some clients may not adapt well to the impairment, denying its presence. Others withdraw from social interactions and contact with others, embarrassed by the problem and the need to wear a hearing aid. Clients show adequate adaptation by obtaining and regularly using a hearing aid.

*Test-Taking Strategy:* The key words in the question are *successful adaptation.* A review of each of the options shows that the only option with positive wording is option 2. The incorrect options indicate a need for further adaptation. Review the psychosocial issues related to the care of the client with a hearing aid if you had difficulty with this question.

*Level of Cognitive Ability:* Analysis
*Client Needs:* Psychosocial Integrity
*Integrated Concept/Process:* Nursing Process/Evaluation
*Content Area:* Adult Health/Ear

*Reference*
Monahan, F., & Neighbors, M. (1998). *Medical-surgical nursing: Foundations for clinical practice* (2nd ed.). Philadelphia: W.B. Saunders, p. 2019.

---

**25.** A nurse is performing an admission assessment on a male child and notes the presence of old and new bruises on the child's back and legs. The nurse suspects physical abuse. The most appropriate nursing action would be to:
1   File charges against the mother and father of the child
2   Report the case to legal authorities
3   Ask the mother to identify the individual who is physically abusing the child
4   Tell the child that he will need to go to a foster home until the situation is straightened out

**Answer: 2**
*Rationale:* The primary legal nursing responsibility when child abuse is suspected is to report the case. All 50 states require health care professionals to report all cases of suspected abuse. It is not appropriate for the nurse to file charges against the father or mother. It is also inappropriate to ask the mother to identify the abuser, because the abuser may be the mother. If so, the possibility exists that the mother may become defensive and leave the emergency department with the child. Option 4 is clearly inappropriate and will produce fear in the child.

*Test-Taking Strategy:* Use the process of elimination, noting the key words *most appropriate.* In addition to the many implications associated with child abuse, abuse is a crime. With this in mind, option 2, reporting the case of abuse, is the primary responsibility of the nurse. If you had difficulty with this question, review the responsibilities of the nurse when child abuse is suspected.

*Level of Cognitive Ability:* Application
*Client Needs:* Psychosocial Integrity
*Integrated Concept/Process:* Nursing Process/Implementation
*Content Area:* Child Health

**Reference**

Wong, D. (1999). *Whaley & Wong's Nursing care of infants and children* (6th ed.). St. Louis: Mosby, p. 765.

---

**26.** An emergency department nurse is performing an assessment on a 7-year-old child with a fractured arm. The child is hesitant to answers questions that the nurse is asking and consistently looks at the parents in a fearful manner. The nurse suspects physical abuse and continues with the assessment procedures. Which of the following assessment findings would most likely assist in verifying the suspicion?

1 Poor hygiene
2 Bald spots on the scalp
3 Lacerations in the anal area
4 Swelling of the genitals

**Answer: 2**

*Rationale:* Bald spots on the scalp are most likely associated with physical abuse. The most likely assessment findings in sexual abuse include difficulty walking or sitting, torn, stained or bloody underclothing, pain, swelling or itching of the genitals, and bruises, bleeding, or lacerations in the genital or anal area. Poor hygiene may be indicative of physical neglect.

*Test-Taking Strategy:* Read the question carefully, noting the key words *physical abuse.* The only option that specifically addresses an assessment finding related to physical abuse is option 2. If you had difficulty with this question, review the assessment findings in a child suspected of abuse.

*Level of Cognitive Ability:* Analysis
*Client Needs:* Psychosocial Integrity
*Integrated Concept/Process:* Nursing Process/Assessment
*Content Area:* Child Health

**Reference**

Ball, J., & Bindler, R. (1999). *Pediatric nursing: Caring for children* (2nd ed.). Stamford, Conn.: Appleton & Lange, p. 994.

---

**27.** A 4-year-old child who was recently hospitalized is brought to the clinic by the mother for a follow-up visit. The mother tells the nurse that the child has begun to wet the bed since the child was brought home from the hospital. The mother is concerned and asks the nurse what to do. The most appropriate nursing response is which of the following?

1 "You need to discipline the child."
2 "This is a normal occurrence following hospitalization."
3 "We will need to discuss this behavior with the physician."
4 "The child probably has developed a urinary tract infection."

**Answer: 2**

*Rationale:* Regression can occur in a preschooler and is most often caused by the stress of the hospitalization. It is best to accept the regression if it occurs. Parents may be overly concerned about the regressive behavior and should be told that regression is normal following hospitalization. It is premature to discuss the situation with the physician. Options 1 and 4 are inappropriate responses to the mother.

*Test-Taking Strategy:* Note the key words *most appropriate* in the stem of the question. Use the process of elimination. Eliminate option 4 first, because there are no data in the question to support this statement. Knowledge regarding the behavior patterns of a preschooler following hospitalization and the use of therapeutic communication techniques will assist in eliminating options 1 and 3. If you had difficulty with this question, review the psychosocial issues related to the hospitalized preschool child.

*Level of Cognitive Ability:* Application
*Client Needs:* Psychosocial Integrity

*Integrated Concept/Process:* Communication and Documentation
*Content Area:* Child Health

### Reference

Wong, D. (1999). *Whaley & Wong's Nursing care of infants and children* (6th ed.). St. Louis: Mosby, p. 680.

---

**28.** During an office visit, a prenatal client with mitral stenosis states that she has been under a lot of stress lately. During the examination, the client questions everything the nurse does and behaves in an anxious manner. The best nursing action at this time would be to:

1  Tell her not to worry
2  Ignore her unfounded concerns and continue with the assessment
3  Explain the purpose of the nursing actions and answer all questions
4  Refer her to a counselor

**Answer: 3**

*Rationale:* In a pregnant cardiac client, stress should be reduced as much as possible. The client should be provided with honest, informed answers to her questions to help alleviate unnecessary fears and emotional stress. Explaining the purpose of nursing actions will assist in decreasing the stress level of the client. Options 1, 2, and 4 are nontherapeutic methods of communication at this time.

*Test-Taking Strategy:* Use the process of elimination and therapeutic communication techniques to answer the question. Always address the client's concerns and feelings. Option 3 is the only option that addresses the client's concerns. Review therapeutic communication techniques if you had difficulty with this question.

*Level of Cognitive Ability:* Application
*Client Needs:* Psychosocial Integrity
*Integrated Concept/Process:* Nursing Process/Implementation
*Content Area:* Maternity

### Reference

Sherwen, L., Scoloveno, M.A., & Weingarten, C. (1999). *Maternity nursing: Care of the childbearing family* (3rd ed.). Stamford, Conn.: Appleton & Lange, p. 595.

---

**29.** A postpartum client with gestational diabetes is scheduled for discharge. During the discharge teaching the client asks the nurse, "Do I have to worry about this diabetes any more?" The best response by the nurse is which of the following?

1  "Your blood glucose level is within normal limits now, you will be all right."
2  "You will only have to worry about the diabetes if you become pregnant again."
3  "You will be at risk for developing gestational diabetes with your next pregnancy and developing overt diabetes mellitus."
4  "Once you have gestational diabetes, you have overt diabetes and must be treated with medication for the rest of your life."

**Answer: 3**

*Rationale:* The client is at risk for developing gestational diabetes with each pregnancy. The client also has an increased risk of developing overt diabetes and needs to comply with follow-up assessments. She also needs to be taught techniques to lower her risk for developing diabetes, such as weight control. A diagnosis of gestational diabetes mellitus indicates that this client has an increased risk for developing overt diabetes; however, with proper care it may not develop.

*Test-Taking Strategy:* Identify the issue of the question: the long-term effect of gestational diabetes. Also, use therapeutic communication techniques to answer the question and direct you to option 3. Review the long-term effects of gestational diabetes if you had difficulty with this question.

*Level of Cognitive Ability:* Application
*Client Needs:* Physiological Integrity
*Integrated Concept/Process:* Communication and Documentation
*Content Area:* Maternity

### Reference

Lowdermilk, D., Perry, S., & Bobak, I. (2000). *Maternity & women's health care* (7th ed.). St. Louis: Mosby, pp. 879-880.

**30.** A nurse is performing an assessment on a 16-year-old female client who has been diagnosed with anorexia nervosa. Which statement, if made by the client, would the nurse identify as a priority requiring further assessment?

1 "I exercise 3 to 4 hours every day to keep my slim figure."
2 "My best friend was in the hospital with this disease a year ago."
3 "I've been told that I am 10% below ideal body weight."
4 "I check my weight every day without fail."

**Answer: 1**

*Rationale:* Exercising 3 to 4 hours every day is excessive physical activity and unrealistic for a 16-year-old. The nurse needs to further assess this statement immediately to find out why the client feels the need to exercise this much to maintain her figure. Although it's unfortunate that her best friend had this disease, this is not considered a major threat to this client's physical well-being. A weight that is more than 15% below the ideal weight is most significant with anorexia nervosa. It is not considered abnormal to check weight every day. Often clients with anorexia nervosa check their weight as many as 20 times a day.

*Test-Taking Strategy:* Note the key word *priority* in the stem of the question. Use the process of elimination. Eliminate options 3 and 4 first, because these client statements are not significant or abnormal. From the remaining options, knowledge regarding the manifestations associated with anorexia nervosa will direct you to option 1. Review these significant manifestations if you had difficulty with this question.

*Level of Cognitive Ability:* Analysis
*Client Needs:* Psychosocial Integrity
*Integrated Concept/Process:* Nursing Process/Analysis
*Content Area:* Mental Health

*Reference*
Leahy, J., & Kizilay, P. (1998). *Foundations of nursing practice: A nursing process approach.* Philadelphia: W.B. Saunders, p.763.

**31.** A physician has written an order to start progressive ambulation as tolerated for a hospitalized client who is experiencing periods of confusion as a result of bed rest and prolonged confinement to the hospital room. Which nursing intervention would be most appropriate when planning to implement the physician's order and in addressing the needs of the client?

1 Ambulate the client in the room for short distances frequently
2 Ambulate the client to the bathroom in the client's room three times a day
3 Progressively ambulate the client in the hall three times a day
4 Assist with range of motion exercises three times a day to increase strength

**Answer: 3**

*Rationale:* The cause of the confusion in this situation is bed rest and decreased sensory stimulation from prolonged confinement. Therefore it is best to ambulate the client in the hall. This will increase sensory stimulation and may decrease confusion. Options 1 and 2 will not address the client's need for sensory stimulation. Option 4 is an action that should have been performed in preparation for ambulation while the client was on bed rest.

*Test-Taking Strategy:* Focus on the issue: confusion as a result of bed rest and prolonged confinement. Eliminate option 4 first, because this action should have been performed in preparation for ambulation while the client was on bed rest. Next, eliminate options 1 and 2, because they are similar in that they both address ambulating the client in the hospital room. Review interventions related to promoting sensory stimulation if you had difficulty with this question.

*Level of Cognitive Ability:* Application
*Client Needs:* Psychosocial Integrity
*Integrated Concept/Process:* Nursing Process/Planning
*Content Area:* Fundamental Skills

*Reference*
Maher, A., Salmond, S., & Pellino, T. (1998). *Orthopaedic nursing* (2nd ed.). Philadelphia: W.B. Saunders, p. 109.

**32.** A nurse is caring for an elderly client who has been placed in Buck's extension traction following a hip fracture. On assessment of the client, the nurse notes that the client is disoriented. The most appropriate nursing intervention is to:

1 Ask the family to stay with the client
2 Apply restraints to the client
3 Ask the laboratory to perform electrolyte studies
4 Reorient the client frequently and place a clock and a calendar in the client's room

**Answer: 4**

*Rationale:* An inactive elderly person may become disoriented from lack of sensory stimulation. The most appropriate nursing intervention would be to frequently reorient the client and to place objects such as a clock and a calendar in the client's room to maintain orientation. The family can assist with orientation of the client, but it is not appropriate to ask the family to stay with the client. It is not within the scope of nursing practice to prescribe laboratory studies. Restraints may cause further disorientation and should not be applied unless specifically prescribed. Agency policies and procedures should be followed before the application of restraints.

*Test-Taking Strategy:* Note the key words *most appropriate*. Eliminate option 3 first, because it is not within the realm of nursing practice to prescribe laboratory studies. Next, eliminate option 2, because restraints may add to the disorientation that the client is experiencing. It is not appropriate to place the responsibility of the client on the family, therefore eliminate option 1. Note the relationship between the words *disoriented* in the question and *reorient* in the correct option. Review the measures related to caring for a client who is disoriented if you had difficulty with this question.

*Level of Cognitive Ability:* Application
*Client Needs:* Psychosocial Integrity
*Integrated Concept/Process:* Nursing Process/Implementation
*Content Area:* Adult Health/Musculoskeletal

*Reference*
Leahy, J., & Kizilay, P. (1998). *Foundations of nursing practice: A nursing process approach.* Philadelphia: W.B. Saunders, p. 1045.

---

**33.** An 8-year-old male child is admitted to the hospital. The child was sexually abused by an adult family member and is withdrawn and appears frightened. Which of the following describes the best plan for the initial nursing encounter to convey concern and support?

1 Introduce self, explain role, and ask the child to act out the sexual encounter with the abuser, using art therapy
2 Introduce self, then ask the child to express how he feels about the events leading up to this admission
3 Introduce self and explain to the child that he is safe now that he is here in the hospital
4 Introduce self and tell the child that the nurse would like to sit with him for a little while

**Answer: 4**

*Rationale:* Victims of sexual abuse may exhibit fear and anxiety over what has just occurred. In addition, they may fear that the abuse could be repeated. On initiating contact with a child victim of sexual abuse who demonstrates fear of others, it is best to convey a willingness to spend time, and move slowly to initiate activities that may be perceived as threatening. Once rapport is established, the nurse may explore the child's feelings or use various therapeutic modalities to encourage recounting the sexual encounter. Option 4 conveys a plan for an initial encounter that establishes trust by sitting with the child in a nonthreatening atmosphere. Options 1 and 2 may be implemented once trust and rapport is established. Option 3 does not convey concern and support by the nurse.

*Test-Taking Strategy:* Use the process of elimination, focusing on the child's experience and that the child is frightened. This will assist in eliminating options 1 and 2. From the remaining options, recalling that rapport needs to be established first will direct you to option 4. Review care of an abused child if you had difficulty with this question.

*Level of Cognitive Ability:* Application
*Client Needs:* Psychosocial Integrity
*Integrated Concept/Process:* Caring
*Content Area:* Child Health

*Reference*
Stuart, G.W., & Laraia, M.T. (1998). *Principles and practice of psychiatric nursing* (6th ed.). St. Louis: Mosby, p. 830.

---

**34.** A female victim of a sexual assault is being seen in the crisis center for a third visit. She states that although the rape occurred nearly 2 months ago, she still feels "as though the rape happened just yesterday." The nurse's best response is:

1    "What can you do to alleviate some of your fears about being assaulted again?"
2    "Tell me more about those aspects of the rape that cause you to feel like the rape just occurred."
3    "In time, our goal will be to help you move on from these strong feelings about your rape."
4    "In reality, the rape did not just occur. It has been over 2 months now."

**Answer: 2**
*Rationale:* Option 2 allows for the client to express her ideas and feelings more fully, and portrays a unhurried, nonjudgmental, supportive attitude. Clients need to be reassured that their feelings are normal and that they may freely express their concerns in a safe care environment. Option 1 places the problem-solving totally on the client. Option 3 places the client's feelings on hold. Although option 4 is true, it immediately blocks communication.

*Test-Taking Strategy:* Use therapeutic communication techniques. Option 2 specifically addresses the client's feelings and concerns. Remember, always address the client's feelings first. Review therapeutic communication techniques if you had difficulty with this question.

*Level of Cognitive Ability:* Application
*Client Needs:* Psychosocial Integrity
*Integrated Concept/Process:* Communication and Documentation
*Content Area:* Mental Health

*Reference*
Stuart, G.W., & Laraia, M.T. (1998). *Principles and practice of psychiatric nursing* (6th ed.). St. Louis: Mosby, p. 35.

---

**35.** A client is admitted to the mental health unit with a diagnosis of schizophrenia. A nursing diagnosis formulated for the client is Altered Thought Process, secondary to paranoia. In formulating the plan of care with the health care team, the nurse includes instruction to the staff to:

1    Avoid laughing or whispering in front of the client
2    Increase socialization of the client with peers
3    Have the client sign a release of information to appropriate parties so that adequate data can be obtained for assessment purposes
4    Begin to educate the client about social supports in the community

**Answer: 1**
*Rationale:* A client experiencing paranoia is distrustful and suspicious of others. The health care team needs to establish rapport and trust with the client. Laughing or whispering in front of the client would increase the client's paranoia. Options 2, 3, and 4 ask the client to trust on a multitude of levels. These options are actions that are too intrusive for a client who is paranoid.

*Test-Taking Strategy:* Focus on the client's problem, paranoia. Recalling that the client with paranoia is distrustful and suspicious of others will direct you to option 1. Review this disorder if you had difficulty with this question.

*Level of Cognitive Ability:* Application
*Client Needs:* Psychosocial Integrity
*Integrated Concept/Process:* Nursing Process/Implementation
*Content Area:* Mental Health

*Reference*
Stuart, G.W., & Laraia, M.T. (1998). *Principles and practice of psychiatric nursing* (6th ed.). St. Louis: Mosby, p. 478.

**36.** A nurse is assessing a male client who has a nursing diagnosis of risk for self-directed violence. The client says, "You won't have to worry about me much longer." The nurse interprets this statement as:

1    An expression of hopelessness
2    An expression of depression
3    The intention for self-mutilation
4    The intention of suicide

**Answer: 4**

*Rationale:* A client with a risk for self-directed violence who says that he will not be around much longer is expressing a suicidal intent. Although hopelessness, depression, and self-mutilation may relate to self-directed violence, the statement that he will not be around is a direct comment about the act of suicide.

*Test-Taking Strategy:* Use the process of elimination. Focus on the client's statement to direct you to option 4. Review the characteristics related to risk for self-directed violence if you had difficulty with this question.

*Level of Cognitive Ability:* Analysis
*Client Needs:* Psychosocial Integrity
*Integrated Concept/Process:* Nursing Process/Analysis
*Content Area:* Mental Health

*Reference*
Stuart, G.W., & Laraia, M.T. (1998). *Principles and practice of psychiatric nursing* (6th ed.). St. Louis: Mosby, p. 389.

---

**37.** A nurse notes that an assigned client is lying tense in bed staring at the cardiac monitor. The client states, " There sure are a lot of wires around there. I sure hope we don't get hit by lightning." The most appropriate nursing response is which of the following?

1    "Would you like a mild sedative to help you relax?"
2    "Oh, don't worry—the weather is supposed to be sunny and clear today."
3    "Yes, all those wires must be a little scary. Did someone explain what the cardiac monitor was for?"
4    "Your family can stay tonight if they wish."

**Answer: 3**

*Rationale:* The nurse should initially validate the client's concern and then assess the client's knowledge regarding the cardiac monitor. This gives the nurse an opportunity to do client education if necessary. Options 1, 2, and 4 do not address the client's concern. Additionally, pharmacological interventions should be considered only if necessary.

*Test-Taking Strategy:* Use therapeutic communication techniques. Remember address the client's feelings first. Option 3 is the only option that addresses the client's feelings. Review therapeutic communication techniques if you had difficulty with this question.

*Level of Cognitive Ability:* Application
*Client Needs:* Psychosocial Integrity
*Integrated Concept/Process:* Communication and Documentation
*Content Area:* Adult Health/Cardiovascular

*Reference*
Sole, M.L., Lamborn, M., & Hartshorn, J. (2001). *Introduction to critical care nursing* (3rd ed.). Philadelphia: W.B. Saunders, p. 15.

**38.** A young adult male client with a spinal cord injury (SCI) tells the nurse, "It's so depressing that I'll never get to have sex again." The nurse replies in a realistic way by making which of the following statements to the client?

1 "You're young, so you'll adapt to this more easily than if you were older."

2 "It must feel horrible to know you can never have sex again."

3 "It is still possible to have a sexual relationship, but it is different."

4 "Because of body reflexes, sexual functioning will be no different than before."

**Answer: 3**

*Rationale:* It is possible to have a sexual relationship after an SCI, but it is different from what the client experienced before the injury. Males may experience reflex erections, although they may not ejaculate. Females can have adductor spasm. Sexual counseling may help the client to adapt to changes in sexuality after an SCI.

*Test-Taking Strategy:* Use the process of elimination, knowledge regarding the effects of an SCI, and therapeutic communication techniques. Option 3 addresses the issue, is accurate, and is a therapeutic response. Review the effects of an SCI if you had difficulty with this question.

*Level of Cognitive Ability:* Application
*Client Needs:* Psychosocial Integrity
*Integrated Concept/Process:* Communication and Documentation
*Content Area:* Adult Health/Neurological

*Reference*
Monahan, F., & Neighbors, M. (1998). *Medical-surgical nursing: Foundations for clinical practice* (2nd ed.). Philadelphia: W.B. Saunders, pp. 826-827.

**39.** A family member of a client with a brain tumor is distraught and feeling guilty for not encouraging the client to seek medical evaluation earlier. The nurse would incorporate which of the following items in formulating a response to the family member's statement?

1 It is true that brain tumors are easily recognizable

2 The symptoms of a brain tumor may be easily attributed to another cause

3 Brain tumors are never detected until very late in their course

4 There are no symptoms of a brain tumor

**Answer: 2**

*Rationale:* Signs and symptoms of a brain tumor vary, depending on location, and may easily be attributed to another cause. Symptoms include headache, vomiting, visual disturbances, and change in intellectual abilities or personality. Seizures occur in some clients. These symptoms can be easily attributed to other causes. The family requires support to assist them in the normal grieving process.

*Test-Taking Strategy:* Use the process of elimination. Eliminate options 3 and 4 first, because they contain the absolute words *never* and *no*, respectively. From the remaining options, recall that the symptoms of a brain tumor may be easily attributed to another cause. Also, note the word *may* in the correct option. Review the symptoms of a brain tumor if you had difficulty with this question.

*Level of Cognitive Ability:* Application
*Client Needs:* Psychosocial Integrity
*Integrated Concept/Process:* Caring
*Content Area:* Adult Health/Neurological

*Reference*
Monahan, F., & Neighbors, M. (1998). *Medical-surgical nursing: Foundations for clinical practice* (2nd ed.). Philadelphia: W.B. Saunders, pp. 828-829.

**40.** A male client is in a hip spica cast because of a fracture of the hip. On the day after the cast was applied, the nurse finds the client surrounded by papers from his briefcase and planning a phone meeting. The nurse's interaction with the client should be based on the knowledge that:
1    Setting limits on a client's behavior is a mandated nursing role
2    Not keeping up with his job will increase his stress level
3    Immediate involvement in his job will keep him from becoming bored while on bed rest
4    Rest is an essential component in bone healing

**Answer: 4**

*Rationale:* Rest is an essential component of bone healing. Nurses can help clients understand the importance of rest and find ways to balance work demands to promote healing. Nurses cannot demand these changes but need to encourage clients to choose them. It may be stress relieving to do work; however, in the immediate postcast period it may not be therapeutic. Stress should be kept at a minimum to promote bone healing. Setting limits on a client's behavior is not a mandated nursing role.

*Test-Taking Strategy:* Use the process of elimination. Eliminate options 2 and 3, because they are similar. From the remaining options, note that option 4 is the most global option and addresses the issue of rest. Review the physiological and psychosocial needs of the client in a hip spica cast if you had difficulty with this question.

*Level of Cognitive Ability:* Analysis
*Client Needs:* Psychosocial Integrity
*Integrated Concept/Process:* Caring
*Content Area:* Adult Health/Musculoskeletal

*Reference*
Black, J., Hawks, J., & Keene, A. (2001). *Medical-surgical nursing: Clinical management for positive outcomes* (6th ed.). Philadelphia: W.B. Saunders, p. 589.

**41.** A charge nurse observes a nursing assistant talking in an unusually loud voice to a client with delirium. The charge nurse takes which action?
1    Speaks to the nursing assistant immediately while in the client's room to solve the problem
2    Informs the client that everything is all right
3    Ascertains the client's safety and calmly asks the nursing assistant to join the nurse outside the room; there the nurse informs the nursing assistant that his or her voice was unusually loud
4    Explains to the nursing assistant that yelling in the client's room is tolerated only if the client is talking loudly

**Answer: 3**

*Rationale:* The nurse must ascertain that the client is safe, and then discuss the matter with the nursing assistant in an area away from the hearing of the client. If the client heard the conversation, the client might become more confused or agitated. Options 1, 2, and 4 are incorrect actions.

*Test-Taking Strategy:* Use Maslow's Hierarchy of Needs theory. Remember when a physiological need is not present, then safety needs are the priority. Review appropriate and therapeutic communication techniques and care of the client with delirium if you had difficulty with this question.

*Level of Cognitive Ability:* Application
*Client Needs:* Psychosocial Integrity
*Integrated Concept/Process:* Nursing Process/Implementation
*Content Area:* Mental Health

*Reference*
Stuart, G.W., & Laraia, M.T. (1998). *Principles and practice of psychiatric nursing* (6th ed.). St. Louis: Mosby, p. 476.

**42.** A teenager who has celiac disease arrives at the emergency department complaining of profuse, watery diarrhea following a pizza party last night. The client states, "I don't want to be different from my friends." The nursing diagnosis that is most appropriate for this client is:
1 Knowledge Deficit
2 Fluid Volume Deficit
3 Risk for Altered Self-esteem
4 Celiac Crisis

**Answer: 3**
*Rationale:* The client expresses concern over being different from friends. Although the question identifies that the client has profuse, watery diarrhea, there are no data that identify an actual fluid volume deficit. Also, the assessment data provided do not support a diagnosis of Knowledge Deficit. Celiac crisis is a medical diagnosis.

*Test-Taking Strategy:* Use the process of elimination, focusing on the data in the question. Eliminate option 4, because it is a medical diagnosis. Next, focus on the client's feelings about "being different." This will direct you to option 3. Review the defining characteristics of risk for altered self-esteem if you had difficulty with this question.

*Level of Cognitive Ability:* Analysis
*Client Needs:* Psychosocial Integrity
*Integrated Concept/Process:* Nursing Process/Analysis
*Content Area:* Child Health

*Reference*
Wong, D. (1999). *Whaley & Wong's Nursing care of infants and children* (6th ed.). St. Louis: Mosby, p. 1568.

**43.** A nurse develops a plan of care for a 1-month-old infant hospitalized for intussusception. Which nursing measure would be most effective to provide psychosocial support for the parent-child relationship?
1 Encourage the parents to go home and get some sleep
2 Encourage the parents to room-in with their infant
3 Provide educational materials
4 Initiate home nutritional support as early as possible

**Answer: 2**
*Rationale:* Rooming-in is effective in reducing separation anxiety and preserving the parent-child relationship. Parents are under stress when a child is ill and hospitalized. Telling a parent to go home and sleep will not relieve this stress. Educational materials may be beneficial but will not provide psychosocial support of the parent-child relationship. Home nutritional support is not usually necessary.

*Test-Taking Strategy:* Focus on the key words *parent-child relationship*. Use the process of elimination, focusing on this concept. The only option that addresses a parent-child relationship is option 2. Review the measures that promote this relationship in a hospitalized infant if you had difficulty with this question.

*Level of Cognitive Ability:* Application
*Client Needs:* Psychosocial Integrity
*Integrated Concept/Process:* Caring
*Content Area:* Child Health

*Reference*
Wong, D. (1999). *Whaley & Wong's Nursing care of infants and children* (6th ed.). St. Louis: Mosby, p. 1566.

**44.** The parent of a male infant who will have a surgical repair of a hernia makes the following comments. Which comment would require follow-up by a nurse?
1 "I understand surgery will repair the hernia."
2 "The day nurse told me to give him sponge baths for a few days after surgery."
3 "I'll need to buy extra diapers, since we need to change them more frequently now."
4 "I don't know if he will be able to father a child."

**Answer: 4**
*Rationale:* The anatomical location of a hernia frequently causes more psychological concern to the parents than does the actual condition or treatment. Options 1, 2, and 3 all indicate accurate understanding. Option 4 is an incorrect comment.

*Test-Taking Strategy:* Focus on the key words *would require follow-up.* Options 1, 2, and 3 do not require follow-up, whereas option 4 reflects parental fear and identifies a need for further assistance. Review parental instructions regarding the effects of a hernia repair if you had difficulty with this question.

*Level of Cognitive Ability:* Analysis
*Client Needs:* Psychosocial Integrity
*Integrated Concept/Process:* Nursing Process/Analysis
*Content Area:* Child Health

*Reference*
Wong, D. (1999). *Whaley & Wong's Nursing care of infants and children* (6th ed.). St. Louis: Mosby, p. 531.

**45.** A nurse is leading a crisis intervention group. The clients are high school students who have experienced the recent death of a classmate. The classmate committed suicide at the school, and the clients are experiencing disbelief. The clients reviewed the details about finding the classmate dead in a bathroom. Initially the nurse would:
1 Inquire how the clients recovered from death in the past
2 Reinforce the clients' sense of growth through this death experience
3 Reinforce the clients' ability to work through this death event
4 Inquire about the clients' perception of their classmate's suicide problem

**Answer: 4**
*Rationale:* It is essential to determine the clients' views. Inquiring about the clients' perceptions of the suicide will specifically identify their appraisal of the suicide and the meaning of their perceptions. Options 2 and 3 are similar in terms of attempts to foster clients' self-esteem. Such an approach is premature at this point. Although option 1 is exploratory, it does not address the "here and now" appraisal in terms of their classmate's suicide. Although the nurse is interested in how clients have coped in the past, this inquiry is not the most immediate assessment.

*Test-Taking Strategy:* Consider the issue of the question and select the option that deals with the "here and now." The nurse must first determine the clients' perceptions or appraisal of the stressful event. Review the phases of crisis if you had difficulty with this question.

*Level of Cognitive Ability:* Analysis
*Client Needs:* Psychosocial Integrity
*Integrated Concept/Process:* Nursing Process/Assessment
*Content Area:* Mental Health

*Reference*
Stuart, G.W., & Laraia, M.T. (1998). *Principles and practice of psychiatric nursing* (6th ed.). St. Louis: Mosby, p. 288.

46. A hospitalized male client has participated in substance abuse therapy group sessions. The nurse is monitoring the client's response to the substance abuse sessions. Which statement by the client would best indicate that the client has assimilated session topics, coping response styles, and has processed information effectively for self-use?

1  "I know I'm ready to be discharged; I feel like I can say 'no' and leave a group of friends if they are drinking. . . . No problem."

2  "This group has really helped a lot. I know it will be different when I go home. But I'm sure that my family and friends will all help me like the people in this group have. They'll all help me. . . . I know they will. . . . They won't let me go back to old ways."

3  "I'm looking forward to leaving here. I know that I will miss all of you. So, I'm happy and I'm sad; I'm excited and I'm scared. I know that I have to work hard to be strong and that everyone isn't going to be as helpful as you people have been. I know it isn't going to be easy. But I'm going to try as hard as I can."

4  "I'll keep all my appointments; I'll do everything I'm supposed to. . . . Nothing will go wrong that way."

**Answer: 3**
*Rationale:* In the defense mechanism of denial, the person denies reality. There can be varying degrees of denial. In option 3 the client is expressing real concern and ambivalence about discharge from the hospital. The client is realistic in the appraisal about the changes he will have to initiate in lifestyle as well as the fact that he has to work hard and develop new friends and meeting places. Option 1 identifies denial. In option 2, the client is relying heavily on others, and his locus of control is external. In option 4, the client's verbalization is concrete and procedure oriented; again, the client verbalizes denial.

*Test-Taking Strategy:* Select the option that identifies the most realistic client verbalization. Recalling that in denial a person is unable to face reality will assist in eliminating options 1, 2, and 4. Review the defense mechanism of denial if you had difficulty with this question.

*Level of Cognitive Ability:* Analysis
*Client Needs:* Psychosocial Integrity
*Integrated Concept/Process:* Nursing Process/Analysis
*Content Area:* Mental Health

*Reference*
Stuart, G.W., & Laraia, M.T. (1998). *Principles and practice of psychiatric nursing* (6th ed.). St. Louis: Mosby, p. 292.

47. A client recovering from a head injury becomes agitated at times. Which action will most likely calm this client?

1  Turn on the television to a musical program

2  Offer the client a favorite object to hold, such as a stuffed animal

3  Assign the client a new task to master

4  Make the client aware that the behavior is undesirable

**Answer: 2**
*Rationale:* Decreasing environmental stimuli aids in reducing agitation for the head injured client. Option 1 increases stimuli. Option 3 does not simplify the environment, because a new task may be frustrating. Option 4 may increase the client's agitation. The correct option helps to distract the client with motor activity, holding the stuffed animal.

*Test-Taking Strategy:* Use the process of elimination, identifying the options that may increase stimuli, agitation, and frustration. Review measures that will relieve agitation if you had difficulty with this question.

*Level of Cognitive Ability:* Application
*Client Needs:* Psychosocial Integrity
*Integrated Concept/Process:* Nursing Process/Implementation
*Content Area:* Adult Health/Neurological

**Reference**
Smeltzer, S., & Bare, B. (2000). *Brunner & Suddarth's Textbook of medical-surgical nursing* (9th ed.). Philadelphia: Lippincott Williams & Wilkins, p. 1683.

**48.** A client recovering from a cerebrovascular accident (CVA) has become irritable and angry regarding limitations. Which of the following is the best nursing approach to help the client regain motivation to succeed?
1    Allow longer and more frequent visitation by the spouse
2    Use supportive statements to correct the client's behavior
3    Tell the client that the nurses are experienced and know how the client feels
4    Ignore the behavior, knowing that the client is grieving

**Answer: 2**
*Rationale:* CVA clients have many and varied needs. The client may need the behavior pointed out so that correction can take place. It is also important to support and praise the client for accomplishments. Spouses of a CVA client are often grieving; therefore more visitation may not be helpful. Additionally, short visits are often encouraged. Stating that the nurse knows how the client feels is inappropriate. The client's behavior should not be ignored.

*Test-Taking Strategy:* Use therapeutic communication techniques to eliminate options 3 and 4. From the remaining options, option 2 is the only option that addresses the client's behavior described in the question. Review the psychosocial aspects related to a CVA if you had difficulty with this question.

*Level of Cognitive Ability:* Application
*Client Needs:* Psychosocial Integrity
*Integrated Concept/Process:* Caring
*Content Area:* Adult Health/Neurological

**Reference**
Smeltzer, S., & Bare, B. (2000). *Brunner & Suddarth's Textbook of medical-surgical nursing* (9th ed.). Philadelphia: Lippincott Williams & Wilkins, p. 30.

**49.** A client is admitted to the hospital with a fractured hip and is experiencing periods of confusion. The nurse reviews the hospital procedures for developing a plan of care for clients with altered thought processes. The nurse develops which psychosocial outcome that has the highest priority in the individualized care plan?
1    Improved sleep patterns
2    Increased ability to concentrate and make decisions
3    Meets self-care needs independently
4    Reduced family fears and anxiety

**Answer: 2**
*Rationale:* The client needs to be able to concentrate and make decisions. Once the client is able to do that, the nurse can work with the client to achieve the other outcomes. The client is the center of the nurse's concern. Options 1 and 3 address physiological needs. Option 4 is a secondary need.

*Test-Taking Strategy:* Use the process of elimination. Select the option that will have the greatest impact on the client's ability to function. Option 4 can be eliminated, because it does not address the client of the question. Options 1 and 3 addresses physiological not psychosocial needs. Review expected outcomes for the client with altered thought process if you had difficulty with this question.

*Level of Cognitive Ability:* Analysis
*Client Needs:* Psychosocial Integrity
*Integrated Concept/Process:* Nursing Process/Planning
*Content Area:* Adult Health/Musculoskeletal

*Reference*
Johnson, M., Bulechek, G., Dochterman, J. Maas, M., Moorhead, S. (2001). *Nursing diagnoses, outcomes, and interventions.* St. Louis: Mosby, p. 332.

---

**50.** A nurse is caring for a young woman dying from breast cancer. The nurse determines that a defining characteristic of anticipatory grief is present when the woman:

1   Verbalizes unrealistic goals and plans for the future
2   Discusses thoughts and feelings related to loss
3   Has prolonged emotional reactions and outbursts
4   Ignores untreated medical conditions that requires treatment

**Answer: 2**

*Rationale:* The nurse can determine the client's stage of grief by observing the client's behavior. This is extremely important, because the appropriate nursing diagnoses need to be developed so that the plan of care is appropriate. Options 1, 3, and 4 are examples of dysfunctional grieving.

*Test-Taking Strategy:* Use the process of elimination. Note the similarity in options 1, 3, and 4. Note the words *unrealistic, prolonged,* and *ignores* in the incorrect options. Review the stages of grief and anticipatory grief if you had difficulty with this question.

*Level of Cognitive Ability:* Analysis
*Client Needs:* Psychosocial Integrity
*Integrated Concept/Process:* Nursing Process/Analysis
*Content Area:* Adult Health/Oncology

*Reference*
Smeltzer, S., & Bare, B. (2000). *Brunner & Suddarth's Textbook of medical-surgical nursing* (9th ed.). Philadelphia: Lippincott Williams & Wilkins, p. 98.

---

**51.** A nurse determines that a gravida 3, para 3 client is beginning to go into shock and is hemorrhaging as a result of a partial inversion of the uterus. The nurse pages the obstetrician STAT and calls for assistance. The client asks in an apprehensive voice, "What is happening to me? I feel so funny, and I know I am bleeding. Am I dying?" The nurse responds to the client, knowing that the client is feeling:

1   Panic secondary to shock
2   Fear and anxiety related to unexpected and ambiguous sensations
3   Anticipatory grieving related to the fear of dying
4   Depression related to postpartum hormonal changes

**Answer: 2**

*Rationale:* Feelings of loss of control are common causes of anxiety. The unknown is the most common cause of fear. Apprehension and feelings of impending doom are also associated with shock, but the case situation does not suggest panic at this point. Anticipatory grieving occurs when there is knowledge of the impending loss, but this is not operative in a sudden situational crisis such as this one. It is far too early for the onset of postpartum depression.

*Test-Taking Strategy:* Focus on the data and the client's statement. Note the relationship between *I feel so funny* in the question and *unexpected and ambiguous sensations* in the correct option. Review client responses when a sudden situational crisis occurs if you had difficulty with this question.

*Level of Cognitive Ability:* Analysis
*Client Needs:* Psychosocial Integrity
*Integrated Concept/Process:* Nursing Process/Analysis
*Content Area:* Maternity

*Reference*
Lowdermilk, D., Perry, S., & Bobak, I. (2000). *Maternity & women's health care* (7th ed.). St. Louis: Mosby, p. 465.

**52.** A perinatal home health nurse has just assessed the fetal status of a client with a diagnosis of partial placental abruption at 20 weeks' gestation. The client is experiencing new bleeding and reports less fetal movement. The nurse informs the client that the physician will be contacted for possible hospital admission. The client begins to cry quietly while holding her abdomen with her hands. She murmurs, " No, no, you can't go, my little man." The nurse recognizes the client's behavior as an indication of:

1    Pain related to abdominal tetany
2    Cognitive confusion secondary to shock
3    Anticipatory grieving related to perceived potential loss
4    Situational crisis, death of fetus, related to fear and loss

**Answer: 3**

*Rationale:* Anticipatory grieving occurs when a client has knowledge of an impending loss. Anticipatory grieving is appropriate when signs of fetal distress accelerate. The first stages of anticipatory grieving may be characterized by shock, emotional numbness, disbelief, and strong emotions, such as tears, screaming, or anger. There are no data that indicate the presence of pain, confusion, or fetal death.

*Test-Taking Strategy:* Use the process of elimination, focusing on the data in the question. Options 1 and 2 can be eliminated, because there is no indication of pain or confusion. Note that in this situation, there is a situational crisis with feelings of grief, but no fetal loss has occurred at this point. Therefore eliminate option 4. Review the defining characteristics of anticipatory grieving if you had difficulty with this question.

*Level of Cognitive Ability:* Analysis
*Client Needs:* Psychosocial Integrity
*Integrated Concept/Process:* Nursing Process/Analysis
*Content Area:* Maternity

*Reference*
Lowdermilk, D., Perry, S., & Bobak, I. (2000). *Maternity & women's health care* (7th ed.). St. Louis: Mosby, p. 1102.

---

**53.** A postoperative client has been vomiting, has absent bowel sounds, and paralytic ileus has been diagnosed. The physician orders insertion of a nasogastric tube. The nurse explains the purpose of the tube and the insertion procedure to the client. The client says to the nurse, "I'm not sure I can take any more of this treatment." The most appropriate response by the nurse is:

1    "It is your right to refuse any treatment. I'll notify the physician."
2    "You are feeling tired and frustrated with your recovery from surgery?"
3    "If you don't have this tube put down, you will just continue to vomit."
4    "Let's just put the tube down so you can get well."

**Answer: 2**

*Rationale:* In option 2, the nurse uses empathy. Empathy, comprehending, and sharing a client's frame of reference constitute an important component in a nurse-client relationship. They assist clients to express and explore feelings, which can lead to problem solving. The other options are examples of barriers to effective communication including defensiveness (option 1), showing disapproval (option 3), and stereotyping (option 4).

*Test-Taking Strategy:* Use therapeutic communication techniques. Option 2 is an open-ended question and is a communication tool. It also focuses on the client's feelings. Review these therapeutic techniques if you had difficulty with this question.

*Level of Cognitive Ability:* Application
*Client Needs:* Psychosocial Integrity
*Integrated Concept/Process:* Communication and Documentation
*Content Area:* Adult Health/Gastrointestinal

*Reference*
Potter, P., & Perry, A. (2001). *Fundamentals of nursing* (5th ed.). St. Louis: Mosby, p. 459.

**54.** A client is admitted to the hospital with a bowel obstruction secondary to a recurrent malignancy. The physician inserts a Miller-Abbott tube. After the procedure the client asks the nurse, "Do you think this is worth all this trouble?" The most appropriate action or response by the nurse is:

1 To stay with the client and be silent
2 "Are you wondering whether you are going to get better?"
3 "Let's give this tube a chance."
4 "I remember a case similar to yours, and the tube relieved the obstruction."

**Answer: 2**

*Rationale:* The nurse uses therapeutic communication tools to assist a client with a chronic terminal illness to express feelings. The nurse listens attentively to the client and uses clarifying and focusing to assist the client in expressing their feelings. Responding with inappropriate silence (option 1), changing the subject (option 3), and offering false reassurance (option 4) are nontherapeutic communication techniques.

*Test-Taking Strategy:* Use therapeutic communications techniques. Option 2 encourages the client to verbalize. Review these techniques if you had difficulty with this question.

*Level of Cognitive Ability:* Application
*Client Needs:* Psychosocial Integrity
*Integrated Concept/Process:* Communication and Documentation
*Content Area:* Adult Health/Oncology

*Reference*
Potter, P., & Perry, A. (2001). *Fundamentals of nursing* (5th ed.). St. Louis: Mosby, p. 459.

---

**55.** A nurse explains to a client receiving total parenteral nutrition (TPN) that intralipids, an intravenous fat emulsion, will also be administered three times per week. The client states to the nurse, "I was always overweight until I had this illness. I'm not sure I want to get that fat. The other IVs are probably enough." Which is the best initial response by the nurse?

1 "Fatty acids are essential for life. You'll develop deficiencies without the fats."
2 "I think you need to discuss this decision with the physician."
3 "Tell me how being ill has affected the way you think of yourself."
4 "I understand what you mean. I've dieted most of my life."

**Answer: 3**

*Rationale:* Clients receiving total parenteral nutrition are at risk for development of essential fatty acid deficiency. However, the client's comment requires more than an informational response initially. Option 3 assists the client to express feelings and deal with aspects of illness and treatment. Option 1 provides an opinion. Option 2 places the client's feelings on hold. Option 4 devalues the client's feelings.

*Test-Taking Strategy:* Note the key words *initial response*. Use therapeutic communication techniques and focus on the client's feelings. Option 3 is the only option that addresses the client's feelings. Review therapeutic communication techniques if you had difficulty with this question.

*Level of Cognitive Ability:* Analysis
*Client Needs:* Psychosocial Integrity
*Integrated Concept/Process:* Communication and Documentation
*Content Area:* Fundamental Skills

*Reference*
Potter, P., & Perry, A. (2001). *Fundamentals of nursing* (5th ed.). St. Louis: Mosby, p. 459.

**56.** A client has terminal cancer and is using narcotic analgesics for pain relief. The client is concerned about becoming addicted to the pain medication. The home health care nurse allays the client's anxiety by:
1 Explaining to the client that his or her fears are justified but should be of no concern in the final stages of care
2 Encouraging the client to hold off as long as possible between doses of pain medication
3 Telling the client to take lower doses of medications even though the pain is not well controlled
4 Explaining to the client that addiction rarely occurs in individuals who are taking medication to relieve pain

**Answer: 4**
*Rationale:* Clients who are receiving narcotics often have well-founded fears about addiction, even in the face of pain. The nurse has a responsibility to provide correct information about the likelihood of addiction while still maintaining adequate pain control. Addiction is rare for individuals who are taking medication to relieve pain. Allowing the client to be in pain, as in options 2 and 3, is not acceptable nursing practice. Option 1 is only partially correct in that it acknowledges the client's fear.

*Test-Taking Strategy:* Use the process of elimination. Eliminate options 2 and 3, because these are not acceptable nursing practices. From the remaining options, eliminate option 1, because it is only partially correct. Review pain management if you had difficulty with this question.

*Level of Cognitive Ability:* Application
*Client Needs:* Psychosocial Integrity
*Integrated Concept/Process:* Caring
*Content Area:* Adult Health/Oncology

*Reference*
Smeltzer, S., & Bare, B. (2000). *Brunner & Suddarth's Textbook of medical-surgical nursing* (9th ed.). Philadelphia: Lippincott Williams & Wilkins, p. 191.

**57.** A client is very anxious about receiving chest physical therapy (CPT) for the first time at home. In planning for the client's care, the home health care nurse proceeds in reassuring the client that:
1 There are no risks associated with this procedure
2 CPT will resolve all of the client's respiratory symptoms
3 CPT will assist in mobilizing secretions to enhance more effective breathing
4 CPT will assist the client to cough more effectively

**Answer: 3**
*Rationale:* There are risks associated with CPT and these include cardiac, gastrointestinal, neurological, and pulmonary. CPT is an intervention to assist in mobilizing and clearing secretions and enhance more effective breathing. It will not resolve all respiratory symptoms. CPT will assist the client to cough, if the secretions have been mobilized and the cough stimulus is present.

*Test-Taking Strategy:* Use the process of elimination. Eliminate options 1 and 2, because they contain the absolute terms *no* and *all*. From the remaining options, focus on the purpose of CPT and recall that coughing will be stimulated once secretions are mobilized. Review the purpose of CPT if you had difficulty with this question.

*Level of Cognitive Ability:* Application
*Client Needs:* Psychosocial Integrity
*Integrated Concept/Process:* Teaching/Learning
*Content Area:* Adult Health/Respiratory

*Reference*
Smeltzer, S., & Bare, B. (2000). *Brunner & Suddarth's Textbook of medical-surgical nursing* (9th ed.). Philadelphia: Lippincott Williams & Wilkins, p. 495.

**58.** A client with cardiomyopathy stops eating, takes long naps, and turns away from the nurse when the nurse talks to the client. The nurse interprets that this client is most likely experiencing:

1    Activity intolerance
2    Intractable pain
3    Noncompliance
4    Depression

**Answer: 4**

*idi'bila,tet/ make someone very weak.*

*Rationale:* Depression is a common problem related to clients who have long-term and debilitating illness. Options 1, 2, and 3 are not related to the symptoms present in the question and therefore are not appropriate interpretations.

*Test-Taking Strategy:* When a question asks for an interpretation of a client's symptoms, focus on the information in the question. Based on the data presented, the only appropriate interpretation is depression. Review the characteristics of depression if you had difficulty with this question.

*Level of Cognitive Ability:* Analysis
*Client Needs:* Psychosocial Integrity
*Integrated Concept/Process:* Nursing Process/Analysis
*Content Area:* Adult Health/Cardiovascular

*Reference*
Johnson, M., Bulechek, G., Dochterman, J. Maas, M., Moorhead, S. (2001). *Nursing diagnoses, outcomes, and interventions.* St. Louis: Mosby, p. 169.

**59.** A nurse is caring for a pregnant client hospitalized for stabilization of diabetes mellitus. The client tells the nurse that her husband is caring for their 2-year-old daughter. The nurse develops which short-term psychosocial outcome for the client?

1    Teach the client and family about diabetes and its implications
2    Provide emotional support and education about altered family processes related to the pregnant woman's hospitalization
3    Protect from risk of injury secondary to convulsions
4    Be alert to the risks of early labor and birth

**Answer: 2**

*Rationale:* The short-term psychosocial well-being of the family is at risk because of the hospitalization of the client. Teaching about diabetes mellitus is a long-term goal related to diabetes. Options 3 and 4 are unrelated to diabetes mellitus and are more related to pregnancy-induced hypertension.

*Test-Taking Strategy:* Use the process of elimination. Eliminate options 3 and 4, because they are unrelated to diabetes mellitus. From the remaining options, note the words *short-term psychosocial outcome* and focus on the data in the question to direct you to option 2. Review outcomes for altered family processes if you had difficulty with this question.

*Level of Cognitive Ability:* Analysis
*Client Needs:* Psychosocial Integrity
*Integrated Concept/Process:* Nursing Process/Planning
*Content Area:* Maternity

*Reference*
Lowdermilk, D., Perry, S., & Bobak, I. (2000). *Maternity & women's health care* (7th ed.). St. Louis: Mosby, p. 874.

**60.** A new parent is trying to make the decision whether or not to have her baby boy circumcised. The nurse makes which statement to assist the mother in making a decision?
   1   "I had my son circumcised, and I am so glad!"
   2   "Circumcision is a difficult decision, but your physician is the best, and you know it's better to get it done now than later!"
   3   "Circumcision is a difficult decision. There are various controversies surrounding circumcision. Here, read this pamphlet that discusses the pros and cons, and we will talk after you read, to answer any questions that you have."
   4   "You know they say it prevents cancer and sexually transmitted diseases, so I would definitely have my son circumcised!"

**Answer: 3**
*Rationale:* Informed decision making is the key point in answering this question. The nurse should provide educational material and answer questions pertaining to the education of the mother. Providing written information to the mother will give her the information she needs to make an educated and informed decision. The nurse's personal thoughts and feelings should not be part of the educational process.

*Test-Taking Strategy:* Use the therapeutic communication techniques and the process of elimination. Options 1, 2, and 4 are communication blocks, because the nurse is providing a personal opinion to the client. Review therapeutic communication techniques if you had difficulty with this question.

*Level of Cognitive Ability:* Application
*Client Needs:* Psychosocial Integrity
*Integrated Concept/Process:* Communication and Documentation
*Content Area:* Maternity

*Reference*
Lowdermilk, D., Perry, S., & Bobak, I. (2000). *Maternity & women's health care* (7th ed.). St. Louis: Mosby, p. 745.

---

**61.** A nurse is planning care for a client who is experiencing anxiety following a myocardial infarction. Which nursing intervention should be included in the plan of care?
   1   Provide detailed explanations of all procedures
   2   Administer cyclobenzaprine (Flexeril) to promote relaxation
   3   Limit family involvement during the acute phase
   4   Answer questions with factual information

**Answer: 4**
*Rationale:* Accurate information reduces fear, strengthens the nurse-client relationship, and assists the client to deal realistically with the situation. Providing detailed information, may increase the client's anxiety. Information should be provided simply and clearly. Flexeril is a skeletal muscle relaxant and is used in the short-term treatment of muscle spasms. Limiting family involvement may or may not be helpful. The client's family may be a source of support for the client.

*Test-Taking Strategy:* Note that the client is experiencing anxiety. Eliminate option 1 because of the word *detailed*. Eliminate option 2, because medication should not be the first intervention to alleviate anxiety. Additionally, this medication is used to relieve muscle spasms. From the remaining options, eliminate option 3, because limiting family involvement is not anxiety reducing in all situations. Review measures to reduce anxiety if you had difficulty with this question.

*Level of Cognitive Ability:* Application
*Client Needs:* Psychosocial Integrity
*Integrated Concept/Process:* Nursing Process/Planning
*Content Area:* Adult Health/Cardiovascular

*Reference*
Black, J., Hawks, J., & Keene, A. (2001). *Medical-surgical nursing: Clinical management for positive outcomes* (6th ed.). Philadelphia: W.B. Saunders, p. 409.

**62.** A client recovering from an acute myocardial infarction will be discharged in 1 day. Which client action on the evening before discharge suggests that the client is in the denial phase of grieving, and a nursing diagnosis of grieving is still applicable for the client?
1   Requests a sedative for sleep at 10:00 P.M.
2   Expresses hesitancy to leave the hospital
3   Walks up and down three flights of stairs unsupervised
4   Consumes 25% of foods and fluids for supper

**Answer: 3**
*Rationale:* Ignoring activity limitations and avoidance of lifestyle changes are signs of denial in the stages of grieving. Walking three flights of stairs should be a supervised activity during this phase of the recovery process. Option 1 is an appropriate client action on the evening before discharge. Option 2, expressing hesitancy to leave, may be a manifestation of anxiety or fear, not of denial. Option 4, anorexia, is a manifestation of depression not denial.

*Test-Taking Strategy:* Note the key word *denial*. Focus on this key word and use the process of elimination. Option 1 is an appropriate client request. Option 2 identifies anxiety or fear. Option 4 identifies depression. Option 3 is the only option that identifies denial. Review the manifestations associated with denial if you had difficulty with this question.

*Level of Cognitive Ability:* Analysis
*Client Needs:* Psychosocial Integrity
*Integrated Concept/Process:* Nursing Process/Analysis
*Content Area:* Adult Health/Cardiovascular

*Reference*
Johnson, M., Bulechek, G., Dochterman, J. Maas, M., Moorhead, S. (2001). *Nursing diagnoses, outcomes, and interventions.* St. Louis: Mosby, p. 97.

**63.** A nurse is caring for a client with Hodgkin's disease who will be receiving radiation and chemotherapy. Which statement by the client indicates a positive coping mechanism to be used during these treatments?
1   "I have selected a wig, even though I will miss my own hair."
2   "I know losing my hair won't bother me."
3   "I will not leave the house bald."
4   "I will be one of the few who doesn't lose their hair."

**Answer: 1**
*Rationale:* A combination of radiation and chemotherapy often causes alopecia in Hodgkin's disease clients. In order to use positive coping mechanisms, the client must identify personal feelings and positive interventions to deal with side effects. Options 2, 3, and 4 are not positive coping mechanisms.

*Test-Taking Strategy:* Focus on the issue: a positive coping mechanism. Options 2, 3, and 4 involve avoidance and denial. Option 1 is the only option that addresses a positive coping mechanism. Review coping mechanisms if you had difficulty with this question.

*Level of Cognitive Ability:* Analysis
*Client Needs:* Psychosocial Integrity
*Integrated Concept/Process:* Nursing Process/Analysis
*Content Area:* Adult Health/Oncology

*Reference*
Black, J., Hawks, J., & Keene, A. (2001). *Medical-surgical nursing: Clinical management for positive outcomes* (6th ed.). Philadelphia: W.B. Saunders, p. 2176.

**64.** A male client is admitted with diabetic ketoacidosis (DKA). His daughter says to the nurse, "My mother died last month, and now this. I've been trying to follow all of the instructions from the doctor; what have I done wrong?" The nurse's best response would be:
1. "Maybe we can keep your father in the hospital for a while longer to give you a rest."
2. "An emotional stress, such as your mother's death, can trigger DKA, even though you are following the prescribed regimen."
3. "You should talk to the social worker about getting you someone at home who is more capable in managing a diabetic's care."
4. "Tell me what you think you did wrong."

**Answer: 2**
*Rationale:* Environment, infection, or an emotional stressor can initiate the physiological mechanism of DKA. Option 1 is not a cost effective intervention. Options 3 and 4 substantiate the daughters' feelings of guilt and incompetence.

*Test-Taking Strategy:* Note that the daughter is the client of the question. This will assist in eliminating option 1 in addition to the fact that this option is not cost effective. Options 3 and 4 devalue the client (the daughter) and block therapeutic communication. Review therapeutic communication techniques if you had difficulty with this question.

*Level of Cognitive Ability:* Application
*Client Needs:* Psychosocial Integrity
*Integrated Concept/Process:* Caring
*Content Area:* Adult Health/Endocrine

*Reference*
Black, J., Hawks, J., & Keene, A. (2001). *Medical-surgical nursing: Clinical management for positive outcomes* (6th ed.). Philadelphia: W.B. Saunders, p. 1172.

**65.** A nurse has been working with a victim of rape in an outpatient setting for the past 4 weeks. The nurse avoids including which of the following short-term goals in the plan of care?
1. The client will resolve feelings of fear and anxiety related to the rape trauma
2. The client will experience physical healing of the wounds that were incurred at the time of the rape
3. The client will verbalize feelings about the rape event
4. The client will participate in the treatment plan by keeping appointments and following through with treatment options

**Answer: 1**
*Rationale:* Short-term goals will include the beginning stages of dealing with the rape trauma. The client will be expected initially to keep appointments, participate in care, begin to explore feelings, and begin to heal physical wounds that were inflicted at the time of the rape.

*Test-Taking Strategy:* Note the key words *avoids* and *short-term*. Use the process of elimination, considering each option and the reality of the option statement being achieved short-term. Note the word *resolve* in option 1; this should provide you with a clue that this option is a long-term goal. Review appropriate goals for the client who is a victim of rape if you had difficulty with this question.

*Level of Cognitive Ability:* Application
*Client Needs:* Psychosocial Integrity
*Integrated Concept/Process:* Nursing Process/Planning
*Content Area:* Mental Health

*Reference*
Stuart, G.W., & Laraia, M.T. (1998). *Principles and practice of psychiatric nursing* (6th ed.). St. Louis: Mosby, p. 835.

**66.** A client is admitted to a surgical unit with a diagnosis of cancer. The client is scheduled for surgery in the morning. When a nurse enters the room and begins surgical preparation, the client states, "I'm not having surgery, you must have the wrong person! My test results were negative. I'll be going home tomorrow." The nurse recognizes that the ego defense mechanism that may be operating here is:

1    Psychosis
2    Denial
3    Delusions
4    Displacement

**Answer: 2**

*Rationale:*  By definition, ego defense mechanisms are operations outside of a person's awareness that the ego calls into play to protect against anxiety. Denial is the defense mechanism that blocks out painful or anxiety-inducing events or feelings. In this case, the client cannot deal with the upcoming surgery for cancer and therefore denies the illness. Psychosis and delusions are not defense mechanisms. Displacement is the discharging of pent-up feelings on persons less dangerous than those who initially aroused the feelings.

*Test-Taking Strategy:*  Focus on the issue: ego defense mechanism. Options 1 and 3 are eliminated first, because these are not ego defense mechanisms. From the remaining options, focus on the client's statement to direct you to option 2. Review ego defense mechanisms if you had difficulty with this question.

*Level of Cognitive Ability:*  Analysis
*Client Needs:*  Psychosocial Integrity
*Integrated Concept/Process:*  Nursing Process/Analysis
*Content Area:*  Adult Health/Oncology

*Reference*
Stuart, G.W., & Laraia, M.T. (1998). *Principles and practice of psychiatric nursing* (6th ed.). St. Louis: Mosby, p. 283.

**67.** A community health nurse working in an industrial setting has received a memo indicating that a large number of employees will be laid off in the next 2 weeks. An analysis of previous layoffs suggested that workers experienced role crises, indecision, and depression. Using these data, the nurse should begin to:

1    Help the workers acquire unemployment benefits to avoid a gap in income
2    Reduce the staff in the occupational health department of the industrial setting
3    Notify the insurance carriers of the upcoming event to assist with potential health alterations
4    Identify referral, counseling, and vocational rehabilitative services for the employees being laid off

**Answer: 4**

*Rationale:*  In preparation for this crisis, the nurse should identify the services that are available to the employees. These resources will provide immediate avenues for the assistance when the layoff occurs. Additional information about the industrial setting is needed to determine whether options 1, 2, or 3 were necessary or possible.

*Test-Taking Strategy:*  Use the steps of the nursing process to direct you to option 4. Additionally, review crisis interventions if you had difficulty with this question.

*Level of Cognitive Ability:*  Analysis
*Client Needs:*  Psychosocial Integrity
*Integrated Concept/Process:*  Nursing Process/Planning
*Content Area:*  Mental Health

*Reference:*
Stuart, G.W., & Laraia, M.T. (1998). *Principles and practice of psychiatric nursing* (6th ed.). St. Louis: Mosby, p. 253.

**68.** A primigravida client comes to the clinic and has been diagnosed with a urinary tract infection. She has repeatedly verbalized concern regarding safety of the fetus. Which of the following nursing diagnoses is most appropriate at this time?
**1** Pain
**2** Impaired Tissue Integrity
**3** Urinary Tract Infection
**4** Fear

**Answer: 4**
*Rationale:* The primary concern for this client is safety of her fetus, not herself. The priority nursing diagnosis at this time is Fear. Option 3 is a medical diagnosis and outside the scope of nursing practice. Pain and Impaired Tissue Integrity are commonly seen in clients experiencing urinary tract infections, but the question includes no data to support either of the options.

*Test-Taking Strategy:* Focus on the data in the question and note the key words *verbalized concern.* Eliminate option 3, because it is a medical diagnosis. Also, note that options 1, 2, and 3 are similar in that they all relate to physiological states. Option 4 addresses the psychosocial issue. Review the defining characteristics of Fear if you had difficulty with this question.

*Level of Cognitive Ability:* Analysis
*Client Needs:* Psychosocial Integrity
*Integrated Concept/Process:* Nursing Process/Analysis
*Content Area:* Maternity

*Reference*
Lowdermilk, D., Perry, S., & Bobak, I. (2000). *Maternity & women's health care* (7th ed.). St. Louis: Mosby. p. 406.

**69.** A nurse is planning interventions for counseling the maternal client newly diagnosed with sickle cell anemia. The most important psychosocial intervention at this time would be which of the following?
**1** Provide all information regarding the disease
**2** Allow the client to be alone if she is crying
**3** Provide emotional support
**4** Avoid the topic of the disease at all costs

**Answer: 3**
*Rationale:* One of the most important nursing functions is providing emotional support to the client and family during the counseling process. Option 1 overwhelms the client with information while the client is trying to cope with the news of the disease. Option 2 is only appropriate if the client requests to be alone. If this is not requested, the nurse is abandoning the client in time of need. Option 4 is similar to option 2 and is nontherapeutic.

*Test-Taking Strategy:* Use the process of elimination. Eliminate options 1 and 4 because of the words *all* and *avoid.* Additionally, these actions are nontherapeutic. From the remaining options, remember that the client's feelings are the priority and an extremely important role of the nurse is to provide emotional support. Review interventions related to providing emotional support if you had difficulty with this question.

*Level of Cognitive Ability:* Application
*Client Needs:* Psychosocial Integrity
*Integrated Concept/Process:* Caring
*Content Area:* Maternity

*Reference*
Lowdermilk, D., Perry, S., & Bobak, I. (2000). *Maternity & women's health care* (7th ed.). St. Louis: Mosby, p. 901.

**70.** A neonatal intensive care nurse is caring for a newborn infant immediately following delivery; the infant has a suspected diagnosis of erythroblastosis fetalis. The nurse would make which of the following statements to the parents at this time?

1   "You must have many concerns. Please ask me any questions as I explain your infant's care."

2   "This is a common neonatal problem; you shouldn't be concerned."

3   "There is no need to worry. We have the most updated equipment in this hospital."

4   "Your infant is very sick. The next 24 hours are most crucial."

**Answer: 1**

*Rationale:* Parental anxiety is expected related to the care of the infant with erythroblastosis fetalis. This anxiety is due to a lack of knowledge regarding the disease process, treatments, and expected outcomes. Parents need to be encouraged to verbalize concerns and participate in care as appropriate.

*Test-Taking Strategy:* Use the therapeutic communication techniques. Eliminate options 2 and 3, because they are similar. Additionally, they are blocks to communication. Eliminate option 4, because it will produce anxiety in the parents. Remember, address clients feelings and concerns. Option 1 is the only option that encourages communication. Review therapeutic communication techniques if you had difficulty with this question.

*Level of Cognitive Ability:* Application
*Clients Needs:* Psychosocial Integrity
*Integrated Concept/Process:* Caring
*Content Area:* Maternity

*Reference*
Lowdermilk, D., Perry, S., & Bobak, I. (2000). *Maternity & women's health care* (7th ed.). St. Louis: Mosby, p. 1073.

**71.** A school nurse is weighing all the high school students. One of the teenagers, who has type 1 diabetes mellitus, has gained 15 pounds since last year, with no gain in height. The nurse also notices this student eating alone in the cafeteria at lunchtime. Based on these data, the nurse is most concerned that the student may have:

1   Bulimia nervosa
2   Self-destructive thoughts
3   An alcohol abuse problem
4   An insulin deficiency

**Answer: 2**

*Rationale:* Diabetic teenagers are at risk for depression and suicide (self-destructive thoughts), which is frequently manifested by changing insulin and eating patterns. Social isolation is another indicator. Weight loss (not gain) is a symptom of type 1 diabetes mellitus, so an insulin deficiency would have the same effect. Bulimics may be of normal weight but control weight gain by purging. Alcohol use is more likely to be related to weight loss.

*Test-Taking Strategy:* Focus on the data in the question and use the process of elimination. Noting the social isolation issue and the age of the client should direct you to option 2. Review the manifestations associated with depression and self-destructive thoughts if you had difficulty with this question.

*Level of Cognitive Ability:* Analysis
*Client Needs:* Psychosocial Integrity
*Integrated Concept/Process:* Nursing Process/Analysis
*Content Area:* Child Health

*Reference*
Wong, D. (1999). *Whaley & Wong's Nursing care of infants and children* (6th ed.). St. Louis: Mosby, p. 922.

**72.** A school nurse is teaching a class of high school students about the risk of sexually transmitted diseases (STD). What opening statement will best encourage participation within the group?

1 "At the end of the class, condoms will be distributed to everyone in the class."

2 "The topic today is very personal. For this reason, anything shared with the group will remain confidential."

3 "Please feel free to share your personal experiences with the group."

4 "Our goal today is to describe ways to prevent acquiring a sexually transmitted disease."

**Answer: 2**

*Rationale:* Option 2 identifies the rules for confidentiality, which will help develop a trust in sharing sensitive issues with the group. Option 1 may be an incentive for those attending to stay, but participation is not required to get the reward. Option 3 provides no protection of confidentiality. Option 4 does not foster trust, especially with those who may already have an STD.

*Test-Taking Strategy:* Focus on the issues, confidentiality, trust-building, and sharing. Option 2 is the only option that addresses the issue of confidentiality. Review the concepts related to group process if you had difficulty with this question.

*Level of Cognitive Ability:* Application
*Client Needs:* Psychosocial Integrity
*Integrated Concept/Process:* Communication and Documentation
*Content Area:* Child Health

*Reference*
Wong, D. (1999). *Whaley & Wong's Nursing care of infants and children* (6th ed.). St. Louis: Mosby, p. 941.

---

**73.** A nurse is planning care for a client with an intrauterine fetal demise. Which of the following is not an appropriate goal for this client?

1 The woman and her family will express their grief about the loss of their desired infant

2 The woman and her family will discuss plans for going home without the infant

3 The woman and her family will contact their Pastor or grief counselor for support following discharge

4 The woman will recognize that thoughts of worthlessness and suicide are normal following a loss

**Answer: 4**

*Rationale:* It is important for the nurse to assess whether the client is undergoing the normal grieving process. Signs that are a cause for concern and are not part of the normal grieving process include thoughts of worthlessness and suicide.

*Test-Taking Strategy:* Use the process of elimination, noting the key words *not an appropriate goal.* These key words should direct you to option 4, because thoughts of worthlessness and suicide are cause for concern. Review care of a client experiencing intrauterine fetal demise if you had difficulty with this client.

*Level of Cognitive Ability:* Analysis
*Client Needs:* Psychosocial Integrity
*Integrated Concept/Process:* Caring
*Content Area:* Maternity

*Reference*
Lowdermilk, D., Perry, S., & Bobak, I. (2000). *Maternity & women's health care* (7th ed.). St. Louis: Mosby, p. 425.

**74.** A client with severe preeclampsia is admitted to the hospital. She is a student at a local college and insists on continuing her studies while in the hospital despite being instructed to rest. The nurse notes she studies about 19 hours a day between numerous visits from fellow students, family, and friends. The nurse plans to:

1 Instruct the client that the health of the baby is more important than her studies at this time

2 Ask her why she is not complying with the order of bed rest

3 Include a significant other in helping the client understand the need for bed rest

4 Develop a routine with the client to balance studies and rest needs

**Answer:** 4

*Rationale:* In options 1 and 2, the nurse is judging the client's opinion and asking probing questions. This will cause a breakdown in communication. Option 3 persuades the client's significant other to disagree with the client's action. This could cause problems with the relationship between the client and significant other and also conflict in communication with the health care workers. Option 4 involves the client in the decision making.

*Test-Taking Strategy:* Use the process of elimination. Eliminate options 1, 2, and 3, because these are blocks to communication and a therapeutic nurse-client relationship. Option 4 is the most thorough nursing action, because it addresses rest, studies, and involves the client in the decision making process. Review care of a client with preeclampsia if you had difficulty with this question.

*Level of Cognitive Ability:* Application
*Client Needs:* Psychosocial Integrity
*Integrated Concept/Process:* Nursing Process/Planning
*Content Area:* Maternity

*References*
Potter, P., & Perry, A. (2001). *Fundamentals of nursing* (5th ed.). St. Louis: Mosby, p. 459.
Lowdermilk, D., Perry, S., & Bobak, I. (2000). *Maternity & women's health care* (7th ed.). St. Louis: Mosby. p. 826

**75.** A pregnant client is newly diagnosed as having gestational diabetes. She cries during the remaining interview and keeps repeating, "What have I done to cause this? If I could only live my life over." Which nursing diagnosis should direct nursing care at this time?

1 Self-Concept Disturbance related to a complication of pregnancy

2 Knowledge Deficit related to diabetic self-care during pregnancy

3 Body Image Disturbance related to complications of pregnancy

4 Risk for Injury to the fetus related to maternal distress

**Answer:** 1

*Rationale:* The client is putting the blame for the diabetes on herself, lowering her self-concept or image. She is expressing fear and grief. Knowledge Deficit is an important nursing diagnosis for this client, but not at this time. The client will not be able to comprehend information at this time. There are no data in question to support the nursing diagnoses in options 3 and 4.

*Test-Taking Strategy:* Use the data presented in the question to direct you to the correct option. The words *what have I done* should assist in eliminating options 2, 3, and 4. Review the defining characteristics of Self-Concept Disturbance if you had difficulty with this question.

*Level of Cognitive Ability:* Analysis
*Client Needs:* Psychosocial Integrity
*Integrated Concept/Process:* Nursing Process/Analysis
*Content Area:* Maternity

*Reference*
Lowdermilk, D., Perry, S., & Bobak, I. (2000). *Maternity & women's health care* (7th ed.). St. Louis: Mosby, p. 877.

**76.** A client says to the nurse, "I 'm going to die, and I wish my family would stop hoping for a cure! I get so angry when they carry on like this! After all, I'm the one who's dying." The most therapeutic response by the nurse is:
1   "You're feeling angry that your family continues to hope for you to be cured?"
2   "I think we should talk more about your anger at your family."
3   "Well, it sounds like you're being pretty pessimistic. After all, years ago people died of pneumonia."
4   "Have you shared your feelings with your family?"

**Answer: 1**
*Rationale:* Reflection is the therapeutic communication technique that redirects the client's feelings back in order to validate what the client is saying. Option 1 uses the therapeutic technique of reflection. In option 2, the nurse attempts to use focusing but the attempt to discuss central issues seems premature. In option 3, the nurse makes a judgment and is nontherapeutic in the one-to-one relationship. In option 4, the nurse is attempting to assess the client's ability to openly discuss feelings with family members. While this is an appropriate communication and assessment for this client, the timing is somewhat premature and closes off facilitation of the client's feelings.

*Test-Taking Strategy:* Use therapeutic communication techniques to answer the question. Option 1 is the only option that uses a therapeutic technique. Also, note the word *angry* in the question and in the correct option. Review the technique of reflection if you had difficulty with this question.

*Level of Cognitive Ability:* Application
*Client Needs:* Psychosocial Integrity
*Integrated Concept/Process:* Caring
*Content Area:* Mental Health

*Reference*
Stuart, G.W., & Laraia, M.T. (1998). *Principles and practice of psychiatric nursing* (6th ed.). St. Louis: Mosby, p. 34.

**77.** A nurse is caring for an older adult client who says, "I don't want to talk with you. You're only a nurse, I'll wait for my doctor." Which of the following would be the most appropriate nursing response?
1   "I understand. I'll leave you now and call your physician."
2   "I'm assigned to work with you. Your doctor placed you in my hands."
3   " You would prefer to speak with your doctor? "
4   "I'm angry with the way you've dismissed me. I am your nurse, not your servant."

**Answer: 3**
*Rationale:* In the correct option, the nurse uses reflection to redirect the client's feelings back for validation and focuses on the client's desire to talk with the physician. Options 2 and 4 are nontherapeutic responses. Option 1 is a response that reinforces the client to continue this behavior. In addition, most nurses wouldn't "understand."

*Test-Taking Strategy:* Use therapeutic communication techniques. Option 3 is the only therapeutic option and uses the technique of reflection. Review therapeutic communication techniques if you had difficulty with this question.

*Level of Cognitive Ability:* Application
*Client Needs:* Psychosocial Integrity
*Integrated Concept/Process:* Communication and Documentation
*Content Area:* Fundamental Skills

*Reference*
Potter, P., & Perry, A. (2001). *Fundamentals of nursing* (5th ed.). St. Louis: Mosby, p. 459.

**78.** A female client and her newborn infant have undergone testing for human immunodeficiency virus (HIV) and both clients were found to be positive. The news is devastating and the mother is crying. Using crisis intervention techniques, which of the following does the nurse interpret that the client needs at this time?

1 Call an HIV counselor and make an appointment for them
2 Describe the progressive stages and treatments for HIV
3 Examine with the mother how she got HIV
4 Listen quietly while the mother talks and cries

**Answer: 4**

*Rationale:* This client has just received devastating news and needs to have someone present with her as she begins to cope with this issue. The nurse needs to sit and actively listen while the mother talks and cries. Calling an HIV counselor may be helpful, but it is not what the client needs at this time. The other options are not appropriate for this stage of coping with the news that both she and the infant are HIV positive.

*Test-Taking Strategy:* Use the process of elimination. Note the key words *the client needs at this time.* Options 2 and 3 can be eliminated first. From the remaining options, remember to address the client's feelings and to support the client. This will direct you to the correct option. The nurse should sit and listen and provide support, because this is the most caring response. Review crisis intervention and the measures that provide support if you had difficulty with this question.

*Level of Cognitive Ability:* Analysis
*Client Needs:* Psychosocial Integrity
*Integrated Concept/Process:* Caring
*Content Area:* Maternity

*Reference*
Potter, P., & Perry, A. (2001). *Fundamentals of nursing* (5th ed.). St. Louis: Mosby, p. 459.

**79.** A community health nurse visits a recently widowed, retired military man who is estranged from his only child, because he was discharged from the service for being "gay." When the nurse visits, the ordinarily immaculate house is in chaos and the client is disheveled and has an alcohol type of odor on his breath. Which of the following nursing statements would be most therapeutic?

1 "You seem to be having a very troubling time."
2 "I can see this isn't a good time to visit."
3 "What are you doing? How much are you drinking and for how long?"
4 "Do you think your wife would want you to behave like this?"

**Answer: 1**

*Rationale:* The most therapeutic statement is the one that facilitates the client to explore his situation and to express his feelings. Reflection, by verbalizing to the client that the nurse feels he is experiencing a troubled or difficult time, is empathic and will assist the client to begin to ventilate. As the client begins to ventilate, the nurse can assist the client to discuss the reasons behind alienation from his only child. Option 2 uses humor to avoid therapeutic intimacy and effective problem solving. Option 3 uses social communication. Option 4 uses admonishment and tries to shame the client, which is not therapeutic or professional. This social communication belittles the client, will cause anger, and may evoke "acting out" by the client.

*Test-Taking Strategy:* Use therapeutic communication techniques. Remember to focus on the client's behavior and feelings. This will direct you to option 1. Review these techniques if you had difficulty with this question.

*Level of Cognitive Ability:* Application
*Client Needs:* Psychosocial Integrity
*Integrated Concept/Process:* Communication and Documentation
*Content Area:* Mental Health

*Reference*
Stuart, G.W., & Laraia, M.T. (1998). *Principles and practice of psychiatric nursing* (6th ed.). St. Louis: Mosby, p. 34.

**80.** A client says to the nurse, "I don't do anything right. I'm such a loser." The most appropriate nursing response is:
1   "You do things right all the time."
2   " Everything will get better."
3   "You don't do anything right?"
4   "You are not a loser, you are sick."

**Answer: 3**
*Rationale:* Option 3 provides the client the opportunity to verbalize. With this statement, the nurse can learn more about what the client really means by the statement. Options 1, 2, and 4 are closed statements and do not encourage the client to explore further.

*Test-Taking Strategy:* Use the process of elimination and therapeutic communication techniques. Option 3 repeats the client's statement and encourages further communication. Review therapeutic communication techniques if you had difficulty with this question.

*Level of Cognitive Ability:* Application
*Client Needs:* Psychosocial Integrity
*Integrated Concept/Process:* Communication and Documentation
*Content Area:* Mental Health

*Reference*
Stuart, G.W., & Laraia, M.T. (1998). *Principles and practice of psychiatric nursing* (6th ed.). St. Louis: Mosby, p. 34.

**81.** A client who is experiencing suicidal thoughts greets the nurse with the following statement: "It just doesn't seem worth it anymore. Why not just end it all." The nurse may further assess the client by making which of the following responses?
1   "I'm sure your family is worried about you."
2   "I know you have had a stressful night."
3   "Did you sleep at all last night?"
4   "Tell me what you mean by that?"

**Answer: 4**
*Rationale:* Option 4 allows the client the opportunity to tell the nurse more about what the current thoughts are. Option 1 is false reassurance and may block communication. While option 2 is offering empathy to the client, it does not further assess. Option 3 changes the subject and may block communication.

*Test-Taking Strategy:* Note the key words *further assess*. Use the nursing process and therapeutic communication techniques to select the correct option. Options 1 and 2 can be eliminated first, because they do not reflect assessment. Both options 3 and 4 relate to assessment, but option 4 is directly related to the issue of the question and is most therapeutic. Review therapeutic communication techniques if you had difficulty with this question.

*Level of Cognitive Ability:* Application
*Client Needs:* Psychosocial Integrity
*Integrated Concept/Process:* Communication and Documentation
*Content Area:* Mental Health

*Reference*
Stuart, G.W., & Laraia, M.T. (1998). *Principles and practice of psychiatric nursing* (6th ed.). St. Louis: Mosby, p. 36.

**82.** A mother says to the nurse, "I am afraid that my child might have another febrile seizure." Which response by the nurse is most therapeutic?
1 "Why worry about something that you cannot control?"
2 "Most children will never experience a second seizure."
3 "Tell me what frightens you the most about seizures."
4 "Tylenol can prevent another seizure from occurring."

**Answer: 3**
*Rationale:* Option 3 is the only response that is an open-ended statement and provides the mother with an opportunity to express feelings. Option 1 is incorrect, because it blocks communication by giving a flippant response to an expressed fear. Options 2 and 4 are incorrect, because the nurse is giving false assurance that a seizure will not recur or can be prevented in this child.

*Test-Taking Strategy:* Note the key words *most therapeutic*. Use the process of elimination seeking the option that is an example of therapeutic communication. Options 1, 2, and 4 violate the principles of therapeutic communication and actually block communication. Review therapeutic communication techniques if you had difficulty with this question.

*Level of Cognitive Ability:* Application
*Client Needs:* Psychosocial Integrity
*Integrated Concept/Process:* Communication and Documentation
*Content Area:* Child Health

*Reference*
Wong, D. (1999). *Whaley & Wong's Nursing care of infants and children* (6th ed.). St. Louis: Mosby, p. 213.

**83.** A mother has just given birth to a baby who has a cleft lip and palate. When planning to talk to the mother, the nurse should recognize that this client must be allowed to work through which of these emotions before maternal bonding can occur?
1 Anger
2 Grief
3 Guilt
4 Depression

**Answer: 2**
*Rationale:* The mother must first be assisted to grieve for the anticipated child that she did not have. Once this is accomplished, the mother can begin to focus on bonding with the baby she gave birth to. Options 1, 3, and 4 are incorrect, because they are only one component of the grief process.

*Test-Taking Strategy:* Use the process of elimination and knowledge of the grief process. Options 1, 3, and 4 are incorrect, because they are only one component of the grief process. Option 2 is the most global option. Review the grief process if you had difficulty with this question.

*Level of Cognitive Ability:* Analysis
*Client Needs:* Psychosocial Integrity
*Integrated Concept/Process:* Nursing Process/Analysis
*Content Area:* Maternity

*Reference*
Wong, D. (1999). *Whaley & Wong's Nursing care of infants and children* (6th ed.). St. Louis: Mosby, p. 477.

**84.** An infant is admitted to the hospital who has been diagnosed with acute chalasia. During the nursing history the mother tells the nurse, "I am concerned that I am somehow causing my infant to vomit after feeding." Considering this statement, which nursing diagnosis is most appropriate?

1 Anxiety related to hospitalization of the infant for chalasia

2 Noncompliance related to denial that chalasia is a physiological defect

3 Knowledge Deficit related to the lack of exposure to feeding an infant with chalasia

4 Altered Parenting related to an unrealistic expectation of self

**Answer: 4**

*Rationale:* The infant is vomiting because of a physiological problem that is not caused by the parent. The misconception that the mother is responsible for the problem may result in a decreased perception of her ability to adequately parent the child. The nurse should assist the parent to understand that she is not responsible for the child's condition. The mother's statement does not reflect symptoms of anxiety regarding the child's hospitalization. The mother states a concern about her behavior. There are no data in the question to support that the mother has ever been told that chalasia is a physiological problem. Again, there are insufficient data to support that the mother has not been instructed on feeding techniques for a child with chalasia.

*Test-Taking Strategy:* Use the process of elimination. Note that the mother is blaming herself for the child's health problem. As a result, the mother is at risk for Altered Parenting. Review the defining characteristics for Altered Parenting if you had difficulty with this question.

*Level of Cognitive Ability:* Analysis
*Client Needs:* Psychosocial Integrity
*Integrated Concept/Process:* Nursing Process/Analysis
*Content Area:* Child Health

*Reference*
Wong, D. (1999). *Whaley & Wong's Nursing care of infants and children* (6th ed.). St. Louis: Mosby, p. 28.

---

**85.** According to standard coronary care unit (CCU) orders, a client with an uncomplicated myocardial infarction (MI) may begin progressive activity after three days. The client who experienced an infarction 4 days ago refuses to dangle at the bedside saying, "If my doctor tells me to do it I will. Otherwise I won't." The nurse determines that the client is likely displaying:

1 Anger

2 Denial

3 Dependency

4 Depression

**Answer: 3**

*Rationale:* Clients may experience numerous emotional and behavioral responses following an MI. Dependency is one response that may be manifested by the client's refusal to perform any tasks or activities unless approved by the physician. There are no data in the question to support denial or depression. Although the client's statement may express anger to some degree, it most specifically addresses dependency.

*Test-Taking Strategy:* Focus on the data in the question to determine the correct option. Begin by eliminating options 2 and 4 first, because the client is not exhibiting signs of denial or depression. From the remaining options, focus on the client's statement to direct you to option 3. Review the characteristics related to dependency if you had difficulty with this question.

*Level of Cognitive Ability:* Analysis
*Client Needs:* Psychosocial Integrity
*Integrated Concept/Process:* Nursing Process/Analysis
*Content Area:* Adult Health/Cardiovascular

*Reference*
Black, J., Hawks, J., & Keene, A. (2001). *Medical-surgical nursing: Clinical management for positive outcomes* (6th ed.). Philadelphia: W.B. Saunders, p. 1598.

**86.** A nurse is assessing a 45-year-old client admitted to the hospital for urinary calculi. The client has received 4 mg of morphine sulfate (MS) approximately 2 hours previously. The client states to the nurse, "I'm scared to death that it'll come back. That was the worst pain I ever had—like a knife going from my right side to my groin." Which of the following nursing diagnoses would be appropriate for the nurse to make regarding this statement?

1 Pain, Acute, related to the presence of calculi in the right ureter
2 Knowledge Deficit related to the lack of information about the disease process
3 Anxiety related to anticipation of recurrent severe pain
4 Urinary Retention related to obstruction of the urinary tract by calculi

**Answer: 3**
*Rationale:* The client has stated, "I'm scared to death that it'll come back." The anticipation of the recurring pain threatens the client's psychological integrity. There is no evidence that the client has a calculus in the right ureter. There is also no evidence that either urinary retention or knowledge deficit exists.

*Test-Taking Strategy:* Use the data presented in the question to assist in answering the question. Note the key statement *I'm scared to death that it'll come back.* This should assist in directing you to the key word *anxiety* in the correct option. Review the defining characteristics of Anxiety if you had difficulty with this question.

*Level of Cognitive Ability:* Analysis
*Client Needs:* Psychosocial Integrity
*Integrated Concept/Process:* Nursing Process/Analysis
*Content Area:* Mental Health

*Reference*
Johnson, M., Bulechek, G., Dochterman, J. Maas, M., Moorhead, S. (2001). *Nursing diagnoses, outcomes, and interventions.* St. Louis: Mosby, p. 132.

**87.** A nurse is observing parents at the bedside of their small-for-gestational-age (SGA) female infant, who is at 27 weeks' gestation. The infant's mother states, "She is so tiny and fragile. I'll never be able to hold her with all those tubes." The nurse interprets the mother's statement as being relevant to which of the following nursing diagnoses?

1 Impaired Adjustment
2 Risk for Caregiver Strain
3 Ineffective Family Coping
4 Risk for Altered Parenting

**Answer: 4**
*Rationale:* One of the nursing diagnoses for the parents of a high-risk neonate, such as a preterm SGA infant, is risk for Altered Parenting. Parent-infant bonding is affected if the infant does not exhibit normal newborn characteristics. Option 1 involves nonacceptance of a health status change or an inability to problem solve or set a goal. Option 2 addresses the strain of a caregiver, which during the initial hospitalization is too early to apply. Option 3 involves identification of ineffective coping. At this time, there are inadequate data for these diagnoses, although they may become relevant at a later time.

*Test-Taking Strategy:* Use the data presented in the question to assist in answering. Eliminate options 1 and 3 first, because these are actual nursing diagnoses. From the remaining options, note the key words *I'll never be able to hold her.* This should assist in directing you to the key words, *Altered Parenting,* in the correct option. Review the defining characteristics of Altered Parenting if you had difficulty with this question.

*Level of Cognitive Ability:* Analysis
*Client Needs:* Psychosocial Integrity
*Integrated Concept/Process:* Nursing Process/Analysis
*Content Area:* Maternity

*Reference*
Johnson, M., Bulechek, G., Dochterman, J. Maas, M., Moorhead, S. (2001). *Nursing diagnoses, outcomes, and interventions.* St. Louis: Mosby, p. 235.

**88.** After vaginal delivery of a large-for-gestational-age (LGA) male infant, the nurse wraps the infant in a warm blanket and hands him to his mother. The mother verbalizes concern over the infant's facial bruising. To enhance attachment, the nurse makes which therapeutic statement?

**1** "Since the bruising is painful, it is advisable that you not touch the baby's face."

**2** "The bruising is caused by polycythemia, which usually leads to jaundice."

**3** "It is a normal finding in large babies and nothing to be concerned about."

**4** "The bruising is temporary and it is important to interact with your infant."

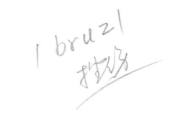

**Answer: 4**

*Rationale:* The mother of an LGA infant with facial bruising may be reluctant to interact with the infant because of concern about causing additional pain to the infant. The bruising is temporary. Option 1 advises the mother not to touch the baby's face, because the bruising is painful. Touch is an important component of the attachment process. Touching the infant gently with fingertips should be encouraged. The LGA infant may have polycythemia, which can contribute to bruising, but the bruising is not actually caused by the polycythemia. Option 3 avoids the mother's verbalized concerns.

*Test-Taking Strategy:* Use the process of elimination and note the issue: to enhance attachment. Eliminate options 2 and 3 first, because they do not specifically address the issue of attachment. From the remaining options, note the relationship of the word *attachment* in the stem of the question and the word *interact* in the correct option. Review the interventions that promote mother-infant bonding if you had difficulty with this question.

*Level of Cognitive Ability:* Application
*Client Needs:* Psychosocial Integrity
*Integrated Concept/Process:* Nursing Process/Implementation
*Content Area:* Maternity

*Reference*
Lowdermilk, D., Perry, S., & Bobak, I. (2000). *Maternity & women's health care* (7th ed.). St. Louis: Mosby p. 729.

---

**89.** A client with myasthenia gravis is ready to return home. The client confides that she is concerned that her husband will no longer find her physically attractive. The nurse would include in the plan of care to:

**1** Encourage the client to start a support group

**2** Insist that the client reach out and face this fear

**3** Tell the client not to dwell on the negative

**4** Encourage the client to share her feelings with her husband

**Answer: 4**

*Rationale:* Sharing feelings with her husband directly addresses the issue of the question. Encouraging the client to start a support group will not address the client's immediate and individual concerns. Options 2 and 3 are blocks to communication and avoid the client's concern.

*Test-Taking Strategy:* Focus on the issue of the question and use therapeutic communication techniques. Option 4 is the only option that addresses the client's immediate concern. Remember, address the client's feelings and concerns first. Review therapeutic communication techniques if you had difficulty with this question.

*Level of Cognitive Ability:* Application
*Client Needs:* Psychosocial Integrity
*Integrated Concept/Process:* Caring
*Content Area:* Adult Health/Neurological

*Reference*
Potter, P., & Perry, A. (2001). *Fundamentals of nursing* (5th ed.). St. Louis: Mosby, p. 459.

**90.** A 9-year-old child is hospitalized for 2 months after an automobile accident. The best way to promote psychosocial development of this child is to plan for:

1    Tutoring to keep the child up with school work
2    A phone to call family and friends
3    Computer games, TV, and videos at the bedside
4    A portable radio and tape player with headphones

**Answer: 1**

*Rationale:* The developmental task of the school-aged child is industry vs. inferiority. The child achieves success by mastering skills and knowledge. Maintaining school work provides for accomplishment and prevents feelings of inferiority from lagging behind the class. The other options provide diversion and are of lesser importance for a child of this age.

*Test-Taking Strategy:* Note the key word *development* in the stem of the question. Note the age of the child and determine the developmental task for this child. Options 2, 3, and 4 address social and diversional issues, whereas option 1 specifically addresses psychosocial development. Review growth and development related to the school-aged child if you had difficulty with this question.

*Level of Cognitive Ability:* Application
*Client Needs:* Psychosocial Integrity
*Integrated Concept/Process:* Nursing Process/Planning
*Content Area:* Child Health

*Reference*
Wong, D. (1999). *Whaley & Wong's Nursing care of infants and children* (6th ed.). St. Louis: Mosby, p. 779.

**91.** A client who is in halo traction, says to the visiting nurse, "I can't get used to this contraption. I can't see properly on the side and I keep misjudging where everything is." The most therapeutic response by the nurse would be:

1    "Halo traction involves many difficult adjustments. Practice scanning with your eyes after standing up, before you move."
2    "No one ever gets used to that thing! It's horrible. Many of our sports people who are in it complain vigorously."
3    "Why do you feel like this when you could have died from a broken neck? This is the way it is for several months. You need to accept it more, don't you think?"
4    "If I were you, I would have had the surgery rather than suffer like this."

**Answer: 1**

*Rationale:* In option 1, the nurse employs empathy and reflection. The nurse then offers a strategy for solving the client's problem, which helps to increase peripheral vision for clients in halo traction. In option 2, the nurse provides a social response that contains emotionally charged language that could increase the client's anxiety. In option 3, the nurse uses excessive questioning and gives advice, which is nontherapeutic. In option 4, the nurse undermines the client's faith in the medical treatment being employed by giving advice that is insensitive and unprofessional.

*Test-Taking Strategy:* Use the process of elimination, seeking the option that represents a therapeutic communication technique. Focus on the client's statement and note that option 1 is the only statement that addresses the client's concern. Review therapeutic communication techniques if you had difficulty with this question.

*Level of Cognitive Ability:* Application
*Client Needs:* Psychosocial Integrity
*Integrated Concept/Process:* Communication and Documentation
*Content Area:* Adult Health/Neurological

*Reference*
Potter, P., & Perry, A. (2001). *Fundamentals of nursing* (5th ed.). St. Louis: Mosby, p. 459.

**92.** An elderly client has been admitted to the hospital with a hip fracture. The nurse prepares a plan of care for the client and identifies desired outcomes related to the alterations in immobility. Which statement by the client most appropriately supports a positive adjustment to the alterations experienced in mobility?

1 "I wish you nurse's would leave me alone! You are always telling me what to do!"
2 "What took you so long. I called for you 30 minutes ago."
3 "Hurry up and go away. I want to be alone."
4 "I find it difficult to concentrate since the doctor talked with me about the surgery tomorrow"

**Answer: 4**

*Rationale:* Option 1 demonstrates acting out by the client. Option 2 is a demanding response. Option 3 demonstrates withdrawal behavior. Demanding, acting out, and withdrawn clients have not coped or adjusted with the injury or disease. Option 4 is reflective of an individual with moderate anxiety by their difficulty to concentrate. It most appropriately supports a positive adjustment.

*Test-Taking Strategy:* Focus on the issue "positive adjustment" and use the process of elimination. You should easily be able to eliminate options 1, 2, and 3. Remember that age and limited mobility, combined with medications often contribute to anxiety and confusion. Review the psychosocial issues related to an elderly client with a hip fracture if you had difficulty with this question.

*Level of Cognitive Ability:* Analysis
*Client Needs:* Psychosocial Integrity
*Integrated Concept/Process:* Nursing Process/Evaluation
*Content Area:* Adult Health/Musculoskeletal

*Reference*
Black, J., Hawks, J., & Keene, A. (2001). *Medical-surgical nursing: Clinical management for positive outcomes* (6th ed.). Philadelphia: W.B. Saunders, p. 614.

**93.** A client who has a spinal cord injury and is paralyzed from the neck down frequently makes lewd sexual suggestions and uses profanity. The nurse interprets that the client is inappropriately using the defense mechanism of displacement and identifies the most appropriate nursing diagnosis for this client to be:

1 Ineffective Individual Coping
2 Risk for Disuse Syndrome
3 Impaired Environmental Interpretation Syndrome
4 Body Image Disturbance

**Answer: 1**

*Rationale:* The definition of Ineffective Individual Coping is the "state in which an individual demonstrates impaired adaptive behaviors and problem-solving abilities in meeting life's demands and roles." By displacing feelings onto the environment instead of in a constructive fashion, this nursing diagnosis clearly applies in this situation. Options 2 and 3 have no relationship to this situation. Option 4 may be appropriate, but it has nothing to do with the displacement that the client is currently using.

*Test-Taking Strategy:* Focus on the data in the question to identify the correct option. Note that the question addresses the defense mechanism of displacement. Focusing on this issue and the definition of displacement will assist in directing you to the correct option. Review this defense mechanism if you had difficulty with this question.

*Level of Cognitive Ability:* Analysis
*Client Needs:* Psychosocial Integrity
*Integrated Concept/Process:* Nursing Process/Analysis
*Content Area:* Mental Health

*Reference*
Johnson, M., Bulechek, G., Dochterman, J. Maas, M., Moorhead, S. (2001). *Nursing diagnoses, outcomes, and interventions.* St. Louis: Mosby, p. 174.

**94.** A nurse in the newborn nursery is caring for a premature infant. The best way to assist the parents to develop attachment behaviors is to:

1　Encourage the parents to touch and speak to their infant
2　Place family pictures in the infant's view
3　Report only positive qualities and progress to the parents
4　Provide information on infant development and stimulation

**Answer: 1**

*Rationale:* Parents' involvement through touch and voice establishes and initiates the bonding process in the parent-infant relationship. Their active participation builds their confidence and supports the parenting role. Providing information and emphasizing only positives are not incorrect, but do not relate to the attachment process. Family pictures are ineffective for an infant.

*Test-Taking Strategy:* Use the process of elimination and focus on the issue: attachment behaviors. The only option that addresses attachment behaviors is option 1. Review measures that promote parent-infant bonding if you had difficulty with this question.

*Level of Cognitive Ability:* Application
*Client Needs:* Psychosocial Integrity
*Integrated Concept/Process:* Nursing Process/Implementation
*Content Area:* Maternity

*Reference*
Lowdermilk, D., Perry, S., & Bobak, I. (2000). *Maternity & women's health care* (7th ed.). St. Louis: Mosby, p. 625.

**95.** A 16-year-old is admitted to the hospital with hyperglycemia from failure to follow the diet, insulin, and glucose monitoring regimen. The client states, "I'm fed up with having my life ruled by doctors' orders and machines!" A priority nursing diagnosis is:

1　Altered Nutrition, greater than body requirements, related to a high blood glucose
2　Altered Family Process related to chronic illness
3　Altered Thought Process related to a personal crisis
4　Ineffective Health Care Management of the therapeutic regimen related to feelings of loss of control

**Answer: 4**

*Rationale:* Adolescents strive for identity and independence and the situation describes a common fear of loss of control. The correct nursing diagnosis relates to the issues of the question, which are not following the prescribed regimen and the feelings of powerlessness. There is no indication of altered family or altered thought processes in the question. Altered nutrition is inaccurate and limited.

*Test-Taking Strategy:* Focus on the information in the question. Eliminate options 1 and 2, because there are no data to support these nursing diagnoses. Eliminate option 3, because although the client may be experiencing a personal crisis, there is no evidence of altered thought process. Review the defining characteristics of Ineffective Health Care Management if you had difficulty with this question.

*Level of Cognitive Ability:* Analysis
*Client Needs:* Psychosocial Integrity
*Integrated Concept/Process:* Nursing Process/Analysis
*Content Area:* Child Health

*Reference*
Wong, D. (1999). *Whaley & Wong's Nursing care of infants and children* (6th ed.). St. Louis: Mosby, p. 898.

**96.** A client angrily tells a nurse that the doctor purposefully provided wrong information. Which of the following responses would hinder therapeutic communication?

1  "I'm certain the doctor would not lie to you."
2  "Can you describe the information that you are referring to?"
3  "I'm not sure what information you are referring to."
4  "Do you think it would be helpful to talk to your doctor about this."

**Answer: 1**

*Rationale:* Option 1 hinders communication by disagreeing with the client. This technique could make the client defensive and block further communication. Options 2 and 3 attempt to clarify what the client is referring to. Option 4 attempts to explore whether the client is comfortable talking to the doctor about this issue and encourages direct confrontation.

*Test-Taking Strategy:* Use the process of elimination and therapeutic communication technique, noting the key word *hinder*. Disagreeing or challenging a client's response will hinder or block therapeutic communication. Review therapeutic communication techniques if you had difficulty with this question.

*Level of Cognitive Ability:* Application
*Client Needs:* Psychosocial Integrity
*Integrated Concept/Process:* Communication and Documentation
*Content Area:* Mental Health

*Reference*
Stuart, G.W., & Laraia, M.T. (1998). *Principles and practice of psychiatric nursing* (6th ed.). St. Louis: Mosby, p. 34.

**97.** A client with major depression says to the nurse, "I should have died. I've always been a failure." The most therapeutic response by the nurse is:

1  "I see a lot of positive things in you."
2  "Feeling like a failure is part of your illness."
3  "You've been feeling like a failure for some time now?"
4  "You still have a great deal to live for."

*restating*

**Answer: 3**

*Rationale:* Responding to the feelings expressed by a client is an effective therapeutic communication technique. The correct option is an example of the use of restating. Options 1, 2, and 4 block communication, because they minimize the client's experience and do not facilitate exploration of the client's expressed feelings.

*Test-Taking Strategy:* Use the techniques that facilitate therapeutic communication to answer this question. Remember to address the client's feelings and concerns. Option 3 is the only option that is stated in the form of a question and is open ended, and thus will encourage the verbalization of feelings. Review therapeutic communication techniques if you had difficulty with this question.

*Level of Cognitive Ability:* Application
*Client Needs:* Psychosocial Integrity
*Integrated Concept/Process:* Communication and Documentation
*Content Area:* Mental Health

*Reference*
Stuart, G.W., & Laraia, M.T. (1998). *Principles and practice of psychiatric nursing* (6th ed.). St. Louis: Mosby, p. 34.

**98.** Two months after a right mastectomy for breast cancer, the client comes to the office for a follow-up appointment. The client was told, after the diagnosis of cancer in the right breast, that the risk for cancer in the left breast existed. When asked about her breast self-examination (BSE) practices since the surgery, the client replies, "I don't need to do that any more." The nurse interprets that this response may indicate:

1   Change in body image
2   Change in role pattern
3   Denial
4   Grief and mourning

**Answer: 3**

*Rationale:* The coping strategy of denying or minimizing a health problem is manifested as anxiety, producing health situations that may be life-threatening. Denial can lead to avoidance of self-care measures such as taking medications or performing BSE. Options 1, 2, and 4 are unrelated to the client's statement.

*Test-Taking Strategy:* Focus on the data in the question. Note the client's statement "I don't need to do that any more." Eliminate options 1, 2, and 4, because they are not directly related to the client's statement. Review the indicators of denial if you had difficulty with this question.

*Level of Cognitive Ability:* Analysis
*Client Needs:* Psychosocial Integrity
*Integrated Concept/Process:* Nursing Process/Analysis
*Content Area:* Adult Health/Oncology

*Reference*
Smeltzer, S., & Bare, B. (2000). *Brunner & Suddarth's Textbook of medical-surgical nursing* (9th ed.). Philadelphia: Lippincott Williams & Wilkins, p. 77.

**99.** In planning for care of the client dying of cancer, one of the goals was that the client would verbalize acceptance of impending death. Which of the following statements indicates to the nurse that this goal has been reached?

1   "I'll be ready to die when my children finish school."
2   "I just want to live until my one-hundredth birthday."
3   "I want to go to my daughter's. Then I'll be ready to die."
4   "I'd like to have my family here when I die."

**Answer: 4**

*Rationale:* Acceptance is often characterized by plans for death. Often the client wants loved ones near. Options 1, 2, and 3 all reflect the bargaining stage of coping, wherein the client tries to negotiate with God or fate.

*Test-Taking Strategy:* Use the process of elimination. Note the similarity in options 1, 2, and 3. These options all demonstrate negotiating for something else to happen before death occurs. Option 4 is the option that is different and the option that reflects acceptance. Review the stages of death and dying if you had difficulty with this question.

*Level of Cognitive Ability:* Analysis
*Client Needs:* Psychosocial Integrity
*Integrated Concept/Process:* Nursing Process/Evaluation
*Content Area:* Adult Health/Oncology

*Reference*
Smeltzer, S., & Bare, B. (2000). *Brunner & Suddarth's Textbook of medical-surgical nursing* (9th ed.). Philadelphia: Lippincott Williams & Wilkins, p. 98.

**100.** A nurse is caring for a client with cancer who has a nursing diagnosis of Body Image Disturbance related to alopecia. The nurse plans to teach the client which of the following related to this nursing diagnosis?
1 Proper dental hygiene with the use of a foam toothbrush
2 The importance of rinsing the mouth after eating
3 The use of wigs, which are often covered by insurance
4 The use of cosmetics to hide drug-induced rashes

**Answer: 3**

*Rationale:* The temporary or permanent thinning or loss of hair, known as alopecia, is common in clients with cancer receiving chemotherapy. This often causes a body image disturbance that can be easily addressed by the use of wigs, hats, or scarves. Options 1, 2, and 4 are all unrelated to alopecia.

*Test-Taking Strategy:* Focus on the definition of alopecia. Recalling that alopecia refers to hair loss will direct you to option 3. Review interventions to treat alopecia if you had difficulty with this question.

*Level of Cognitive Ability:* Application
*Client Needs:* Psychosocial Integrity
*Integrated Concept/Process:* Teaching/Learning
*Content Area:* Adult Health/Oncology

*Reference*
Smeltzer, S., & Bare, B. (2000). *Brunner & Suddarth's Textbook of medical-surgical nursing* (9th ed.). Philadelphia: Lippincott Williams & Wilkins, p. 298.

---

**101.** A client with aldosteronism has developed renal failure and says to the nurse, "This means that I will die very soon." The most appropriate nursing response is:
1 "What are you thinking about?"
2 "You will do just fine."
3 "You sound discouraged today."
4 "I read that death is a beautiful experience"

**Answer: 3**

*Rationale:* Option 3 uses the therapeutic communication technique of reflection, and clarifies and encourages further expression of the client's feelings. Option 1 requests an explanation and does not encourage expression of feelings. Options 2 and 4 denies the client's concerns and provides false reassurance.

*Test-Taking Strategy:* Use the therapeutic communication techniques. Note that option 3 facilitates the client's expression of feelings. Remember to focus on the client's feelings. Review therapeutic communication techniques if you had difficulty with this question.

*Level of Cognitive Ability:* Application
*Client Needs:* Psychosocial Integrity
*Integrated Concept/Process:* Communication and Documentation
*Content Area:* Adult Health/Endocrine

*Reference*
Potter, P., & Perry, A. (2001). *Fundamentals of nursing* (5th ed.). St. Louis: Mosby, p. 276.

**102.** A client with diabetes mellitus has expressed frustration in learning the diabetic regimen and insulin administration. The home health care nurse would initially:
1 Identify the cause of the frustration
2 Continue with diabetic teaching, knowing that the client will overcome any frustrations
3 Call the physician to discuss termination from home health care services
4 Offer to administer the insulin on a daily basis until the client is ready to learn

**Answer: 1**
*Rationale:* The home health care nurse must determine what is causing the client's frustration. Continuing to teach may only further block the learning process. Terminating the client from home care services achieves nothing and is considered abandonment unless other follow-up care is arranged. Administering insulin only provides a short-term solution.

*Test-Taking Strategy:* Use the process of elimination and the steps of the nursing process. Assessment is the first step. Of the options presented, options 2, 3, and 4 represent implementation phases of the nursing process. The only assessment option is option 1. Review teaching/learning principles if you had difficulty with this question.

*Level of Cognitive Ability:* Application
*Client Needs:* Psychosocial Integrity
*Integrated Concept/Process:* Teaching/Learning
*Content Area:* Adult Health/Endocrine

*Reference*
Smeltzer, S., & Bare, B. (2000). *Brunner & Suddarth's Textbook of medical-surgical nursing* (9th ed.). Philadelphia: Lippincott Williams & Wilkins, p. 41.

**103.** A client with cancer is placed on permanent total parenteral nutrition (TPN). The nurse includes psychosocial support when planning care for this client, because:
1 Death is imminent
2 TPN requires disfiguring surgery for permanent port implantation
3 The client will need to adjust to the idea of living without eating by the usual route
4 Nausea and vomiting occur regularly with this type of treatment and will prevent the client from engaging in social activities

**Answer: 3**
*Rationale:* Permanent TPN is indicated for clients who can no longer absorb nutrients via the enteral route. These clients will no longer take nutrition orally. Options 1, 2, and 4 are inaccurate. There is no indication in the question that death is imminent. Permanent port implantation is not disfiguring. TPN does not cause nausea and vomiting.

*Test-Taking Strategy:* Note the key word *permanent* in the question. Note the relationship between the key word and option 3. Option 3 states *living without eating.* These are similar thoughts. Also, knowledge regarding TPN therapy will assist in eliminating options 1, 2, and 4. Review care of a client receiving permanent TPN if you had difficulty with this question.

*Level of Cognitive Ability:* Application
*Client Needs:* Psychosocial Integrity
*Integrated Concept/Process:* Nursing Process/Planning
*Content Area:* Adult Health/Oncology

*Reference*
Black, J., Hawks, J., & Keene, A. (2001). *Medical-surgical nursing: Clinical management for positive outcomes* (6th ed.). Philadelphia: W.B. Saunders, p. 671.

**104.** A client who is to be discharged to home with a temporary colostomy, says to the nurse, "I know I've changed this thing once but I just don't know how I'll do it by myself when I'm home alone. Can't I stay here until the doctor puts it back?" Which of the following is the most therapeutic nursing response?
 1 "So you're saying that while you've practiced changing your colostomy bag once, you don't feel comfortable on your own yet?"
 2 "Well, your insurance will not pay for a longer stay just to practice changing your colostomy so you'll have to fight it out with them."
 3 "Going home to care for yourself still feels pretty overwhelming? I will schedule you for home visits until you're feeling more comfortable."
 4 "This is only temporary but you need to hire a nurse companion until your surgery."

**Answer: 3**
*Rationale:* The client is expressing feelings of fear and helplessness. Option 3 assists in meeting this need. Option 1 is restating, but this response could cause the client to feel more helpless because the client's fears are reflected back to the client. Option 2 provides what is probably accurate information but the words *just to practice* can be interpreted by the client as belittling. Option 4 provides information that the client already knows and then problem solves by using a client-centered action, which would probably overwhelm the client.

*Test-Taking Strategy:* Use therapeutic communication techniques and focus on the issue of the question, fear and helplessness. This will easily eliminate options 2 and 4. From the remaining options, remember the issue of the question and address the client's feelings and concerns. Option 1 is restating, but this intervention could cause the client to feel more helpless. Option 3 addresses the client's fear and dependency (helplessness) needs. Review therapeutic communication techniques if you had difficulty with this question.

*Level of Cognitive Ability:* Application
*Client Needs:* Psychosocial Integrity
*Integrated Concept/Process:* Communication and Documentation
*Content Area:* Adult Health/Gastrointestinal

*Reference*
Black, J., Hawks, J., & Keene, A. (2001). *Medical-surgical nursing: Clinical management for positive outcomes* (6th ed.). Philadelphia: W.B. Saunders, p. 785.

**105.** The parents of a newborn infant with congenital hypothyroidism and Down's syndrome tells the nurse how sad they are that their child was born with these problems. They had many plans for a normal child, and now these will need to be adjusted. Based on these statements, the nurse plans to address which nursing diagnosis?
 1 Anticipatory Grieving
 2 Dysfunctional Grieving
 3 Impaired Adjustment
 4 Ineffective Family Coping

**Answer: 1**
*Rationale:* Anticipatory Grieving is the intellectual and emotional responses and behaviors by which individuals and families work through the process of modifying self-concept based on the perception of potential loss. Defining characteristics include expressions of sorrow and distress at potential loss. Dysfunctional Grieving or Impaired Adjustment are abnormal responses to changes in health status. The nursing diagnosis of Ineffective Family Coping is used when a usually supportive person is providing insufficient, ineffective, or compromised support, comfort, assistance, or encouragement.

*Test-Taking Strategy:* Focus on the data in the question. Noting the key words *how sad they are* should lead you to one of the options related to grieving. Recalling the defining characteristics of Anticipatory Grieving will direct you to this option. Review these two forms of grieving if you had difficulty with this question.

*Level of Cognitive Ability:* Analysis
*Client Needs:* Psychosocial Integrity
*Integrated Concept/Process:* Nursing Process/Analysis
*Content Area:* Maternity

*Reference*
Lowdermilk, D., Perry, S., & Bobak, I. (2000). *Maternity & women's health care* (7th ed.). St. Louis: Mosby, p. 1102.

**106.** A nurse is caring for a client who is diagnosed as having schizophrenia. The client is unable to speak although there is no known pathological dysfunction of the organs of communication. The nurse documents that this client is experiencing:
1    Pressured speech
2    Verbigeration
3    Poverty of speech
4    Mutism

**Answer: 4**

*Rationale:* Mutism is the absence of verbal speech. The client does not communicate verbally, despite an intact physical structural ability to speak. Pressured speech refers to rapidity of speech reflecting the client's racing thoughts. Verbigeration is the purposeless repetition of words or phrases. Poverty of speech means diminished amounts of speech or monotonic replies.

*Test-Taking Strategy:* Use the process of elimination. Focus on the issue "unable to speak." This should assist in easily eliminating options 1 and 2. From the remaining options, recalling that poverty of speech indicates a diminished amount of speech will assist in eliminating option 3. If you had difficulty with this question, review altered thought and speech patterns.

*Level of Cognitive Ability:* Analysis
*Client Needs:* Psychosocial Integrity
*Integrated Concept/Process:* Communication and Documentation
*Content Area:* Mental Health

*Reference*
Stuart, G.W., & Laraia, M.T. (1998). *Principles and practice of psychiatric nursing* (6th ed.). St. Louis: Mosby, p. 409.

**107.** A client tells the nurse, "I am a spy for the FBI. I am an eye, an eye in the sky." The nurse recognizes that this is an example of:
1    Loosened associations
2    Echolalia
3    Clang associations
4    Word salad

**Answer: 3**

*Rationale:* Repetition of words or phrases that are similar in sound and in no other way (rhyming) is one altered thought and language pattern seen in schizophrenia. Clang associations often take the form of rhyming. Loosened associations occur when the individual speaks with frequent changes of subject, and the content is only obliquely related. Echolalia is the involuntary parrotlike repetition of words spoken by others. Word salad is the use of words with no apparent meaning attached to them or to their relationship to one another.

*Test-Taking Strategy:* Use the process of elimination, focusing on the client's statement. Recalling that clang associations often take the form of rhyming will direct you to option 3 Review altered thought and language patterns if you had difficulty with this question.

*Level of Cognitive Ability:* Analysis
*Client Needs:* Psychosocial Integrity
*Integrated Concept/Process:* Nursing Process/Analysis
*Content Area:* Mental Health

*Reference*
Stuart, G.W., & Laraia, M.T. (1998). *Principles and practice of psychiatric nursing* (6th ed.). St. Louis: Mosby, p. 118.

**108.** A nurse is planning the discharge of a young, newly diagnosed male client with type 1 diabetes mellitus. The client tells the nurse that he is concerned about self-administering insulin while in school with other students around. Which statement by the nurse best supports the client's need at this time?

  1  "You could contact the school nurse who could provide a private area for you to administer your insulin."
  2  "You could leave school early and take your insulin at home."
  3  "You shouldn't be embarrassed by your diabetes. Lots of people have this disease."
  4  "Oh, don't worry about that! You'll do fine!"

**Answer: 1**

*Rationale:* In planning this client's role transition, the nurse functions in the role of a problem solver in assisting the client to adapt to his illness. In option 1, the nurse offers information that addresses the client's need and promotes or assists the client to reach a decision that optimizes a sense of well-being. Option 2 requires a change in lifestyle. Options 3 and 4 are inappropriate statements and are similar in that they are both blocks to communication.

*Test-Taking Strategy:* Use therapeutic communication techniques. Focus on the issue: a concern of self-administering insulin while in school. Eliminate options 3 and 4 first, because they are nontherapeutic. From the remaining options, select option 1, because it promotes the client's ability to continue the present lifestyle whereas option 2 changes the lifestyle. Review measures that will assist the client in making a role transition if you had difficulty with this question.

*Level of Cognitive Ability:* Application
*Client Needs:* Psychosocial Integrity
*Integrated Concept/Process:* Communication and Documentation
*Content Area:* Adult Health/Endocrine

*Reference*
Potter, P., & Perry, A. (2001). *Fundamentals of nursing* (5th ed.). St. Louis: Mosby, p. 452.

**109.** A nurse is preparing a client for a parathyroidectomy. The client states, "I guess I'll have to learn to love wearing a scarf after this surgery!" Which nursing diagnosis would be appropriate to identify in the plan of care that addresses this client's need?

  1  Alteration in Comfort related to surgical interruption of body tissue
  2  Body Image Disturbance related to perceived negative effect of the surgical incision
  3  High Risk for Impaired Mobility related to limited movement secondary to neck surgery
  4  Denial related to poor coping mechanisms

**Answer: 2**

*Rationale:* The client's statement reflects a psychosocial concern regarding his or her appearance after surgery. Therefore Body Image Disturbance is the correct option. Options 1 and 3 identify physiological nursing diagnoses and option 4 is inappropriate, because the client is addressing a concern, rather than avoiding one.

*Test-Taking Strategy:* Use the process of elimination. Note that the client is expressing a concern. Keeping that in mind, eliminate option 4, because denial is a way of avoiding concerns. From the remaining options, focus on the client's statement to direct you to option 2. Review the psychosocial concerns following parathyroidectomy if you had difficulty with this question.

*Level of Cognitive Ability:* Analysis
*Client Needs:* Psychosocial Integrity
*Integrated Concept/Process:* Nursing Process/Analysis
*Content Area:* Fundamental Skills

*Reference*
Potter, P., & Perry, A. (2001). *Fundamentals of nursing* (5th ed.). St. Louis: Mosby, p. 459.

**110.** A husband of a client with Graves' disease expresses concern regarding his wife's health, because during the past 3 months she has been experiencing bursts of temper, nervousness, and inability to concentrate, even on trivial tasks. Based on this information, which of the following nursing diagnoses would be the most appropriate for the client?

1   Ineffective Individual Coping
2   Alteration in Sensory Perception
3   Social Isolation
4   Grieving

**Answer: 1**

*Rationale:* A client with Graves' disease may become irritable or depressed, especially on discharge from the hospital. The signs and symptoms in the question support the nursing diagnosis of Ineffective Individual Coping. The information in the question does not support options 2, 3, and 4.

*Test-Taking Strategy:* Use the process of elimination. Focusing on the data in the question will direct you to option 1. Review the defining characteristics related to Ineffective Individual Coping if you had difficulty with this question.

*Level of Cognitive Ability:* Analysis
*Client Needs:* Psychosocial Integrity
*Integrated Concept/Process:* Nursing Process/Analysis
*Content Area:* Adult Health/Endocrine

*Reference*
Johnson, M., Bulechek, G., Dochterman, J. Maas, M., Moorhead, S. (2001). *Nursing diagnoses, outcomes, and interventions.* St. Louis: Mosby, p. 175.

**111.** A female client who was admitted to the hospital for recurrent thyroid storm is preparing for discharge. The client is anxious about her illness and at times emotionally labile. Which of the following approaches would be most appropriate for the nurse to include in the discharge plan of care for this client?

1   Avoid teaching the client anything about the disease until she is emotionally stable
2   Assist the client in identifying coping skills, support systems, and potential stressors
3   Reassure the client that everything will be fine once she is in the home environment
4   Confront the client and explain that she must control her anxiety if she wants to go home

**Answer: 2**

*Rationale:* It is normal for clients who experience thyroid storm (hyperthyroidism) to continue to be anxious and emotionally labile at the time of discharge. Confrontation in option 4 will only heighten their anxiety. In addition, options 1 and 3 block communication by either avoiding the issue or providing false reassurance. The best intervention is to help the client cope with these changes in behavior and anticipate potential stressors so that symptoms will not be as severe.

*Test-Taking Strategy:* Use the process of elimination and therapeutic communication techniques. Eliminate options 3 and 4, because they are blocks to communication. From the remaining options, note the key words *anxious about her illness.* Eliminate option 1, because it is unrelated to addressing the client's anxiety and is a communication block. When confronted with psychosocial issues, always select the option that addresses the client's feelings and concerns. Review therapeutic communication techniques if you had difficulty with this question.

*Level of Cognitive Ability:* Application
*Client Needs:* Psychosocial Integrity
*Integrated Concept/Process:* Nursing Process/Planning
*Content Area:* Adult Health/Endocrine

*Reference*
Potter, P., & Perry, A. (2001). *Fundamentals of nursing* (5th ed.). St. Louis: Mosby, p. 459.

**112.** A nurse is caring for a client admitted to the hospital for subclavian line placement. Which psychosocial area of assessment should the nurse address with the client?

1  Strict restrictions of neck mobility
2  Loss of ability to ambulate as tolerated
3  Possible body image disturbance
4  Continuous pain related to ongoing placement of the subclavian line

**Answer: 3**

*Rationale:* When a client has a central line placed in the subclavian area, the client is able to move as tolerated with no restriction of movement. The client may have pain when the catheter is placed, but the pain will not last continuously. The client may, however, be self-conscious about the IV altering body image.

*Test-Taking Strategy:* Use the process of elimination, noting the key words *psychosocial area*. Pain, altered mobility, and restricted neck movements are physical concerns. Review the psychosocial effects of a subclavian line if you had difficulty with this question.

*Level of Cognitive Ability:* Analysis
*Client Needs:* Psychosocial Integrity
*Integrated Concept/Process:* Nursing Process/Assessment
*Content Area:* Fundamental Skills

*Reference*
Smeltzer, S., & Bare, B. (2000). *Brunner & Suddarth's Textbook of medical-surgical nursing* (9th ed.). Philadelphia: Lippincott Williams & Wilkins, p. 852.

---

**113.** A 12-year-old child is seen in the health care clinic. During the assessment, which of the following findings would suggest to the nurse that the child is experiencing a disruption in the development of self-concept?

1  The child has a part-time baby sitting job
2  The child enjoys playing chess and mastering new skills with this game
3  The child has many friends
4  The child has an intimate relationship with a significant other

**Answer: 4**

*Rationale:* A sense of industry is appropriate for this age group and may be exhibited by having a part-time job. The increase in self-esteem associated with skill mastery is an important part of development for the school-aged child. Friends are also important and appropriate in this age group. The formation of an intimate relationship would not be expected until young adulthood.

*Test-Taking Strategy:* Use the process of elimination, focusing on normal growth and development. Note the age of the child in the question. This will assist in eliminating options 1, 2, and 3. Review normal growth and development and developmental tasks associated with this age group if you had difficulty with this question.

*Level of Cognitive Ability:* Analysis
*Client Needs:* Psychosocial Integrity
*Integrated Concept/Process:* Nursing Process/Assessment
*Content Area:* Child Health

*Reference*
Wong, D. (1999). *Whaley & Wong's Nursing care of infants and children* (6th ed.). St. Louis: Mosby, p. 895.

**114.** A client newly diagnosed with tuberculosis (TB) is hospitalized and will be on respiratory isolation for at least 2 weeks. Which of the following would be most important in preventing psychosocial distress in the client?

1 Remove the calendar and clock in the room so that the client will not obsess about time
2 Note whether the client has visitors
3 Give the client a roommate with TB who persistently tries to talk
4 Instruct all staff not to touch the client

**Answer: 2**

*Rationale:* The nurse should note whether the client has visitors and social contacts, since the presence of others can offer positive stimulation. The calendar and clock are needed to promote orientation to time. A roommate who insists on talking could create sensory overload. Additionally, the client in respiratory isolation should be in a private room. Touch may be important in order to help the client feel socially acceptable.

*Test-Taking Strategy:* Use the process of elimination. Note the key words *preventing psychosocial distress*. Eliminate option 3 first, because the client should be in a private room. From the remaining options, noting that the client will be on respiratory isolation for at least 2 weeks and recalling the basic principles related to sensory overload will direct you to option 2. Review the psychosocial concerns related to isolation if you had difficulty with this question.

*Level of Cognitive Ability:* Application
*Client Needs:* Psychosocial Integrity
*Integrated Concept/Process:* Nursing Process/Assessment
*Content Area:* Adult Health/Respiratory

*Reference*
Potter, P., & Perry, A. (2001). *Fundamentals of nursing* (5th ed.). St. Louis: Mosby, p. 1663.

**115.** A nurse is interviewing a client with chronic obstructive pulmonary disease (COPD), who has a respiratory rate of 35 breaths/min and is experiencing extreme dyspnea. Which of the following nursing diagnoses would be most appropriate for this client?

1 Impaired Verbal Communication related to a physical barrier
2 Ineffective Individual Coping related to the client's inability to handle a situational crisis
3 Altered Body Image related to a neurological deficit
4 Knowledge Deficit related to COPD

**Answer: 1**

*Rationale:* A client may suffer physical or psychological alterations that impair communication. To speak spontaneously and clearly, a person must have an intact respiratory system. Extreme dyspnea is a physical alteration affecting speech. There are no data in the question that support options 2, 3, and 4.

*Test-Taking Strategy:* Use the process of elimination, focusing on the data in the question. Option 1 clearly addresses the problem that the client is experiencing. Option 2 is judgmental and inappropriate. There is nothing to indicate that the client has a neurological deficit. Option 4 identifies a medical diagnosis. Review the defining characteristics associated with Impaired Verbal Communication if you had difficulty with this question.

*Level of Cognitive Ability:* Analysis
*Client Needs:* Psychosocial Integrity
*Integrated Concept/Process:* Nursing Process/Analysis
*Content Area:* Adult Health/Respiratory

*Reference*
Smeltzer, S., & Bare, B. (2000). *Brunner & Suddarth's Textbook of medical-surgical nursing* (9th ed.). Philadelphia: Lippincott Williams & Wilkins, p. 31.

**116.** A client was injured as a result of passing out from drinking alcohol and falling into the coals of a fire. A fourth degree circumferential burn wound to the left leg resulted from this accident. In report, the nurse is told that the client just signed an informed consent for amputation of the limb and the procedure is scheduled for tomorrow. During the nursing assessment, the client seems upset and withdrawn. What is the most appropriate nursing action at this time?

1   Let the client have some time alone to grieve over the future loss of the limb
2   Teach the client that the injury was a result of alcohol abuse and refer the client for counseling
3   Inform the physician of the client's behavior and request medication to assist the client in coping with the diagnosis
4   Reflect back to the client that he or she appears upset

**Answer: 4**
*Rationale:* Reflection statements tend to elicit deeper awareness of feelings. A well-timed reflection can reveal an emotion that has escaped the client's notice. Additionally, option 4 validates the perception that the client is upset. Option 2 is inappropriate and a block to communication. Options 1 and 3 jump to interventions before assessing the situation.

*Test-Taking Strategy:* Use therapeutic communication techniques. Focus on the client's feelings. Select the option that encourages the client to express feelings and talk more. This will direct you to option 4. Review therapeutic communication techniques if you had difficulty with this question.

*Level of Cognitive Ability:* Application
*Client Needs:* Psychosocial Integrity
*Integrated Concept/Process:* Nursing Process/Implementation
*Content Area:* Mental Health

*Reference*
Smeltzer, S., & Bare, B. (2000). *Brunner & Suddarth's Textbook of medical-surgical nursing* (9th ed.). Philadelphia: Lippincott Williams & Wilkins, p. 32.

---

**117.** A nurse is caring for a client with left-sided Bell's palsy. Which statement by the client requires further exploration by the nurse?

1   "My left eye is tearing a lot."
2   "I have trouble closing my left eyelid."
3   "I can't taste anything on the left side."
4   "I don't know how I'll live with the effects of this stroke for the rest of my life."

**Answer: 4**
*Rationale:* Bell's palsy is an inflammatory condition involving the facial nerve (cranial nerve VII). Although it results in facial paralysis, it is not the same as a stroke or cerebrovascular accident (CVA). Many clients fear that they have had a CVA when the symptoms of Bell's palsy appear and they commonly believe that the paralysis is permanent. Symptoms resolve, although it may take several weeks to months. Options 1, 2, and 3 are expected assessment findings in the client with Bell's palsy.

*Test-Taking Strategy:* Use the process of elimination. Note the key words *requires further exploration*. Recalling that this disorder is a temporary condition will direct you to option 4. Option 4 identifies an inaccurate understanding of the disorder and requires further exploration. Review this disorder if you had difficulty with this question.

*Level of Cognitive Ability:* Analysis
*Client Needs:* Physiological Integrity
*Integrated Concept/Process:* Nursing Process/Evaluation
*Content Area:* Adult Health/Neurological

*Reference*
Smeltzer, S., & Bare, B. (2000). *Brunner & Suddarth's Textbook of medical-surgical nursing* (9th ed.). Philadelphia: Lippincott Williams & Wilkins, p. 1754.

**118.** A client newly diagnosed with diabetes mellitus has a nursing diagnosis of Altered Health Maintenance related to anxiety regarding the self-administration of insulin. Initially, the nurse should plan to:

1  Teach the family member to give the client the insulin

2  Use an orange for the client to inject into until he or she is less anxious

3  Insert the needle and have the client push in the plunger and remove the needle

4  Give the injection until the client feels confident enough to do so by himself or herself

**Answer: 3**

*Rationale:* Some clients find it difficult to insert a needle into their own skin. For these clients, the nurse might assist by selecting the site and inserting the needle. Then, as a first step in self-injection, the client can push in the plunger and remove the needle. Options 1 and 4 place the client into a dependent role. Option 2 is not realistic, considering the issue of the question.

*Test-Taking Strategy:* Use the process of elimination, focusing on the issue: anxiety regarding self-administration of insulin. Eliminate options 1 and 4, because they place the client in a dependent position. From the remaining options, select option 3, because it addresses the issue of self-administration. Review teaching learning principles related to an anxious client if you had difficulty with this question.

*Level of Cognitive Ability:* Application
*Client Needs:* Psychosocial Integrity
*Integrated Concept/Process:* Teaching/Learning
*Content Area:* Adult Health/Endocrine

*Reference*
Smeltzer, S., & Bare, B. (2000). *Brunner & Suddarth's Textbook of medical-surgical nursing* (9th ed.). Philadelphia: Lippincott Williams & Wilkins, p. 995.

**119.** A client in labor has human immunodeficiency virus (HIV) and says to the nurse, "I know I will have a sick looking baby." Which of the following would be the most appropriate nursing response?

1  "There is no reason to worry. Our neonatal unit offers the latest treatments available."

2  "You have concerns about how HIV will affect your baby?"

3  "You are very sick, but your baby may not be."

4  "All babies are beautiful. I am sure your baby will be too."

**Answer: 2**

*Rationale:* Option 2 is the most therapeutic response and the response that will elicit the best information. It addresses the therapeutic communication technique of paraphrasing. Parents need to know that their baby will not look sick from HIV at birth and that there will be a period of uncertainty before it is known whether the baby has acquired the infection. The client should not be told "there is no reason to worry." Options 3 and 4 provide false reassurances. Option 2 is an open-ended response that will provide an opportunity to the client to verbalize concerns.

*Test-Taking Strategy:* Use therapeutic communication techniques. Remember to address the client's feelings and concerns. Review these techniques if you had difficulty with this question.

*Level of Cognitive Ability:* Analysis
*Client Needs:* Psychosocial Integrity
*Integrated Concept/Process:* Communication and Documentation
*Content Area:* Maternity

*Reference*
Lowdermilk, D., Perry, S., & Bobak, I. (2000). *Maternity & women's health care* (7th ed.). St. Louis: Mosby, p. 104.

**120.** A client who is scheduled for an abdominal peritoneoscopy, states to the visiting nurse, "The doctor told me to restrict food and liquids for at least 8 hours before this procedure and to use a Fleet enema 4 hours before entering the hospital. Do people ever get into trouble after this procedure?" Which of the following is the most therapeutic response by the nurse?

1    "Any invasive procedure brings risk with it. You need to report any shoulder pain immediately."

2    "There are relatively few problems, especially if you are having local anesthesia, but any bleeding should be reported immediately."

3    "Trouble? There is never any trouble with this procedure. That's why the surgeon will use local anesthesia."

4    "You seem to understand the preparation very well. Are you having any concerns about the procedure?"

**Answer: 4**
*Rationale:* Abdominal peritoneoscopy is performed to directly visualize the liver, gallbladder, spleen, and stomach after the insufflation of nitrous oxide. During the procedure, a rigid laparoscope is inserted through a small incision in the abdomen. A microscope in the endoscope allows visualization of the organs and provides a way to collect a specimen for biopsy or to remove small tumors. The most therapeutic response is the one that facilitates the client's expression of feelings. Option 1 may increase the client's anxiety. In option 3, the nurse states that there are no problems associated with this procedure. This is an absolute and is incorrect. Although option 2 contains accurate information, the word *immediately* can increase the client's anxiety.

*Test-Taking Strategy:* Use the process of elimination. Remember to focus on the client's feelings and concerns. Option 4 is the most therapeutic response, because it provides an opportunity for the client to verbalize concerns. Review therapeutic communication techniques if you had difficulty with this question.

*Level of Cognitive Ability:* Application
*Client Needs:* Psychosocial Integrity
*Integrated Concept/Process:* Communication and Documentation
*Content Area:* Adult Health/Gastrointestinal

*Reference*
Smeltzer, S., & Bare, B. (2000). *Brunner & Suddarth's Textbook of medical-surgical nursing* (9th ed.). Philadelphia: Lippincott Williams & Wilkins, p. 32.

**121.** A nurse is caring for a client during a precipitate labor. In assessing the client's emotional needs, the nurse can anticipate the client having:

1    Less pain and anxiety than with a normal labor

2    A need for support in maintaining a sense of control

3    Fewer fears regarding the effect on the infant

4    A sense of satisfaction regarding the quick labor

**Answer: 2**
*Rationale:* The client experiencing a precipitate labor may have more difficulty maintaining control due to the abrupt onset and quick progression of the labor. This may be very different from previous labor experiences; therefore the client needs support from the nurse to understand and adapt to the rapid progression. The contractions often increase in intensity quickly, adding to the pain, anxiety, and lack of control. The client may also have an increased amount of concern about the effect of the labor on the baby. Lack of control over the situation combined with increased pain and anxiety can result in a decreased level of satisfaction with the labor and delivery experience.

*Test-Taking Strategy:* Use the process of elimination. Focus on the client's condition, a precipitate labor. Note the key words *emotional needs* in the question, and the key words *a need for support* in the correct option. Review care of a client with a precipitate labor if you had difficulty with this question.

*Level of Cognitive Ability:* Analysis
*Client Needs:* Psychosocial Integrity
*Integrated Concept/Process:* Nursing Process/Assessment
*Content Area:* Maternity

*Reference*
Lowdermilk, D., Perry, S., & Bobak, I. (2000). *Maternity & women's health care* (7th ed.). St. Louis: Mosby p. 988.

**122.** A nurse is planning care for a client who presents in active labor with a history of a previous cesarean delivery. The client complains of a "tearing" sensation in the lower abdomen, is upset, and expresses concern for the safety of her baby. The most appropriate nursing response would be:
1  "Don't worry, you are in good hands."
2  "I can understand that you are fearful. We are doing everything possible for your baby."
3  "You'll have to talk to your doctor about that."
4  "I don't have time to answer questions now. We'll talk later."

**Answer: 2**
*Rationale:* Clients have a concern for the safety of their baby during labor and delivery, especially when a problem arises. Empathy and a calm attitude with realistic reassurances are an important aspect of client care. Dismissing or ignoring the client's concerns can lead to increased fear and lack of cooperation. Option 1 uses a cliché and false reassurance. Options 3 and 4 attempt to place the client's feelings "on hold."

*Test-Taking Strategy:* Use therapeutic communication techniques. Options 3 and 4 place the client's feelings "on hold." The client should not be told "Don't worry." Review therapeutic communication techniques if you had difficulty with this question.

*Level of Cognitive Ability:* Application
*Client Needs:* Psychosocial Integrity
*Integrated Concept/Process:* Communication and Documentation
*Content Area:* Maternity

*Reference*
Lowdermilk, D., Perry, S., & Bobak, I. (2000). *Maternity & women's health care* (7th ed.). St. Louis: Mosby, p. 538.

**123.** A newborn male infant is diagnosed with an undescended testicle (cryptorchidism) and these findings are shared with the parents. The parents ask questions about the condition. The nurse responds knowing that if this condition is not corrected, which of the following could have a psychosocial impact?
1  Infertility
2  Malignancy
3  Feminization
4  Atrophy

**Answer: 1**
*Rationale:* Infertility can occur in this condition, because proper function of the testes depends on a temperature cooler than 98.6° F. The psychological effects of an "empty scrotum" could affect the client's perception of self and the ability to reproduce. Options 2 and 4 are possible physical consequences of failure to treat cryptorchidism, not psychosocial consequences. Since all hormones responsible for secondary sex characteristics continue to be secreted directly into bloodstream, option 3 is not correct.

*Test-Taking Strategy:* Use the process of elimination. Focusing on the issue: psychosocial impact, will assist in eliminating options 2 and 4. From the remaining options, it is necessary to know that infertility can occur if the condition is uncorrected. Review this disorder if you had difficulty with this question.

*Level of Cognitive Ability:* Analysis
*Client Needs:* Psychosocial Integrity
*Integrated Concept/Process:* Nursing Process/Analysis
*Content Area:* Maternity

*Reference*
Wong, D. (1999). *Whaley & Wong's Nursing care of infants and children* (6th ed.). St. Louis: Mosby, p. 539.

**124.** A mother of an infant with hydrocephalus is concerned about the complication of mental retardation. The mother states to the nurse, "I'm not sure if I can care for my baby at home." The most appropriate response by the nurse would be which of the following?

1  "There is no reason to worry. You have a good pediatrician."

2  "Mothers instinctively know what is best for their babies."

3  "You have concerns about your baby's condition and care?"

4  "All babies have individual needs."

**Answer: 3**

*Rationale:* Paraphrasing is restating the mother's message in the nurse's own words. Option 3 addresses the therapeutic technique of paraphrasing. In options 1 and 2, the nurse is offering a false reassurance and these types of responses will block communication. In option 4, the nurse is minimizing the social needs involved with the baby's diagnosis, which is harmful for the nurse-parent relationship.

*Test-Taking Strategy:* Use therapeutic communication techniques and the process of elimination to answer the question. Option 3 is the only therapeutic response and addresses paraphrasing. This is the only option that will provide the client an opportunity to verbalize concerns. Review therapeutic communication techniques if you had difficulty with this question.

*Level of Cognitive Ability:* Application
*Client Needs:* Psychosocial Integrity
*Integrated Concept/Process:* Communication and Documentation
*Content Area:* Maternity

*Reference*
Potter, P., & Perry, A. (2001). *Fundamentals of nursing* (5th ed.). St. Louis: Mosby, p. 459.

---

**125.** A preschooler has just been diagnosed with impetigo. The child's mother tells the nurse, "But my children take baths every day." The most appropriate response by the nurse is which of the following?

1  "You are concerned about how your child got impetigo?"

2  "There is no need to worry, we will not tell daycare why your child is absent."

3  "Not only do you have to do a better job in keeping the children clean, you must also wash your hands more frequently."

4  "You should have seen the doctor before the wound became infected; then you would not have had to worry about the child having impetigo."

**Answer: 1**

*Rationale:* By paraphrasing what the parent tells the nurse, the nurse is addressing the parent's thoughts. Option 1 is the therapeutic technique of paraphrasing. Options 2, 3, and 4 are blocks to communication, because they make the parent feel guilty for the child's illness.

*Test-Taking Strategy:* Use therapeutic communication techniques and the process of elimination to answer the question. Option 1 is the only therapeutic technique and addresses paraphrasing. This is the only option that will provide the client an opportunity to verbalize concerns. Options 2, 3, and 4 are blocks to communication. Review therapeutic communication techniques if you had difficulty with this question.

*Level of Cognitive Ability:* Application
*Client Needs:* Psychosocial Integrity
*Integrated Concept/Process:* Communication and Documentation
*Content Area:* Child Health

*Reference*
Potter, P., & Perry, A. (2001). *Fundamentals of nursing* (5th ed.). St. Louis: Mosby, p. 459.

**126.** A nurse is preparing to care for a child from a different culture. What is the best way to address the cultural needs of the child and family when the child is admitted to the health care facility?

1  Ask questions about the culture and explain to the family why the questions are being asked

2  Explain to the family that while the child is being treated, they need to discontinue cultural practices, because they may be harmful to the child

3  Ignore cultural needs, because they are not important to health care professionals

4  Only address those issues that directly affect the nurse's care of the child

**Answer: 1**

*Rationale:* When caring for individuals from a different culture, it is important to ask questions about their specific cultural needs and means of treatment. An understanding of the family's beliefs and health practices is essential to successful interventions for that particular family. Options 2, 3, and 4 ignore the cultural beliefs and values of the client.

*Test-Taking Strategy:* Use the process of elimination, focusing on the issue: cultural needs. Options 2, 3, and 4 are judgmental. Additionally, these options are all similar in that they ignore the cultural practices and values of the client. Review nursing interventions related to cultural diversity if you had difficulty with this question.

*Level of Cognitive Ability:* Application
*Client Needs:* Psychosocial Integrity
*Integrated Concept/Process:* Cultural Awareness
*Content Area:* Child Health

*Reference*
Wong, D. (1999). *Whaley & Wong's Nursing care of infants and children* (6th ed.). St. Louis: Mosby, p. 34.

**127.** A client with a T1 spinal cord injury has just learned that the cord was completely severed. The client says, "I'm no good to anyone. I might as well be dead." The most appropriate response by the nurse is:

1  "It makes me uncomfortable when you talk this way."

2  "I'll ask the psychologist to see you about this."

3  "You're not a useless person at all."

4  "You are feeling pretty bad about things right now."

**Answer: 4**

*Rationale:* Restating and reflecting keeps the lines of communication open and encourages the client to expand on current feelings of unworthiness and loss that require exploration. The nurse can block communication by showing discomfort, disapproval, or by postponing discussion of issues. Grief is a common reaction to loss of function. The nurse facilitates grieving through open communication.

*Test-Taking Strategy:* Use therapeutic communication techniques and the process of elimination. Options 1, 2, and 3 block communication. Option 4 identifies the therapeutic communication technique of restating and reflecting. Review therapeutic communication if you had difficulty with this question.

*Level of Cognitive Ability:* Application
*Client Needs:* Psychosocial Integrity
*Integrated Concept/Process:* Communication and Documentation
*Content Area:* Adult Health/Neurological

*Reference*
Smeltzer, S., & Bare, B. (2000). *Brunner & Suddarth's Textbook of medical-surgical nursing* (9th ed.). Philadelphia: Lippincott Williams & Wilkins, p. 31.

**128.** A nurse enters the room of a client with myocardial infarction (MI) and finds the client quietly crying. After determining that there is no physiological reason for the client's distress, the nurse replies:

1   "Do you want me to call your daughter?"
2   "Can you tell me a little about what has you so upset?"
3   "I understand how you feel. I'd cry too if I had a major heart attack."
4   "Try not to be so upset. Psychological stress is bad for your heart."

**Answer: 2**

*Rationale:* Clients with an MI often have a nursing diagnosis of Anxiety or Fear. The nurse allows the client to express concerns by showing genuine interest and concern, and by facilitating communication using therapeutic communication techniques. Option 2 provides the client an opportunity to express concerns. Options 1, 3, and 4 do not address the client's feelings or promote client verbalization.

*Test-Taking Strategy:* Use the process of elimination. Select an option that has an exploratory approach, since the question does not identify why the client is upset. This technique helps you eliminate each of the incorrect options. Review therapeutic communication techniques if you had difficulty with this question.

*Level of Cognitive Ability:* Analysis
*Client Needs:* Psychosocial Integrity
*Integrated Concept/Process:* Communication and Documentation
*Content Area:* Adult Health/Cardiovascular

*References*
Potter, P., & Perry, A. (2001). *Fundamentals of nursing* (5th ed.). St. Louis: Mosby, p. 459.

---

**129.** A client with a recent complete T4 spinal cord transection tells the nurse that he will walk as soon as the spinal shock resolves. Which of the following will provide the most accurate basis for planning a response?

1   To speed acceptance, the client needs reinforcement that he will not walk again
2   The client needs to move through the grieving process rapidly to benefit from rehabilitation
3   The client is projecting by insisting that walking is the rehabilitation goal
4   Denial can be protective while the client deals with the anxiety created by the new disability

**Answer: 4**

*Rationale:* In the adjustment period during the first few weeks after spinal cord injury, clients may use denial as a defense mechanism. Denial may decrease anxiety temporarily, and is a normal part of grieving. After the spinal shock resolves, prolonged or excessive use of denial may impair rehabilitation. However, rehabilitation programs include psychological counseling to deal with denial and grief.

*Test-Taking Strategy:* Use the process of elimination and knowledge of the physiological effects of a T4 spinal injury. The words *speed acceptance, move through the grieving process rapidly,* and *walking is the rehabilitation goal* should be indicators that these are incorrect options. Focus on the client's statement, which is an indication of denial, to direct you to option 4. Review the defining characteristics of denial if you had difficulty with this question.

*Level of Cognitive Ability:* Analysis
*Client Needs:* Psychosocial Integrity
*Integrated Concept/Process:* Nursing Process/Planning
*Content Area:* Adult Health/Neurological

*Reference*
Smeltzer, S., & Bare, B. (2000). *Brunner & Suddarth's Textbook of medical-surgical nursing* (9th ed.). Philadelphia: Lippincott Williams & Wilkins, p. 77.

**130.** A nurse is developing a plan of care for a client scheduled for an above-the-knee leg amputation. The nurse should include which action in the plan when addressing psychosocial needs of the client?

1    Explain to the client that open grieving is abnormal
2    Discourage sharing feelings with others that have had similar experiences
3    Encourage the client to express feelings about body changes
4    Advise the client to seek psychological treatment after surgery

**Answer: 3**

*Rationale:* Surgical incisions or loss of a body part can alter a client's body image. The onset of problems with coping with these changes may occur in the immediate or extended postoperative stage. Nursing interventions primarily involve providing psychological support. The nurse should encourage clients to express how they feel these postoperative changes will affect their lives. Option 1 is an incorrect statement, because open grieving in normal. Option 2 indicates disapproval and in option 4, the nurse is giving advice.

*Test-Taking Strategy:* Use therapeutic communication techniques. Remember, always focus on the client's feelings first. This will direct you to option 3. Review therapeutic communication techniques if you had difficulty with this question.

*Level of Cognitive Ability:* Application
*Client Needs:* Psychosocial Integrity
*Integrated Concept/Process:* Caring
*Content Area:* Mental Health

*Reference:*
Johnson, M., Bulechek, G., Dochterman, J. Maas, M., Moorhead, S. (2001). *Nursing diagnoses, outcomes, and interventions.* St. Louis: Mosby, p. 58.

**131.** A client with pulmonary edema exhibits severe anxiety. The nurse is preparing to carry out the medically prescribed orders. Which approach should the nurse plan to best meet the needs of the client in a holistic manner?

1    Leave the client alone while gathering required equipment and medications
2    Give the client the call bell and encourage its use if the client feels worse
3    Ask a family member to stay with the client
4    Stay with the client and ask another nurse to gather equipment and supplies not already in the room

**Answer: 4**

*Rationale:* Pulmonary edema is accompanied by extreme fear and anxiety. Since the client typically experiences a sense of impending doom, the nurse should remain with the client as much as possible. Options 1 and 2 do not provide for the psychological needs of the client in distress. Family members (option 3) can emotionally support the client but are not able to respond to physiological needs and symptoms. In fact, they are typically in psychological distress themselves.

*Test-Taking Strategy:* Use the process of elimination. The word *holistic* in the stem of the question guides you to consider both physical and emotional well being of the client. Option 4 is the only option that addresses both needs. Review the psychosocial aspects of care for the client in pulmonary edema if you had difficulty with this question.

*Level of Cognitive Ability:* Application
*Client Needs:* Psychosocial Integrity
*Integrated Concept/Process:* Nursing Process/Planning
*Content Area:* Adult Health/Respiratory

*Reference*
Smeltzer, S., & Bare, B. (2000). *Brunner & Suddarth's Textbook of medical-surgical nursing* (9th ed.). Philadelphia: Lippincott Williams & Wilkins, p. 670.

**132.** Family members of a client with a myocardial infarction complicated by cardiogenic shock are visibly anxious and upset about the client's condition. A nurse would plan to do which of the following to provide the best support to the family?

1   Insist they go home to sleep at night to keep up their own strength
2   Provide flexibility with visiting times according to the client's condition and family needs
3   Offer them coffee and other beverages on a regular basis
4   Ask the hospital chaplain to sit with them until the client's condition stabilizes

**Answer: 2**
*Rationale:* The use of flexible visiting hours meets the needs of both the client and family in reducing the anxiety levels of both. Insisting that the family go home is nontherapeutic. Offering the family beverages does not provide support. Although the chaplain may provide support, it is unrealistic for the chaplain to stay until the client stabilizes.

*Test-Taking Strategy:* Note the issue: the best method of providing support. Options 1 and 4 may or may not be helpful, depending on the client and family situation. Coffee and beverages, while probably helpful to many, do not provide the best support and can also be obtained in the hospital cafeteria. Review measures to provide support to the family of a client with a critical disorder if you had difficulty with this question.

*Level of Cognitive Ability:* Application
*Client Needs:* Psychosocial Integrity
*Integrated Concept/Process:* Caring
*Content Area:* Adult Health/Cardiovascular

*Reference*
Smeltzer, S., & Bare, B. (2000). *Brunner & Suddarth's Textbook of medical-surgical nursing* (9th ed.). Philadelphia: Lippincott Williams & Wilkins, p. 670.

**133.** A client with premature ventricular contractions says to the nurse, "I'm so afraid something bad will happen." Which action by the nurse would be of most immediate help to the client?

1   Giving reassurance that nothing will happen to the client
2   Telephoning the client's family
3   Having a staff member stay with the client
4   Using television to distract the client

**Answer: 3**
*Rationale:* When a client experiences fear, the nurse can provide a calm, safe environment by offering appropriate reassurance, the therapeutic use of touch, and by having someone remain with the client as much as possible. Option 1 provides false reassurance. Options 2 and 4 do not address the client's fear.

*Test-Taking Strategy:* Use the process of elimination. Noting the key words *most immediate help* will direct you to option 3. Review measures to reduce a client's fear if you had difficulty with this question.

*Level of Cognitive Ability:* Application
*Client Needs:* Psychosocial Integrity
*Integrated Concept/Process:* Caring
*Content Area:* Adult Health/Cardiovascular

*Reference*
Potter, P., & Perry, A. (2001). *Fundamentals of nursing* (5th ed.). St. Louis: Mosby, p. 460.

**134.** A client with Raynaud's disease tells the nurse that she has a stressful job and does not handle stressful situations well. The nurse most appropriately guides the client to:

1 Change jobs
2 Consider a stress management program
3 Seek help from a psychologist
4 Use earplugs to minimize environmental noise

**Answer: 2**

*Rationale:* Stress can trigger the vasospasm that occurs with Raynaud's disease, so referral to stress management programs or the use of biofeedback training may be helpful. Option 1 is unrealistic. Option 3 is not necessarily required at this time. Option 4 does not specifically address the issue.

*Test-Taking Strategy:* Use the process of elimination, focusing on the issue: stress. Note the relationship between this issue and option 2. Review measures that reduce stress if you had difficulty with this question.

*Level of Cognitive Ability:* Application
*Client Needs:* Psychosocial Integrity
*Integrated Concept/Process:* Nursing Process/Implementation
*Content Area:* Adult Health/Cardiovascular

**Reference**
Smeltzer, S., & Bare, B. (2000). *Brunner & Suddarth's Textbook of medical-surgical nursing* (9th ed.). Philadelphia: Lippincott Williams & Wilkins, p. 704.

---

**135.** A client with a history of pulmonary emboli is scheduled for insertion of an inferior vena cava filter. The nurse checks on the client 1 hour after the physician has explained the procedure and obtained consent from the client. The client is lying in bed, wringing his hands, and says to the nurse, "I'm not sure about this. What if it doesn't work, and I'm just as bad off as before?" The nurse formulates which of the following nursing diagnoses for the client?

1 Fear related to the potential risks and outcome of surgery
2 Anxiety related to the fear of death
3 Ineffective Individual Coping related to the treatment regimen
4 Knowledge Deficit related to the surgical procedure

**Answer: 1**

*Rationale:* The North American Nursing Diagnosis Association (NANDA) defines Fear as "a feeling of dread related to an identifiable source that the person validates." This client has identified the surgical procedure and its outcome as the object of fear. Anxiety is used when the client cannot identify the source of the uneasy feelings. Ineffective Individual Coping is appropriate when the client is not making needed adaptations to deal with daily life. Knowledge Deficit is characterized by a lack of appropriate information.

*Test-Taking Strategy:* Focus on the data in the question and on the client's statement. Note the relationship between the client's statement and option 1. Review the defining characteristics of Fear if you had difficulty with this question.

*Level of Cognitive Ability:* Analysis
*Client Needs:* Psychosocial Integrity
*Integrated Concept/Process:* Nursing Process/Analysis
*Content Area:* Adult Health/Respiratory

**Reference**
Johnson, M., Bulechek, G., Dochterman, J. Maas, M., Moorhead, S. (2001). *Nursing diagnoses, outcomes, and interventions.* St. Louis: Mosby, p. 98.

**136.** A client has an oral endotracheal tube attached to a mechanical ventilator and is about to begin the weaning process. The nurse interprets that which of the following items should now be limited, which was previously useful in minimizing the client's anxiety?
1   Radio
2   Television
3   Family visitors
4   Antianxiety medications

**Answer: 4**
*Rationale:* Antianxiety medications and narcotic analgesics are used cautiously in the client being weaned from a mechanical ventilator. These medications may interfere with the weaning process by suppressing the respiratory drive. The client may exhibit anxiety during the weaning process as well for a variety of reasons, and therefore distractions such as radio, television, and visitors are still very useful.

*Test-Taking Strategy:* Use the process of elimination. Think about the items that could interfere with the client's strength, endurance, and respiratory drive in maintaining independent ventilation. Using this as the guideline, the only possible option is option 4. The side effects of these medications could include sedation, which could interfere with optimal respiratory function. Review care of a client who is weaning from a mechanical ventilator if you had difficulty with this question.

*Level of Cognitive Ability:* Analysis
*Client Needs:* Psychosocial Integrity
*Integrated Concept/Process:* Nursing Process/Analysis
*Content Area:* Adult Health/Respiratory

*Reference*
Smeltzer, S., & Bare, B. (2000). *Brunner & Suddarth's Textbook of medical-surgical nursing* (9th ed.). Philadelphia: Lippincott Williams & Wilkins, p. 511.

**137.** A client scheduled for pulmonary angiography is fearful about the procedure and asks the nurse if the procedure involves significant pain and radiation exposure. The nurse provides a response to the client that provides reassurance, based on the understanding that:
1   The procedure is somewhat painful, but there is minimal exposure to radiation
2   Discomfort may occur with needle insertion, and there is minimal exposure to radiation
3   There is absolutely no pain, although a moderate amount of radiation must be used to get accurate results
4   There is very mild pain throughout the procedure, and the exposure to radiation is negligible

**Answer: 2**
*Rationale:* Pulmonary angiography involves minimal exposure to radiation. The procedure is painless, although the client may feel discomfort with insertion of the needle for the catheter that is used for dye injection. Options 1, 3, and 4 are incorrect.

*Test-Taking Strategy:* Focus on the diagnostic procedure. Eliminate option 3 because of the absolute word *no*. From the remaining options, recalling that discomfort occurs with needle insertion will direct you to option 2. Review this procedure if you had difficulty with this question.

*Level of Cognitive Ability:* Analysis
*Client Needs:* Psychosocial Integrity
*Integrated Concept/Process:* Nursing Process/Analysis
*Content Area:* Adult Health/Respiratory

*Reference*
Smeltzer, S., & Bare, B. (2000). *Brunner & Suddarth's Textbook of medical-surgical nursing* (9th ed.). Philadelphia: Lippincott Williams & Wilkins, p. 577.

**138.** A nurse is caring for an anxious client who has an open pneumothorax and a sucking chest wound. An occlusive dressing has been applied to the site. Which intervention by the nurse would be the best to relieve the client's anxiety?
1  Encouraging the client to cough and deep breathe
2  Staying with the client
3  Interpreting the arterial blood gas report
4  Distracting the client with television

**Answer: 2**
*Rationale:* Staying with the client has a twofold benefit. First, it relieves the client's anxiety. In addition, the nurse must stay with the client to observe respiratory status after application of the occlusive dressing. It is possible that the dressing could convert the open pneumothorax to a closed (tension) pneumothorax, resulting in a sudden decline in respiratory status and mediastinal shift. If this occurs, the nurse is present and able to remove the dressing immediately. Coughing and deep breathing have no immediate benefit for the client who is in distress. Option 4 is nontherapeutic.

*Test-Taking Strategy:* Focus on the issue: relieving the client's anxiety. Eliminate option 4 first, since the client is in distress. From the remaining options, use therapeutic nursing measures to direct you to option 2. Review the measures to relieve anxiety if you had difficulty with this question.

*Level of Cognitive Ability:* Application
*Client Needs:* Psychosocial Integrity
*Integrated Concept/Process:* Nursing Process/Implementation
*Content Area:* Adult Health/Respiratory

**Reference**
Smeltzer, S., & Bare, B. (2000). *Brunner & Suddarth's Textbook of medical-surgical nursing* (9th ed.). Philadelphia: Lippincott Williams & Wilkins, p. 485.

**139.** A client with acquired immunodeficiency syndrome (AIDS) shares with the nurse feelings of social isolation since the diagnosis was made. The nurse plans to suggest which of the following strategies as the most useful way to decrease the client's stated loneliness?
1  Using the Internet on the computer to facilitate communication
2  Use of the television and newspapers to maintain a feeling of being "in touch" with the world
3  Contacting a support group available in the local region for clients with AIDS
4  Reinstituting contact with the client's family, who live in a distant city

**Answer: 3**
*Rationale:* The nurse encourages the client to maintain social contact and support, and assists the client in reducing barriers to social contact. This can include educating the client's family about the disease and transmission, and suggesting utilization of community resources and support groups. Options 1 and 2 will not decrease the client's loneliness. Option 4, although feasible, is a solution that is less likely to address the client's current feelings of loneliness.

*Test-Taking Strategy:* Use the process of elimination. Eliminate options 1 and 2 first, because they do not actually decrease the client's isolation and loneliness. These options maintain a measure of distance between the client and others. From the remaining options, note that the wording of option 4 implies that contact has been lost over time, and the logistics of distance make this the less likely solution to the client's current feelings of isolation. Review the strategies related to reducing social isolation if you had difficulty with this question.

*Level of Cognitive Ability:* Application
*Client Needs:* Psychosocial Integrity
*Integrated Concept/Process:* Nursing Process/Planning
*Content Area:* Adult Health/Immune

**Reference**
Smeltzer, S., & Bare, B. (2000). *Brunner & Suddarth's Textbook of medical-surgical nursing* (9th ed.). Philadelphia: Lippincott Williams & Wilkins, p. 1385.

**140.** A client has an initial positive result of an enzyme-linked immunosorbent assay (ELISA) test for human immunodeficiency virus (HIV). The client begins to cry, and asks the nurse what this means. The nurse is able to provide support to the client by using knowledge that:

1   The client is HIV positive, but the disease has been detected early

2   The client is HIV positive, but the client's CD4 cell count is high

3   There is a high rate of false-positive results with this test, and more testing is needed before diagnosing the client's status as HIV positive

4   There are occasional false-positive readings with this test, which can be cleared up by repeating it

**Answer: 3**

*Rationale:* If the client's test results are positive with the ELISA, the test is repeated. If the results are positive a second time, the Western blot (a more specific test) is done to confirm the finding. The client is not diagnosed as HIV positive unless results of the Western blot test are positive. (Some laboratories also run the Western blot a second time with a new specimen before making a final determination.) The ELISA is fast and relatively inexpensive, but it carries a high false-positive rate. This is because it is not as specific, although it is a very sensitive test.

*Test-Taking Strategy:* Recall that HIV is not diagnosed with a single laboratory test. With this in mind, eliminate options 1 and 2 first. From the remaining options, knowing that the ELISA would be repeated, and then a Western blot would be done to confirm these results, will direct you to option 3. Review the methods of diagnosing HIV if you had difficulty with this question.

*Level of Cognitive Ability:* Analysis
*Client Needs:* Psychosocial Integrity
*Integrated Concept/Process:* Nursing Process/Implementation
*Content Area:* Adult Health/Immune

*Reference*
Smeltzer, S., & Bare, B. (2000). *Brunner & Suddarth's Textbook of medical-surgical nursing* (9th ed.). Philadelphia: Lippincott Williams & Wilkins, p. 1359.

---

**141.** In performing a lethality assessment with a suicidal client, the nurse most appropriately asks the client:

1   "Do you ever think about ending it all?"

2   "Do you have any thoughts of killing yourself?"

3   "Do you wish your life was over?"

4   "Do you have a death wish?"

**Answer: 2**

*Rationale:* A lethality assessment requires direct communication between the client and the nurse concerning the client's intent. It is important to provide a question that is directly related to lethality. Euphemisms should be avoided.

*Test-Taking Strategy:* Use the process of elimination. Note the relationship between *suicidal* in the question and *killing* in the correct option. Although options 1, 3, and 4 infer a suicide intent, option 2 is most direct. If you had difficulty with this question, review assessment for suicide risk.

*Level of Cognitive Ability:* Application
*Client Needs:* Psychosocial Integrity
*Integrated Concept/Process:* Nursing Process/Assessment
*Content Area:* Mental Health

*Reference*
Stuart, G.W., & Laraia, M.T. (1998). *Principles and practice of psychiatric nursing* (6th ed.). St. Louis: Mosby, p. 389.

**142.** A client diagnosed with cancer of the bladder has a nursing diagnosis of "Fear related to the uncertain outcome of the upcoming cystectomy and urinary diversion." The nurse assesses that this diagnosis still applies if the client makes which of the following statements?

1 "I'm so afraid I won't live through all this."

2 "What if I have no help at home after going through this awful surgery?"

3 "I'll never feel like myself if I can't go to the bathroom normally."

4 "I wish I'd never gone to the doctor at all."

**Answer: 1**

*Rationale:* For Fear to be an actual diagnosis, the client must be able to identify the object of fear. In this question, the client is expressing a fear of death related to cancer. The statement in option 2 reflects risk for impaired home maintenance management. Option 3 reflects a body image disturbance. Option 4 is vague and nonspecific. Further exploration would be required to associate the statement in option 4 with a nursing diagnosis.

*Test-Taking Strategy:* Note that the diagnostic statement includes wording about the uncertain outcome of surgery. Since option 4 is a general statement, it should be eliminated first. Options 2 and 3 focus on the self after surgery but do not contain statements about an uncertain outcome. In option 1, the client expresses a fear of dying after enduring the ordeal of surgery. Review the defining characteristics of Fear if you had difficulty with this question.

*Level of Cognitive Ability:* Analysis
*Client Needs:* Psychosocial Integrity
*Integrated Concept/Process:* Nursing Process/Assessment
*Content Area:* Adult Health/Renal

*Reference*
Johnson, M., Bulechek, G., Dochterman, J. Maas, M., Moorhead, S. (2001). *Nursing diagnoses, outcomes, and interventions.* St. Louis: Mosby, p. 91.

**143.** A client with nephrotic syndrome asks the nurse, "Why should I even bother trying to control my diet and the edema? It doesn't really matter what I do, if I can never get rid of this kidney problem anyway!" The nurse selects which of the following most appropriate nursing diagnoses?

1 Powerlessness

2 Ineffective Individual Coping

3 Anxiety

4 Body Image Disturbance

**Answer: 1**

*Rationale:* Powerlessness is used when the client believes that personal actions will not affect an outcome in any significant way. Ineffective Individual Coping is used when the client has impaired adaptive abilities or behaviors in meeting the demands or roles expected. Anxiety is used when the client has a feeling of unease with a vague or undefined source. Body Image Disturbance occurs when there is an alteration in the way the client perceives body image.

*Test-Taking Strategy:* Focus on the data in the question and the client's statement. Note the statement "It doesn't really matter what I do." This implies that the client has a sense of "no control" over the situation. This will direct you to option 1. Review the defining characteristics of Powerlessness if you had difficulty with this question.

*Level of Cognitive Ability:* Analysis
*Client Needs:* Psychosocial Integrity
*Integrated Concept/Process:* Nursing Process/Analysis
*Content Area:* Adult Health/Renal

*Reference*
Johnson, M., Bulechek, G., Dochterman, J. Maas, M., Moorhead, S. (2001). *Nursing diagnoses, outcomes, and interventions.* St. Louis: Mosby, p. 248.

**144.** A client with renal cell carcinoma of the left kidney is scheduled for nephrectomy. The right kidney appears normal at this time. The client is anxious about whether dialysis will ultimately be a necessity. The nurse would plan to use which of the following information in discussions with the client?

1 There is absolutely no chance of needing dialysis due to the nature of the surgery

2 Dialysis could become likely, but it depends on how well the client complies with fluid restriction after surgery

3 One kidney is adequate to meet the needs of the body as long as it has normal function

4 There is a strong likelihood that the client will need dialysis within 5 to 10 years

**Answer: 3**

*Rationale:* Fears about having only one functioning kidney are common in clients who must undergo nephrectomy for renal cancer. These clients need emotional support and reassurance that the remaining kidney should be able to fully meet the body's metabolic needs, as long as it has normal function.

*Test-Taking Strategy:* Use the process of elimination. Eliminate option 1 because of the words *absolutely no chance.* Knowing that there is no need for fluid restriction with a functioning kidney guides you to eliminate option 2 next. From the remaining options, recalling that an individual can donate a kidney without adverse consequences or the need for dialysis will direct you to option 3. Review the psychosocial aspects related to nephrectomy if you had difficulty with this question.

*Level of Cognitive Ability:* Application
*Client Needs:* Psychosocial Integrity
*Integrated Concept/Process:* Nursing Process/Planning
*Content Area:* Adult Health/Oncology

*Reference*
Smeltzer, S., & Bare, B. (2000). *Brunner & Suddarth's Textbook of medical-surgical nursing* (9th ed.). Philadelphia: Lippincott Williams & Wilkins, p. 1125.

---

**145.** A charge nurse is supervising a new registered nurse (RN) providing care to a client with end-stage heart failure. The client is withdrawn, reluctant to talk, and shows little interest in participating in hygienic care or activities. Which statement if made by the new RN to the client indicates that the new RN needs further teaching in the use of therapeutic communication techniques?

1 "Many clients with end-stage heart failure fear death."

2 "Why don't you feel like getting up for your bath?"

3 "What are your feelings right now?"

4 "These dreams you mentioned, what are they like?"

**Answer: 2**

*Rationale:* When the nurse asks a "why" question of the client, the nurse is requesting an explanation for feelings and behaviors when the client may not know the reason. Requesting an explanation is a nontherapeutic communication technique. In option 1, the nurse is using the therapeutic communication technique of giving information. Imparting the common fear of death of client's with end-stage heart failure may encourage the client to voice concerns. In option 3, the nurse is encouraging verbalization of emotions or feelings, which is a therapeutic communication technique. In option 4, the nurse is using the therapeutic communication technique of exploring. Exploring is asking the client to describe something in more detail or to discuss it more fully.

*Test-Taking Strategy:* Note the key words *needs further teaching in the use of therapeutic communication techniques.* Use the process of elimination, seeking the option that is a block to communication. The word *why* in option 2 should guide you to this option. Review therapeutic communication techniques if you had difficulty with this question.

*Level of Cognitive Ability:* Analysis
*Client Needs:* Psychosocial Integrity
*Integrated Concept/Process:* Teaching/Learning
*Content Area:* Adult Health/Cardiovascular

*Reference*
Potter, P., & Perry, A. (2001). *Fundamentals of nursing* (5th ed.). St. Louis: Mosby, p. 459.

**146.** A nurse is caring for a client with acute pulmonary edema. The nurse should include strategies for which of the following in the care of the client?
1    Decreasing cardiac output
2    Increasing fluid volume
3    Promoting a positive body image
4    Reducing anxiety

**Answer: 4**
*Rationale:* When cardiac output falls as a result of acute pulmonary edema, the sympathetic nervous system is stimulated. Stimulation of the sympathetic nervous system results in the flight or fight reaction, which further impairs cardiac function. The goal of treatment is to increase cardiac output and decrease fluid volume. An alteration in body image is not a common problem experienced by clients with acute pulmonary edema.

*Test-Taking Strategy:* Use the process of elimination. Thinking about the physiological occurrences of this condition will assist in eliminating options 1, 2, and 3. Also recalling that severe dyspnea occurs, should assist in directing you to the correct option. Review care of a client with pulmonary edema if you had difficulty with this question.

*Level of Cognitive Ability:* Application
*Client Needs:* Psychosocial Integrity
*Integrated Concept/Process:* Nursing Process/Implementation
*Content Area:* Adult Health/Cardiovascular

*Reference*
Smeltzer, S., & Bare, B. (2000). *Brunner & Suddarth's Textbook of medical-surgical nursing* (9th ed.). Philadelphia: Lippincott Williams & Wilkins, p. 662.

**147.** A client with acute renal failure (ARF) is having trouble remembering information and instructions as a result of altered laboratory values. The nurse avoids doing which of the following when communicating with this client?
1    Giving simple, clear directions
2    Explaining treatments using understandable language
3    Including the family in discussions related to care
4    Giving thorough, complete explanations of treatment options

**Answer: 4**
*Rationale:* The client with ARF may have difficulty remembering information and instructions due to anxiety and due to altered laboratory values. Communications should be clear, simple, and understandable. The family is included whenever possible. It is the physician's responsibility to explain treatment options.

*Test-Taking Strategy:* Use the process of elimination and note the key word *avoids*. Recalling the basic principles of effective communication would lead you to recognize that options 1, 2, and 3 are helpful in maintaining effective communication. Review the basic principles of effective communication if you had difficulty with this question.

*Level of Cognitive Ability:* Application
*Client Needs:* Psychosocial Integrity
*Integrated Concept/Process:* Nursing Process/Implementation
*Content Area:* Adult Health/Renal

*Reference*
Black, J., Hawks, J., & Keene, A. (2001). *Medical-surgical nursing: Clinical management for positive outcomes* (6th ed.). Philadelphia: W.B. Saunders, p. 877.

**148.** A rehabilitation nurse witnessed a postoperative coronary artery bypass graft client and spouse arguing after a rehabilitation session. The most appropriate statement by the nurse in identifying the feelings of the client would be:

1   "You seem upset.."
2   "You shouldn't get upset. It'll affect your heart."
3   "Oh, don't let this get you down."
4   "It will seem better tomorrow, smile."

**Answer: 1**

*Rationale:* Acknowledging the client's feelings without inserting your own values or judgments is a method of therapeutic communication. Therapeutic communication techniques assist the flow of communication and always focus on the client. Option 1 is an open-ended statement that allows the client to verbalize, which gives the nurse a direction or clarification of the true feelings. Options 2, 3, and 4 do not encourage verbalization by the client.

*Test-Taking Strategy:* Use therapeutic communication techniques. Focusing on the issue: identifying the feelings of the client, will direct you to option 1. Review therapeutic communication techniques if you had difficulty with this question.

*Level of Cognitive Ability:* Application
*Client Needs:* Psychosocial Integrity
*Integrated Concept/Process:* Communication and Documentation
*Content Area:* Adult Health/Cardiovascular

*Reference*
Potter, P., & Perry, A. (2001). *Fundamentals of nursing* (5th ed.). St. Louis: Mosby, p. 459.

**149.** An acutely psychotic client displays increased psychomotor activity. Which of the following medications, if prescribed for the client, would the nurse administer?

1   Sertraline hydrochloride (Zoloft)
2   Haloperidol (Haldol)
3   Chloral hydrate
4   Isocarboxazid (Marplan)

**Answer: 2**

*Rationale:* Antipsychotics are used to treat acute and chronic psychosis, especially when the client has increased psychomotor activity. A fast-acting, injectable agent would be the medication of choice. Antidepressants (Zoloft and Marplan) and hypnotics (chloral hydrate) are not indicated for the presenting condition.

*Test-Taking Strategy:* Use the process of elimination, focusing on the issue: increased psychomotor activity. Eliminate options 1 and 4, because they are both antidepressants. From the remaining options, recalling that haloperidol is an antipsychotic will direct you to option 2. Review these medications if you had difficulty with this question.

*Level of Cognitive Ability:* Application
*Client Needs:* Psychosocial Integrity
*Integrated Concept/Process:* Nursing Process/Implementation
*Content Area:* Pharmacology

*Reference*
Stuart, G.W., & Laraia, M.T. (1998). *Principles and practice of psychiatric nursing* (6th ed.). St. Louis: Mosby, pp. 291; 312.

**150.** A client is admitted to the mental health unit with a diagnosis of panic disorder. The nurse anticipates that the physician will prescribe a benzodiazepine and checks the physician's order sheet for which medication order?

1 Imipramine (Tofranil)
2 Alprazolam (Xanax)
3 Buproprion (Wellbutrin)
4 Doxepin (Sinequan)

**Answer: 2**

*Rationale:* Options 1, 3, and 4 are classified as antidepressants and act by stimulating the central nervous system (CNS) to elevate mood. Xanax, a benzodiazepine antianxiety agent, depresses the CNS and induces relaxation in panic disorders.

*Test-Taking Strategy:* Knowledge regarding panic disorders and the classification of the medications identified in the options is required to answer this question. Recalling these classifications will assist in eliminating options 1, 3, and 4, because they are antidepressants. Review these medications if you had difficulty with this question.

*Level of Cognitive Ability:* Analysis
*Client Needs:* Psychosocial Integrity
*Integrated Concept/Process:* Nursing Process/Analysis
*Content Area:* Pharmacology

*Reference*
Stuart, G.W., & Laraia, M.T. (1998). *Principles and practice of psychiatric nursing* (6th ed.). St. Louis: Mosby, pp. 291, 373.

**151.** A client with empyema is to undergo decortication to remove the inflamed tissue, pus, and debris. The nurse offers emotional support to the client based on the understanding that:

1 The client is likely to be in excruciating pain after surgery
2 The client will probably have chronic dyspnea after the surgery
3 Chest tubes will be in place after surgery for some time, and the healing process is slow
4 This problem may decrease the client's life expectancy

**Answer: 3**

*Rationale:* The client undergoing decortication to treat empyema needs ongoing support by the nurse. This is especially true because the client will have chest tubes in place after surgery, which must remain until the former pus-filled space is completely obliterated. This usually takes a considerable amount of time, and may be discouraging to the client. Progress is monitored by chest x-ray. Options 1, 2, and 4 are not accurate.

*Test-Taking Strategy:* Use the process of elimination. Option 4 is the least likely response and is eliminated first. Option 1 is eliminated next, because no client should be in "excruciating pain" postoperatively. From the remaining options, it is necessary to know that the client will need chest tubes, and that it may take some time for full healing to occur. Recalling that the client has chest tubes after thoracic surgery may be sufficient to help you select between these last two options. Review the psychosocial aspects of care following decortication if you had difficulty with this question.

*Level of Cognitive Ability:* Analysis
*Client Needs:* Psychosocial Integrity
*Integrated Concept/Process:* Caring
*Content Area:* Adult Health/Respiratory

*Reference*
Black, J., Hawks, J., & Keene, A. (2001). *Medical-surgical nursing: Clinical management for positive outcomes* (6th ed.). Philadelphia: W.B. Saunders, Philadelphia: W.B. Saunders, p. 1743.

**152.** A client who has never been hospitalized before is having trouble initiating the stream of urine. Knowing that there is no pathological reason for this difficulty, the nurse avoids which of the following as the least helpful method of assisting the client?

1   Running tap water in the sink
2   Instructing the client to pour warm water over the perineal area
3   Assisting the client to a commode behind a closed curtain
4   Closing the bathroom door and instructing the client to pull the call bell when done

**Answer: 3**

*Rationale:* Lack of privacy is a key issue that may inhibit the ability of the client to void in the absence of known pathology. Using a commode behind a curtain may inhibit voiding in some people. Use of a bathroom is preferable, and may be supplemented with the use of running water, or pouring water over the perineum as needed.

*Test-Taking Strategy:* Use the process of elimination and note the key words *least helpful*. Think about the issue related to decreased privacy and its effects on elimination. Review measures to assist in promoting elimination if you had difficulty with this question.

*Level of Cognitive Ability:* Application
*Client Needs:* Psychosocial Integrity
*Integrated Concept/Process:* Nursing Process/Implementation
*Content Area:* Adult Health/Renal

*Reference*
Black, J., Hawks, J., & Keene, A. (2001). *Medical-surgical nursing: Clinical management for positive outcomes* (6th ed.). Philadelphia: W.B. Saunders, Philadelphia: W.B. Saunders, p. 747.

**153.** A client tells the nurse, "My doctor says I can have the surgery and go home the same day but I'm afraid. My husband's dead and my son is 3,000 miles away. I'm alone and what happens if something goes wrong? I'm not supposed to be up walking unless absolutely necessary." Which of the following responses would be most therapeutic for the nurse to employ?

1   "I know, I know. They say, Managed Care is no Care! Have you got an alarm system so if you fall, it will alert someone to come? If worst comes to worst, call me and I'll come immediately."
2   "Don't worry. This procedure is done all the time without any problems. You'll be fine!"
3   "Your concern is well voiced. I advise you to call your son and insist he come home immediately! You can't be too careful."
4   "You seem very concerned about going home without help. Have you discussed your concerns with your doctor?"

**Answer: 4**

*Rationale:* The client has verbalized concerns. In option 4, the nurse uses reflection to direct the client's feelings and concerns. In option 1, the nurse is ventilating the nurse's own anger, frustration, and powerlessness. In addition, the nurse is trying to problem solve for the client but is overly controlling and takes the decision making out of the client's hands. In option 2, the nurse provides false reassurance and then minimizes the client's concerns. In option 3, the nurse is projecting the client's own fears, and the problem solving suggested by the nurse will increase fear and anxiety in the client.

*Test-Taking Strategy:* Use therapeutic communication techniques. Remember that the priority is to address the client's feelings. Option 4 is the only option that addresses the feelings and concerns of the client. Review therapeutic communication techniques if you had difficulty with this question.

*Level of Cognitive Ability:* Application
*Client Needs:* Psychosocial Integrity
*Integrated Concept/Process:* Communication and Documentation
*Content Area:* Mental Health

*Reference*
Stuart, G.W., & Laraia, M.T. (1998). *Principles and practice of psychiatric nursing* (6th ed.). St. Louis: Mosby, p. 34.

**154.** During the nursing assessment, the client says, "My doctor just told me that my cancer has spread and that I have less than 6 months to live." Which of the following nursing responses would be most therapeutic?
1  "I know it seems desperate, but there have been a lot of break-throughs. Something might come along in a month or so to change your status drastically."
2  "I hope you'll focus on the fact that your doctor says you have 6 months to live and that you'll think of how you'd like to live."
3  "I am sorry. There are no easy answers in times like this, are there?"
4  "I am sorry. Would you like to discuss this with me some more?"

**Answer: 4**
*Rationale:* The client has received very distressing news. The client is most likely still in the stage of shock and denial. In the correct option, the nurse invites the client to ventilate. Option 1 provides a social communication and false hope. Option 2 is patronizing and stereotypical. Option 3 is social and expresses the nurse's feelings rather than the client's feelings.

*Test-Taking Strategy:* Use therapeutic communication techniques. Note that option 4 is providing the opportunity for the client to express feelings. Remember to focus on the client's feelings. Review therapeutic communication techniques if you had difficulty with this question.

*Level of Cognitive Ability:* Application
*Client Needs:* Psychosocial Integrity
*Integrated Concept/Process:* Communication and Documentation
*Content Area:* Adult Health/Oncology

*Reference*
Potter, P., & Perry, A. (2001). *Fundamentals of nursing* (5th ed.). St. Louis: Mosby, p. 459.

**155.** A client with an endotracheal tube gets easily frustrated when trying to communicate personal needs to the nurse. The nurse determines that which of the following methods for communication may be the easiest for the client?
1  Have the family interpret needs
2  Use a picture or word board
3  Use a pad and pencil
4  Devise a system of hand signals

**Answer: 2**
*Rationale:* The client with an endotracheal tube in place cannot speak. The nurse devises an alternative communication system with the client. Use of a picture or word board is the simplest method of communication, because it requires only pointing at the word or object. A pad and pencil is an acceptable alternative, but it requires more client effort and more time. The use of hand signals may not be a reliable method, because it may not meet all needs, and is subject to misinterpretation. The family does not need to bear the burden of communicating the client's needs, and they may not understand them either.

*Test-Taking Strategy:* Note the key words *frustrated* and *easiest*. Options 3 and 4 are not the "easiest" and are therefore eliminated first. Since the family may not necessarily know what the client is trying to communicate, this option could cause added frustration for the client. Review alternative methods of communication if you had difficulty with this question.

*Level of Cognitive Ability:* Analysis
*Client Needs:* Psychosocial Integrity
*Integrated Concept/Process:* Nursing Process/Planning
*Content Area:* Adult Health/Respiratory

*Reference*
Black, J., Hawks, J., & Keene, A. (2001). *Medical-surgical nursing: Clinical management for positive outcomes* (6th ed.). Philadelphia: W.B. Saunders, Philadelphia: W.B. Saunders, p. 1750.

**156.** A community health nurse visits a client who is receiving total parenteral nutrition (TPN) in the home. The client states, "I really miss eating with my family at dinner." Which is the best response by the nurse?

1  "It is normal to miss something as basic as eating."
2  "I think in a few weeks you will probably be allowed to eat a little."
3  "Tell me more about how you feel about dinner time?"
4  "You could sit with your family at dinner time anyway even if you do not eat."

**Answer: 3**

*Rationale:* The nurse assists the client to express feelings and deal with the aspects of illness and treatment. In option 3, the nurse uses clarifying and focusing to encourage the client to explore concerns. Blocks to communication such as giving opinions and changing the subject will stop the client from verbalizing feelings.

*Test-Taking Strategy:* Use therapeutic communication techniques. Always focus on client feelings first. This will direct you to option 3. Review therapeutic communication techniques if you had difficulty with this question.

*Level of Cognitive Ability:* Application
*Client Needs:* Psychosocial Integrity
*Integrated Concept/Process:* Communication and Documentation
*Content Area:* Fundamental Skills

*Reference*
Potter, P., & Perry, A. (2001). *Fundamentals of nursing* (5th ed.). St. Louis: Mosby, p. 459.

---

**157.** A client has been receiving maprotiline (Ludiomil). The nurse notifies the health care provider if which of the following adverse client responses to the medication is noted?

1  Increased sense of well-being
2  Reported decrease in anxiety
3  Increased drowsiness
4  Increased appetite

**Answer: 3**

*Rationale:* Maprotiline is a tetracyclic antidepressant used to treat various forms of depression and anxiety. The client is also often in psychotherapy while on this medication. Expected effects of the medication include improved sense of well-being, appetite, and sleep, as well as a reduced sense of anxiety. Common side effects to report to the health care provider include drowsiness, lethargy, and fatigue.

*Test-Taking Strategy:* Focus on the issue: an adverse response. Recall that this medication is an antidepressant. It would seem reasonable to expect options 1, 2, and 4 to occur as a positive response to this medication. Review this medication if you had difficulty with this question.

*Level of Cognitive Ability:* Analysis
*Client Needs:* Psychosocial Integrity
*Integrated Concept/Process:* Nursing Process/Evaluation
*Content Area:* Pharmacology

*Reference*
Hodgson, B., & Kizior, R. (2001). *Saunders Nursing drug handbook 2001.* Philadelphia: W.B. Saunders, p. 1103.

**158.** A client who is to undergo thoracentesis is afraid of not being able to tolerate the procedure. The nurse interprets that the client needs honest support and reassurance, which can best be accomplished by which of the following statements?

1    "The procedure takes only 1 to 2 minutes, so you might try to get through it by mentally counting up to 120."

2    "The needle is a little uncomfortable going in, but this is controlled by rhythmically breathing in and out. I'll be with you to coach your breathing."

3    "The needle hurts when it goes in and you must remain still. I'll stay with you throughout the entire procedure and help you hold your position."

4    "I'll be right by your side, but the procedure will be totally painless as long as you don't move."

**Answer: 3**

*Rationale:* The needle insertion for thoracentesis is painful for the client. The nurse tells the client how important it is to remain still during the procedure, so the needle doesn't injure visceral pleura or lung tissue. The nurse reassures the client during the procedure and helps the client hold the proper position.

*Test-Taking Strategy:* Use the process of elimination and therapeutic communication techniques. Recalling that the client must remain still during the procedure helps you to eliminate option 2 first. Knowing that the procedure may be painful for the client and takes longer than 1 to 2 minutes helps you to eliminate options 1 and 4. Review this procedure if you had difficulty with this question.

*Level of Cognitive Ability:* Application
*Client Needs:* Psychosocial Integrity
*Integrated Concept/Process:* Communication and Documentation
*Content Area:* Adult Health/Respiratory

*Reference*

Black, J., Hawks, J., & Keene, A. (2001). *Medical-surgical nursing: Clinical management for positive outcomes* (6th ed.). Philadelphia: W.B. Saunders, Philadelphia: W.B. Saunders, p. 1648.

**159.** A client with chronic respiratory failure is dyspneic. The client becomes anxious, which worsens the feelings of dyspnea. The nurse teaches the client which of the following methods to best interrupt the dyspnea-anxiety-dyspnea cycle?

1    Relaxation and breathing techniques

2    Biofeedback and coughing techniques

3    Guided imagery and limiting fluids

4    Distraction and increased dietary carbohydrates

**Answer: 1**

*Rationale:* The anxious client with dyspnea should be taught interventions to decrease anxiety, which include relaxation, biofeedback, guided imagery, and distraction. This will stop the escalation of feelings of anxiety and dyspnea. The dyspnea can be further controlled by teaching the client respiratory techniques, which include pursed lip and diaphragmatic breathing. Coughing techniques are useful, but breathing techniques are more effective. Limiting fluids will thicken secretions and increased dietary carbohydrates will increase production of $CO_2$ by the body.

*Test-Taking Strategy:* Focus on the issue: relieving anxiety and dyspnea. Limiting fluids and increasing carbohydrates are contraindicated, and are therefore eliminated. From the remaining options, recall that breathing techniques are more effective than coughing techniques. This will direct you to option 1. Review measures to relieve anxiety and dyspnea in the client with respiratory failure if you had difficulty with this question.

*Level of Cognitive Ability:* Application
*Client Needs:* Psychosocial Integrity
*Integrated Concept/Process:* Teaching/Learning
*Content Area:* Adult Health/Respiratory

*Reference*

Black, J., Hawks, J., & Keene, A. (2001). *Medical-surgical nursing: Clinical management for positive outcomes* (6th ed.). Philadelphia: W.B. Saunders, Philadelphia: W.B. Saunders, p. 452.

**160.** A client who has had drainage of a pleural effusion is in pain. The nurse avoids which of the following interventions in providing support to this client?
1 Offering verbal support and reassurance
2 Assisting the client to find positions of comfort
3 Leaving the client alone for an extended rest period
4 Providing pain medication for the client

**Answer: 3**
*Rationale:* The pain associated with drainage of pleural effusion is minimized by positioning the client for comfort and administering analgesics for relief of pain. The nurse also offers verbal support and reassurance. All of these measures help the client to cope with the pain and discomfort associated with this problem. It is least helpful to leave the client alone for extended periods, because the client may experience continued pain, which may be augmented by isolation.

*Test-Taking Strategy:* Use the process of elimination, noting the key word *avoids* in the stem of the question. Noting the words *alone* and *extended* in option 3 will direct you to this option. Review the psychosocial measures that provide support to a client in pain if you had difficulty with this question.

*Level of Cognitive Ability:* Application
*Client Needs:* Psychosocial Integrity
*Integrated Concept/Process:* Caring
*Content Area:* Fundamental Skills

**Reference**
Black, J., Hawks, J., & Keene, A. (2001). *Medical-surgical nursing: Clinical management for positive outcomes* (6th ed.). Philadelphia: W.B. Saunders, Philadelphia: W.B. Saunders, p. 1742.

---

**161.** A nurse is caring for a client who has just experienced a pulmonary embolism. The client is restless and very anxious. The nurse uses which approach in communicating with this client?
1 Explaining each treatment in great detail
2 Having the family reinforce the nurse's directions
3 Giving simple, clear directions and explanations
4 Speaking very little to the client until the crisis is over

**Answer: 3**
*Rationale:* The client who has suffered pulmonary embolism is fearful and apprehensive. The nurse effectively communicates with this client by staying with the client, providing simple, clear, and accurate information, and displaying in a calm, efficient manner. Options 1, 2, and 4 will produce more anxiety for the client and family.

*Test-Taking Strategy:* Use the process of elimination. Eliminate option 1 because of the words *great detail*. Next eliminate option 4 because of the words *speaking very little*. From the remaining options, having the family reinforce the directions may place stress on the family and provide too much sensory input for the client. This will direct you to option 3. Review communication strategies for the client who is restless and anxious if you had difficulty with this question.

*Level of Cognitive Ability:* Application
*Client Needs:* Psychosocial Integrity
*Integrated Concept/Process:* Nursing Process/Implementation
*Content Area:* Adult Health/Respiratory

**Reference**
Black, J., Hawks, J., & Keene, A. (2001). *Medical-surgical nursing: Clinical management for positive outcomes* (6th ed.). Philadelphia: W.B. Saunders, Philadelphia: W.B. Saunders, p. 1425.

**162.** A nurse in the emergency department is admitting a client with carbon monoxide poisoning from a suicide attempt. The nurse plans to ensure that which of the following most needed services is put in place for the client?

1 Pulmonary rehabilitation
2 Occupational therapy
3 Psychiatric consultation
4 Neurological consultation

**Answer: 3**

*Rationale:* The client with carbon monoxide poisoning as a result of a suicide attempt should have a psychiatric consultation. The necessity of a neurological consultation would depend on the sequelae to the nervous system from the carbon monoxide poisoning, and there are no data in the question indicating this need. Occupational therapy and pulmonary rehabilitation are not indicated.

*Test-Taking Strategy:* Focus on the client's diagnosis and note the key words *most needed.* Eliminate occupational therapy first, because there is no indication of the need for that service. The client will need respiratory therapy, but not pulmonary rehabilitation, so option 1 is eliminated next. A neurological consult could be beneficial, but only if the client suffers long- term central nervous system (CNS) damage from this suicide attempt. Review care of a client who attempted suicide if you had difficulty with this question.

*Level of Cognitive Ability:* Application
*Client Needs:* Psychosocial Integrity
*Integrated Concept/Process:* Nursing Process/Planning
*Content Area:* Mental Health

*Reference*
Stuart, G.W., & Laraia, M.T. (1998). *Principles and practice of psychiatric nursing* (6th ed.). St. Louis: Mosby, p. 399.

**163.** A nurse is caring for a young adult diagnosed with sarcoidiosis. The client is angry and tells the nurse there is no point in learning disease management, since there is no possibility of ever being cured. The nurse formulates which of the following nursing diagnoses for this client?

1 Impaired Thought Processes
2 Altered Health Maintenance
3 Anxiety
4 Powerlessness

**Answer: 4**

*Rationale:* The client with Powerlessness expresses feelings of having no control over a situation or outcome. Altered Health Maintenance involves the inability to seek out help that is needed to maintain health. Anxiety is a vague sense of unease. Impaired Thought Processes involves disruption in cognitive abilities or thought.

*Test-Taking Strategy:* Use the process of elimination and note the data in the question. Focusing on the issue: anger over a situation in which the client has little control, will direct you to option 4. If this question was difficult review the definitions of these nursing diagnoses.

*Level of Cognitive Ability:* Analysis
*Client Needs:* Psychosocial Integrity
*Integrated Concept/Process:* Nursing Process/Analysis
*Content Area:* Adult Health/Respiratory

*Reference*
Johnson, M., Bulechek, G., Dochterman, J. Maas, M., Moorhead, S. (2001). *Nursing diagnoses, outcomes, and interventions.* St. Louis: Mosby, p. 248.

**164.** A client immobilized in skeletal leg traction complains of being bored and restless. Based on these complaints, the nurse formulates which of the following nursing diagnoses for this client?

1  Diversional Activity Deficit
2  Powerlessness
3  Self-Care Deficit
4  Impaired Physical Mobility

**Answer: 1**

*Rationale:* A major defining characteristic of Diversional Activity Deficit is expression of boredom by the client. The question does not identify difficulties with coordination, range of motion, or muscle strength, which would indicate Impaired Physical Mobility. The question also does not identify client feelings of inability to perform activities of daily living (Self-Care Deficit) or lack of control (Powerlessness).

*Test-Taking Strategy:* Use the process of elimination, focusing on the data in the question. Noting the key words *bored and restless* will direct you to option 1. Review the defining characteristics of Diversional Activity Deficit if you had difficulty with this question.

*Level of Cognitive Ability:* Analysis
*Client Needs:* Psychosocial Integrity
*Integrated Concept/Process:* Nursing Process/Analysis
*Content Area:* Adult Health/Musculoskeletal

*Reference*
Johnson, M., Bulechek, G., Dochterman, J. Maas, M., Moorhead, S. (2001). *Nursing diagnoses, outcomes, and interventions.* St. Louis: Mosby, p. 129.

**165.** A client being mechanically ventilated after experiencing a fat embolus is visibly anxious. The nurse should:

1  Encourage the client to sleep until arterial blood gas results improve
2  Ask a family member to stay with the client at all times
3  Ask the physician for an order for succinylcholine
4  Provide reassurance to the client and give small doses of intravenous morphine sulfate as prescribed

**Answer: 4**

*Rationale:* The nurse always speaks to the client calmly and provides reassurance to the anxious client. Morphine sulfate is often prescribed for pain and anxiety for the client receiving mechanical ventilation. In option 1, the nurse does nothing to reassure or help the client. It is not beneficial to ask the family to take on the burden of remaining with the client at all times. Succinylcholine is a paralyzing agent, but has no antianxiety properties.

*Test-Taking Strategy:* Use the process of elimination. Note that the client is anxious. Option 4 is the only option in which the nurse interacts with the client. Also note the words *provide reassurance* in the correct option. Review measures to relieve anxiety if you had difficulty with this question.

*Level of Cognitive Ability:* Application
*Client Needs:* Psychosocial Integrity
*Integrated Concept/Process:* Nursing Process/Implementation
*Content Area:* Adult Health/Respiratory

*Reference*
Smeltzer, S., & Bare, B. (2000). *Brunner & Suddarth's Textbook of medical-surgical nursing* (9th ed.). Philadelphia: Lippincott Williams & Wilkins, p. 506.

**166.** A nurse is assessing a confused elderly client admitted to the hospital with a hip fracture. Which of the following data obtained by the nurse would not place the client at more risk for Altered Thought Processes?

1    Stress induced by the fracture
2    Hearing aid available and in working order
3    Unfamiliar hospital setting
4    Eyeglasses left at home

**Answer: 2**

*Rationale:* Confusion in the elderly client with a hip fracture could result from the unfamiliar hospital setting, stress due to the fracture, concurrent systemic diseases, cerebral ischemia, or side effects of medications. Use of eyeglasses and hearing aids enhance the client's interaction with the environment, and can reduce disorientation.

*Test-Taking Strategy:* Note the key words *would not*. The wording asks you to look for an option that will keep the client at the highest possible level of functioning from a cognitive perspective. Stress from the fracture (option 1) and an unfamiliar setting (option 3) is not likely to help the client's functional level, and are eliminated. Eyeglasses and hearing aids are both useful adjuncts in communicating with a client. Since the eyeglasses were left at home, they are of no use at the current time. Review the factors that place a hospitalized client at risk for Altered Thought Processes if you had difficulty with this question.

*Level of Cognitive Ability:* Analysis
*Client Needs:* Psychosocial Integrity
*Integrated Concept/Process:* Nursing Process/Assessment
*Content Area:* Fundamental Skills

*Reference*
Black, J., Hawks, J., & Keene, A. (2001). *Medical-surgical nursing: Clinical management for positive outcomes* (6th ed.). Philadelphia: W.B. Saunders, Philadelphia: W.B. Saunders, p. 612.

---

**167.** A client is admitted to the nursing unit after a left below-the-knee amputation following a crush injury to the foot and lower leg. The client tells the nurse, "I think I'm going crazy. I can feel my left foot itching." The nurse interprets the client's statement to be:

1    A normal response, and indicates the presence of phantom limb sensation
2    A normal response, and indicates the presence of phantom limb pain
3    An abnormal response, and indicates that the client needs more psychological support
4    An abnormal response, and indicates that the client is in denial about the limb loss

**Answer: 1**

*Rationale:* Phantom limb sensations are felt in the area of the amputated limb. These can include itching, warmth, and cold. The sensations are due to intact peripheral nerves in the area amputated. Whenever possible, clients should be prepared that they may experience these sensations. The client may also feel painful sensations in the amputated limb, called phantom limb pain. The origin of the pain is less well understood, but the client should be prepared for this, too, whenever possible. This is not an abnormal response.

*Test-Taking Strategy:* Focus on the client's complaint, itching. Recalling that sensation and pain may be felt in the residual limb eliminates options 3 and 4 first, because the sensations are not abnormal responses. From the remaining options, select option 1 because the client has complained of an itching sensation, but has not complained of pain in the residual limb. Review the expected findings in a client who had an amputation if you had difficulty with this question.

*Level of Cognitive Ability:* Analysis
*Client Needs:* Psychosocial Integrity
*Integrated Concept/Process:* Nursing Process/Analysis
*Content Area:* Adult Health/Neurological

### Reference
Black, J., Hawks, J., & Keene, A. (2001). *Medical-surgical nursing: Clinical management for positive outcomes* (6th ed.). Philadelphia: W.B. Saunders, Philadelphia: W.B. Saunders, p. 1410.

---

**168.** A client who has had a spinal fusion with insertion of hardware is extremely concerned with the perceived lengthy rehabilitation period. The client expresses concerns about finances and the ability to return to prior employment. The nurse understands that the client's needs could best be addressed by referral to the:

1 Surgeon
2 Clinical nurse specialist
3 Social worker
4 Physical therapist

**Answer: 3**
*Rationale:* Following spinal surgery, concerns about finances and employment are best handled by referral to a social worker. This individual is able to provide information about resources available to the client. The physical therapist has the best knowledge of techniques for increasing mobility and endurance. The clinical nurse specialist and surgeon would not have the necessary information related to financial resources.

*Test-Taking Strategy:* Use the process of elimination. Focusing on the client's concern about finances, and thinking about the role of each health care worker identified in the options will direct you to option 3. Review the roles of these health care workers if you had difficulty with this question.

*Level of Cognitive Ability:* Analysis
*Client Needs:* Psychosocial Integrity
*Integrated Concept/Process:* Nursing Process/Planning
*Content Area:* Fundamental Skills

### Reference
Potter, P., & Perry, A. (2001). *Fundamentals of nursing* (5th ed.). St. Louis: Mosby, p. 395.

---

**169.** A client is fearful about having an arm cast removed. Which of the following actions by the nurse would be the most helpful?

1 Telling the client that the saw makes a frightening noise
2 Reassuring the client that no one has had an arm lacerated yet
3 Stating that the hot cutting blades have rarely caused burns
4 Showing the client the cast cutter and explaining how it works

**Answer: 4**
*Rationale:* Clients may be fearful of having a cast removed because of the cast-cutting blade. The nurse should show the cast cutter to the client before it is used, and explain that the client may feel heat, vibration, and pressure. The cast cutter resembles a small electric saw with a circular blade. The nurse should reassure the client that the blade does not cut like a saw, but instead cuts the cast by vibrating side to side. Options 1, 2, and 3 are inappropriate and may increase the client's fear.

*Test-Taking Strategy:* Use the process of elimination, noting the key words *most helpful*. Focusing on the issue: the client's fear, will direct you to option 4. Option 4 gives the client the most reassurance because it best prepares the client for what will occur when the cast is removed. Review measures to relieve fear in a client preparing for a procedure if you had difficulty with this question.

*Level of Cognitive Ability:* Application
*Client Needs:* Psychosocial Integrity
*Integrated Concept/Process:* Nursing Process/Implementation
*Content Area:* Adult Health/Musculoskeletal

*Reference*

Black, J., Hawks, J., & Keene, A. (2001). *Medical-surgical nursing: Clinical management for positive outcomes* (6th ed.). Philadelphia: W.B. Saunders, Philadelphia: W.B. Saunders, p. 602.

---

**170.** A client has several fractures of the lower leg and has been placed in an external fixation device. The client is upset about the appearance of the leg, which is very edematous. The nurse formulates which of the following nursing diagnoses for the client?

1    Body Image Disturbance
2    Activity Intolerance
3    Risk for Impaired Physical Mobility
4    Social Isolation

**Answer: 1**

*Rationale:* The client is at risk for Body Image Disturbance related to a change in the structure and function of the affected leg. There are no data in the question to support a diagnosis of (actual) Activity Intolerance or Social Isolation. The client has an actual (not a risk for) Impaired Mobility because of the fixation device.

*Test-Taking Strategy:* Use the process of elimination, focusing on the data in the question. Noting the key words *upset about the appearance of the leg* will direct you to option 1. Review the defining characteristics for Body Image Disturbance if you had difficulty with this question.

*Level of Cognitive Ability:* Analysis
*Client Needs:* Psychosocial Integrity
*Integrated Concept/Process:* Nursing Process/Analysis
*Content Area:* Adult Health/Musculoskeletal

*Reference*

Johnson, M., Bulechek, G., Dochterman, J. Maas, M., Moorhead, S. (2001). *Nursing diagnoses, outcomes, and interventions.* St. Louis: Mosby, p. 54.

---

**171.** A client and her husband are being discharged from the hospital after giving birth to a fetal demise. They ask about the possibility of attending a bereavement support group in the community. The nurse is aware that this is an indication of:

1    Denial
2    Prolonged sadness
3    Normal grieving
4    Anger

**Answer: 3**

*Rationale:* A perinatal bereavement support group can help the parents' work through their pain by nonjudgmental sharing of feelings. It is a necessary part of normal grieving. The parents request is not indicative of denial, prolonged sadness, or anger.

*Test-Taking Strategy:* Use the process of elimination, focusing on the issue of the question. Focus on the parents' request to assist in directing you to option 3. Review the normal grieving process if you had difficulty with this question.

*Level of Cognitive Ability:* Analysis
*Client Needs:* Psychosocial Integrity
*Integrated Concept/Process:* Nursing Process/Assessment
*Content Area:* Maternity

*Reference*

Sherwen, L., Scoloveno, M.A., & Weingarten, C. (1999). *Maternity nursing: Care of the childbearing family* (3rd ed.). Stamford, Conn.: Appleton & Lange, pp. 329-333.

**172.** A client was just told by her primary care physician that she will have an exercise stress test to evaluate the client's status after recent episodes of more severe chest pain. As a nurse enters the examining room, the client states, "Maybe I shouldn't bother going. I wonder if I should just take more medication instead." The nurse's best response would be:
1 "Can you tell me more about how you're feeling?"
2 "Don't worry. Emergency equipment is available if it should be needed."
3 "Most people tolerate the procedure well without any complications."
4 "Don't you really want to control your heart disease?"

**Answer: 1**
*Rationale:* Anxiety and fear are often present before stress testing. The nurse should explore a client's feelings if concerns are expressed. Options 2, 3, and 4 are inappropriate statements and limit communication. Option 1 is open ended and is the only one of the options that is phrased to engender trust and sharing of concerns by the client.

*Test-Taking Strategy:* Use therapeutic communication techniques and the process of elimination. Remember to focus on the client's feelings. This will direct you to option 1. Review therapeutic communication techniques if you had difficulty with this question.

*Level of Cognitive Ability:* Application
*Client Needs:* Psychosocial Integrity
*Integrated Concept/Process:* Communication and Documentation
*Content Area:* Adult Health/Cardiovascular

*Reference*
Potter, P., & Perry, A. (2001). *Fundamentals of nursing* (5th ed.). St. Louis: Mosby, p. 459.

**173.** A nurse is giving a client with heart failure home care instructions for use after hospital discharge. The client interrupts, saying, "What's the use? I'll never remember all of this, and I'll probably die anyway!" The nurse interprets that the client's response is most likely the result of:
1 The teaching strategies used by the nurse
2 Anger about the new medical regimen
3 Insufficient financial resources to pay for the medications
4 Anxiety about the ability to manage the disease process at home

**Answer: 4**
*Rationale:* Anxiety and fear often develop after heart failure and can further tax the failing heart. The client's statement is made in the middle of receiving self-care instructions. There is no evidence in the question to support options 1, 2, or 3.

*Test-Taking Strategy:* Use the process of elimination. Focus on the data in the question. Note that the client's comment is made when preparing for self-care at home, which implies anxiety about disease self-management. Review the psychosocial concerns for a client with heart failure if you had difficulty with this question.

*Level of Cognitive Ability:* Analysis
*Client Needs:* Psychosocial Integrity
*Integrated Concept/Process:* Nursing Process/Analysis
*Content Area:* Adult Health/Cardiovascular

*Reference*
Johnson, M., Bulechek, G., Dochterman, J. Maas, M., Moorhead, S. (2001). *Nursing diagnoses, outcomes, and interventions.* St. Louis: Mosby, p. 90.

**174.** Before initiating intravenous (IV) therapy, the nurse notes nonverbal signs of anxiety in the client. In order to help relieve the anxiety, the nurse should explain the procedure of IV initiation to the client. Which of the following would be most appropriate for the nurse to say to the client?

1  "I'll be starting an IV that will add fluid directly to your bloodstream."
2  "I will be starting an IV and it should not hurt much."
3  "A number 18 angiocatheter will be inserted into your arm so fluid can be administered."
4  "Try not to worry. This procedure won't take long and will be over with before you know it."

**Answer: 1**

*Rationale:* Option 1 explains what an IV is in simple terms. Option 2 is incorrect and gives the client unwarranted reassurance because initiating an IV can be painful. Eliminate option 3 because the terminology of a number 18 gauge angiocatheter is medical and will not be understood by the client. Suggesting the client not worry is a cliché and blocks client communication of fears and feelings.

*Test Taking Strategy:* Use therapeutic communication techniques. Remembering to avoid the use of medical jargon and terminology that clients will not understand will eliminate option 3. Eliminate option 4, because the client should not be told not to worry. Eliminate option 2 because inserting an IV is painful. Review this procedure and therapeutic communication techniques if you had difficulty with this question.

*Level of Cognitive Ability:* Application
*Client Needs:* Psychosocial Integrity
*Integrated Concept/Process:* Communication and Documentation
*Content Area:* Fundamental Skills

*Reference*
Potter, P., & Perry, A. (2001). *Fundamentals of nursing* (5th ed.). St. Louis: Mosby, p. 459.

**175.** A client scheduled for the insertion of an implanted port for intermittent chemotherapy treatments says, "I'm not sure if I can handle having a tube coming out of me all the time. What will my friends think?" Based on the client's statements, the nurse plans to do which of the following first?

1  Show the client various central line tubes and catheters
2  Explain that an implanted port is placed under the skin and is not visible
3  Notify the physician of the client's concerns
4  Explain that the client's friends probably will not see the tube under the clothing

**Answer: 2**

*Rationale:* An implanted port is placed under the skin and is not visible. There is no tubing external to the body. Tubing is used only when the port is accessed intermittently and the IV line is connected. Showing the client various other tubes will not be beneficial because the client will not be using them. It is premature to notify the physician. Option 4 does not correct the client's confusion regarding the implanted port.

*Test-Taking Strategy:* Use the process of elimination. Note the key words *implanted port* in the question and the relationship to option 2. Review the concepts related to implanted catheters and the teaching/learning process if you had difficulty with this question.

*Level of Cognitive Ability:* Application
*Client Needs:* Psychosocial Integrity
*Integrated Concept/Process:* Nursing Process/Planning
*Content Area:* Fundamental Skills

*Reference*
Black, J., Hawks, J., & Keene, A. (2001). *Medical-surgical nursing: Clinical management for positive outcomes* (6th ed.). Philadelphia: W.B. Saunders, Philadelphia: W.B. Saunders, p. 386.

**176.** A client displays signs of anxiety when the nurse explains that the intravenous (IV) line will need to be discontinued due to an infiltration. The nurse makes which appropriate statement to the client?

1  "This will be a totally painless experience. It is nothing to worry about."

2  "I'm sure it will be a real relief for you just as soon as I discontinue this IV for good."

3  "Just relax and take a deep breath. This procedure will not take long and will be over soon."

4  "I can see that you're anxious. Removal of the IV shouldn't be painful; however, the IV will need to be restarted in another location."

**Answer: 4**

*Rationale:* While discontinuing an IV is a painless experience, it is not therapeutic to tell a client not to worry. Option 2 does not acknowledge the client's feelings and does not tell the client that an infiltrated IV may need to be restarted. Option 3 does not address the client's feelings. Option 4 addresses the client's anxiety and honestly informs the client that the IV will need to be restarted. This option uses the therapeutic technique of giving information as well as acknowledging the client's feelings.

*Test-Taking Strategy:* Use therapeutic communication techniques recalling that an infiltrated IV may need to be restarted. This will direct you to option 4. Also note that the correct option acknowledges the client's feelings. Review therapeutic communication techniques if you had difficulty with this question.

*Level of Cognitive Ability:* Application
*Client Needs:* Psychosocial Integrity
*Integrated Concept/Process:* Communication and Documentation
*Content Area:* Fundamental Skills

*Reference*
Potter, P., & Perry, A. (2001). *Fundamentals of nursing* (5th ed.). St. Louis: Mosby, p. 459.

---

**177.** A toddler with suspected conjunctivitis is crying and refuses to sit still during the eye examination. Which of the following is the most appropriate nursing statement to the child?

1  "If you will sit still, the examination will be over soon."

2  "Would you like to see my flashlight?"

3  "I know you are upset. We can do this examination later."

4  "Don't be scared, the light won't hurt you."

**Answer: 2**

*Rationale:* Fears in this age group can be decreased by getting the child actively involved in the examination. Option 1 ignores the toddler's feelings. Option 3, although acknowledging feelings, falsely puts off the inevitable. Option 4 tells the toddler how to feel.

*Test-Taking Strategy:* Use knowledge regarding the stages of growth and development noting that the child is a toddler. Also, the use of therapeutic communication techniques will direct you to option 2. Review growth and development related to the toddler if you had difficulty with this question.

*Level of Cognitive Ability:* Application
*Client Needs:* Psychosocial Integrity
*Integrated Concept/Process:* Communication and Documentation
*Content Area:* Child Health

*Reference*
Wong, D. (1999). *Whaley & Wong's Nursing care of infants and children* (6th ed.). St. Louis: Mosby, p. 238.

**178.** A client with acute pyelonephritis is scheduled for a voiding cystourethrogram. The client is very shy and modest. The nurse interprets that this client would most likely benefit from increased support and teaching about the procedure because:

1 Radiopaque contrast is injected into the bloodstream
2 Radioactive material is inserted into the bladder
3 The client must lie on an x-ray table in a cold, barren room
4 The client must void while the voiding process is filmed

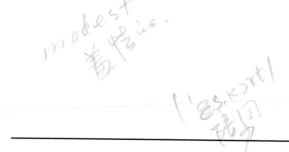

**Answer: 4**

*Rationale:* Having to void in the presence of others can be very embarrassing for clients, and may actually interfere with the client's ability to void. The nurse teaches the client about the procedure to try to minimize stress from lack of preparation, and gives the client encouragement and emotional support. Screens may be used in the radiology department to try to provide an element of privacy during this procedure.

*Test-Taking Strategy:* Use the process of elimination and knowledge regarding this procedure. Noting the key words *shy* and *modest* will direct you to option 4. Review this procedure if you had difficulty with this question.

*Level of Cognitive Ability:* Analysis
*Client Needs:* Psychosocial Integrity
*Integrated Concept/Process:* Nursing Process/Analysis
*Content Area:* Adult Health/Renal

*Reference*
Black, J., Hawks, J., & Keene, A. (2001). *Medical-surgical nursing: Clinical management for positive outcomes* (6th ed.). Philadelphia: W.B. Saunders, Philadelphia: W.B. Saunders, p. 759.

---

**179.** A female client in a manic state emerges from her room. She is topless and is making sexual remarks and gestures toward staff and peers. The best initial nursing action is to:

1 Quietly approach the client, escort her to her room, and assist her in getting dressed
2 Approach the client in the hallway and insist that she go to her room
3 Confront the client about the inappropriateness of her behavior and offer her a time-out
4 Ask the other clients to ignore her behavior; eventually she will return to her room

**Answer: 1**

*Rationale:* A person who is experiencing mania lacks insight and judgment, has poor impulse control, and is highly excitable. The nurse must take control without creating increased stress or anxiety to the client. "Insisting" the client go to her room may meet with a great deal of resistance. Confronting the client and offering her a consequence of "time-out" may be meaningless to her. Asking other clients to ignore her is inappropriate. A quiet, firm approach while distracting the client (walking her to her room and assisting her to get dressed) achieves the goal of having her dressed appropriately and preserving her psychosocial integrity.

*Test-Taking Strategy:* Use the process of elimination, noting that the client is in a "manic state." Recalling that the nurse must take control to protect the client will direct you to option 1. Review care of a client with mania if you had difficulty with this question.

*Level of Cognitive Ability:* Application
*Client Needs:* Psychosocial Integrity
*Integrated Concept/Process:* Nursing Process/Implementation
*Content Area:* Mental Health

*Reference*
Stuart, G.W., & Laraia, M.T. (1998). *Principles and practice of psychiatric nursing* (6th ed.). St. Louis: Mosby, p. 354.

**180.** Both the client who had cardiac surgery and the client's family express anxiety about how to cope with the recuperative process once they are home alone after discharge. The nurse plans to tell the client and family about which available resource?

1 Local library
2 United Way
3 American Heart Association Mended Hearts Club
4 American Cancer Society Reach for Recovery

**Answer: 3**

*Rationale:* Most clients and families benefit from knowing there are available resources to help them cope with the stress of self-care management at home. These can include telephone contact with the surgeon, cardiologist, and nurse; postcardiac surgery sponsored cardiac rehabilitation programs; and community support groups such as the American Heart Association Mended Hearts Club (a nationwide program with local chapters). The United Way provides a wide variety of services to people who might otherwise not afford them. The American Cancer Society Reach for Recovery helps women recover after mastectomy.

*Test-Taking Strategy:* Use the process of elimination. Note that the options identify three organizations and a library. Eliminate the library first because the client and family need resources to cope, implying the need for interactive processes. From the remaining options, noting that the client had cardiac surgery will direct you to option 3. Review the support services for clients who had cardiac surgery if you had difficulty with this question.

*Level of Cognitive Ability:* Application
*Client Needs:* Psychosocial Integrity
*Integrated Concept/Process:* Nursing Process/Planning
*Content Area:* Adult Health/Cardiovascular

*Reference*
Smeltzer, S., & Bare, B. (2000). *Brunner & Suddarth's Textbook of medical-surgical nursing* (9th ed.). Philadelphia: Lippincott Williams & Wilkins, p. 630.

**181.** An elderly client who has never been hospitalized before is to have a 12 lead electrocardiogram (ECG). The nurse could best plan to alleviate the client's anxiety about the test by giving which of the following explanations?

1 "The ECG can give the doctor information about what might be wrong with your heart."
2 "It's important to lie still during the procedure."
3 "It should take only about 20 minutes to complete the ECG tracings."
4 "The ECG electrodes are painless and will record the electrical activity of the heart."

**Answer: 4**

*Rationale:* The ECG uses painless electrodes, which are applied to the chest and limbs. It takes less than 5 minutes to complete, and requires the client to lie still. The ECG measures the heart's electrical activity to determine rate, rhythm, and a variety of abnormalities. Options 1 and 2 are factual statements and are not stated to reduce anxiety.

*Test-Taking Strategy:* Use the process of elimination and focus on the issue: alleviating the client's anxiety. Eliminate option 3 because it is inaccurate. Next, eliminate options 1 and 2 because they will not alleviate anxiety. Review this diagnostic test and measures to alleviate anxiety if you had difficulty with this question.

*Level of Cognitive Ability:* Application
*Client Needs:* Psychosocial Integrity
*Integrated Concept/Process:* Communication and Documentation
*Content Area:* Adult Health/Cardiovascular

*Reference*
Smeltzer, S., & Bare, B. (2000). *Brunner & Suddarth's Textbook of medical-surgical nursing* (9th ed.). Philadelphia: Lippincott Williams & Wilkins, p. 566.

**182.** A spouse of a client scheduled for insertion of an automatic implantable cardioverter-defibrillator (AICD) expresses anxiety about what would happen if the device discharges during physical contact. The nurse tells the spouse that:

1    Physical contact should be avoided whenever possible

2    A warning device sounds before countershock so there is time to move away

3    The spouse would not feel or be harmed by the countershock

4    The shock would be felt, but it would not cause the spouse any harm

**Answer: 4**

*Rationale:* Clients and families are often fearful about activation of the AICD. Their fears are about the device itself, and also the occurrence of life-threatening dysrhythmias that triggers its function. Family members need reassurance that even if the device activates while touching the client, the level of the charge is not high enough to harm the family member, although it will be felt. The AICD emits a warning beep when the client is near magnetic fields, which could possibly deactivate it, but does not beep before countershock.

*Test-Taking Strategy:* Focus on the issue, anxiety, and use knowledge of the function of the AICD to answer this question. This will direct you to option 4. Review the concepts related to this device if you had difficulty with this question.

*Level of Cognitive Ability:* Application
*Client Needs:* Psychosocial Integrity
*Integrated Concept/Process:* Nursing Process/Implementation
*Content Area:* Adult Health/Cardiovascular

**Reference**
Smeltzer, S., & Bare, B. (2000). *Brunner & Suddarth's Textbook of medical-surgical nursing* (9th ed.). Philadelphia: Lippincott Williams & Wilkins, p. 583.

**183.** A client who is scheduled for permanent transvenous pacemaker insertion says to the nurse, "I know I need it, but I'm not sure this surgery is the best idea." Which of the following responses will best help the nurse assess the client's preoperative concerns?

1    "Has anyone taught you about the procedure yet?"

2    "You sound uncertain about the procedure. Can you tell me more about what has you concerned?"

3    "You sound unnecessarily worried. Has anyone told you that the technology is quite advanced now?"

4    "How does your family feel about the surgery?"

**Answer: 2**

*Rationale:* Anxiety is common in the client with the need for pacemaker insertion. This can be related to fear of life-threatening dysrhythmias, or related to the surgical procedure. Options 1 and 3 are closed-ended and not exploratory. Option 4 is not indicated because it asks about the family, and deflects attention away from the client's concerns. Option 2 is open-ended and uses clarification as a communication technique to explore the client's concerns.

*Test-Taking Strategy:* Use therapeutic communication techniques, focusing on the issue: addressing the client's preoperative concerns. Option 4 can be eliminated first because it addresses the family, not the client. From the remaining options, the only option that addresses the client's concerns is option 2. Review therapeutic communication techniques if you had difficulty with this question.

*Level of Cognitive Ability:* Application
*Client Needs:* Psychosocial Integrity
*Integrated Concept/Process:* Communication and Documentation
*Content Area:* Adult Health/Cardiovascular

**Reference**
Smeltzer, S., & Bare, B. (2000). *Brunner & Suddarth's Textbook of medical-surgical nursing* (9th ed.). Philadelphia: Lippincott Williams & Wilkins, p. 583.

**184.** A client with superficial varicose veins says to the nurse, "I hate these things. They're so ugly; I wish I could get them to go away." The nurse's best response would be:

1  "You should try sclerotherapy. It's great."
2  "What have you been told about varicose veins and their management?"
3  "There's not much you can do once you get them."
4  "I understand how you feel, but you know, they really don't look too bad."

**Answer: 2**
*Rationale:* The client is expressing distress about physical appearance, and has a risk for Body Image Disturbance. The nurse assesses self-management of the condition as a means of empowering the client, and helping in adapting to the body change. Options 1, 3, and 4 are nontherapeutic.

*Test-Taking Strategy:* Use the process of elimination. With questions that deal with client's feelings, select the option that facilitates sharing of information and concerns by the client. Options 1, 3, and 4 cut off or limit further comments by the client. Additionally, option 2 addresses assessment, the first step of the nursing process. Review therapeutic communication techniques if you had difficulty with this question.

*Level of Cognitive Ability:* Application
*Client Needs:* Psychosocial Integrity
*Integrated Concept/Process:* Communication and Documentation
*Content Area:* Adult Health/Cardiovascular

*Reference*
Johnson, M., Bulechek, G., Dochterman, J. Maas, M., Moorhead, S. (2001). *Nursing diagnoses, outcomes, and interventions.* St. Louis: Mosby, p. 54.

**185.** A client who has been diagnosed with chronic renal failure has been told that hemodialysis will be required. The client becomes angry and withdrawn, and states, "I'll never be the same now." The nurse formulates which of the following nursing diagnoses for this client?

1  Altered Thought Processes
2  Body Image Disturbance
3  Anxiety
4  Noncompliance

**Answer: 2**
*Rationale:* A client with a renal disorder, such as renal failure, may become angry and depressed due to the permanence of the alteration. Due to the physical change and the change in lifestyle that may be required to manage a severe renal condition, the client may experience Body Image Disturbance. Anxiety is not appropriate because the client is able to identify the cause of concern. The client is not cognitively impaired (option 1) or stating refusal to undergo therapy (option 4).

*Test-Taking Strategy:* Use the process of elimination. Focus on the client's statement. Note that the client's statement focuses on self, which is consistent with Body Image Disturbance. Review the defining characteristics of Body Image Disturbance if you had difficulty with this question.

*Level of Cognitive Ability:* Analysis
*Client Needs:* Psychosocial Integrity
*Integrated Concept/Process:* Nursing Process/Analysis
*Content Area:* Adult Health/Renal

*Reference*
Johnson, M., Bulechek, G., Dochterman, J. Maas, M., Moorhead, S. (2001). *Nursing diagnoses, outcomes, and interventions.* St. Louis: Mosby, p. 54.

**186.** A client with the diagnosis of hyperparathyroidism says to the nurse, "I can't stay on this diet. It is too difficult for me." When intervening in this situation, the nurse should respond:

1   "It is very important that you stay on this diet to avoid forming renal calculi."
2   "It really isn't difficult to stick to this diet. Just avoid milk products."
3   "Why do you think you find this diet plan difficult to adhere to?"
4   "You are having a difficult time staying on this plan. Lets discuss this."

**Answer: 4**

*Rationale:* By paraphrasing the client's statement, the nurse can encourage the client to verbalize emotions. The nurse also sends feedback to the client that the message was understood. An open-ended statement or question such as this, prompts a lengthy response from the client. Option 1 is giving advice, which blocks communication. Option 2 devalues the client's feelings. Option 3 is requesting information that the client may not be able to express.

*Test-Taking Strategy:* Use therapeutic communication techniques. Focus on the client's statement. Note that option 4 paraphrases the client's statement. Review therapeutic communication techniques if you had difficulty with this question.

*Level of Cognitive Ability:* Application
*Client Needs:* Psychosocial Integrity
*Integrated Concept/Process:* Communication and Documentation
*Content Area:* Adult Health/Endocrine

*Reference*
Potter, P., & Perry, A. (2001). *Fundamentals of nursing* (5th ed.). St. Louis: Mosby, p. 459.

**187.** A nurse is caring for a male client with newly diagnosed type 1 diabetes mellitus. To develop an effective teaching plan, it would be most important for the nurse to assess the client for:

1   Knowledge of the diabetic diet
2   Expressions of denial of having diabetes
3   Fear of performing insulin administration
4   Feelings of depression about lifestyle changes

**Answer: 2**

*Rationale:* When diabetes mellitus is first diagnosed, the client may go through the phases of grief-denial, fear, anger, bargaining, depression, and acceptance. Denial is the phase that is most detrimental to the teaching/learning process. If the client is denying the fact that he has diabetes, the client probably will not listen to discussions about the disease or how to manage it. Denial must be identified before the nurse can develop a teaching plan.

*Test-Taking Strategy:* Use the process of elimination, noting the key words *most important*. All of the options may be appropriate to assess, however note that options 1, 3, and 4 relate to very specific components of the teaching. Option 2 is the most global option, and considering the principles of teaching and learning, this aspect needs to be assessed before the implementation of teaching. Review teaching/learning principles if you had difficulty with this question.

*Level of Cognitive Ability:* Application
*Client Needs:* Psychosocial Integrity
*Integrated Concept/Process:* Teaching/Learning
*Content Area:* Adult Health/Endocrine

*Reference*
Potter, P., & Perry, A. (2001). *Fundamentals of nursing* (5th ed.). St. Louis: Mosby, p. 496.

**188.** A client with newly diagnosed type 1 diabetes mellitus has been seen for 3 consecutive days in the emergency department with hyperglycemia. During the assessment the client says to the nurse, "I'm sorry to keep bothering you every day, but I just can't give myself those awful shots." The nurse's best response is:

1   "You must learn to give yourself the shots."
2   "I couldn't give myself a shot either."
3   "I'm sorry you are having trouble with your injections. Has someone given you instructions on them?"
4   "Let me see if the doctor can change your medication."

**Answer: 3**
*Rationale:* It is important to determine and deal with a client's underlying fear of self-injection. The nurse should determine whether a knowledge deficit exists. Demanding a behavior or skill is inappropriate (option 1). Positive reinforcement is necessary instead of focusing on negative behaviors (option 2). The nurse should not offer a change in regimen that can't be accomplished (option 4).

*Test-Taking Strategy:* Use therapeutic communication techniques. Options 1, 2, and 4 are nontherapeutic. Additionally, option 4 may provide false reassurance regarding a change in medications. Review therapeutic communication techniques if you had difficulty with this question.

*Level of Cognitive Ability:* Application
*Client Needs:* Psychosocial Integrity
*Integrated Concept/Process:* Communication and Documentation
*Content Area:* Adult Health/Endocrine

*Reference*
Potter, P., & Perry, A. (2001). *Fundamentals of nursing* (5th ed.). St. Louis: Mosby, p. 459.

---

**189.** A nurse requests that a client with diabetes mellitus ask their significant other(s) to attend an educational conference on self-administration of insulin. The client questions why significant others need to be included. The nurse's best response would be:

1   "Clients and families often work together to develop strategies for the management of diabetes."
2   "Family members can take you to the doctor."
3   "Family members are at risk of developing diabetes."
4   "Nurses need someone to call and check on a client's progress."

**Answer: 1**
*Rationale:* Families and/or significant others may be included in diabetes education to assist with adjustment to the diabetic regimen. Although option 2 and option 3 may be accurate, they are not the most appropriate response. Option 4 devalues the client and disregards the issue of independence and promotes powerlessness.

*Test-Taking Strategy:* Use the process of elimination and therapeutic communication techniques. Eliminate option 4 first because it devalues the client. From the remaining options, note that option 1 is the most global. Review therapeutic communication techniques if you had difficulty with this question.

*Level of Cognitive Ability:* Application
*Client Needs:* Psychosocial Integrity
*Integrated Concept/Process:* Communication and Documentation
*Content Area:* Adult Health/Endocrine

*Reference*
Johnson, M., Bulechek, G., Dochterman, J. Maas, M., Moorhead, S. (2001). *Nursing diagnoses, outcomes, and interventions.* St. Louis: Mosby, p. 248.

**190.** A 22-year-old woman has recently been diagnosed with polycystic kidney disease. A nurse has a series of discussions with the client, which are intended to help her adjust to the disorder. The nurse plans to include which of the following items as part of one of these discussions?

1    Ongoing fluid restriction
2    Depression about massive edema
3    Risk of hypotensive episodes
4    Need for genetic counseling

**Answer: 4**

*Rationale:* Adult polycystic kidney disease is a hereditary disorder that is inherited as an autosomal dominant trait. Because of this, the client should have genetic counseling, as should the extended family. The client is likely to have hypertension, not hypotension. Massive edema is not part of the clinical picture for this disorder. Ongoing fluid restriction is unnecessary.

*Test-Taking Strategy:* Use the process of elimination. Since massive edema and the need for fluid restriction are not part of the clinical picture for the client with polycystic kidney disease, eliminate options 1 and 2. From the remaining options, recalling either that this disorder is hereditary in nature or that the client would exhibit hypertension, not hypotension will direct you to option 4. Review psychosocial aspects related to polycystic kidney disease if you had difficulty with this question.

*Level of Cognitive Ability:* Application
*Client Needs:* Psychosocial Integrity
*Integrated Concept/Process:* Nursing Process/Planning
*Content Area:* Adult Health/Renal

*Reference*
Black, J., Hawks, J., & Keene, A. (2001). *Medical-surgical nursing: Clinical management for positive outcomes* (6th ed.). Philadelphia: W.B. Saunders, Philadelphia: W.B. Saunders, p. 871.

**191.** A nurse is admitting a client to the hospital who is to undergo ureterolithotomy for urinary calculi removal. The nurse understands that it is unnecessary to assess which of the following in determining the client's readiness for surgery?

1    Understanding of the surgical procedure
2    Knowledge of postoperative activities
3    Feelings or anxieties about the surgical procedure
4    Need for a visit from a support group

**Answer: 4**

*Rationale:* Ureterolithotomy is removal of a calculus from the ureter using either a flank or abdominal incision. Since there is no urinary diversion created during this procedure, the client has no need for a visit from a member of a support group. The client should have an understanding of the same items as for any surgery, which includes knowledge of the procedures, expected outcome, and postoperative routines and discomfort. The client should also be assessed for any concerns or anxieties before surgery.

*Test-Taking Strategy:* Use the process of elimination noting the key word *unnecessary*. Eliminate options 1, 2, and 3, because they are assessments that should be performed before any surgery. Also, recalling that a urinary diversion is not needed in this type of surgery will direct you to option 4. Review preoperative assessments if you had difficulty with this question.

*Level of Cognitive Ability:* Application
*Client Needs:* Psychosocial Integrity
*Integrated Concept/Process:* Nursing Process/Assessment
*Content Area:* Adult Health/Renal

*Reference*
Black, J., Hawks, J., & Keene, A. (2001). *Medical-surgical nursing: Clinical management for positive outcomes* (6th ed.). Philadelphia: W.B. Saunders, Philadelphia: W.B. Saunders, p. 828.

**192.** The spouse of a client who is dying says to the nurse, "I don't think I can come anymore and watch her die. It's chewing me up too much!" The most therapeutic nursing response is:

1   "I wish you'd focus on your wife's pain rather than yours. I know it's hard but this isn't about what's happening to you, you know."

2   "I know it's hard for you but she would know if you're not there and you'd feel guilty all the rest of your days."

3   "It's hard to watch someone you love die. You've been here with your wife every day. Are you taking any time for yourself?"

4   "I think you're making the right decision. Your wife knows you love her. You don't have to come. I'll take care of her."

**Answer: 3**

*Rationale:* The most therapeutic response is the one that is empathic and reflects the nurse's understanding of the client's (the husband) stress and emotional pain. In the correct option, the nurse suggests that the client take time for himself. Option 1 is an example of a nontherapeutic, judgmental attitude that places blame. Option 2 makes statements that the nurse cannot know are true (the wife may, in fact, not know if the husband visits) and predicts guilt feelings, which is inappropriate. Option 4 fosters dependency and gives advice, which is nontherapeutic.

*Test-Taking Strategy:* Use therapeutic communication techniques to answer the question. Note that the client of the question is the husband. Option 3 is the only option that is therapeutic and addresses the husband's feelings. Review therapeutic communication techniques if you had difficulty with this question.

*Level of Cognitive Ability:* Application
*Client Needs:* Psychosocial Integrity
*Integrated Concept/Process:* Communication and Documentation
*Content Area:* Mental Health

*Reference*
Stuart, G.W., & Laraia, M.T. (1998). *Principles and practice of psychiatric nursing* (6th ed.). St. Louis: Mosby, p. 34.

---

**193.** An older adult client at the Retirement Center spits her food out and throws it on the floor at a Thanksgiving dinner held in the community dining room. The client yells, "This turkey is dry and cold! I can't stand the food here!" The most therapeutic nursing response is which of the following?

1   "Let me get you another serving that is more to your liking. Would you like to come visit the chef and select your own serving?"

2   "I think you had better return to your apartment where a new meal will be served to you there."

3   "Now look what you've done! You're ruining this meal for the whole community. Aren't you ashamed of yourself?"

4   "One of the things that the residents of this group agreed was that anyone who did not use appropriate behavior would be asked to leave the dining room. Please leave now."

**Answer: 1**

*Rationale:* Asking the client to accompany the nurse to the kitchen respects the client's need for control, removes the angry client from the dining room, and may offer the nurse an opportunity to assess what is happening to the client. Option 2 could provoke a regressive struggle between the nurse and client and cause more anger in the client. Option 3 is angry and aggressive and nontherapeutic. In option 4, the nurse is authoritative and it would not be appropriate to ask the client to leave. This action might set up an aggressive struggle between the nurse and the client.

*Test-Taking Strategy:* Use therapeutic communication techniques and knowledge about care of an angry client. Option 1 is the only option that addresses the client's angry feelings. It also provides the nurse an opportunity to further assess the client. Review therapeutic communication techniques if you had difficulty with this question.

*Level of Cognitive Ability:* Application
*Client Needs:* Psychosocial Integrity
*Integrated Concept/Process:* Communication and Documentation
*Content Area:* Mental Health

*Reference*
Stuart, G.W., & Laraia, M.T. (1998). *Principles and practice of psychiatric nursing* (6th ed.). St. Louis: Mosby, p. 34.

**194.** A physician orders a follow-up home care visit for an older adult client with emphysema. When the home health nurse arrives, the client is smoking. Which of the following statements made by the nurse would be most therapeutic?
1 "Well, I can see you never got to the Stop Smoking clinic!"
2 "I notice that you are smoking. Did you explore the Stop Smoking Program at the Senior Citizens?"
3 "I wonder if you realize that you are slowly killing yourself? Why prolong the agony? You can just jump off the bridge!"
4 "I'm glad I caught you smoking! Now that your secret is out, let's decide what you are going to do?"

**Answer: 2**
*Rationale:* Emphysema clients need to avoid smoking and all airborne irritants. The nurse who observes a maladaptive behavior in a client should not make judgmental comments and should explore an adaptive strategy with the client without being overly controlling. This will place the decision making in the client's hands, and provide an avenue for the client to share what may be expressions of frustration at an inability to stop what is essentially a physiological addiction. Option 1 is an intrusive use of sarcastic humor that is degrading to the client. In Option 3, the nurse preaches and is judgmental. Option 4 is a disciplinary remark and places a barrier between the nurse and client within the therapeutic relationship.

*Test-Taking Strategy:* Use therapeutic communication techniques. Option 2 recognizes and addresses the client's behavior and explores an avenue to deal with the behavior. Review therapeutic communication techniques if you had difficulty with this question.

*Level of Cognitive Ability:* Application
*Client Needs:* Psychosocial Integrity
*Integrated Concept/Process:* Communication and Documentation
*Content Area:* Adult Health/Respiratory

*Reference*
Potter, P., & Perry, A. (2001). *Fundamentals of nursing* (5th ed.). St. Louis: Mosby, p. 459.

**195.** A client is to have arterial blood gases drawn. While the nurse is performing the Allen test, the client says to the nurse, "What are you doing? No one else has done that!" The most therapeutic nursing response would be:
1 "This is a routine precautionary step that simply makes certain your circulation is intact before obtaining a blood sample."
2 "Oh? You have questions about this? You should insist that they all do this procedure before drawing up your blood."
3 "I assure you that I am doing the correct procedure. I cannot account for what others do."
4 "This step is crucial to safe blood withdrawal. I would not let anyone take my blood until they did this."

**Answer: 1**
*Rationale:* The Allen test is performed to assess collateral circulation in the hand before drawing a radial artery blood specimen. The most therapeutic response provides information to the client. Option 2 is aggressive and controlling as well as nontherapeutic in its disapproving stance. Option 3 is defensive and nontherapeutic in offering false reassurance. Option 4 identifies client advocacy, but is overly controlling and quite aggressive and undermining of treatment.

*Test-Taking Strategy:* Use therapeutic communication techniques and the process of elimination. Option 1 addresses the issue of the question and provides information to the client. Review therapeutic communication techniques if you had difficulty with this question.

*Level of Cognitive Ability:* Application
*Client Needs:* Psychosocial Integrity
*Integrated Concept/Process:* Communication and Documentation
*Content Area:* Adult Health/Cardiovascular

*References*
Potter, P., & Perry, A. (2001). *Fundamentals of nursing* (5th ed.). St. Louis: Mosby, p. 459.

**196.** A client is complaining of difficulty concentrating, having outbursts of anger, and feeling "keyed up" all the time. The nurse obtaining the client's history discovers that the symptoms started about 6 months ago. The client reveals that a best friend was killed in a drive-by shooting while they were sitting on the porch talking. The nurse suspects that the client is experiencing:

1 Obsessive-compulsive disorder (OCD)
2 Panic disorder
3 Posttraumatic stress disorder (PTSD)
4 Social phobia

**Answer: 3**

*Rationale:* PTSD is a response to an event that would be markedly distressing to almost anyone. Characteristic symptoms include sustained level of anxiety, difficulty sleeping, irritability, difficulty concentrating, or outbursts of anger. Obsessive-compulsive disorder refers to some repetitive thoughts or behaviors. Panic disorders and social phobia are characterized by a specific fear of an object or situation.

*Test-Taking Strategy:* Focus on the data in the question and use the process of elimination. Eliminate options 2 and 4 first because they are similar. From the remaining options, recalling that OCD relates to a repetitive thought or behavior will direct you to option 3. Review this disorder if you had difficulty with this question.

*Level of Cognitive Ability:* Analysis
*Client Needs:* Psychosocial Integrity
*Integrated Concept/Process:* Nursing Process/Analysis
*Content Area:* Mental Health

*Reference*
Stuart, G.W., & Laraia, M.T. (1998). *Principles and practice of psychiatric nursing* (6th ed.). St. Louis: Mosby, p. 286.

**197.** A client who is reported by the staff to be very demanding, says to the nurse, "I can't get any help with my care! I call and call but the nurses never answer my light. Last night one of them told me she had other patients besides me! I'm very sick, but the nurses don't care!" Which of the following would be the most therapeutic response by the nurse?

1 "I think you are being very impatient. The nurses work very hard and come as quickly as they can."
2 "I can hear your anger. That nurse had no right to speak to you that way. I will report her to the Director. It won't happen again."
3 "It's hard to be in bed and have to ask for help. You ring for a nurse who never seems to answer?"
4 "You poor thing! I'm so sorry this happened to you. That nurse should be fired."

**Answer: 3**

*Rationale:* Empathy is a term that describes the nurse's capacity to enter into the life of another person and to perceive how the client is feeling and what meaning this has for the client. In option 3, the nurse displays empathy and shares perceptions. Sharing perceptions asks the client to validate the nurse's understanding of what the client is feeling and thinking. It opens the door for the client to share concerns, fears, and anxieties. In option 1, the nurse is assertive and certainly defends the nursing staff as well. In option 2, the nurse expresses the client's frustration by labeling the client's feelings as "angry" and disapproving of the nursing staff. This is splitting and is nontherapeutic. Option 4 is a social response and is demeaning to the client.

*Test-Taking Strategy:* Use therapeutic communication techniques and the process of elimination. Focus on the client's statement in the question. Note the relationship between the client's statement and option 3. Also, in this option the nurse validates the client's feelings. Review therapeutic communication techniques if you had difficulty with this question.

*Level of Cognitive Ability:* Application
*Client Needs:* Psychosocial Integrity
*Integrated Concept/Process:* Communication and Documentation
*Content Area:* Mental Health

*Reference*
Stuart, G.W., & Laraia, M.T. (1998). *Principles and practice of psychiatric nursing* (6th ed.). St. Louis: Mosby, p. 32.

**198.** An English-speaking Hispanic male with a newly applied long leg cast has a right proximal fractured tibia. During rounds that night, the nurse finds the client restless, withdrawn, and quiet. Which of the following initial nurse statements would be most appropriate?

1    "Are you uncomfortable?"
2    "Tell me what you are feeling?"
3    "I'll get you pain medication right away."
4    "You'll feel better in the morning."

**Answer: 2**

*Rationale:* Option 2 is open-ended and makes no assumptions about the client's psychological or emotional state. Option 1 is incorrect because males in traditional standard Hispanic cultures practice "machismo," in which stoicism is valued, so this client may deny any pain when asked. Option 3 is incorrect because an assessment is necessary before administering medication for pain. False reassurance is never therapeutic, which makes option 4 incorrect.

*Test-Taking Strategy:* Use therapeutic communication techniques. Recalling that the client's feelings are the priority will direct you to option 2. Review therapeutic communication techniques if you had difficulty with this question.

*Level of Cognitive Ability:* Application
*Client Needs:* Psychosocial Integrity
*Integrated Concept/Process:* Cultural Awareness
*Content Area:* Adult Health/Musculoskeletal

*Reference*
Potter, P., & Perry, A. (2001). *Fundamentals of nursing* (5th ed.). St. Louis: Mosby, p. 459.

---

**199.** A client was started on oral anticoagulant therapy while hospitalized. The client is now being discharged to home and is intermittently confused. The nurse would evaluate that the client has the best support system for successful anticoagulant therapy monitoring if the client:

1    Has a good friend living next door who would take the client to the doctor
2    Has a home health aide coming to the house for 9 weeks
3    Was going to stay with a daughter in the daughter's home indefinitely
4    Was going to have blood work drawn in the home by a local laboratory

**Answer: 3**

*Rationale:* The client taking anticoagulant therapy should be informed about the medication, its purpose, and the necessity of taking the proper dose at the specified times. If the client is unwilling or unable to comply with the medication regimen, the continuance of the regime should be questioned. Clients may need support systems in place to enhance compliance with therapy. Option 1 facilitates medical care, option 2 facilitates reminding the client to take the medication, and option 4 facilitates blood work only.

*Test-Taking Strategy:* Use the process of elimination. Note the issue: the best support system. Note that option 3 is the only option that indicates direct support for the client. Review the concepts surrounding support systems for the client if you had difficulty with this question.

*Level of Cognitive Ability:* Analysis
*Client Needs:* Psychosocial Integrity
*Integrated Concept/Process:* Nursing Process/Evaluation
*Content Area:* Adult Health/Cardiovascular

*Reference*
Smeltzer, S., & Bare, B. (2000). *Brunner & Suddarth's Textbook of medical-surgical nursing* (9th ed.). Philadelphia: Lippincott Williams & Wilkins, p. 735.

**200.** A client who has undergone successful femoral-popliteal bypass grafting to the leg says to the nurse, "I hope everything goes well after this, and I don't lose my leg. I'm so afraid that I'll have gone through this for nothing." The nurse's best response would be:
1   "I can understand what you mean. I'd be nervous too, if I were in your shoes."
2   "Stress isn't helpful for you. You should probably just relax and try not to worry unless something actually happens."
3   "Complications are possible, but you have a good deal of control if you make the lifestyle adjustments we talked about."
4   "This surgery is so successful, that I wouldn't be concerned at all if I were you."

**Answer: 3**
*Rationale:* Clients frequently fear that they will ultimately lose a limb or become debilitated in some other way. Option 1 feeds into the client's anxiety and is not therapeutic. Option 4 gives false reassurance. Option 2 is meant to be reassuring, but offers no suggestions to empower the client. Option 3 acknowledges the client's concerns, and empowers the client to improve health, which will ultimately reduce concern about the risk of complications.

*Test-Taking Strategy:* Use the process of elimination and therapeutic communication techniques. Option 3 is the only option that acknowledges the client's concerns and addresses the client's control over the situation. Review therapeutic communication techniques if you had difficulty with this question.

*Level of Cognitive Ability:* Application
*Client Needs:* Psychosocial Integrity
*Integrated Concept/Process:* Communication and Documentation
*Content Area:* Adult Health/Cardiovascular

*Reference*
Black, J., Hawks, J., & Keene, A. (2001). *Medical-surgical nursing: Clinical management for positive outcomes* (6th ed.). Philadelphia: W.B. Saunders, Philadelphia: W.B. Saunders, 1406.

**201.** A client in the coronary care unit is about to have a pericardiocentesis done for a rapidly accumulating pericardial effusion. The nurse could best plan to alleviate the apprehension of the client by:
1   Staying beside the client and giving information and encouragement during the procedure
2   Talking to the client from the foot of the bed to be available to get added supplies
3   Telling the client that the nurse will take care of another assigned client at this time, so as to be available once the procedure is complete
4   Telling the client to watch television during the procedure as a distraction

**Answer: 1**
*Rationale:* Clients who develop sudden complications are in situational crisis and need therapeutic intervention. Staying with the client, and giving information and encouragement is part of building and maintaining trust in the nurse-client relationship. Options 3 and 4 distance the nurse from the client in the psychosocial as well as physical sense. The nurse should ask another care giver to be available to get extra supplies if needed.

*Test-Taking Strategy:* Use the process of elimination and therapeutic communication techniques. Option 1 is the only option that provides direct contact and assistance to the client. Review therapeutic communication techniques if you had difficulty with this question.

*Level of Cognitive Ability:* Application
*Client Needs:* Psychosocial Integrity
*Integrated Concept/Process:* Caring
*Content Area:* Adult Health/Cardiovascular

*Reference*
Black, J., Hawks, J., & Keene, A. (2001). *Medical-surgical nursing: Clinical management for positive outcomes* (6th ed.). Philadelphia: W.B. Saunders, Philadelphia: W.B. Saunders, 1490.

**202.** A nurse has formulated a nursing diagnosis of Body Image Disturbance for the male client taking spironolactone (Aldactone). The nurse based this diagnosis on assessment of which of the following side effects of the medication?

1 Edema
2 Hair loss
3 Alopecia
4 Decreased libido

**Answer: 4**

*Rationale:* The nurse should be alert to the fact that the client taking spironolactone may experience body image changes as a result of threatened sexual identity. These are related to decreased libido, gynecomastia in males, and hirsuitism in females. Edema and hair loss are not specifically associated with the use of this medication.

*Test-Taking Strategy:* Use the process of elimination and knowledge regarding the side effects of spironolactone. Eliminate options 2 and 3 because they are similar. From the remaining options, focusing on the nursing diagnosis in the question will direct you to option 4. Review the side effects of this medication if you had difficulty with this question.

*Level of Cognitive Ability:* Analysis
*Client Needs:* Psychosocial Integrity
*Integrated Concept/Process:* Nursing Process/Analysis
*Content Area:* Pharmacology

*Reference*
Hodgson, B., & Kizior, R. (2001). *Saunders Nursing drug handbook 2001.* Philadelphia: W.B. Saunders, pp. 942-944.

---

**203.** A nurse is caring for a client who is recovering from the signs and symptoms of autonomic dysreflexia (hyperreflexia). The nurse makes which therapeutic statement to the client?

1 "I'm sure you now understand the importance of preventing this from occurring."
2 "Now that this problem is taken care of, I'm sure you'll be fine."
3 "How could your home care nurse let this happen?"
4 "I have some time if you would like to talk about what happened to you."

**Answer: 4**

*Rationale:* Option 4 encourages the client to discuss feelings. Options 1 and 3 show disapproval and option 2 provides false reassurance. These are nontherapeutic techniques.

*Test-Taking Strategy:* Use the process of elimination and therapeutic communication techniques. Remembering to always address the client's concerns and feelings first will direct you to option 4. Review therapeutic communication techniques if you had difficulty with this question.

*Level of Cognitive Ability:* Application
*Client Needs:* Psychosocial Integrity
*Integrated Concept/Process:* Communication and Documentation
*Content Area:* Adult Health/Neurological

*Reference*
Potter, P., & Perry, A. (2001). *Fundamentals of nursing* (5th ed.). St. Louis: Mosby, p. 459.

---

**204.** While assisting a spinal cord injury client with activities of daily living, the client states, "I can't do this; I wish I were dead." The nurse's best response would be which of the following?

1 "Lets wash your back now."
2 "You wish you were dead?"
3 "I'm sure you are frustrated, but things will work out just fine for you."
4 "Why do you say that?"

**Answer: 2**

*Rationale:* Clarifying is a therapeutic technique involving restating what was said to obtain additional information. Option 1 changes the subject. In option 3, false reassurance is offered. By asking why (option 4), the nurse puts the client on the defensive. Options 1, 3, and 4 are nontherapeutic and block communication.

*Test-Taking Strategy:* Use the process of elimination and therapeutic communication techniques. Remember, focus on the client's feelings. Option 2 identifies clarifying and restating and is the only option that will encourage the client to verbalize feelings and concerns. Review therapeutic communication techniques if you had difficulty with this question.

*Level of Cognitive Ability:* Application
*Client Needs:* Psychosocial Integrity
*Integrated Concept/Process:* Communication and Documentation
*Content Area:* Adult Health/Neurological

*Reference*
Potter, P., & Perry, A. (2001). *Fundamentals of nursing* (5th ed.). St. Louis: Mosby, p. 459.

---

**205.** Family members who are awaiting the outcome of a suicide attempt are tearful. Which statement by the nurse would be most therapeutic to the family at this time?

1 "Don't worry, you have nothing to feel guilty about."
2 "Everything possible is being done."
3 "Let me check to see how long it will be before you can see your loved one."
4 "I can see you are worried."

**Answer: 4**
*Rationale:* Options 1, 2, and 3 are communication blocks. Option 1 labels the family's behavior without their validation. Option 2 uses clichés and false reassurance. Option 3 does not address the family's feelings. Option 4 addresses the family's feelings and displays empathy.

*Test-Taking Strategy:* Use the process of elimination and therapeutic communication techniques. Option 4 identifies clarifying and is the only option that will encourage the family to verbalize feelings and concerns. Review therapeutic communication techniques if you had difficulty with this question.

*Level of Cognitive Ability:* Application
*Client Needs:* Psychosocial Integrity
*Integrated Concept/Process:* Communication and Documentation
*Content Area:* Mental Health

*Reference*
Stuart, G.W., & Laraia, M.T. (1998). *Principles and practice of psychiatric nursing* (6th ed.). St. Louis: Mosby, p. 32.

---

**206.** A nurse is caring for an 11-year-old child who has been abused. Which of the following is most important to include in the plan of care?

1 Encourage the child to fear the abuser
2 Provide a care environment that allows for the development of trust
3 Teach the child to make wise choices when confronted with an abusive situation
4 Have the child point out the abuser if they should visit while the child is hospitalized

**Answer: 2**
*Rationale:* The abused child usually requires long-term therapeutic support. The environment provided during the child's healing must include one in which trust and empathy are modeled and provided for the child. Option 1 reinforces fear, which although it is a legitimate response to abuse, should not be encouraged. Options 3 and 4 ask the child to behave with a maturity beyond that which would be expected for an 11-year-old. Option 2 is the option that is most appropriate because it provides the child with a nurturing and supportive environment in which to begin the healing process.

*Test-Taking Strategy:* Use the process of elimination and therapeutic communication techniques. Option 2 is the only option that provides support to the child. Review therapeutic interventions for a child who has been abused if you had difficulty with this question.

*Level of Cognitive Ability:* Application
*Client Needs:* Psychosocial Integrity
*Integrated Concept/Process:* Caring
*Content Area:* Child Health

*Reference*
Stuart, G.W., & Laraia, M.T. (1998). *Principles and practice of psychiatric nursing* (6th ed.). St. Louis: Mosby, p. 830.

---

**207.** A nurse assesses an elderly client for signs of potential abuse. Which of the following psychosocial factors obtained during the assessment place the client at risk for abuse?
1    The client is completely dependent on family members for receiving food and medicine
2    The client shows signs and symptoms of depression
3    The client resides in a low income neighborhood
4    The client has a chronic illness

**Answer: 1**
*Rationale:* Elder abuse is sometimes the result of frustrated adult children who find themselves caring for dependent parents. Increasing demands by parents for care and financial support can cause resentment and burden. Option 2 relates to depression rather than the risk for abuse. Option 4 relates to a physical factor not a psychosocial factor. The issues of abuse are not bound to socioeconomic status.

*Test-Taking Strategy:* Use the process of elimination. Note the key words *psychosocial factors* and focus on the issue: at risk for abuse. Noting the key words *completely dependent* in option 1 will direct you to this option. If you had difficulty with this question review the risk factors associated with elder abuse.

*Level of Cognitive Ability:* Application
*Client Needs:* Psychosocial Integrity
*Integrated Concept/Process:* Nursing Process/Assessment
*Content Area:* Mental Health

*Reference*
Stuart, G.W., & Laraia, M.T. (1998). *Principles and practice of psychiatric nursing* (6th ed.). St. Louis: Mosby, p. 833.

---

**208.** A nurse is caring for a dying client who says, " What would you say if I asked you to be the executor for my will?" Which of the following nursing responses would be most therapeutic?
1    "Why, I'd be honored to be the executor of your will."
2    "Is there any money in it? I adore money but I am honest."
3    "Your confidence in me is an honor, but I would like to understand more about your thinking."
4    "I'd say, great! No worries. I'll carry out your will just as you want me to."

**Answer: 3**
*Rationale:* In option 3, this nurse is seeking clarification and empathy. The client's question reflects the fact that the client has been thinking about the will and how best to obtain an executor. What is unknown is why the client is asking the nurse to be executor of the will and other specific and important information. In addition, the nurse would want to investigate the legal ramifications, which could arise if such a position was accepted. In option 1, the nurse responds with a social communication with no assessment of the consequences, which is lacking critical thinking and exploration of motivation or client needs. In option 2, the nurse uses histrionic language and crass ideation. In option 4, the nurse provides false reassurance, which is nontherapeutic.

*Test-Taking Strategy:* Use therapeutic communication techniques and the process of elimination. Option 3 is the only option that addresses the client's thoughts and feelings. Review therapeutic communication techniques if you had difficulty with this question.

*Level of Cognitive Ability:* Application
*Client Needs:* Psychosocial Integrity
*Integrated Concept/Process:* Communication and Documentation
*Content Area:* Fundamental Skills

### Reference

Potter, P., & Perry, A. (2001). *Fundamentals of nursing* (5th ed.). St. Louis: Mosby, p. 459.

---

**209.** A client who is suffering from urticaria (hives) and pruritus, says to the nurse, "What am I going to do? I'm getting married next week and I'll probably be covered in this rash and itching like crazy." Which of the following is the most therapeutic nursing response?

1  "You're very troubled that this will extend into your wedding?"
2  "It's probably just from prewedding jitters."
3  "The antihistamine will help a great deal, just you wait and see."
4  "I hope your husband-to-be has a sense of humor."

**Answer: 1**

*Rationale:* The therapeutic communication technique that the nurse uses in option 1 is reflection. In option 2, the nurse minimizes the client's anxiety and fears. In option 3, the nurse talks about antihistamines and asks the client to "wait and see." This is nontherapeutic because the nurse is making promises that may not be kept and because the response is close-ended and shuts off the client's expression of feelings. In option 4, the nurse uses humor inappropriately and with insensitivity.

*Test-Taking Strategy:* Use the process of elimination and therapeutic communication techniques. Options 2, 3, and 4 are nontherapeutic responses. Option 1 addresses the client's feelings. Use therapeutic communication techniques if you had difficulty with this question.

*Level of Cognitive Ability:* Application
*Client Needs:* Psychosocial Integrity
*Integrated Concept/Process:* Communication and Documentation
*Content Area:* Mental Health

### Reference

Stuart, G.W., & Laraia, M.T. (1998). *Principles and practice of psychiatric nursing* (6th ed.). St. Louis: Mosby, p. 34.

---

**210.** A client with a spinal cord injury makes the following comments. Which comment warrants additional intervention by the nurse?

1  "I'm so angry this happened to me."
2  "I know I will have to make major adjustments in my life."
3  "I would like my family members to be here for my teaching sessions."
4  "I'm really looking forward to going home."

**Answer: 1**

*Rationale:* It is important to allow the client with a spinal cord injury to verbalize their feelings. If the client indicates a desire to discuss feelings, the nurse should respond therapeutically. Options 2 and 3 indicate that the client understands changes that will be occurring and that family involvement is best. There are no data in the question that indicates that the client will not be going home, therefore this comment does not require further intervention.

*Test-Taking Strategy:* Use the process of elimination, noting the key words *warrants additional intervention*. Noting the word *angry* in option 1 will direct you to this option. Review psychosocial issues related to the care of a client with a spinal cord injury if you had difficulty with this question.

*Level of Cognitive Ability:* Analysis
*Client Needs:* Psychosocial Integrity
*Integrated Concept/Process:* Nursing Process/Analysis
*Content Area:* Adult Health/Neurological

*Reference*

Black, J., Hawks, J., & Keene, A. (2001). *Medical-surgical nursing: Clinical management for positive outcomes* (6th ed.). Philadelphia: W.B. Saunders, Philadelphia: W.B. Saunders, p. 2049.

---

**211.** A nurse is caring for a client with a grade II cerebral aneurysm rupture. The client becomes restless and anxious before visiting hours. The nurse determines that the client's behavior is likely related to:

1   Fear
2   Ineffective Family Coping
3   Body Image Disturbance
4   Spiritual Distress

**Answer: 3**
*Rationale:* A grade II cerebral aneurysm rupture is a mild bleed in which the client remains alert but has nuchal rigidity with possible neurological deficits, depending on the area of the bleed. Because these clients remain alert, they are acutely aware of the neurological deficits and frequently have some degree of body image disturbance.

*Test-Taking Strategy:* Focus on the client's behavior and note the key words *before visiting hours*. Using knowledge of the effects of this disorder and focusing on the client's behavior will direct you to option 3. Review the effects of a grade II cerebral aneurysm rupture if you had difficulty with this question.

*Level of Cognitive Ability:* Analysis
*Client Needs:* Psychosocial Integrity
*Integrated Concept/Process:* Nursing Process/Analysis
*Content Area:* Adult Health/Neurological

*Reference*

Johnson, M., Bulechek, G., Dochterman, J. Maas, M., Moorhead, S. (2001). *Nursing diagnoses, outcomes, and interventions.* St. Louis: Mosby, p. 115.

---

**212.** In planning care for the client with thromboangiitis obliterans (Buerger's disease), the nurse incorporates measures to help the client cope with the lifestyle changes needed to control the disease process. The nurse can best accomplish this by recommending a:

1   Smoking cessation program
2   Pain management clinic
3   Consult with a dietician
4   Referral to a medical social worker

**Answer: 1**
*Rationale:* Smoking is highly detrimental to the client with Buerger's disease, and clients are recommended to stop completely. Since smoking is a form of chemical dependency, referral to a smoking cessation program may be helpful for many clients. For many clients, symptoms are relieved or alleviated once smoking stops. Options 2, 3, and 4 are not directly related to the physiology associated with this condition.

*Test-Taking Strategy:* Use the process of elimination and focus on the client's diagnosis. Recalling that the treatment goals are the same as for peripheral vascular disease will direct you to option 1. Review the treatment goals for this disorder if you had difficulty with this question.

*Level of Cognitive Ability:* Application
*Client Needs:* Psychosocial Integrity
*Integrated Concept/Process:* Self-Care
*Content Area:* Adult Health/Cardiovascular

### Reference

Black, J., Hawks, J., & Keene, A. (2001). *Medical-surgical nursing: Clinical management for positive outcomes* (6th ed.). Philadelphia: W.B. Saunders, Philadelphia: W.B. Saunders, p. 1421.

---

**213.** A nurse is performing an assessment on a 14-year-old client. On assessment, the nurse notes bruises and bleeding in the genital area, cigarette burns on the chest, rope burns on the buttocks, and multiple old fractures. The client states, "I'm afraid to go home! My stepfather will be angry with me for telling on him!" The most therapeutic nursing response to the client is:

1  "I am sorry that this has happened to you but you will be safe here. Your physician has admitted you until further plans can be made."

2  "You can't go back there with that man. How do you think your mother will react?"

3  "You must know that your presence in the house will only tease your step-father more."

4  "Let's keep this between you, me, and the physician until we can formulate further plans to assist you."

**Answer: 1**
*Rationale:* A child who has been physically and sexually abused should be admitted to the hospital. This will provide time for a more comprehensive evaluation while protecting the child from further abusiveness. The correct option also provides an empathic statement that supports the client to appropriately perceive himself or herself as the victim, while assuring the client of protection from abuse. In option 2, the nurse does not respond with a calm and reassuring communication style, nor does the nurse maintain a professional attitude. Option 3, which holds an innuendo, appears to accuse the victim of teasing the stepfather, and is incorrect. It is also judgmental, controlling, and demeaning. The nurse's suggestion in option 4 is not only incorrect, but is passive in its stance.

*Test-Taking Strategy:* Use the process of elimination, therapeutic communication techniques, and knowledge of care of the child who has been physically abused. Recalling that the priority is safety to the victim will direct you to option 1. Review care of a child who has been abused if you had difficulty with this question.

*Level of Cognitive Ability:* Application
*Client Needs:* Psychosocial Integrity
*Integrated Concept/Process:* Communication and Documentation
*Content Area:* Mental Health

### Reference

Stuart, G.W., & Laraia, M.T. (1998). *Principles and practice of psychiatric nursing* (6th ed.). St. Louis: Mosby, p. 32.

**214.** A nurse is caring for a 12-year-old female client admitted to the hospital with a diagnosis of physical and sexual abuse by her father. That evening, the father angrily approaches the nurse and says, "I'm taking my daughter home. She's told me what you people are up to and we're out of here!" Which of the following would be the most therapeutic nursing response?

1    "Over my dead body you will! She's here and here she stays until the doctor says different. So get off my floor or I'll call hospital security and the police!"

2    "Listen to me. If you attempt to take your daughter from this unit, the police will only bring her back."

3    "Your daughter is ill and needs to be here. I know you want to help her to recover and that you will work to help everyone straighten out the circumstances that caused this. Go to the Chapel and pray for your daughter and for your soul."

4    "You seem very upset. Let's talk at the nurse's station. I want to help you. I know you're very concerned and want to help your daughter. It will be best if you agree to let your daughter stay here for now."

**Answer: 4**

*Rationale:* When a suspected abused child is admitted to the hospital for further evaluation and protection, the physician will usually work with the parents so that they will agree to the admission. If the parents refuse to agree to the admission, the hospital can request an immediate court order to retain the child for a specific length of time. In option 1, the nurse is angry and verbally abusive. It is clear that the nurse has decided that the father is guilty of child abuse. In addition, the nurse is so aggressive and challenging, she may antagonize the father and become a victim of violence as well. In option 2, the command to listen is somewhat demanding. Option 3 seems somewhat pompous and lecturing.

*Test-Taking Strategy:* Use the process of elimination and therapeutic communication techniques. Note that the client of the question is the child's father. Note that option 4 addresses the father's behavior yet protects the child. Review psychosocial issues related to child abuse if you had difficulty with this question.

*Level of Cognitive Ability:* Application
*Client Needs:* Psychosocial Integrity
*Integrated Concept/Process:* Communication and Documentation
*Content Area:* Mental Health

*Reference*
Stuart, G.W., & Laraia, M.T. (1998). *Principles and practice of psychiatric nursing* (6th ed.). St. Louis: Mosby, p. 828.

---

**215.** A client with peripheral arterial disease is being discharged to home. The client is occasionally forgetful about medication, exercise, and diet instructions; needs daily dressing changes to a small open area on the leg; has limited endurance for activities of daily living (ADLs); and lives alone in a one-story house. To best assist the client to adapt to self-care and disease management, the nurse initiates a request to the physician for which follow-up services to be provided in the home?

1    Nursing, home health aide, physical therapy

2    Nursing, home health aide, speech therapy

3    Home health aide, physical therapy, and occupational therapy

4    Nursing, physical therapy, and occupational therapy

**Answer: 1**

*Rationale:* Home health care agencies provide a variety of services to clients, depending on the individual need. The multidisciplinary team includes nurses, home health aides, social workers, and physical, occupational, and speech therapists. Nurses provide skilled nursing services including assessments. Home health aides can assist clients with ADLs, and physical therapists assist in rehabilitation and increasing musculoskeletal endurance. The occupational therapist would train clients to adapt to physical handicaps through new vocational skills and adaptive techniques for ADLs. A speech therapist trains the client to speak.

*Test-Taking Strategy:* Use the process of elimination and focus on the client's needs identified in the question. Recalling the role of each of these health care members and focusing on the client's needs will direct you to option 1. Review the roles of these health care members if you had difficulty with this question.

*Level of Cognitive Ability:* Application
*Client Needs:* Psychosocial Integrity

*Integrated Concept/Process:* Nursing Process/Implementation
*Content Area:* Fundamental Skills

*Reference*
Potter, P., & Perry, A. (2001). *Fundamentals of nursing* (5th ed.). St. Louis: Mosby, p. 395.

---

**216.** A client with chronic arterial leg ulcers complains of pain and tells the nurse, "I'm so discouraged. I have had this pain for over a year now. The pain never seems to go away. I can't do anything, and I feel as though I'll never get better." The nurse would formulate which of the following nursing diagnoses for this client?
1  Acute Pain related to the effects of leg ischemia
2  Chronic Pain related to the non-healing arterial ulcerations
3  Fatigue related to lack of sleep and frustration with illness
4  Ineffective Individual Coping related to chronic illness

**Answer: 2**
*Rationale:* The major focus of the client's complaint is the experience of pain. Pain that has a duration of greater than 6 months is defined as chronic pain, not acute pain. The North American Nursing Diagnosis Association (NANDA) defines Fatigue as "a sense of exhaustion and decreased capacity for physical and mental work." NANDA defines Ineffective Individual Coping as "impairment of adaptive behaviors and abilities of a person in meeting life's demands and roles."

*Test-Taking Strategy:* Use the process of elimination. Focus on the client's statement "I have had this pain for over a year now." This statement and noting the key word *chronic* in the question will direct you to option 2. Review the defining characteristics for this nursing diagnosis if you had difficulty with this question.

*Level of Cognitive Ability:* Analysis
*Client Needs:* Psychosocial Integrity
*Integrated Concept/Process:* Nursing Process/Analysis
*Content Area:* Adult Health/Cardiovascular

*Reference*
Johnson, M., Bulechek, G., Dochterman, J. Maas, M., Moorhead, S. (2001). *Nursing diagnoses, outcomes, and interventions.* St. Louis: Mosby, p. 224.

---

**217.** A client with valvular heart disease is being considered for mechanical valve replacement. Which of the following items does the nurse know is essential to assess before the surgery is done?
1  The likelihood of the client experiencing body image problems
2  The ability to participate in a cardiac rehabilitation program
3  The physical demands of the client's lifestyle
4  The ability to comply with anticoagulant therapy for life

**Answer: 4**
*Rationale:* Mechanical valves carry the associated risk of thromboemboli, which requires long-term anticoagulation with warfarin (Coumadin). There are no data in the question that indicate that physical demands in the client's lifestyle exist. Body image problems are important, but not critical. Not all clients who undergo cardiac surgery need cardiac rehabilitation.

*Test-Taking Strategy:* Use the process of elimination, focusing on the key word *essential*. Recalling that mechanical valves are thrombogenic will direct you to option 4. Review care of a client undergoing a mechanical valve replacement if you had difficulty with this question.

*Level of Cognitive Ability:* Application
*Client Needs:* Physiological Integrity

*Integrated Concept/Process:* Nursing Process/Assessment
*Content Area:* Adult Health/Cardiovascular

*Reference*

Black, J., Hawks, J., & Keene, A. (2001). *Medical-surgical nursing: Clinical management for positive outcomes* (6th ed.). Philadelphia: W.B. Saunders, Philadelphia: W.B. Saunders, p. 1527.

---

**218.** A client who has a history of depression has been prescribed nadolol (Corgard) in the management of angina pectoris. Which of the following items is a priority when the nurse plans to counsel this client about the effects of this medication?
1    High incidence of hypoglycemia
2    Possible exacerbation of depression
3    Risk of tachycardia
4    Probability of fatigue

**Answer: 2**
*Rationale:* Clients with depression or a history of depression have experienced an exacerbation of depression after beginning therapy with beta-adrenergic blocking agents. These clients should be monitored carefully if these agents are prescribed. The medication would cause bradycardia, not tachycardia. Fatigue is a possible side effect, but is not a "priority" item. Hypoglycemia is a sign that is masked with beta-blockers.

*Test-Taking Strategy:* Use the process of elimination. Noting the relationship between the client's history and option 2 will direct you to this option. Review this medication if you had difficulty with this question.

*Level of Cognitive Ability:* Application
*Client Needs:* Psychosocial Integrity
*Integrated Concept/Process:* Teaching/Learning
*Content Area:* Pharmacology

*Reference*

Hodgson, B., & Kizior, R. (2001). *Saunders Nursing drug handbook 2001.* Philadelphia: W.B. Saunders, pp. 712-714.

---

**219.** A nurse is caring for a client with terminal cancer of the throat. The family approaches the nurse and tells that nurse that they have spoken to the physician regarding taking their loved one home. The nurse plans to coordinate discharge planning. Which of the following services would be most supportive to the client and family?
1    American Cancer Society
2    Lung Association
3    Hospice care
4    Local religious and social organizations

**Answer: 3**
*Rationale:* Hospice care provides an environment that emphasizes caring rather than curing. The emphasis is on palliative care. One of the major goals of hospice care is that the client is free of pain and other symptoms that do not allow clients to maintain the quality of their lives. A interdisciplinary approach is utilized. Options 1, 2, and 4 would be helpful but are not the most supportive of the options provided.

*Test-Taking Strategy:* Knowledge regarding the goals and services provided by hospice care will assist in answering the question. Think about what each support service presented in the options will provide in meeting this client's needs. This will assist in directing you to option 3. Review the goals of these support services and hospice care if you had difficulty with this question.

*Level of Cognitive Ability:* Analysis
*Client Needs:* Psychosocial Integrity

*Integrated Concept/Process:* Caring
*Content Area:* Adult Health/Oncology

### Reference
Black, J., Hawks, J., & Keene, A. (2001). *Medical-surgical nursing: Clinical management for positive outcomes* (6th ed.). Philadelphia: W.B. Saunders, Philadelphia: W.B. Saunders, p. 401.

---

**220.** A home health care nurse is caring for a client with acute cancer pain. The most appropriate assessment of the client's pain would include which of the following?
1   The client's pain rating
2   The nurse's impression of the client's pain
3   Verbal and nonverbal clues from the client
4   Pain relief after appropriate nursing intervention

**Answer: 1**
*Rationale:* The client's perception of pain is the hallmark of pain assessment. Usually noted by the client rating on a scale of 1 to 10, the assessment is documented and followed with appropriate medical and nursing intervention. The nurse's impression and the verbal and nonverbal clues are subjective data. Pain relief following intervention is appropriate but relates to evaluation.

*Test-Taking Strategy:* Use the process of elimination. Eliminate option 4 first because it relates to evaluation. Next, eliminate options 2 and 3 because they relate to subjective data. Also, option 1 is client focused. Review the techniques of pain assessment if you had difficulty with this question.

*Level of Cognitive Ability:* Application
*Client Needs:* Physiological Integrity
*Integrated Concept/Process:* Caring
*Content Area:* Adult Health/Oncology

### Reference
Ignatavicius, D., Workman, M., & Mishler, M. (1999). *Medical-surgical nursing across the health care continuum* (3rd ed.). Philadelphia: W.B. Saunders, p. 123.

---

**221.** A prenatal client has been told during a physician office visit that she is positive for human immunodeficiency virus (HIV). The client cried and was significantly distressed regarding this news. Which of the following nursing diagnoses would these data best support?
1   Pain
2   Noncompliance
3   High Risk for Infection
4   Anticipatory Grieving

**Answer: 4**
*Rationale:* A life-threatening diagnosis such as HIV will stimulate the anticipatory grief response. Anticipatory grief occurs when the client, family, and loved ones know that the client will die. The prenatal HIV client is forced to make important changes in her life, frequently resulting in grief related to lost future dreams, and diminished self-esteem resulting from inability to achieve life goals.

*Test-Taking Strategy:* Use the process of elimination, focusing on the data in the question. Noting that the client is distressed and is crying provides supporting data for the nursing diagnosis of Anticipatory Grieving. Review this nursing diagnosis if you had difficulty with this question.

*Level of Cognitive Ability:* Analysis
*Client Needs:* Psychosocial Integrity
*Integrated Concept/Process:* Caring
*Content Area:* Adult Health/Immune

### Reference
Lowdermilk, D., Perry, S., & Bobak, I. (2000). *Maternity & women's health care* (7th ed.). St. Louis: Mosby, p. 1102.

**222.** A nurse is assessing a client's suicide potential. The most important nursing inquiry is:
1    "Why do you want to hurt yourself?"
2    "Can you describe how you are feeling right now?"
3    "Has anyone in your family committed suicide?"
4    "Do you have a plan to commit suicide?"

**Answer: 4**
*Rationale:* When assessing for suicide risk, the nurse must evaluate if the client has a suicide plan. Clients who have a definitive plan pose a greater risk for suicide.

*Test-Taking Strategy:* Use the process of elimination, noting the key words *most important*. Recalling the importance of assessing for a suicide plan will direct you to option 4. If you are unfamiliar with assessment of suicide potential, review this content.

*Level of Cognitive Ability:* Application
*Client Needs:* Psychosocial Integrity
*Integrated Concept/Process:* Communication and Documentation
*Content Area:* Mental Health

*Reference*
Stuart, G.W., & Laraia, M.T. (1998). *Principles and practice of psychiatric nursing* (6th ed.). St. Louis: Mosby, p. 389.

---

**223.** A nurse is caring for a client who is receiving electroconvulsive therapy (ECT) for a major depressive disorder. Which assessment finding would the nurse identify as an unexpected side effect of ECT requiring notifying the physician?
1    Memory loss
2    Disorientation
3    Confusion
4    Hypertension

**Answer: 4**
*Rationale:* The major side effects of ECT are confusion, disorientation, and memory loss. A change in blood pressure would not be an anticipated side effect and would be a cause for concern. If hypertension occurred following ECT, the physician should be notified.

*Test-Taking Strategy:* Use the process of elimination, focusing on the issue: an unexpected side effect. Recall the side effects of ECT and note that options 1, 2, and 3 are similar. Review the expected and unexpected side effects of ECT if you had difficulty with this question.

*Level of Cognitive Ability:* Analysis
*Client Needs:* Psychosocial Integrity
*Integrated Concept/Process:* Nursing Process/Assessment
*Content Area:* Mental Health

*Reference*
Stuart, G.W., & Laraia, M.T. (1998). *Principles and practice of psychiatric nursing* (6th ed.). St. Louis: Mosby, p. 609.

---

**224.** During the admission assessment of a client admitted to the hospital for esophageal varices, the client says, "I deserve this. I brought it on myself." The nurse's most appropriate response is:
1    "Would you like to talk to the chaplain?"
2    "Not all esophageal varices are caused by alcohol."
3    "Is there some reason you feel you deserve this?"
4    "That is something to think about when you leave the hospital."

**Answer: 3**
*Rationale:* Ruptured esophageal varices are often a complication of cirrhosis of the liver and the most common type of cirrhosis is caused by chronic alcohol abuse. It is important to obtain an accurate history of alcohol intake from the client. If the client is ashamed or embarrassed, he or she may not respond accurately. Option 3 is open-ended and allows the client to discuss feelings about drinking. Option 1 blocks the nurse/client communication process. Options 2 and 4 are somewhat judgmental.

*Test-Taking Strategy:* Use the process of elimination and therapeutic communication techniques to direct you to option 3. Remember that the client's feelings should be addressed first.

Review therapeutic communication techniques if you had difficulty with this question.

*Level of Cognitive Ability:* Application
*Client Needs:* Psychosocial Integrity
*Integrated Concept/Process:* Communication and Documentation
*Content Area:* Adult Health/Gastrointestinal

*Reference*
Smeltzer, S., & Bare, B. (2000). *Brunner & Suddarth's Textbook of medical-surgical nursing* (9th ed.). Philadelphia: Lippincott Williams & Wilkins, p. 928.

---

**225.** A nurse is performing a neurological assessment on a client with dementia and is assessing the function of the frontal lobes of the brain. Assessment of which of the following items by the nurse would yield the best information about this area of functioning?
1 Level of consciousness
2 Insight, judgment, and planning
3 Feelings or emotions
4 Eye movements

**Answer: 2**
*Rationale:* Insight, judgment, and planning are part of the function of the frontal lobe. Level of consciousness is controlled by the reticular activating system. Feelings are part of the role of the limbic system. Eye movements are under the control of cranial nerves III, IV, and VI.

*Test-Taking Strategy:* A specific understanding of the function of the frontal lobe of the brain will direct you to option 2. Review the function of this lobe if you had difficulty with this question.

*Level of Cognitive Ability:* Application
*Client Needs:* Psychosocial Integrity
*Integrated Concept/Process:* Nursing Process/Assessment
*Content Area:* Adult Health/Neurological

*Reference*
Smeltzer, S., & Bare, B. (2000). *Brunner & Suddarth's Textbook of medical surgical nursing* (9th ed.). Philadelphia: Lippincott Williams & Wilkins, p. 1611.

## CRITICAL THINKING: FREE-TEXT ENTRY

**1.** A clinic nurse is performing a physical assessment on an 8-year-old child. During the assessment, the nurse notes the presence of swelling and lacerations in the genital area. The child is hesitant to answers questions that the nurse is asking and consistently looks at the mother in a fearful manner. The nurse suspects that the child is a victim of which type of abuse?

**Answer:** Sexual abuse
*Rationale:* The most likely assessment findings in sexual abuse include difficulty walking or sitting, torn, stained or bloody underclothing, pain, swelling or itching of the genitals, and bruises, and bleeding or lacerations in the genital or anal area.

*Test-Taking Strategy:* Focus on the assessment findings noted in the question and focus on the issue: the type of abuse suspected. Noting the key words *swelling and lacerations in the genital area* will assist you in answering the question. If you had difficulty with this question, review the assessment findings in a child suspected of sexual abuse.

*Level of Cognitive Ability:* Analysis
*Client Needs:* Psychosocial Integrity
*Integrated Concept/Process:* Nursing Process/Assessment
*Content Area:* Child Health

### Reference
Ball, J., & Bindler, R. (1999). *Pediatric nursing: Caring for children* (2nd ed.). Stamford, Conn.: Appleton & Lange, p. 994.

---

**2.** A nurse is monitoring a client who is diagnosed as having schizophrenia. The client continuously repeats words or phrases that are purposeless. The nurse documents that the client is exhibiting what type of speech pattern?

**Answer:** Verbigeration

*Rationale:* Verbigeration is the purposeless repetition of words or phrases. It is a type of speech pattern that may be noted in a client with schizophrenia.

*Test-Taking Strategy:* Focus on the key words *repeats words or phrases that are purposeless.* Use knowledge of the descriptions of the various types of speech patterns noted in a client with schizophrenia to answer this question. If you had difficulty with this question, review altered speech patterns in the client with schizophrenia.

*Level of Cognitive Ability:* Analysis
*Client Needs:* Psychosocial Integrity
*Integrated Concept/Process:* Nursing Process/Assessment
*Content Area:* Mental Health

### Reference
Stuart, G.W., & Laraia, M.T. (1998). *Principles and practice of psychiatric nursing* (6th ed.). St. Louis: Mosby, p. 409.

---

**3.** A nurse is performing an assessment on a client admitted to the mental health unit who is at risk for self-harm. In performing a lethality assessment, the nurse asks the client what most appropriate question?

**Answer:** "Do you have any thoughts of killing yourself and a specific plan?"

*Rationale:* A lethality assessment requires direct communication between the client and the nurse concerning the client's intent. It is important to provide a question that is directly related to lethality. The nurse should ask the client about the presence of thoughts or a plan related to self-harm.

*Test-Taking Strategy:* Note the key words *at risk for self-harm* and the issue: a lethality assessment. Recall that assessing for thoughts of self-harm and a suicide plan is the priority during a lethality assessment. If you had difficulty with this question, review assessment for suicide risk.

*Level of Cognitive Ability:* Application
*Client Needs:* Psychosocial Integrity
*Integrated Concept/Process:* Nursing Process/Assessment
*Content Area:* Mental Health

### Reference
Stuart, G.W., & Laraia, M.T. (1998). *Principles and practice of psychiatric nursing* (6th ed.). St. Louis: Mosby, p. 389.

**4.** A nurse is caring for a client who is receiving lithium carbonate (Lithium) for the treatment of bipolar disorder. A lithium level is performed on the client and the results indicate a level of 1.0 mEq/L. The nurse documents what interpretation regarding this laboratory result?

**Answer:** The lithium level is within normal limits
*Rationale:* The therapeutic level for lithium is 0.8 to 1.2 mEq/L. A level of 1.0 mEq/L indicates a therapeutic level.

*Test-Taking Strategy:* Knowledge regarding the therapeutic lithium level is required to answer this question. If you are unfamiliar with this level, review this content.

*Level of Cognitive Ability:* Analysis
*Client Needs:* Psychosocial Integrity
*Integrated Concept/Process:* Nursing Process/Analysis
*Content Area:* Pharmacology

*Reference*
Hodgson, B., & Kizior, R. (2001). *Saunders Nursing drug handbook 2001.* Philadelphia: W.B. Saunders, pp. 598-600.

# REFERENCES

Ball, J., & Bindler, R. (1999). *Pediatric nursing: Caring for children* (2nd ed.). Stamford, Conn.: Appleton & Lange.

Black, J., Hawks, J., & Keene, A. (2001). *Medical-surgical nursing: Clinical management for positive outcomes* (6th ed.). Philadelphia: W.B. Saunders.

Hodgson, B., & Kizior, R. (2001). *Saunders Nursing drug handbook 2001.* Philadelphia: W.B. Saunders.

Ignatavicius, D., Workman, M., & Mishler, M. (1999). *Medical-surgical nursing across the health care continuum* (3rd ed.). Philadelphia: W.B. Saunders.

Johnson, M., Bulechek, G., Dochterman, J. Maas, M., Moorhead, S. (2001). *Nursing diagnoses, outcomes, and interventions.* St. Louis: Mosby.

Leahy, J., & Kizilay, P. (1998). *Foundations of nursing practice: A nursing process approach.* Philadelphia: W.B. Saunders.

Lowdermilk, D., Perry, S., & Bobak, I. (2000). *Maternity & women's health care* (7th ed.). St. Louis: Mosby.

Maher, A., Salmond, S., & Pellino, T. (1998). *Orthopaedic nursing* (2nd ed.). Philadelphia: W.B. Saunders.

Monahan, F., & Neighbors, M. (1998). *Medical-surgical nursing: Foundations for clinical practice* (2nd ed.). Philadelphia: W.B. Saunders.

Potter, P., & Perry, A. (2001). *Fundamentals of nursing* (5th ed.). St. Louis: Mosby.

Sherwen, L., Scoloveno, M.A., & Weingarten, C. (1999). *Maternity nursing: Care of the childbearing family* (3rd ed.). Stamford, Conn.: Appleton & Lange.

Smeltzer, S., & Bare, B. (2000). *Brunner & Suddarth's Textbook of medical-surgical nursing* (9th ed.). Philadelphia: Lippincott Williams & Wilkins.

Sole, M.L., Lamborn, M., & Hartshorn, J. (2001). *Introduction to critical care nursing* (3rd ed.). Philadelphia: W.B. Saunders.

Stuart, G.W., & Laraia, M.T. (1998). *Principles and practice of psychiatric nursing* (6th ed.). St. Louis: Mosby.

Wong, D. (1999). *Whaley & Wong's Nursing care of infants and children* (6th ed.). St. Louis: Mosby.

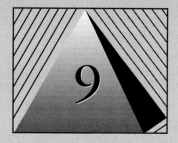

# Health Promotion and Maintenance

**1.** A mother of a teenage client with an anxiety disorder is concerned about her daughter's progress after discharge. She states that her daughter "stashes food, eats all the wrong things that make her hyperactive," and "hangs out with the wrong crowd." In helping the mother prepare for her daughter's discharge, the nurse advises the mother to:

1   Restrict the daughter's socializing time with her friends

2   Consider taking time from work to help her daughter readjust to the home environment

3   Limit the amount of chocolate and caffeine products in the home

4   Keep her daughter out of school until she can adjust to the school environment

**Answer: 3**

*Rationale:* Clients with anxiety disorder are advised to limit their intake of caffeine, chocolate, and alcohol. These products have the potential of increasing anxiety. Options 1 and 4 are unreasonable and are an unhealthy approach. It may not be realistic for a family member to take time from work.

*Test-Taking Strategy:* Use the process of elimination. Options 1, 2, and 4 are similar and are concerned with monitoring or curtailing the client's physical activities, while option 3 addresses preparation of the environment. Option 3 also focuses on the issue of the question. Review home care measures for the client with anxiety disorder if you had difficulty with this question.

*Level of Cognitive Ability:* Application
*Client Needs:* Health Promotion and Maintenance
*Integrated Concept/Process:* Teaching/Learning
*Content Area:* Mental Health

*Reference*
Stuart, G.W., & Laraia, M.T. (1998). *Principles and practice of psychiatric nursing.* (6th ed.). St. Louis: Mosby, p. 646.

**2.** A nurse caring for the client with hepatic encephalopathy assesses for asterixis. To appropriately test for asterixis the nurse:
1 Asks the client to extend an arm, dorsiflex the wrist, and extend the fingers
2 Checks the stools for clay-colored pigmentation
3 Asks the client to sign his or her name on a piece of paper and note for any deterioration in hand movements
4 Reviews laboratory serum levels of bilirubin and alkaline phosphatase for elevation

**Answer: 1**
*Rationale:* Asterixis is an abnormal muscle tremor often associated with hepatic encephalopathy. Asterixis is sometimes called "liver flap." Options 2, 3, and 4 are associated with hepatitis but are not signs of asterixis.

*Test-Taking Strategy:* Recalling the signs and symptoms of hepatic encephalopathy will direct you to option 1. Also, focus on the definition of asterixis. If you are unfamiliar with assessment for asterixis, review this technique.

*Level of Cognitive Ability:* Application
*Client Needs:* Health Promotion and Maintenance
*Integrated Concept/Process:* Nursing Process/Assessment
*Content Area:* Adult Health/Gastrointestinal

*Reference*
Smeltzer, S., & Bare, B. (2000). *Brunner & Suddarth's Textbook of medical-surgical nursing* (9th ed.). Philadelphia: Lippincott Williams & Wilkins, p. 938.

**3.** A nurse assesses the twelfth cranial nerve in the client who sustained a cerebrovascular accident (CVA). When assessing the twelfth cranial nerve, the nurse asks the client to:
1 Extend the arms
2 Turn the head toward the nurse's arm
3 Extend the tongue
4 Focus the eyes on the object held by the nurse

**Answer: 3**
*Rationale:* To assess the function of the twelfth cranial (hypoglossal) nerve, the nurse would assess the client's ability to extend the tongue. Impairment of the twelfth cranial nerve can occur with a CVA. Options 1, 2, and 4 do not test the function of the twelfth cranial nerve.

*Test-Taking Strategy:* Recalling that the twelfth cranial nerve is the hypoglossal nerve will direct you to option 3. Review the cranial nerves and the method of testing these nerves if you had difficulty with this question.

*Level of Cognitive Ability:* Application
*Client Needs:* Health Promotion and Maintenance
*Integrated Concept/Process:* Nursing Process/Assessment
*Content Area:* Adult Health/Neurological

*Reference*
Ignatavicius, D., Workman, M., & Mishler, M. (1999). *Medical-surgical nursing across the health care continuum* (3rd ed.). Philadelphia: W.B. Saunders, p. 1009.

**4.** A client with diabetes mellitus is being discharged from the hospital after an occurrence of hyperglycemic hyperosmolar nonketotic syndrome (HHNS). The nurse develops a discharge teaching plan for the client and identifies which of the following as the priority?
1 Exercise routines
2 Signs and symptoms of dehydration
3 The need to keep follow-up appointments
4 How to control dietary intake

**Answer: 2**
*Rationale:* Clients at risk for HHNS should immediately report signs and symptoms of dehydration to health care providers. Dehydration can be severe and may progress rapidly. Although options 1, 3, and 4 are a component of the teaching plan, in the client with HHNS, dehydration is the priority.

*Test-Taking Strategy:* Use the process of elimination, noting the key word *priority*. Look at each option in terms of its seriousness and recall that dehydration can rapidly progress to HHNS. Review HHNS if you had difficulty with this question.

*Level of Cognitive Ability:* Application
*Client Needs:* Health Promotion and Maintenance

*Integrated Concept/Process:* Teaching/Learning
*Content Area:* Adult Health/Endocrine

**Reference**
Smeltzer, S., & Bare, B. (2000). *Brunner & Suddarth's Textbook of medical-surgical nursing* (9th ed.). Philadelphia: Lippincott Williams & Wilkins, p. 1007.

**5.** A nurse develops a plan of care for an elderly client with diabetes mellitus. The nurse plans to first:

1   Teach with videotapes showing insulin administration to ensure competence

2   Assess the client's ability to read label markings on syringes and blood glucose monitoring equipment

3   Structure menus for adherence to diet

4   Encourage dependence to prepare the client for the chronicity of the disease

**Answer: 2**
*Rationale:* The nurse first assesses the client's ability to care for self. Allowing the client "hands on" experience rather than teaching with videos is more effective. Independence should be encouraged. Structuring menus for the client promotes dependence.

*Test-Taking Strategy:* Use the steps of the nursing process. Option 2 reflects assessment, the first step of the nursing process. Review teaching/learning principles and the teaching/learning needs of the elderly if you had difficulty with this question.

*Level of Cognitive Ability:* Application
*Client Needs:* Health Promotion and Maintenance
*Integrated Concept/Process:* Teaching/Learning
*Content Area:* Adult Health/Endocrine

**Reference**
Smeltzer, S., & Bare, B. (2000). *Brunner & Suddarth's Textbook of medical-surgical nursing* (9th ed.). Philadelphia: Lippincott Williams & Wilkins, p. 1020.

**6.** A nurse is conducting a health screening on a client with a family history of hypertension. Which assessment finding would alert the nurse to the need for teaching related to cerebrovascular accident (CVA) prevention?

1   Eats two bowls of high-fiber grain cereal with skim milk for breakfast

2   Works as the manager of a busy medical-surgical unit yet jogs 2 miles daily

3   Uses oral contraceptives and condoms for pregnancy and disease prevention

4   Has a blood pressure (BP) of 136/86 mmHg and has lost ten pounds recently

**Answer: 3**
*Rationale:* Obesity, hypertension, hypercholesterolemia, smoking, and the use of oral contraceptives are all modifiable risk factors for CVA. Oral contraceptive use is discouraged in some clients due to the side effect of clot formation. A low-fat diet and stress reduction methods are encouraged and identified in options 1 and 2. Although option 4 identifies a borderline BP, the client has made a change in eating habits.

*Test-Taking Strategy:* Use the process of elimination, noting the issue: a need for teaching related to CVA prevention. Recalling the risk factors related to CVA will direct you to option 3. If you had difficulty with this question and are unfamiliar with the risk factors related to CVA, review this content.

*Level of Cognitive Ability:* Analysis
*Client Needs:* Health Promotion and Maintenance
*Integrated Concept/Process:* Nursing Process/Assessment
*Content Area:* Adult Health/Neurological

**Reference**
Ignatavicius, D., Workman, M., & Mishler, M. (1999). *Medical-surgical nursing across the health care continuum* (3rd ed.). Philadelphia: W.B. Saunders, p. 1110.

**7.** A nurse is reviewing assessment data on a clinic client. Which assessment data would be most important for the client to modify to lessen the risk for coronary artery disease (CAD)?

1 Elevated high-density lipoprotein (HDL) levels

2 Elevated low-density lipoprotein (LDL) levels

3 Elevated triglyceride levels

4 Elevated serum lipase levels

**Answer: 2**

*Rationale:* LDL is more directly associated with CAD than other lipoproteins. LDL levels, along with cholesterol, have a higher predictive association for CAD than triglycerides. Additionally, HDL is inversely associated with the risk of CAD. Lipase is a digestive enzyme that breaks down ingested fats in the gastrointestinal tract.

*Test-Taking Strategy:* Knowledge regarding the risk factors related to CAD will direct you to option 2. If you are unfamiliar with these risk factors, review this content.

*Level of Cognitive Ability:* Analysis
*Client Needs:* Health Promotion and Maintenance
*Integrated Concept/Process:* Nursing Process/Assessment
*Content Area:* Adult Health/Cardiovascular

*Reference*
Smeltzer, S., & Bare, B. (2000). *Brunner & Suddarth's Textbook of medical-surgical nursing* (9th ed.). Philadelphia: Lippincott Williams & Wilkins, p. 595.

---

**8.** A nurse is taking a history from a client suspected of having testicular cancer. Which of the following data will be most helpful in determining risk factors of this type of cancer?

1 Number of sexual partners

2 Age and race

3 Geographic location

4 Marital status and number of children

**Answer: 2**

*Rationale:* Two basic but important risk factors for testicular cancer are age and race. The disease occurs most frequently in Caucasian males between the ages of 18 and 40 years. Other risk factors include a history of undescended testis and a family history of testicular cancer. Marital status and number of children do not pose a risk factor for males and cancer.

*Test-Taking Strategy:* Use the process of elimination and knowledge of the risk factors associated with this type of cancer. Recalling that testicular cancer most often occurs between ages 18 and 40 will help to eliminate other options. If you had difficulty with this question, review the risk factors related to testicular cancer.

*Level of Cognitive Ability:* Analysis
*Client Needs:* Health Promotion and Maintenance
*Integrated Concept/Process:* Nursing Process/Assessment
*Content Area:* Adult Health/Oncology

*Reference*
Smeltzer, S., & Bare, B. (2000). *Brunner & Suddarth's Textbook of medical-surgical nursing* (9th ed.). Philadelphia: Lippincott Williams & Wilkins, p. 1319.

**9.** A client with a history of ear problems is going on vacation by aircraft. The nurse advises the client to avoid which of the following to prevent barotrauma during ascent and descent of the airplane?
1  Sucking hard candy
2  Swallowing
3  Yawning
4  Keeping the mouth motionless

**Answer: 4**
*Rationale:* Clients who are prone to barotrauma should perform any of a variety of mouth movements to equalize pressure in the ear, particularly during ascent and descent of an aircraft. These can include yawning, swallowing, drinking, chewing, or sucking on hard candy. Valsalva maneuver may also be helpful. The client should avoid sitting with the mouth motionless during this time, because this aggravates pressure build-up behind the tympanic membrane.

*Test-Taking Strategy:* Use the process of elimination and note the key word *avoid*. Eliminate options 1, 2, and 3, because they are similar and involve movement of the mouth. Review the measures that will prevent barotrauma of the ear if you had difficulty with this question.

*Level of Cognitive Ability:* Application
*Client Needs:* Health Promotion and Maintenance
*Integrated Concept/Process:* Teaching/Learning
*Content Area:* Adult Health/Ear

*Reference*
Beare, P., & Myers, J. (1998). *Adult health nursing* (3rd ed.). St. Louis: Mosby, p. 1176.

**10.** A community health nurse is working with food services in a rural school setting. A goal for the school dietary program is to avoid nutritional deficiencies and enhance children's nutritional status through healthy dietary practices. In implementing interventions by levels of prevention, which of the following would be a primary prevention intervention that the nurse could use?
1  Case finding in the school to identify dietary practices
2  School screening programs for early detection of children with poor eating habits
3  Providing educational programs, literature, and posters to promote awareness of healthy eating
4  Conducting a community-wide dietary screening activity to detect community dietary trends

**Answer: 3**
*Rationale:* Primary prevention interventions are those measures that keep illness, injury, or potential problems from occurring, therefore option 3 is correct. Options 1, 2, and 4 are secondary prevention measures that seek to detect existing health problems or trends.

*Test-Taking Strategy:* Note the issue of the question, primary prevention intervention. Knowledge that primary prevention interventions are those measures that keep illness from occurring will direct you to option 3. If you had difficulty with this question, review the levels of prevention.

*Level of Cognitive Ability:* Application
*Client Needs:* Health Promotion and Maintenance
*Integrated Concept/Process:* Nursing Process/Implementation
*Content Area:* Fundamental Skills

*Reference*
Craven, R., & Hirnle, C. (2000). *Fundamentals of nursing: Human health and function* (3rd ed.). Philadelphia: Lippincott, p. 665.

**11.** A nursing instructor asks a nursing student to identify situations that indicate a secondary level of prevention in health care. Which situation if identified by the student would indicate a need for further study of the levels of prevention?

1  Teaching a stroke client how to use a walker

2  Encouraging a client to take antihypertensive medications as prescribed

3  Screening for hypertension in a community

4  Encouraging a woman over 40 years of age to obtain periodic mammograms

**Answer: 1**

*Rationale:* Secondary prevention focuses on the early diagnosis and prompt treatment of disease. Tertiary prevention is represented by rehabilitation services. Options 3 and 4 identify screening procedures and option 2 identifies a treatment of a disease. Option 1 identifies a rehabilitative service.

*Test-Taking Strategy:* Note the key words *indicate a need for further study.* Use knowledge regarding the characteristics of the various levels of prevention to assist in directing you to the correct option. Review the levels of prevention if you had difficulty with this question.

*Level of Cognitive Ability:* Analysis
*Client Needs:* Health Promotion and Maintenance
*Integrated Concept/Process:* Teaching/Learning
*Content Area:* Fundamental Skills

*Reference*
Craven, R., & Hirnle, C. (2000). *Fundamentals of nursing: Human health and function* (3rd ed.). Philadelphia: Lippincott, p. 665.

**12.** A substance abuse clinic nurse is providing dietary instructions to clients. A client asks the nurse about the foods that are high in thiamine. The nurse tells the client that which food is especially rich in this vitamin?

1  Chicken

2  Broccoli

3  Pork

4  Milk

**Answer: 3**

*Rationale:* Thiamine is present in a variety of foods of plant and animal origin. Pork products are especially rich in this vitamin. Other good sources include nuts, whole-grain cereals, and legumes.

*Test-Taking Strategy:* Note the key words *especially rich* in the stem of the question. This may indicate that more than one option may contain thiamine. Use the process of elimination and knowledge regarding food items high in thiamine to answer this question. If you are unfamiliar with these foods, review this content.

*Level of Cognitive Ability:* Application
*Client Needs:* Health Promotion and Maintenance
*Integrated Concept/Process:* Teaching/Learning
*Content Area:* Mental Health

*Reference*
Harkreader. H. (2000). *Fundamentals of nursing: Caring and clinical judgment.* Philadelphia: W.B. Saunders, p. 683.

**13.** A nurse provides home care instructions to a mother of an infant with a diagnosis of hydrocephalus. Which statement, if made by the mother, indicates an understanding of the care of the infant?

  **1**    "I need to keep my infant's head in a pushed back position during sleep."

  **2**    "I need to feed my infant in a flat, side-lying position."

  **3**    "I need to place my infant on its stomach with a towel under the neck for sleep."

  **4**    "I need to support my infant's neck and head."

**Answer: 4**

*Rationale:* Hydrocephalus is a condition characterized by an enlargement of the cranium due to an abnormal accumulation of cerebrospinal fluid within the cerebral ventricular system. This characteristic causes an increase in the weight of the infant's head. The infant's head becomes top heavy. Supporting the infant's head and neck when picking the infant up will prevent the hyperextension of the neck area and the infant from falling backwards. Hyperextension of the infant's head can put pressure on the neck vertebrae causing injury. Options 1 and 3 will cause hyperextension. The infant should be fed with the head elevated for proper motility of food processing.

*Test-Taking Strategy:* Note the key words *indicates an understanding*. Use the process of elimination and eliminate option 2 first, because feeding any infant in this position is unsafe. Note the similarity between options 1 and 3. Both of these positions will cause hyperextension of the infant's neck. If you had difficulty with this question, review care of an infant with hydrocephalus.

*Level of Cognitive Ability:* Analysis
*Client Needs:* Health Promotion and Maintenance
*Integrated Concept/Process:* Teaching/Learning
*Content Area:* Child Health

*Reference*
Wong, D. (1999). *Whaley & Wong's Nursing care of infants and children* (6th ed.). St. Louis: Mosby, p. 499.

**14.** A nurse is preparing a teaching plan for the parents of an infant with a ventricular peritoneal shunt. The nurse plans to include which of the following instructions in the plan of care?

  **1**    Call the physician if the infant is fussy

  **2**    Position the infant on the side of the shunt when the infant is put to bed

  **3**    Expect an increased urine output from the shunt

  **4**    Call the physician if the infant has a high-pitched cry

**Answer: 4**

*Rationale:* If the shunt is broken or malfunctioning, the fluid from the ventricle part of the brain will not be diverted to the peritoneal cavity. The cerebrospinal fluid will build up in the cranial area. The result is intracranial pressure, which then causes a high-pitched cry in the infant. The infant should not be positioned on the side of the shunt, because this will cause pressure on the shunt and skin breakdown. This type of shunt affects the gastrointestinal system, not the genitourinary system, and an increased urinary output is not expected. Option 1 is only a concern if other signs indicative of a complication are occurring.

*Test-Taking Strategy:* Use the process of elimination. Remember that a high-pitched cry in an infant indicates a concern or problem. If you had difficulty with this question, review significant assessment findings and home care instructions for the parents of an infant with a shunt.

*Level of Cognitive Ability:* Application
*Client Needs:* Health Promotion and Maintenance
*Integrated Concept/Process:* Teaching/Learning
*Content Area:* Child Health

*Reference*
Ball, J., & Bindler, R. (1999). *Pediatric nursing: Caring for children* (2nd ed.). Stamford, Conn.: Appleton & Lange, pp. 758; 783.

**15.** A home health nurse visits a child with Reye's syndrome and plans to provide instructions to the mother regarding care of the child. The nurse plans to instruct the mother to:

1   Increase the stimuli in the environment

2   Give the child frequent, small meals if vomiting occurs

3   Avoid daytime naps so that the child will sleep at night

4   Check the child's skin and eyes every day for a yellow discoloration

**Answer: 4**

*Rationale:* Checking for jaundice will assist in identifying the presence of liver complications that are characteristic of Reye's syndrome. If vomiting occurs in Reye's syndrome, it is caused by cerebral edema, is a sign of increased intracranial pressure, and needs to be reported. Decreasing stimuli and providing rest decreases stress on the brain tissue. Options 1 and 3 do not promote a restful environment for the child.

*Test-Taking Strategy:* Read each option carefully and think about the manifestations and complications associated with Reye's syndrome. Recalling that increased intracranial pressure is a concern will assist in eliminating option 2. Eliminate options 1 and 3, because they are similar in that they do not promote a restful environment for the child. Review care of a child with Reye's syndrome if you had difficulty with this question.

*Level of Cognitive Ability:* Application
*Client Needs:* Health Promotion and Maintenance
*Integrated Concept/Process:* Teaching/Learning
*Content Area:* Child Health

*Reference*
Bowden, V., Dickey, S., & Greenberg, C. (1998). *Children and their families: The continuum of care.* Philadelphia: W.B. Saunders, p. 1403.

---

**16.** A nurse in the well baby clinic has provided instructions regarding dental care to a mother of a 10-month-old child. Which statement if made by the mother indicates a need for further instructions?

1   "I need to start dental hygiene as soon as the primary teeth erupt."

2   "I need to use fluoride supplements if the water is not fluoridated."

3   "I can coat a pacifier with honey during the day as long as I do not give my child a bottle at nap or bedtime."

4   "I need to limit the amount of concentrated sweets."

**Answer: 3**

*Rationale:* The practice of coating pacifiers with honey or using commercially available hard-candy pacifiers is discouraged. Besides being cariogenic, honey may also cause botulism, and parts of the candy pacifier may be aspirated. Additionally, a bottle at nap or bedtime that contains sweet milk or other fluids such as juice, bathes the teeth, producing caries. Fluoride, an essential mineral for building caries-resistant teeth, is needed beginning at 6 months of age if the infant does not receive adequate fluoride content. A diet that is low in sweets and high in nutritious food promotes dental health.

*Test-Taking Strategy:* Note the key words *indicates a need for further instructions.* Use the process of elimination and keep in mind that the issue relates to the prevention of dental caries. Recalling that honey is cariogenic and may also cause botulism will direct you to option 3. Review dental care measures if you had difficulty with this question.

*Level of Cognitive Ability:* Analysis
*Client Needs:* Health Promotion and Maintenance
*Integrated Concept/Process:* Teaching/Learning
*Content Area:* Child Health

*Reference*
Wong, D. (1999). *Whaley & Wong's Nursing care of infants and children* (6th ed.). St. Louis: Mosby, p. 594.

**17.** A 7-year-old is hospitalized with a fracture of the femur and is placed in traction. In meeting the psychosocial needs of the child, the nurse most appropriately selects which of the following play activities for the child?

1   A coloring book with crayons
2   A finger-painting set
3   A large puzzle
4   A board game

**Answer: 4**

*Rationale:* The school-aged child becomes organized with more direction with play activities. Such activities include collections, drawing, construction, dolls, pets, guessing games, board games, riddles, hobbies, competitive games, and listening to the radio or television. Options 1 and 2 are most appropriate for a pre-schooler. Option 3 is most appropriate for a toddler.

*Test-Taking Strategy:* Note the age and the diagnosis of the child to answer this question. Knowledge regarding the toys and specific types of age-related play activities that are appropriate for the school-aged child will assist in directing you to option 4. If you had difficulty with this question, review the age appropriate activities for the school-aged child.

*Level of Cognitive Ability:* Application
*Client Needs:* Health Promotion and Maintenance
*Integrated Concept/Process:* Nursing Process/Implementation
*Content Area:* Child Health

*Reference*
Wong, D. (1999). *Whaley & Wong's Nursing care of infants and children* (6th ed.). St. Louis: Mosby, p. 791.

**18.** A clinic nurse has provided information to the mother of a toddler regarding toilet-training. Which statement if made by the mother would indicate a need for further instructions?

1   "I should wait until my child is between 18 and 24 months old."
2   "I know that my child will develop bowel control before bladder control."
3   "I should have my child sit on the potty until the child urinates."
4   "I know my child is ready to begin toilet training if my child is walking."

**Answer: 3**

*Rationale:* The child should not be forced to sit on the potty for long periods of time. The physical ability to control the anal and urethral sphincters is achieved sometime after the child is walking, probably between ages 18 and 24 months. Bowel control is usually achieved before bladder control.

*Test-Taking Strategy:* Note the key words *a need for further instructions* in the stem of the question. Use the process of elimination, recalling that forcing a child to develop this behavior will result in a negative response. Review the task of toilet-training if you had difficulty with this question.

*Level of Cognitive Ability:* Analysis
*Client Needs:* Health Promotion and Maintenance
*Integrated Concept/Process:* Teaching/Learning
*Content Area:* Child Health

*Reference*
Wong, D. (1999). *Whaley & Wong's Nursing care of infants and children* (6th ed.). St. Louis: Mosby, p. 673.

**19.** A clinic nurse is performing an assessment on a 12-month-old infant. The nurse determines that the infant is demonstrating the highest level of developmental achievement if the 12-month-old is able to:

1 Produce cooing sounds
2 Produce babbling sounds
3 Obey simple commands
4 Begin to use simple words

**Answer: 4**

*Rationale:* Simple words as "mama" and the use of gestures to communicate begins between 9 and 12 months of age. A 1 to 3 month old infant will produce cooing sounds. Babbling is common in a 3 to 4 month old infant. Between 8 and 9 months, the infant begins to understand and obey simple commands such as "wave bye-bye." Using single consonant babbling occurs between 6 and 8 months.

*Test-Taking Strategy:* Note that the infant is 12 months of age and note the key words *highest level.* Use the process of elimination and knowledge of language and communication developmental milestones to answer the question. Review these milestones if you had difficulty with this question.

*Level of Cognitive Ability:* Analysis
*Client Needs:* Health Promotion and Maintenance
*Integrated Concept/Process:* Nursing Process/Assessment
*Content Area:* Child Health

*Reference*
Wong, D. (1999). *Whaley & Wong's Nursing care of infants and children* (6th ed.). St. Louis: Mosby, p. 680.

---

**20.** A nurse is instructing a maternity client how to keep a fetal activity diary. Which of the following instructions would the nurse provide to the client?

1 "Schedule the counting periods about 1 hour before eating."
2 "Lie on your stomach when you prepare to count the fetal movement."
3 "You should expect the baby to move at least 35 times in 3 hours."
4 "You need to contact the physician if the baby's movements are less than 10 times in 3 hours."

**Answer: 4**

*Rationale:* Most healthy fetuses move at least 10 times in 3 hours. Slowing or stopping of fetal movement may be an indication that the fetus needs some attention and evaluation. In general, women are advised to count fetal movements for 30 to 60 minutes three times a day usually after meals when the fetus is more active. The client should lie on the left side during the procedure because it provides optimal circulation to the uterus-placenta-fetus unit.

*Test-Taking Strategy:* Use the process of elimination. Think about the purpose of this procedure to direct you to option 4. If you had difficulty with this question, review content regarding normal fetal activity.

*Level of Cognitive Ability:* Application
*Client Needs:* Health Promotion and Maintenance
*Integrated Concept/Process:* Teaching/Learning
*Content Area:* Maternity

*Reference*
Gorrie, T., McKinney, E., & Murray, S. (1998). *Foundations of maternal newborn nursing* (2nd ed.) Philadelphia: W.B. Saunders, p. 241.

**21.** A nurse is assessing the status of the prenatal client. Following the assessment, the nurse determines that which piece of data places the client into the high-risk category for contracting human immunodeficiency virus (HIV)?
1   Living in an area where HIV infections are minimal
2   A history of IV drug use in the past year
3   A history of one sexual partner within the past 10 years
4   A spouse who is heterosexual and had only one sexual partner in the past 10 years

**Answer: 2**
*Rationale:* HIV is transmitted by intimate sexual contact and the exchange of body fluids, exposure of infected blood, and transmission from an infected woman to her fetus. Women who fall into the high-risk category for HIV infection include those with persistent and recurrent sexually transmitted diseases, those with a history of multiple sexual partners, and those who have used IV drugs. A heterosexual partner, particularly a partner who has had only one sexual partner in 10 years, is not a high risk factor for developing HIV.

*Test-Taking Strategy:* Use the process of elimination, recalling that that exchange of blood and body fluids places the client at high risk for HIV infection. This will assist in directing you to the correct option. If you had difficulty with this question, review the risk factors for HIV.

*Level of Cognitive Ability:* Analysis
*Client Needs:* Health Promotion and Maintenance
*Integrated Concept/Process:* Nursing Process/Assessment
*Content Area:* Adult Health/Immune

*Reference*
Gorrie, T., McKinney, E., & Murray, S. (1998). *Foundations of maternal newborn nursing* (2nd ed.) Philadelphia: W.B. Saunders, p. 738.

**22.** A nurse instructs a perinatal client about measures to prevent urinary tract infections. Which statement if made by the client would indicate an understanding of these measures?
1   "I can take a bubble bath as long as the soap doesn't contain any oils."
2   "I should always use scented toilet paper."
3   "I can wear my tight-fitting jeans."
4   "I should choose underwear with a cotton panel liner."

**Answer: 4**
*Rationale:* Wearing items with a cotton panel liner allows for air movement in and around the genital area. Bubble bath or other bath oils should be avoided, because these may be irritating to the urethra. Harsh, scented, or printed toilet paper may cause irritation. Wearing tight clothes irritates the genital area and does not allow for air circulation.

*Test-Taking Strategy:* Use the process of elimination. Note the key words *indicate an understanding*. Eliminate option 2 because of the absolute term *always* and option 3 because of the words *tight-fitting*. From the remaining options, recall that bubble baths need to be avoided. Review measures to prevent urinary tract infections if you had difficulty with this question.

*Level of Cognitive Ability:* Analysis
*Client Need:* Health Promotion and Maintenance
*Integrated Concept/Process:* Teaching/Learning
*Content Area:* Maternity

*Reference*
Lowdermilk, D., Perry, S., & Bobak, I. (2000). *Maternity & women's health care* (7th ed.). St. Louis: Mosby, p. 406.

**23.** A nurse instructs a client with mild preeclampsia about home care measures. The nurse evaluates that the teaching has been effective concerning assessment of complications when the client states:

1 "As long as the home health care nurse is visiting me daily I do not have to keep my next physician's appointment."

2 "I need to take my blood pressure each morning and alternate arms each time."

3 "I need to check my weight every day at different times during the day."

4 "I need to check my urine with a dipstick every day for protein and call the physician if it is 2+ or more."

**Answer: 4**

*Rationale:* The client needs to be instructed to report any increases in blood pressure, 2+ proteinuria, weight gain greater than 1 lb per week, presence of edema, and decreased fetal activity to the physician or health care provider immediately to prevent worsening of the preeclamptic condition. It is important to keep physician appointments even if the client is receiving visits from a home health care nurse. Blood pressures need to be taken in the same arm, in a sitting position, every day in order to obtain a consistent and accurate reading. The weight needs to be checked at the same time each day, wearing the same clothes, after voiding, and before breakfast in order to obtain reliable weights.

*Test-Taking Strategy:* Use the process of elimination, noting the key words *teaching has been effective.* Basic principles related to health care teaching and focusing on the specific issue of the question, mild preeclampsia, will assist in directing you to option 4. Review home care teaching points for the client with preeclampsia if you had difficulty with this question.

*Level of Cognitive Ability:* Analysis
*Client Needs:* Health Promotion and Maintenance
*Integrated Concept/Process:* Teaching/Learning
*Content Area:* Maternity

*Reference*
Lowdermilk, D., Perry, S., & Bobak, I. (2000). *Maternity & women's health care* (7th ed.). St. Louis: Mosby, p. 828.

**24.** A nurse is providing instructions to a client and family regarding home care following left eye cataract removal. The nurse would plan to teach the client which of the following pieces of information about positioning in the postoperative period?

1 Lower the head between the knees three times a day

2 Bend below the waist as frequently as able

3 Do not sleep on the left side

4 Sleep only on the left side

**Answer: 3**

*Rationale:* Following cataract surgery, the client should not sleep on the side of the body that was operated on. The client should also avoid bending below the level of the waist or lowering the head, because these actions will increase intraocular pressure.

*Test-Taking Strategy:* Use the process of elimination. Remember that options that are similar are not likely to be correct. With this in mind, eliminate options 1 and 2 first. Remembering that the client needs to be instructed to remain off of the operative side will direct you to option 3. Review postoperative instructions for the client following cataract surgery if you had difficulty with this question.

*Level of Cognitive Ability:* Application
*Client Needs:* Health Promotion and Maintenance
*Integrated Concept/Process:* Teaching/Learning
*Content Area:* Adult Health/Eye

*Reference*
Ignatavicius, D., Workman, M., & Mishler, M. (1999). *Medical-surgical nursing across the health care continuum* (3rd ed.). Philadelphia: W.B. Saunders, p. 1178.

**25.** A nurse has provided instructions to a new mother with a urinary tract infection regarding foods and fluids to consume that will acidify the urine. Which of the following fluids, if identified by the mother, indicates a need for further education regarding the fluids that will acidify the urine?

1   Apricot juice
2   Carbonated drinks
3   Prune juice
4   Cranberry juice

**Answer: 2**

*Rationale:* Acidification of the urine inhibits multiplication of bacteria. Fluids that acidify the urine include apricot, plum, prune, and cranberry juice. Carbonated drinks should be avoided, because they increase urine alkalinity.

*Test-Taking Strategy:* Use the process of elimination, noting the key words *need for further education.* Note the similarity between options 1, 3, and 4 in that all of these items are fruit juices. This will assist in directing you to option 2. Review foods and fluids that cause urine acidification if you had difficulty with this question.

*Level of Cognitive Ability:* Analysis
*Client Needs:* Health Promotion and Maintenance
*Integrated Concept/Process:* Teaching/Learning
*Content Area:* Maternity

*Reference*
Gorrie, T., McKinney, E., & Murray, S. (1998). *Foundations of maternal-newborn nursing* (2nd ed.). Philadelphia: W.B. Saunders, p. 800.

---

**26.** A postpartum nurse has instructed a new mother on how to bathe her newborn infant. The nurse demonstrates the procedure to the mother and on the following day, asks the mother to perform the procedure. Which observation, if made by the nurse, indicates that the mother is performing the procedure correctly?

1   The mother cleans the ears and then moves to the eyes and the face
2   The mother begins to wash the newborn infant by starting with the eyes and face
3   The mother washes the arms, chest, and back, followed by the neck, arms and face
4   The mother washes the entire newborn infant's body and then washes the eyes, face, and scalp

**Answer: 2**

*Rationale:* Bathing should start at the eyes and face and with the cleanest area first. Next, the external ears and the area behind the ears are cleaned. The newborn infant's neck should be washed, because formula, lint, or breast milk will often accumulate in the folds of the neck. Hands and arms are then washed. The newborn infant's legs are washed next, with the diaper area washed last.

*Test-Taking Strategy:* Use the process of elimination. Remember the basic techniques of bathing a client to assist in answering this question. Always start with the cleanest area of the body first and proceed to the dirtiest area. Use techniques related to washing an adult to assist in answering this question. If you had difficulty with this question, review home care measures related to the care of a newborn infant.

*Level of Cognitive Ability:* Analysis
*Client Needs:* Health Promotion and Maintenance
*Integrated Concept/Process:* Teaching/Learning
*Content Area:* Maternity

*Reference*
Olds, S., London. M., & Ladewig, P. (2000). *Maternal-newborn nursing: A family and community-based approach* (6th ed.). Upper Saddle River, N.J.: Prentice Hall Health, pp. 996-997.

**27.** A nurse is teaching cord care to a new mother. The nurse tells the mother that:

1    Cord care is done only at birth to control bleeding

2    Alcohol is the best agent used to clean the cord

3    The process of keeping the cord clean and dry will decrease bacterial growth

4    It takes 21 days for the cord to dry up and fall off

**Answer: 3**

*Rationale:* The cord should be kept clean and dry to decrease bacterial growth. The cord should be cleansed 2 to 3 times a day using alcohol or other agents. Cord care is required until the cord dries up and falls off between 7 to 14 days. Additionally, the diaper should be folded below the cord to keep urine away from the cord.

*Test-Taking Strategy:* Use the process of elimination. Recalling the purpose of cord care will easily direct you to the correct option. Review concepts related to cord care if you had difficulty with this question.

*Level of Cognitive Ability:* Application
*Client Needs:* Health Promotion and Maintenance
*Integrated Concept/Process:* Teaching/Learning
*Content Area:* Maternity

*Reference*
Gorrie, T., McKinney, E., & Murray, S. (1998). *Foundations of maternal-newborn nursing* (2nd ed.). Philadelphia: W.B. Saunders, p. 574.

**28.** The parents of a male newborn infant who is not circumcised are instructed on how to clean the newborn's penis. Which statement by the parents indicates an understanding of the instructions?

1    "I should retract the foreskin to clean the penis."

2    "I should not retract the foreskin to clean the penis, because this may cause adhesions."

3    "I should retract the foreskin no farther than it will go to clean the penis."

4    "I should retract the foreskin for cleaning every morning and evening."

**Answer: 2**

*Rationale:* In male newborn infants, the prepuce is continuous with the epidermis of the gland and is not retractable. If retraction is forced, this may cause adhesions to develop. The parents should be told to allow separation to occur naturally, which usually occurs between 3 years and puberty. Most foreskins are retractable by 3 years of age and should be pushed back gently at this time for cleaning once a week. Options 1, 3, and 4 identify an action that addresses retraction of the foreskin.

*Test-Taking Strategy:* Use the process of elimination. Note that options 1, 3, and 4 are similar in that they all identify retracting the foreskin. Option 2 is the option that is different. If you had difficulty with this question, review teaching points related to cleaning the male penis who is uncircumcised.

*Level of Cognitive Ability:* Analysis
*Client Needs:* Health Promotion and Maintenance
*Integrated Concept/Process:* Teaching/Learning
*Content Area:* Maternity

*Reference*
Olds, S., London. M., & Ladewig, P. (2000). *Maternal-newborn nursing: A family and community-based approach* (6th ed.). Upper Saddle River, N.J.: Prentice Hall Health, p. 967.

**29.** A nurse prepares a teaching plan regarding the administration of ear drops for the parents of a 6-year-old-child. The nurse tells the parents that when administering the drops to:

1  Pull the ear up and back
2  Wear gloves when administering the medication
3  Hold the child in a sitting position when administering the ear drops
4  Pull the ear down and back

**Answer: 1**

*Rationale:* To administer ear drops in a child older than 3 years of age, the ear is pulled upward and back. The ear is pulled down and back in children younger than 3 years of age. Gloves do not need to be worn by the parents but handwashing before and after the procedure needs to be performed. The child needs to be in a side-lying position with the affected ear facing upward to facilitate the flow of medication down the ear canal by gravity.

*Test-Taking Strategy:* Use the process of elimination, visualizing this procedure. Options 2 and 3 can then be eliminated first. From the remaining options, recalling the anatomy of the child's ear canal and noting the age of the child will direct you to option 1. Review this procedure if you had difficulty with this question.

*Level of Cognitive Ability:* Application
*Client Needs:* Health Promotion and Maintenance
*Integrated Concept/Process:* Teaching/Learning
*Content Area:* Child Health

*Reference*
Wong, D. (1999). *Whaley & Wong's Nursing care of infants and children* (6th ed.). St. Louis: Mosby, p. 1270.

**30.** A nurse is providing discharge instructions to the mother of an 8-year-old child who had a tonsillectomy. The mother tells the nurse that the child loves tacos and asks when the child can safely eat one. The most appropriate response is:

1  "In 1 week."
2  "In 3 weeks."
3  "Two days after surgery."
4  "When the physician says it's okay."

**Answer: 2**

*Rationale:* Rough or scratchy foods or spicy foods are to be avoided for 3 weeks following a tonsillectomy. Citrus juices that irritate the throat need to be avoided for 10 days. Red liquids are avoided, because they will give the appearance of blood if the child vomits. The mother is instructed to add full liquids on the second day and soft foods as the child tolerates them.

*Test-Taking Strategy:* Use the process of elimination and knowledge regarding the specific instructions related to food and fluids following tonsillectomy. Review these dietary instructions if you had difficulty with this question.

*Level of Cognitive Ability:* Application
*Client Needs:* Health Promotion and Maintenance
*Integrated Concept/Process:* Teaching/Learning
*Content Area:* Child Health

*Reference*
Wong, D. (1999). *Whaley & Wong's Nursing care of infants and children* (6th ed.). St. Louis: Mosby, p. 1466.

**31.** Following a cleft lip repair, the nurse instructs the parents regarding cleaning of the lip repair site. The nurse uses which solution in demonstrating this procedure to the parents?
1   Tap water
2   Sterile water
3   Full-strength hydrogen peroxide
4   Half-strength hydrogen peroxide

**Answer: 2**
*Rationale:* The lip repair site is cleansed with sterile water using a cotton swab, after feeding and as prescribed. The parents should be instructed to use a rolling motion from the suture line out. Tap water is not a sterile solution. Peroxide may disrupt the integrity of the site.

*Test-Taking Strategy:* Use the process of elimination. Eliminate options 3 and 4 first, because they are similar. From the remaining options, recall the importance of asepsis to a surgical site to direct you to option 2. Review this procedure if you had difficulty with this question.

*Level of Cognitive Ability:* Application
*Client Needs:* Health Promotion and Maintenance
*Integrated Concept/Process:* Teaching/Learning
*Content Area:* Child Health

*Reference*
Wong, D. (1999). *Whaley & Wong's Nursing care of infants and children* (6th ed.). St. Louis: Mosby, p. 518.

**32.** A child with a diagnosis of umbilical hernia has been scheduled for surgical repair in 2 weeks. The clinic nurse instructs the parents about the signs of possible hernial strangulation. The nurse tells the parents that which sign would require physician notification?
1   Fussiness
2   Diarrhea
3   Constipation
4   Vomiting

**Answer: 4**
*Rationale:* The parents of a child with an umbilical hernia need to be instructed in the signs of strangulation. These signs include vomiting, pain, and irreducible mass at the umbilicus. The parents should be instructed to contact the physician immediately if strangulation is suspected.

*Test-Taking Strategy:* Use the process of elimination and the definition of the word *strangulation* to assist in eliminating options 1 and 2. From the remaining options, use knowledge regarding these signs to direct you to option 4. Review the signs of strangulation if you had difficulty with this question.

*Level of Cognitive Ability:* Application
*Client Needs:* Health Promotion and Maintenance
*Integrated Concept/Process:* Teaching/Learning
*Content Area:* Child Health

*Reference*
Bowden, V., Dickey, S., & Greenberg, C. (1998). *Children and their families: The continuum of care.* Philadelphia: W.B. Saunders, p. 1066.

**33.** A client with a compound fracture of the radius has a plaster of Paris cast applied in the emergency room. The nurse provides discharge instructions and instructs the client to seek medical attention if which of the following occurs?

1  The cast feels heavy and damp after 24 hours of application

2  Numbness and tingling occur in the fingers

3  Any bloody drainage is noted on the cast during the first 6 hours after application

4  If the entire cast feels warm in the first 24 hours after application

**Answer: 2**

*Rationale:* A limb encased in a cast is at risk for nerve damage and diminished circulation from increased pressure due to edema. Signs of increased pressure from the cast include numbness, tingling, and increased pain. A plaster of Paris cast can take up to 48 hours to dry and generates heat while drying. Some drainage may occur initially with a compound (open) fracture.

*Test-Taking Strategy:* Note the key word *compound* in the question. This key word and use of the ABCs: airway, breathing, and circulation, will assist in directing you to option 2. Review teaching points for the client with a plaster cast if you had difficulty with this question.

*Level of Cognitive Ability:* Application
*Client Needs:* Health Promotion and Maintenance
*Integrated Concept/Process:* Teaching/Learning
*Content Area:* Adult Health/Musculoskeletal

*Reference*
Monahan, F., & Neighbors, M. (1998). *Medical-surgical nursing: Foundations for clinical practice* (2nd ed.). Philadelphia: W.B Saunders, p. 857.

**34.** A mother of a child with celiac disease asks the nurse how long a special diet is necessary. The nurse tells the mother that:

1  A gluten-free diet will need to be followed for life

2  Adequate nutritional status will help prevent celiac crisis

3  Supplemental vitamins, iron, and folate will prevent complications

4  A lactose-free diet will need to be followed temporarily

**Answer: 1**

*Rationale:* The main nursing consideration with celiac disease is helping the child adhere to dietary management. Treatment of celiac disease consists primarily of dietary management with a gluten-free diet. Options 2, 3, and 4 are all true statements, but do not answer the question the client is asking. Children with untreated celiac disease may have lactose intolerance, which usually improves with gluten withdrawal. Nutritional deficiencies resulting from malabsorption are treated with appropriate supplements.

*Test-Taking Strategy:* Focus on the issue of the question, the length of time a special diet is necessary. Option 1 directly relates to this issue. If you had difficulty with this question, review dietary requirements for celiac disease.

*Level of Cognitive Ability:* Application
*Client Needs:* Health Promotion and Maintenance
*Integrated Concept/Process:* Teaching/Learning
*Content Area:* Child Health

*Reference*
Wong, D. (1999). *Whaley & Wong's Nursing care of infants and children* (6th ed.). St. Louis: Mosby, p. 1567

**35.** A nurse teaches a mother of a newly circumcised infant about postcircumcision care. Which statement by the mother indicates an understanding of the care required?

1   "I need to check for bleeding every hour for the first 12 hours."
2   "I need to clean the penis every hour with baby wipes."
3   "I need to wrap the penis completely in dry sterile gauze, making sure it is dry when I change his diaper."
4   "The baby will not urinate for the next 24 hours because of swelling."

**Answer: 1**

*Rationale:* The mother needs to be taught to observe for bleeding, and to assess the site hourly for 8 to 12 hours following the circumcision. Voiding needs to be assessed. The mother should call the physician if the baby has not urinated within 24 hours. Swelling or damage may obstruct urine output. When the diaper is changed, vaseline gauze should be reapplied. Frequent changing prevents contamination of the site. Water is used for cleaning, because soap or baby wipes may irritate the area and cause discomfort.

*Test-Taking Strategy:* Use the process of elimination. Eliminate option 2, because baby wipes will cause stinging in the newly circumcised penis. Eliminate option 3, because gauze will stick to the penis if it is completely dry. Eliminate option 4, because penile swelling that prevents voiding needs to be reported to the physician. Review postcircumcision care if you had difficulty answering the question.

*Level of Cognitive Ability:* Analysis
*Client Needs:* Health Promotion and Maintenance
*Integrated Concept/Process:* Teaching/Learning
*Content Area:* Maternity

*Reference*
Lowdermilk, D., Perry, S., & Bobak, I. (2000). *Maternity & women's health care* (7th ed.). St. Louis: Mosby, p. 749.

---

**36.** A nurse is developing a teaching plan for a client who will be receiving phenelzine sulfate (Nardil). The nurse plans to tell the client to avoid:

1   Aged cheeses
2   Cherries and blueberries
3   Digitalis preparations
4   Vasodilators

**Answer: 1**

*Rationale:* Nardil is in the monoamine oxidase inhibitor (MAOI) class of antidepressant medications. An individual on a MAOI must avoid aged cheeses, alcoholic beverages, avocados, bananas, and caffeine drinks. There are also other food items to avoid. These include chocolate, meat tenderizers, pickled herring, raisins, sour cream, yogurt, and soy sauce. Medications that should be avoided include amphetamines, antiasthmatic, and certain antidepressants. They should also avoid antiasthmatics, antihypertensive medications, Levodopa, and meperidine (Demerol).

*Test-Taking Strategy:* Use the process of elimination and note the key word *avoid*. Recalling that phenelzine sulfate is a MAOI and recalling the foods that need to be avoided will direct you to option 1. If you had difficulty with this question, review this medication.

*Level of Cognitive Ability:* Application
*Client Needs:* Health Promotion and Maintenance
*Integrated Concept/Process:* Teaching/Learning
*Content Area:* Pharmacology

*Reference*
Hodgson, B., & Kizior, R. (2001). *Saunders Nursing drug handbook 2001.* Philadelphia: W.B. Saunders, p. 813.

**37.** A nurse is providing home care instructions to the parents of an infant who had a surgical repair of an inguinal hernia. The nurse instructs the parents to do which of the following to prevent infection at the surgical site?

  1   Change the diapers as soon as they become damp
  2   Report a fever immediately
  3   Soak the infant in a tub bath twice a day for the next 5 days
  4   Restrict the infant's physical activity

**Answer: 1**

*Rationale:* Changing diapers as soon as they become damp helps prevent infection at the surgical site. Parents are instructed to change diapers more frequently than usual during the day and once or twice during the night. Parents are instructed to give the infant sponge baths instead of tub baths for 2 to 5 days. There are no restrictions placed on the infant's activity. A fever could indicate the presence of an infection.

*Test-Taking Strategy:* Focus on the issue, to prevent infection, to eliminate options 2 and 3 From the remaining options, thinking about the anatomical location of an inguinal hernia will direct you to option 1. Review measures to prevent infection following inguinal hernia repair if you had difficulty with this question.

*Level of Cognitive Ability:* Application
*Client Needs:* Health Promotion and Maintenance
*Integrated Concept/Process:* Teaching/Learning
*Content Area:* Child Health

*Reference*
Wong, D. (1999). *Whaley & Wong's Nursing care of infants and children* (6th ed.). St. Louis: Mosby, p. 538

**38.** A client is experiencing difficulty using an incentive spirometer. The nurse teaches the client that which of the following may interfere with effective use of the device?

  1   Breathing through the nose
  2   Forming a tight seal around the mouthpiece with the lips
  3   Inhaling slowly
  4   Removing the mouthpiece to exhale

**Answer: 1**

*Rationale:* Incentive spirometry is not effective if the client breathes through the nose. The client should exhale, form a tight seal around the mouthpiece, inhale slowly, hold to the count of 3, and remove the mouthpiece to exhale. The client should repeat the exercise approximately 10 times every hour for best results.

*Test-Taking Strategy:* Note the key words *may interfere with effective use.* Visualize the use of this device to direct you to option 1. If this question was difficult, review this procedure.

*Level of Cognitive Ability:* Application
*Client Needs:* Health Promotion and Maintenance
*Integrated Concept/Process:* Teaching/Learning
*Content Area:* Adult Health/Respiratory

*Reference*
Smeltzer, S., & Bare, B. (2000). *Brunner & Suddarth's Textbook of medical-surgical nursing* (9th ed.). Philadelphia: Lippincott Williams & Wilkins, p. 354.

**39.** A client with chronic obstructive pulmonary disease (COPD) has a knowledge deficit related to positions used to breathe more easily. The nurse plans to teach the client to:

1   Lie on the side with the head of the bed at a 45-degree angle
2   Sit bolt upright in bed with the arms crossed over the chest
3   Sit on the edge of the bed with the arms leaning on an overbed table
4   Sit in a reclining chair tilted slightly back with the feet elevated

**Answer: 3**

*Rationale:* Proper positioning can decrease episodes of dyspnea in a client. These include sitting upright while leaning on an overbed table, sitting upright in a chair with the arms resting on the knees, and leaning against a wall while standing. Option 1 restricts expansion of the lateral wall of the lungs. Option 2 restricts movement of the anterior and posterior walls. Option 4 restricts posterior lung expansion.

*Test-Taking Strategy:* Use the process of elimination. Visualize each of the positions described in the options. Think about how each position affects lung expansion to direct you to option 3. Review positions that relieve dyspnea in the client with COPD if you had difficulty with this question.

*Level of Cognitive Ability:* Application
*Client Needs:* Health Promotion and Maintenance
*Integrated Concept/Process:* Teaching/Learning
*Content Area:* Adult Health/Respiratory

*Reference*
Ignatavicius, D., Workman, M., & Mishler, M. (1999). *Medical-surgical nursing across the health care continuum* (3rd ed.). Philadelphia: W.B. Saunders, p. 630.

**40.** A nurse has taught a client with pleurisy about measures to promote comfort during recuperation. The nurse determines that the client has understood the instructions if the client states an intention to:

1   Try to take only small, shallow breaths
2   Splint the chest wall during coughing and deep breathing
3   Lie as much as possible on the unaffected side
4   Take as much pain medication as possible

**Answer: 2**

*Rationale:* The client with pleurisy should splint the chest wall during coughing and deep breathing. The client may also lie on the affected side to minimize movement of the affected chest wall. Taking small, shallow breaths promotes atelectasis. The client should take medication prudently so that adequate coughing and deep breathing is performed and an adequate level of comfort is maintained.

*Test-Taking Strategy:* Focus on the issue: to promote comfort. Eliminate option 1 because of the word *only*. From the remaining options, noting the word *splint* in option 2 will direct you to this option. Review the measures that will promote comfort in a client with pleurisy if you had difficulty with this question.

*Level of Cognitive Ability:* Analysis
*Client Needs:* Health Promotion and Maintenance
*Integrated Concept/Process:* Teaching/Learning
*Content Area:* Adult Health/Respiratory

*Reference*
Smeltzer, S., & Bare, B. (2000). *Brunner & Suddarth's Textbook of medical-surgical nursing* (9th ed.). Philadelphia: Lippincott Williams & Wilkins, p. 444.

**41.** A client with a diagnosis of trigeminal neuralgia is started on a regimen of carbamazepine (Tegretol). The nurse provides instructions to the client about the medication and determines that the client understands if the client states:

1  "I will report a fever or sore throat to my doctor."

2  "If I notice a pink color to my urine, I will stop the medication and call my doctor."

3  "I must brush my teeth frequently to avoid damage to my gums."

4  "If I notice ringing in my ears that doesn't stop, I'll seek medical attention."

**Answer: 1**

*Rationale:* Agranulocytosis is an adverse effect of carbamazepine and places the client at risk for infection. If the client develops a fever or a sore throat, the physician should be notified. Pink-colored urine, gum damage, and ringing in the ears is not related to this medication.

*Test-Taking Strategy:* Use the process of elimination. Recalling that agranulocytosis is an adverse effect will direct you to option 1. If you had difficulty with this question review the adverse effects of this medication and the laboratory tests that need monitoring.

*Level of Cognitive Ability:* Analysis
*Client Needs:* Health Promotion and Maintenance
*Integrated Concept/Process:* Teaching/Learning
*Content Area:* Pharmacology

*Reference*
Hodgson, B., & Kizior, R. (2001). *Saunders Nursing drug handbook 2001.* Philadelphia: W.B. Saunders, p. 144.

**42.** A nurse teaches a preoperative client about the nasogastric (NG) tube that will be inserted in preparation for surgery. The nurse determines that the client understands when the tube will be removed in the postoperative period when the client states:

1  "When my gastrointestinal (GI) system is healed."

2  "When I can tolerate food without vomiting."

3  "When my bowels begin to function again, and I begin to pass gas."

4  "When the doctor says so."

**Answer: 3**

*Rationale:* NG tubes are discontinued when normal function returns to the GI tract. The tube will be removed before GI healing. Food would not be administered unless bowel function returns. Although the physician determines when the NG tube will be removed, option 4 does not determine effectiveness of teaching.

*Test-Taking Strategy:* Use the process of elimination. Option 4 can be easily eliminated first. Eliminate option 1, considering the time factor associated with healing of the GI tract. From the remaining options, recalling that food would not be administered unless bowel function returns will assist in eliminating option 2. If you had difficulty with this question, review the use and care of an NG tube.

*Level of Cognitive Ability:* Analysis
*Client Needs:* Health Promotion and Maintenance
*Integrated Concept/Process:* Teaching/Learning
*Content Area:* Adult Health/Gastrointestinal

*Reference*
Smeltzer, S., & Bare, B. (2000). *Brunner & Suddarth's Textbook of medical-surgical nursing* (9th ed.). Philadelphia: Lippincott Williams & Wilkins, p. 840.

**43.** A client receives Intralipids intravenously in the home. The client's spouse manages the infusion. The community health nurse discusses potential adverse reactions and side effects of the therapy with the client and the spouse. Following the discussion, the nurse expects the spouse to verbalize, that in case of a suspected adverse reaction, the priority action is to:

1   Take a blood pressure
2   Stop the infusion
3   Contact the nurse
4   Contact the local area emergency response team

**Answer: 2**

*Rationale:* Intravenous fat emulsions (Intralipids) can cause overloading syndrome (focal seizures, fever, shock) and adverse effects including chest pain, chills, and shock. The priority action is to stop the infusion and limit the adverse response before obtaining additional assistance.

*Test-Taking Strategy:* Note the key words *suspected adverse reaction* and *priority*. Remembering that the priority action when an adverse reaction occurs is to stop the infusion will direct you to the correct option. If you had difficulty with this question review the adverse reactions of fat emulsion therapy and the priority actions if an adverse reaction occurs.

*Level of Cognitive Ability:* Analysis
*Client Needs:* Health Promotion and Maintenance
*Integrated Concept/Process:* Teaching/Learning
*Content Area:* Fundamental Skills

*Reference*
Smeltzer, S., & Bare, B. (2000). *Brunner & Suddarth's Textbook of medical-surgical nursing* (9th ed.). Philadelphia: Lippincott Williams & Wilkins, p. 850.

---

**44.** A home health care nurse suspects that a client's spouse is experiencing caregiver strain. The nurse most appropriately assesses for this occurrence by:

1   Obtaining feedback from the client as to the coping abilities of the caregiver
2   Gathering subjective and objective data from the caregiver and client
3   Waiting until the caregiver expresses concern about the significant responsibility in caring for the client
4   Making a referral to the home health care agency social worker to complete the assessment

**Answer: 2**

*Rationale:* Caregiver strain can occur when a client is significantly dependent on someone for their personal and health care needs. Option 1 is not appropriate. The nurse should not expect the client to assess the coping abilities of the caregiver. Although a social worker may be helpful, the nurse needs to perform the assessment of the situation before making the referral. Waiting for the caregiver to express concern is not appropriate. The caregiver may be exhausted or incapable of caring for the client by this time.

*Test-Taking Strategy:* Use the steps of the nursing process to eliminate options 3 and 4. From the remaining options, select option 2, because it addresses both the client and the caregiver. Review the concepts of caregiver strain if you had difficulty with this question.

*Level of Cognitive Ability:* Application
*Client Needs:* Health Promotion and Maintenance
*Integrated Concept/Process:* Nursing Process/Assessment
*Content Area:* Fundamental Skills

*Reference*
Potter, P., & Perry, A. (2001). *Fundamentals of nursing* (5th ed.). St. Louis: Mosby, p. 251.

**45.** A client being discharged from the hospital will be taking warfarin sodium (Coumadin) at home on a daily basis. The nurse has provided instructions to the client about the medication and determines that further teaching is needed if the client states:

1. "This medicine thins my blood and allows me to clot slower."
2. "I need to have my prothrombin level checked in 2 weeks."
3. "If I notice any increased bleeding or bruising, I need to call my doctor."
4. "I need to increase foods high in vitamin K in my diet."

**Answer: 4**

*Rationale:* Warfarin sodium (Coumadin) is an oral anticoagulant that is used mainly to prevent thromboembolitic events, such as thrombophlebitis, pulmonary embolism, and embolism formation caused by atrial fibrillation. Oral anticoagulants prolong the clotting time and are monitored by the prothrombin time (PT) and the International Normalized Ratio (INR). Client education should include signs and symptoms of adverse effects and dietary restrictions such as limiting foods high in vitamin K (leafy green vegetables, liver, cheese, and egg yolk), since these increase clotting times.

*Test-Taking Strategy:* Note the key words *further teaching is needed.* Recalling that warfarin sodium is an anticoagulant will assist in eliminating options 1, 2, and 3. Also, remembering the role vitamin K plays in the clotting mechanism will direct you to option 4. If you had difficulty with this question, review client education points related to this medication.

*Level of Cognitive Ability:* Analysis
*Client Needs:* Health Promotion and Maintenance
*Integrated Concept/Process:* Teaching/Learning
*Content Area:* Pharmacology

*Reference*
Hodgson, B., & Kizior, R. (2001). *Saunders Nursing drug handbook 2001.* Philadelphia: W.B. Saunders, p. 10

---

**46.** A teenager returns to the gynecological (GYN) clinic for a follow-up visit for a sexually transmitted disease (STD). Which of the following statements, if made by the teenager, indicates the need for further teaching?

1. "I always make sure my boyfriend uses a condom."
2. "I know you won't tell my parents I'm sick."
3. "My boyfriend doesn't have to come in for treatment, does he?"
4. "I finished all the antibiotic, just like you said."

**Answer: 3**

*Rationale:* In treating STDs, all the sexual contacts must be contacted and treated with medication. Clients should always use a condom with any sexual contact. Any treatment at a teenager GYN clinic is confidential and parents will not be contacted, even if the client is under 18 years of age. Any client should always finish the course of antibiotics prescribed by the health care provider.

*Test-Taking Strategy:* Use the process of elimination, noting the key words *need for further teaching.* Recalling the concepts related to safe sex, the treatment of STDs in the teenager, and the principles related to antibiotic therapy will direct you to option 3. Review this content if you had difficulty with this question.

*Level of Cognitive Ability:* Analysis
*Client Needs:* Health Promotion and Maintenance
*Integrated Concept/Process:* Teaching/Learning
*Content Area:* Child Health

*Reference*
Wong, D. (1999). *Whaley & Wong's Nursing care of infants and children* (6th ed.). St. Louis: Mosby, p. 917.

**47.** A nurse is preparing to teach a client newly diagnosed with diabetes mellitus about blood glucose monitoring. The nurse plans to teach the client to report glucose levels that exceed:

1   150 mg/dL
2   200 mg/dL
3   250 mg/dL
4   350 mg/dL

**Answer: 3**

*Rationale:* The client should be taught to report blood glucose levels that exceed 250 mg/dL, unless otherwise instructed by the physician. Options 1 and 2 are levels that do not require physician notification. Option 4 is a high value.

*Test-Taking Strategy:* Use the process of elimination. Recalling the basic principles related to diabetic home care instructions will direct you to option 3. Review this common area of teaching for clients with diabetes mellitus if you had difficulty with this question.

*Level of Cognitive Ability:* Application
*Client Needs:* Health Promotion and Maintenance
*Integrated Concept/Process:* Teaching/Learning
*Content Area:* Adult Health/Endocrine

*Reference*
Smeltzer, S., & Bare, B. (2000). *Brunner & Suddarth's Textbook of medical-surgical nursing* (9th ed.). Philadelphia: Lippincott Williams & Wilkins, p. 985.

---

**48.** A client with gastritis asks the nurse at a screening clinic about analgesics that will not cause epigastric distress. The nurse tells the client to take which of the following medications?

1   Bufferin
2   Acetaminophen (Tylenol)
3   Ecotrin
4   Ascriptin

**Answer: 2**

*Rationale:* Aspirin is irritating to the gastrointestinal (GI) tract of the client with a history of gastritis. The client should be advised to take analgesics that do not contain aspirin, such as acetaminophen. The other medications listed have aspirin in them. Another category of medications that is irritating to the GI tract is the nonsteroidal antiinflammatory drugs (NSAIDs).

*Test-Taking Strategy:* Use the process of elimination. Note that options 1, 3 and 4 are similar and are aspirin-containing medications. Review these medications if you had difficulty with this question.

*Level of Cognitive Ability:* Application
*Client Needs:* Health Promotion and Maintenance
*Integrated Concept/Process:* Teaching/Learning
*Content Area:* Pharmacology

*Reference*
Hodgson, B., & Kizior, R. (2001). *Saunders Nursing drug handbook 2001.* Philadelphia: W.B. Saunders, p. 6.

---

**49.** A client is diagnosed with thromboangiitis obliterans (Buerger's disease). The nurse places highest priority on teaching the client about modifications of which of the following risk factors related to this disorder?

1   Exposure to cold
2   Exposure to heat
3   Diet low in vitamin C
4   Cigarette smoking

**Answer: 4**

*Rationale:* Buerger's disease occurs predominantly in men between 25 to 40 years of age who smoke cigarettes. A familial tendency is noted, but cigarette smoking is consistently a risk factor. Symptoms of the disease improve with smoking cessation. Options 1, 2, and 3 are not risk factors.

*Test-Taking Strategy:* Use the process of elimination. Note the key words *highest priority* and *risk factors*. Although avoiding environmental extremes in temperature may be a component of treatment, they are not risk factors. Review the risk factors of this disorder if you had difficulty with this question.

*Level of Cognitive Ability:* Application
*Client Needs:* Health Promotion and Maintenance
*Integrated Concept/Process:* Teaching/Learning
*Content Area:* Adult Health/Cardiovascular

*Reference*
Smeltzer, S., & Bare, B. (2000). *Brunner & Suddarth's Textbook of medical-surgical nursing* (9th ed.). Philadelphia: Lippincott Williams & Wilkins, p. 699.

---

**50.** A client has a new prescription for timolol (Betimol). The nurse determines that the client has not fully understood instructions given about the medication if the client stated to:
1 Take the pulse daily and hold the dose if the pulse is less than 60 beats/min
2 To change positions slowly
3 Taper or discontinue the medication once the client feels well
4 Have enough medication on hand to last through weekends and vacations

**Answer: 3**
*Rationale:* Common client teaching points about beta-adrenergic blocking agents include taking the pulse daily and holding the dose if the pulse is below 60 beats/min (and notify the physician). The client should not discontinue or change the medication dose. The client is also instructed to keep enough medication on hand so as not to run out, to change positions slowly, not to take over-the-counter medications (especially decongestants, cough and cold preparations) without consulting the physician, and to carry medical identification stating a beta-blocker is being taken.

*Test-Taking Strategy:* Use the process of elimination, noting the key words *has not fully understood.* Noting the word *discontinue* in option 3 will direct you to this option. Review client teaching points related to this medication if you had difficulty with this question.

*Level of Cognitive Ability:* Analysis
*Client Needs:* Health Promotion and Maintenance
*Integrated Concept/Process:* Teaching/Learning
*Content Area:* Pharmacology

*Reference*
Hodgson, B., & Kizior, R. (2001). *Saunders Nursing drug handbook 2001.* Philadelphia: W.B. Saunders, p. 994.

---

**51.** A nurse has completed giving medication instructions to the client receiving benazepril (Lotensin). The nurse determines that the client needs further instruction if the client states to:
1 Change positions slowly
2 Report signs and symptoms of infection immediately
3 Monitor the blood pressure every week
4 Use salt substitutes and eat foods high in potassium

**Answer: 4**
*Rationale:* The client taking an angiotensin-converting enzyme (ACE) inhibitor is instructed to take the medication exactly as prescribed, monitor blood pressure weekly, and continue with other lifestyle changes to control hypertension. The client should change positions slowly to avoid orthostatic hypotension, report fever, mouth sores, sore throat to the physician (neutropenia), and avoid salt substitutes and high-potassium foods. Salt substitutes contain potassium, as do high-potassium foods, and place the client at risk for hyperkalemia.

*Test-Taking Strategy:* Use the process of elimination, noting the key words *needs further instruction.* Noting the name of the medication "Lotensin" will assist in determining that the medication is an antihypertensive. This will assist in eliminating options 1 and 3. Recalling that neutropenia and hyperkalemia are side effects will assist in eliminating option 2. Review this medication if you had difficulty with this question.

*Level of Cognitive Ability:* Analysis
*Client Needs:* Health Promotion and Maintenance
*Integrated Concept/Process:* Teaching/Learning
*Content Area:* Pharmacology

*Reference*
Hodgson, B., & Kizior, R. (2001). *Saunders Nursing drug handbook 2001.* Philadelphia: W.B. Saunders, p. 100.

---

**52.** A nurse has conducted medication instructions with a client receiving lovastatin (Mevacor). The nurse determines that the client understands the effects of the medication if the client stated the need to adhere to the periodic evaluation of serum:

1    Triglyceride levels
2    Liver function studies
3    Blood glucose levels
4    Bleeding times

**Answer: 2**

*Iri'dnk,tes* (?)

*Rationale:* Lovastatin is a reductase inhibitor. It results in an increase in the high-density lipoprotein (HDL) cholesterol, and a decrease in the triglycerides and low density lipoprotein (LDL) cholesterol. This medication is converted by the liver to active metabolites, and therefore is not used in clients with active hepatic disease or elevated transaminase levels. For this reason, clients are recommended to have periodic liver function studies. Periodic cholesterol levels are also needed to monitor the effectiveness of therapy.

*Test-Taking Strategy:* Use the process of elimination. Recalling that this medication is used to lower the blood cholesterol level and that cholesterol is synthesized in the liver, will direct you to option 2. Review this medication if you had difficulty with this question.

*Level of Cognitive Ability:* Analysis
*Client Needs:* Health Promotion and Maintenance
*Integrated Concept/Process:* Teaching/Learning
*Content Area:* Pharmacology

*Reference*
Hodgson, B., & Kizior, R. (2001). *Saunders Nursing drug handbook 2001.* Philadelphia: W.B. Saunders, p. 612.

---

**53.** A home health nurse visits a client at home. Clonazepam (Klonopin) has been prescribed for the client and the nurse teaches the client about the medication. Which of the following statements, if made by the client, indicates that further teaching is necessary?

1    "I can take my medicine at bedtime if it tends to make me feel drowsy."
2    "My drowsiness will decrease over time with continued treatment."
3    "I should take my medicine with food to decrease stomach problems."
4    "If I experience slurred speech, it will disappear in about 8 weeks."

**Answer: 4**

*Rationale:* Clients who are experiencing signs and symptoms of toxicity with the administration of clonazepam exhibit slurred speech, sedation, confusion, respiratory depression, hypotension, and eventually coma. Some drowsiness may occur but will decrease with continued use. The medication may be taken with food to decrease gastrointestinal irritation. Options 1, 2, and 3 are all correct and represent an accurate understanding of the medication.

*Test-Taking Strategy:* Use the process of elimination, noting the key words *further teaching is necessary.* Recalling the toxic effects that can occur will direct you to option 4. If you had difficulty with this question, review this medication.

*Level of Cognitive Ability:* Analysis
*Client Needs:* Health Promotion and Maintenance

*Integrated Concept/Process:* Teaching/Learning
*Content Area:* Pharmacology

*Reference*
Hodgson, B., & Kizior, R. (2001). *Saunders Nursing drug handbook 2001.* Philadelphia: W.B. Saunders, p. 238.

---

**54.** The home health nurse visits a client at home. Persantine (Dipyridamole) taken orally daily has been prescribed for the client and the nurse teaches the client about the medication. Which of the following statements, if made by the client, indicates that the client understands the instructions?
1 "If I take this medicine with my warfarin sodium (Coumadin), it will protect my artificial heart valve."
2 "This medication will prevent a heart attack."
3 "This medication will prevent a stroke."
4 "This medication will help me to keep my blood pressure down."

**Answer: 1**
*Rationale:* Persantine (Dipyridamole) combined with warfarin sodium is prescribed to protect the client's artificial heart valves. Persantine does not prevent heart attacks, strokes, or hypertension.

*Test-Taking Strategy:* Use the process of elimination. Recalling that this medication is an antiplatelet will assist in eliminating option 4. Noting the word *prevent* in option 2 and 3 will assist in eliminating these options. Review the use of this medication, if you had difficulty with this question.

*Level of Cognitive Ability:* Analysis
*Client Needs:* Health Promotion and Maintenance
*Integrated Concept/Process:* Teaching/Learning
*Content Area:* Pharmacology

*Reference*
Hodgson, B., & Kizior, R. (2001). *Saunders Nursing drug handbook 2001.* Philadelphia: W.B. Saunders, p. 335.

---

**55.** A nurse is preparing to care for the mother of a preterm infant. The nurse plans to begin discharge planning for the preterm infant:
1 When the discharge date is set
2 When the parents feel comfortable with and can demonstrate adequate care of their infant
3 When the mother is in labor
4 After stabilization of the infant in the early stages of hospitalization

**Answer: 4**
*Rationale:* Discharge planning begins at admission. Determination of the services, needs, supplies, and equipment requirements should not be determined on the day of discharge. Option 1 and 2 are incorrect, because it is much too late to make the plans that need to be made. Option 3 is incorrect, because the outcome of the delivery in not known.

*Test-Taking Strategy:* Use the process of elimination, remembering that discharge planning always begins at admission to the hospital. Noting the key words *early stages of hospitalization* will direct you to option 4. Review the guidelines related to discharge planning if you had difficulty with this question.

*Level of Cognitive Ability:* Application
*Client Needs:* Health Promotion and Maintenance
*Integrated Concept/Process:* Nursing Process/Planning
*Content Area:* Maternity

*Reference*
Olds, S., London. M., & Ladewig, P. (2000). *Maternal-newborn nursing: A family and community-based approach* (6th ed.). Upper Saddle River, N.J.: Prentice-Hall, p. 831.

**56.** A nurse is providing home care instructions to a client recovering from an acute inferior myocardial infarction (MI) with recurrent angina. The nurse teaches the client to:

1   Avoid sexual intercourse for at least 4 months
2   Replace sublingual nitroglycerin tablets yearly
3   Recognize the side effects of acetylsalicylic acid (aspirin), which include tinnitus and hearing loss
4   Participate in an exercise program that includes overhead lifting and reaching

**Answer: 3**

*Rationale:* After an acute MI, many clients are instructed to take one aspirin daily. Side effects include tinnitus, hearing loss, epigastric distress, gastrointestinal bleeding, and nausea. In regard to option 1, sexual intercourse may be resumed in 4 to 8 weeks after an MI if the physician agrees. Clients should be advised to purchase a new supply of nitroglycerin tablets every 6 to 9 months. Expiration dates on the medication bottle should be checked. Activities that include lifting and reaching over the head should be avoided, because they reduce cardiac output.

*Test-Taking Strategy:* Use the process of elimination and focus on the client's diagnosis. Noting the time limits in options 1 and 2, "4 months" and "yearly," will assist in eliminating these options. From the remaining options, "overhead lifting and reaching" in option 4 should indicate that this is incorrect. If you had difficulty with this question, review client teaching points following an MI.

*Level of Cognitive Ability:* Application
*Client Needs:* Health Promotion and Maintenance
*Integrated Concept/Process:* Teaching/Learning
*Content Area:* Adult Health/Cardiovascular

*Reference*
Smeltzer, S., & Bare, B. (2000). *Brunner & Suddarth's Textbook of medical-surgical nursing* (9th ed.). Philadelphia: Lippincott Williams & Wilkins, p. 632.

**57.** A nurse is reviewing home care instructions with an elderly client who has type 1 diabetes mellitus and a history of diabetic ketoacidosis (DKA). The client's spouse is present when the instructions are given. Which of the following statements, if made by the spouse, indicates that further teaching is necessary?

1   "If the grandchildren are sick they probably shouldn't come to visit."
2   "I should call the doctor if he has nausea and/or abdominal pain lasting for more than 1 or 2 days."
3   "If he is vomiting I shouldn't give him any insulin."
4   "I should bring him to the physician's office if he develops a cough."

**Answer: 3**

*Rationale:* Infection and stopping insulin are precipitating factors for DKA. Nausea and abdominal pain that last more than 1 or 2 days need to be reported, because these signs may be indicative of DKA.

*Test-Taking Strategy:* Note the key words *history of diabetic ketoacidosis*. Eliminate options 1 and 4 first, because both relate to infection. From the remaining options, recalling the causes of DKA will direct you to option 3. If you had difficulty with this question review the precipitating factors associated with DKA.

*Level of Cognitive Ability:* Analysis
*Client Needs:* Health Promotion and Maintenance
*Integrated Concept/Process:* Teaching/Learning
*Content Area:* Adult Health/Endocrine

*Reference*
Smeltzer, S., & Bare, B. (2000). *Brunner & Suddarth's Textbook of medical-surgical nursing* (9th ed.). Philadelphia: Lippincott Williams & Wilkins, p. 1004.

**58.** A home care nurse provides self-care instructions to a client with chronic venous insufficiency due to deep vein thrombosis. Which statement by the client indicates a need for further instructions?

1    "I can cross my legs at the knee, but not the ankle."
2    "I need to elevate the foot of the bed during sleep."
3    "I need to avoid prolonged standing or sitting."
4    "I should continue to wear elastic hose for at least 6 to 8 weeks."

**Answer: 1**

*Rationale:* Clients with chronic venous insufficiency are advised to avoid crossing the legs, sitting in chairs where the feet don't touch the floor, and wearing garters or sources of pressure above the legs (such as girdles). The client should wear elastic hose for 6 to 8 weeks, and in some situations for life. The client should sleep with the foot of the bed elevated to promote venous return during sleep. Venous problems are characterized by insufficient drainage of blood from the legs returning to the heart. Thus, interventions need to be aimed at promoting flow of blood out of the legs and back to the heart.

*Test-Taking Strategy:* Use the concept of gravity when answering questions that relate to peripheral vascular problems. Option 1 is the only action that does not promote venous drainage. Review home care instructions for the client with venous insufficiency if you had difficulty with this question.

*Level of Cognitive Ability:* Analysis
*Client Needs:* Health Promotion and Maintenance
*Integrated Concept/Process:* Teaching/Learning
*Content Area:* Adult Health/Cardiovascular

*Reference*
Smeltzer, S., & Bare, B. (2000). *Brunner & Suddarth's Textbook of medical-surgical nursing* (9th ed.). Philadelphia: Lippincott Williams & Wilkins, p. 709.

---

**59.** A nurse is providing home care discharge instructions to a client who had varicose vein stripping and ligation and is being discharged from the ambulatory care unit. The nurse tells the client to:

1    Maintain bed rest for the first 3 days
2    Ambulate for 5 to 10 minutes twice a day beginning the day after surgery
3    Elevate the foot of the bed while in bed
4    Remove elastic hose after 24 hours

**Answer: 3**

*Rationale:* Standard postoperative care following vein ligation and stripping consists of bed rest for 24 hours, with ambulation for 5 to 10 minutes every 2 hours thereafter. Continuous elastic compression of the leg is maintained for 1 week following the procedure, followed by long-term use of elastic hose. The foot of the bed should be elevated to promote venous drainage.

*Test-Taking Strategy:* Use knowledge of the concepts related to blood flow and immobility to answer this question. Options 1 and 4 will promote venous stasis, so they are eliminated first. From the remaining options, noting the words *twice a day* in option 2 will eliminate this option. Review postoperative teaching points following varicose vein stripping and ligation if you had difficulty with this question.

*Level of Cognitive Ability:* Application
*Client Needs:* Health Promotion and Maintenance
*Integrated Concept/Process:* Teaching/Learning
*Content Area:* Adult Health/Cardiovascular

*Reference*
Smeltzer, S., & Bare, B. (2000). *Brunner & Suddarth's Textbook of medical-surgical nursing* (9th ed.). Philadelphia: Lippincott Williams & Wilkins, p. 713.

**60.** A nurse is developing a teaching plan for the client with Raynaud's disease. The nurse plans to tell the client that the symptoms may improve with:

1   A high-protein diet, which will minimize tissue malnutrition
2   Vitamin K administration, which will prevent tendencies toward bleeding
3   Keeping the hands and feet warm and dry, which will prevent vasoconstriction
4   Daily cool baths, which will provide an analgesic effect

**Answer: 3**

*Rationale:* Use of measures to prevent vasoconstriction are helpful in managing Raynaud's disease. The hands and feet should be kept dry. Gloves and warm fabrics should be worn in cold weather, and the client should avoid exposure to nicotine and caffeine. Avoidance of situations that trigger stress is also helpful. Options 1, 2, and 4 are not components of the treatment for this disorder.

*Test-Taking Strategy:* Use the process of elimination. Recalling the need to promote vasodilation will direct you to option 3. Review teaching points related to Raynaud's disease if you had difficulty with this question.

*Level of Cognitive Ability:* Application
*Client Needs:* Health Promotion and Maintenance
*Integrated Concept/Process:* Teaching/Learning
*Content Area:* Adult Health/Cardiovascular

*Reference*
Smeltzer, S., & Bare, B. (2000). *Brunner & Suddarth's Textbook of medical-surgical nursing* (9th ed.). Philadelphia: Lippincott Williams & Wilkins, p. 704.

**61.** A client with peripheral arterial disease has received instructions from the nurse about how to limit progression of the disease. The nurse determines that the client needs further instructions if which of the following statements was made by the client?

1   "I should walk daily to increase the circulation to my legs."
2   "A hot heating pad on my leg will help to soothe the leg pain."
3   "I need to take special care of my feet to prevent injury."
4   "I need to eat a balanced diet."

**Answer: 2**

*Rationale:* Long-term management of peripheral arterial disease consists of measures that increase peripheral circulation (exercise), promote vasodilatation (warmth), relieve pain, and maintain tissue integrity (foot care and nutrition). Application of heat directly to the extremity is contraindicated. The limb may have decreased sensitivity and be more at risk for burns. Additionally, direct application of heat raises oxygen and nutritional requirements of the tissue even further.

*Test-Taking Strategy:* Use the process of elimination. Focus on the client's diagnosis and note the key words *needs further instructions.* Noting the key word *hot* in option 2 will direct you to the correct option. Review the teaching points related to peripheral arterial disease if you had difficulty with this question.

*Level of Cognitive Ability:* Analysis
*Client Needs:* Health Promotion and Maintenance
*Integrated Concept/Process:* Teaching/Learning
*Content Area:* Adult Health/Cardiovascular

*Reference*
Smeltzer, S., & Bare, B. (2000). *Brunner & Suddarth's Textbook of medical-surgical nursing* (9th ed.). Philadelphia: Lippincott Williams & Wilkins, p. 691.

**62.** A nurse is planning to teach a client with hypertension about nonfood items that contain sodium and develops a written list for the client. The nurse avoids placing which of the following items on the list?

1    Demineralized water
2    Antacids
3    Laxatives
4    Toothpaste

**Answer: 1**

*Rationale:* Sodium intake can be increased by the use of several types of products, including toothpaste and mouthwashes; over-the-counter medications such as analgesics, antacids, cough remedies, laxatives, and sedatives; and softened water, as well as some mineral waters. Water that is bottled, distilled, deionized, or demineralized may be used for drinking and cooking. Clients are highly advised to read labels for sodium content.

*Test-Taking Strategy:* Use the process of elimination, noting the key word *avoids*. Look for the item that is low in sodium. Noting the word *demineralized*, which means having the minerals taken out of, will direct you to option 1. Review items that are low and high in sodium content if you had difficulty with this question.

*Level of Cognitive Ability:* Application
*Client Needs:* Health Promotion and Maintenance
*Integrated Concept/Process:* Teaching/Learning
*Content Area:* Adult Health/Cardiovascular

*Reference*
Peckenpaugh, N., & Poleman, C. (1999). *Nutrition essentials and diet therapy* (8th ed.). Philadelphia: W.B. Saunders, p. 190.

---

**63.** A school nurse provides several teaching sessions to a group of high school students regarding the hazards of smoking. Which comment by a student indicates the need for further teaching?

1    "Inhalation of tobacco smoke from active smoking, and passive smoke inhaled from other people smoking, are both public health issues."
2    "Chewing tobacco is a safer method of tobacco use than is smoking the tobacco."
3    "My health is at risk when my parents smoke."
4    "Smoking during pregnancy increases the risk of stillbirth and miscarriages."

**Answer: 2**

*Rationale:* All forms of tobacco use are health hazards. Options 1, 3, and 4 are accurate regarding the health hazards of tobacco use.

*Test-Taking Strategy:* Note the key words *need for further teaching*. This should direct you to option 2. If you had difficulty with this question review the hazards of tobacco use.

*Level of Cognitive Ability:* Analysis
*Client Needs:* Health Promotion and Maintenance
*Integrated Concept/Process:* Teaching/Learning
*Content Area:* Fundamental Skills

*Reference*
Smeltzer, S., & Bare, B. (2000). *Brunner & Suddarth's Textbook of medical-surgical nursing* (9th ed.). Philadelphia: Lippincott Williams & Wilkins. p. 268.

---

**64.** A nurse is developing goals for the postpartum client who is at risk for infection. Which of the following goals would be most appropriate for this client?

1    The client will verbalize a reduction of pain
2    The client will no longer have a positive Homans' sign
3    The client will report how to treat an infection
4    The client will be able to identify measures to prevent infection

**Answer: 4**

*Rationale:* The uterus is theoretically sterile during pregnancy, and until the membranes rupture. It is capable of being invaded by pathogens after rupture. Options 1 and 2 are unrelated to the issue of infection. Option 3 indicates that an infection is present. Option 4 is a goal for the client "at risk" for infection.

*Test-Taking Strategy:* Focus on the key words *at risk for infection*. Noting the word *prevent* in option 4 will direct you to this option. Option 3 implies that an infection has been diagnosed. Options 1 and 2 are unrelated to the issue of the question. Review the goals for a client at risk for infection if you had difficulty with this question.

*Level of Cognitive Ability:* Analysis
*Client Needs:* Health Promotion and Maintenance
*Integrated Concept/Process:* Nursing Process/Planning
*Content Area:* Maternity

**Reference**
Olds, S., London. M., & Ladewig, P. (2000). *Maternal-newborn nursing: A family and community-based approach* (6th ed.). Upper Saddle River, N.J.: Prentice Hall, p. 980.

---

**65.** A neonatal intensive care unit (NICU) nurse teaches handwashing techniques to parents before their handling of an infant who is receiving antibiotic treatment for a neonatal infection. The nurse determines that the parents understand the purpose of handwashing if they state that this is primarily done to:

1   Reduce their own fears
2   Minimize the spread of infection to other siblings
3   Reduce the possibility of environmental infection for their infant
4   Allow them an opportunity to communicate with each other and staff

**Answer: 3**
*Rationale:* Appropriate handwashing by staff and parents has been effective in the prevention of nosocomial infections in nursery units. This action also promotes parents' taking an active part in the care of their infant. Options 1 and 4 are not the primary reason to perform handwashing. Since the infant has the infection and is in the NICU, option 2 is incorrect.

*Test-Taking Strategy:* Note the key word *primarily* to assist in eliminating options 1 and 4. Noting that the infant is in the NICU will assist in eliminating option 2. Review the purposes of handwashing if you had difficulty with this question.

*Level of Cognitive Ability:* Analysis
*Clients Needs:* Health Promotion and Maintenance
*Integrated Concept/Process:* Teaching/Learning
*Content Area:* Maternity

**Reference**
Olds, S., London. M., & Ladewig, P. (2000). *Maternal-newborn nursing: A family and community-based approach* (6th ed.). Upper Saddle River, N.J.: Prentice Hall, p. 765.

---

**66.** A client is receiving rehabilitative services during pregnancy for alcohol abuse. The nurse would provide supportive care by:

1   Encouraging the client to participate in care and identifying supportive strategies that are helpful
2   Avoiding discussion of the alcohol problem and recovery with the client
3   Minimizing communication with supportive family members
4   Encouraging the client to stop counseling once the infant is born

**Answer: 1**
*Rationale:* The nurse provides supportive care by encouraging the client to participate in care. The nurse should not avoid discussing the client's problem with the client, and communication with family members is important. Counseling needs to continue after the infant is born.

*Test-Taking Strategy:* Use the process of elimination, noting the key words *supportive care*. Option 1 provides the client with an active role in care. Options 2, 3, and 4 create barriers for long-term success in dealing with the problem. Review measures that provide supportive nursing care for the pregnant client who abuses alcohol if you had difficulty with this question.

*Level of Cognitive Ability:* Application
*Clients Needs:* Health Promotion and Maintenance

*Integrated Concept/Process:* Nursing Process/Implementation
*Content Area:* Maternity

*Reference*
Olds, S., London. M., & Ladewig, P. (2000). *Maternal-newborn nursing: A family and community-based approach* (6th ed.). Upper Saddle River, N.J.: Prentice Hall, p. 351.

---

**67.** A client with active pulmonary tuberculosis (TB) has been receiving multi-drug chemotherapy for the past month. The client is being prepared for discharge from the hospital to home. The nurse determines respiratory isolation is no longer required and that medication therapy has been effective when:

1  Nausea and vomiting has stopped
2  The Mantoux test (PPD) is negative
3  Sputum cultures are negative
4  Stools are clay colored

**Answer: 3**
*Rationale:* The primary diagnostic tool for pulmonary tuberculosis is a sputum culture. A negative culture indicates effectiveness of treatment. Nausea and vomiting and clay-colored stools are side effects of the medication used to treat tuberculosis. Their presence or absence does not measure the therapeutic effectiveness of the medication. The Mantoux test is a screening tool, not a diagnostic test for tuberculosis. Since the Mantoux test indicates exposure to the organism but not active disease, the test results will remain positive.

*Test-Taking Strategy:* Use the process of elimination, noting the key words *therapy has been effective*. Remember, the absence of infectious organisms is a desired outcome in communicable diseases. The sputum is the only diagnostic test that will determine the absence of infectious organisms. If you had difficulty with this question, review the diagnostic tests related to TB.

*Level of Cognitive Ability:* Analysis
*Client Needs:* Health Promotion and Maintenance
*Integrated Concept/Process:* Nursing Process/Evaluation
*Content Area:* Adult Health/Respiratory

*Reference*
Smeltzer, S., & Bare, B. (2000). *Brunner & Suddarth's Textbook of medical-surgical nursing* (9th ed.). Philadelphia: Lippincott Williams & Wilkins. p. 438.

---

**68.** A nurse has conducted a class for pregnant clients with diabetes mellitus on signs and symptoms of potential complications. The nurse determines that the teaching was effective if a client made which of the following statements?

1  "I'm glad I don't have to worry about developing hypoglycemia while I am pregnant."
2  "I need to watch my weight for any sudden gains, since I am prone to pregnancy-induced hypertension."
3  "My insulin needs should decrease in the last 2 months, because I will be using some of the baby's insulin supply."
4  "I should not have ultrasonography done since I am diabetic."

**Answer: 2**
*Rationale:* Hypoglycemia is a problem during pregnancy and needs to be assessed. A diabetic pregnant client has a higher incidence of pregnancy-induced hypertension than the nondiabetic pregnant client. Insulin needs will increase during the last trimester because of increased placenta degradation. Ultrasonography is performed frequently during a diabetic pregnancy to check for congenital anomalies and determine appropriate growth patterns.

*Test-Taking Strategy:* Use the process of elimination, focusing on the issue: a pregnant client with diabetes mellitus. Options 1 and 4 can be easily eliminated. Remembering that insulin needs will increase during the last trimester of pregnancy will assist in eliminating option 3. If you had difficulty with this question, review the complications associated with diabetes and pregnancy.

*Level of Cognitive Ability:* Analysis
*Client Needs:* Health Promotion and Maintenance

*Integrated Concept/Process:* Teaching/Learning
*Content Area:* Maternity

*Reference*
Olds, S., London. M., & Ladewig, P. (2000). *Maternal-newborn nursing: A family and community-based approach* (6th ed.). Upper Saddle River, N.J.: Prentice-Hall, p. 257.

---

**69.** A postpartum client recovering from disseminated intravascular coagulopathy is to be discharged on low dosages of an anticoagulant medication. The nurse includes which priority safety instruction regarding this medication in the home care instructions?

1   Avoid activities, because bruising injuries can occur
2   Avoid walking long distances and climbing stairs
3   Avoid taking acetylsalicylic acid (aspirin)
4   Avoid brushing teeth

**Answer: 3**
*Rationale:* Aspirin can interact with the anticoagulant medication and increase clotting time beyond therapeutic ranges. Avoiding aspirin is a priority. Not all activities need to be avoided. Walking and climbing stairs constitute acceptable activity. The client does not need to avoid brushing the teeth; however, the client should be instructed to use a soft toothbrush.

*Test-Taking Strategy:* Note the key word *priority* in the question. Recalling the safety measures related to the administration of anticoagulants will direct you to the correct option. If you had difficulty with this question, review teaching points related to anticoagulants.

*Level of Cognitive Ability:* Application
*Client Needs:* Health Promotion and Maintenance
*Integrated Concept/Process:* Teaching/Learning
*Content Area:* Pharmacology

*Reference*
Hodgson, B., & Kizior, R. (2001). *Saunders Nursing drug handbook 2001.* Philadelphia: W.B. Saunders, p. 1062.

---

**70.** A client with a diagnosis of depression admits that one reason for the depression is that too many demands drain her energy. The client also admits that, in part, the situation is as bad as it is because the word *no* is not part of her vocabulary when it comes to the requests and needs of others. After 7 days of hospitalization, another client asks for assistance in cleaning the unit immediately. The client with depression says, "No, I can't help you now. I am enjoying the movie." The nurse interprets this response as:

1   A shirking of responsibility
2   Withdrawal from peers
3   Increased control over decisions
4   Decreased cooperation with others

**Answer: 3**
*Rationale:* The client has been unable to refuse requests in the past. Saying "no" now indicates that the client is trying to meet her own needs. "No" is being said now without guilt and apology. During the treatment process, the client has learned how to meet her own needs, and this can help to maintain health after discharge. Options 1, 2, and 4 are incorrect interpretations.

*Test-Taking Strategy:* Use the process of elimination. Focusing on the data in the question will direct you to option 3. Review measures that assist in increasing control in the client with depression if you had difficulty with this question.

*Level of Cognitive Ability:* Analysis
*Client Needs:* Health Promotion and Maintenance
*Integrated Concept/Process:* Nursing Process/Analysis
*Content Area:* Mental Health

*Reference*
Stuart, G.W., & Laraia, M.T. (1998). *Principles and practice of psychiatric nursing.* (6th ed.). St. Louis: Mosby, 331.

**71.** A suicidal client who was admitted to the mental health unit approximately 7 days ago is preparing for discharge. The nurse is evaluating the coping strategies learned during hospitalization. The nurse determines that further teaching needs to occur if the client makes which of the following statements?

1   "I think this has been a very positive experience in my life."
2   "I know I must continue to take my medications just as prescribed."
3   "I now know that I can't be all things to all people."
4   "I know that I probably won't have depression in the future."

**Answer: 4**

*Rationale:* Depression may be a recurring illness for some people. The client needs to understand the symptoms of depression and recognize when or if treatment needs to begin again. The other statements indicate that the client has learned some coping skills, such as setting limits, taking medications, and reframing an unpleasant experience into a more positive one.

*Test-Taking Strategy:* Use the process of elimination, noting the key words *further teaching needs to occur*. Recalling that depression may reoccur will direct you to option 4. Review the characteristics of depression if you had difficulty with this question.

*Level of Cognitive Ability:* Analysis
*Client Needs:* Health Promotion and Maintenance
*Integrated Concept/Process:* Teaching/Learning
*Content Area:* Mental Health

*Reference*
Stuart, G.W., & Laraia, M.T. (1998). *Principles and practice of psychiatric nursing.* (6th ed.). St. Louis: Mosby, p. 352.

**72.** A nurse demonstrates to a mother how to correctly take an axillary temperature to determine whether the child has a fever. Which action by the mother would indicate a need for further teaching?

1   She selects a mercury thermometer with a slender tip
2   She holds the thermometer in the axilla for 1 minute
3   She records the actual temperature reading and route
4   She places the thermometer in the center of the axilla

**Answer: 2**

*Rationale:* Taking an axillary temperature for at least 5 minutes is most accurate. Options 1, 3, and 4 are correct steps for taking an axillary temperature.

*Test-Taking Strategy:* Note the key words *a need for further teaching*. Visualize the procedure. Noting the words *1 minute* in option 2 will direct you to this option. If you had difficulty with this question, review the procedure for obtaining an axillary temperature.

*Level of Cognitive Ability:* Analysis
*Client Needs:* Health Promotion and Maintenance
*Integrated Concept/Process:* Teaching/Learning
*Content Area:* Child Health

*Reference*
Wong, D. (1999). *Whaley & Wong's Nursing care of infants and children* (6th ed.). St. Louis: Mosby. pp. 243, 246.

**73.** A school nurse is teaching an athletic coach how to prevent dehydration in athletes during football practice. Which action by the coach during football practice would indicate that the teaching was ineffective?

1 Schedules fluid breaks every 30 minute throughout practice
2 Weighs athletes before, during, and after football practice
3 Asks the athletes to take a salt tablet before football practice
4 Tells the athletes to drink 16 oz of fluid per pound lost during practice

**Answer: 3**

*Rationale:* Salt tablets should not be taken, because they can contribute to dehydration. Frequent fluid breaks should be taken to prevent dehydration. Early detection of decreased body weight alerts an individual to drink fluids before becoming dehydrated. Sixteen ounces of fluid should be consumed for every pound lost to prevent dehydration.

*Test-Taking Strategy:* Note the key word *ineffective*. Recalling the principles of fluid and electrolyte balance and the causes of dehydration will direct you to option 3. Options 1, 2, and 4 are measures that prevent the occurrence of dehydration in athletes. If you had difficulty with this question, review these measures.

*Level of Cognitive Ability:* Analysis
*Client Needs:* Health Promotion and Maintenance
*Integrated Concept/Process:* Teaching/Learning
*Content Area:* Fundamental Skills

*Reference*
Wong, D. (1999). *Whaley & Wong's Nursing care of infants and children* (6th ed.). St. Louis: Mosby. p. 1286.

---

**74.** A nurse instructs a client in a low-fat diet. The client indicates an understanding of this diet by choosing which of the following from the menu?

1 Liver, potato salad, sherbet
2 Shrimp and bacon salad
3 Turkey breast, boiled rice, and angel food cake
4 Lean hamburger steak, macaroni and cheese

**Answer: 3**

*Rationale:* Major sources of fats include meats, salad dressings, eggs, butter, cheese, and bacon. Options 1, 2, and 4 contain high-fat foods.

*Test-Taking Strategy:* Use the process of elimination. Eliminate options 2 and 4 first, because both a hamburger steak and bacon are high in fat. From the remaining options, look at the foods closely. Option 3 does not contain any high fat foods. Potato salad (option 1) will contain mayonnaise, which is high in fat. If you had difficulty with this question, review those foods that contain fat.

*Level of Cognitive Ability:* Analysis
*Client Needs:* Health Promotion and Maintenance
*Integrated Concept/Process:* Teaching/Learning
*Content Area:* Fundamental Skills

*Reference*
Peckenpaugh, N., & Poleman, C. (1999). *Nutrition essentials and diet therapy* (8th ed.). Philadelphia: W.B. Saunders, p. 145.

**75.** A nurse has provided discharge instructions regarding nitroglycerin therapy to the client with angina. Which statement by the client indicates an understanding of home use of the nitroglycerin?

1 "When I have chest pain, I should put a tablet under my tongue. If I have a burning sensation, I should call my doctor immediately."

2 "When I experience chest pain, I can continue what I'm doing. If it doesn't go away in 10 minutes, I should use a nitroglycerin."

3 "When I have pain, I should lie down and place a tablet under my tongue. If the pain is unrelieved in 5 minutes, I should take another tablet."

4 "If I use a nitroglycerin tablet and the pain does not subside in 15 minutes, I should go to the hospital."

**Answer: 3**

*Rationale:* The client taking sublingual nitroglycerin should lie down after taking the medication, because lightheadedness and dizziness may occur as a result of postural hypotension. The client should use up to three tablets at 5-minute intervals before seeking medical attention. Options 1, 2, and 4 are incorrect regarding the use of nitroglycerin. A burning sensation is a common side effect of nitroglycerin. Nitroglycerin should be used with the onset of anginal pain. The client should repeat nitroglycerin if relief is not obtained with the first or second dose.

*Test-Taking Strategy:* Use the process of elimination. Recalling that nitroglycerin may be taken at 5 minute intervals times three, will direct you to option 3. If you had difficulty with this question, review client teaching related to nitroglycerin.

*Level of Cognitive Ability:* Analysis
*Client Needs:* Health Promotion and Maintenance
*Integrated Concept/Process:* Teaching/Learning
*Content Area:* Adult Health/Cardiovascular

*Reference*
Hodgson, B., & Kizior, R. (2001). *Saunders Nursing drug handbook 2001.* Philadelphia: W.B. Saunders, p. 750.

**76.** A client has urinary calculi composed of uric acid. The nurse is teaching the client dietary measures to prevent further development of urolithiasis. Which of the following statements would indicate that the client understands these dietary measures?

1 "I would avoid milk and dairy products."

2 "I would avoid foods, such as spinach, chocolate, and tea."

3 "I would avoid foods, such as fish with fine bones and organ meats."

4 "I need to drink cranberry juice."

**Answer: 3**

*Rationale:* With a uric acid stone, the client should limit intake of foods high in purines. Organ meats, sardines, herring, and other high-purine foods are eliminated from the diet. Foods with moderate levels of purines, such as red and white meats and some seafood, are also limited. Options 1 and 2 are recommended dietary changes for calculi composed of calcium phosphate or calcium oxalate. Cranberry juice is commonly recommended to help lower the pH of urine, rendering it more acid to prevent the development of urinary tract infections. However, uric acid stones form most readily in acid urine, and cranberry juice would be contraindicated in this client with uric acid stone formation.

*Test-Taking Strategy:* Note the key words *uric acid*. Remembering that organ meats are high in purines will assist in directing you to the correct option. If you had difficulty with this question, review foods to avoid with uric acid calculi.

*Level of Cognitive Ability:* Analysis
*Client Needs:* Health Promotion and Maintenance
*Integrated Concept/Process:* Teaching/Learning
*Content Area:* Adult Health/Renal

*Reference*
Smeltzer, S., & Bare, B. (2000). *Brunner & Suddarth's Textbook of medical-surgical nursing* (9th ed.). Philadelphia: Lippincott Williams & Wilkins, p. 1164.

**77.** A nurse is teaching a mother with diabetes mellitus who delivered a large for gestational age (LGA) male infant about care of the infant. The nurse tells the mother that LGA infants appear to be more mature because of their large size, and in reality, these infants frequently need to be aroused to facilitate nutritional intake and attachment. Which statement, if made by the mother, indicates further teaching is necessary?

1   "I will talk to my baby when he is in a quiet alert state."
2   "I will watch my baby closely, because I know he may not be as mature in motor development."
3   "I will breastfeed my baby every 2½ to 3 hours, and will implement arousing techniques."
4   "I will allow my baby to sleep throughout the night, because he needs his rest."

**Answer: 4**

**Rationale:** LGA infants tend to be more difficult to arouse and therefore will need to be aroused to facilitate nutritional intake and attachment opportunities. These infants also have problems maintaining a quiet alert state. It is beneficial for the mother to interact with the infant during this time to enhance and lengthen the quiet alert state. Even though the infant is large, motor function is not usually as mature as in the term infant. LGA infants need to be aroused for feedings, usually every 2½ to 3 hours for breastfeeding.

**Test-Taking Strategy:** Note that the question asks for the option that indicates the need for further teaching. Note the key words *frequently need to be aroused* in the question. Focusing on the key words will direct you to option 4. Options 1, 2, and 3 address observation and arousal whereas, option 4 does not. Review care of an LGA infant if you had difficulty with this question.

**Level of Cognitive Ability:** Analysis
**Client Needs:** Health Promotion and Maintenance
**Integrated Concept/Process:** Teaching/Learning
**Content Area:** Maternity

**Reference**
Olds, S., London. M., & Ladewig, P. (2000). *Maternal-newborn nursing: A family and community-based approach* (6th ed.). Upper Saddle River, N.J.: Prentice-Hall, p. 812.

**78.** A client has been experiencing muscle weakness over a period of several months. The physician suspects polymyositis. Which statement, if made by the client, correctly identifies a confirmation of test results and this diagnosis?

1   "The physician said if the muscle fibers were thickened, I would have polymyositis."
2   "If I have polymyositis, there will be a decrease in elastic tissue."
3   "I will know I have polymyositis if the muscle fibers are inflamed."
4   "The physician said there would be more fibers and tissue with polymyositis."

**Answer: 3**

**Rationale:** In polymyositis, necrosis and inflammation is seen in muscle fibers and myocardial fibers. Option 1 is an opposite of what is noted in this disorder. Option 2 refers to the decreased elastic tissue in the aorta seen in Marfan's syndrome. Option 4 refers to increased fibrous tissue seen in ankylosis.

**Test-Taking Strategy:** Note that the issue of the question is polymyositis. "Itis" indicates inflammation. The only option that addresses inflammation is option 3. If you had difficulty with this question, review the description of polymyositis.

**Level of Cognitive Ability:** Analysis
**Client Needs:** Health Promotion and Maintenance
**Integrated Concept/Process:** Teaching/Learning
**Content Area:** Adult Health/Musculoskeletal

**Reference**
Smeltzer, S., & Bare, B. (2000). *Brunner & Suddarth's Textbook of medical-surgical nursing* (9th ed.). Philadelphia: Lippincott Williams & Wilkins, p. 1427.

**79.** A client has two chest tubes inserted in the right pleural space following thoracic surgery, which are attached to Pleu-revac drainage systems. The nurse instructs the client in measures that will promote optimal respiratory functioning and plans to:

1 Milk and strip the chest tubes once a shift
2 Maintain the client on bed rest until the chest tubes are removed
3 Position the client only on the back and on the right side
4 Encourage the client to cough and deep breathe every hour

**Answer: 4**

*Rationale:* The client who has chest tubes following thoracic surgery should be encouraged to cough and deep breathe every 1 to 2 hours after surgery. This helps to facilitate drainage of fluid from the pleural space, as well as facilitate the clearance of secretions from the respiratory tract. Milking and stripping of the chest tube is done only when there is an occlusion, such as with a small clot. Even then, it is done only with a physician's order or when allowed by agency policy. The client is maintained in semi-Fowler's position, and may lie on the back or on the nonoperative side. The client may be allowed to lie on the operative side according to surgeon preference, but care must be taken not to compress the chest tube or attached drainage tubing. Ambulation is generally allowed within a day or two, and also facilitates optimal respiratory function.

*Test-Taking Strategy:* Focus on the issue: to promote optimal respiratory functioning. Option 1 is somewhat controversial and is eliminated first. Bed rest does not promote respiratory function, and is eliminated next. From the remaining options, recalling that positioning is done according to surgeon preference directs you to option 4. Review the measures that promote optimal respiratory function in the client with a chest tube if you had difficulty with this question.

*Level of Cognitive Ability:* Application
*Client Needs:* Health Promotion and Maintenance
*Integrated Concept/Process:* Nursing Process/Planning
*Content Area:* Adult Health/Respiratory

*Reference*
Smeltzer, S., & Bare, B. (2000). *Brunner & Suddarth's Textbook of medical-surgical nursing* (9th ed.). Philadelphia: Lippincott Williams & Wilkins, p. 515.

**80.** A nurse in an ambulatory clinic administers a Mantoux skin test to a client on a Monday. The nurse plans to have the client return to the clinic to have the results read on:

1 Tuesday or Wednesday
2 Wednesday or Thursday
3 Thursday or Friday
4 The following Monday

**Answer: 2**

*Rationale:* The Mantoux skin test for tuberculosis is read in 48 to 72 hours. The client should return to the clinic on Wednesday or Thursday.

*Test-Taking Strategy:* Use the process of elimination. Recalling that this test is read within 48 to 72 hours will direct you to option 2. Review the procedure for this test if you had difficulty with this question.

*Level of Cognitive Ability:* Application
*Client Needs:* Health Promotion and Maintenance
*Integrated Concept/Process:* Nursing Process/Planning
*Content Area:* Adult Health/Respiratory

*Reference*
Smeltzer, S., & Bare, B. (2000). *Brunner & Suddarth's Textbook of medical-surgical nursing* (9th ed.). Philadelphia: Lippincott Williams & Wilkins, p. 439.

**81.** A client with chronic airflow limitation (CAL) is admitted to the hospital with exacerbation, and has a nursing diagnosis of Ineffective Airway Clearance. The nurse assesses the client with regard to which of the following prehospitalization factors that could have contributed most to this nursing diagnosis?
1   Anxiety level
2   Amount of sleep
3   Fat intake
4   Fluid intake

**Answer: 4**
*Rationale:* The client with Ineffective Airway Clearance has ineffective coughing and excess sputum in the airways. The nurse assesses for contributing factors, such as dehydration and lack of knowledge of proper coughing techniques. Reduction of these factors helps to limit exacerbations of the disease. Options 1, 2, and 3 are not directly associated with this nursing diagnosis.

*Test-Taking Strategy:* Note the nursing diagnosis, Ineffective Airway Clearance. This calls to mind the concept of sputum production and clearance. Evaluate each of the options in terms of their potential ability to inhibit sputum production or clearance. The fluid intake is the only factor that could affect the viscosity of secretions, thus affecting airway clearance. Review the defining characteristics of Ineffective Airway Clearance if you had difficulty with this question.

*Level of Cognitive Ability:* Analysis
*Client Needs:* Health Promotion and Maintenance
*Integrated Concept/Process:* Nursing Process/Assessment
*Content Area:* Adult Health/Respiratory

*Reference*
Smeltzer, S., & Bare, B. (2000). *Brunner & Suddarth's Textbook of medical-surgical nursing* (9th ed.). Philadelphia: Lippincott Williams & Wilkins, p. 456.

**82.** A client with acquired immunodeficiency syndrome (AIDS) gets recurrent *Candida* infections (thrush) of the mouth. The nurse has given instructions to the client to minimize the occurrence of thrush, and evaluates that the client understands the material if which of the following statements is made by the client?
1   "I should brush my teeth and rinse my mouth once a day."
2   "I should use a strong mouthwash at least once a week."
3   "Increasing red meat in my diet will keep this from recurring."
4   "Eating 8 oz of yogurt that contains live cultures helps to control this."

**Answer: 4**
*Rationale: Candida* infections can be controlled by eating 8 oz of yogurt that contains live cultures *(Lactobacillus acidophilus)*. Careful routine skin and mouth care are also helpful in preventing recurrence. Red meat will not prevent thrush. In options 1 and 2 the timeframes for oral hygiene are too infrequent.

*Test-Taking Strategy:* Use the process of elimination. Eliminate options 1 and 2, because they are similar. From the remaining options, recalling that red meat is not likely to minimize the occurrence of thrush will direct you to option 4. Review teaching points related to the prevention of *Candida* infections if you had difficulty with this question.

*Level of Cognitive Ability:* Analysis
*Client Needs:* Health Promotion and Maintenance
*Integrated Concept/Process:* Self-Care
*Content Area:* Adult Health/Immune

*Reference*
Smeltzer, S., & Bare, B. (2000). *Brunner & Suddarth's Textbook of medical-surgical nursing* (9th ed.). Philadelphia: Lippincott Williams & Wilkins, p. 1365.

**83.** A nurse is teaching a client with acquired immunodeficiency syndrome (AIDS) how to avoid food-borne illnesses. The nurse instructs the client to avoid acquiring infection from food by avoiding which of the following items?

1   Raw oysters
2   Pasteurized milk
3   Products with sorbitol
4   Bottled water

**Answer: 1**

*Rationale:* The client is taught to avoid raw or undercooked seafood, meat, poultry, and eggs. The client should also avoid unpasteurized milk and dairy products. Fruits that the client peels are safe, as are bottled beverages. The client may be taught to avoid sorbitol, but this is to diminish diarrhea, and has nothing to do with food-borne illnesses.

*Test-Taking Strategy:* Use the process of elimination, focusing on the issue: food-borne illness. Sorbitol gives diarrhea, but is unrelated to food-borne illness, so option 3 is eliminated first. Eliminate option 2, because products that are pasteurized are free of microbes. From the remaining options, noting the key word *raw* in option 1 will direct you to this option. Review dietary teaching for the client with AIDS if you had difficulty with this question.

*Level of Cognitive Ability:* Application
*Client Needs:* Health Promotion and Maintenance
*Integrated Concept/Process:* Teaching/Learning
*Content Area:* Adult Health/Immune

*Reference*
Smeltzer, S., & Bare, B. (2000). *Brunner & Suddarth's Textbook of medical-surgical nursing* (9th ed.). Philadelphia: Lippincott Williams & Wilkins, pp. 1367-1368.

**84.** A client with histoplasmosis has an order for ketoconazole (Nizoral). The nurse teaches the client to do which of the following while taking this medication?

1   Take the medication on an empty stomach
2   Take the medication with an antacid
3   Avoid exposure to sunlight
4   Limit alcohol intake to 2 oz per day

**Answer: 3**

*Rationale:* The client should be taught that ketoconazole is an antifungal medication. It should be taken with food or milk. Antacids should be avoided for 2 hours after it is taken, because gastric acid is needed to activate the medication. The client should avoid concurrent use of alcohol, since the medication is hepatotoxic. The client should also avoid exposure to sunlight, since the medication increases photosensitivity.

*Test-Taking Strategy:* Use the process of elimination and general guidelines related to medication administration to eliminate options 2 and 4. From the remaining options, it is necessary to know that the medication causes a photosensitivity reaction, and should be taken with food or milk. Review this medication if you had difficulty with this question.

*Level of Cognitive Ability:* Application
*Client Needs:* Health Promotion and Maintenance
*Integrated Concept/Process:* Teaching/Learning
*Content Area:* Pharmacology

*Reference*
Hodgson, B., & Kizior, R. (2001). *Saunders Nursing drug handbook 2001.* Philadelphia: W.B. Saunders, p. 565.

**85.** A nurse is planning to teach a teenage client about sexuality. The nurse would begin the instruction by:
1   Establishing a relationship and determining prior knowledge
2   Providing written information about sexually transmitted diseases
3   Informing the teenager of the dangers of pregnancy
4   Advising the teenager to maintain sexual abstinence until marriage

**Answer: 1**
*Rationale:* The first step in effective communication is establishing a relationship. By exploring the client's interest and prior knowledge, rapport is established and learning needs are assessed. The other options may be later steps depending on the data obtained.

*Test-Taking Strategy:* Use the nursing process and select an assessment option. This will direct you to option 1. When teaching, assessing motivation, interest, and level of knowledge comes before providing information. If you had difficulty with this question review the principles of teaching and learning.

*Level of Cognitive Ability:* Application
*Client Needs:* Health Promotion and Maintenance
*Integrated Concept/Process:* Teaching/Learning
*Content Area:* Child Health

*Reference*
Ball, J., & Bindler, R. (1999). *Pediatric nursing: Caring for children* (2nd ed.). Stamford, Conn.: Appleton & Lange, p. 185.

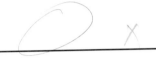

**86.** A nurse provides home care instructions to a client with Cushing's syndrome. The nurse determines that the client understands the hospital discharge instructions if the client makes which of these statements?
1   "I need to eat foods low in potassium."
2   "I need to take aspirin rather than Tylenol for a headache."
3   "I need to check the color of my stools."
4   "I need to check the temperature of my legs."

**Answer: 3**
*Rationale:* Cortisol stimulates the secretion of gastric acid and this can result in the development of peptic ulcers and gastrointestinal bleeding. Potassium rich foods should be encouraged to correct hypokalemia that occurs in this disorder. Aspirin can increase the risk for gastric bleeding and skin bruising. Cushing's syndrome does not affect temperature changes in lower extremities.

*Test-Taking Strategy:* Note the key word *understands*. Recalling the pathophysiology in this disorder and that cortisol stimulates the secretion of gastric acid will direct you to option 3. If you had difficulty with this question, review Cushing's syndrome.

*Level of Cognitive Ability:* Analysis
*Client Needs:* Health Promotion and Maintenance
*Integrated Concept/Process:* Teaching/Learning
*Content Area:* Adult Health/Endocrine

*Reference*
Smeltzer, S., & Bare, B. (2000). *Brunner & Suddarth's Textbook of medical-surgical nursing* (9th ed.). Philadelphia: Lippincott Williams & Wilkins, p. 1060.

**87.** A client with congestive heart failure and secondary hyperaldosteronism is started on spironolactone (Aldactone) to manage this disorder. The nurse anticipates the need to instruct the client regarding dosage adjustment of which of the following medications, if it is also being taken by the client?

1. Warfarin sodium (Coumadin)
2. Alprazolam (Xanax)
3. Verapamil hydrochloride (Calan)
4. Potassium chloride

**Answer: 4**

*Rationale:* Spironolactone (Aldactone) is a potassium-sparing diuretic. If the client is taking potassium chloride or another potassium supplement, the risk for hyperkalemia exists. Potassium doses would need to be adjusted while on this medication. A dosage adjustment would not be necessary if the client is taking either of the medications identified in options 1, 2, or 3.

*Test-Taking Strategy:* Focus on the issue: a dosage adjustment. Recalling that spironolactone is a potassium-sparing diuretic will direct you to option 4. If you had difficulty with this question, review those diuretics that are potassium-sparing.

*Level of Cognitive Ability:* Analysis
*Client Needs:* Health Promotion and Maintenance
*Integrated Concept/Process:* Nursing Process/Analysis
*Content Area:* Adult Health/Cardiovascular

**Reference**
Smeltzer, S., & Bare, B. (2000). *Brunner & Suddarth's Textbook of medical-surgical nursing* (9th ed.). Philadelphia: Lippincott Williams & Wilkins, p. 218.

**88.** A nurse is teaching health education classes to a group of expectant parents and the topic is preventing mental retardation caused by congenital hypothyroidism. The nurse tells the parents that the most effective means of preventing mental retardation caused by this disorder is by:

1. Adequate protein intake
2. Limiting alcohol consumption
3. Genetic testing
4. Neonatal screening

**Answer: 4**

*Rationale:* Congenital hypothyroidism is the most common preventable cause of mental retardation. Neonatal screening is the only means of early diagnosis. Newborn infants are screened for congenital hypothyroidism before discharge from the nursery and before 7 days of life.

*Test-Taking Strategy:* Focus on the issue: preventing mental retardation caused by congenital hypothyroidism. Options 1 and 2 are appropriate measures to prevent all birth defects. Genetics is only one factor related to the development of congenital hypothyroidism. Neonatal screening is the most global option. If you had difficulty with this question, review congenital hypothyroidism.

*Level of Cognitive Ability:* Application
*Client Needs:* Health Promotion and Maintenance
*Integrated Concept/Process:* Teaching/Learning
*Content Area:* Maternity

**Reference**
Lowdermilk, D., Perry, S., & Bobak, I. (2000). *Maternity & women's health care* (7th ed.). St. Louis: Mosby, p. 884.

**89.** A nurse in an outpatient diabetes clinic is monitoring a client with type 1 diabetes mellitus. Today's blood work reveals a glycosylated hemoglobin (HbA1c) of 10%. The nurse interprets this blood work as indicating which of the following?

1   A normal value, indicating that the client is managing blood glucose control well

2   A low value, indicating that the client is not managing blood glucose control very well

3   A high value, indicating that the client is not managing blood glucose control very well

4   The value does not offer information regarding client management of their disease

**Answer: 3**

*Rationale:* Glycosylated hemoglobin is a measure of glucose control during the past 6 to 8 weeks before the test. It is a reliable measure to determine the degree of glucose control in diabetic clients over a period of time and is not influenced by good glucose or dietary management a day or two before the test is done. The normal range for HbA1c is 4% to 7% with elevated levels indicating poor glucose control.

*Test-Taking Strategy:* Specific knowledge regarding the normal values for this test will direct you to option 3. If you had difficulty with this question, review this test.

*Level of Cognitive Ability:* Analysis
*Client Needs:* Health Promotion and Maintenance
*Integrated Concept/Process:* Nursing Process/Analysis
*Content Area:* Adult Health/Endocrine

*Reference*
Smeltzer, S., & Bare, B. (2000). *Brunner & Suddarth's Textbook of medical-surgical nursing* (9th ed.). Philadelphia: Lippincott Williams & Wilkins, p. 986.

---

**90.** A nurse is instructing a client with type 1 diabetes mellitus about management of hypoglycemic reactions. The nurse instructs the client that hypoglycemia most likely occurs during what time interval after insulin administration?

1   Onset

2   Peak

3   Duration

4   Anytime

**Answer: 2**

*Rationale:* Insulin reactions are most likely to occur during the peak time of the insulin, when the medication is at its maximum action. Peak action depends on the type of insulin, the amount administered, the injection site, and other factors.

*Test-Taking Strategy:* Use the process of elimination. Remember that insulin is a hypoglycemic agent. The word "peak" means the "highest point." Remembering this should assist in directing you to the correct option. If you had difficulty with this question, review the occurrence of hypoglycemia when a client is taking insulin.

*Level of Cognitive Ability:* Application
*Client Needs:* Health Promotion and Maintenance
*Integrated Concept/Process:* Teaching/Learning
*Content Area:* Adult Health/Endocrine

*Reference*
Smeltzer, S., & Bare, B. (2000). *Brunner & Suddarth's Textbook of medical-surgical nursing* (9th ed.). Philadelphia: Lippincott Williams & Wilkins, p. 991.

**91.** A nurse is caring for a client who is scheduled to have a thyroidectomy and provides instructions to the client about the surgical procedure. Which of the following statements by the client would indicate an understanding of the nurse's instructions?

1 "I will definitely have to continue taking antithyroid medications after this surgery."
2 "I need to place my hands behind my neck when I have to cough or change positions."
3 "I need to turn my head and neck front, back, and laterally every hour for the first 12 hours after surgery."
4 "I expect to experience some tingling of my toes, fingers, and lips after surgery."

**Answer: 2**

*Rationale:* The client is taught that tension needs to be avoided on the suture line; otherwise, hemorrhage may develop. One way of reducing incisional tension is to teach the client how to support their neck when coughing or being repositioned. Likewise, during the postoperative period, the client should avoid any unnecessary movement of the neck. That is why sandbags and pillows are frequently used to support the head and neck. Removal of the thyroid does not mean that the client will be taking antithyroid medications postoperatively. If a client experiences tingling in the fingers, toes, and lips, it is probably due to injury to the parathyroid gland during surgery resulting in hypocalcemia. These signs and symptoms need to be reported immediately.

*Test-Taking Strategy:* Use the process of elimination. Focusing on the type of surgery and the anatomical location of the surgical procedure will assist in eliminating options 1, 3, and 4. If you had difficulty with this question review postoperative care following thyroidectomy.

*Level of Cognitive Ability:* Analysis
*Client Needs:* Health Promotion and Maintenance
*Integrated Concept/Process:* Teaching/Learning
*Content Area:* Adult Health/Endocrine

*Reference*
Ignatavicius, D., Workman, M., & Mishler, M. (1999). *Medical-surgical nursing across the health care continuum* (3rd ed.). Philadelphia: W.B. Saunders, p. 1619.

**92.** A nurse has been preparing a client with chronic obstructive pulmonary disease (COPD) for discharge to home. Which statement by the client indicates a need for further teaching in relation to nutrition?

1 "I will certainly try to drink 3 L of fluid every day."
2 "It's best to eat three large meals a day so I will get all my nutrients."
3 "I will not eat as much cabbage as I once did."
4 "I will rest a few minutes before I eat."

**Answer: 2**

*Rationale:* Adequate fluid intake helps to liquefy pulmonary secretions. Large meals distend the abdomen and elevate the diaphragm, which may interfere with breathing. Gas-forming foods may cause bloating, which interferes with normal diaphragmatic breathing. Resting before eating may decrease the fatigue that is often associated with COPD.

*Test-Taking Strategy:* Use the process of elimination, noting the key words *need for further teaching*. Focusing on the client's diagnosis and recalling the activities that produce dyspnea will direct you to option 2. If you had difficulty with this question, review nutrition and the client with a chronic respiratory disorder.

*Level of Cognitive Ability:* Analysis
*Client Needs:* Health Promotion and Maintenance
*Integrated Concept/Process:* Teaching/Learning
*Content Area:* Adult Health/Respiratory

*Reference*
Ignatavicius, D., Workman, M., & Mishler, M. (1999). *Medical-surgical nursing across the health care continuum* (3rd ed.). Philadelphia: W.B. Saunders, p. 633.

**93.** A nurse is preparing a client with pneumonia for discharge to home. Which statement by the client would alert the nurse to the fact that the client is in need of further discharge teaching?

1   "I will take all of my antibiotics, even if I do feel 100% better."
2   "I understand that it may be weeks before my usual sense of well-being returns."
3   "It is a good idea for me to take a nap every afternoon for the next couple of weeks."
4   "You can toss out that incentive spirometry as soon as I leave for home."

**Answer: 4**

*Rationale:* Deep breathing and coughing exercises and use of incentive spirometry should be practiced for 6 to 8 weeks after the client is discharged from the hospital to keep the alveoli expanded and promote the removal of lung secretions. If the entire regimen of antibiotics is not taken, the client may suffer a relapse. Adequate rest is needed to maintain progress toward recovery. The period of convalescence with pneumonia is often lengthy and it may be weeks before the client feels a sense of well-being.

*Test-Taking Strategy:* Note the key words *further discharge teaching*. Focusing on the client's diagnosis and recalling the need to promote removal of lung secretions will direct you to option 4. If you had difficulty with this question, review teaching points for the client with pneumonia.

*Level of Cognitive Ability:* Analysis
*Client Needs:* Health Promotion and Maintenance
*Integrated Concept/Process:* Teaching/Learning
*Content Area:* Adult Health/Respiratory

*Reference*
Smeltzer, S., & Bare, B. (2000). *Brunner & Suddarth's Textbook of medical-surgical nursing* (9th ed.). Philadelphia: Lippincott Williams & Wilkins. p. 433.

---

**94.** A community health nurse provides an educational session to members of the local community regarding breast self-examination (BSE). Which statement, if made by a client, indicates a need for further education?

1   "I should perform the BSE when I have my period."
2   "It is easiest to perform when I am in the shower when my hands are soapy."
3   "I need to perform the BSE every month."
4   "I'll use the pads of my three middle fingers to feel for lumps and thickening."

**Answer: 1**

*Rationale:* The best time to perform BSE is after (not during) the monthly period when the breasts are not tender and swollen. Options 2, 3, and 4 identify accurate information regarding this self-examination.

*Test-Taking Strategy:* Use the process of elimination, focusing on the issue: BSE. Visualizing this procedure will direct you to option 1. If you had difficulty with this question, review this procedure.

*Level of Cognitive Ability:* Analysis
*Client Needs:* Health Promotion and Maintenance
*Integrated Concept/Process:* Self-Care
*Content Area:* Adult Health/Oncology

*Reference*
Smeltzer, S., & Bare, B. (2000). *Brunner & Suddarth's Textbook of medical-surgical nursing* (9th ed.). Philadelphia: Lippincott Williams & Wilkins. p. 1263.

**95.** A nurse makes a home care visit to a client with Bell's palsy. Which of the following statements by the client requires clarification by the nurse?

1  "I have been wearing a facial sling during the daytime."
2  "I wear dark glasses when I go out."
3  "I have started to actively exercise my face a few times a day."
4  "I am staying on a liquid diet."

**Answer: 4**

*Rationale:* It is not necessary for a client with Bell's palsy to stay on a liquid diet. These clients should be encouraged to chew on the unaffected side. Options 1, 2, and 3 identify accurate statements related to managing Bell's palsy.

*Test-Taking Strategy:* Use the process of elimination, focusing on the client's diagnosis. Recalling that Bell's palsy relates to the face will assist in eliminating options 1, 2, and 3. If you had difficulty with this question, review interventions associated with this disorder.

*Level of Cognitive Ability:* Analysis
*Client Needs:* Health Promotion and Maintenance
*Integrated Concept/Process:* Nursing Process/Analysis
*Content Area:* Adult Health/Neurological

*Reference*
Smeltzer, S., & Bare, B. (2000). *Brunner & Suddarth's Textbook of medical-surgical nursing* (9th ed.). Philadelphia: Lippincott Williams & Wilkins, p. 1754.

---

**96.** A home care nurse is evaluating a client's understanding of self-management of trigeminal neuralgia. Which client statement requires further teaching by the nurse?

1  "Wearing a facial sling will help relieve my symptoms."
2  "I should chew on my good side."
3  "I should use warm mouth wash for oral hygiene."
4  "Taking carbamazepine (Tegretol) will help control my pain."

**Answer: 1**

*Rationale:* Facial slings help the paralysis of Bell's palsy and are not useful with trigeminal neuralgia. It is recommended that clients chew on the unaffected side and use warm mouth wash or a water jet for oral hygiene. Medications such as carbamazepine (Tegretol) help control the pain of trigeminal neuralgia.

*Test-Taking Strategy:* Use the process of elimination, noting the key words *requires further teaching*. Recalling the manifestations associated with trigeminal neuralgia will direct you to option 1. If you had difficulty with this question, review this disorder.

*Level of Cognitive Ability:* Analysis
*Client Needs:* Health Promotion and Maintenance
*Integrated Concept/Process:* Teaching/Learning
*Content Area:* Adult Health/Neurological

*Reference*
Smeltzer, S., & Bare, B. (2000). *Brunner & Suddarth's Textbook of medical-surgical nursing* (9th ed.). Philadelphia: Lippincott Williams & Wilkins, p. 1751.

---

**97.** A nurse is caring for a client with type 1 diabetes mellitus. Because the client is at risk for hypoglycemia, the nurse teaches the client to:

1  Omit the evening NPH insulin if the client is exercising
2  Monitor the urine for acetone
3  Assess for signs of drowsiness and coma
4  Keep glucagon subcutaneously available

**Answer: 4**

*Rationale:* Glucagon is administered subcutaneously or intramuscularly to release glycogen stores and raise blood glucose levels in hypoglycemia. This medication is useful if the client loses consciousness and is unable to take glucose by mouth. Family members can be taught to administer this medication and possibly prevent an emergency room visit. The nurse would not instruct a client to omit insulin. Acetone in the urine may indicate hyperglycemia. Although signs of hypoglycemia need to be taught to the client, drowsiness and coma are not the initial and key signs of this disorder.

*Test-Taking Strategy:* Use the process of elimination. Eliminate option 1 first, because the nurse would not instruct a client to omit insulin doses. Options 2 and 3 can be eliminated next, because they are not related to the issue of hypoglycemia. If you had difficulty with this question, review the signs of hypoglycemia and the appropriate interventions.

*Level of Cognitive Ability:* Application
*Client Needs:* Health Promotion and Maintenance
*Integrated Concept/Process:* Teaching/Learning
*Content Area:* Adult Health/Endocrine

*Reference*
Hodgson, B., & Kizior, R. (2001). *Saunders Nursing drug handbook 2001.* Philadelphia: W.B. Saunders, p. 469.

---

**98.** A nurse is caring for a client with a precipitate labor. The nurse tells the client that in this type of labor:
1   The labor will last less than 3 hours
2   A lengthy period of pushing may be necessary
3   The onset of contractions is gradual
4   Induction may be necessary

**Answer: 1**
*Rationale:* Precipitate labor is defined as that which lasts 3 or fewer hours for the entire labor and delivery. It usually has an abrupt, not a gradual onset. Induction, particularly with an oxytocic agent, is contraindicated because of the enhanced stimulatory effects on the uterine muscle and an increased risk for fetal hypoxia.

*Test-Taking Strategy:* Use the process of elimination, The word *precipitate* should assist in defining this condition. Note the relationship between this word and *less than 3 hours* in option 1. Review information related to precipitate labor if you had difficulty answering this question.

*Level of Cognitive Ability:* Application
*Client Needs:* Health Promotion and Maintenance
*Integrated Concept/Process:* Teaching/Learning
*Content Area:* Maternity

*Reference*
Olds, S., London. M., & Ladewig, P. (2000). *Maternal-newborn nursing: A family and community-based approach* (6th ed.). Upper Saddle River, N.J.: Prentice-Hall, p. 501.

---

**99.** A nurse is instructing a pregnant client on measures to prevent a recurrent episode of preterm labor. Which statement by the client indicates a need for further teaching?
1   "I will report any feeling of pelvic pressure."
2   "I will adhere to the limitations in activity and stay off my feet."
3   "I will avoid sexual intercourse at this time."
4   " I will limit my fluid intake to three 8-oz glasses of fluid a day."

**Answer: 4**
*Rationale:* Risks for preterm labor include dehydration. A client should not restrict fluids (except for those containing alcohol and caffeine). A sign of preterm labor may be pelvic pressure, without the perception of a "contraction." A decrease in activity and bed rest is often prescribed in an attempt to decrease pressure on the cervix and increase uterine blood flow. Mechanical stimulation of the cervix during intercourse can stimulate contractions.

*Test-Taking Strategy:* Note the key words *indicates a need for further teaching* in the stem of the question. Focusing on the issue, preventing preterm labor, will direct you to option 4. It is generally not a good practice for the client to limit fluid intake to three 8-oz glasses of fluid a day. Review this content if you had difficulty answering the question.

*Level of Cognitive Ability:* Analysis
*Client Needs:* Health Promotion and Maintenance
*Integrated Concept/Process:* Teaching/Learning
*Content Area:* Maternity

**Reference**
Olds, S., London. M., & Ladewig, P. (2000). *Maternal-newborn nursing: A family and community-based approach* (6th ed.). Upper Saddle River, N.J.: Prentice-Hall, p. 252.

---

**100.** A nurse has completed discharge teaching with the parents of a child with glomerulonephritis. Which statement by the parents indicates that further teaching is necessary?

1  "We'll check our child's blood pressure every day."
2  "We'll be sure that our child eats a lot of vegetables and does not add extra salt to food."
3  "It'll be so good to have my child back in karate next week."
4  "We'll test our child's urine for albumin every week."

**Answer: 3**
*Rationale:* After discharge, parents should allow the child to return to his or her normal routine and activities, with adequate periods allowed for rest. Karate 1 week after discharge would be a too rapid increase in activity and unrealistic. Options 1, 2 and 4 are correct home care measures.

*Test-Taking Strategy:* Use the process of elimination, noting the key words *further teaching is necessary.* These key words will direct you to option 3, because karate is an aggressive exercise. If you had difficulty with this question, review home care measures for glomerulonephritis.

*Level of Cognitive Ability:* Analysis
*Client Needs:* Health Promotion and Maintenance
*Integrated Concept/Process:* Teaching/Learning
*Content Area:* Child Health

**Reference**
Wong, D. (1999). *Whaley & Wong's Nursing care of infants and children* (6th ed.). St. Louis: Mosby, p. 1380.

---

**101.** A nurse is planning discharge teaching for parents of a child who had sustained a head injury and is now on tapering doses of dexamethasone sodium phosphate (Decadron). The nurse plans to include which of the following statements in the parent teaching?

1  "This medication decreases chances of infections."
2  "This medication is tapered to minimize side effects."
3  "If your child's face becomes puffy, the medication dose needs to be increased."
4  "This medication is tapered to decrease the chance of recurring swelling in the brain."

**Answer: 4**
*Rationale:* Rebounding of cerebral edema is a side effect of dexamethasone sodium phosphate (Decadron) withdrawal if done abruptly. Tapering the medication is not done for the purpose of decreasing side effects. Dexamethasone sodium phosphate decreases inflammation not infection. Facial edema is a common side effect that disappears when the medication is discontinued.

*Test-Taking Strategy:* Focus on the name of the medication and recall that it is a corticosteroid. Remember that tapering is required with corticosteroids to prevent a rebound effect as a result of adrenal insufficiency. If you had difficulty with this question, review this medication.

*Level of Cognitive Ability:* Application
*Client Needs:* Health Promotion and Maintenance
*Integrated Concept/Process:* Teaching/Learning
*Content Area:* Pharmacology

**Reference**
Hodgson, B., & Kizior, R. (2001). *Saunders Nursing drug handbook 2001.* Philadelphia: W.B. Saunders, pp. 296-299.

**102.** A nurse has implemented a plan of care for a client with a C5 spinal cord injury. Which of the following client outcomes would indicate effectiveness of the interventions?

1. Regains bladder and bowel control
2. Performs activities of daily living independently
3. Maintains intact skin
4. Independently transfers self to and from the wheelchair

**Answer: 3**
*Rationale:* A C5 spinal cord injury results in quadriplegia with no sensation below the clavicle, including most of the arms and hands. The client maintains partial movement of the shoulders and elbows. Maintaining intact skin is an outcome for spinal cord injury clients. The remaining options are inappropriate for this type of client.

*Test-Taking Strategy:* Focus on the key words *C5 spinal cord injury*. Eliminate option 2 and 4 first, because they are similar. Knowledge of a C5 spinal cord injury will assist in eliminating option 1, because it is unrealistic. If you are unfamiliar with this type of injury, review this content.

*Level of Cognitive Ability:* Analysis
*Client Needs:* Health Promotion and Maintenance
*Integrated Concept/Process:* Nursing Process/Evaluation
*Content Area:* Adult Health/Neurological

*Reference*
Ignatavicius, D., Workman, M., & Mishler, M. (1999). *Medical-surgical nursing across the health care continuum* (3rd ed.). Philadelphia: W.B. Saunders, p. 1071.

**103.** A home health nurse visits a child who is being treated with penicillin for scarlet fever. The mother tells the nurse that the child has only voided a small amount of tea-colored urine since the previous day. The mother also reports that the child's appetite has decreased and the child's face was swollen this morning. The nurse interprets that these new symptoms are:

1. Signs of the normal progression of scarlet fever
2. Nothing to be concerned about
3. The symptoms of acute glomerulonephritis
4. Symptoms of an allergic reaction to penicillin

**Answer: 3**
*Rationale:* The symptoms identified in the question indicate glomerulonephritis. Although the child is on penicillin, these are not symptoms of an allergic reaction. These symptoms are not normal and should not be ignored.

*Test-Taking Strategy:* Use the process of elimination. Eliminate options 1 and 2, because they are similar. From the remaining options, recalling the complications of scarlet fever and the symptoms of an allergic reaction will direct you to option 3. If you had difficulty with this question, review the complications of scarlet fever and the symptoms of glomerulonephritis.

*Level of Cognitive Ability:* Analysis
*Client Needs:* Health Promotion and Maintenance
*Integrated Concept/Process:* Nursing Process/Analysis
*Content Area:* Child Health

*Reference*
Wong, D. (1999). *Whaley & Wong's Nursing care of infants and children* (6th ed.). St. Louis: Mosby, p. 1380.

**104.** A client who sustained a thoracic cord injury a year ago returns to the clinic with a small reddened area on the coccyx. The client is not aware of the reddened area. After counseling the client to relieve pressure on the area according to a turning schedule, which action by the nurse is most appropriate?
1   Ask a family member to assess the skin daily
2   Schedule the client to return to the clinic daily for a skin check
3   Teach the client to feel for reddened areas
4   Teach the client to use a mirror for skin assessment

**Answer: 4**

*Rationale:* The client should be encouraged to be as independent as possible. The most effective way of skin self-assessment for this client is with the use of mirror.

*Test-Taking Strategy:* Use the process of elimination, recalling that independence is the key in rehabilitation of clients. Options 1 and 2 involve others in performing a task that the client can do independently. Option 3 is an inaccurate assessment technique, since redness cannot be felt. Option 4 is the only option that addresses client self assessment. Review home care measures for the client with a thoracic cord injury if you had difficulty with this question.

*Level of Cognitive Ability:* Analysis
*Client Needs:* Health Promotion and Maintenance
*Integrated Concept/Process:* Self-Care
*Content Area:* Adult Health/Neurological

*Reference*
Smeltzer, S., & Bare, B. (2000). *Brunner & Suddarth's Textbook of medical-surgical nursing* (9th ed.). Philadelphia: Lippincott Williams & Wilkins, p. 1692.

**105.** A nurse has given instructions to a client returning home following an arthroscopy of the knee. The nurse determines that the client understands the instructions if the client stated to:
1   Stay off the leg entirely for the rest of the day
2   Resume strenuous exercise the following day
3   Refrain from eating food for the remainder of the day
4   Report fever or site inflammation to the physician

**Answer: 4**

*Rationale:* After arthroscopy, the client can usually walk carefully on the leg once sensation has returned. The client is instructed to avoid strenuous exercise for at least a few days. The client may resume the usual diet. Signs and symptoms of infection should be reported to the physician.

*Test-Taking Strategy:* Use the process of elimination, focusing on the procedure, arthroscopy. Recalling that the procedure is invasive will direct you to option 4. Additionally, the client is always taught the signs and symptoms of infection to report to the physician. Review home care instructions for the client following arthroscopy if you had difficulty with this question.

*Level of Cognitive Ability:* Analysis
*Client Needs:* Health Promotion and Maintenance
*Integrated Concept/Process:* Teaching/Learning
*Content Area:* Adult Health/Musculoskeletal

*Reference*
Smeltzer, S., & Bare, B. (2000). *Brunner & Suddarth's Textbook of medical-surgical nursing* (9th ed.). Philadelphia: Lippincott Williams & Wilkins, p. 1775.

**106.** A client has been prescribed allopurinol (Zyloprim) in the treatment of gouty arthritis. The nurse teaches the client to anticipate which of the following prescriptions during an acute attack?
1   Add colchicine or a nonsteroidal antiinflammatory drug (NSAID)
2   Double the dose of the allopurinol
3   Stop the allopurinol and take an NSAID
4   Stop the allopurinol and take acetylsalicylic acid (aspirin)

**Answer: 1**
*Rationale:* Allopurinol helps to prevent an attack of gouty arthritis, but it does not relieve the pain. Therefore, another medication such as colchicine or an NSAID must be added during this time. Because acute attacks may occur more frequently early in the course of therapy with allopurinol, some physicians recommend taking the two products concurrently during the first 3 to 6 months.

*Test-Taking Strategy:* Use the process of elimination. Eliminate options 3 and 4 first, because it is unlikely that medication will be stopped. Recalling that an acute attack of gouty arthritis is painful will assist in selecting option 1 because of the antiinflammatory action of the NSAID. If you had difficulty with this question, review interventions for an acute attack of gouty arthritis.

*Level of Cognitive Ability:* Application
*Client Needs:* Health Promotion and Maintenance
*Integrated Concept/Process:* Teaching/Learning
*Content Area:* Pharmacology

*Reference*
Smeltzer, S., & Bare, B. (2000). *Brunner & Suddarth's Textbook of medical-surgical nursing* (9th ed.). Philadelphia: Lippincott Williams & Wilkins, p. 1424.

**107.** A client is taking propranolol (Inderal) to treat hypertension. The nurse teaches the client that concurrent use of which of the following items may aggravate the hypertension?
1   Alcohol
2   Insulin
3   Ephedrine
4   Digoxin (Lanoxin)

**Answer: 3**
*Rationale:* Ephedrine is an ingredient in some commonly used nasal decongestant products. Clients on beta-adrenergic blocking agents such as propranolol should avoid concurrent use of this medication, because it could cause rebound hypertension and bradycardia. Alcohol has an additive hypotensive effect. Digoxin has an additive bradycardic effect. The insulin effect may be altered by propranolol, requiring dosage adjustments of the insulin.

*Test-Taking Strategy:* Focus on the client's diagnosis and the issue of the effect on the hypertension. Recalling the effects of the items listed in the options on the cardiovascular system will direct you to option 3. If you are unfamiliar with these medications and their effects on hypertension, review this content.

*Level of Cognitive Ability:* Application
*Client Needs:* Health Promotion and Maintenance
*Integrated Concept/Process:* Teaching/Learning
*Content Area:* Pharmacology

*Reference*
Hodgson, B., & Kizior, R. (2001). *Saunders Nursing drug handbook 2001.* Philadelphia: W.B. Saunders, p. 877.

**108.** A client has received a prescription for lisinopril (Prinivil). The nurse teaches the client that which of the following frequent side effects may occur?

　1　Hypertension
　2　Polyuria
　3　Hypothermia
　4　Cough

*[handwritten: benazepril (Lotensin)]*
*[handwritten: ACE]*
*[handwritten: "ril"]*
*[handwritten: avoid salt and potassium]*

**Answer: 4**

*Rationale:* Cough is a frequent side effect of therapy with any of the angiotensin converting enzyme (ACE) inhibitors. Hypertension is the reason to administer the medication, not a side effect. Fever is an occasional side effect. Proteinuria is another common side effect, but not polyuria.

*Test-Taking Strategy:* Use the process of elimination. Recalling that lisinopril is an ACE inhibitor will assist in eliminating option 1. From the remaining options, it is necessary to know that cough is a frequent side effect. If this question was difficult, review the side effects of this medication.

*Level of Cognitive Ability:* Application
*Client Needs:* Health Promotion and Maintenance
*Integrated Concept/Process:* Teaching/Learning
*Content Area:* Pharmacology

*Reference*

Hodgson, B., & Kizior, R. (2001). *Saunders Nursing drug handbook 2001.* Philadelphia: W.B. Saunders, p. 596.

---

**109.** A nurse has provided home care instructions to a client taking lithium carbonate (Eskalith). Which of the following statements indicates that the client understands the prescribed regimen?

　1　" I make sure that my diet contains salt."
　2　"I keep my medication next to the milk in the refrigerator so that I can remember to take it every day."
　3　"It is not difficult to restrict my water intake."
　4　"I am careful to avoid eating foods high in potassium."

**Answer: 1**

*Rationale:* Lithium replaces sodium ions in the cells and induces excretion of sodium and potassium from the body. Client teaching includes maintenance of sodium in the daily diet and increased fluid intake (at least 1 to 1.5 L/day) during maintenance therapy. Lithium is stored at room temperature and protected from light and moisture.

*Test-Taking Strategy:* Note the key word *understands*. Recalling that lithium is a salt that replaces sodium ions and induces excretion of sodium will direct you to the correct option. If you had difficulty with this question, review this medication.

*Level of Cognitive Ability:* Analysis
*Client Needs:* Health Promotion and Maintenance
*Integrated Concept/Process:* Teaching/Learning
*Content Area:* Pharmacology

*Reference*

Hodgson, B., & Kizior, R. (2001). *Saunders Nursing drug handbook 2001.* Philadelphia: W.B. Saunders, pp. 598-600.

**110.** An elderly client is given a prescription for haloperidol (Haldol). The nurse instructs the client and family to report any signs of pseudoparkinsonism and tells the family to monitor for:

1   Stooped posture and a shuffling gait
2   Muscle weakness and decreased salivation
3   Tremors and hyperreflexia
4   Motor restlessness and aphasia

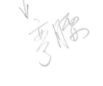

**Answer: 1**

*Rationale:* Pseudoparkinsonism is a common extrapyramidal side effect (EPS) of antipsychotic medications. This condition is characterized by a stooped posture, shuffling gait, mask-like facial appearance, drooling, tremors, and pill-rolling motions of the fingers. Hyperpyrexia is characteristic of another EPS, neuroleptic malignant syndrome (NMS). Aphasia is not a characteristic of pseudoparkinsonism.

*Test-Taking Strategy:* Focus on the issue: pseudoparkinsonism. Recalling the characteristics of pseudoparkinsonism will direct you to option 1. Review the characteristics and the effects of antipsychotic medications if you had difficulty with this question.

*Level of Cognitive Ability:* Application
*Client Needs:* Health Promotion and Maintenance
*Integrated Concept/Process:* Teaching/Learning
*Content Area:* Pharmacology

*Reference*
Hodgson, B., & Kizior, R. (2001). *Saunders Nursing drug handbook 2001.* Philadelphia: W.B. Saunders, p. 486.

---

**111.** A client on tranylcypromine (Parnate) requests information on foods that are acceptable to eat, while on this medication. The nurse tells the client that it is safe to eat:

1   Raisins
2   Smoked fish
3   Yogurt
4   Oranges

**Answer: 4**

*Rationale:* Parnate is classified as a MAO inhibitor, and as such, tyramine-containing food should be avoided. Types of food to be avoided include, but is not limited to options 1, 2, and 3. Additionally, beer, wine, caffeine beverages, pickled meats, yeast preparations, avocados, bananas, and plums are to be avoided. Oranges are permissible.

*Test-Taking Strategy:* Use the process of elimination. Note the similarity in options 1, 2, and 3. Options 1, 2, and 3 are processed or contain some type of additive. The only natural food is option 4. Bear in mind, however, that if option 4 were bananas, avocados, or plums, it would be an incorrect answer. If you had difficulty with this question, review foods high in tyramine.

*Level of Cognitive Ability:* Application
*Client Needs:* Health Promotion and Maintenance
*Integrated Concept/Process:* Teaching/Learning
*Content Area:* Pharmacology

*Reference*
Hodgson, B., & Kizior, R. (2001). *Saunders Nursing drug handbook 2001.* Philadelphia: W.B. Saunders, pp. 1012-1014.

**112.** A client is being discharged to home with a Heimlich (flutter) valve. The nurse teaches the client that if the valve needs to be changed, it is done:

1   On inspiration
2   On expiration
3   During a Valsalva maneuver
4   Between inspiration and expiration

**Answer: 3**

*Rationale:* A Heimlich valve is a one-way valve that is used instead of underwater chest drainage in some clients. The client is taught to change the valve during a Valsalva maneuver while the stopcock is turned off. The client is also instructed how to do dressing changes, to keep the dressing and tubing airtight, and to recognize the signs of infection.

*Test-Taking Strategy:* Specific knowledge regarding the purpose of the Heimlich valve is required to answer this question. Recalling the purpose will enable you to apply the same principles that relate to the care of a client with a chest tube. Review this procedure if you had difficulty with this question.

*Level of Cognitive Ability:* Application
*Client Needs:* Health Promotion and Maintenance
*Integrated Concept/Process:* Self-Care
*Content Area:* Adult Health/Respiratory

*Reference*
Monahan, F., & Neighbors, M. (1998). *Medical surgical nursing: Foundations for clinical practice* (2nd ed.). Philadelphia: W.B. Saunders, pp. 579-580.

---

**113.** A nurse is providing instructions about foot care to a client with chronic arterial insufficiency. The nurse tells the client to:

1   Wear shoes that are snugly fitting
2   Clean the feet daily, drying them well
3   Apply moisturizer to feet, especially between toes
4   Cut the toenails very short to prevent scratching

**Answer: 2**

*Rationale:* Foot care for the client with vascular disease is the same as for clients who have diabetes mellitus. This includes daily cleansing of the feet; drying well especially between the toes; applying lotion to dry areas except between the toes; wearing shoes that fit well without pressure areas; and keeping the toenails trimmed short.

*Test-Taking Strategy:* Recall that diabetes mellitus and vascular disease both result in impairment of the tissues of the feet. Using the principles involved in diabetic foot care, eliminate options 1, 3, and 4. Review foot care for the client with vascular disease if you had difficulty with this question.

*Level of Cognitive Ability:* Application
*Client Needs:* Health Promotion and Maintenance
*Integrated Concept/Process:* Teaching/Learning
*Content Area:* Adult Health/Cardiovascular

*Reference*
Monahan, F., & Neighbors, M. (1998). *Medical surgical nursing: Foundations for clinical practice* (2nd ed.). Philadelphia: W.B. Saunders, p. 355.

**114.** A nurse is giving instructions to a client with peptic ulcer disease about symptom management. The nurse tells the client to:
1   Eat slowly and chew food thoroughly
2   Eat large meals to absorb gastric acid
3   Limit the intake of water
4   Use acetylsalicylic acid (aspirin) to relieve gastric pain

**Answer: 1**
*Rationale:* The client with a peptic ulcer is taught to eat smaller, more frequent meals to help keep the gastric secretions neutralized. The client should eat slowly and chew thoroughly to prevent excess gastric acid secretion. The client should consume fluids of 6 to 8 glasses of water per day to dilute gastric acid. The use of aspirin is avoided, because it is irritating to gastric mucosa.

*Test-Taking Strategy:* Use the process of elimination. Recalling the concepts related to digestion, and knowledge of substances that are known gastric irritants will direct you to option 1. Review teaching points related to the client with peptic ulcer disease if you had difficulty with this question.

*Level of Cognitive Ability:* Application
*Client Needs:* Health Promotion and Maintenance
*Integrated Concept/Process:* Teaching/Learning
*Content Area:* Adult Health/Gastrointestinal

*Reference*
Monahan, F., & Neighbors, M. (1998). *Medical surgical nursing: Foundations for clinical practice* (2nd ed.). Philadelphia: W.B. Saunders, p. 1032.

**115.** A client with hiatal hernia asks the nurse for something to drink. The nurse offers the client which of the following items stocked in the nursing unit kitchen?
1   Tomato juice
2   Orange juice
3   Grapefruit juice
4   Apple juice

**Answer: 4**
*Rationale:* Substances that are irritating to the client with hiatal hernia include tomato products and citrus fruits, which should be avoided. Since caffeine stimulates gastric acid secretion, beverages that contain caffeine, such as coffee, tea, cola and cocoa, are also eliminated from the diet.

*Test-Taking Strategy:* Use the process of elimination. Eliminate options 1, 2, and 3, because they are similar and are citrus products. Additionally, option 4 is the least irritating to the stomach. Review dietary measures for the client with hiatal hernia if you had difficulty with this question.

*Level of Cognitive Ability:* Application
*Client Needs:* Health Promotion and Maintenance
*Integrated Concept/Process:* Nursing Process/Implementation
*Content Area:* Adult Health/Gastrointestinal

*Reference*
Monahan, F., & Neighbors, M. (1998). *Medical surgical nursing: Foundations for clinical practice* (2nd ed.). Philadelphia: W.B. Saunders, p. 1044.

**116.** A client with a spinal cord injury (SCI) experiences bladder spasms and reflex incontinence. In preparing for discharge to home, the nurse instructs the client to:

1    Limit fluid intake to 1000 mL in 24 hours
2    Take own temperature every day
3    Catheterize self every 2 hours PRN to prevent spasm
4    Avoid caffeine in the diet

**Answer: 4**

*Rationale:* Caffeine in the diet can contribute to bladder spasms and reflex incontinence. This should be eliminated in the diet of the client with an SCI. Limiting fluid intake does not prevent spasm, and could place the client at further risk of urinary tract infection. Self-monitoring of temperature would be useful in detecting infection, but does nothing to alleviate bladder spasms. Self catheterization every 2 hours is too frequent, and serves no useful purpose.

*Test-Taking Strategy:* Focus on the issue: preventive measures for bladder spasm and reflex incontinence. Eliminate options 1 and 3 first, because they place the client at increased risk of urinary tract infection, and are therefore not appropriate. From the remaining options, eliminate option 2, because this action would detect infection but does not deal with spasm and incontinence. Review measures to prevent bladder spasms and reflex incontinence if you had difficulty with this question.

*Level of Cognitive Ability:* Application
*Client Needs:* Health Promotion and Maintenance
*Integrated Concept/Process:* Self-Care
*Content Area:* Adult Health/Neurological

*Reference*
Monahan, F., & Neighbors, M. (1998). *Medical-surgical nursing: Foundations for clinical practice* (2nd ed.). Philadelphia: W.B. Saunders, p. 826.

**117.** A client seeks treatment in an ambulatory care center for symptoms of Raynaud's disease. The nurse instructs the client to:

1    Wear protective items, such as gloves and warm socks as necessary
2    Alternate exposures to both heat and cold
3    Decrease cigarette smoking by half
4    Continue activity during vasospasm for more rapid relief of symptoms

**Answer: 1**

*Rationale:* Treatment for Raynaud's disease includes avoidance of precipitating factors such as cold or damp weather, stress, and cigarettes. The client should get sufficient rest and sleep, protect the extremities by wearing protective clothing, and stop activity during vasospasm.

*Test-Taking Strategy:* Use the process of elimination. Recall that the symptoms of Raynaud's disease are caused by vasospasm. Eliminate options 2, 3, and 4, because these actions will cause vasospasm. Review client teaching points related to Raynaud's disease if you had difficulty with this question.

*Level of Cognitive Ability:* Application
*Client Needs:* Health Promotion and Maintenance
*Integrated Concept/Process:* Teaching/Learning
*Content Area:* Adult Health/Cardiovascular

*Reference*
Monahan, F., & Neighbors, M. (1998). *Medical-surgical nursing: Foundations for clinical practice* (2nd ed.). Philadelphia: W.B. Saunders, p. 356.

**118.** A client with atherosclerosis asks the nurse about dietary modifications to lower the risk of heart disease. The nurse instructs the client to eat which of the following foods?

1   Baked chicken with skin
2   Fresh cantaloupe
3   Broiled cheeseburger
4   Mashed potato with gravy

**Answer: 2**

*Rationale:* To lower the risk of heart disease, the diet should be low in saturated fat with the appropriate number of total calories. The diet should include fewer red meats and more white meat, with the skin removed. Dairy products used should be low in fat, and foods with high amounts of empty calories should be avoided.

*Test-Taking Strategy:* Focus on the issue: lower the risk of heart disease. Use fat content of the foods in the options as a guide to answering this question. Eliminate options 1 and 3 first because of the fat content of the described meats. From the remaining options, eliminate option 4, because fresh fruits and vegetables are naturally low in fat. Review dietary measures that will lower the risk of heart disease if you had difficulty with this question.

*Level of Cognitive Ability:* Application
*Client Needs:* Health Promotion and Maintenance
*Integrated Concept/Process:* Teaching/Learning
*Content Area:* Adult Health/Cardiovascular

*Reference*
Monahan, F., & Neighbors, M. (1998). *Medical-surgical nursing: Foundations for clinical practice* (2nd ed.). Philadelphia: W.B. Saunders, p. 363.

---

**119.** A client is being discharged to home after angioplasty using the right femoral area as the catheter insertion site. The nurse instructs the client that which of the following signs and symptoms may be expected after the procedure?

1   Coolness or discoloration of the right foot
2   Temperature as high as 101° F
3   Large area of bruising in the right groin area
4   Mild discomfort in the right groin area

**Answer: 4**

*Rationale:* The client may feel some mild discomfort at the catheter insertion site following angioplasty. This is usually well relieved by analgesics such as acetaminophen (Tylenol). The client is taught to report to the physician any neurovascular changes to the affected leg, bleeding or bruising at the insertion site, and signs of local infection, such as drainage at the site or increased temperature.

*Test-Taking Strategy:* Use the process of elimination, noting the key word *expected.* Knowing that bleeding and infection are complications of the procedure guides you to eliminate options 2 and 3. From the remaining options, eliminate option 1 knowing that neurovascular status should not be impaired by the procedure, or by knowing that the area may be mildly uncomfortable. Review the complications associated with angioplasty if you had difficulty with this question.

*Level of Cognitive Ability:* Application
*Client Needs:* Health Promotion and Maintenance
*Integrated Concept/Process:* Teaching/Learning
*Content Area:* Adult Health/Cardiovascular

*Reference*
Monahan, F., & Neighbors, M. (1998). *Medical-surgical nursing: Foundations for clinical practice* (2nd ed.). Philadelphia: W.B. Saunders, p. 344.

**120.** A nurse is teaching dietary modifications to a client with hypertension. The nurse instructs the client to eat which of the following snack foods?

1 Cheese and crackers
2 Honeydew melon slices
3 Frozen pizza
4 Canned tomato soup

**Answer: 2**

*Rationale:* Sodium should be avoided by a client with hypertension. Fresh fruits and vegetables are naturally low in sodium. Hypertensive clients are also advised to keep fat intake to less than 30% of total calories as part of prudent heart living. Each of the incorrect options contain increased amounts of sodium, and options 1 and 3 are likely to be also higher in fat.

*Test-Taking Strategy:* Focus on the issue: the dietary modifications needed with hypertension. Eliminate options 1, 3, and 4, because they are similar and are all processed food items. Review dietary measures for the client with hypertension if you had difficulty with this question.

*Level of Cognitive Ability:* Application
*Client Needs:* Health Promotion and Maintenance
*Integrated Concept/Process:* Teaching/Learning
*Content Area:* Adult Health/Cardiovascular

*Reference*
Monahan, F., & Neighbors, M. (1998). *Medical-surgical nursing: Foundations for clinical practice* (2nd ed.). Philadelphia: W.B. Saunders, p. 382.

---

**121.** A nurse is teaching a client with hypertension to recognize the signs and symptoms that may occur during periods of an elevated blood pressure (BP). The nurse avoids telling the client that which of the following will occur?

1 Early morning headaches
2 Epistaxis
3 Feeling of fullness in the head
4 Blurred vision

**Answer: 3**

*Rationale:* Cerebrovascular symptoms of hypertension include early morning headaches, occipital headaches, blurred vision, lightheadedness and vertigo, dizziness, and epistaxis. The client should be aware of these symptoms and report them if they occur. The client should also be taught self-monitoring of blood pressure. Feelings of fullness in the head is more likely associated with a sinus condition.

*Test-Taking Strategy:* Use the process of elimination, focusing on the issue: signs of an elevated BP. Option 3 is the most vague option whereas options 1, 2, and 4 are specific and related to hypertension. If this question was difficult, review the signs and symptoms of hypertension.

*Level of Cognitive Ability:* Application
*Client Needs:* Health Promotion and Maintenance
*Integrated Concept/Process:* Teaching/Learning
*Content Area:* Adult Health/Cardiovascular

*Reference*
Monahan, F., & Neighbors, M. (1998). *Medical-surgical nursing: Foundations for clinical practice* (2nd ed.). Philadelphia: W.B. Saunders, p. 375.

**122.** A client is taking iron supplements to correct iron-deficiency anemia (IDA). The nurse teaches the client which of the following special considerations while on iron therapy?
1   Avoid taking iron with milk or antacids
2   Limit intake of meat, fish, and poultry
3   Eat a low-fiber diet
4   Limit intake of fluids

**Answer: 1**
*Rationale:* The client should avoid taking iron with milk or antacids, because these items decrease absorption of iron. The client should also avoid taking iron with food if possible. The client should increase natural sources of iron, such as meats, fish, and poultry. Finally, the client should take in sufficient fiber and fluids to prevent constipation as a side effect of therapy.

*Test-Taking Strategy:* Use the process of elimination. Begin to answer this question by eliminating options 3 and 4, knowing that constipation is a common side effect of iron therapy. Recalling that meat products contain iron would guide you to eliminate option 2 next. Remember, several medications have impaired absorption with milk products or antacids. Review home care measures for the client with IDA if you had difficulty with this question.

*Level of Cognitive Ability:* Application
*Client Needs:* Health Promotion and Maintenance
*Integrated Concept/Process:* Teaching/Learning
*Content Area:* Pharmacology

*Reference*
Monahan, F., & Neighbors, M. (1998). *Medical-surgical nursing: Foundations for clinical practice* (2nd ed.). Philadelphia: W.B. Saunders, p. 470.

**123.** A client with a colostomy complains to the nurse of appliance odor. The nurse recommends that the client take in which of the following deodorizing foods?
1   Yogurt
2   Mushrooms
3   Cucumbers
4   Eggs

**Answer: 1**
*Rationale:* Foods that help to eliminate odor with a colostomy include yogurt, buttermilk, spinach, beet greens, and parsley. Foods that cause odor are many, and include alcohol, beans, turnips, radishes, asparagus, onions, cucumbers, mushrooms, cabbage, asparagus, eggs, and fish.

*Test-Taking Strategy:* Use the process of elimination. Remember that foods that cause gas in the client with normal gastrointestinal (GI) function also form gas in the GI tract of the client with a colostomy. Use basic nutritional knowledge to eliminate options 2, 3, and 4. Review foods that are gas forming if you had difficulty with this question.

*Level of Cognitive Ability:* Application
*Client Needs:* Health Promotion and Maintenance
*Integrated Concept/Process:* Teaching/Learning
*Content Area:* Adult Health/Gastrointestinal

*Reference*
Monahan, F., & Neighbors, M. (1998). *Medical-surgical nursing: Foundations for clinical practice* (2nd ed.). Philadelphia: W.B. Saunders, p. 1009.

**124.** A nurse is demonstrating colostomy care to a client with a newly created colostomy. The nurse demonstrates correct cutting of the appliance by making the circle how much larger than the client's stoma?

1   $^1/_{16}$ inch
2   $^1/_8$ inch
3   $^1/_4$ inch
4   $^1/_2$ inch

**Answer: 2**

*Rationale:* The size of the opening for the appliance is generally cut $^1/_8$ inch larger than the size of the client's stoma. This minimizes the amount of exposed skin, but does not cause pressure on the stoma itself. Option 1 is an extremly small size that would cause irritation to the stoma. Options 3 and 4 leave too much skin area exposed for possible irritation by gastrointestinal contents.

*Test-Taking Strategy:* Use the process of elimination. Visualizing each of the appliance sizes in the options will direct you to option 2. Review home care instructions for a client with a colostomy if you had difficulty with this question.

*Level of Cognitive Ability:* Application
*Client Needs:* Health Promotion and Maintenance
*Integrated Concept/Process:* Teaching/Learning
*Content Area:* Adult Health/Gastrointestinal

*Reference*
Monahan, F., & Neighbors, M. (1998). *Medical-surgical nursing: Foundations for clinical practice* (2nd ed.). Philadelphia: W.B. Saunders, p. 1009.

**125.** A nurse teaches a client with a spinal cord injury about measures to prevent autonomic dysreflexia (hyperreflexia). Which of the following statements made by the client would indicate the need for additional teaching?

1   "I need to pay close attention to how frequently my bowels move."
2   "It is best if I avoid tight clothing and lumpy bed clothes."
3   "I should watch for headache, congestion, and flushed skin."
4   "Symptoms I should watch for include fever and chest pain."

**Answer: 4**

*Rationale:* Symptoms of autonomic dysreflexia include headache, congestion, flushed skin above the injury and cold skin below it, diaphoresis, nausea, and anxiety. Fever and chest pain are not associated with this condition.

*Test-Taking Strategy:* Use the process of elimination, noting the key words *need for additional teaching*. Recalling the signs and symptoms and causes of autonomic dysreflexia will direct you to option 4. If you are unfamiliar with this syndrome, review this content.

*Level of Cognitive Ability:* Analysis
*Client Needs:* Health Promotion and Maintenance
*Integrated Concept/Process:* Self-Care
*Content Area:* Adult Health/Neurological

*Reference*
Smeltzer, S., & Bare, B. (2000). *Brunner & Suddarth's Textbook of medical-surgical nursing* (9th ed.). Philadelphia: Lippincott Williams & Wilkins, p.1693.

**126.** A nurse is discharging a female client from the hospital who has a diagnosis of T11 fracture with cord transection. The nurse has reinforced home care instructions with the client. Which of the following would indicate the need for further discharge teaching?

1   The client states she will have to be careful not to eat as many dairy products

2   The client states she will wash her hands, perineum, and catheter with soap and water before performing self-catheterization

3   The client jokes about no longer needing to worry about birth control

4   The client verbalizes the need to eat her meals close to the same time every day

**Answer: 3**

*Rationale:* Female spinal cord trauma clients in their reproductive years remain fertile. Contraception is necessary for these clients who are sexually active. Oral contraceptives may increase the risk for thrombophlebitis. Clients with paralysis should avoid dairy products to control the formation of urinary calculi. Clients who lack bladder control are taught to self-catheterize using clean technique. Meals should be at the same time every day and include fiber and warm solid and liquid foods to promote evacuation of the bowel.

*Test-Taking Strategy:* Note the key words *need for further discharge teaching*. Remember, key aspects of dealing with a spinal cord injury client are nutrition and elimination. Options 1, 2, and 4 address these key areas. If you had difficulty with this question, review teaching points for a client with transection of the cord.

*Level of Cognitive Ability:* Analysis
*Client Needs:* Health Promotion and Maintenance
*Integrated Concept/Process:* Teaching/Learning
*Content Area:* Adult Health/Neurological

*Reference*
Smeltzer, S., & Bare, B. (2000). *Brunner & Suddarth's Textbook of medical-surgical nursing* (9th ed.). Philadelphia: Lippincott Williams & Wilkins, p. 1692.

**127.** A client has been started on a monoamine oxidase (MAO) inhibitor. Which of the following should the nurse include when teaching the client about the medication?

1   The medication will begin to alleviate symptoms of depression almost immediately

2   The medication is associated with a high rate of abuse

3   This medication can cause severe drowsiness

4   The client must avoid foods containing tyramine

**Answer: 4**

*Rationale:* Although MAO inhibitors usually produce hypotension as a side effect, potentially lethal hypertension can occur if the client eats foods that contain tyramine. Such foods include aged cheeses, hot dogs, and beer, among others. Options 1, 2, and 3 are incorrect statements.

*Test-Taking Strategy:* Recalling that MAO inhibitors are associated with a food-medication interaction will direct you to option 4. If you had difficulty with this question, review these interactions.

*Level of Cognitive Ability:* Application
*Client Needs:* Health Promotion and Maintenance
*Integrated Concept/Process:* Teaching/Learning
*Content Area:* Pharmacology

*Reference*
Fortinash, K., & Holoday-Worret, P. (2000). *Psychiatric mental health nursing* (2nd ed.). St. Louis: Mosby, p. 289.

**128.** A nurse is developing a plan of care for an elderly client with dementia and formulates a nursing diagnosis of Self-Care Deficit. The nurse develops which realistic outcome for the client?

1  The client will be admitted to a nursing home to have activities of daily living (ADL) needs met

2  The client will function at the highest level of independence possible

3  The client will complete all ADLs independently within a 1- to 1½-hour time frame

4  The nursing staff will attend to all the client's ADL needs during the hospital stay

**Answer: 2**

*Rationale:* All clients, regardless of age, need to be encouraged to perform at the highest level of independence possible. This contributes to the client's sense of control and sense of well-being. Options 1 and 4 are not client centered goals. A 1- to 1½-hour time frame may not be realistic for an elderly client with dementia.

*Test-Taking Strategy:* Use the process of elimination, focusing on the key words *realistic outcome for the client.* Eliminate options 1 and 4 first, because they are not client-centered. From the remaining options, eliminate option 3 because of the unrealistic time frame. Review care of a client with dementia if you had difficulty with this question.

*Level of Cognitive Ability:* Analysis
*Client Needs:* Health Promotion and Maintenance
*Integrated Concept/Process:* Nursing Process/Planning
*Content Area:* Mental Health

*Reference*

Smeltzer, S., & Bare, B. (2000). *Brunner & Suddarth's Textbook of medical-surgical nursing* (9th ed.). Philadelphia: Lippincott Williams & Wilkins, p. 161.

**129.** A client who is on haloperidol (Haldol) at bedtime also receives benztropine (Cogentin) at the same time. The nurse instructs the client that the benztropine is given to:

1  Combat extrapyramidal side effects (EPS)

2  Enhance sleep

3  Enhance the effects of haloperidol

4  Enhance the anticholinergic effects of the medications

**Answer: 1**

*Rationale:* Haloperidol is a neuroleptic medication that may cause the client to experience EPS. Antiparkinsonian medications such as benztropine are given to decrease the symptoms of EPS. Options 2, 3, and 4 are incorrect

*Test-Taking Strategy:* Use the process of elimination. Recalling that EPS is a concern with the use of neuroleptic medications will direct you to option 1. If you had difficulty with this question, review the purposes of these medications.

*Level of Cognitive Ability:* Application
*Client Needs:* Health Promotion and Maintenance
*Integrated Concept/Process:* Teaching/Learning
*Content Area:* Pharmacology

*Reference*

Hodgson, B., & Kizior, R. (2001). *Saunders Nursing drug handbook 2001.* Philadelphia: W.B. Saunders, pp. 102-104, 486-488.

**130.** A client is newly diagnosed with chronic obstructive pulmonary disease (COPD). The client returns home after a short hospitalization. The home health nurse visits the client, and, most important, plans teaching strategies that are designed to:

1   Encourage the client to become a more active person
2   Improve oxygenation and minimize carbon dioxide retention
3   Identify irritants in the home that interfere with breathing
4   Promote membership in support groups

**Answer: 2**

*Rationale:* Improving oxygenation and minimizing carbon dioxide retention is the primary objective. The other options are interventions that will help to achieve this primary goal.

*Test-Taking Strategy:* Note the key words *most important.* Use the ABCs: airway, breathing, and circulation, to direct you to option 2. Review care of a client with COPD if you had difficulty with this question.

*Level of Cognitive Ability:* Application
*Client Needs:* Health Promotion and Maintenance
*Integrated Concept/Process:* Nursing Process/Planning
*Content Area:* Adult Health/Respiratory

*Reference*
Smeltzer, S., & Bare, B. (2000). *Brunner & Suddarth's Textbook of medical-surgical nursing* (9th ed.). Philadelphia: Lippincott Williams & Wilkins, p. 447.

---

**131.** A client is being discharged from the hospital following a bronchoscopy that was performed yesterday. In performing the discharge planning, the client makes all of the following statements to the nurse. Which statement would the nurse identify as indicating a need for further teaching?

1   "I can expect to cough up bright red blood."
2   "I will stop smoking my cigarettes."
3   "I will get help immediately if I start having trouble breathing."
4   "I will use the throat lozenges as directed by the physician until my sore throat goes away."

**Answer: 1**

*Rationale:* After the procedure, the client should be observed for signs of respiratory distress, including dyspnea, changes in respiratory rate, use of accessory muscles, and changes in or absent lung sounds. Expectorated secretions are inspected for hemoptysis. The client needs to avoid smoking. A sore throat is common and lozenges would be helpful to alleviate the sore throat.

*Test-Taking Strategy:* Use the process of elimination, noting the key words *need for further teaching.* Option 2 and 3 can be easily eliminated first. From the remaining options, remember that bright red bleeding indicates active bleeding. Thus, bright red blood and any signs of distress would need to be reported to the physician. Review care to the client following bronchoscopy if you had difficulty with this question.

*Level of Cognitive Ability:* Analysis
*Client Needs:* Health Promotion and Maintenance
*Integrated Concept/Process:* Teaching/Learning
*Content Area:* Adult Health/Respiratory

*Reference*
Smeltzer, S., & Bare, B. (2000). *Brunner & Suddarth's Textbook of medical-surgical nursing* (9th ed.). Philadelphia: Lippincott Williams & Wilkins, p. 397.

**132.** A client who is on chlorpromazine (Thorazine) is preparing for discharge. In developing a plan of care for the client, the nurse instructs the client:

1 To adhere to a strict tyramine restricted diet

2 On the signs and symptoms of relapse of depression

3 To avoid prolonged exposure to the sun

4 To have the therapeutic blood levels drawn, because there is a narrow range between the therapeutic and toxic levels of the medication

**Answer: 3**

*Rationale:* Chlorpromazine is an antipsychotic medication often used in the treatment of psychosis. Photosensitivity is sometimes a side effect of the phenothiazine class of antipsychotic medications to which chlorpromazine (Thorazine) belongs. Options 1, 2, and 4 are unrelated to the administration of this medication.

*Test-Taking Strategy:* Use the process of elimination. Since chlorpromazine is an antipsychotic medication, option 2 can be eliminated. Eliminate option 1, because this option relates to medications that are monoamine oxidase inhibitors. There is not a narrow range between therapeutic and toxic levels such as with lithium; therefore eliminate option 4. If you had difficulty with this question, review this medication.

*Level of Cognitive Ability:* Application
*Client Needs:* Health Promotion and Maintenance
*Integrated Concept/Process:* Teaching/Learning
*Content Area:* Pharmacology

*Reference*
Hodgson, B., & Kizior, R. (2001). *Saunders Nursing drug handbook 2001.* Philadelphia: W.B. Saunders, pp. 210-213.

**133.** A nurse is instructing a client with hepatitis about measures to control fatigue. The nurse avoids telling the client to:

1 Plan rest periods after meals

2 Rest in-between activities

3 Perform personal hygiene if not fatigued

4 Complete all daily activities in the morning when the client is most rested

**Answer: 4**

*Rationale:* A client with hepatitis has tremendous metabolic demands that lead to fatigue and interfere with activities of daily living (ADLs). The nurse encourages ADLs unless they cause excessive fatigue. The client is advised to plan rest periods after activities, such as meals. Activities should be spaced throughout the day with frequent planned rest periods. Clients who engage in excessive activity too early in the recovery stage may experience a relapse.

*Test-Taking Strategy:* Note the key word *avoids*. Use the basic principles associated with a balance of rest and activities to answer the question. By the process of elimination, the only option that does not provide this balance is option 4. Review measures to alleviate fatigue in the client with hepatitis if you had difficulty with this question.

*Level of Cognitive Ability:* Application
*Client Needs:* Health Promotion and Maintenance
*Integrated Concept/Process:* Self-Care
*Content Area:* Adult Health/Gastrointestinal

*Reference*
Smeltzer, S., & Bare, B. (2000). *Brunner & Suddarth's Textbook of medical-surgical nursing* (9th ed.). Philadelphia: Lippincott Williams & Wilkins, p. 944.

**134.** A nurse provides home care instructions to a client with multiple sclerosis (MS). The nurse tells the client to:

1   Avoid pregnancy
2   Restrict fluid intake to 1000 mL/day
3   Maintain a low-fiber diet
4   Avoid taking hot baths or showers

**Answer: 4**

*Rationale:* Because fatigue can be precipitated by warm temperatures, the client is instructed to take cool baths and maintain a cool environmental temperature. A high-fiber diet and an adequate fluid intake of 2000 mL daily is encouraged to prevent alterations in elimination and bowel patterns. The client should not be told to avoid pregnancy, but the nurse should assist the client to make informed decisions regarding pregnancy.

*Test-Taking Strategy:* Use the process of elimination and knowledge regarding the effects of MS in answering the question. Eliminate option 1 first, because it is inappropriate to tell a client to avoid pregnancy. Eliminate options 2 and 3 next, because these measures are unhealthy in this client and would promote alterations in elimination patterns. Review teaching points related to the client with MS if you had difficulty with this question.

*Level of Cognitive Ability:* Application
*Client Needs:* Health Promotion and Maintenance
*Integrated Concept/Process:* Self-Care
*Content Area:* Adult Health/Musculoskeletal

*Reference*
Smeltzer, S., & Bare, B. (2000). *Brunner & Suddarth's Textbook of medical-surgical nursing* (9th ed.). Philadelphia: Lippincott Williams & Wilkins, p. 1721.

**135.** A home care nurse provides instructions to the client with a halo vest. The nurse tells the client to:

1   Have the spouse use the metal frame to assist the client to sit up
2   Perform pin care three times a week using hydrogen peroxide or alcohol
3   Loosen the bolts once a day for bathing
4   Carry the correct size wrench to loosen the bolts in an emergency

**Answer: 4**

*Rationale:* The metal frame is never used or pulled on for turning or lifting. Pin care should be performed at least once a day using soap and water with cotton tipped swabs or alcohol swabs. The bolts should never be loosened except in an emergency. In fact, the physician should be notified if the bolts loosen. The client is instructed to carry the correct size wrench in case of an emergency requiring cardiopulmonary resuscitation (CPR). In such a situation, the anterior portion of the vest including the anterior bolts will need to be loosened and the posterior portion should remain in place to provide stability for the spine during CPR.

*Test-Taking Strategy:* Try to visualize the appearance of a halo vest. Recall that the purpose of this vest is to stabilize a cervical fracture. Eliminate option 2 first, because pin care should be done at least once a day. Eliminate option 1, because pulling on the frame will disrupt the stabilization of the fracture and possibly lead to serious complications. Remember, bolts should never be loosened except in an emergency situation. Review home care instructions for a client with a halo vest if you had difficulty with this question.

*Level of Cognitive Ability:* Application
*Client Needs:* Health Promotion and Maintenance
*Integrated Concept/Process:* Self-Care
*Content Area:* Adult Health/Neurological

*Reference*
Smeltzer, S., & Bare, B. (2000). *Brunner & Suddarth's Textbook of medical-surgical nursing* (9th ed.). Philadelphia: Lippincott Williams & Wilkins, p. 1693.

**136.** Haloperidol (Haldol) has been prescribed for a client with Tourette's syndrome. The nurse instructs the client about the medication. Which of the following statements, if made by the client, indicates the need for further education?

1    "It may take 6 weeks before the medication works."
2    "The drowsiness will probably go away as I continue the medication."
3    "I should stop the medication if my vision becomes blurred."
4    "I need to avoid alcohol while taking this medication."

**Answer: 3**

*Rationale:* The client needs to be instructed not to abruptly stop the medication therapy. The client is informed that if visual disturbances occur, the physician should be notified. Options 1, 2, and 4 are accurate statements regarding the medication.

*Test-Taking Strategy:* Use the process of elimination, focusing on the key words *need for further education.* Eliminate option 4 first, because this is a general principle with most medications. Knowledge that this medication is an antipsychotic will assist in eliminating options 1 and 2. Additionally, knowing that the medication should not be abruptly stopped, will assist in directing you to option 3. Review this medication if you had difficulty with this question.

*Level of Cognitive Ability:* Analysis
*Client Needs:* Health Promotion and Maintenance
*Integrated Concept/Process:* Teaching/Learning
*Content Area:* Pharmacology

*Reference*
Hodgson, B., & Kizior, R. (2001). *Saunders Nursing drug handbook 2001.* Philadelphia: W.B. Saunders, p. 488.

**137.** A client with diabetes mellitus has received instructions about foot care. Which of the following statements would indicate that the client needs further instruction?

1    "The best time to cut my nails is after bathing."
2    "Cotton stockings should be worn to absorb excess moisture."
3    "The cuticles of my nails must be cut to prevent overgrowth."
4    "My feet should be inspected daily using a mirror."

**Answer: 3**

*Rationale:* Trimming or cutting the cuticles of the nails can lead to injury to the foot by scratching the skin. Even small injuries can be dangerous to the client with diabetes mellitus who has decreased peripheral vascular circulation. A manicure stick can be used to gently push the cuticle back under the nail. Nails can be cut straight across, and after a bath is the best time, since the nails are softest then. White cotton stockings are best, and the client needs to inspect the feet daily.

*Test-Taking Strategy:* Use the process of elimination, noting the key words *needs further instruction.* Look for the option that could result in altered skin integrity. Using this principle, eliminate options 1, 2, and 4. Review diabetic foot care if you had difficulty with this question.

*Level of Cognitive Ability:* Analysis
*Client Needs:* Health Promotion and Maintenance
*Integrated Concept/Process:* Self-Care
*Content Area:* Adult Health/Endocrine

*Reference*
Smeltzer, S., & Bare, B. (2000). *Brunner & Suddarth's Textbook of medical-surgical nursing* (9th ed.). Philadelphia: Lippincott Williams & Wilkins, p. 1017.

**138.** A nurse has taught a client about the signs and symptoms of hyperglycemia. Which statement by the client best reflects accurate understanding?
1 "I may become diaphoretic and faint."
2 "I need to take an extra diabetic pill if my blood glucose level is greater than 300."
3 "I may notice signs of fatigue, dry skin, and increased urination and thirst."
4 "I should restrict my fluid intake if my blood glucose level is greater than 250 mg."

**Answer: 3**
*Rationale:* Fatigue, dry skin, polyuria, and polydipsia are classic symptoms of hyperglycemia. Fatigue occurs because of lack of energy from inability of the body to utilize glucose. Dry skin occurs secondary to dehydration related to the polyuria. Polydipsia occurs secondary to fluid loss. Diaphoresis is associated with hypoglycemia. Clients should not take extra oral hypoglycemic agents to reduce an elevated blood glucose level. Rather, Regular insulin is used for its rapid response to reduce hyperglycemia. A client with hyperglycemia becomes dehydrated secondary to the osmotic effect of elevated glucose. Therefore the client must increase fluid intake.

*Test-Taking Strategy:* Note the key words *reflects accurate understanding* and focus on the issue: hyperglycemia. Recalling that polyuria and polydipsia are signs of hyperglycemia will direct you to option 3. Review these signs if you had difficulty with this question.

*Level of Cognitive Ability:* Analysis
*Client Needs:* Health Promotion and Maintenance
*Integrated Concept/Process:* Self-Care
*Content Area:* Adult Health/Endocrine

*Reference*
Smeltzer, S., & Bare, B. (2000). *Brunner & Suddarth's Textbook of medical-surgical nursing* (9th ed.). Philadelphia: Lippincott Williams & Wilkins, p. 1009.

**139.** A client taking famotidine (Pepcid) asks the home health nurse what would be the best medication to take for a headache. The nurse tells the client that it would be best to take:
1 Aspirin (acetylsalicylic acid [ASA])
2 Ibuprofen (Motrin)
3 Acetaminophen (Tylenol)
4 Naproxen (Naprosyn)

**Answer: 3**
*Rationale:* The client is taking famotidine, a histamine receptor antagonist. This implies that the client has a disorder characterized by gastrointestinal irritation. The only medication of the ones listed in the options that is not irritating to the gastrointestinal (GI) tract is acetaminophen. The other medications could aggravate an already existing GI problem.

*Test-Taking Strategy:* Note the medication that the client is taking. Recalling that this medication is used for GI irritation will direct you to option 3. Review these medications if you had difficulty with this question.

*Level of Cognitive Ability:* Application
*Client Needs:* Health Promotion and Maintenance
*Integrated Concept/Process:* Teaching/Learning
*Content Area:* Pharmacology

*Reference*
Hodgson, B., & Kizior, R. (2001). *Saunders Nursing drug handbook 2001.* Philadelphia: W.B. Saunders, p. 402.

**140.** A nurse is teaching the client taking cyclosporine (Sandimmune) after renal transplant about the medication. The nurse tells the client to be especially alert for:
1. Signs of infection
2. Hypotension
3. Weight loss
4. Hair loss

**Answer: 1**
*Rationale:* Cyclosporine is an immunosuppressant medication used to prevent transplant rejection. The client should be especially alert for signs and symptoms of infection while taking this medication, and report them to the physician if experienced. The client is also taught about other side effects of the medication, including hypertension, increased facial hair, tremors, gingival hyperplasia, and gastrointestinal complaints.

*Test-Taking Strategy:* Recalling that cyclosporine is an immunosuppressant and that the client is at risk for infection while taking this medication will direct you to option 1. Review this information if you had difficulty with this question, because this is a major concern with transplant medication therapy.

*Level of Cognitive Ability:* Application
*Client Needs:* Health Promotion and Maintenance
*Integrated Concept/Process:* Self-Care
*Content Area:* Pharmacology

*Reference*
Hodgson, B., & Kizior, R. (2001). *Saunders Nursing drug handbook 2001.* Philadelphia: W.B. Saunders, p. 272.

**141.** A client has undergone surgery for glaucoma. The nurse provides which discharge instructions to the client?
1. Wound healing usually takes 12 weeks
2. Expect that vision will be permanently impaired
3. A shield or eye patch should be worn to protect the eye
4. The sutures are removed after 1 week

**Answer: 3**
*Rationale:* After ocular surgery, the client should wear an eye patch or eyeglasses for protection of the eye. Healing takes place in about 6 weeks. Once the postoperative inflammation subsides, the client's vision should return to the preoperative level of acuity. Sutures may be either absorbable or nonabsorbable, but in either case, they are not removed.

*Test-Taking Strategy:* Use the process of elimination, focusing on the issue: ocular surgery. Recalling that the eye requires protection after surgery will direct you to option 3. If you had difficulty with this question, review postoperative teaching points following eye surgery.

*Level of Cognitive Ability:* Application
*Client Needs:* Health Promotion and Maintenance
*Integrated Concept/Process:* Self-Care
*Content Area:* Adult Health/Eye

*Reference*
Smeltzer, S., & Bare, B. (2000). *Brunner & Suddarth's Textbook of medical-surgical nursing* (9th ed.). Philadelphia: Lippincott Williams & Wilkins, p. 1554.

**142.** A client has undergone surgery for cataracts. The nurse instructs the client to call the physician for which of the following complaints?
  1   A sudden decrease in vision
  2   Eye pain relieved by acetaminophen (Tylenol)
  3   Small amounts of dried matter on the eyelashes after sleep
  4   Gradual resolution of eye redness

**Answer: 1**
*Rationale:* The client should report a noticeable or sudden decrease in vision to the physician. The client is taught to take acetaminophen, which is usually effective in relieving discomfort. The eye may be slightly reddened postoperatively, but this should gradually resolve. Small amounts of dried material may be present on the lashes after sleep. This is expected, and should be removed with a warm facecloth.

*Test-Taking Strategy:* Use the process of elimination, noting the key words *call the physician*. Noting the key words *sudden decrease* in option 1 will direct you to this option. If this question was difficult, review home care instructions following eye surgery.

*Level of Cognitive Ability:* Application
*Client Needs:* Health Promotion and Maintenance
*Integrated Concept/Process:* Teaching/Learning
*Content Area:* Adult Health/Eye

*Reference*
Smeltzer, S., & Bare, B. (2000). *Brunner & Suddarth's Textbook of medical-surgical nursing* (9th ed.). Philadelphia: Lippincott Williams & Wilkins, p. 1557.

**143.** A home health nurse visits a client with a diagnosis of cirrhosis and ascites. The nurse provides dietary instructions and tells the client to:
  1   Decrease fat intake
  2   Decrease carbohydrate intake
  3   Restrict calories to 1500/day
  4   Restrict sodium intake

**Answer: 4**
*Rationale:* If the client has ascites, sodium and possibly fluids should be restricted in the diet. Fat restriction is not necessary. Total daily calories should range between 2000 and 3000. The diet should supply sufficient carbohydrates to maintain weight and spare protein. The diet should provide ample protein to rebuild tissue but not enough protein to precipitate hepatic encephalopathy.

*Test-Taking Strategy:* Focus on the client's diagnosis, cirrhosis and ascites. Recalling that ascites indicates the accumulation of fluid will direct you to option 4. If you had difficulty with this question, review dietary measures for the client with cirrhosis and ascites.

*Level of Cognitive Ability:* Analysis
*Client Needs:* Health Promotion and Maintenance
*Integrated Concept/Process:* Teaching/Learning
*Content Area:* Adult Health/Gastrointestinal

*Reference*
Smeltzer, S., & Bare, B. (2000). *Brunner & Suddarth's Textbook of medical-surgical nursing* (9th ed.). Philadelphia: Lippincott Williams & Wilkins, p. 949.

**144.** A nurse is preparing a client with a diagnosis of multiple myeloma for discharge. The nurse tells the client to:
1   Restrict fluid intake to 1500 mL/day
2   Maintain bed rest
3   Maintain a high-calorie, low-fiber diet
4   Notify the physician if anorexia and nausea persist

**Answer:** 4

*Rationale:* Clients with multiple myeloma need to be taught to monitor for signs of hypercalcemia and to report them immediately to the physician. Anorexia, nausea, vomiting, polyuria, weakness and fatigue, constipation, and signs of dehydration are signs of moderate hypercalcemia. A fluid intake of 3000 mL/day is required to dilute the calcium overload and prevent protein from precipitating in the renal tubules. Activity is encouraged. Although a high calorie diet is encouraged, a diet low in fiber can lead to constipation.

*Test-Taking Strategy:* Recall that hypercalcemia is a concern in multiple myeloma. Eliminate option 2, because bed rest will promote hypercalcemia. Next, eliminate option 1, because this amount of fluid is rather low. Finally, eliminate option 3, because a low fiber diet can lead to constipation. Review the signs of hypercalcemia if you had difficulty in selecting the correct option.

*Level of Cognitive Ability:* Analysis
*Client Needs:* Health Promotion and Maintenance
*Integrated Concept/Process:* Self-Care
*Content Area:* Adult Health/Oncology

*Reference*
Smeltzer, S., & Bare, B. (2000). *Brunner & Suddarth's Textbook of medical-surgical nursing* (9th ed.). Philadelphia: Lippincott Williams & Wilkins, p. 766.

---

**145.** A nurse provides discharge instructions to the client who had a mastectomy and axillary lymph node dissection. The nurse tells the client to:
1   Avoid the use of insect repellent
2   Cut cuticles on the nails carefully using clean cuticle scissors
3   Wear protective gloves when doing the dishes
4   Avoid the use of lanolin hand cream on the affected arm

**Answer:** 3

*Rationale:* Following axillary node dissection, the affected arm may swell and is less able to fight infection. The client needs to be instructed in the several measures required to prevent complications, such as using insect repellent to avoid bites and stings; never picking at or cutting cuticles; applying lanolin hand cream a few times daily; and wearing protective gloves while doing dishes and cleaning.

*Test-Taking Strategy:* Note the client's diagnosis and focus on the issue: preventing altered skin integrity and thus infection. Keeping this in mind will assist in eliminating options 1, 2, and 4, which could potentially lead to a skin alteration. Review the client education teaching points related to mastectomy and lymph node dissection if you had difficulty with this question.

*Level of Cognitive Ability:* Application
*Client Needs:* Health Promotion and Maintenance
*Integrated Concept/Process:* Self-Care
*Content Area:* Adult Health/Oncology

*Reference*
Ignatavicius, D., Workman, M., & Mishler, M. (1999). *Medical-surgical nursing across the health care continuum* (3rd ed.). Philadelphia: W.B. Saunders, p. 1975.

**146.** A camp nurse provides instructions regarding skin protection from the sun to the parents who are preparing their children for a camping adventure. The nurse avoids telling the parents:

1    To obtain a sunscreen product with an SPF of 15 or more

2    That sunscreen will not be required on cloudy days

3    To pack a hat, long-sleeved shirt, and long pants for the child

4    To select tightly woven materials for greater protection from sun rays

**Answer: 2**
*Rationale:* The sun's rays are as damaging to the skin on cloudy hazy days as they are on sunny days. Sunscreens with an SPF of 15 or more are recommended and should be applied before exposure to the sun and reapplied frequently and liberally at least every 2 hours. A hat, long sleeved shirt, and long pants should be worn when out in the sun. Tightly woven materials provide greater protection from the sun's rays.

*Test-Taking Strategy:* Use the process of elimination. Recalling the concept that the ultraviolet rays can be damaging regardless of cloudiness or haziness will assist in directing you to option 2. Eliminate options 1, 3, and 4, because these measures provide the greatest protection from the sun. Review guidelines that protect the skin from the damaging rays of the sun if you had difficulty with this question.

*Level of Cognitive Ability:* Application
*Client Needs:* Health Promotion and Maintenance
*Integrated Concept/Process:* Teaching/Learning
*Content Area:* Fundamental Skills

*Reference*
Ignatavicius, D., Workman, M., & Mishler, M. (1999). *Medical-surgical nursing across the health care continuum* (3rd ed.). Philadelphia: W.B. Saunders. p. 487.

**147.** A client is receiving a course of chemotherapy on an outpatient basis for the diagnosis of lung cancer. Which of the following home care instructions would the nurse provide to the client?

1    A bathroom can be shared with any members of the family

2    Urinary and bowel excreta is not considered contaminated

3    Disposable plates and plastic utensils must be used during the entire course of chemotherapy

4    Contaminated linens should be washed separately and then washed a second time with other laundry if necessary

**Answer: 4**
*Rationale:* The client may excrete the chemotherapeutic agent for 48 hours or more after administration, depending on the medication administered. Blood, emesis, and excreta may be considered contaminated during this time. The client should not share a bathroom with children or pregnant women during this time. Any contaminated linens or clothing should be washed separately and then washed a second time with other laundry if necessary. All contaminated disposable items should be sealed in plastic bags and disposed of as hazardous waste.

*Test-Taking Strategy:* Use the process of elimination. Eliminate options 1 and 2 first, because they are similar. Eliminate option 3 next, because it would seem unreasonable to have to use disposable utensils for the "entire" course of therapy. Review client teaching points related to chemotherapy if you had difficulty with this question.

*Level of Cognitive Ability:* Application
*Client Needs:* Health Promotion and Maintenance
*Integrated Concept/Process:* Teaching/Learning
*Content Area:* Adult Health/Oncology

*Reference*
Smeltzer, S., & Bare, B. (2000). *Brunner & Suddarth's Textbook of medical-surgical nursing* (9th ed.). Philadelphia: Lippincott Williams & Wilkins, p. 281.

**148.** A home care nurse visits a client with bowel cancer who recently received a course of chemotherapy. The client has developed stomatitis. The nurse avoids telling the client to:
1 Drink foods and liquids that are cold
2 Eat foods without spices
3 Maintain a diet of soft foods
4 Drink juices that are not citrus

**Answer: 1**
*Rationale:* Stomatitis is a term used to describe inflammation and ulceration of the mucosal lining of the mouth. Dietary modifications for this condition include avoiding extremely hot or cold foods, spices, and citrus fruits and juices. The client should be instructed to eat soft foods and take nutritional supplements as prescribed.

*Test-Taking Strategy:* Note the word *avoids* in the stem of the question. Recalling that stomatitis is an inflammation of the mucosal lining of the mouth will assist in eliminating options 2, 3, and 4, because these measures will alleviate further irritation and prevent discomfort. Review client teaching points for stomatitis if you had difficulty with this question.

*Level of Cognitive Ability:* Application
*Client Needs:* Health Promotion and Maintenance
*Integrated Concept/Process:* Self-Care
*Content Area:* Adult Health/Oncology

*Reference*
Smeltzer, S., & Bare, B. (2000). *Brunner & Suddarth's Textbook of medical-surgical nursing* (9th ed.). Philadelphia: Lippincott Williams & Wilkins, pp. 283-284.

**149.** A home health nurse provides instructions to a postpartum client who has developed breast engorgement. The nurse tells the mother to:
1 Feed the infant less frequently, every 4 to 6 hours, using bottle feeding in between
2 Apply cool packs to both breasts 20 minutes before a feeding
3 Avoid the use of a bra during engorgement
4 Gently massage the breast from the outer areas to the nipple during feeding

**Answer: 4**
*Rationale:* The client with breast engorgement should be advised to feed frequently, at least every 2½ hours for 15 to 20 minutes per side. Moist heat should be applied to both breasts for about 20 minutes before a feeding. Between feedings, the mother should wear a supportive bra. During a feeding, it is helpful to gently massage the breast from the outer areas to the nipple to stimulate the letdown and flow of milk.

*Test-Taking Strategy:* Note the client's diagnosis. Think about the manifestations that occur with engorgement and recall that measures are initiated to facilitate the flow of milk. With this concept in mind, eliminate options 1, 2, and 3, because they will not facilitate the flow of milk. If you had difficulty with this question, review the measures used for breast engorgement.

*Level of Cognitive Ability:* Application
*Client Needs:* Health Promotion and Maintenance
*Integrated Concept/Process:* Teaching/Learning
*Content Area:* Maternity

*Reference*
Lowdermilk, D., Perry, S., & Bobak, I. (2000). *Maternity & women's health care* (7th ed.). St. Louis: Mosby, p. 609.

**150.** A client in the third trimester of pregnancy arrives at the clinic and tells the nurse that she frequently has a backache. Which instruction would the nurse provide to the client to alleviate the backache?
1   Sleep in a supine position and on a firm mattress
2   Wear a maternity girdle
3   Eat small meals frequently
4   Elevate the legs when sitting

**Answer: 2**
*Rationale:* To provide relief from backache, the nurse would advise the client to use good posture and body mechanics, perform pelvic rock exercises, and to wear flat supportive shoes. The client is also instructed to wear a maternity girdle, avoid overexertion, and sleep in the lateral position on a firm mattress. Back massage is also helpful. Eating small meals would more specifically assist in the relief of dyspnea. Leg elevation assists the client who has varicosities.

*Test-Taking Strategy:* Use the process of elimination, keeping in mind that the issue of the question is backache. This should assist in eliminating option 3 and 4, because they are unrelated to the relief of backache. From the remaining options, knowledge that the lateral position is most appropriate for the pregnant client will assist in directing you to option 2. Review relief measures for backache if you had difficulty with this question.

*Level of Cognitive Ability:* Application
*Client Needs:* Health Promotion and Maintenance
*Integrated Concept/Process:* Self-Care
*Content Area:* Maternity

*Reference*
Lowdermilk, D., Perry, S., & Bobak, I. (2000). *Maternity & women's health care* (7th ed.). St. Louis: Mosby, p. 410.

**151.** A nurse provides dietary instructions to the client receiving spironolactone (Aldactone). Which of the following foods would the nurse instruct the client to avoid while taking this medication?
1   Crackers
2   Shrimp
3   Apricots
4   Popcorn

**Answer: 3**
*Rationale:* Aldactone is a potassium-sparing diuretic and the client needs to avoid foods high in potassium, such as whole-grain cereals, legumes, meat, bananas, apricots, orange juice, potatoes, and raisins. Option 3 provides the highest source of potassium and should be avoided.

*Test-Taking Strategy:* Use the process of elimination and note the key word *avoid*. Recall that this medication is a potassium-sparing diuretic. Eliminate options 1 and 4, because they are food items that are similar. Remembering that fruits, vegetables, and fresh meats are high in potassium will direct you to option 3 as the food to avoid. Review this medication if you had difficulty with this question.

*Level of Cognitive Ability:* Application
*Client Needs:* Health Promotion and Maintenance
*Integrated Concept/Process:* Teaching/Learning
*Content Area:* Pharmacology

*Reference*
Hodgson, B., & Kizior, R. (2001). *Saunders Nursing drug handbook 2001.* Philadelphia: W.B. Saunders, p. 944.

**152.** Oral lactulose (Chronulac) is prescribed for a client with a hepatic disorder. The home health nurse provides instructions to the client regarding this medication. The nurse avoids telling the client to:
1 Take the medication with milk
2 Increase fluid intake
3 Increase fiber in the diet
4 Notify the physician immediately if nausea occurs

**Answer: 4**

*Rationale:* Lactulose retains ammonia in the colon and promotes increased peristalsis and bowel evacuation, expelling ammonia from the colon. It should be taken with water, juice, or milk to aid in softening the stool. An increased fluid intake and a high fiber diet will promote defecation. If nausea occurs, the client should be instructed to drink cola, or eat unsalted crackers or dry toast. Notifying the physician is not necessary.

*Test-Taking Strategy:* Use the process of elimination, noting the key word *avoids*. Eliminate options 2 and 3 first, because they are similar in that they will both promote defecation. From the remaining options, recall that there are measures that can be provided to the client to relieve nausea before notifying the physician. Review client teaching points related to this medication if you had difficulty with question.

*Level of Cognitive Ability:* Application
*Client Needs:* Health Promotion and Maintenance
*Integrated Concept/Process:* Teaching/Learning
*Content Area:* Pharmacology

*Reference*
Hodgson, B., & Kizior, R. (2001). *Saunders Nursing drug handbook 2001.* Philadelphia: W.B. Saunders, p. 944.

**153.** A client with leukemia receives a course of chemotherapy. The home care nurse scheduled to visit the client receives a telephone call from the client's physician. The physician informs the nurse that the neutrophil count is 600/mm$^3$. Which of the following instructions will the nurse provide to the client during the home care visit?
1 Avoid eating any raw fruits or vegetables
2 Avoid aspirin or medications containing aspirin
3 Avoid straining at bowel movements
4 Use an electric shaver for shaving

**Answer: 1**

*Rationale:* Neutrophil counts should range between 3000 and 5800/mm$^3$. A low neutrophil count places the client at risk for infection. When the client is at risk for infection, the client should avoid exposure to individuals with colds or infections. All live plants, flowers, or objects that harbor bacteria should be removed from the client's environment. The client should be on a low bacteria diet and avoid eating any raw fruits and vegetables. Options 2, 3, and 4 are measures that would be implemented if the client was at risk for bleeding.

*Test-Taking Strategy:* Use the process of elimination. Recalling that a low neutrophil count places the client at risk for infection will direct you to option 1. Also, bearing in mind that the issue of the question relates to infection will assist in eliminating options 2, 3, and 4, because these options identify measures that reduce the risk of bleeding. Review care of a client with a low neutrophil count if you had difficulty with this question.

*Level of Cognitive Ability:* Application
*Client Needs:* Health Promotion and Maintenance
*Integrated Concept/Process:* Teaching/Learning
*Content Area:* Adult Health/Oncology

*Reference*
Smeltzer, S., & Bare, B. (2000). *Brunner & Suddarth's Textbook of medical-surgical nursing* (9th ed.). Philadelphia: Lippincott Williams & Wilkins, p. 280.

**154.** A nurse provides instructions to a client who received cryosurgery for a local stage 0 cervical tumor. The nurse tells the client:
1 To call the physician if a watery discharge occurs
2 To call the physician if the discharge remains odorous in 1 week
3 To avoid tub baths
4 That pain indicates a complication of the procedure

**Answer: 3**
*Rationale:* Mild pain may occur and continue for several days following this procedure. A clear watery discharge is expected. For about 14 days, this is followed by discharge containing debris, which may be malodorous. If the discharge continues longer than 8 weeks, an infection is suspected. Healing takes about 10 weeks. Showers or sponge baths should be taken during this time. Tub baths and sitz baths need to be avoided.

*Test-Taking Strategy:* Use the process of elimination. Think about the anatomical area of the body in terms of where this procedure is performed. It would seem likely that the client would be instructed to avoid tub baths following this procedure. Review teaching points related to this procedure if you had difficulty with this question.

*Level of Cognitive Ability:* Application
*Client Needs:* Health Promotion and Maintenance
*Integrated Concept/Process:* Teaching/Learning
*Content Area:* Adult Health/Oncology

*Reference*
Smeltzer, S., & Bare, B. (2000). *Brunner & Suddarth's Textbook of medical-surgical nursing* (9th ed.). Philadelphia: Lippincott Williams & Wilkins, p. 1488.

**155.** A home care nurse provides instructions to the client taking digoxin (Lanoxin) 25 mg daily. Which of the following client statements would indicate a need for further education?
1 "I will take my prescribed antacid if I become nauseated."
2 "It is important to have my blood drawn when prescribed."
3 "I will check my pulse before I take my medication."
4 "I will carry a medication identification (ID) card with me."

**Answer: 1**
*Rationale:* Digoxin is an antidysrhythmic. The most common early manifestations of toxicity are gastrointestinal (GI) disturbances, such as anorexia, nausea, and vomiting. Digoxin blood levels need to be obtained as prescribed to monitor for therapeutic plasma levels (0.5 to 2.0 ng/mL). The client is instructed to take the pulse, hold the medication if the pulse is below 60 beats/min, and notify the physician. The client is instructed to wear or carry an ID bracelet or card.

*Test-Taking Strategy:* Use the process of elimination, recalling that toxicity can occur with the use of this medication. Also, note the key words *a need for further education*. Remembering that GI disturbances are the earliest signs of digoxin toxicity will assist in directing you to option 1. Review this medication if you had difficulty with this question.

*Level of Cognitive Ability:* Analysis
*Client Needs:* Health Promotion and Maintenance
*Integrated Concept/Process:* Teaching/Learning
*Content Area:* Pharmacology

*Reference*
Hodgson, B., & Kizior, R. (2001). *Saunders Nursing drug handbook 2001.* Philadelphia: W.B. Saunders, pp. 324-326

**156.** A nurse is providing immediate postprocedure care to a client who had a thoracentesis to relieve a tension pneumothorax that resulted from rib fractures. The goal is that the client will exhibit normal respiratory functioning. The nurse provides instructions to assist the client toward this goal. Which statement by the client indicates to the nurse that further instructions are needed?
1 "I will let you know at once if I have trouble breathing."
2 "I will lie on the affected side for an hour."
3 "I can expect a chest x-ray to be done shortly."
4 "I will notify you if I feel a crackling sensation on my chest."

**Answer: 2**
*Rationale:* After the procedure, the client is usually turned onto the unaffected side for 1 hour to facilitate lung expansion. Tachypnea, dyspnea, cyanosis, retractions, or diminished breath sounds, which may indicate pneumothorax, should be reported to the physician. A chest x-ray may be performed to evaluate the degree of lung reexpansion or pneumothorax. Subcutaneous emphysema may follow this procedure, because air in the pleural cavity leaks into subcutaneous tissues. The tissues feel like lumpy paper and crackle when palpated (crepitus). Usually subcutaneous emphysema causes no problems unless it is increasing and constricting vital organs, such as the trachea.

*Test-Taking Strategy:* Use the process of elimination, noting the key words *further instructions are needed.* Focus on the issue: postprocedure care following thoracentesis. Note that option 2 states "the affected side for an hour." Recall that facilitating lung expansion is important. Noting the words *affected side* in option 2 will direct you to this option. Review postprocedure care for a thoracentesis if you had difficulty with this question.

*Level of Cognitive Ability:* Analysis
*Client Needs:* Health Promotion and Maintenance
*Integrated Concept/Process:* Teaching/Learning
*Content Area:* Adult Health/Respiratory

**Reference**
Smeltzer, S., & Bare, B. (2000). *Brunner & Suddarth's Textbook of medical-surgical nursing* (9th ed.). Philadelphia: Lippincott Williams & Wilkins, p. 398.

**157.** An elderly client with coronary artery disease is scheduled for hospital discharge and lives alone. The client states, "I don't know how I'll be able to remember all these instructions and take care of myself once I get home." The nurse plans which of the following actions to assist the client?
1 Ask an out of town relative to stay with the client for a day or so
2 Ask the physician to delay the discharge until the client is better able to manage self-care
3 Ask the social worker to follow-up with a telephone call after discharge to assure the client is progressing
4 Ask the physician for a referral to a home health agency for nursing and home health aide support

**Answer: 4**
*Rationale:* With earlier hospital discharge, clients may require support from a home health agency until they are independent in functioning. Option 1 does not ensure that the client will receive continued care until able to be independent in managing his or her own care. Option 3 does nothing to actively assist the client, and option 2 is not realistic in the current health care environment. Option 4 is the method of ensuring the client necessary assistance for as long as required.

*Test-Taking Strategy:* Use the process of elimination, focusing on the key words *lives alone.* Note that option 4 is the global option and assures client assistance at home. Review home care resources following hospital discharge if you had difficulty with this question.

*Level of Cognitive Ability:* Application
*Client Needs:* Health Promotion and Maintenance
*Integrated Concept/Process:* Nursing Process/Planning
*Content Area:* Fundamental Skills

**Reference**
Black, J., Hawks, J., & Keene, A. (2001). *Medical-surgical nursing: Clinical management for positive outcomes* (6th ed.). Philadelphia: W.B. Saunders, p. 110.

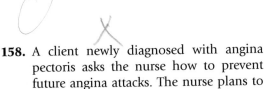

**158.** A client newly diagnosed with angina pectoris asks the nurse how to prevent future angina attacks. The nurse plans to incorporate which of the following instructions in a teaching session?

1. Eat fewer, larger meals for more efficient digestion
2. Plan all activities for early in the morning, when the client is most rested
3. Adjust medication doses freely until symptoms do not recur
4. Dress appropriately in very cold or very hot weather

**Answer: 4**

*Rationale:* Anginal episodes are triggered by events such as eating heavy meals, straining during bowel movements, smoking, overexertion, and experiencing emotional upset, or temperature extremes. Medication therapy is monitored and regulated by the physician.

*Test-Taking Strategy:* Use the process of elimination, focusing on the issue: preventing angina attacks. Recalling the causes of chest pain and principles of medication therapy will direct you to option 4. If you had difficulty with this question, review teaching points for the client with angina.

*Level of Cognitive Ability:* Application
*Client Needs:* Health Promotion and Maintenance
*Integrated Concept/Process:* Teaching/Learning
*Content Area:* Adult Health/Cardiovascular

*Reference*
Smeltzer, S., & Bare, B. (2000). *Brunner & Suddarth's Textbook of medical-surgical nursing* (9th ed.). Philadelphia: Lippincott Williams & Wilkins, p. 600.

---

**159.** A nurse has performed a nutritional assessment on a client with cystitis. The nurse tells the client to consume which of the following beverages to minimize recurrence of cystitis?

1. Coffee
2. Tea
3. Water
4. White wine

**Answer: 3**

*Rationale:* Caffeine and alcohol can irritate the bladder. Therefore, alcohol and caffeine containing beverages such as coffee, tea, and cocoa are avoided to minimize risk. Water helps flush bacteria out of the bladder, and an intake of 6 to 8 glasses per day is encouraged.

*Test-Taking Strategy:* Use the process of elimination. Option 4 is eliminated first, since alcohol intake is not encouraged for any disorder. Options 1 and 2 are similar to each other in that they both contain caffeine. Thus, it is unlikely that either of these are correct options. Review client teaching points related to preventing cystitis if you had difficulty with this question.

*Level of Cognitive Ability:* Application
*Client Needs:* Health Promotion and Maintenance
*Integrated Concept/Process:* Teaching/Learning
*Content Area:* Adult Health/Renal

*Reference*
Smeltzer, S., & Bare, B. (2000). *Brunner & Suddarth's Textbook of medical-surgical nursing* (9th ed.). Philadelphia: Lippincott Williams & Wilkins, p. 1141.

**160.** A home care nurse has given instructions to a female client with cystitis about measures to prevent recurrence. The nurse determines that the client needs further instruction if the client verbalizes an intention to:

1 Take bubble baths for more effective hygiene
2 Wear underwear made of cotton or with cotton panels
3 Drink a glass of water and void after intercourse
4 Avoid wearing pantyhose while wearing slacks

**Answer: 1**

*Rationale:* Measures to prevent cystitis include increasing fluid intake to 3 L/day; eating an acid-ash diet; wiping front to back after urination; taking showers instead of tub baths; drinking water and voiding after intercourse; avoiding bubble baths, feminine hygiene sprays, or perfumed toilet tissue or sanitary pads; and wearing clothes that "breathe" (cotton pants, no tight jeans, no pantyhose under slacks). Other measures include teaching pregnant women to void every 2 hours, and teaching menopausal women to use estrogen vaginal creams to restore vaginal pH.

*Test-Taking Strategy:* Use the process of elimination, noting the key words *needs further instruction.* Eliminate option 3 first, knowing that drinking water is a basic measure to prevent cystitis. Next, eliminate options 2 and 4, because they are similar. Review teaching measures to prevent cystitis if you had difficulty with this question.

*Level of Cognitive Ability:* Analysis
*Client Needs:* Health Promotion and Maintenance
*Integrated Concept/Process:* Teaching/Learning
*Content Area:* Adult Health/Renal

*Reference*
Smeltzer, S., & Bare, B. (2000). *Brunner & Suddarth's Textbook of medical-surgical nursing* (9th ed.). Philadelphia: Lippincott Williams & Wilkins. p. 1141.

---

**161.** A client with pyelonephritis is being discharged from the hospital. The nurse provides the client with discharge instructions to prevent recurrence. The nurse determines that the client understands the information that was given if the client states an intention to:

1 Report signs and symptoms of urinary tract infection (UTI) if they persist for more than 1 week
2 Take the prescribed antibiotics until all symptoms subside
3 Return to the physician's office for scheduled follow-up urine cultures
4 Modify fluid intake for the day based on the previous day's output

**Answer: 3**

*Rationale:* The client with pyelonephritis should take the full course of antibiotic therapy that has been prescribed, and return to the physician's office for follow-up urine cultures if so instructed. The client should learn the signs and symptoms of UTI, and report them immediately if they occur. The client should use all measures that are used to prevent cystitis, which includes forcing fluids to 3 liters per day.

*Test-Taking Strategy:* Use the process of elimination. Eliminate option 1 since UTI symptoms should never go unreported for a week. Option 2 is eliminated next, because antibiotics should be taken for the full course of treatment for adequate elimination of the infection. From the remaining options, recalling the importance of increased fluids will direct you to option 3. Review client teaching points related to pyelonephritis if you had difficulty with this question.

*Level of Cognitive Ability:* Analysis
*Client Needs:* Health Promotion and Maintenance
*Integrated Concept/Process:* Teaching/Learning
*Content Area:* Adult Health/Renal

*Reference*
Smeltzer, S., & Bare, B. (2000). *Brunner & Suddarth's Textbook of medical-surgical nursing* (9th ed.). Philadelphia: Lippincott Williams & Wilkins, p. 1141.

**162.** A client with nephrotic syndrome needs dietary teaching about how diet can help counteract the effects of altered renal function. The nurse plans to include which of the following statements in instructions to the client?

1   "Plan to drink at least 10 to 12 glasses of water a day."
2   "Add salt during cooking to replace sodium lost in the urine."
3   "Increase your intake of fish, meat, and eggs."
4   "Increase your intake of fatty foods to prevent protein loss."

**Answer: 3**
*Rationale:* The diet in nephrotic syndrome is limited in sodium. This is done to help control edema, which is a predominant part of the clinical picture. Fluids are not limited unless hyponatremia is present. On the other hand, the client is not encouraged to force fluids. Protein is increased, unless the glomerular filtration rate is impaired. This helps to replace protein lost in the urine, and ultimately helps in controlling edema also. A part of the clinical picture in nephrotic syndrome is hyperlipidemia, which results from the liver's synthesis of lipoproteins in response to hypoalbuminemia. Increasing fatty food intake would not be helpful in this circumstance.

*Test-Taking Strategy:* Use the process of elimination. Recalling that nephrotic syndrome is characterized by fluid retention and hypoalbuminemia will eliminate options 1 and 2. From the remaining options, knowing that hyperlipidemia accompanies this disorder will direct you to option 3. Review home care instructions for the client with nephrotic syndrome if you had difficulty with this question.

*Level of Cognitive Ability:* Application
*Client Needs:* Health Promotion and Maintenance
*Integrated Concept/Process:* Teaching/Learning
*Content Area:* Adult Health/Renal

*Reference*
Smeltzer, S., & Bare, B. (2000). *Brunner & Suddarth's Textbook of medical-surgical nursing* (9th ed.). Philadelphia: Lippincott Williams & Wilkins p. 1142.

**163.** A nurse is giving a client with polycystic kidney disease instructions in replacing elements lost in the urine as a result of impaired kidney function. The nurse instructs the client to increase intake of which of the following in the diet?

1   Sodium and potassium
2   Sodium and water
3   Water and phosphorus
4   Calcium and phosphorus

**Answer: 2**
*Rationale:* Clients with polycystic kidney disease waste sodium rather than retain it, and therefore need an increase in sodium and water in the diet. Potassium, calcium, and phosphorus need no special attention.

*Test-Taking Strategy:* Use the process of elimination. Recalling that this disorder causes sodium (not phosphorus) to be wasted, will assist in eliminating options 3 and 4. From the remaining options, recall that when the kidney excretes sodium, water is carried with it. This will direct you to option 2. Review care of a client with polycystic kidney disease if you had difficulty with this question.

*Level of Cognitive Ability:* Application
*Client Needs:* Health Promotion and Maintenance
*Integrated Concept/Process:* Teaching/Learning
*Content Area:* Adult Health/Renal

*Reference*
Ignatavicius, D., Workman, M., & Mishler, M. (1999). *Medical-surgical nursing across the health care continuum* (3rd ed.). Philadelphia: W.B. Saunders, p. 1857.

**164.** A client with acquired immunodeficiency syndrome (AIDS) is being treated for tuberculosis with isoniazid (INH). The nurse plans to teach the client which of the following regarding the administration of the medication?

1 Administer with an antacid to prevent gastrointestinal (GI) distress
2 Administer at least 1 hour before administering an aluminum containing antacid to prevent a medication interaction
3 Administer with food to prevent rapid absorption of INH
4 Administer with a corticosteroid to potentiate the effects of INH

**Answer: 2**

*Rationale:* Aluminum hydroxide, a common ingredient in antacids, significantly decreases INH absorption. INH should be administered at least 1 hour before aluminum-containing antacids. Food affects the rate of absorption of rifampin (Rifadin), not INH. INH administration with a corticosteroid decreases INH's effects and increases the corticosteroids effects.

*Test-Taking Strategy:* Use the process of elimination. Recall the general principles related to medication administration. In general, you would not usually administer a medication with an antacid, because it would decrease absorption of the medication. Review this medication to treat tuberculosis if you had difficulty with this question.

*Level of Cognitive Ability:* Application
*Client Needs:* Health Promotion and Maintenance
*Integrated Concept/Process:* Teaching/Learning
*Content Area:* Adult Health/Immune

*Reference*
Hodgson, B., & Kizior, R. (2001). *Saunders Nursing drug handbook 2001.* Philadelphia: W.B. Saunders, p. 550.

---

**165.** A nurse has provided dietary instructions to a client to minimize the risk of osteoporosis. The nurse determines that the client understands the recommended changes if the client verbalized to increase intake of which foods?

1 Rice
2 Yogurt
3 Sardines
4 Chicken

**Answer: 2**

*Rationale:* The major dietary source of calcium is from dairy foods, including milk, yogurt, and a variety of cheeses. Calcium may also be added to certain products, such as orange juice, which are then advertised as being 'fortified' with calcium. Calcium supplements are available and recommended for those with typically low calcium intake. Rice, sardines, and chicken are not high calcium foods.

*Test-Taking Strategy:* Use the process of elimination. Recalling that dairy products are high in calcium, and that yogurt is a dairy product will direct you to option 2. Review osteoporosis and the foods high in calcium if you had difficulty with this question.

*Level of Cognitive Ability:* Analysis
*Client Needs:* Health Promotion and Maintenance
*Integrated Concept/Process:* Teaching/Learning
*Content Area:* Adult Health/Musculoskeletal

*Reference*
Ignatavicius, D., Workman, M., & Mishler, M. (1999). *Medical-surgical nursing across the health care continuum* (3rd ed.). Philadelphia: W.B. Saunders, p. 1250.

**166.** A nurse is conducting a health screening clinic for osteoporosis. The nurse determines that which of the following clients seen in the clinic is at greatest risk of developing this disorder?

1   A 36-year-old man who has asthma
2   A 25-year-old woman who jogs
3   A sedentary 65-year-old woman who smokes cigarettes
4   A 70-year-old man who consumes excess alcohol

**Answer: 3**

*Rationale:* Risk factors for osteoporosis include being female, postmenopausal, of advanced age, low calcium diet, excessive alcohol intake, being sedentary, and smoking cigarettes. Long-term use of corticosteroids, anticonvulsants, and furosemide (Lasix) also increases the risk.

*Test-Taking Strategy:* Use the process of elimination, thinking about the risk factors associated with osteoporosis. Option 2 is eliminated first. The 25-year-old female who jogs (exercise using the long bones) has negligible risk. The 36-year-old male with asthma is eliminated next, because the only risk factor may be long-term corticosteroid use prescribed for asthma. From the remaining options, the 65-year-old female has more risk (age, gender, postmenopausal, sedentary, smoking) than the 70-year-old male (age, alcohol consumption). Review the risk factors associated with osteoporosis if you had difficulty with this question.

*Level of Cognitive Ability:* Analysis
*Client Needs:* Health Promotion and Maintenance
*Integrated Concept/Process:* Nursing Process/Assessment
*Content Area:* Adult Health/Musculoskeletal

*Reference*
Ignatavicius, D., Workman, M., & Mishler, M. (1999). *Medical-surgical nursing across the health care continuum* (3rd ed.). Philadelphia: W.B. Saunders, p. 1244.

**167.** A client with right-sided weakness needs to learn how to use a cane. The nurse plans to teach the client to position the cane by holding it with the:

1   Left hand, and placing the cane in front of the left foot
2   Right hand, and placing the cane in front of the right foot
3   Left hand, and 6 inches lateral to the left foot
4   Right hand, and 6 inches lateral to the right foot

**Answer: 3**

*Rationale:* The client is taught to hold the cane on the opposite side of the weakness. This is because, with normal walking, the opposite arm and leg move together (called reciprocal motion). The cane is placed 6 inches lateral to the fifth toe.

*Test-Taking Strategy:* Use the process of elimination and visualize this procedure. Knowing that the cane is held at the client's side, not in front, helps to eliminate options 1 and 2. Recalling that the preferred method is to have the cane positioned on the stronger side helps you choose option 3 over option 4. Remember client teaching points related to the use of a cane if you had difficulty with this question.

*Level of Cognitive Ability:* Application
*Client Needs:* Health Promotion and Maintenance
*Integrated Concept/Process:* Self-Care
*Content Area:* Adult Health/Musculoskeletal

*Reference*
Potter, P., & Perry, A. (2001). *Fundamentals of nursing* (5th ed.). St. Louis: Mosby, p. 1007.

**168.** A nurse has taught a client with a below-the-knee amputation about prosthesis and stump care. The nurse determines that the client has understood the instructions if the client stated an intention to:

1 Wear a clean nylon stump sock every day
2 Toughen the skin of the stump by rubbing it with alcohol
3 Prevent cracking of the skin of the stump by applying lotion daily
4 Use a mirror to inspect all areas of the stump each day

**Answer: 4**

*Rationale:* The client should wear a clean woolen stump sock each day. The stump is cleansed daily with a gentle soap and water, and is dried carefully. Alcohol is avoided, because it could cause drying or cracking of the skin. Oils and creams are also avoided, because they are too softening to the skin for safe prosthesis use. The client should inspect all surfaces of the stump daily for irritation, blisters, or breakdown.

*Test-Taking Strategy:* Use the process of elimination. Recall that nylon is a synthetic material that does not allow the best air circulation and holds in moisture. For this reason, option 1 is incorrect. Either alcohol or lotion can interfere with the natural condition of the skin, increasing the likelihood of breakdown either from drying or from excess moisture. For these reasons, eliminate options 2 and 3. Review client teaching points related to stump care following amputation if you had difficulty with this question.

*Level of Cognitive Ability:* Analysis
*Client Needs:* Health Promotion and Maintenance
*Integrated Concept/Process:* Self-Care
*Content Area:* Adult Health/Musculoskeletal

*Reference*
Smeltzer, S., & Bare, B. (2000). *Brunner & Suddarth's Textbook of medical-surgical nursing* (9th ed.). Philadelphia: Lippincott Williams & Wilkins, p. 1859.

**169.** A nurse is ambulating a client with a right leg fracture who has an order for partial weight-bearing status. The nurse determines that the client demonstrates compliance with this restriction if the client:

1 Does not bear weight on the right leg
2 Allows the right leg to touch the floor only
3 Puts 30% to 50% of the weight on the right leg
4 Puts 60% to 80% of the weight on the right leg

**Answer: 3**

*Rationale:* The client who has partial weight-bearing status places 30% to 50% of the body weight on the affected limb. Full weight-bearing status is placing full weight on the limb. Non-weight-bearing status does not allow the client to let the limb touch the floor. Touch-down weight-bearing allows the client to let the limb touch the floor, but not bear weight. There is no classification for 60% to 80% weight-bearing status.

*Test-Taking Strategy:* Use the process of elimination, focusing on the key words *partial weight-bearing status.* Option 3 is the only option that fits the description of partial weight bearing. Review the categories related to weight bearing if you had difficulty with this question.

*Level of Cognitive Ability:* Analysis
*Client Needs:* Health Promotion and Maintenance
*Integrated Concept/Process:* Nursing Process/Evaluation
*Content Area:* Adult Health/Musculoskeletal

*Reference*
Black, J., Hawks, J., & Keene, A. (2001). *Medical-surgical nursing: Clinical management for positive outcomes* (6th ed.). Philadelphia: W.B. Saunders, p. 614.

**170.** A nurse is planning measures to increase bed mobility for a client in skeletal leg traction. Which of the following items would the nurse consider to be most helpful for this client?
1   Television
2   Reading materials
3   Overhead trapeze
4   Fracture bedpan

**Answer: 3**
*Rationale:* The use of an overhead trapeze is extremely helpful in assisting a client to move about in bed, and to get on and off the bedpan. This device has the greatest value in increasing overall bed mobility. A fracture bedpan is useful in reducing discomfort with elimination. Television and reading materials are helpful in reducing boredom and providing distraction.

*Test-Taking Strategy:* Note the key words *most helpful* and focus on the issue: increase bed mobility. While all options are useful to the client in skeletal traction, the only one that helps with bed mobility is the trapeze. Review care of a client in traction if you had difficulty with this question.

*Level of Cognitive Ability:* Analysis
*Client Needs:* Health Promotion and Maintenance
*Integrated Concept/Process:* Nursing Process/Planning
*Content Area:* Adult Health/Musculoskeletal

*Reference*
Smeltzer, S., & Bare, B. (2000). *Brunner & Suddarth's Textbook of medical-surgical nursing* (9th ed.). Philadelphia: Lippincott Williams & Wilkins, p. 1791.

---

**171.** A nurse has given medication instructions to a client beginning anticonvulsant therapy with carbamazepine (Tegretol). The nurse determines that the client understands the use of the medication if the client stated to:
1   Drive as long as it is not at night
2   Use sunscreen when out of doors
3   Keep tissues handy because of excess salivation
4   Discontinue the medication if fever or sore throat occurs

**Answer: 2**
*Rationale:* Carbamazepine acts by depressing synaptic transmission in the central nervous system (CNS). Because of this, the client should avoid driving or doing other activities that require mental alertness until the effect on the client is known. The client should use protective clothing and sunscreen to avoid photosensitivity reactions. The medication may cause dry mouth, and the client should be instructed to provide good oral hygiene, and use sugarless candy or gum as needed. The medication should not be abruptly discontinued, because it could cause the return of seizures. Fever and sore throat should be reported to the physician (leukopenia).

*Test-Taking Strategy:* Use the process of elimination. Recalling that this is an anticonvulsant medication with CNS depressant properties will assist in eliminating option 1 first. Option 4 is eliminated next, because an anticonvulsant is not just discontinued, because side effects or infection occur. Rather, the physician should be called. From the remaining options, remembering that carbamazepine causes dry mouth will assist in eliminating option 3. Review client teaching points related to this medication if you had difficulty with this question.

*Level of Cognitive Ability:* Analysis
*Client Needs:* Health Promotion and Maintenance
*Integrated Concept/Process:* Teaching/Learning
*Content Area:* Pharmacology

*Reference*
Hodgson, B., & Kizior, R. (2001). *Saunders Nursing drug handbook 2001.* Philadelphia: W.B. Saunders, p. 144.

**172.** A nurse provides discharge instructions to a client with rheumatoid arthritis (RA). The instructions focus on measures to lessen discomfort and provide joint protection and the nurse tells the client to:

**1** Change positions every hour
**2** Lift items rather than sliding them
**3** Perform prescribed exercises even if the joints are inflamed
**4** Avoid stooping, bending, or overreaching

**Answer: 4**

*Rationale:* The client with RA should avoid remaining in one position and should change positions or stretch every 20 minutes. To reduce efforts by joints, the client's should slide objects rather than lift them. The client should avoid exercises and activities other than gentle range of motion when the joints are inflamed. The client is instructed to avoid stooping, bending, or overreaching.

*Test-Taking Strategy:* Use the process of elimination. Eliminate option 1, because with RA, remaining in one position for 1 hour is rather lengthy. Eliminate option 3 based on the basic principle that joints should be rested if inflamed. From the remaining options, use the principles related to body mechanics to direct you to option 4. Review principles for joint protection in RA if you had difficulty with this question.

*Level of Cognitive Ability:* Application
*Client Needs:* Health Promotion and Maintenance
*Integrated Concept/Process:* Self-Care
*Content Area:* Adult Health/Musculoskeletal

*Reference*
Black, J., Hawks, J., & Keene, A. (2001). *Medical-surgical nursing: Clinical management for positive outcomes* (6th ed.). Philadelphia: W.B. Saunders, p. 2147.

**173.** A home health nurse visits an elderly client with arthritis. The client complains of difficulty instilling glaucoma eye drops because of shaking hands due to the arthritis. Which of the following instructions would the nurse provide to the client to alleviate this problem?

**1** Keep the drops in the refrigerator so they will thicken and be easier to instill
**2** Lie down on a bed or sofa to instill the eye drops
**3** Tilt the head back to instill the eye drops
**4** Inform the client that a family member will have to instill the eye drops

**Answer: 2**

*Rationale:* Elderly clients with arthritis or shaking hands have difficulty instilling their own eye drops. An elderly client is instructed to lie down on a bed or sofa. Tilting the head back can lead to loss of balance. Eye drops should not be kept in a refrigerator unless specifically prescribed. Eye drop regimen for glaucoma requires accurate timing and it is unreasonable to expect a family member to instill the drops. Additionally, this discourages client independence.

*Test-Taking Strategy:* Use the process of elimination. Eliminate option 1 first, because eye medication should not be refrigerated unless specifically prescribed. Considering the issue of promoting client independence, and the fact that the question does not provide data regarding family, eliminate option 4. From the remaining options, select option 2, because it provides greater safety for the elderly client. Review procedures for instilling eye drops if you had difficulty with this question.

*Level of Cognitive Ability:* Application
*Client Needs:* Health Promotion and Maintenance
*Integrated Concept/Process:* Self-Care
*Content Area:* Adult Health/Eye

*Reference*
Black, J., Hawks, J., & Keene, A. (2001). *Medical-surgical nursing: Clinical management for positive outcomes* (6th ed.). Philadelphia: W.B. Saunders, p. 1813.

**174.** A scleral buckling procedure is performed on a client with retinal detachment and the nurse provides home care instructions to the client. Which statement by the client indicates a need for further instructions?
1 "I need to clean the eye daily with sterile water and a clean washcloth."
2 "I need to wear an eye shield during naps and at night."
3 "I need to avoid vigorous activity."
4 "I need to avoid heavy lifting."

**Answer: 1**
*Rationale:* In a scleral buckling procedure, the sclera is compressed from the outside by Silastic sponges or silicone bands that are sutured in place permanently. In addition, an intraocular injection of air or a gas bubble, or both, may be used to apply pressure on the retina from the inside of the eye to hold the retina in place. If an air or gas bubble has been injected, it may take several weeks to absorb. Vigorous activities and heavy lifting is avoided. An eye shield or glasses should be worn during the day and a shield should be worn during naps and at night. The client is instructed to clean the eye with warm tap water using a clean wash cloth.

*Test-Taking Strategy:* Use the process of elimination, noting the key words *a need for further instructions.* It is not necessary to use sterile water to clean the eye. In fact, it does not make sense to use a sterile solution with a clean washcloth. Review client teaching points following scleral buckling if you had difficulty with this question.

*Level of Cognitive Ability:* Analysis
*Client Needs:* Health Promotion and Maintenance
*Integrated Concept/Process:* Teaching/Learning
*Content Area:* Adult Health/Eye

*Reference*
Black, J., Hawks, J., & Keene, A. (2001). *Medical-surgical nursing: Clinical management for positive outcomes* (6th ed.). Philadelphia: W.B. Saunders, p. 1818.

**175.** A nurse provides dietary instruction to the parents of a child with a diagnosis of cystic fibrosis (CF). The nurse tells the parents that the diet should be:
1 Low in protein
2 Low in fat
3 High in calories
4 Low in sodium

**Answer: 3**
*Rationale:* Children with CF are managed with a high calorie, high protein diet, pancreatic enzyme replacement therapy, fat soluble vitamin supplements, and if nutritional problems are severe, night time gastrostomy feedings or total parental nutrition. Fats are not restricted unless steatorrhea cannot be controlled by pancreatic enzyme replacement therapy. Sodium intake is unrelated to this disorder.

*Test-Taking Strategy:* Use the process of elimination and knowledge regarding the digestive problems and the dietary management in children with CF. If you are unfamiliar with this content, select option 3, because children do require calories for growth and development and because this option is global and different from the others. Review this content if you had difficulty with this question.

*Level of Cognitive Ability:* Application
*Client Needs:* Health Promotion and Maintenance
*Integrated Concept/Process:* Teaching/Learning
*Content Area:* Child Health

*Reference*
Wong, D. (1999). *Whaley & Wong's Nursing care of infants and children* (6th ed.). St. Louis: Mosby. p. 1526.

**176.** A clinic nurse instructs an adolescent with iron deficiency anemia about the administration of oral iron preparations. The nurse instructs the adolescent that it is best to take the iron with:

1 Water
2 Soda
3 Tomato juice
4 Cola

**Answer: 3**

*Rationale:* Iron should be administered with vitamin C rich fluids, because vitamin C enhances the absorption of the iron preparation. Tomato juice contains a high content of ascorbic acid (vitamin C). Water, soda, and cola do not contain vitamin C.

*Test-Taking Strategy:* Use the process of elimination. Eliminate options 2 and 4 first, because they are similar. From the remaining options recall that vitamin C increases the absorption of iron to direct you to option 3. Review the administration of oral iron if you had difficulty with this question.

*Level of Cognitive Ability:* Application
*Client Needs:* Health Promotion and Maintenance
*Integrated Concept/Process:* Teaching/Learning
*Content Area:* Child Health

*Reference*
Wong, D. (1999). *Whaley & Wong's Nursing care of infants and children* (6th ed.). St. Louis: Mosby, p. 1665.

**177.** A nurse is conducting a home visit for a client who started taking a sustained release preparation of procainamide hydrochloride (Pronestyl SR). The nurse plans on teaching the client which of the following items about this medication?

1 Not to crush, chew, or break the sustained-release preparations
2 The presence of a tablet wax matrix in the stool indicates poor medication absorption
3 A double dose may be taken if a dose is missed
4 Monitoring the pulse rate is not necessary once this medication is begun

**Answer: 1**

*Rationale:* Procainamide (Pronestyl) is an antidysrhythmic that is available in a sustained-release (SR) form. The sustained-release preparations should not be broken, chewed, or crushed. The SR form has a wax matrix that may be noted in the stool and is not significant. If a dose is missed, a sustained-release tablet may be taken if remembered within 4 hours (2 hours for regular acting form); otherwise the dose should be omitted. The client or family member should be taught to monitor the client's pulse, and report any change in rate or rhythm.

*Test-Taking Strategy:* Use the process of elimination. Note the key words sustained-release to direct you to option 1. Review the administration of this type of medication if you had difficulty with this question.

*Level of Cognitive Ability:* Application
*Client Needs:* Health Promotion and Maintenance
*Integrated Concept/Process:* Teaching/Learning
*Content Area:* Pharmacology

*Reference*
Hodgson, B., & Kizior, R. (2001). *Saunders Nursing drug handbook 2001.* Philadelphia: W.B. Saunders. p. 861.

**178.** A nurse has given a client with a nephrostomy tube instructions to follow after hospital discharge. The nurse determines that the client understands the instructions if the client verbalizes to drink at least how many glasses of water per day?

1   2 to 4
2   6 to 8
3   10 to 12
4   14 to 16

**Answer: 2**
*Rationale:* The client with a nephrostomy tube needs to have adequate fluid intake to dilute urinary particles that could cause calculus, and to provide good mechanical flushing of the kidney and tube. The nurse encourages the client to take in at least 2000 mL of fluid per day, which is roughly equivalent to 6 to 8 glasses of water. Option 1 is an inadequate amount. Options 3 and 4 are amounts that could distend the renal pelvis.

*Test-Taking Strategy:* Use the process of elimination, noting that the client has a nephrostomy tube. Recall that the client needs at least 2 L of fluid per day. This will direct you to option 2. Also, avoid options in the much higher range, because these are unnecessary, and could possibly cause undue distention of the renal pelvis. Review care of a client with a nephrostomy tube if you had difficulty with this question.

*Level of Cognitive Ability:* Analysis
*Client Needs:* Health Promotion and Maintenance
*Integrated Concept/Process:* Teaching/Learning
*Content Area:* Adult Health/Renal

*Reference*
Smeltzer, S., & Bare, B. (2000). *Brunner & Suddarth's Textbook of medical-surgical nursing* (9th ed.). Philadelphia: Lippincott Williams & Wilkins. p. 1127.

**179.** A clinic nurse is providing home care instructions to a female client who has been diagnosed with recurrent trichomoniasis. Which statement by the client indicates a need for further instructions?

1   "I need to perform good perineal hygiene."
2   "I need to refrain from sexual intercourse."
3   "I need to discontinue treatment if my menstrual period begins."
4   "I need to take metronidazole (Flagyl) for 7 days."

**Answer: 3**
*Rationale:* Treatment for a recurrent infection should be continued through the menstrual period, because the vagina is more alkaline during this time, and a flare-up is likely to occur. The client should refrain from sexual intercourse while the infection remains active. If this is not possible a condom is recommended. Options 1, 2, and 4 are correct.

*Test-Taking Strategy:* Use the process of elimination, noting the key words *need for further instructions*. Recalling basic principles related to taking prescribed medications will direct you to option 3. If you had difficulty with this question, review treatment for this infection.

*Level of Cognitive Ability:* Analysis
*Client Needs:* Health Promotion and Maintenance
*Integrated Concept/Process:* Teaching/Learning
*Content Area:* Fundamental Skills

*Reference*
Black, J., Hawks, J., & Keene, A. (2001). *Medical-surgical nursing: Clinical management for positive outcomes* (6th ed.). Philadelphia: W.B. Saunders, p. 1054.

**180.** A nurse is providing home care instructions to a client recovering from a radical vulvectomy. Which statement by the client indicates a need for further instructions?

1    "I need to take showers rather than tub baths."

2    "I need to wipe from front to back after a bowel movement."

3    "I need to monitor for foul-smelling perineal discharge."

4    "I need to notify the physician if swelling of the groin or genital area persists for longer than 1 week."

**Answer: 4**

*Rationale:* The physician needs to be notified if any swelling of the groin or genital area occurs. The client should not wait 1 week before notifying the physician. Options 1, 2 and 3 are accurate instructions. Additionally, the client should monitor for pain, redness, or tenderness in the calves and for any signs of infection.

*Test-Taking Strategy:* Use the process of elimination, noting the key words *need for further instructions*. Basic hygiene principles will assist in eliminating options 1 and 2. From the remaining options, select option 4 noting the time frame in this option. Review client teaching points related to a radical vulvectomy if you had difficulty with this question.

*Level of Cognitive Ability:* Analysis
*Client Needs:* Health Promotion and Maintenance
*Integrated Concept/Process:* Teaching/Learning
*Content Area:* Adult Health/Oncology

*Reference*
Black, J., Hawks, J., & Keene, A. (2001). *Medical-surgical nursing: Clinical management for positive outcomes* (6th ed.). Philadelphia: W.B. Saunders, p. 1006.

---

**181.** A client with major depression is considering cognitive therapy. The client says to the nurse, "How does this treatment work?" The nurse makes which statement to the client?

1    "This type of treatment helps you examine how your thoughts and feelings contribute to your difficulties."

2    "This type of treatment helps you examine how your past life has contributed to your problems."

3    "This type of treatment helps you confront your fears by gradually exposing you to them."

4    "This type of treatment will help you relax and develop new coping skills."

**Answer: 1**

*Rationale:* Cognitive therapy is frequently used with clients who have depression. This type of therapy is based on exploring the client's subjective experience. It includes examining the client's thoughts and feelings about situations as well as how these thoughts and feelings contribute and perpetuate the client's difficulties and mood.

*Test-Taking Strategy:* Focusing on the key word *cognitive* will direct you to option 1. Option 1 uses the word *thoughts* in describing the treatment. Review this form of therapy if you had difficulty with this question.

*Level of Cognitive Ability:* Application
*Client Needs:* Health Promotion and Maintenance
*Integrated Concept/Process:* Nursing Process/Implementation
*Content Area:* Mental Health

*Reference*
Stuart, G.W., & Laraia, M.T. (1998). *Principles and practice of psychiatric nursing.* (6th ed.). St. Louis: Mosby, p. 648.

**182.** A client with acquired immunodeficiency syndrome (AIDS) has a nursing diagnosis of Altered Nutrition: Less Than Body Requirements. The nurse has instructed the client about methods to maintain and increase weight. The nurse determines that the client would benefit from further instruction if the client stated to:

1   Eat low-calorie snacks between meals

2   Eat small, frequent meals throughout the day

3   Consume nutrient-dense foods and beverages

4   Keep easy-to-prepare foods available in the home

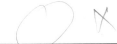

**Answer: 1**

*Rationale:*  The client should eat small, frequent meals throughout the day. The client also should take in nutrient-dense and high-calorie meals and snacks. The client is encouraged to eat favorite foods to keep intake up, and plan meals that are easy to prepare. The client can also avoid taking fluids with meals to increase food intake before satiety sets in.

*Test-Taking Strategy:*  Use the process of elimination. Note the key words *would benefit from further instruction*. Recalling that the client should choose snacks that are high in calories (not low in calories) will direct you to option 1. Review care of a client with Altered Nutrition if you had difficulty with this question.

*Level of Cognitive Ability:*  Analysis
*Client Needs:*  Health Promotion and Maintenance
*Integrated Concept/Process:*  Teaching/Learning
*Content Area:*  Adult Health/Immune

*Reference*
Black, J., Hawks, J., & Keene, A. (2001). *Medical-surgical nursing: Clinical management for positive outcomes* (6th ed.). Philadelphia: W.B. Saunders, p. 2210.

---

**183.** A nurse has given the postoperative thoracotomy client instructions about how to perform arm and shoulder exercises after discharge from the hospital. The nurse evaluates that the client has not learned the proper techniques if the client is observed doing which of the following movements on the affected side?

1   Moving the arm up over the head and back down

2   Holding the hands crossed in front and raising them over the head

3   Holding the upper arm straight out while moving the forearm up and down

4   Making circles with the wrist

**Answer: 4**

*Rationale:*  A variety of exercises that involve moving the shoulder and elbow joints are indicated after thoracotomy. These include shrugging the shoulders and moving them back and forth; moving the arms up and down, forward, and backward; holding the hands crossed in front of the waist and then raising them over the head; and holding the upper arm straight out while moving the lower arm up and down. Exercises that move only the wrist joint are of no use after this surgery.

*Test-Taking Strategy:*  Use the process of elimination, noting the key words *has not learned* and focus on the issue: arm and shoulder exercises. Note that options 1 and 2 move the shoulder joint. Option 3 moves the shoulder and elbow joint. Option 4 moves only the wrist joint. Review arm and shoulder exercises after thoracotomy if you had difficulty with this question.

*Level of Cognitive Ability:*  Analysis
*Client Needs:*  Health Promotion and Maintenance
*Integrated Concept/Process:*  Nursing Process/Evaluation
*Content Area:*  Adult Health/Respiratory

*Reference*
Smeltzer, S., & Bare, B. (2000). *Brunner & Suddarth's Textbook of medical-surgical nursing* (9th ed.). Philadelphia: Lippincott Williams & Wilkins, p. 520.

**184.** A nurse is teaching a client with histoplasmosis infection about prevention of future exposure to infectious sources. The nurse evaluates that the client needs further instruction if the client states that potential infectious sources include:

1. Grape arbors
2. Mushroom cellars
3. Floors of chicken houses
4. Bird droppings

**Answer: 1**

*Rationale:* A client with histoplasmosis is taught to avoid exposure to potential sources of the fungus, which includes bird droppings (especially starlings and blackbirds), floors of chicken houses and bat caves, and mushroom cellars.

*Test-Taking Strategy:* Use the process of elimination. Eliminate options 3 and 4 first, because they are similar. Since histoplasmosis is a fungus, recall that there is increased exposure to areas where the fungus thrives. By the process of elimination, the least likely option is the grape arbor, which is above ground and is not in a dark and damp area. Review the source of histoplasmosis infection if you had difficulty with this question.

*Level of Cognitive Ability:* Analysis
*Client Needs:* Health Promotion and Maintenance
*Integrated Concept/Process:* Nursing Process/Evaluation
*Content Area:* Adult Health/Respiratory

*Reference*
Smeltzer, S., & Bare, B. (2000). *Brunner & Suddarth's Textbook of medical-surgical nursing* (9th ed.). Philadelphia: Lippincott Williams & Wilkins, p. 1871.

---

**185.** A nurse is teaching a client with pulmonary sarcoidosis about long-term ongoing management. The nurse plans to include which of the following in the instructions?

1. Need for daily corticosteroid therapy
2. Usefulness of home oxygen equipment
3. Need for follow-up chest x-ray evaluation every 6 months
4. Importance of using incentive spirometer daily

**Answer: 3**

*Rationale:* The client with pulmonary sarcoidosis needs to have follow-up chest x-rays every 6 months to monitor disease progression. If an exacerbation occurs, treatment is initiated with systemic corticosteroids, which tend to provide rapid improvement in symptoms. Home oxygen and ongoing use of incentive spirometer are not indicated.

*Test-Taking Strategy:* Use the process of elimination and focus on the client's diagnosis. Eliminate option 2 first, since there is no specific information in the question to indicate a need for its use. Recalling that corticosteroids are used for exacerbation helps you to eliminate this option as well. From the remaining options, it is necessary to know that serial monitoring with x-ray is needed to track progression of the disease. Review the treatment for pulmonary sarcoidosis if you had difficulty with this question.

*Level of Cognitive Ability:* Application
*Client Needs:* Health Promotion and Maintenance
*Integrated Concept/Process:* Teaching/Learning
*Content Area:* Adult Health/Respiratory

*Reference*
Black, J., Hawks, J., & Keene, A. (2001). *Medical-surgical nursing: Clinical management for positive outcomes* (6th ed.). Philadelphia: W.B. Saunders, p. 1726.

**186.** A nurse has taught a client with silicosis about situations to avoid to prevent self-exposure to silica dust. The nurse evaluates that the client understands the instructions if the client verbalizes giving up or wearing a mask for which of the following hobbies?
1   Pottery making
2   Woodworking
3   Painting
4   Gardening

**Answer: 1**
*Rationale:* Exposure to silica dust occurs with activities such as pottery making and doing stone masonry. Exposure to finely ground silica, such as is used with soaps, polishes, and filters, is also dangerous. Silica is not a pesticide and is not found in the average soil. Silica is not inhaled in fumes, such as in woodworking or painting.

*Test-Taking Strategy:* Use the process of elimination, focusing on the issue: silica dust. Think about the materials that could give off silica dust. Recalling that pottery is made from clay will direct you to option 1. Review the sources of silica dust if you had difficulty with this question.

*Level of Cognitive Ability:* Analysis
*Client Needs:* Health Promotion and Maintenance
*Integrated Concept/Process:* Self-Care
*Content Area:* Adult Health/Respiratory

*Reference*
Smeltzer, S., & Bare, B. (2000). *Brunner & Suddarth's Textbook of medical-surgical nursing* (9th ed.). Philadelphia: Lippincott Williams & Wilkins, p. 476.

**187.** A nurse is conducting dietary teaching with a client who is hypocalcemic. The nurse encourages the client to increase intake of which of the following foods?
1   Apples
2   Chicken breast
3   Cheese
4   Cooked pasta

**Answer: 3**
*Rationale:* Products that are naturally high in calcium are dairy products, including milk, cheese, ice cream, and yogurt. High-calcium foods generally have greater than 100 mg of calcium per serving. The other options are foods that are low in calcium, which means that they have less than 25 mg of calcium per serving.

*Test-Taking Strategy:* Use the process of elimination, focusing on the client's diagnosis. Recalling that dairy products are naturally high in calcium will direct you to option 3. Review foods high in calcium if you had difficulty with this question.

*Level of Cognitive Ability:* Application
*Client Needs:* Health Promotion and Maintenance
*Integrated Concept/Process:* Teaching/Learning
*Content Area:* Fundamental Skills

*Reference*
Smeltzer, S., & Bare, B. (2000). *Brunner & Suddarth's Textbook of medical-surgical nursing* (9th ed.). Philadelphia: Lippincott Williams & Wilkins, p. 222.

**188.** A client is diagnosed with hyperphosphatemia. The nurse encourages the client to limit intake of which of the following items that exacerbates the condition?
1   Bananas
2   Grapes
3   Coffee
4   Carbonated beverages

**Answer: 4**
*Rationale:* Food items and liquids that are naturally high in phosphates should be avoided by the client with hyperphosphatemia. These include fish, eggs, milk products, vegetables, whole grains, and carbonated beverages.

*Test-Taking Strategy:* Focus on the client's diagnosis and note the key words *exacerbates the condition*. Recalling the phosphate content of foods and fluids will direct you to option 4. Review these foods and fluids if you had difficulty with this question.

*Level of Cognitive Ability:* Application
*Client Needs:* Health Promotion and Maintenance
*Integrated Concept/Process:* Teaching/Learning
*Content Area:* Fundamental Skills

*Reference*
Smeltzer, S., & Bare, B. (2000). *Brunner & Suddarth's Textbook of medical-surgical nursing* (9th ed.). Philadelphia: Lippincott Williams & Wilkins, p. 227.

---

**189.** A nurse is caring for a client with a burn injury who has sustained thoracic burns and smoke inhalation, and is at risk for Impaired Gas Exchange. The nurse avoids which of the following actions in caring for this client?

1. Reposition the client from side to side every 2 hours
2. Position the client on the back with the head of the bed at a 45-degree angle only
3. Suction the airway PRN
4. Provide humidified oxygen and incentive spirometry

**Answer: 2**
*Rationale:* Aggressive pulmonary measures are used to prevent respiratory complications in the client who has Impaired Gas Exchange as a result of a burn injury. These include turning and repositioning, positioning for comfort, using humidified oxygen, providing incentive spirometry, and suctioning the client on an as needed basis. The least helpful measure is to keep the client in one single position. This will ultimately lead to atelectasis and possible pneumonia.

*Test-Taking Strategy:* Note the key word *avoids*. This tells you that the answer to the question is an incorrect nursing action. Use basic nursing knowledge of respiratory support measures to eliminate each of the incorrect options. Also, note the word *only* in option 2. Review care of a client with Impaired Gas Exchange if you had difficulty with this question.

*Level of Cognitive Ability:* Application
*Client Needs:* Health Promotion and Maintenance
*Integrated Concept/Process:* Nursing Process/Implementation
*Content Area:* Adult Health/Integumentary

*Reference*
Smeltzer, S., & Bare, B. (2000). *Brunner & Suddarth's Textbook of medical-surgical nursing* (9th ed.). Philadelphia: Lippincott Williams & Wilkins, p. 1506.

---

**190.** A community health nurse provides an educational session on the risk factors of cervical cancer to the women in a local community. The nurse determines that further teaching is needed if a woman attending the session identifies which of the following as a risk factor of this type of cancer?

1. Caucausian race
2. Early age of first pregnancy
3. Prostitution
4. Sexually transmitted disease

**Answer: 1**
*Rationale:* Risk factors for cervical cancer include African-American and Native American individuals, prostitution, early first pregnancy, untreated chronic cervicitis, sexually transmitted diseases, postpartum lacerations, partners with a history of penile or prostate cancer, and infection with human papillomavirus. Options 2, 3, and 4 identify risk factors.

*Test-Taking Strategy:* Note the key words *further teaching is needed* and use knowledge regarding the risk factors for cervical cancer to answer this question. Review these risk factors if you had difficulty with this question.

*Level of Cognitive Ability:* Analysis
*Client Needs:* Health Promotion and Maintenance

*Integrated Concept/Process:* Teaching/Learning
*Content Area:* Adult Health/Oncology

*Reference*
Black, J., Hawks, J., & Keene, A. (2001). *Medical-surgical nursing: Clinical management for positive outcomes* (6th ed.). Philadelphia: W.B. Saunders, p. 370.

---

**191.** A high school nurse teaches the female students how to prevent pelvic inflammatory disease (PID). The nurse tells the students:
1  That single sexual partners should be avoided
2  To consult with a gynecologist regarding placement of an intrauterine device (IUD)
3  To douche monthly
4  To avoid unprotected intercourse

**Answer: 4**
*Rationale:* Primary prevention for PID includes avoiding unprotected intercourse, avoiding multiple sexual partners, avoiding the use of an IUD, and avoiding douching.

*Test-Taking Strategy:* Use the process of elimination and the principle of exposure of the pelvic area to factors that cause infection. With this concept in mind, eliminate options 1, 2, and 3. Review preventive measures for PID if you had difficulty with this question.

*Level of Cognitive Ability:* Application
*Client Needs:* Health Promotion and Maintenance
*Integrated Concept/Process:* Self-Care
*Content Area:* Fundamental Skills

*Reference*
Black, J., Hawks, J., & Keene, A. (2001). *Medical-surgical nursing: Clinical management for positive outcomes* (6th ed.). Philadelphia: W.B. Saunders, p. 986.

---

**192.** A nurse provides discharge teaching to a client following a vasectomy. Which of the following statements, if made by the client, would indicate a need for further teaching?
1  "If I have pain or swelling I can use an ice bag and take Tylenol."
2  "I can use a scrotal support if I need to."
3  "I can resume sexual intercourse whenever I want."
4  "I don't need to practice birth control any longer."

**Answer: 4**
*Rationale:* Following vasectomy, the client must continue to practice a method of birth control until the follow-up semen analysis shows azoospermia. Live sperm may be present in the ampulla of vas following this procedure. Options 1, 2, and 3 are appropriate client statements.

*Test-Taking Strategy:* Use the process of elimination. Considering the purpose of a vasectomy will direct you to option 4. Options 1 and 2 can be eliminated, because these measures assist in alleviating discomfort or swelling following the procedure. Option 3 can be eliminated, because there would be no reason to avoid sexual intercourse unless the client was experiencing discomfort. Review client teaching following a vasectomy if you had difficulty with this question.

*Level of Cognitive Ability:* Analysis
*Client Needs:* Health Promotion and Maintenance
*Integrated Concept/Process:* Teaching/Learning
*Content Area:* Fundamental Skills

*Reference*
Black, J., Hawks, J., & Keene, A. (2001). *Medical-surgical nursing: Clinical management for positive outcomes* (6th ed.). Philadelphia: W.B. Saunders, p. 967.

**193.** A physician in a community clinic diagnoses a client with prostatitis. A nurse provides home care instructions to the client. Which of the following statements, if made by the client, would indicate a need for further education?

1. "I need to take the antiinflammatory medications as prescribed."
2. "The sitz baths will help my condition."
3. "I need to avoid sexual activity for 1 week."
4. "There are no restrictions in my diet."

**Answer: 3**

*Rationale:* Interventions for prostatitis include antiinflammatory agents or short-term antimicrobial medication. Sitz baths and normal sexual activity are recommended. Dietary restrictions are not necessary unless the person finds that certain foods are associated with manifestations.

*Test-Taking Strategy:* Use the process of elimination, noting the key words *need for further education.* Eliminate option 1 first, using the general principles associated with medication prescriptions. Option 4 can be eliminated next, because there is no specific relationship of diet to this disorder. From the remaining options, eliminate option 2, because it would seem reasonable that sitz baths would provide comfort. Review home care instructions for the client with prostatitis if you had difficulty with this question.

*Level of Cognitive Ability:* Analysis
*Client Needs:* Health Promotion and Maintenance
*Integrated Concept/Process:* Teaching/Learning
*Content Area:* Fundamental Skills

*Reference*
Black, J., Hawks, J., & Keene, A. (2001). *Medical-surgical nursing: Clinical management for positive outcomes* (6th ed.). Philadelphia: W.B. Saunders, p. 963.

---

**194.** A nursing instructor asks a student to identify the risk factors and methods of preventing prostate cancer. Which of the following, if stated by the student, would indicate a need to review this information?

1. Men older than 50 years of age should be monitored with a yearly digital rectal examination
2. Men older than 50 years of age should be monitored with a prostate-specific antigen (PSA) assay
3. A high-fat diet will assist in preventing this type of cancer
4. Employment in fertilizer, textile, or rubber industries increase the risk of prostate cancer

**Answer: 3**

*Rationale:* A high intake of dietary fat is a risk factor for prostate cancer. Options 1, 2, and 4 are accurate statements regarding the risks and prevention measures related to this type of cancer.

*Test-Taking Strategy:* Use the process of elimination, noting the key words *a need to review this information.* Recalling the general principles related to cancer prevention will direct you to option 3. Review these measures if you had difficulty with this question.

*Level of Cognitive Ability:* Analysis
*Client Needs:* Health Promotion and Maintenance
*Integrated Concept/Process:* Teaching/Learning
*Content Area:* Fundamental Skills

*Reference*
Black, J., Hawks, J., & Keene, A. (2001). *Medical-surgical nursing: Clinical management for positive outcomes* (6th ed.). Philadelphia: W.B. Saunders, p. 370.

**195.** A clinic nurse provides information to a married couple regarding measures to prevent infertility. Which statement made by the husband indicates a need for providing further information?
1   "We need to avoid excessive intake of alcohol."
2   "We need to decrease exposure to environmental hazards."
3   "We need to eat a nutritious diet."
4   "I need to maintain warmth to the scrotum."

**Answer: 4**

*Rationale:* Keeping the testes cool by avoiding hot baths and tight clothing appears to improve the sperm count. Avoiding factors that depress spermatogenesis such as the use of drugs, alcohol, marijuana, and exposure to occupational or environmental hazards, and maintaining good nutrition are key components to prevent infertility.

*Test-Taking Strategy:* Use the process of elimination, noting the key words *a need for providing further information*. Eliminate option 3 first, because maintenance of a nutritious diet is important in all situations. From the remaining options, recalling that heat decreases motility of sperm will assist in directing you to the correct option. Review the measures that prevent infertility, if you have difficulty with this question.

*Level of Cognitive Ability:* Application
*Client Needs:* Health Promotion and Maintenance
*Integrated Concept/Process:* Teaching/Learning
*Content Area:* Fundamental Skills

**Reference**
Black, J., Hawks, J., & Keene, A. (2001). *Medical-surgical nursing: Clinical management for positive outcomes* (6th ed.). Philadelphia: W.B. Saunders, p. 1047.

---

**196.** A nurse teaches a client preparing for discharge from the hospital about home care measures following a total hip replacement. Which of the following statements, if made by the client, would indicate a need for further education?
1   "I need to place a pillow between my knees when I lie down."
2   "I need to wear a support stocking on my unaffected leg."
3   "I should not sit in one position for longer than 4 hours."
4   "I cannot drive a car for 6 weeks."

**Answer: 3**

*Rationale:* The client needs to be instructed not to sit continuously for longer than 1 hour. The client should be instructed to stand, stretch, and take a few steps periodically. The client cannot drive a car for 6 weeks after surgery unless allowed by a physician. A support stocking should be worn on the unaffected leg and an Ace bandage on the affected leg until there is no swelling in the legs and feet, and until full activities are resumed. The legs are abducted by placing a pillow between them when the client lies down.

*Test-Taking Strategy:* Use the process of elimination, noting the key words *a need for further education*. Recalling standard measures related to the postoperative period will assist in eliminating option 4. Knowing that leg abduction is maintained postoperatively during hospitalization may assist in eliminating option 1. From the remaining options, note the time frame of 4 hours in option 3. This is a rather lengthy time period for the client to remain in one position. Review teaching points following total hip replacement if you had difficulty with this question.

*Level of Cognitive Ability:* Analysis
*Client Needs:* Health Promotion and Maintenance
*Integrated Concept/Process:* Self-Care
*Content Area:* Adult Health/Musculoskeletal

**Reference**
Black, J., Hawks, J., & Keene, A. (2001). *Medical-surgical nursing: Clinical management for positive outcomes* (6th ed.). Philadelphia: W.B. Saunders, p. 558.

**197.** A client is diagnosed with hypothyroidism and is to begin on thyroid supplements. The nurse instructs the client about the medication. Which of the following statements, if made by the client, would indicate the need for further education?

1 "I need to take my daily dose every night at bedtime."
2 "I need to call my physician if I develop any chest pain."
3 "I need to speak to my physician when I begin to plan for parenthood."
4 "My appetite may increase because of the medication."

**Answer: 1**

*Rationale:* The client is instructed to take the medication in the morning to prevent insomnia. If the client experiences any chest pain it may indicate overdose and the physician needs to be notified. The dose needs to be adjusted if the client is pregnant or plans to get pregnant. Gastrointestinal complaints from thyroid supplements include increased appetite, nausea, and diarrhea.

*Test-Taking Strategy:* Use the process of elimination, noting the key words *need for further education*. Eliminate options 2 and 3 based on general principles related to medication therapy. Chest pain warrants follow-up and pregnancy would require a review of the medication dosage. Considering the disorder, hypothyroidism, you would expect that thyroid hormone would have an effect on increasing body metabolism. This should assist in directing you to option 1. Review client teaching points related to thyroid supplements if you had difficulty with this question.

*Level of Cognitive Ability:* Analysis
*Client Needs:* Health Promotion and Maintenance
*Integrated Concept/Process:* Teaching/Learning
*Content Area:* Adult Health/Endocrine

*Reference*
Black, J., Hawks, J., & Keene, A. (2001). *Medical-surgical nursing: Clinical management for positive outcomes* (6th ed.). Philadelphia: W.B. Saunders, p. 1098.

**198.** A clinic nurse instructs a client with diabetes mellitus about how to prevent diabetic ketoacidosis (DKA) on days when the client is feeling ill. Which statement, if made by the client, indicates a need for further education?

1 "I need to stop my insulin if I am vomiting."
2 "I need to call my physician if I am ill for more than 24 hours."
3 "I need to eat 10 to 15 g of carbohydrates every 1 to 2 hours."
4 "I need to drink small quantities of fluid every 15 to 30 minutes."

**Answer: 1**

*Rationale:* The client needs to be instructed to take insulin even if they are vomiting and unable to eat. It is important to self monitor blood glucose more frequently during illness (every 2 to 4 hours). If the premeal blood glucose is greater than 250 mg/dL, the client should test for urine ketones and contact the physician. Options 2, 3, and 4 are accurate interventions.

*Test-Taking Strategy:* Use the process of elimination, noting the key words *need for further education*. Recalling that insulin needs to be taken every day will assist in directing you to option 1. Review sick day rules for the client with diabetes mellitus if you had difficulty with this question.

*Level of Cognitive Ability:* Analysis
*Client Needs:* Health Promotion and Maintenance
*Integrated Concept/Process:* Self-Care
*Content Area:* Adult Health/Endocrine

*Reference*
Black, J., Hawks, J., & Keene, A. (2001). *Medical-surgical nursing: Clinical management for positive outcomes* (6th ed.). Philadelphia: W.B. Saunders, p. 1176.

**199.** A nurse is instructing a client with diabetes mellitus regarding hypoglycemia. Which of the following statements, if made by the client, would indicate a need for further education?

1  "Hypoglycemia can occur at anytime of the day or night."
2  "If hypoglycemia occurs, I need to take my Regular insulin as prescribed."
3  "If I feel sweaty or shaky I might be experiencing hypoglycemia."
4  "I can drink 8 oz of 2% milk if hypoglycemia occurs."

**Answer: 2**

*Rationale:* If a hypoglycemia reaction occurs, the client will need to consume 10 to 15 g of carbohydrate. Six to 8 oz of 2% milk contains this amount of carbohydrate. Tremors and diaphoresis are signs of mild hypoglycemia. Insulin is not taken as a treatment for hypoglycemia, because the insulin will lower the blood glucose. Hypoglycemic reactions can occur at anytime of the day or night.

*Test-Taking Strategy:* Use the process of elimination, noting the key words *need for further education*. Think about the concept that in hypoglycemia, the blood glucose in lowered. Insulin also lowers blood glucose, therefore it would seem reasonable that insulin is not a treatment for this condition. Review the signs of hypoglycemia and the appropriate interventions if you had difficulty with this question.

*Level of Cognitive Ability:* Analysis
*Client Needs:* Health Promotion and Maintenance
*Integrated Concept/Process:* Teaching/Learning
*Content Area:* Adult Health/Endocrine

*Reference*
Black, J., Hawks, J., & Keene, A. (2001). *Medical-surgical nursing: Clinical management for positive outcomes* (6th ed.). Philadelphia: W.B. Saunders, p. 1177.

---

**200.** A client with nephrolithiasis arrives at the clinic for a follow-up visit. The laboratory analysis of the stone that the client passed 1 week ago indicates that the stone is composed of calcium oxalate. Based on this analysis, the nurse tells the client to avoid:

1  Lentils
2  Spinach
3  Lettuce
4  Pasta

[akso, let] 草酸盐

**Answer: 2**

*Rationale:* Many kidney stones are composed of calcium oxalate. Foods that raise urinary oxalate excretion include spinach, rhubarb, strawberries, chocolate, wheat bran, nuts, beets, and tea.

*Test-Taking Strategy:* Note the key word *avoid* and focus on the type of stone. Recalling the foods that raise urinary oxalate excretion will direct you to option 2. If you had difficulty identifying this food, review this content.

*Level of Cognitive Ability:* Application
*Client Needs:* Health Promotion and Maintenance
*Integrated Concept/Process:* Teaching/Learning
*Content Area:* Adult Health/Renal

*Reference*
Black, J., Hawks, J., & Keene, A. (2001). *Medical-surgical nursing: Clinical management for positive outcomes* (6th ed.). Philadelphia: W.B. Saunders, p. 825.

**201.** A nurse provides instructions to a new mother who is about to breastfeed her newborn infant. The nurse avoids telling the mother to:

1 Turn the newborn infant on his or her side facing the mother

2 When the newborn opens the mouth, draw the newborn the rest of the way onto the breast

3 Tilt up the nipple or squeeze the areola, pushing it into the newborn's mouth

4 Place a clean finger in the side of the newborn's mouth to break the suction before removing the newborn from the breast

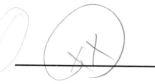

**Answer: 3**

*Rationale:* The mother is instructed to avoid tilting up the nipple or squeezing the areola and pushing it into the newborn's mouth. Options 1, 2, and 4 are correct procedures for breastfeeding.

*Test-Taking Strategy:* Note the key word *avoids*. Attempt to visualize the descriptions in each of the options. This will eliminate options 1, 2, and 4. Careful reading of option 3, noting the word *pushing* suggests force or resistance and should assist in directing you to this option. Review the procedure for breastfeeding if you had difficulty with this question.

*Level of Cognitive Ability:* Application
*Client Needs:* Health Promotion and Maintenance
*Integrated Concept/Process:* Teaching/Learning
*Content Area:* Maternity

*Reference*
Lowdermilk, D., Perry, S., & Bobak, I. (2000). *Maternity & women's health care* (7th ed.). St. Louis: Mosby, p. 766.

---

**202.** A clinic nurse provides instructions to a mother regarding the care of her child who is diagnosed with croup. Which of the following statements, if made by the mother, indicates a need for further education?

1 "I will place a cool mist humidifier next to my child's bed."

2 "Sips of warm fluids during a croup attack will help."

3 "I will give acetaminophen (Tylenol) for the fever."

4 "I will give cough syrup every night at bed time."

**Answer: 4**

*Rationale:* The mother needs to be instructed that cough syrup and cold medicines are not to be administered, because they may dry and thicken secretions. Sips of warm fluid will relax the vocal cords and thin mucus. A cool mist humidifier rather than a steam vaporizer is recommended because of the danger of the child pulling the machine over and causing a burn. Tylenol will reduce the fever.

*Test-Taking Strategy:* Use the process of elimination, noting the key words *need for further education*. Option 3 can be easily eliminated. Remembering that warm fluids will thin secretions will assist in eliminating option 2. From the remaining options, recalling that cough syrup will dry secretions will assist in directing you to option 4. Review home care instructions for the child with croup if you had difficulty with this question.

*Level of Cognitive Ability:* Analysis
*Client Needs:* Health Promotion and Maintenance
*Integrated Concept/Process:* Teaching/Learning
*Content Area:* Child Health

*Reference*
Wong, D. (1999). *Whaley & Wong's Nursing care of infants and children* (6th ed.). St. Louis: Mosby, p. 1474.

**203.** A client with anxiety disorder is taking buspirone (BuSpar) orally. The client tells the nurse that it is difficult to swallow the tablets. Which of the following would be the best instruction to provide to the client?

1  To purchase the liquid preparation with the next refill
2  To crush the tablets before taking them
3  To call the physician for a change in medication
4  To mix the tablet uncrushed in applesauce

**Answer: 2**

*Rationale:* BuSpar may be administered without regard to meals and the tablets may be crushed. This medication is not available in liquid form. It is premature to advise the client to call the physician for a change in medication without first trying alternative interventions. Mixing the tablet uncrushed in applesauce will not assure ease in swallowing.

*Test-Taking Strategy:* Use the process of elimination. Eliminate option 3 first, because in most situations there is a nursing intervention that can be instituted before calling the physician. Next, eliminate option 4, because this instruction will not ensure ease in swallowing. From the remaining options, it is necessary to know that this medication is not available in liquid form. Additionally, many tablets can be crushed. Review client instructions for administering this medication if you had difficulty with this question.

*Level of Cognitive Ability:* Application
*Client Needs:* Health Promotion and Maintenance
*Integrated Concept/Process:* Teaching/Learning
*Content Area:* Pharmacology

*Reference*
Hodgson, B., & Kizior, R. (2001). *Saunders Nursing drug handbook 2001.* Philadelphia: W.B. Saunders, p. 131.

**204.** A nurse caring for a child with congestive heart failure provides instructions to the parents regarding the administration of digoxin (Lanoxin). Which of the following statements, if made by the mother indicates a need for further education?

1  "If my child vomits after I give the medication, I will not repeat the dose."
2  "I will check my child's pulse before giving the medication."
3  "I will check the dose of the medication with my husband before I give the medication."
4  "I will mix the medication with food."

**Answer: 4**

*Rationale:* The medication should not be mixed with food or formula, because this method would not assure that the child receives the entire dose of medication. Options 1, 2, and 3 are correct. Additionally, if a dosage is missed and is not identified until 4 or more hours later, the dose is not administered. If more than one consecutive dose is skipped, the physician needs to be notified.

*Test-Taking Strategy:* Use the process of elimination, noting the key words *a need for further education.* General principles regarding medication administration to children should assist in directing you to the correct option. Mixing medications with formula or food may alter the effectiveness of the medication and, more importantly, if the child does not consume the entire formula or food, the total dosage would not be administered. Review parental instructions regarding administering digoxin if you had difficulty with this question.

*Level of Cognitive Ability:* Analysis
*Client Needs:* Health Promotion and Maintenance
*Integrated Concept/Process:* Teaching/Learning
*Content Area:* Pharmacology

*Reference*
Wong, D. (1999). *Whaley & Wong's Nursing care of infants and children* (6th ed.). St. Louis: Mosby, p. 1261.

**205.** A nurse provides discharge instructions to the mother of a child who was hospitalized for heart surgery. The nurse tells the mother that:

1 The child may return to school 1 week after hospital discharge
2 After bathing, rub lotion and sprinkle powder on the incision
3 The child can play outside for short periods of time
4 The physician is to be notified if the child develops a fever greater than 100.5° F

**Answer: 4**

*Rationale:* Following heart surgery, the child should not return to school until 3 weeks after hospital discharge at which time they should go to school for half days for the first few days. No creams, lotions, or powders should be placed on the incision until it is completely healed and without scabs. The mother is instructed to omit play outside for several weeks. The physician needs to be notified if the child develops a fever greater than 100.5° F.

*Test-Taking Strategy:* Use the process of elimination, bearing in mind the potential for infection in this child. Eliminate option 1 because of the time frame of 1 week. Eliminate option 3, because outside play can expose the child to infection and the risk of injury. Basic principles related to incision care should assist in eliminating option 2. Review home care instructions for the child following heart surgery if you had difficulty with this question.

*Level of Cognitive Ability:* Application
*Client Needs:* Health Promotion and Maintenance
*Integrated Concept/Process:* Teaching/Learning
*Content Area:* Child Health

**Reference**
Ball, J., & Bindler, R. (1999). *Pediatric nursing: Caring for children* (2nd ed.). Stamford, Conn.: Appleton & Lange, p. 494.

**206.** A clinic nurse provides instructions to a client who will begin on oral contraceptives. Which of the following statements, if made by the client, would indicate the need for further education?

1 "I will take one pill daily at the same time every day."
2 "I will not need to use an additional birth control method once I start these pills."
3 "If I miss a pill I need to take it as soon as I remember."
4 "If I miss two pills I will take them both as soon as I remember and I will take two pills the next day also."

**Answer: 2**

*Rationale:* The client needs to be instructed to use a second birth control method during the first pill cycle. Options 1, 3, and 4 are correct. Additionally, the client needs to be instructed that if she misses three pills, she will need to discontinue use for that cycle and use another birth control method.

*Test-Taking Strategy:* Use the process of elimination, noting the key words *need for further education.* It would seem reasonable that during the first pill cycle, a second birth control method would need to be used to prevent conception. Review these guidelines if you had difficulty with this question.

*Level of Cognitive Ability:* Analysis
*Client Needs:* Health Promotion and Maintenance
*Integrated Concept/Process:* Self-Care
*Content Area:* Pharmacology

**Reference**
Lowdermilk, D., Perry, S., & Bobak, I. (2000). *Maternity & women's health care* (7th ed.). St. Louis: Mosby, p. 195.

**207.** A nurse is providing dietary instructions to the client hospitalized for pancreatitis. Which of the following foods would the nurse instruct the client to avoid?
1    Lentil soup
2    Bagel
3    Chili
4    Watermelon

**Answer: 3**
*Rationale:* The client needs to avoid alcohol, coffee and tea, spicy foods, and heavy meals, which stimulate pancreatic secretions and produces attacks of pancreatitis. The client is instructed in the benefit of eating small frequent meals that are high in protein, low in fat, and moderate to high in carbohydrates.

*Test-Taking Strategy:* Use the process of elimination, noting that options 1, 2, and 4 are foods that are moderately bland. Option 3 is different in that chili is a spicy food. Review dietary measures for the client with pancreatitis if you had difficulty with this question.

*Level of Cognitive Ability:* Application
*Client Needs:* Health Promotion and Maintenance
*Integrated Concept/Process:* Teaching/Learning
*Content Area:* Adult Health/Gastrointestinal

*Reference*
Black, J., Hawks, J., & Keene, A. (2001). *Medical-surgical nursing: Clinical management for positive outcomes* (6th ed.). Philadelphia: W.B. Saunders, p. 1196.

**208.** A home health care nurse visits a client who was recently diagnosed with cirrhosis. The nurse provides home care management instructions to the client. Which of the following statements, if made by the client, indicates a need for further education?
1    "I will take acetaminophen (Tylenol) if I get a headache."
2    "I will obtain adequate rest."
3    "I do not need to restrict fat in my diet."
4    "I should monitor my weight on a regular basis."

**Answer: 1**
*Rationale:* Tylenol is avoided, because it can cause fatal liver damage in the client with cirrhosis. Adequate rest and nutrition are important. Fat restriction is not necessary and the diet should supply sufficient carbohydrates with a total daily calorie intake of 2000 to 3000. The client's weight should be monitored on a regular basis.

*Test-Taking Strategy:* Use the process of elimination, noting the key words *need for further education*. Recalling that Tylenol is a hepatotoxic agent will assist in directing you to the correct option. Review medications that are restricted or are avoided in clients with cirrhosis if you had difficulty with this question.

*Level of Cognitive Ability:* Analysis
*Client Needs:* Health Promotion and Maintenance
*Integrated Concept/Process:* Teaching/Learning
*Content Area:* Adult Health/Gastrointestinal

*Reference*
Black, J., Hawks, J., & Keene, A. (2001). *Medical-surgical nursing: Clinical management for positive outcomes* (6th ed.). Philadelphia: W.B. Saunders, p. 1325.

**209.** A client who has a history of gout is also diagnosed with urolithiasis. The stones are determined to be of the uric acid type. The nurse gives the client instructions in foods to limit, which include:

1    Liver
2    Apples
3    Carrots
4    Milk

**Answer: 1**

*Rationale:* Foods containing high amounts of purines should be avoided in the client with uric acid stones. This includes limiting or avoiding organ meats, such as liver, brain, heart, and kidney. Other foods to avoid include sweetbreads, herring, sardines, anchovies, meat extracts, consommés, and gravies. Foods that are low in purines include all fruits, many vegetables, milk, cheese, eggs, refined cereals, coffee, tea, chocolate, and carbonated beverages.

*Test-Taking Strategy:* Use the process of elimination, focusing on the client's diagnosis and noting the key word *limit.* Since purines are end-products of protein metabolism, eliminate options 2 and 3 first. From the remaining options, recall that organ meats such as liver provide a greater quantity of protein than milk. Review dietary instructions for the client with uric acid stones if you had difficulty with this question.

*Level of Cognitive Ability:* Application
*Client Needs:* Health Promotion and Maintenance
*Integrated Concept/Process:* Teaching/Learning
*Content Area:* Fundamental Skills

**Reference**

Black, J., Hawks, J., & Keene, A. (2001). *Medical-surgical nursing: Clinical management for positive outcomes* (6th ed.). Philadelphia: W.B. Saunders, p. 825.

**210.** A client tells the nurse that he gets dizzy and lightheaded with each use of the incentive spirometer. The nurse asks the client to demonstrate the use of the device, expecting that the client is:

1    Not forming a tight seal around the mouthpiece
2    Inhaling too slowly
3    Not resting adequately between breaths
4    Exhaling too slowly

**Answer: 3**

*Rationale:* If the client does not breathe normally between incentive spirometer breaths, then hyperventilation and fatigue can result. Hyperventilation is the most common cause of respiratory alkalosis, which is characterized by lightheadedness and dizziness. Options 1, 2, and 4 would not be a cause of lightheadedness and dizziness.

*Test-Taking Strategy:* Focus on the issue: the cause of lightheadedness and dizziness. Think about each of the actions in the options to direct you to option 3. Options 1, 2, and 4 would result in ineffective use, but would not cause dizziness and lightheadedness. Review the procedure for the use of the incentive spirometer if you had difficulty with this question.

*Level of Cognitive Ability:* Analysis
*Client Needs:* Health Promotion and Maintenance
*Integrated Concept/Process:* Nursing Process/Evaluation
*Content Area:* Adult Health/Respiratory

**Reference**

Black, J., Hawks, J., & Keene, A. (2001). *Medical-surgical nursing: Clinical management for positive outcomes* (6th ed.). Philadelphia: W.B. Saunders, p. 308.

**211.** A nurse is conducting a health screening clinic. The nurse interprets that which of the following clients participating in the screening has the greatest need for instruction to lower the risk of developing respiratory disease?

1   A 50-year-old smoker with cracked asbestos lining on basement pipes in the home
2   A 40-year-old smoker who works in a hospital
3   A 36-year-old who works with pesticides
4   A 25-year-old whose hobby is woodworking

**Answer: 1**
*Rationale:* Smoking greatly enhances the client's risk of developing some form of respiratory disease. Other risk factors include exposure to harmful chemicals, airborne toxins, and dust or fumes. The client at greatest risk has two identified risk factors, one of which is smoking.

*Test-Taking Strategy:* Use the process of elimination. Eliminate options 3 and 4, since the most harmful risk factor for the respiratory system is smoking. From the remaining options, select option 1, because asbestos is a substance that is toxic to the lungs, if particles are inhaled. Also, there are two risk factors identified in option 1, which makes this client at greater risk than the others who have one factor identified. Review the risk factors associated with respiratory disease if you had difficulty with this question.

*Level of Cognitive Ability:* Analysis
*Client Needs:* Health Promotion and Maintenance
*Integrated Concept/Process:* Nursing Process/Assessment
*Content Area:* Adult Health/Respiratory

*Reference*
Black, J., Hawks, J., & Keene, A. (2001). *Medical-surgical nursing: Clinical management for positive outcomes* (6th ed.). Philadelphia: W.B. Saunders, p. 354.

**212.** A nurse has conducted teaching with a client who has experienced pulmonary embolism about methods to prevent recurrence after discharge from the hospital. The nurse evaluates that the instructions have been effective if the client states an intention to:

1   Continue to wear supportive hose
2   Limit intake of fluids
3   Cross the legs only at the ankle, but not at the knees
4   Sit down whenever possible

**Answer: 1**
*Rationale:* Recurrence of pulmonary embolism can be minimized by wearing elastic or supportive hose, which enhances venous return. The client can also enhance venous return by avoiding crossing the legs at the knees or ankles, interspersing periods of sitting with walking, and performing active foot and ankle exercises. The client should also take in sufficient fluids to prevent hemoconcentration and hypercoagulability.

*Test-Taking Strategy:* Use the process of elimination, noting the key words *instructions have been effective.* Recalling that promoting venous return will prevent pulmonary embolism will direct you to option 1. Review the measures that will prevent recurrence of pulmonary embolism if you had difficulty with this question.

*Level of Cognitive Ability:* Analysis
*Client Needs:* Health Promotion and Maintenance
*Integrated Concept/Process:* Nursing Process/Evaluation
*Content Area:* Adult Health/Respiratory

*Reference*
Black, J., Hawks, J., & Keene, A. (2001). *Medical-surgical nursing: Clinical management for positive outcomes* (6th ed.). Philadelphia: W.B. Saunders, p. 1425.

**213.** A female client is being discharged from the hospital to home with an indwelling urinary catheter following surgical repair of the bladder following trauma. The nurse evaluates that the client understands the principles of catheter management if the client states to:

1    Cleanse the perineal area with soap and water once a day
2    Keep the drainage bag lower than the level of the bladder
3    Limit fluid intake so the bag won't become full so quickly
4    Coil the tubing and place under the thigh when sitting to avoid tugging on the bladder

**Answer: 2**

*Rationale:* The perineal area should be cleansed twice daily and following each bowel movement with soap and water. The drainage bag should be lower than the level of the bladder, and the tubing should be free of kinks and compression. Adequate fluid intake is necessary to prevent infection and to provide natural irrigation of the catheter from increased urine flow.

*Test-Taking Strategy:* Use the process of elimination, noting the key words *understands the principles.* Option 4 is eliminated first, because sitting on coiled tubing could cause compression and obstruct drainage. Option 3 is eliminated next, knowing that increased fluids are important. From the remaining options, noting the words *once a day* in option 1 will assist in eliminating this option. Review the principles related to catheter care if you had difficulty with this question.

*Level of Cognitive Ability:* Analysis
*Client Needs:* Health Promotion and Maintenance
*Integrated Concept/Process:* Self-Care
*Content Area:* Adult Health/Renal

*Reference*
Black, J., Hawks, J., & Keene, A. (2001). *Medical-surgical nursing: Clinical management for positive outcomes* (6th ed.). Philadelphia: W.B. Saunders, p. 831.

**214.** A 24-year-old female with a familial history of heart disease presents to the physician's office asking to begin oral contraceptive therapy for birth control. The nurse would next inquire whether the client:

1    Has taken oral contraceptives before
2    Exercises regularly
3    Eats a low cholesterol diet
4    Is currently a smoker

**Answer: 4**

*Rationale:* Oral contraceptive use is a risk factor for heart disease, particularly when it is combined with cigarette smoking. Regular exercise and keeping total cholesterol levels under 200 mg/dL are general measures to decrease cardiovascular risk.

*Test-Taking Strategy:* Use the process of elimination, noting the key words *familial history of heart disease.* Remember, smoking is the item that is linked to oral contraceptive use to make it a risk factor for cardiovascular disease. This will direct you to option 4. Review the risks associated with the use of oral contraceptives if you had difficulty with this question.

*Level of Cognitive Ability:* Analysis
*Client Needs:* Health Promotion and Maintenance
*Integrated Concept/Process:* Nursing Process/Assessment
*Content Area:* Adult Health/Cardiovascular

*Reference*
Black, J., Hawks, J., & Keene, A. (2001). *Medical-surgical nursing: Clinical management for positive outcomes* (6th ed.). Philadelphia: W.B. Saunders, p. 918.

**215.** A nurse is implementing measures to maintain adequate peripheral tissue perfusion in a postcardiac surgery client. The nurse avoids which of the following in giving care to this client?
1  Range-of-motion (ROM) exercises to the feet
2  Application of compression stockings
3  Leg elevation while sitting in chair
4  Use of the knee gatch

**Answer: 4**
*Rationale:* After surgery, measures are taken to prevent venous stasis. They include applying elastic stockings or leg wraps, use of pneumatic compression boots, discouraging leg crossing, avoiding use of the knee gatch, performing passive and active ROM exercise, and avoiding the use of pillows in the popliteal space. Leg elevation while sitting will promote venous drainage and help prevent postoperative edema.

*Test-Taking Strategy:* Focus on the issue, postcardiac surgery, and note the key word *avoids*. Select the option that will impede venous return. The use of the knee gatch puts pressure on blood vessels in the popliteal area, impeding venous return. Review care of a client following cardiac surgery if you had difficulty with this question.

*Level of Cognitive Ability:* Application
*Client Needs:* Health Promotion and Maintenance
*Integrated Concept/Process:* Nursing Process/Implementation
*Content Area:* Adult Health/Cardiovascular

*Reference*
Black, J., Hawks, J., & Keene, A. (2001). *Medical-surgical nursing: Clinical management for positive outcomes* (6th ed.). Philadelphia: W.B. Saunders, p. 308.

**216.** A nurse is planning to teach a client with atrial fibrillation about the need to begin long-term anticoagulant therapy. Which of the following explanations would the nurse use to best describe the reasoning for this therapy?
1  "Because of this dysrhythmia, blood backs up in the legs, and puts you at risk for blood clots, also called deep vein thrombosis."
2  "The antidysrhythmic medications you are taking cause blood clots as a side effect, so you need this medication to prevent them."
3  "Because the atria are 'quivering,' blood flows sluggishly through them, and clots can form along the heart wall, which could then loosen and travel to the lungs or brain."
4  "This dysrhythmia decreases the amount of blood flow coming from the heart, which can lead to blood clots forming in the brain."

**Answer: 3**
*Rationale:* A severe complication of atrial fibrillation is the development of mural thrombi. The blood stagnates in the "quivering" atria, due to the loss of organized atrial muscle contraction and "atrial kick." The blood that pools in the atria can then clot, which increases the risk of pulmonary and cerebral emboli.

*Test-Taking Strategy:* Use the process of elimination. Note the relationship between the client's diagnosis, atrial fibrillation, and the words *atria are quivering* in option 3. Review the pathophysiology of atrial fibrillation if you had difficulty with this question.

*Level of Cognitive Ability:* Application
*Client Needs:* Health Promotion and Maintenance
*Integrated Concept/Process:* Teaching/Learning
*Content Area:* Adult Health/Cardiovascular

*Reference*
Black, J., Hawks, J., & Keene, A. (2001). *Medical-surgical nursing: Clinical management for positive outcomes* (6th ed.). Philadelphia: W.B. Saunders, p. 1556.

**217.** A clinic nurse is providing instructions to a client in the third trimester of pregnancy regarding relief measures related to heartburn. Which of the following instructions would the nurse provide to the client?

1 Eat fatty foods only once a day in the morning
2 Avoid milk and hot tea
3 Take frequent sips of water
4 Use antacids that contain sodium

**Answer: 3**

**Rationale:** Measures to provide relief of heartburn include small frequent meals, and avoiding fatty fried foods, coffee, and cigarettes. Mild antacids can be used if they do not contain aspirin or sodium. Frequent sips of milk, hot tea, or water is helpful. Gum is also helpful in the relief of heart burn.

**Test-Taking Strategy:** Use the process of elimination. Eliminate option 4 first, because sodium will lead to edema and edema should be avoided. Eliminate option 1 next based on basic nutritional principles that fatty and fried foods should be avoided. From the remaining options, recalling that milk and hot tea can be soothing to the gastrointestinal tract will assist in eliminating option 2. Review the measures that relieve heartburn if you had difficulty with this question.

**Level of Cognitive Ability:** Application
**Client Needs:** Health Promotion and Maintenance
**Integrated Concept/Process:** Teaching/Learning
**Content Area:** Maternity

**Reference**
Lowdermilk, D., Perry, S., & Bobak, I. (2000). *Maternity & women's health care* (7th ed.). St. Louis: Mosby, p. 350.

---

**218.** A nurse provides instructions regarding home care to the parents of a 3-year old child hospitalized with hemophilia. Which of the following home care measures would not be included in the teaching plan?

1 Do not leave the child unattended
2 Pad table corners in the home
3 Remove household items that can tip over
4 Avoid immunizations and dental hygiene

**Answer: 4**

**Rationale:** The nurse needs to stress the importance of immunizations, dental hygiene, and routine well-child care. Options 1, 2, and 3 are appropriate. The parents are also instructed in measures to implement if blunt trauma occurs especially trauma involving the joints, and how to apply prolonged pressure to superficial wounds until the bleeding has stopped.

**Test-Taking Strategy:** Use the process of elimination, noting the key word *not*. Knowledge that bleeding is a concern in this disorder will assist in eliminating options 1, 2, and 3, which include measures of protection and safety for the child. Also, recalling the importance of immunizations and dental hygiene care will direct you to option 4. If you had difficulty with this question, review care of a child with hemophilia.

**Level of Cognitive Ability:** Application
**Client Needs:** Health Promotion and Maintenance
**Integrated Concept/Process:** Teaching/Learning
**Content Area:** Child Health

**Reference**
Wong, D. (1999). *Whaley & Wong's Nursing care of infants and children* (6th ed.). St. Louis: Mosby, p. 1684.

**219.** A nurse provides instructions to the client taking clorazepate (Tranxene) for management of an anxiety disorder. The nurse tells the client that:
1   Drowsiness is a side effect that usually disappears with continued therapy
2   If dizziness occurs, call the physician
3   Smoking increases the effectiveness of the medication
4   If gastrointestinal (GI) disturbances occur, discontinue the medication

**Answer: 1**
*Rationale:* Dizziness is a common side effect of this medication and usually disappears with continued use. The client should be instructed that if dizziness occurs, changing positions slowly from lying, to sitting, to standing will help. Smoking reduces medication effectiveness. GI disturbance is an occasional side effect and the medication can be given with food if this occurs.

*Test-Taking Strategy:* Use the process of elimination. Eliminate option 4 first, because the client should not be instructed to discontinue medication. Eliminate option 2 next, because episodes of dizziness commonly occur with antianxiety medications and interventions to alleviate the dizziness should be told to the client. From the remaining options, recall that drowsiness is commonly associated with antianxiety medications and normally disappears with continued therapy. Review client teaching points related to this medication if you had difficulty with this question.

*Level of Cognitive Ability:* Application
*Client Needs:* Health Promotion and Maintenance
*Integrated Concept/Process:* Teaching/Learning
*Content Area:* Mental Health

*Reference*
Hodgson, B., & Kizior, R. (2001). *Saunders Nursing drug handbook 2001.* Philadelphia: W.B. Saunders, p. 243.

**220.** A client with chlamydia infection has received instructions on self-care and prevention of further infection. The nurse evaluates that the client needs further reinforcement if the client states to:
1   Reduce the chance of reinfection by limiting the number of sexual partners
2   Use latex condoms to prevent disease transmission
3   Return to the clinic as requested for follow-up culture in 1 week
4   Use antibiotics prophylactically to prevent symptoms of chlamydia

**Answer: 4**
*Rationale:* Antibiotics are not taken prophylactically to prevent chlamydia. The risk of reinfection can be reduced by limiting the number of sexual partners, and by the use of condoms. In some instances, follow-up culture is requested in 4 to 7 days to confirm a cure.

*Test-Taking Strategy:* Use the process of elimination, noting the key words *needs further reinforcement*. Recalling the basic principles of antibiotic therapy will direct you to option 4, since antibiotics are not used intermittently for prophylaxis of this infection. Review the treatment measures for chlamydia infection if you had difficulty with this question.

*Level of Cognitive Ability:* Analysis
*Client Needs:* Health Promotion and Maintenance
*Integrated Concept/Process:* Teaching/Learning
*Content Area:* Fundamental Skills

*Reference*
Black, J., Hawks, J., & Keene, A. (2001). *Medical-surgical nursing: Clinical management for positive outcomes* (6th ed.). Philadelphia: W.B. Saunders, p. 1047.

**221.** A client with prostatitis asks the nurse, "Why do I need to take a stool softener? The problem is with my urine, not my bowels!" Which of the following is the best response by the nurse?

1  "Being constipated puts you at more risk for developing complications of prostatitis."
2  "This is a standard medication order for anyone with an abdominal problem."
3  "This will keep the bowel free of feces, which will help decrease the swelling inside."
4  "This will help you avoid constipation, because straining is painful with prostatitis."

**Answer: 4**

*Rationale:* Stool softeners are ordered for the client with prostatitis to prevent constipation, which is painful. It has no direct effect on decreasing swelling. Constipation does not cause complications of prostatitis. Stool softeners are not standardly prescribed for "anyone with an abdominal problem."

*Test-Taking Strategy:* Use the process of elimination. Recalling the purpose and use of stool softeners, to prevent constipation, will direct you to option 4. Review care of a client with prostatitis if you had difficulty with this question.

*Level of Cognitive Ability:* Application
*Client Needs:* Health Promotion and Maintenance
*Integrated Concept/Process:* Teaching/Learning
*Content Area:* Adult Health/Renal

*Reference*
Black, J., Hawks, J., & Keene, A. (2001). *Medical-surgical nursing: Clinical management for positive outcomes* (6th ed.). Philadelphia: W.B. Saunders, p. 963.

**222.** A client with Parkinson's disease has begun therapy with levodopa (L-dopa). The nurse determines that the client understands the action of the medication if the client verbalizes that results may not be apparent for:

1  24-hours
2  5 to 7 days
3  1 week
4  2 to 3 weeks

**Answer: 4**

*Rationale:* Signs and symptoms of Parkinson's disease usually begin to resolve within 2 to 3 weeks of starting therapy, although in some clients marked improvement may not be seen for up to 6 months. Clients need to understand this concept to aid in compliance with medication therapy.

*Test-Taking Strategy:* Use the process of elimination and knowledge regarding this medication. Eliminate options 2 and 3, because they are similar. From the remaining options, eliminate option 1, because it is unlikely that results would be noted in 24 hours. If this question was difficult, review this medication.

*Level of Cognitive Ability:* Analysis
*Client Needs:* Health Promotion and Maintenance
*Integrated Concept/Process:* Teaching/Learning
*Content Area:* Pharmacology

*Reference*
Spratto, G., & Woods, A. (2001). *PDR Nurse's drug handbook.* Montvale, N.J.: Medical Economics. p. 807.

**223.** A nurse in the physician's office is reviewing the results of a client's phenytoin (Dilantin) level drawn that morning. The nurse determines that the client had a therapeutic drug level if the client's result was:

1    3 µg/mL
2    8 µg/mL
3    15 µg/mL
4    24 µg/mL

**Answer: 3**
*Rationale:* The therapeutic range for serum phenytoin levels is 10 to 20 µg/mL in clients with normal serum albumin levels and renal function. A level below this range indicates that the client is not receiving sufficient medication, and is at risk for seizure activity. In this case, the medication dose should be adjusted upward. A level above the normal range indicates that the client is entering the toxic range and is at risk for toxic side effects of the medication. In this case, the dose should be adjusted downward.

*Test-Taking Strategy:* Recalling the therapeutic drug serum level for phenytoin will direct you to option 3. Review this level if you had difficulty with this question.

*Level of Cognitive Ability:* Analysis
*Client Needs:* Health Promotion and Maintenance
*Integrated Concept/Process:* Nursing Process/Evaluation
*Content Area:* Pharmacology

*Reference*
Hodgson, B., & Kizior, R. (2001). *Saunders Nursing drug handbook 2001.* Philadelphia: W.B. Saunders, p. 823.

**224.** A nurse is conducting a prostate screening clinic. The nurse interprets that a client understands the educational information that was shared if the nurse overhears the client tell another participant that:

1    Increased intake of green, leafy vegetables is helpful
2    A daily supplement of vitamin E will prevent prostate problems
3    An annual prostate exam after age 40 is best for early detection
4    Cigarette smoking triples the chance of developing prostate problems

**Answer: 3**
*Rationale:* Increasing age is the major risk factor for developing benign prostatic hyperplasia (BPH). Increased intake of yellow vegetables and some elements of the Japanese diet may be helpful in reducing risk. Vitamin E and cigarette smoking have no known relationship with BPH. Early detection is the only method of prevention (and is actually secondary prevention). This is accomplished by an annual prostate exam after the age of 40.

*Test-Taking Strategy:* Focus on the issue: prostate screening. Use knowledge regarding measures to prevent BPH and focus on the issue to direct you to option 3. Review the screening measures for BPH if you had difficulty with this question.

*Level of Cognitive Ability:* Analysis
*Client Needs:* Health Promotion and Maintenance
*Integrated Concept/Process:* Teaching/Learning
*Content Area:* Adult Health/Renal

*Reference*
Black, J., Hawks, J., & Keene, A. (2001). *Medical-surgical nursing: Clinical management for positive outcomes* (6th ed.). Philadelphia: W.B. Saunders, p. 946.

**225.** A client is being discharged to home without a Foley catheter following prostatectomy. The nurse plans to teach the client which of the following points as part of discharge teaching?
1 Drink 15 glasses of water a day to minimize clot formation
2 Mowing the lawn is allowed after 1 week
3 Notify the physician if fever, increased pain, or inability to void occurs
4 Avoid lifting more than 50 lb for 4 to 6 weeks after surgery

**Answer: 3**
*Rationale:* The client should notify the physician if there are any signs of infection, bleeding, or urinary obstruction. Lifting more than 20 lb is prohibited for 4 to 6 weeks after surgery. Other strenuous activities that could increase intraabdominal tension are also restricted, such as mowing the lawn. The client should drink 6 to 8 glasses of water or nonalcoholic beverages per day to minimize the risk of clot formation.

*Test-Taking Strategy:* Focus on the client's diagnosis. Eliminate option 1 as an excessive fluid intake. Noting that the activities identified in options 2 and 4 are excessive assists in eliminating these options. Review home care instructions following prostatectomy if you had difficulty with this question.

*Level of Cognitive Ability:* Application
*Client Needs:* Health Promotion and Maintenance
*Integrated Concept/Process:* Teaching/Learning
*Content Area:* Adult Health/Renal

*Reference*
Black, J., Hawks, J., & Keene, A. (2001). *Medical-surgical nursing: Clinical management for positive outcomes* (6th ed.). Philadelphia: W.B. Saunders, p. 957.

**226.** A nurse is teaching a client with acute renal failure (ARF) to include proteins in the diet that are considered high quality. Which of the following foods would the nurse discourage, since it is a low-quality protein source?
1 Eggs
2 Broccoli
3 Chicken
4 Fish

**Answer: 2**
*Rationale:* High-quality proteins come from animal sources, and include such foods as eggs, chicken, meat, and fish. Low-quality proteins derive from plant sources and include vegetables and foods made from grains. Since a renal diet is limited in protein, it is important that the proteins ingested are of high quality.

*Test-Taking Strategy:* Use the process of elimination, noting the key words *low-quality protein source*. In comparing the options, note that option 2 (broccoli) is the only item that does not derive from a living source. Chicken, eggs, and fish derive from animal sources, while the broccoli is a plant. Review food items that are high and low protein if you had difficulty with this question.

*Level of Cognitive Ability:* Application
*Client Needs:* Health Promotion and Maintenance
*Integrated Concept/Process:* Teaching/Learning
*Content Area:* Adult Health/Renal

*Reference*
Black, J., Hawks, J., & Keene, A. (2001). *Medical-surgical nursing: Clinical management for positive outcomes* (6th ed.). Philadelphia: W.B. Saunders, p. 879.

**227.** A home care nurse visits a client with a cerebrovascular accident (CVA) with unilateral neglect who was recently discharged from the hospital. The nurse provides instructions to the family regarding care and tells the family to:

1. Place personal items directly in front of the client
2. Assist the client from the affected side
3. Assist the client to groom the unaffected side first
4. Discourage the client from scanning the environment

**Answer: 2**

*Rationale:* Unilateral neglect is a pattern of lack of awareness of body parts such as paralyzed arms or legs. Initially, the environment is adapted to the deficit by focusing on the client's unaffected side and the client's personal items are placed on the unaffected side. Gradually, the client's attention is focused to the affected side. The client is assisted from the affected side and the client grooms the affected side first. The client needs to scan the entire environment.

*Test-Taking Strategy:* Note the client's diagnosis, unilateral neglect, and note the issue, home care instructions. Recalling the physiological alteration that occurs in unilateral neglect will direct you to option 2. Review interventions associated with unilateral neglect if you had difficulty with this question.

*Level of Cognitive Ability:* Application
*Client Needs:* Health Promotion and Maintenance
*Integrated Concept/Process:* Teaching/Learning
*Content Area:* Adult Health/Neurological

*Reference*
Black, J., Hawks, J., & Keene, A. (2001). *Medical-surgical nursing: Clinical management for positive outcomes* (6th ed.). Philadelphia: W.B. Saunders, p. 1957.

---

**228.** A nurse has completed discharge teaching for a client who has had surgery for lung cancer. The nurse determines that the client has not understood all of the essential elements of home management if the client verbalizes to:

1. Sit up and lean forward to breathe more easily
2. Deal with any increases in pain independently
3. Avoid exposure to crowds
4. Call the physician for increased temperature or shortness of breath

**Answer: 2**

*Rationale:* Health teaching includes using positions that facilitate respiration, such as sitting up and leaning forward. Health teaching also includes avoiding exposure to crowds or persons with respiratory infections; and reporting signs and symptoms of respiratory infection or increases in pain. The client should not be expected to deal with increases in pain independently.

*Test-Taking Strategy:* Use the process of elimination, focusing on the client's diagnosis, lung cancer. Noting the key words *has not understood* will direct you to option 2. Review home care measures for the client with lung cancer if you had difficulty with this question.

*Level of Cognitive Ability:* Analysis
*Client Needs:* Health Promotion and Maintenance
*Integrated Concept/Process:* Self-Care
*Content Area:* Adult Health/Oncology

*Reference*
Black, J., Hawks, J., & Keene, A. (2001). *Medical-surgical nursing: Clinical management for positive outcomes* (6th ed.). Philadelphia: W.B. Saunders, p. 1731.

**229.** A nurse is evaluating the nutritional status of a client after radical neck dissection. The nurse determines that the client has maintained adequate nutritional status if the client maintains what percentage of body weight?

1   100
2   95
3   90
4   80

**Answer: 3**

*Rationale:* The nurse determines that the client has maintained adequate nutritional status if the client does not lose more than 10% of body weight. Mathematically, this is the same as maintaining 90% of body weight.

*Test-Taking Strategy:* Specific knowledge regarding nutritional status and body weight is required to answer this question. Recalling that in maintaining adequate nutritional status in this client, that the standard maximal weight loss is 10% will direct you to option 3. Review these nutritional principles if you had difficulty with this question.

*Level of Cognitive Ability:* Analysis
*Client Needs:* Health Promotion and Maintenance
*Integrated Concept/Process:* Nursing Process/Evaluation
*Content Area:* Fundamental Skills

*Reference*
Black, J., Hawks, J., & Keene, A. (2001). *Medical-surgical nursing: Clinical management for positive outcomes* (6th ed.). Philadelphia: W.B. Saunders, p. 1668.

**230.** A nurse has given the client with a nonplaster (fiberglass) leg cast instructions on cast care at home. The nurse determines that the client needs further instruction if the client makes which of the following statements?

1   "I should avoid walking on wet, slippery floors."
2   "It's OK to wipe dirt off the top of the cast with a damp cloth."
3   "I'm not supposed to scratch the skin underneath the cast."
4   "If the cast gets wet, I can dry it with a hair dryer turned to the warmest setting."

**Answer: 4**

*Rationale:* The client is instructed to avoid walking on wet, slippery floors to prevent falls. Surface soil on a cast may be removed with a damp cloth. If the cast gets wet, it can be dried with a hair dryer set to a cool setting. If the skin under the cast itches, cool air from a hair dryer may be used to relieve it. The client should never scratch under a cast due to the risk of skin breakdown and infection.

*Test-Taking Strategy:* Use the process of elimination, noting the key words *needs further instruction*. Noting the words *warmest setting* in option 4 will direct you to this option. Review home care instructions for a client with a cast if you had difficulty with this question.

*Level of Cognitive Ability:* Analysis
*Client Needs:* Health Promotion and Maintenance
*Integrated Concept/Process:* Self-Care
*Content Area:* Adult Health/Musculoskeletal

*Reference*
Black, J., Hawks, J., & Keene, A. (2001). *Medical-surgical nursing: Clinical management for positive outcomes* (6th ed.). Philadelphia: W.B. Saunders, p. 606.

**231.** A child is seen in the health care clinic and initial testing for human immunodeficiency virus (HIV) is performed because of the child's exposure to HIV infection. Which of the following home care instructions would the nurse provide to the parents of the child?
1   Avoid all immunizations until the diagnosis is established
2   Avoid sharing toothbrushes
3   Wipe up any blood spills with soap and water and allow to air dry
4   Wash hands with half-strength bleach if they come in contact with the child's blood

**Answer: 2**
*Rationale:* Immunizations must be kept up to date. Blood spills are wiped up with a paper towel. The area is then washed with soap and water, rinsed with bleach and water, and allowed to air dry. Hands are washed with soap and water if they come in contact with blood. Parents are instructed that toothbrushes are not to be shared.

*Test-Taking Strategy:* Use the process of elimination. Eliminate option 1 first because of the word *all*. Eliminate option 3 next based on the knowledge that blood spills need to be cleaned with a bleach solution. Eliminate option 4, because bleach would be very irritating and caustic to the skin. If you had difficulty with this question, review home care instructions for the child exposed to HIV infection.

*Level of Cognitive Ability:* Application
*Client Needs:* Health Promotion and Maintenance
*Integrated Concept/Process:* Teaching/Learning
*Content Area:* Child Health

*Reference*
Wong, D. (1999). *Whaley & Wong's Nursing care of infants and children* (6th ed.). St. Louis: Mosby, p. 1696.

**232.** A client is ready to be discharged to home health care for continued intravenous (IV) therapy in the home. Home care instructions regarding care of the IV have been given to the client. The best way to evaluate the client's ability to care for the IV site is to:
1   Ask the client to verbalize IV site care
2   Ask the client to change the IV dressing
3   Review the entire discharge plan with the client again
4   Demonstrate the dressing change again for the client one last time before discharge

**Answer: 2**
*Rationale:* Acquisition of psychomotor skills is best evaluated by observing how a client can carry out a procedure. The client may be able to verbalize how to do the procedure, but may not be able to actually perform the psychomotor function. Reviewing the entire plan again, and demonstrating it again will not evaluate the client's ability. Actively demonstrating is always the best method of evaluating a psychomotor skill.

*Test-Taking Strategy:* Use teaching/learning principles to answer the question and note the key word *best*. The correct option needs to identify some type of client active participation. This concept will direct you to option 2. Review teaching/learning principles if you had difficulty with this question.

*Level of Cognitive Ability:* Analysis
*Client Needs:* Health Promotion and Maintenance
*Integrated Concept/Process:* Teaching/Learning
*Content Area:* Fundamental Skills

*Reference*
Potter, P., & Perry, A. (2001). *Fundamentals of nursing* (5th ed.). St. Louis: Mosby, p. 473.

**233.** A nurse provides home care instructions to a client with an implanted vascular access port. Which statement by the client indicates a need for further instructions?
1 "If the site becomes red, I will notify my physician."
2 "I should keep the site clean and dry."
3 "I should pump the port daily to maintain patency."
4 "The port will need to be flushed with saline solution to maintain patency."

**Answer: 3**
*Rationale:* An implanted port does not need to be pumped in order to maintain patency. The site will need to be kept clean and dry and the physician would need to be notified of signs and symptoms of infection. Saline is used to flush the site to maintain patency.

*Test-Taking Strategy:* Use the process of elimination, noting the key words *need for further instructions.* Using principles related to IV care will direct you to option 3. Review these principles if you had difficulty with this question.

*Level of Cognitive Ability:* Analysis
*Client Needs:* Health Promotion and Maintenance
*Integrated Concept/Process:* Teaching/Learning
*Content Area:* Fundamental Skills

*Reference*
Potter, P., & Perry, A. (2001). *Fundamentals of nursing* (5th ed.). St. Louis: Mosby, p. 1219.

**234.** A nurse is planning to teach a client with a below-the-knee amputation about skin care to prevent breakdown. Which of the following points would the nurse include while developing the teaching plan?
1 A stump sock must be worn at all times and changed twice a week
2 The residual limb (stump) is washed gently and dried every other day
3 The socket of the prosthesis is washed with a harsh bactericidal agent daily
4 The socket of the prosthesis must be dried carefully before using it

**Answer: 4**
*Rationale:* A stump sock must be worn at all times to absorb perspiration and is changed daily. The residual limb is washed, dried, and inspected for breakdown twice each day. The socket of the prosthesis is cleansed with a mild detergent, and rinsed and dried carefully each day. A harsh bactericidal agent would not be used.

*Test-Taking Strategy:* Use the process of elimination. Recalling the procedures related to care of the stump will assist in eliminating option 1 and 2. From the remaining options, noting the key word *harsh* in option 3 will assist in eliminating this option. Review home care instructions following amputation if you had difficulty with this question.

*Level of Cognitive Ability:* Application
*Client Needs:* Health Promotion and Maintenance
*Integrated Concept/Process:* Self-Care
*Content Area:* Adult Health/Musculoskeletal

*Reference*
Smeltzer, S., & Bare, B. (2000). *Brunner & Suddarth's Textbook of medical-surgical nursing* (9th ed.). Philadelphia: Lippincott Williams & Wilkins, p. 1862.

**235.** A nurse has completed instructions on diet and fluid restriction for the client with chronic renal failure. The nurse would evaluate that the client best understands the information presented if the client selected which of the following desserts from the dietary menu?
1   Angel food cake
2   Ice cream
3   Sherbet
4   Jell-O

**Answer: 1**
*Rationale:* Dietary fluid includes anything that is liquid at room temperature. This includes items such as ice cream, sherbet, and Jell-O. With clients on a fluid restricted diet, it is helpful to avoid "hidden" fluids to whatever extent is possible. This allows the client more fluid for drinking, which can help alleviate thirst.

*Test-Taking Strategy:* Use the process of elimination, noting the key words *fluid restriction*. Recalling that dietary fluid includes anything liquid at room temperature will direct you to option 1. Review this type of dietary restriction if you had difficulty with this question.

*Level of Cognitive Ability:* Analysis
*Client Needs:* Health Promotion and Maintenance
*Integrated Concept/Process:* Nursing Process/Evaluation
*Content Area:* Adult Health/Renal

*Reference*
Smeltzer, S., & Bare, B. (2000). *Brunner & Suddarth's Textbook of medical-surgical nursing* (9th ed.). Philadelphia: Lippincott Williams & Wilkins, p. 1156.

**236.** A nurse has given instructions to a client with chronic renal failure about reducing pruritis from uremia. The nurse evaluates that the client needs further information if the client states to use which of the following items for skin care?
1   Mild soap
2   Oil in the bath water
3   Alcohol cleansing pads
4   Lanolin-based lotion

**Answer: 3**
*Rationale:* The client with chronic renal failure often has dry skin, accompanied by itching (pruritis) from uremia. The client should use mild soaps, lotions, and bath water oils to reduce dryness without increasing skin irritation. Products that contain perfumes or alcohol increase dryness and pruritis and should be avoided.

*Test-Taking Strategy:* Focus on the issue: reducing pruritis, and note the key words *needs further information*. Eliminate options 2 and 4 first, because they are similar. From the remaining options, select option 3, knowing that the client should avoid irritating products on the skin. Review measures to treat pruritis if you had difficulty with this question.

*Level of Cognitive Ability:* Analysis
*Client Needs:* Health Promotion and Maintenance
*Integrated Concept/Process:* Nursing Process/Evaluation
*Content Area:* Adult Health/Renal

*Reference*
Smeltzer, S., & Bare, B. (2000). *Brunner & Suddarth's Textbook of medical-surgical nursing* (9th ed.). Philadelphia: Lippincott Williams & Wilkins, p. 1458.

**237.** A client who is scheduled for implantation of an automatic internal defibrillator-cardioverter (AICD) asks the nurse why there is a need to keep a diary, and what to put in it. In formulating a reply, the nurse understands that the primary purpose of the diary is to:

1 Provide a count of the number of shocks delivered
2 Document events that precipitate a countershock
3 Record a variety of data useful for the physician in medical management
4 Analyze which activities to avoid

**Answer: 3**

*Rationale:* The client with an AICD maintains a log or diary of a variety of data. This includes recording date, time, activity before the shock and any symptoms experienced, number of shocks delivered, and how the client felt after the shock. The information is used by the physician to adjust the medical regimen, especially medication therapy, which must be maintained after AICD insertion.

*Test-Taking Strategy:* Use the process of elimination, noting the key word *primary*. Each of the incorrect options lists one of the items that should be logged in the diary, but the correct option is the only one that could be considered a "primary" purpose. Option 3 is the global option. Review home care instructions for the client with an AICD if you had difficulty with this question.

*Level of Cognitive Ability:* Application
*Client Needs:* Health Promotion and Maintenance
*Integrated Concept/Process:* Teaching/Learning
*Content Area:* Adult Health/Cardiovascular

*Reference*
Smeltzer, S., & Bare, B. (2000). *Brunner & Suddarth's Textbook of medical-surgical nursing* (9th ed.). Philadelphia: Lippincott Williams & Wilkins, p. 586.

**238.** A nurse is evaluating a hypertensive client's understanding of dietary modifications to control the disease process. The nurse would evaluate the client's understanding as satisfactory if the client made which of the following meal selections?

1 Scallops, French fries, salad with bleu cheese dressing
2 Corned beef, fresh carrots, boiled potato
3 Hot dog in a bun, sauerkraut, baked beans
4 Turkey, baked potato, salad with oil and vinegar

**Answer: 4**

*Rationale:* The client with hypertension should avoid foods high in sodium. Foods from the meat group that are higher in sodium include bacon, hot dogs, luncheon meat, chipped or corned beef, Kosher meat, smoked or salted meat or fish, peanut butter, and a variety of shellfish.

*Test-Taking Strategy:* Use the process of elimination, focusing on the client's diagnosis. Eliminate options 2 and 3, because they are highly processed meats, which would be high in sodium. From the remaining options, recalling that shellfish and commercial dressing are high in sodium will assist in eliminating option 1. Review foods high in sodium if you had difficulty with this question.

*Level of Cognitive Ability:* Analysis
*Client Needs:* Health Promotion and Maintenance
*Integrated Concept/Process:* Nursing Process/Evaluation
*Content Area:* Adult Health/Cardiovascular

*Reference*
Peckenpaugh, N., & Poleman, C. (1999). *Nutrition essentials and diet therapy* (8th ed.). Philadelphia: W.B. Saunders, p. 189.

**239.** A nurse has provided teaching to a client who will be taking warfarin sodium (Coumadin) indefinitely. Which statement by the client indicates a need for further teaching?
1 "I need to use a soft toothbrush."
2 "I need to avoid drinking alcohol while taking this medication."
3 "I need to carry identification about the medication being taken."
4 "I need to use a straight razor for shaving."

**Answer: 4**
*Rationale:* Client instructions for oral anticoagulant therapy include taking the medication only as prescribed and at the same time each day; avoiding other medications (including over-the-counter medications) without physician approval; avoiding alcohol; notifying all care givers about the medication; carrying a Medic-Alert bracelet or card; reporting any signs of bleeding and implementing measures to prevent bleeding; and adhering to the schedule for follow-up blood work.

*Test-Taking Strategy:* Note the key words *need for further teaching.* Recalling that warfarin sodium is an anticoagulant and that the client is at risk for bleeding will direct you to option 4. Review home care instructions for the client on an anticoagulant if you had difficulty with this question.

*Level of Cognitive Ability:* Analysis
*Client Needs:* Health Promotion and Maintenance
*Integrated Concept/Process:* Teaching/Learning
*Content Area:* Pharmacology

*Reference*
Hodgson, B., & Kizior, R. (2001). *Saunders Nursing drug handbook 2001.* Philadelphia: W.B. Saunders, p. 1064.

---

**240.** A home care nurse has given instructions to a client recently discharged from the hospital with an arterial ischemic leg ulcer. The nurse determines that further instruction is needed if the client made which of the following statements?
1 "I should wear shoes and socks."
2 "I should cut my toenails straight across."
3 "I should raise my legs above the level of my heart periodically."
4 "I should inspect my feet daily."

**Answer: 3**
*Rationale:* Foot care instructions for the client with peripheral arterial ischemia are the same instructions given to the client with diabetic mellitus. The client with arterial disease, however, should avoid raising the legs above heart level, unless instructed to do so as part of an exercise program (such as Buerger-Allen exercises), or unless venous stasis is also present. Options 1, 2, and 4 are accurate client statements.

*Test-Taking Strategy:* Use the process of elimination, noting the key words *further instruction is needed.* Also, note that the client has an arterial disorder. Recalling the anatomy of the blood vessels and the pattern of blood flow in the arteries will direct you to option 3. Review home care instructions for the client with an arterial disorder if you had difficulty with this question.

*Level of Cognitive Ability:* Analysis
*Client Needs:* Health Promotion and Maintenance
*Integrated Concept/Process:* Teaching/Learning
*Content Area:* Adult Health/Cardiovascular

*Reference*
Smeltzer, S., & Bare, B. (2000). *Brunner & Suddarth's Textbook of medical-surgical nursing* (9th ed.). Philadelphia: Lippincott Williams & Wilkins, p. 710.

**241.** A client with chronic renal failure is about to begin hemodialysis therapy. The client asks the nurse about the frequency and scheduling of hemodialysis treatments. The nurse's response is based on an understanding that the typical schedule is:

1 5 hours of treatment 2 days/week
2 3 to 4 hours of treatment 3 days/week
3 2 to 3 hours of treatment 5 days/week
4 2 hours of treatment 6 days/week

**Answer: 2**

*Rationale:* The typical schedule for hemodialysis is 3 to 4 hours of treatment 3 days per week. Individual adjustments may be made according to variables, such as the size of the client, type of dialyzer, the rate of blood flow, personal client preferences, and others.

*Test-Taking Strategy:* Focus on the issue: the *typical* dialysis schedule. Recalling that the client receives dialysis 3 days per week will direct you to option 2. Review the typical dialysis schedule if you had difficulty with this question.

*Level of Cognitive Ability:* Application
*Client Needs:* Health Promotion and Maintenance
*Integrated Concept/Process:* Teaching/Learning
*Content Area:* Adult Health/Renal

*Reference*
Smeltzer, S., & Bare, B. (2000). *Brunner & Suddarth's Textbook of medical-surgical nursing* (9th ed.). Philadelphia: Lippincott Williams & Wilkins, p. 1112.

---

**242.** A client is being discharged with a peripheral intravenous (IV) site for continued home IV therapy. In planning for the discharge, the nurse teaches the client which of the following to help prevent phlebitis and infiltration?

1 Gently massage the area around the site daily
2 Cleanse the site daily with alcohol
3 Keep the cannula stabilized or anchored properly with tape
4 Immobilize the extremity until the IV is discontinued

**Answer: 3**

*Rationale:* The principles of maintaining IV therapy at home are the same as in the hospital. It is extremely important to assure that the IV site is anchored properly in order to reduce the risk of phlebitis and infiltration. Massaging the site may actually contribute to catheter movement and tissue damage. Dressings surrounding peripheral IV sites are changed and cleansed at various times (usually every 2 to 5 days) depending on facility protocols. Immobilizing the extremity is not routinely necessary for peripheral IV sites.

*Test-Taking Strategy:* Use the process of elimination, focusing on the issue: preventing phlebitis and infiltration. Eliminate options 1, 2, and 4 because of the words *massage, alcohol,* and *immobilize* respectively. Review interventions related to the prevention of phlebitis and infiltration if you had difficulty with this question.

*Level of Cognitive Ability:* Application
*Client Needs:* Health Promotion and Maintenance
*Integrated Concept/Process:* Teaching/Learning
*Content Area:* Fundamental Skills

*Reference*
Smeltzer, S., & Bare, B. (2000). *Brunner & Suddarth's Textbook of medical-surgical nursing* (9th ed.). Philadelphia: Lippincott Williams & Wilkins, p. 242.

**243.** A nurse is teaching a client how to stand on crutches. The nurse tells the client to place the crutches:

1   8 inches to the front and side of the toes
2   3 inches to the front and side of the toes
3   20 inches to the front and side of the toes
4   15 inches to the front and side of the toes

**Answer: 1**

*Rationale:*  The classic tripod position is taught to the client before giving instructions on gait. The crutches are placed anywhere from 6 to 10 inches in front and to the side of the client's toes, depending on the client's body size. This provides a wide enough base of support to the client and improves balance.

*Test-Taking Strategy:*  Use the process of elimination. Three inches (option 2) and 20 inches (option 3) seem excessively short and long respectively, and these options should be eliminated first. From the remaining options, visualize this procedure. Eight inches seems more in keeping with the normal length of a stride than 15 inches. Review this procedure if you had difficulty with this question.

*Level of Cognitive Ability:*  Application
*Client Needs:*  Health Promotion and Maintenance
*Integrated Concept/Process:*  Self-Care
*Content Area:*  Adult Health/Musculoskeletal

*Reference*
Potter, P., & Perry, A. (2001). *Fundamentals of nursing* (5th ed.). St. Louis: Mosby, p. 1008.

---

**244.** A nurse is giving instructions to a client who is beginning therapy with digoxin (Lanoxin). The nurse teaches the client to:

1   Monitor the blood pressure once a week
2   Measure weight each morning before breakfast
3   Take the pulse daily
4   Have electrolyte levels drawn weekly

**Answer: 3**

*Rationale:*  Clients taking digoxin should take the pulse each day and notify the physician if the heart rate is below 60 beats/min or above 100 beats/min. Options 1, 2, and 4 are not necessary interventions for the client taking digoxin.

*Test-Taking Strategy:*  Use the process of elimination, focusing on the medication identified in the question. Recalling that digoxin is a cardiac medication will direct you to option 3. Review client instructions regarding this medication if you had difficulty with this question.

*Level of Cognitive Ability:*  Application
*Client Needs:*  Health Promotion and Maintenance
*Integrated Concept/Process:*  Teaching/Learning
*Content Area:*  Pharmacology

*Reference*
Hodgson, B., & Kizior, R. (2001). *Saunders Nursing drug handbook 2001.* Philadelphia: W.B. Saunders, p. 325.

**245.** A nurse has completed client teaching with a hemodialysis client about self monitoring of fluid status between hemodialysis treatments. The nurse determines that the client best understands the information given if the client states to record which of the following on a daily basis?
1   Pulse and respiratory rate
2   Intake and output and weight
3   Blood urea nitrogen and creatinine levels
4   Activity log

**Answer: 2**
*Rationale:* The client on hemodialysis should monitor fluid status between hemodialysis treatments. This can be done by recording intake and output, and measuring weight on a daily basis. Ideally, the hemodialysis client should not gain more than 0.5 kg of weight per day. Options 1, 3, and 4 are not necessary.

*Test-Taking Strategy:* Use the process of elimination, and note the key words *daily basis*. Focusing on the key words and the issue, fluid status, will direct you to option 2. Review self-care instructions for the hemodialysis client if you had difficulty with this question.

*Level of Cognitive Ability:* Analysis
*Client Needs:* Health Promotion and Maintenance
*Integrated Concept/Process:* Self-Care
*Content Area:* Adult Health/Renal

*Reference*
Smeltzer, S., & Bare, B. (2000). *Brunner & Suddarth's Textbook of medical-surgical nursing* (9th ed.). Philadelphia: Lippincott Williams & Wilkins, p. 1112.

---

**246.** Diltiazem hydrochloride (Cardizem) is prescribed for the client with Prinzmetal's angina. A nurse provides instructions to the client regarding this medication. Which statement by the client indicates a need for further instructions?
1   "I will call the physician if shortness of breath occurs."
2   "I will rise slowly when getting out of bed in the morning."
3   "I will take the medication after meals."
4   "I will avoid activities that require alertness until my body gets used to the medication."

**Answer: 3**
*Rationale:* Cardizem is a calcium-channel blocker. It is administered before meals and at bed time as prescribed. Hypotension can occur and the client is instructed to rise slowly. The client should avoid tasks that require alertness until a response to the medication is established. The client should call the physician if an irregular heartbeat, shortness of breath, pronounced dizziness, nausea, or constipation occurs.

*Test-Taking Strategy:* Note the key words *need for further instructions*. Focusing on the client's diagnosis will assist in eliminating options 1, 2, and 4. Review home care instructions regarding this medication if you had difficulty with this question.

*Level Cognitive Ability:* Analysis
*Client Needs:* Health Promotion and Maintenance
*Integrated Concept/Process:* Teaching/Learning
*Content Area:* Pharmacology

*Reference*
Hodgson, B., & Kizior, R. (2001). *Saunders Nursing drug handbook 2001.* Philadelphia: W.B. Saunders, pp. 327-328.

**247.** A nurse has provided instructions to a client being discharged from the hospital to home after an abdominal aortic aneurysm (AAA) resection. The nurse determines that the client understands the instructions if the client stated that an appropriate activity would be to:
1 Lift objects up to 30 lb
2 Walk as tolerated, including stairs and out of doors
3 Mow the lawn
4 Play a game of 18-hole golf

**Answer: 2**
*Rationale:* The client can walk as tolerated after repair or resection of an AAA, including climbing stairs and walking outdoors. The client should not lift objects that weight more than 15 to 20 lb for 6 to 12 weeks, or engage in any activities that involve pushing, pulling, or straining. Driving is also prohibited for several weeks.

*Test-Taking Strategy:* Use the process of elimination, noting the key words *understands the instructions.* Evaluate each option in terms of the strain it could put on the sutured graft. This will direct you to option 2. Review discharge instructions following AAA if you had difficulty with this question.

*Level of Cognitive Ability:* Analysis
*Client Needs:* Health Promotion and Maintenance
*Integrated Concept/Process:* Teaching/Learning
*Content Area:* Adult Health/Cardiovascular

*Reference*
Black, J., Hawks, J., & Keene, A. (2001). *Medical-surgical nursing: Clinical management for positive outcomes* (6th ed.). Philadelphia: W.B. Saunders, p. 1416.

**248.** A nurse is planning dietary counseling for the client taking triamterene (Dyrenium). The nurse plans to include which of the following in a list of foods that are acceptable?
1 Baked potato
2 Bananas
3 Oranges
4 Pears canned in water

**Answer: 4**
*Rationale:* Triamterene is a potassium-sparing diuretic and clients taking this medication should be cautioned against eating foods that are high in potassium. Foods high in potassium include many vegetables, fruits, and fresh meats. Since potassium is very water-soluble, foods that are prepared in water are often lower in potassium.

*Test-Taking Strategy:* Focus on the medication, noting the key words *foods that are acceptable.* Recall that triamterene is a potassium-sparing diuretic. Next, review the options identifying the food item lowest in potassium. Review high-potassium foods and this medication if you had difficulty with this question.

*Level of Cognitive Ability:* Application
*Client Needs:* Health Promotion and Maintenance
*Integrated Concept/Process:* Nursing Process/Planning
*Content Area:* Pharmacology

*Reference*
Peckenpaugh, N., & Poleman, C. (1999). *Nutrition essentials and diet therapy* (8th ed.). Philadelphia: W.B. Saunders, p. 147.

**249.** Cyclophosphamide (Cytoxan) is prescribed for a client with breast cancer and
the nurse provides instructions to the
client regarding the medication. Which of
the following statements, if made by the
client, would indicate a need for further
education?
1    "I need to avoid contact with anyone who recently recieved a live
virus vaccine."
2    "If I lose my hair, it will grow back."
3    "If I develop a sore throat, I should
notify the physician."
4    "I need to limit my fluid intake
while taking this medication."

**Answer: 4**
*Rationale:* Hemorrhagic cystitis is an adverse reaction associated
with this medication. The client needs to be instructed to consume
copious amounts of fluid during therapy. Avoiding contact with
anyone who recently received a live virus vaccine is important,
because cyclophosphamide produces immunosuppression placing the client at risk for infection. Hair will grow back although it
may have a different color and texture. A sore throat may be an
indication of an infection and needs to be reported to the
physician.

*Test-Taking Strategy:* Use the process of elimination, noting the
key words *need for further education.* Eliminate options 1 and 3,
because they are similar in that they both relate to the risk of
infection. From the remaining options, recalling that hemorrhagic
cystitis is an adverse effect of this medication will direct you to
option 4. Review the adverse effects of this medication if you had
difficulty with this question.

*Level of Cognitive Ability:* Analysis
*Client Needs:* Health Promotion and Maintenance
*Integrated Concept/Process:* Teaching/Learning
*Content Area:* Pharmacology

*Reference*
Hodgson, B., & Kizior, R. (2001). *Saunders Nursing drug handbook 2001.*
Philadelphia: W.B. Saunders, pp. 273-274.

**250.** A community health nurse has reviewed
information on the population in a local
community. The nurse determines that
there are groups in the population that are
at high risk for infection with tuberculosis
(TB). The nurse targets which of the
following groups for screening?
1    White, Anglo-Saxon Americans
2    Adolescents 13 to 17 years of age
3    French Canadians in rural America
4    Elders in long-term care facilities

**Answer: 4**
*Rationale:* Elderly persons, particularly those in long-term care
facilities, are at high risk for infection with TB. Almost half of all
new cases of tuberculosis occur in this age group. Other people at
risk include children 5 years of age or less; individuals who are
malnourished, immunosuppressed, and/or economically disad-
vantaged; foreign born persons, and persons of a minority race
who formerly lived in a place where TB is common, such as Asia
and the Pacific Islands.

*Test-Taking Strategy:* Use the process of elimination. Recalling
the risk factors associated with TB will direct you to option 4.
Remember that the very young and the very old often fall into a
high-risk category. Review the risk factors associated with TB if you
had difficulty with this question.

*Level of Cognitive Ability:* Analysis
*Client Needs:* Health Promotion and Maintenance
*Integrated Concept/Process:* Nursing Process/Assessment
*Content Area:* Adult Health/Respiratory

*Reference*
Smeltzer, S., & Bare, B. (2000). *Brunner & Suddarth's Textbook of medical-surgical
nursing* (9th ed.). Philadelphia: Lippincott Williams & Wilkins, p. 437.

# CRITICAL THINKING: FREE-TEXT ENTRY

**1.** A client is treated in the physician's office after a fall, which sprained the ankle. An x-ray examination has ruled out a fracture. Before sending the client home, the nurse instructs the client to implement which measure during the next 24 hours to prevent edema and pain in the injured area?

**Answer:** Rest, ice, compression, elevation (RICE)
*Rationale:* Soft tissue injuries such as sprains are treated by RICE for the first 24 hours after the injury to prevent edema and pain at the injured site. Ice is applied intermittently for 20 to 30 minutes at a time. Heat is not used in the first 24 hours, because it could increase venous congestion, which would increase edema and pain.

*Test-Taking Strategy:* Focus on the type of injury identified in the question and note the key words *during the next 24 hours.* Recalling the concept RICE will assist in answering the question. Review home care measures for the client with a sprained ankle if you had difficulty with this question.

*Level of Cognitive Ability:* Application
*Client Needs:* Health Promotion and Maintenance
*Integrated Concept/Process:* Teaching/Learning
*Content Area:* Adult Health/Musculoskeletal

*Reference*
Ignatavicius, D., Workman, M., & Mishler, M. (1999). *Medical-surgical nursing across the health care continuum* (3rd ed.). Philadelphia: W.B. Saunders, p. 1308.

**2.** A client with myasthenia gravis reports the occurrence of difficulty chewing. The physician prescribes pyridostigmine bromide (Mestinon) to increase muscle strength for this activity. The nurse instructs the client to take the medication at what time, in relation to meals?

**Answer:** 30 minutes before meals
*Rationale:* Pyridostigmine is a cholinergic medication used to increase muscle strength for the client with myasthenia gravis. For the client who has difficulty chewing, the medication should be administered 30 minutes before meals to enhance the client's ability to eat.

*Test-Taking Strategy:* Focus on the issue: difficulty chewing. Knowing that the medication increases muscle strength will assist in determining that administering the medication 30 minutes before meals will provide the client the ability to chew the food. Review client teaching points related to this medication if you had difficulty with this question.

*Level of Cognitive Ability:* Application
*Client Needs:* Health Promotion and Maintenance
*Integrated Concept/Process:* Self-Care
*Content Area:* Pharmacology

*Reference*
Hodgson, B., & Kizior, R. (2001). *Saunders Nursing drug handbook 2001.* Philadelphia: W.B. Saunders, p. 888.

**3.** A school nurse is performing health screening for scoliosis on children ages 9 through ages 15. What specific instructions are provided to the child and what technique would the nurse use to perform this screening procedure?

**Answer:** The child should be asked to unclothe or wear underpants only for this screening procedure so that the chest, back, and hips can be clearly seen. The child is asked to stand with weight equally on both feet with the legs straight, and the arms hanging loosely at both sides. The nurse assesses the child's posture, spinal column, shoulder height, and leg lengths.

*Rationale:* Having the child unclothe and stand with the weight equally on both feet, and with the legs straight and the arms hanging loosely at both sides allows the nurse to adequately assess the child's posture and spinal column. Additionally, shoulder heights are observed for unequal alignment. Observation for equal leg lengths is also done.

*Test-Taking Strategy:* Recall the anatomical location of this disorder and then attempt to visualize the screening procedure and the preparation required to adequately assess for this disorder. If you had difficulty with this question, review this screening procedure.

*Level of Cognitive Ability:* Application
*Client Needs:* Health Promotion and Maintenance
*Integrated Concept/Process:* Nursing Process/Assessment
*Content Area:* Child Health

**Reference**
Wong, D. (1999). *Whaley & Wong's Nursing care of infants and children* (6th ed.). St. Louis: Mosby, p. 1941.

**4.** A client with a history of rheumatic heart disease asks the nurse why the dentist needs to know about this condition before dental cleaning or other work. What would the nurse tell the client?

**Answer:** The client is at risk for infection; therefore, prophylactic antibiotic therapy is given before any invasive procedure treatment.

*Rationale:* The client with a history of rheumatic fever is at risk for developing infective endocarditis. The client notifies all physicians and dentists about the history so prophylactic antibiotic therapy can be given before any invasive procedure, or when there is risk of bleeding.

*Test-Taking Strategy:* Focus on the client's diagnosis, rheumatic heart disease. Recalling that the client is a risk for developing infective endocarditis will assist in answering the question. Review client teaching points related to rheumatic heart disease if you had difficulty with this question.

*Level of Cognitive Ability:* Application
*Client Needs:* Health Promotion and Maintenance
*Integrated Concept/Process:* Teaching/Learning
*Content Area:* Adult Health/Cardiovascular

**Reference**
Smeltzer, S., & Bare, B. (2000). *Brunner & Suddarth's Textbook of medical-surgical nursing* (9th ed.). Philadelphia: Lippincott Williams & Wilkins, p. 651.

## REFERENCES

Ball, J., & Bindler, R. (1999). *Pediatric nursing: Caring for children* (2nd ed.). Stamford, Conn.: Appleton & Lange.

Ball, J., & Bindler, R. (1999). *Quick reference to pediatric clinical skills.* Stamford, Conn.: Appleton & Lange.

Beare, P., & Myers, J. (1998). *Adult health nursing* (3rd ed.). St. Louis: Mosby.

Black, J., Hawks, J., & Keene, A. (2001). *Medical-surgical nursing: Clinical management for positive outcomes* (6th ed.). Philadelphia: W.B. Saunders.

Bowden, V., Dickey, S, & Greenberg, C. (1998). *Children and their families: The continuum of care.* Philadelphia: W.B. Saunders.

Craven, R., & Hirnle, C. (2000). *Fundamentals of nursing: Human health and function* (3rd ed.). Philadelphia: Lippincott.

Fortinash, K., & Holoday-Worret, P. (2000). *Psychiatric mental health nursing* (2nd ed.). St. Louis: Mosby.

Gorrie, T., McKinney, E., & Murray, S. (1998). *Foundations of maternal-newborn nursing* (2nd ed.). Philadelphia: W.B. Saunders.

Harkreader, H. (2000). *Fundamentals of nursing: Caring and clinical judgment.* Philadelphia: W.B. Saunders.

Hodgson, B., & Kizior, R. (2001). *Saunders Nursing drug handbook 2001.* Philadelphia: W.B. Saunders.

Ignatavicius, D., Workman, M., & Mishler, M. (1999). *Medical-surgical nursing across the health care continuum* (3rd ed.). Philadelphia: W.B. Saunders.

Lowdermilk, D., Perry, S., & Bobak, I. (2000). *Maternity & women's health care* (7th ed.). St. Louis: Mosby.

Monahan, F., & Neighbors, M. (1998). *Medical-surgical nursing: Foundations for clinical practice* (2nd ed.). Philadelphia: W.B. Saunders.

Olds, S., London. M., & Ladewig, P. (2000). *Maternal-newborn nursing: A family and community-based approach* (6th ed.). Upper Saddle River, N.J.: Prentice-Hall.

Peckenpaugh, N., & Poleman, C. (1999). *Nutrition essentials and diet therapy* (8th ed.). Philadelphia: W.B. Saunders.

Potter, P., & Perry, A. (2001). *Fundamentals of nursing* (5th ed.). St. Louis: Mosby.

Smeltzer, S., & Bare, B. (2000). *Brunner & Suddarth's Textbook of medical-surgical nursing* (9th ed.). Philadelphia: Lippincott Williams & Wilkins.

Spratto, G., & Woods, A. (2001). *PDR Nurse's drug handbook.* Montvale, N.J.: Medical Economics.

Stuart, G.W., & Laraia, M.T. (1998). *Principles and practice of psychiatric nursing.* (6th ed.). St. Louis: Mosby.

Wong, D. (1999). *Whaley & Wong's Nursing care of infants and children* (6th ed.). St. Louis: Mosby.

# Integrated Concepts and Processes

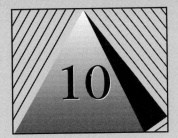

# Integrated Concepts and Processes and the NCLEX-RN Test Plan

In the new Test Plan implemented in April 2001, the National Council of State Boards of Nursing has identified a test plan framework based on Client Needs. This framework was selected on the basis of the analysis of the findings in a practice analysis study of newly licensed registered nurses in the United States. This study identified the nursing activities performed by entry-level nurses across all settings for all clients. The National Council of State Boards of Nursing identifies four major categories of Client Needs. The Client Needs categories, which are described in Chapter 5, include Safe, Effective Care Environment; Health Promotion and Maintenance; Psychosocial Integrity; and Physiological Integrity.

The 2001 NCLEX-RN Test Plan also identifies six concepts and processes that are fundamental to the practice of nursing. These concepts and processes are integrated throughout the four major categories of Client Needs. The Test Plan for NCLEX-RN refers to these components as Integrated Concepts and Processes. The Integrated Concepts and Processes include Nursing Process; Caring; Communication and Documentation; Cultural Awareness; Self-Care; and Teaching/Learning (Box 10-1).

## NURSING PROCESS

The steps of the Nursing Process provide a systematic and organized method of problem solving and providing care to clients. These steps include Assessment, Analysis, Planning, Implementation, and Evaluation (Box 10-2).

### Assessment

Assessment is the first step of the nursing process. It involves a systematic method of collecting data about a client in order to identify actual and potential client health problems and establish a database. The database provides the foundation for the remaining steps of the nursing process; therefore, a thorough and adequate database is essential.

Data collection begins with the first contact with the client. During all successive contacts, the nurse continues to collect information that is significant and relevant to the needs of the client.

During the assessment process, the nurse collects data about the client from a variety of sources. The client is the primary source of data. Family members and significant others are secondary sources of assessment data, and these sources may supplement or verify information provided by the client. Data may also be obtained from the client's record through the medical history, laboratory results, and diagnostic reports. Med-

---

**BOX 10-1**

**Integrated Concepts and Processes**

Nursing Process
Caring
Communication and Documentation
Cultural Awareness
Self-Care
Teaching/Learning

---

**BOX 10-2**

**Steps of the Nursing Process**

Assessment
Analysis
Planning
Implementation
Evaluation

ical records from previous admissions may provide additional information about the client. The nurse may also obtain information through consultation with other health care team members who have had contact with the client.

A thorough database is obtained through a health history and physical assessment. The information collected by the nurse includes both subjective and objective data. Subjective data include the information that the client states. Objective data are the observable, measurable pieces of information about the client. Objective data include measurements, such as vital signs and laboratory findings, and information obtained from observing the client. Objective data also include clinical manifestations, such as the signs and symptoms of an illness or disease.

The process of assessment also consists of confirming and verifying client data, communicating information obtained through the assessment process, and documenting assessment findings in a thorough and accurate manner.

On the NCLEX-RN, remember that assessment is the first step in the nursing process. When answering these types of questions, focus on the data in the question and select the option that addresses an assessment action. Also, use skills of prioritizing and the ABCs—airway, breathing, and circulation—to answer the question (Box 10-3).

## Analysis

Analysis is the second step of the nursing process. In this step, the nurse focuses on the data gathered during the assessment process and identifies actual or potential health care needs or problems, or both.

During this process, the nurse summarizes and interprets the assessment data, organizes and validates the data, and determines the need for additional data. Client assessment data are compared with the normal expected findings and behaviors for the client's age, education, and cultural background. The nurse then draws conclusions regarding the client's unique needs and health care risks or problems.

Client health problems are categorized as potential problems requiring prevention or actual problems being managed or requiring interventions. The nurse reports the results of analysis to relevant members of the health care team and documents the client's unique health care problems or needs, or both.

On the NCLEX-RN, questions that address the process of analysis are difficult questions because they require an understanding of the principles of physiological responses and require the interpretation of the data on the basis of assessment findings. Analysis questions require critical thinking and determining the rationale for therapeutic interventions that may be addressed in the case situation. Analysis questions may address the formulation of a nursing diagnosis and the communication and documentation of the results of the process of analysis (Box 10-4).

## Planning

Planning is the third step of the nursing process. This step involves the functions of setting priorities, determining goals of care, planning actions, collaborating with other health team members, establishing evaluative criteria, and communicating the plan of care.

Setting priorities assists the nurse in organizing and planning care that solves the most urgent problems. Priorities may change as the client's level of wellness changes. Both actual and potential problems should be

---

**BOX 10-3**

### Nursing Process: Assessment

A child with hemophilia is brought into the emergency room after being hit on the neck with a baseball. The nurse immediately assesses the child for:
1. Spontaneous hematuria
2. Airway obstruction
3. Headache and slurred speech
4. Factor VIII deficiency

**Answer: 2**

**Rationale:** Trauma to the neck may cause bleeding into the tissues of the neck, which may compromise the airway. Though hematuria is a symptom of hemophilia, it is not associated with a neck injury. Headache and slurred speech are associated with head trauma. Factor VIII deficiency is not a symptom of hemophilia but rather a common form of the disease. Use the ABCs—airway, breathing, and circulation—to answer this question. Airway assessment is always a first priority!

---

**BOX 10-4**

### Nursing Process: Analysis

A client is admitted to the cardiac unit and is placed on telemetry. A nurse reviews the client's laboratory values and notes that the client's potassium level is 6.3 mEq/L. In analyzing the cardiac rhythm, the nurse would expect to note which electrocardiogram (ECG) finding?
1. A sinus rhythm with a depressed ST segment
2. A sinus tachycardia with a prolonged QT interval
3. A sinus tachycardia with an extra U wave
4. A sinus rhythm with a peaked T wave

**Answer: 4**

**Rationale:** A potassium level greater than 5.1 mEq/L indicates hyperkalemia, which can be detected on the ECG by the presence of a tall, peaked T wave. A U wave and a depressed ST segment are present with hypokalemia. A prolonged QT interval is indicative of hypocalcemia. In this question, it is necessary to know that the client is experiencing hyperkalemia. Once this has been determined, it is necessary to know the ECG changes that occur with hyperkalemia.

considered in establishing priorities. Actual problems are usually more important than potential problems. However, potential problems may at times take precedence over actual problems.

Once priorities are established, the client and the nurse mutually decide on the expected goals. The selected goals serve as a guide in the selection of nursing interventions and in the determination of the criteria for evaluation. Before nursing actions are implemented, mechanisms to define goal achievement and to determine the effectiveness of nursing interventions are established. Unless criteria have been predetermined, it is difficult to know whether a goal has been achieved and the problem has been resolved.

It is important for the nurse both to identify health or social resources available to the client and to collaborate with other health care team members when planning the delivery of care. The nurse needs to communicate the plan of care, review the plan of care with the client, and document the plan of care thoroughly and accurately.

When answering questions on the NCLEX-RN, remember that this is a nursing examination and that the answer to the question most likely involves something that is included in the nursing care plan, rather than the medical plan. Also remember that actual problems are usually more important than potential problems and that physiological needs are usually the priority (Box 10-5).

## Implementation

Implementation is the fourth step of the nursing process. It includes initiating and completing nursing actions required to accomplish the defined goals. This step is the action phase, which involves counseling, teaching, organizing and managing client care, providing care to achieve established goals, supervising and coordinating the delivery of client care, and communicating and documenting the nursing interventions and client responses.

During implementation, the nurse uses intellectual skills, interpersonal skills, and technical skills. Intellectual skills involve critical thinking, problem solving, and making judgments. Interpersonal skills involve the ability to communicate, listen, and convey compassion. Technical skills relate to the performance of treatments and procedures and the use of necessary equipment in providing care to the client.

The nurse independently implements actions that do not require a physician's order. The nurse also implements actions collaboratively on the basis of the physician's orders. Sound nursing judgment and working with other health care members are incorporated into the process of implementation. The implementation step concludes when the nurse's actions are completed and these actions, including their effects and the client's response, are communicated and documented.

The NCLEX-RN is an examination about nursing, so focus on the nursing action rather than on the medical action, unless the question is asking what prescribed medical action is anticipated (Box 10-6).

## Evaluation

Evaluation is the fifth and final step of the nursing process. The process of evaluation identifies the degree to which the nursing diagnoses, plans for care, and interventions have been successful.

Although evaluation is the final step of the nursing process, it is an ongoing and integral component of each step. The process of data collection and assessment is

---

**BOX 10-5**

### Nursing Process: Planning

A nurse is caring for a client with dementia who has a nursing diagnosis of Self-Care Deficit. The nurse plans for which most appropriate goal for this client?
1. Client will be oriented to place by the time of discharge
2. Client will correctly identify objects in his or her room by the time of discharge
3. Client will be free of hallucinations
4. Client will feed self with cuing within 24 hours

**Answer: 4**

**Rationale:** Option 4 identifies a goal that is directly related to the client's ability to care for self. Options 1, 2, and 3 are not related to the nursing diagnosis of Self-Care Deficit. Remember, according to Maslow's Hierarchy of Needs theory, physiological needs take precedence. Option 4 is the only option that addresses a physiological need.

---

**BOX 10-6**

### Nursing Process: Implementation

A client with heart failure is receiving furosemide (Lasix) and digoxin (Lanoxin) daily. When a nurse enters the room to administer the morning doses, the client complains of anorexia, nausea, and yellow vision. The nurse should do which of the following first?
1. Administer the medications
2. Give the digoxin only
3. Check the morning serum potassium level
4. Check the morning serum digoxin level

**Answer: 4**

**Rationale:** The nurse should check for the result of the digoxin level that was drawn, since the symptoms are compatible with digoxin toxicity. Because a low potassium level may contribute to digoxin toxicity, checking the serum potassium level may give useful additive information, but the digoxin level is checked first. The digoxin should be withheld until the level is known. Noting the key word *first* will assist in determining that the nurse's action is to further investigate the cause of the client's complaints.

---

**BOX 10-7**

**Nursing Process: Evaluation**

A home care nurse visits a child with a diagnosis of celiac disease. Which of these findings would best indicate that a gluten-free diet is being maintained and has been effective?
1. The child is free of diarrhea
2. The child is free of bloody stools
3. The child tolerates dietary wheat and rye
4. A balanced fluid and electrolyte status is noted in the laboratory results

**Answer: 1**

**Rationale:** This question addresses the child's response to prescribed dietary measures for celiac disease. Watery diarrhea is a frequent clinical manifestation of celiac disease. The absence of diarrhea indicates effective treatment. The grains of wheat and rye contain gluten and are not allowed. A balance in fluids and electrolytes does not necessarily demonstrate improved status of celiac disease. Remember, an evaluation type of question addresses a client's response to a treatment measure.

---

**BOX 10-8**

**Caring**

A female client and her newborn infant have undergone testing for human immunodeficiency virus (HIV), and both clients have been found to be positive. The news is devastating, and the mother is crying. Using crisis intervention techniques, the nurse interprets that the mother needs which of the following at this time?
1. Call an HIV counselor and make an appointment for mother and child
2. Describe the progressive stages and treatments for HIV
3. Examine with the mother how she got HIV
4. Listen quietly while the mother talks and cries

**Answer: 4**

**Rationale:** This mother has just received devastating news and needs to have someone present with her as she begins to cope with this issue. The nurse needs to sit and actively listen while the mother talks and cries. Calling an HIV counselor may be helpful, but it is not what the client needs at this time. The other options are not appropriate for this stage of coping with the news that both she and the baby are HIV positive. Remember to address the client's feelings and to support the client. The nurse should sit and listen and provide support because this is the most caring response.

---

reviewed to determine whether sufficient information was obtained and whether the information obtained was specific and appropriate. The nursing diagnoses are evaluated for accuracy and completeness on the basis of the specific needs of the client. The plan and expected outcomes are examined to determine whether they are realistic, achievable, measurable, and effective. Interventions are examined to determine their effectiveness in achieving the expected outcomes.

Because evaluation is an ongoing process, it is vital to all steps of the nursing process. It is the continuous process of comparing actual outcomes with expected outcomes of care, and provides the means for determining the need to modify the plan of care. Inherent in this step of the nursing process is the communication of evaluation findings and the process of documenting the client's response to treatment, care, and/or teaching. Evaluation-type questions on the NCLEX-RN may be written to address a client's response to treatment measures, or to determine a client's understanding of the prescribed treatment measures (Box 10-7).

## CARING

Caring is the essence of nursing and is basic to any helping relationship. Caring is central to every encounter that a nurse may have with a client. Through caring, the nurse humanizes the client. Treating the client with respect and dignity is a true expression of caring. In the technological environment of health care, emphasizing the client's individuality counteracts any potential process of depersonalization. Caring is an Integrated Concept and Process of the Test Plan for NCLEX-RN.

This means that this concept is essential to all Client Needs components of the test plan.

On the NCLEX-RN, the concept of caring is primary. It is very easy to become involved with looking at a question from a technological viewpoint. The concept of caring needs to be addressed when you are reading a test question and selecting an option. Always address the client's feelings and provide support. Remember, this examination is all about nursing, and that nursing is caring (Box 10-8).

## COMMUNICATION AND DOCUMENTATION

The process of communication occurs as a nurse interacts either verbally or nonverbally with a client. Therapeutic communication techniques are key to an effective nurse-client relationship. Communication-type test questions are integrated throughout the NCLEX-RN test plan and may address a client situation in any health care setting. When you are answering a question on the NCLEX-RN, use of communication tools indicates a correct option and use of a communication block indicates an incorrect option. In addition, some communication-type questions may focus on psychosocial issues or issues related to client anxiety, fears, or concerns. In communication-type questions, always focus on the client's feelings FIRST. If an option reflects the client's feelings, anxiety, or concerns, select that option.

BOX 10-9

## Communication and Documentation

### COMMUNICATION

A client says to a nurse, "I 'm going to die, and I wish my family would stop hoping for a cure! I get so angry when they carry on like this! After all, I'm the one who's dying." The most therapeutic response by the nurse is:
1. "You're feeling angry that your family continues to hope for you to be cured?"
2. "I think we should talk more about your anger toward your family."
3. "Well, it sounds like you're being pretty pessimistic. After all, years ago people died of pneumonia."
4. "Have you shared your feelings with your family?"

**Answer: 1**

**Rationale:** Reflection is the therapeutic communication technique that redirects the client's feelings back in order to validate what the client is saying. Option 1 uses the therapeutic technique of reflection. In option 2, the nurse attempts to use focusing, but the attempt to discuss central issues seems premature. In option 3, the nurse makes a judgment and is nontherapeutic in the one-to-one relationship. In option 4, the nurse is attempting to assess the client's ability to openly discuss feelings with family members. Although this is an appropriate assessment of this client, the timing is somewhat premature and closes off facilitation of the client's feelings.

Remember, the use of communication tools indicates a correct option.

### DOCUMENTATION

A nurse hears a client calling out for help. The nurse hurries down the hallway to the client's room and finds the client lying on the floor. The nurse performs a thorough assessment and assists the client back to bed. The nurse notifies the physician of the incident and completes an incident report. Which of the following would the nurse document on the incident report?
1. The client was found lying on the floor
2. The client climbed over the side rails
3. The client fell out of bed
4. The client became restless and tried to get out of bed

**Answer: 1**

**Rationale:** The incident report should contain the client's name, age, and diagnosis. It should contain a factual description of the incident, any injuries experienced by those involved, and the outcome of the situation. Option 1 is the only option that describes the facts as observed by the nurse. Options 2, 3, and 4 are interpretations of the situation and are not factual data as observed by the nurse. Remember to focus on factual information when documenting, and avoid including interpretations.

Documentation is a critical component of a nurse's responsibility. The process of documentation serves many purposes and provides a comprehensive representation of the client's health status and the care given by all members of the health care team. There are many methods for documenting, but the responsibilities surrounding this practice remain the same.

When answering a question on the NCLEX-RN related to documenting, consider the ethical and legal responsibilities related to documentation, and the specific guidelines related to both narrative and computerized documentation systems (Box 10-9).

## CULTURAL AWARENESS

Cultural awareness is a concept and process that is fundamental to the practice of nursing. Often, nurses care for clients who come from ethnic, cultural, or religious backgrounds different from their own. Awareness of and sensitivity to unique health and illness beliefs and practices are essential in the delivery of safe and effective care. Acknowledgment and acceptance of cultural differences with a nonjudgmental attitude are essential in providing culturally sensitive care.

The belief underlying the NCLEX-RN Test Plan is that people are unique individuals and define their own systems of daily living, which reflect their values, motives, and lifestyles. On the NCLEX-RN, look for data in the question that relate to the issue of cultural awareness (Box 10-10).

BOX 10-10

### Cultural Awareness

A nurse is providing discharge instructions to a Chinese client regarding prescribed dietary modifications. During the teaching session, the client continuously turns away from the nurse. Which nursing action is most appropriate?
1. Continue with the instructions, verifying client understanding
2. Tell the client about the importance of the instructions for the maintenance of health care
3. Walk around the client so that you continuously face the client
4. Give the client a dietary booklet and return later to continue with the instructions

**Answer: 1**

**Rationale:** Most Chinese maintain a formal distance with others, which is a form of respect. Many Chinese are uncomfortable with face-to-face communications, especially when there is direct eye contact. If the client turns away from the nurse during a conversation, the most appropriate action is to continue with the conversation. Walking around to the client so that the nurse faces the client is in direct conflict with the cultural practice. Telling the client about the importance of the instructions for the maintenance of health care may be viewed as degrading. The client may view returning later to continue with the explanation as a rude gesture. Remember, awareness of and sensitivity to unique health and illness beliefs and practices is essential in the delivery of safe and effective care.

---

### BOX 10-11
#### Self-Care

A 9-year-old child is newly diagnosed with type 1 diabetes mellitus. A nurse is planning for home care with the child and family and determines that an age-appropriate activity for this child for health maintenance is:
1. Independently self-administer insulin
2. Make independent decisions regarding sliding-scale coverage of insulin
3. Have an adult assist in the administration of insulin and glucose monitoring
4. Administer insulin drawn up by an adult

**Answer: 1**

**Rationale:** School-aged children have the cognitive and motor skills to independently administer insulin with adult supervision. Developmentally, they do not yet have the maturity to make situational decisions without adult validation. Options 3 and 4 suppress the maximum level of independence appropriate to the level of this child. Remember, use concepts related to growth and development when selecting an answer.

---

### BOX 10-12
#### Teaching/Learning

A nurse provides instructions to a client about administering nitroglycerin ointment (Nitrobid). The nurse determines that the client is using correct technique when applying the ointment if the client:
1. Applies additional ointment if chest pain occurs
2. Applies the ointment directly to the skin, and then gently rubs the ointment into the skin
3. Applies the ointment to any nonhairy area of the body
4. Washes the ointment off when bathing and reapplies after the bath

**Answer: 3**

**Rationale:** Nitroglycerin ointment is used on a scheduled basis and is not prescribed specifically for the occurrence of chest pain. The ointment is not rubbed into the skin. It is reapplied only as directed. The correct client action (option 3) indicates the acquisition of knowledge in regard to administering the prescribed medication.

---

## SELF-CARE

The ability to care for oneself promotes an overall sense of well-being in the client. When a client's health is compromised, it is necessary for the nurse to provide the needed care to the client. Whenever possible, or as soon as the client is able, the nurse should promote the client's ability to perform self-care. When promoting independence in the client, the nurse needs to provide information to the client regarding safety measures related to personal needs, prescribed treatment measures, and medication administration. Nursing care involves promoting growth and development throughout the life span, promoting self-care, providing support systems, and the measures related to the prevention and early treatment of disease. The nurse is instrumental as a teacher in promoting self-care through client and family education, and by facilitating the coordination of support services for the client and family.

When answering questions on the NCLEX-RN, remember to promote independence in the client. Use concepts related to growth and development when selecting an answer (Box 10-11).

## TEACHING/LEARNING

Client and family education is a primary nursing responsibility. The National Council of State Boards of Nursing describes this concept as facilitating the acquisition of knowledge, skills, and attitudes that lead to a change in behavior.

The principles related to the teaching/learning process are used when the nurse functions in the role of a teacher. The nurse needs to remember that assessment of the client's readiness and motivation to learn is the initial step in the teaching/learning process.

When answering a question on the NCLEX-RN related to the teaching/learning process, use the principles related to Teaching/Learning Theory. If a test question addresses client education, remember that client motivation and client readiness to learn are the FIRST priority (Box 10-12).

## REFERENCES

Hertz, J., Yocom, C., & Gawel, S. (2000). *Linking the NCLEX-RN examination to practice: 1999 practice analysis of newly licensed registered nurses in the United States.* Chicago: National Council of State Boards of Nursing.

Hodgson, B., & Kizior, R. (2001). *Saunders nursing drug handbook 2001.* Philadelphia: W.B. Saunders.

National Council of State Boards of Nursing (eds.) (2000). *The NCLEX Process: Serving as an anchor for the NCLEX Examination.* Chicago: Author.

National Council of State Boards of Nursing (eds.) (2000). *Test Plan for the National Council Licensure Examination for Registered Nurses.* Chicago: Author.

National Council of State Boards of Nursing. Web Site: http://www.ncsbn.org/files/boards/boardscontact.asp

Potter, P., & Perry, A. (2001). *Fundamentals of nursing* (5th ed.). St. Louis: Mosby.

Riley, J. (2000). *Communication in nursing* (4th ed.). St. Louis: Mosby.

Smeltzer, S., & Bare, B. (2000). *Brunner & Suddarth's Textbook of medical-surgical nursing* (9th ed.). Philadelphia: Lippincott Williams & Wilkins.

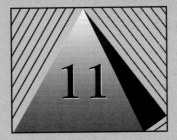

# Integrated Concepts and Processes

## NURSING PROCESS
### Nursing Process: Assessment

1. A nurse reviews the record of a client receiving external radiation therapy and notes documentation of a skin finding referred to as moist desquamation. The nurse expects to observe which of the following on assessment of the client?
   1. Reddened skin
   2. A rash
   3. Weeping of the skin
   4. Dermatitis

**Answer: 3**

*[deskwə meʃən] 脱痂*

*Rationale:* Moist desquamation occurs when the basal cells of the skin are destroyed. The dermal level is exposed, which results in the leakage of serum. Reddened skin, a rash, and dermatitis may occur with external radiation but are not described as moist desquamation.

*Test-Taking Strategy:* Use the process of elimination. Noting the key word *moist* will direct you to option 3. Options 1, 2, and 4 are eliminated because they are similar and describe a dry rather than a moist skin alteration. Review the signs associated with moist desquamation if you had difficulty with this question.

*Level of Cognitive Ability:* Analysis
*Client Needs:* Physiological Integrity
*Integrated Concept/Process:* Nursing Process/Assessment
*Content Area:* Adult Health/Oncology

*Reference*
Monahan, F., & Neighbors, M. (1998). *Medical-surgical nursing: Foundations for clinical practice* (2nd ed.). Philadelphia: W.B. Saunders, p. 1520.

2. A nurse is performing an assessment on a pregnant client with a history of cardiac disease and is assessing for venous congestion. The nurse assesses which of the following body areas, knowing that venous congestion is most commonly noted in this area?
   1. Vulva
   2. Fingers of the hands
   3. Around the eyes
   4. Around the abdomen

**Answer: 1**

*Rationale:* Assessment of the cardiovascular system includes observation for venous congestion that can develop into varicosities. Venous congestion is most commonly noted in the legs, vulva, or rectum. It would be difficult to assess for edema in the abdominal area of a client who is pregnant. Although edema may be noted in the fingers and around the eyes, edema in these areas would not be directly associated with venous congestion.

*Test-Taking Strategy:* Use the process of elimination. Focusing on the key words *venous congestion* will direct you to option 1. Review physical assessment of the cardiovascular system in a pregnant client if you had difficulty with this question.

*Level of Cognitive Ability:* Application
*Client Needs:* Physiological Integrity
*Integrated Concept/Process:* Nursing Process/Assessment
*Content Area:* Maternity

*Reference*
Gorrie, T., McKinney, E., & Murray, S. (1998). *Foundations of maternal-newborn nursing* (2nd ed.). Philadelphia: W.B. Saunders, p. 143.

---

**3.** A client who has been receiving long-term diuretic therapy is admitted to the hospital with a diagnosis of dehydration. A nurse would assess for which sign or symptom that correlates with this fluid imbalance?
1   Increased blood pressure
2   Decreased pulse
3   Decreased central venous pressure (CVP)
4   Bibasilar crackles

**Answer: 3**
*Rationale:* A client with dehydration has a low CVP. The normal CVP is between 4 and 11 mm H$_2$O. Other assessment findings with fluid volume deficit are increased pulse and respirations, weight loss, poor skin turgor, dry mucous membranes, decreased urine output, concentrated urine with increased specific gravity, increased hematocrit, and altered level of consciousness. The assessment signs in options 1, 2, and 4 occur with fluid volume excess.

*Test-Taking Strategy:* Use the process of elimination, focusing on the client's diagnosis. Remember that central venous pressure reflects the pressure under which blood is returned to the right atrium, and that pressure (volume) decreases with fluid volume deficit. If you had difficulty with this question, review the signs and symptoms of fluid volume deficit.

*Level of Cognitive Ability:* Analysis
*Client Needs:* Physiological Integrity
*Integrated Concept/Process:* Nursing Process/Assessment
*Content Area:* Fundamental Skills

*Reference*
Smeltzer, S., & Bare, B. (2000). *Textbook of medical-surgical nursing* (9th ed.). Philadelphia: Lippincott Williams & Wilkins, p. 209.

---

**4.** A nurse is preparing a plan of care for a child with Reye's syndrome. The nurse prioritizes the nursing interventions included in the plan and monitors for:
1   Signs of increased intracranial pressure (ICP)
2   The presence of protein in the urine
3   Signs of a bacterial infection
4   Signs of hyperglycemia

**Answer: 1**
*Rationale:* Intracranial pressure, encephalopathy, and hepatic dysfunction are major symptoms of Reye's syndrome. Protein is not present in the urine. Reye's syndrome is related to a history of viral infections, and hypoglycemia is a symptom of this disease.

*Test-Taking Strategy:* Use the process of elimination and focus on the diagnosis. Note the key word *prioritizes*. Recalling that increased ICP is a major symptom of Reyes's syndrome will direct you to option 1. If you had difficulty with this question, review the care of the child with Reye's syndrome.

*Level of Cognitive Ability:* Application
*Client Needs:* Physiological Integrity
*Integrated Concept/Process:* Nursing Process/Assessment
*Content Area:* Child Health

*Reference*
Bowden, V., Dickey, S., & Greenberg, C. (1998). *Children and their families: The continuum of care.* Philadelphia: W.B. Saunders, p. 1403.

---

**5.** A clinic nurse reads the chart of a client who was seen by a physician and notes that the physician has documented that the client has Lyme disease, stage III. On assessment of the client, which of the following clinical manifestations would the nurse expect to note?
1  A generalized skin rash
2  A cardiac dysrhythmia
3  Enlarged and inflamed joints
4  Palpitations

**Answer: 3**
*Rationale:* Stage III develops within a month to several months after initial infection. It is characterized by arthritic symptoms, such as arthralgias and enlarged or inflamed joints, which can persist for several years after the initial infection. Cardiac and neurological dysfunction occurs in stage II. A rash occurs in stage I.

*Test-Taking Strategy:* Use the process of elimination. Eliminate options 2 and 4 first because they are both cardiac related. Recalling that a rash occurs in stage I will direct you to option 3. If you had difficulty with this question, review the clinical manifestations associated with Lyme disease.

*Level of Cognitive Ability:* Analysis
*Client Needs:* Physiological Integrity
*Integrated Concept/Process:* Nursing Process/Assessment
*Content Area:* Adult Health/Integumentary

*Reference*
Phipps, W., Sands, J., & Marek, J. (1999). *Medical-surgical nursing: Concepts & clinical practice* (6th ed.). St. Louis: Mosby, p. 1993.

---

**6.** A female client with narcolepsy has been prescribed dextroamphetamine (Dexedrine). The client complains to a nurse that she cannot sleep well anymore at night and does not want to take the medication any longer. The nurse asks the client if the medication is taken at which of the following appropriate times?
1  At least 6 hours before bedtime
2  Two hours before bedtime
3  Before a bedtime snack
4  Just before going to sleep

**Answer: 1**
*Rationale:* Dextroamphetamine is a central nervous system (CNS) stimulant that acts by releasing norepinephrine from nerve endings. The client should take the medication at least 6 hours before going to bed at night to prevent disturbances with sleep.

*Test-Taking Strategy:* Use the process of elimination. Evaluate each of the options in terms of how far removed the scheduled dose is from the client's bedtime. Recalling that this medication causes CNS stimulation and interferes with sleep will direct you to option 1. Review this medication if you had difficulty with this question.

*Level of Cognitive Ability:* Application
*Client Needs:* Physiological Integrity
*Integrated Concept/Process:* Nursing Process/Assessment
*Content Area:* Pharmacology

*Reference*
Hodgson, B., & Kizior, R. (2001). *Saunders nursing drug handbook 2001.* Philadelphia: W.B. Saunders, p. 304.

**7.** A nurse is assessing the level of consciousness of a child with a head injury and documents that the child is obtunded. On the basis of this documentation, which of the following observations did the nurse note?
1  The child is unable to recognize place or person *disorientation*
2  The child is unable to think clearly and rapidly *confusion*
3  The child requires considerable stimulation for arousal *Stupor*
4  The child sleeps unless aroused and once aroused has limited interaction with the environment *obtunded*

**Answer: 4**
*Rationale:* If the child is obtunded, the child sleeps unless aroused and once aroused has limited interaction with the environment. Option 1 describes disorientation. Option 2 describes confusion. Option 3 describes stupor.

*Test-Taking Strategy:* Use the process of elimination, noting the key word *obtunded*. Knowledge of the standard terms used to identify level of consciousness will direct you to option 4. If you are unfamiliar with assessment of level of consciousness, review this content.

*Level of Cognitive Ability:* Analysis
*Client Needs:* Physiological Integrity
*Integrated Concept/Process:* Nursing Process/Assessment
*Content Area:* Child Health

*Reference*
Wong, D. (1999). *Whaley & Wong's Nursing care of infants and children* (6th ed.). St. Louis: Mosby, p. 1769.

**8.** A nurse is assessing a client with Addison's disease for signs of hyperkalemia. The nurse expects to note which of the following if hyperkalemia is present?
1  Polyuria
2  Dry mucous membranes
3  Cardiac dysrhythmias
4  Prolonged bleeding time

**Answer: 3**
*Rationale:* The inadequate production of aldosterone in Addison's disease causes inadequate excretion of potassium and results in hyperkalemia. The clinical manifestations of hyperkalemia are the result of altered nerve transmission. The most harmful consequence of hyperkalemia is its effect on cardiac function. Options 1, 2, and 4 are not manifestations associated with Addison's disease or hyperkalemia.

*Test-Taking Strategy:* Use the process of elimination. Recalling the effects of hyperkalemia will direct you to option 3. If you had difficulty with this question, review the pathophysiology associated with Addison's disease and the effects of hyperkalemia.

*Level of Cognitive Ability:* Analysis
*Client Needs:* Physiological Integrity
*Integrated Concept/Process:* Nursing Process/Assessment
*Content Area:* Adult Health/Endocrine

*Reference*
Smeltzer, S., & Bare, B. (2000). *Brunner & Suddarth's Textbook of medical-surgical nursing* (9th ed.). Philadelphia: Lippincott Williams & Wilkins, p. 214.

**9.** A client goes into respiratory distress, and an arterial blood gas (ABG) specimen is drawn from the radial artery. The nurse performs the Allen test prior to the ABGs to determine the adequacy of the:
1  Femoral circulation
2  Brachial circulation
3  Carotid circulation
4  Ulnar circulation

**Answer: 4**
*Rationale:* Before radial puncture for obtaining an arterial specimen for ABGs, an Allen test should be performed to determine adequate ulnar circulation. Failure to assess collateral circulation could result is severe ischemic injury to the hand, if damage to the radial artery occurs with arterial puncture. The other options are incorrect.

*Test-Taking Strategy:* Use the process of elimination and note the key words *radial artery*. Using knowledge of anatomy of the cardiovascular system, eliminate options 1, 2, and 3. Review the purpose and procedure of the Allen test if you had difficulty with this question.

*Level of Cognitive Ability:* Application
*Client Needs:* Physiological Integrity
*Integrated Concept/Process:* Nursing Process/Assessment
*Content Area:* Fundamental Skills

*Reference*
Lewis, S., Heitkemper, M., & Dirksen, S. (2000). *Medical-surgical nursing: Assessment and management of clinical problems* (5th ed.). St. Louis: Mosby, p. 1920.

---

**10.** A pregnant client with diabetes mellitus arrives at the health care clinic for a follow-up visit. In this client, the nurse most importantly monitors:
1   Urine for glucose and ketones
2   Blood pressure, pulse, and respirations
3   Urine for specific gravity
4   For the presence of edema

**Answer: 1**
*Rationale:* The nurse assesses the pregnant client with diabetes mellitus for glucose and ketones in the urine at each prenatal visit because the physiological changes of pregnancy can drastically alter insulin requirements. Assessment of blood pressure, pulse, respirations, urine for specific gravity, and the presence of edema are more related to the client with pregnancy-induced hypertension.

*Test-Taking Strategy:* Use the process of elimination, focusing on the client's diagnosis. The only option that specifically addresses diabetes mellitus is option 1. If you had difficulty with this question, review prenatal care of the client with diabetes mellitus.

*Level of Cognitive Ability:* Application
*Client Needs:* Physiological Integrity
*Integrated Concept/Process:* Nursing Process/Assessment
*Content Area:* Maternity

*Reference*
Lowdermilk, D., Perry, S., & Bobak, I. (2000). *Maternity & women's health care* (7th ed.). St. Louis: Mosby, p. 872.

---

**11.** A home care nurse is visiting a client who is in a body cast. The nurse is performing an assessment, including the psychosocial adjustment of the client to the cast. In this regard, the nurse would most appropriately assess:
1   The type of transportation available for follow-up care
2   The ability to perform activities of daily living
3   The need for sensory stimulation
4   The amount of home care support available

**Answer: 3**
*Rationale:* A psychosocial assessment of a client who is immobilized would most appropriately include the need for sensory stimulation. This assessment should also include such factors as body image, past and present coping skills, and the coping methods used during the period of immobilization. Although transportation, home care support, and the ability to perform activities of daily living are components of an assessment, they are not as specifically related to psychosocial adjustment as is the need for sensory stimulation.

*Test-Taking Strategy:* Use the process of elimination and focus on the key words *psychosocial* and *most appropriately*. Option 2 can be eliminated first because it relates to physiological integrity rather than psychosocial integrity. Next eliminate options 1 and 4 because they are most closely related to physical supports rather than psychosocial needs of the client. Review the components of a psychosocial assessment, if you had difficulty with this question.

*Level of Cognitive Ability:* Analysis
*Client Needs:* Psychosocial Integrity
*Integrated Concept/Process:* Nursing Process/Assessment
*Content Area:* Adult Health/Musculoskeletal

*Reference*
Smeltzer, S., & Bare, B. (2000). *Brunner & Suddarth's Textbook of medical-surgical nursing* (9th ed.). Philadelphia: Lippincott Williams & Wilkins, p. 1791.

12. A nurse is caring for a client with acquired immunodeficiency syndrome (AIDS). Which finding noted in the client indicates the presence of an opportunistic respiratory infection?
   1 White plaques located on the oral mucosa
   2 Fever, exertional dyspnea, and non-productive cough
   3 Ophthalmic nerve involvement causing blindness
   4 Colitis and ulcerated perirectal lesions

**Answer: 2**
*Rationale:* Fever, exertional dyspnea, and a nonproductive cough are signs of *Pneumocystis* pneumonia, a common, life-threatening opportunistic infection afflicting those with AIDS. Options 1, 3, and 4 are not associated with a respiratory infection. Option 1 describes the fungal infection oral candidiasis *(Candida albicans)*, called thrush. Option 3 describes the viral infection herpes zoster (shingles), when it has spread to involve the ophthalmic nerve. Option 4 describes herpes simplex, which occurs in homosexual men.

*Test-Taking Strategy:* Use the process of elimination and focus on the issue, respiratory infection. Option 2 is the only option that identifies symptoms related to the respiratory system. Review the signs of respiratory infection if you had difficulty with this question.

*Level of Cognitive Ability:* Analysis
*Client Needs:* Physiological Integrity
*Integrated Concept/Process:* Nursing Process/Assessment
*Content Area:* Adult Health/Immune

*Reference*
Smeltzer, S., & Bare, B. (2000). *Brunner & Suddarth's Textbook of medical-surgical nursing* (9th ed.). Philadelphia: Lippincott Williams & Wilkins, p. 1998.

13. An adult client seeks treatment in an ambulatory care clinic for complaints of a left earache, nausea, and a full feeling in the left ear. The client has an elevated temperature. A nurse first questions the client about:
   1 A history of a recent brain abscess
   2 A history of a recent upper respiratory infection (URI)
   3 Whether acetaminophen (Tylenol) relieves the pain
   4 Whether hearing is magnified in that ear

**Answer: 2**
*Rationale:* Otitis media in the adult is typically one sided, and presents as an acute process with earache, nausea and possible vomiting, fever, and fullness in the ear. The client may complain of diminished hearing in that ear. The nurse takes a client history first, assessing whether the client has had a recent URI. It is unnecessary to question the client about a brain abscess. The nurse may ask the client if anything relieves the pain, but ear infection pain is usually not relieved until antibiotic therapy is initiated.

*Test-Taking Strategy:* Use the process of elimination. Note the key word *first*. Recalling the relationship between a URI and otitis media will direct you to option 2. Review otitis media if you had difficulty with this question.

*Level of Cognitive Ability:* Analysis
*Client Needs:* Physiological Integrity
*Integrated Concept/Process:* Nursing Process/Assessment
*Content Area:* Adult Health/Ear

*Reference*
Beare, P., & Myers, J. (1998). *Adult health nursing* (3rd ed.). St. Louis, Mosby, pp. 1172-1173.

---

**14.** A home care nurse is making home visits to an elderly client with urinary incontinence who is very disturbed by the incontinent episodes. The nurse assesses the client's home situation to determine environmental barriers to normal voiding. The nurse determines that which of the following items may be contributing to the client's problem?
1 Presence of hand railings in the bathroom
2 Having one bathroom on each floor of the home
3 Night-light present in the hall between the bedroom and the bathroom
4 Bathroom located on the second floor, bedroom on the first floor

**Answer: 4**
*Rationale:* Having the bathroom on the second floor and the bedroom on the first floor may pose a problem for the elderly client with incontinence. The need to negotiate the stairs and the distance may interfere with reaching the bathroom in a timely fashion. It is more helpful to the incontinent client to have a bathroom on the same floor as the bedroom, or to have a commode rented for use. The presence of night-lights and hand railings is helpful to the client in reaching the bathroom quickly and safely.

*Test-Taking Strategy:* Focus on the issue, an environmental barrier to normal voiding. Note that options 1, 2, and 3 are similar in that they all are helpful and safe. Review measures that promote normal voiding if you had difficulty with this question.

*Level of Cognitive Ability:* Analysis
*Client Needs:* Health Promotion and Maintenance
*Integrated Concept/Process:* Nursing Process/Assessment
*Content Area:* Fundamental Skills

*Reference*
Smeltzer, S., & Bare, B. (2000). *Brunner & Suddarth's Textbook of medical-surgical nursing* (9th ed.). Philadelphia: Lippincott Williams & Wilkins, p. 1105.

---

**15.** A nurse is preparing to administer continuous intravenous (IV) fluid replacement to a client with a diagnosis of dehydration. Which of the following is essential for the nurse to assess prior to initiating the IV fluid?
1 Usual sleep patterns
2 Ability to ambulate
3 Body weight
4 Intake and output

**Answer: 3**
*Rationale:* Body weight is an accurate indicator of fluid status. As a client is hydrated with IV fluids, the nurse monitors for increasing body weight. Accurate body weight is a better measurement of gains and losses than intake and output records. An IV should not greatly alter sleep patterns, and clients will still be able to ambulate with a peripheral IV site.

*Test-Taking Strategy:* Use the process of elimination. Focus on the client's diagnosis to direct you to option 3. Remember, body weight is an accurate measurement of gains and losses. Review care of the dehydrated client, if you had difficulty with this question.

*Level of Cognitive Ability:* Analysis
*Client Needs:* Physiological Integrity
*Integrated Concept/Process:* Nursing Process/Assessment
*Content Area:* Fundamental Skills

*Reference*
Potter, P., & Perry, A. (2001). *Fundamentals of nursing* (5th ed.). St. Louis: Mosby, p. 1220.

---

**16.** A client is scheduled for an arteriogram using a radiopaque dye. A nurse assesses which most critical item before the procedure?

1. Intake and output
2. Vital signs
3. Height and weight
4. Allergy to iodine or shellfish

**Answer: 4**

*Rationale:* This procedure requires a signed informed consent, because it involves injection of a radiopaque dye into the blood vessel. Although options 1, 2, and 3 are components of the preprocedure assessment, the risk of allergic reaction and possible anaphylaxis is most critical.

*Test-Taking Strategy:* Use the process of elimination, noting the key words *most critical*. Recalling the risk of anaphylaxis related to the dye will direct you to option 4. If you had difficulty with this question, review preprocedure care for angiography.

*Level of Cognitive Ability:* Application
*Client Needs:* Physiological Integrity
*Integrated Concept/Process:* Nursing Process/Assessment
*Content Area:* Fundamental Skills

*Reference*
Fischbach, F. (2000). *A manual of laboratory & diagnostic tests* (6th ed.). Philadelphia: Lippincott Williams & Wilkins, p. 752.

---

**17.** A nurse is performing a cardiovascular assessment. Which of the following items would the nurse assess to obtain information about the client's right-sided heart function?

1. Status of breath sounds
2. Presence of peripheral edema
3. Presence of dyspnea
4. Rate of respirations

**Answer: 2**

*Rationale:* The client with heart failure may present different symptoms, depending on whether the right or the left side of the heart is failing. Options 1, 3, and 4 identify assessments for left-sided heart failure. Assessment of breath sounds provides information about right-sided heart function.

*Test-Taking Strategy:* Use the process of elimination and focus on the issue, the status of right-sided heart function. Remember "left" and "lungs." Options 1, 3, and 4 reflect left-sided heart failure. Review the signs of right- and left-sided heart failure, if you had difficulty with this question.

*Level of Cognitive Ability:* Application
*Client Needs:* Physiological Integrity
*Integrated Concept/Process:* Nursing Process/Assessment
*Content Area:* Adult Health/Cardiovascular

*Reference*
Smeltzer, S., & Bare, B. (2000). *Brunner & Suddarth's Textbook of medical-surgical nursing* (9th ed.). Philadelphia: Lippincott Williams & Wilkins, p. 548.

**18.** A nurse is obtaining a history on a client admitted to the hospital with a thrombotic cerebrovascular accident (CVA). The nurse assesses the client, knowing that prior to the CVA, the client most likely experienced:
1 Transient hemiplegia and loss of speech
2 Throbbing headaches
3 Unexplained episodes of loss of consciousness
4 No symptoms at all

**Answer: 1**
*Rationale:* Cerebral thrombosis does not occur suddenly. In the few hours or days preceding a thrombotic CVA, the client may experience a transient loss of speech, hemiplegia, or paresthesias on one side of the body. Other signs and symptoms of thrombotic CVA vary, but may include dizziness, cognitive changes, or seizures. Headache is rare, and loss of consciousness is not likely to occur.

*Test-Taking Strategy:* Use the process of elimination. Option 4 is eliminated first. From the remaining options, focus on the type of stroke addressed in the question to direct you to option 1. If you had difficulty with this question, review the signs and symptoms of a thrombotic CVA.

*Level of Cognitive Ability:* Application
*Client Needs:* Physiological Integrity
*Integrated Concept/Process:* Nursing Process/Assessment
*Content Area:* Adult Health/Neurological

*Reference*
Smeltzer, S., & Bare, B. (2000). *Brunner & Suddarth's Textbook of medical-surgical nursing* (9th ed.). Philadelphia: Lippincott Williams & Wilkins, p. 1651.

---

**19.** A client in a long-term-care facility has had a series of gastrointestinal (GI) diagnostic tests, including an upper GI series and endoscopies. Upon the client's return to the long-term-care facility, the priority nursing assessment should focus on:
1 Level of consciousness
2 Activity tolerance
3 Hydration and nutrition status
4 Comfort level

**Answer: 3**
*Rationale:* Many of the diagnostic studies to identify GI disorders require that the GI tract be cleaned (usually with laxatives and enemas) prior to testing. In addition, the client is most often NPO prior to and during the testing period. Because the studies may be done over a period exceeding 24 hours, the client may become dehydrated and/or malnourished. Although options 1, 2, and 4 may be components of the assessment, option 3 is the priority.

*Test-Taking Strategy:* Use the process of elimination. Note the key words *priority nursing assessment.* Use Maslow's Hierarchy of Needs theory to direct you to option 3. Review care of a client after diagnostic GI tests, if you had difficulty with this question.

*Level of Cognitive Ability:* Application
*Client Needs:* Physiological Integrity
*Integrated Concept/Process:* Nursing Process/Assessment
*Content Area:* Adult Health/Gastrointestinal

*Reference*
Smeltzer, S., & Bare, B. (2000). *Brunner & Suddarth's Textbook of medical-surgical nursing* (9th ed.). Philadelphia: Lippincott Williams & Wilkins, p. 798.

**20.** A nurse plans to assess a client for the vegetative signs of depression. The nurse assesses for these signs by determining the client's:

1  Ability to think, concentrate, and make decisions
2  Appetite, weight, sleep patterns, and psychomotor activity
3  Level of self-esteem
4  Level of suicidal ideation

**Answer: 2**

*Rationale:* The vegetative signs of depression are changes in physiological functioning during depression. These include changes in appetite, weight, sleep patterns, and psychomotor activity. Options 1, 3, and 4 represent psychological assessment categories.

*Test-Taking Strategy:* Use the process of elimination. Recalling that the vegetative signs of depression refer to physiological changes directs you to option 2. Review assessment of depression, if you had difficulty with this question.

*Level of Cognitive Ability:* Analysis
*Client Needs:* Physiological Integrity
*Integrated Concept/Process:* Nursing Process/Assessment
*Content Area:* Mental Health

*Reference*
Stuart, G.W., & Laraia, M.T. (1998). *Principles and practice of psychiatric nursing.* (6th ed.). St. Louis: Mosby, p. 352.

---

**21.** A nurse is caring for a client diagnosed with cirrhosis of the liver. The client is receiving spironolactone (Aldactone), 50 mg PO daily. Which of the following would indicate to the nurse that the client is experiencing a side effect related to the medication?

1  Hypokalemia
2  Hyperkalemia
3  Constipation
4  Dry skin

**Answer: 2**

*Rationale:* Spironolactone (Aldactone) is a potassium-sparing diuretic. Side effects include hyperkalemia, dehydration, hyponatremia, and lethargy. Although the concern with most diuretics is hypokalemia, this medication is potassium sparing, which means that the concern with the administration of this medication is hyperkalemia. Additional side effects include nausea, vomiting, cramping, diarrhea, headache, ataxia, drowsiness, confusion, and fever.

*Test-Taking Strategy:* Use the process of elimination. Recalling that this medication is potassium sparing will direct you to option 2. If you had difficulty with this question, review those medications in the classification of potassium-sparing diuretics.

*Level of Cognitive Ability:* Analysis
*Client Needs:* Physiological Integrity
*Integrated Concept/Process:* Nursing Process/Assessment
*Content Area:* Pharmacology

*Reference*
Hodgson, B., & Kizior, R. (2001). *Saunders nursing drug handbook 2001.* Philadelphia: W.B. Saunders, p. 943.

---

**22.** A nurse is preparing a woman in labor for an amniotomy. The nurse would assess which priority data prior to the procedure?

1  Maternal blood pressure
2  Maternal heart rate
3  Fetal heart rate
4  Fetal scalp sampling

**Answer: 3**

*Rationale:* Fetal well-being must be confirmed before and after amniotomy. Fetal heart rate should be checked by Doppler or by the application of the external fetal monitor. Although maternal vital signs may be assessed, fetal heart rate is the priority. A fetal scalp sampling cannot be done when the membranes are intact.

*Test-Taking Strategy:* Note the key word *priority*. Eliminate option 4 first, knowing that a fetal scalp sampling cannot be done prior to an amniotomy. Eliminate options 1 and 2 next, noting that they are similar and address maternal vital signs. Option 3 addresses fetal well-being. Review preprocedure care for amniotomy if you had difficulty with this question.

*Level of Cognitive Ability:* Application
*Client Needs:* Physiological Integrity
*Integrated Concept/Process:* Nursing Process/Assessment
*Content Area:* Maternity

*Reference*
Lowdermilk, D., Perry, S., & Bobak, I. (2000). *Maternity & women's health care* (7th ed.). St. Louis: Mosby, p. 995.

---

**23.** A nurse is monitoring a client who is receiving an oxytocin (Pitocin) infusion for the induction of labor. The nurse would suspect water intoxication if which of the following were noted?

1   Bradycardia
2   Lethargy
3   Tachycardia
4   Fatigue

**Answer: 3**
*Rationale:* During an oxytocin infusion, the woman is monitored closely for water intoxication. Signs of water intoxication include tachycardia, cardiac dysrhythmias, shortness of breath, nausea, and vomiting.

*Test-Taking Strategy:* Focus on the issue of the question, water intoxication. Think about the physiological response that occurs when fluid overload exists to direct you to option 3. Review the signs of water intoxication if you had difficulty with this question.

*Level of Cognitive Ability:* Analysis
*Client Needs:* Physiological Integrity
*Integrated Concept/Process:* Nursing Process/Assessment
*Content Area:* Maternity

*Reference*
Lowdermilk, D., Perry, S., & Bobak, I. (2000). *Maternity & women's health care* (7th ed.). St. Louis: Mosby, p. 572.

---

**24.** A clinic nurse of a well-baby clinic is collecting data regarding the motor development of a 15-month-old child. Which of the following is the highest level of development that the nurse would expect to observe in this child?

1   The child builds a tower of two blocks
2   The child opens a door knob
3   The child unzips a large zipper
4   The child puts on simple clothes independently

**Answer: 1**
*Rationale:* At age 15 months, the nurse would expect that the child could build a tower of two blocks. A 24-month-old would be able to open a door knob and unzip a large zipper. At age 30 months, a child would be able to put on simple clothes independently.

*Test-Taking Strategy:* Note the age of the child and the key words *highest level of development*. Visualize each of the motor skills presented in the options to assist in selecting the correct option. Review these developmental milestones if you had difficulty with this question.

*Level of Cognitive Ability:* Analysis
*Client Needs:* Health Promotion and Maintenance
*Integrated Concept/Process:* Nursing Process/Assessment
*Content Area:* Child Health

*Reference*
Wong, D. (1999). *Whaley & Wong's Nursing care of infants and children* (6th ed.). St. Louis: Mosby, p. 132.

**25.** A nurse is admitting a child with a diagnosis of irritable bowel syndrome to the hospital. Which of the following data would the nurse expect to obtain on assessment of the child?
1. Reports of frothy diarrhea
2. Reports of profuse, watery diarrhea and vomiting
3. Reports of foul-smelling ribbon stools
4. Reports of diffuse abdominal pain unrelated to meals or activity

**Answer: 4**
*Rationale:* Irritable bowel syndrome causes diffuse abdominal pain unrelated to meals or activity. Alternating constipation and diarrhea with the presence of undigested food and mucus in the stools may also be noted. Option 1 is a clinical manifestation of lactose intolerance. Option 2 is a clinical manifestation of celiac disease. Option 3 is a clinical manifestation of Hirschsprung's disease.

*Test-Taking Strategy:* Focus on the child's diagnosis. Noting the name of the syndrome will direct you to option 4 because you would expect abdominal pain in such a disorder. Review the clinical manifestations associated with this disorder, if you had difficulty with this question.

*Level of Cognitive Ability:* Analysis
*Client Needs:* Physiological Integrity
*Integrated Concept/Process:* Nursing Process/Assessment
*Content Area:* Child Health

*Reference*
Wong, D. (1999). *Whaley & Wong's Nursing care of infants and children* (6th ed.). St. Louis: Mosby, p. 1550.

**26.** A nurse is caring for a child diagnosed with rubeola (measles). The nurse notes that the physician has documented the presence of Koplik spots. On the basis of this documentation, which of the following would the nurse expect to note on assessment of the child?
1. Petechiae spots that are reddish and pinpoint on the soft palate
2. Whitish vesicles located across the chest
3. Small, blue-white spots with a red base, found on the buccal mucosa
4. Pinpoint petechiae on both legs

**Answer: 3**
*Rationale:* Koplik spots appear approximately 2 days before the appearance of the rash. These are small, blue-white spots with a red base, found on the buccal mucosa. The spots last approximately 3 days, after which time they slough off. Options 1, 2, and 4 are incorrect.

*Test-Taking Strategy:* Knowledge regarding the characteristics associated with rubeola and the characteristics of Koplik spots is required to answer this question. If you are unfamiliar with these characteristics, review this content.

*Level of Cognitive Ability:* Analysis
*Client Needs:* Physiological Integrity
*Integrated Concept/Process:* Nursing Process/Assessment
*Content Area:* Child Health

*Reference*
Wong, D. (1999). *Whaley & Wong's Nursing care of infants and children* (6th ed.). St. Louis: Mosby, p. 726.

**27.** A child is hospitalized with a diagnosis of nephrotic syndrome. Which of the following assessment findings would a nurse expect to note in the child?
1. Weight loss
2. Hypotension
3. Abdominal pain
4. Constipation

**Answer: 3**
*Rationale:* Clinical manifestations associated with nephrotic syndrome include edema, anorexia, fatigue, and abdominal pain from the presence of extra fluid in the peritoneal cavity. Diarrhea resulting from edema of the bowel occurs and may cause decreased absorption of nutrients. Increased weight and a normal blood pressure are noted.

*Test-Taking Strategy:* Recalling that edema is a clinical manifestation associated with nephrotic syndrome will direct you to option

3. If you had difficulty with this question or are unfamiliar with the clinical manifestations associated with this disorder, review this content.

*Level of Cognitive Ability:* Analysis
*Client Needs:* Physiological Integrity
*Integrated Concept/Process:* Nursing Process/Assessment
*Content Area:* Child Health

*Reference*
Wong, D. (1999). *Whaley & Wong's Nursing care of infants and children* (6th ed.). St. Louis: Mosby, p. 1385.

---

**28.** A child is admitted to the hospital with a suspected diagnosis of von Willbrand's disease. On assessment of the child, which of the following symptoms would most likely be noted?

1  Bleeding from the mucous membranes
2  Presence of hemarthrosis
3  Hematuria
4  Presence of hematomas

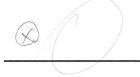

*Von Willbrand's
Hemophilia .*

**Answer: 1**
*Rationale:* The primary clinical manifestations of von Willebrand's disease are bruising and mucous membrane bleeding from the nose, mouth, and gastrointestinal tract. Prolonged bleeding after trauma and surgery, including tooth extraction, may be the first evidence of abnormal hemostasis in those with mild disease. In females, menorrhagia may occur. Bleeding associated with von Willbrand's disease may be severe and lead to anemia and shock, but unlike the situation in hemophilia, deep bleeding into joints and muscles is rare. Options 2, 3, and 4 are characteristic of those signs found in hemophilia.

*Test-Taking Strategy:* Specific knowledge regarding the clinical manifestations associated with von Willbrand's disease is required to answer this question. Recalling that options 2, 3, and 4 are characteristic of hemophilia will assist in directing you to option 1. If you are unfamiliar with this disorder, review this content.

*Level of Cognitive Ability:* Analysis
*Client Needs:* Physiological Integrity
*Integrated Concept/Process:* Nursing Process/Assessment
*Content Area:* Child Health

*Reference*
Bowden, V., Dickey, S., & Greenberg, C. (1998). *Children and their families: The continuum of care.* Philadelphia: W.B. Saunders, pp. 1540, 1553-1554.

---

**29.** A nurse is assigned to care for a child with a basilar skull fracture. The nurse reviews the child's record and notes that the physician has documented the presence of Battle sign. Which of the following would the nurse expect to note in the child?

1  Bruising behind the ear
2  Edematous periorbital area
3  Bruised periorbital area
4  Presence of epistaxis

**Answer: 1**
*Rationale:* The most serious type of skull fracture is a basilar skull fracture. Two classic findings associated with this type of skull fracture are Battle sign and raccoon eyes. Battle sign is the presence of bruising or ecchymosis behind the ear as a result of leaking of blood into the mastoid sinuses. Raccoon eyes occur as a result of blood leaking into the frontal sinus, which causes an edematous and bruised periorbital area.

*Test-Taking Strategy:* Use the process of elimination. Eliminate options 2 and 3 first because they are similar. From the remaining options, recalling the description of Battle sign will direct you to option 1. If you are unfamiliar with this sign and its description, review this content.

*Level of Cognitive Ability:* Analysis
*Client Needs:* Physiological Integrity
*Integrated Concept/Process:* Nursing Process/Assessment
*Content Area:* Child Health

*Reference*
Bowden, V., Dickey, S., & Greenberg, C. (1998). *Children and their families: The continuum of care.* Philadelphia: W.B. Saunders, p. 1411.

---

**30.** A mother brings a child to a health care clinic. The child has been complaining of severe headaches and has been vomiting. The child has a high fever, and a nurse notes the presence of nuchal rigidity in the child. The nurse suspects a diagnosis of bacterial meningitis. The nurse continues to assess the child for the presence of Kernig's sign. Which of the following findings would indicate the presence of this sign?

1   Inability of the child to extend the legs fully when lying supine
2   Flexion of the hips when the neck is flexed from a lying position
3   Pain when the chin is pulled down to the chest
4   Calf pain when the foot is dorsiflexed

**Answer: 1**
*Rationale:* Kernig's sign is the inability of the child to extend the legs fully when lying supine. Brudzinski's sign is flexion of the hips when the neck is flexed from a supine position. Both of these signs are frequently present in bacterial meningitis. Nuchal rigidity is also present in bacterial meningitis and occurs when pain prevents the child from touching the chin to the chest. Homans' sign is elicited when pain occurs in the calf region when the foot is dorsiflexed. Homans' sign is present in thrombophlebitis.

*Test-Taking Strategy:* Use the process of elimination, focusing on the child's diagnosis. Option 4 is eliminated first because this is an assessment test for the presence of thrombophlebitis, not meningitis. Next eliminate option 3 because this option identifies the presence of nuchal rigidity. From the remaining options, it is necessary to be able to distinguish between Kernig's sign and Brudzinski's sign. If you had difficulty with this question, review the assessment findings in meningitis.

*Level of Cognitive Ability:* Analysis
*Client Needs:* Physiological Integrity
*Integrated Concept/Process:* Nursing Process/Assessment
*Content Area:* Child Health

*Reference*
Bowden, V., Dickey, S., & Greenberg, C. (1998). *Children and their families: The continuum of care.* Philadelphia: W.B. Saunders, p. 1387.

## Nursing Process: Analysis

---

**1.** A nonstress test is performed on a client, and the results are documented in the chart. The results are documented as "two or more fetal heart rate (FHR) accelerations of 15 beats per minute, lasting 15 seconds, in association with fetal movement." A nurse interprets these findings as:

1   A reactive nonstress test
2   A nonreactive nonstress test
3   Unclear for accurate interpretation
4   Unsatisfactory

**Answer: 1**
*Rationale:* A reactive nonstress test (normal/negative) indicates a healthy fetus. It is described as two or more FHR accelerations of at least 15 beats per minute, lasting at least 15 seconds from the beginning of the acceleration to the end, in association with fetal movement, during a 20-minute period. A nonreactive nonstress test (abnormal) is described as no accelerations or accelerations of less than 15 beats per minute or lasting less than 15 seconds throughout any fetal movement during the testing period. An unsatisfactory test cannot be interpreted because of the poor quality of the FHR.

*Test-Taking Strategy:* Use the process of elimination. Eliminate options 3 and 4 first because they are similar. From the remaining options, remembering that a reactive nonstress test is a normal or negative test will assist in directing you to option 1. If you had difficulty answering this question, review the nonstress test.

*Level of Cognitive Ability:* Analysis
*Client Needs:* Physiological Integrity
*Integrated Concept/Process:* Nursing Process/Analysis
*Content Area:* Maternity

### Reference
Lowdermilk, D., Perry, S., & Bobak, I. (2000). *Maternity & women's health care* (7th ed.). St. Louis: Mosby, p. 810.

---

**2.** A nurse is developing a plan of care for a client in Buck's traction regarding measures to prevent complications. The nurse determines that the priority nursing diagnosis to be included in the plan is which of the following?

1. Diversional Activity Deficit related to bed rest
2. Self-Care Deficit related to the need for traction
3. Impaired Physical Mobility related to traction
4. Potential for Infection at pin sites

**Answer: 3**
*Rationale:* The priority nursing diagnosis for the client in Buck's traction is Impaired Physical Mobility. Options 1 and 2 may also be appropriate for the client in traction, but immobility presents the greatest risk for the development of complications. Buck's traction is a skin traction, and there are no pin sites.

*Test-Taking Strategy:* Use the process of elimination, and eliminate option 4 first because there are no pin sites with Buck's traction. From the remaining options, focus on the key word *priority* to assist in directing you to option 3. Review care of the client in Buck's traction if you had difficulty with this question.

*Level of Cognitive Ability:* Analysis
*Client Needs:* Physiological Integrity
*Integrated Concept/Process:* Nursing Process/Analysis
*Content Area:* Adult Health/Musculoskeletal

### Reference
Smeltzer, S., & Bare, B. (2000). *Brunner & Suddarth's Textbook of medical-surgical nursing* (9th ed.). Philadelphia: Lippincott Williams & Wilkins, pp. 1788-1789.

---

**3.** A pregnant client with mitral valve prolapse is receiving anticoagulant therapy during pregnancy. A nurse performs an assessment on the client and expects that the client will indicate that which of the following medications is prescribed?

1. Oral intake of 15 mg of warfarin (Coumadin) daily
2. Intravenous infusion of heparin sodium, 5000 units daily
3. Subcutaneous administration of heparin sodium, 5000 units daily
4. Subcutaneous administration of terbutaline (Brethine) daily

**Answer: 3**
*Rationale:* Pregnant women with mitral valve prolapse are frequently given anticoagulant therapy during pregnancy, since they are at greater risk for thromboembolic disease during the antenatal, intrapartal, and postpartum periods. Warfarin (Coumadin) is contraindicated during pregnancy because it passes the placental barrier, causing potential fetal malformations and hemorrhagic disorders. Heparin, which does not pass the placental barrier, is safe for anticoagulant therapy during pregnancy and would be administered by the subcutaneous route. Terbutaline is indicated for preterm labor management only.

*Test-Taking Strategy:* Use the process of elimination and knowledge regarding the medications that are safe during pregnancy to assist in answering the question. Eliminate options 1 and 4 first, since warfarin is contraindicated and terbutaline is indicated for preterm labor management only. From the remaining options, select option 3 because of the word *subcutaneous.* Review the treatment measures for the pregnant client with mitral valve prolapse if you had difficulty with this question.

*Level of Cognitive Ability:* Analysis
*Client Needs:* Health Promotion and Maintenance
*Integrated Concept/Process:* Nursing Process/Analysis
*Content Area:* Maternity

*Reference*
Gorrie, T., McKinney, E., & Murray, S. (1998). *Foundations of maternal newborn nursing* (2nd ed.). Philadelphia: W.B. Saunders, pp. 722-727.

---

**4.** A nurse continues to assess a client who is in the late first stage of labor for progress and fetal well-being. At the last vaginal exam, the client was fully effaced, 8 centimeters dilated, vertex presentation, and station 1. Which observation would indicate that the fetus was in distress?

**1** Vaginal exam continues to reveal some old meconium staining of the liquid, and the fetal monitor demonstrates a U-shaped pattern of deceleration during contractions, recovering to a baseline of 140 beats per minute

**2** Fresh, thick meconium is passed with a small gush of liquid, and the fetal monitor shows late decelerations with a variable descending baseline

**3** Fresh meconium is found on the examiner's gloved fingers after a vaginal exam, and the fetal monitor pattern remains essentially unchanged

**4** The fetal heart rate slowly drops to 110 beats per minute during strong contractions, recovering to 138 beats per minute immediately afterward

**Answer: 2**
*Rationale:* Meconium staining alone is not a sign of fetal distress. Meconium passage is a normal physiological function, frequent in a fetus over 38 weeks' gestation. Old meconium staining may be the result of prenatal trauma that is resolved. It is not unusual for the fetal heart rate to drop below the 140 to 160 beats per minute range in late labor during contractions, and in a healthy fetus the fetal heart rate will recover between contractions. Fresh meconium in combination with late decelerations and a variable descending baseline is an ominous signal of fetal distress resulting from fetal hypoxia.

*Test-Taking Strategy:* Use the process of elimination, noting the issue, fetal distress. Eliminate options 1 and 4 first because they both indicate a recovering fetal heart rate. From the remaining options, eliminate option 3 because of the key words *fetal monitor pattern remains essentially unchanged.* Review signs of fetal distress if you had difficulty with this question.

*Level of Cognitive Ability:* Analysis
*Client Needs:* Physiological Integrity
*Integrated Concept/Process:* Nursing Process/Analysis
*Content Area:* Maternity

*Reference*
Lowdermilk, D., Perry, S., & Bobak, I. (2000). *Maternity & women's health care* (7th ed.). St. Louis: Mosby, p. 537.

---

**5.** A nurse is caring for a child with complex partial seizures who is being treated with carbamazepine (Tegretol). The nurse reviews the laboratory report for the results of the drug plasma level and determines that the plasma level is in a therapeutic range if which of the following is noted?

**1** 1 µg/mL
**2** 10 µg/mL
**3** 18 µg/mL
**4** 20 µg/mL

**Answer: 2**
*Rationale:* When carbamazepine is administered, plasma levels of the medication need to be monitored periodically to check for the child's absorption of the medication. The amount of the medication prescribed is based on the results of this laboratory test. The therapeutic plasma level of carbamazepine is 3 to 14 µg/mL.

*Test-Taking Strategy:* Use the process of elimination and knowledge of the therapeutic plasma level of carbamazepine to answer the question. Recalling that the therapeutic plasma level is 3 to 14 µg/mL will direct you to option 2. If you had difficulty with this question, review the therapeutic plasma level of carbamazepine.

*Level of Cognitive Ability:* Analysis
*Client Needs:* Physiological Integrity
*Integrated Concept/Process:* Nursing Process/Analysis
*Content Area:* Pharmacology

**Reference**
Hodgson, B., & Kizior, R. (2000). *Saunders nursing drug handbook 2000.* Philadelphia: W.B. Saunders, pp. 144-146.

---

**6.** A nurse performs an assessment of a client with a history of congestive heart failure. The client has been taking diuretics on a long-term basis. The nurse reviews the medication record, knowing that which of the following medications, if prescribed for this client, would place the client at risk for hypokalemia?
1   Spironolactone (Aldactone)
2   Bumetanide (Bumex)
3   Triamterene (Dyrenium)
4   Amiloride HCl (Midamor)

**Answer: 2**
*Rationale:* Bumetanide (Bumex) is a loop diuretic. A client who is taking this medication would be at risk for hypokalemia. Spironolactone (Aldactone), triamterene (Dyrenium), and amiloride HCl (Midamor) are potassium-sparing diuretics.

*Test-Taking Strategy:* Use the process of elimination and knowledge regarding the diuretics that are in the classification of potassium-sparing. Recalling that bumetanide is a loop diuretic will direct you to option 2. Review these medications if you had difficulty with this question.

*Level of Cognitive Ability:* Analysis
*Client Needs:* Physiological Integrity
*Integrated Concept/Process:* Nursing Process/Analysis
*Content Area:* Pharmacology

**Reference**
Hodgson, B., & Kizior, R. (2000). *Saunders nursing drug handbook 2000.* Philadelphia: W.B. Saunders, pp. 41-43, 126-128, 494-496, 942-944, 1021-1022.

---

**7.** A home care nurse is preparing to visit a client with a diagnosis of Meniere's disease. The nurse reviews the physician's orders and expects to note that which of the following dietary measures will be prescribed?
1   Low-fiber diet with decreased fluids
2   Low-sodium diet and fluid restriction
3   Low-carbohydrate diet and elimination of red meats
4   Low-fat diet with restriction of citrus fruits

**Answer: 2**
*Rationale:* Dietary changes, such as salt and fluid restrictions, that reduce the amount of endolymphatic fluid are sometimes prescribed for clients with Meniere's disease. Options 1, 3, and 4 are not prescribed for this disorder.

*Test-Taking Strategy:* Use the process of elimination, and focus on the client's diagnosis. Recalling that salt and fluid restrictions are sometimes necessary to reduce the amount of endolymphatic fluid will assist in directing you to option 2. Review the pathophysiology related to this condition and the treatment, if you had difficulty with this question.

*Level of Cognitive Ability:* Analysis
*Client Needs:* Health Promotion and Maintenance
*Integrated Concept/Process:* Nursing Process/Analysis
*Content Area:* Adult Health/Ear

**Reference**
Ignatavicius, D., Workman, M., & Mishler, M. (1999). *Medical-surgical nursing across the health care continuum* (3rd ed.). Philadelphia: W.B. Saunders, p. 1217.

**8.** A nurse is caring for a client diagnosed with tuberculosis. The client is receiving rifampin (Rifadin), 600 mg PO daily. Which of the following would indicate to the nurse that the client is experiencing an adverse reaction?

1    A white blood cell count of 6000/μl
2    An alkaline phosphatase of 25 units/dL
3    A sedimentation rate of 15 mm/hr
4    A total bilirubin of 0.5 mg/dL

**Answer: 2**

*Rationale:* Adverse reactions or toxic effects of rifampin include hepatotoxicity, hepatitis, blood dyscrasias, Stevens-Johnson syndrome, and antibiotic-related colitis. The nurse monitors for increased liver function, bilirubin, blood urea nitrogen, and uric acid because elevations indicate an adverse reaction. A normal white blood cell count is 4500 to 11,000/μl. The normal sedimentation rate is 0 to 30 mm/hr. The normal total bilirubin level is less than 1.5 mg/dL. The normal alkaline phosphatase is 4.5 to 13 King-Armstrong units/dL.

*Test-Taking Strategy:* Use the process of elimination. Knowing that the medication is metabolized in the liver will assist in eliminating options 1 and 3 because these laboratory studies are not directly related to assessing liver function. From the remaining options, knowledge of normal laboratory values will direct you to option 2. If you are unfamiliar with this medication or these laboratory values, review this content.

*Level of Cognitive Ability:* Analysis
*Client Needs:* Physiological Integrity
*Integrated Concept/Process:* Nursing Process/Analysis
*Content Area:* Pharmacology

*Reference*
Hodgson, B., & Kizior, R. (2001). *Saunders nursing drug handbook 2001.* Philadelphia: W.B. Saunders, p. 907.

**9.** A home health nurse is assessing a client who is taking prazosin (Minipres). Which of the following statements by the client would support the nursing diagnosis of Noncompliance with medication therapy?

1    "I don't understand why I have to keep taking the pills when my blood pressure is normal."
2    "I can't see the numbers on the label to know how much salt is in food."
3    'If I feel dizzy, I'll skip my dose for a few days."
4    "If I have a cold, I shouldn't take any over-the-counter remedies without consulting my doctor."

**Answer: 3**

*Rationale:* Side effects of prazosin are dizziness and impotence. The client needs to be instructed to call the physician if these side effects occur. Holding (skipping) medication will cause an abrupt rise of blood pressure. Option 1 indicates a knowledge deficit. Option 2 indicates a self-care deficit. Option 4 indicates client understanding regarding the medication.

*Test-Taking Strategy:* Focus on the nursing diagnosis, Noncompliance, to select the correct option. Noting the key words *I'll skip my dose* will direct you to option 3. Review the defining characteristics of Noncompliance if you had difficulty with this question.

*Level of Cognitive Ability:* Analysis
*Client Needs:* Health Promotion and Maintenance
*Integrated Concept/Process:* Nursing Process/Analysis
*Content Area:* Pharmacology

*Reference*
Hodgson, B., & Kizior, R. (2001). *Saunders nursing drug handbook 2001.* Philadelphia: W.B. Saunders, p. 851.

**10.** A client with a history of self-managed peptic ulcer disease has frequently used excessive amounts of oral antacids. A nurse interprets that this client is most at risk for which acid-base disturbance?
1. Metabolic acidosis
2. Metabolic alkalosis
3. Respiratory alkalosis
4. Respiratory acidosis

**Answer: 2**
*Rationale:* Oral antacids commonly contain bicarbonate or other alkaline components. These bind onto the hydrochloric acid in the stomach to neutralize the acid. Excessive use of oral antacids containing bicarbonate can cause a metabolic alkalosis over time. Options 1, 3, and 4 are incorrect.

*Test-Taking Strategy:* Note that the question indicates that the problem is not respiratory in nature. With this in mind, eliminate options 3 and 4 first. Choose correctly from the remaining options, knowing that an antacid must work against acids. Review the causes of metabolic alkalosis if you had difficulty with the question.

*Level of Cognitive Ability:* Analysis
*Client Needs:* Physiological Integrity
*Integrated Concept/Process:* Nursing Process/Analysis
*Content Area:* Fundamental Skills

*Reference*
Ignatavicius, D., Workman, M., & Mishler, M. (1999). *Medical-surgical nursing across the health care continuum* (3rd ed.). Philadelphia: W.B. Saunders, p. 301.

**11.** A nurse is assessing a 39-year-old Caucasian female client. The client has a blood pressure (BP) of 152/92 mm Hg at rest, total cholesterol of 190 mg/dL, and a fasting blood glucose level of 114 mg/dL. The nurse would place priority on which risk factor for coronary artery disease (CAD) in this client?
1. Age
2. Hyperlipidemia
3. Hypertension
4. Glucose intolerance

**Answer: 3**
*Rationale:* Hypertension, cigarette smoking, and hyperlipidemia are major risk factors for CAD. Glucose intolerance, obesity, and response to stress are also contributing factors. Age greater than 40 is a nonmodifiable risk factor. A cholesterol level of 190 mg/dL and a blood glucose level of 114 mg/dL are within the normal ranges. The nurse places priority on major risk factors that need modification.

*Test-Taking Strategy:* Focus on the data in the question and note the key word *priority*. Note that the only abnormal value is the BP. Review the risk factors associated with CAD if you had difficulty with this question.

*Level of Cognitive Ability:* Analysis
*Client Needs:* Health Promotion and Maintenance
*Integrated Concept/Process:* Nursing Process/Analysis
*Content Area:* Adult Health/Cardiovascular

*Reference*
Smeltzer, S., & Bare, B. (2000). *Brunner & Suddarth's Textbook of medical-surgical nursing* (9th ed.). Philadelphia: Lippincott Williams & Wilkins, p. 541.

**12.** A nurse is caring for a client who has just returned to the nursing unit after an intravenous pyelogram (IVP). The nurse determines that which of the following is a priority in the postprocedure care of this client?

1 Encouraging increased intake of oral fluids
2 Ambulating the client in the hallway
3 Encouraging the client to try to void frequently
4 Maintaining the client on bed rest

**Answer: 1**

*Rationale:* After IVP, the client should take in increased fluids to aid in clearance of the dye used for the procedure. It is unnecessary to void frequently after the procedure. The client is usually allowed activity as tolerated, without any specific activity guidelines.

*Test-Taking Strategy:* Use the process of elimination and note the key word *priority*. Option 3 has no useful purpose, and is eliminated first. From the remaining options, recall that there are no activity guidelines after this procedure. Also, recall that fluids are necessary to promote clearance of the dye from the client's system. Review this procedure if you had difficulty with this question.

*Level of Cognitive Ability:* Analysis
*Client Needs:* Physiological Integrity
*Integrated Concept/Process:* Nursing Process/Analysis
*Content Area:* Adult Health/Renal

*Reference*
Smeltzer, S., & Bare, B. (2000). *Brunner & Suddarth's Textbook of medical-surgical nursing* (9th ed.). Philadelphia: Lippincott Williams & Wilkins, p. 1095.

**13.** A client has had arterial blood gases drawn. The results are as follows: pH of 7.34, $Paco_2$ of 37 mm Hg, $Pao_2$ of 79, $HCO_3$ of 19 mEq/L. A nurse interprets that the client is experiencing:

1 Respiratory acidosis
2 Respiratory alkalosis
3 Metabolic acidosis
4 Metabolic alkalosis

**Answer: 3**

*Rationale:* Metabolic acidosis occurs when the pH falls below 7.35 and the bicarbonate level falls below 22 mEq/L. With respiratory acidosis, the pH drops below 7.35 and the carbon dioxide level rises above 45 mm Hg. With respiratory alkalosis, the pH rises above 7.45 and the carbon dioxide level falls below 35 mm Hg. With metabolic alkalosis, the pH rises above 7.45 and the bicarbonate level rises above 26 mEq/L.

*Test-Taking Strategy:* Use the process of elimination. Knowing that a pH of 7.34 is acidotic helps to eliminate options 2 and 4 first. From the remaining options, knowing that a metabolic condition exists when the bicarbonate follows the same up or down pattern as the pH helps you to choose option 3 over option 1. Review the analysis of arterial blood gas results if you had difficulty with this question.

*Level of Cognitive Ability:* Analysis
*Client Needs:* Physiological Integrity
*Integrated Concept/Process:* Nursing Process/Analysis
*Content Area:* Adult Health/Respiratory

*Reference*
Monahan, F., & Neighbors, M. (1998). *Medical-surgical nursing: Foundations for clinical practice* (2nd ed.). Philadelphia: W.B Saunders, p. 104.

**14.** A client with advanced cirrhosis of the liver is not tolerating protein well, as evidenced by abnormal laboratory values. A nurse anticipates that which of the following medications will be prescribed for the client?

**1**   Lactulose (Chronulac)
**2**   Ethacrynic acid (Edecrin)
**3**   Folic acid (Folvite)
**4**   Thiamine (vitamin $B_1$)

**Answer:** 1

*Rationale:* The client with cirrhosis has impaired ability to metabolize protein because of liver dysfunction. Administration of lactulose aids in the clearance of ammonia via the gastrointestinal (GI) tract. Ethacrynic acid is a diuretic. Folic acid and thiamine are vitamins, which may be used in clients with liver disease as supplemental therapy.

*Test-Taking Strategy:* To answer this question correctly, it is necessary to know that ammonia levels are elevated with advanced liver disease, and that lactulose is a standard form of medication therapy for this condition. Review this disorder and the purpose of this medication, if you had difficulty with this question.

*Level of Cognitive Ability:* Analysis
*Client Needs:* Physiological Integrity
*Integrated Concept/Process:* Nursing Process/Analysis
*Content Area:* Pharmacology

*References*
Hodgson, B., & Kizior, R. (2001). *Saunders nursing drug handbook 2001.* Philadelphia: W.B. Saunders, pp. 573-574.

---

**15.** A nurse is caring for a child with renal disease and is analyzing the laboratory results. The nurse notes a sodium level of 148 mEq/L. On the basis of this finding, which clinical manifestation would the nurse expect to note in the child?

**1**   Increased heart rate
**2**   Cold clammy skin
**3**   Dry sticky mucous membranes
**4**   Lethargy

**Answer:** 3

*Rationale:* Hypernatremia occurs when the sodium level is greater that 145 mEq/L. Clinical manifestations include intense thirst, oliguria, agitation and restlessness, flushed skin, peripheral and pulmonary edema, dry sticky mucous membranes, and nausea and vomiting. Options 1, 2, and 4 are not associated with the clinical manifestations of hypernatremia.

*Test-Taking Strategy:* First, determine that the sodium level is elevated and that the child is experiencing hypernatremia. Next, recalling the clinical manifestations associated with hypernatremia will direct you to option 3. If you had difficulty with this question, review the normal sodium level and the clinical manifestations associated with an imbalance.

*Level of Cognitive Ability:* Analysis
*Client Needs:* Physiological Integrity
*Integrated Concept/Process:* Nursing Process/Analysis
*Content Area:* Child Health

*Reference*
Wong, D. (1999). *Whaley & Wong's Nursing care of infants and children* (6th ed.). St. Louis: Mosby, p. 1288.

**16.** A nurse is caring for an infant who is admitted to the hospital with a diagnosis of hemolytic disease. The nurse reviews the laboratory results, expecting to note which of the following in this infant?

1. Decreased red blood cell count
2. Decreased bilirubin count
3. Elevated blood glucose level
4. Decreased white blood cell count

**Answer: 1**

*Rationale:* The two primary pathophysiological alterations associated with hemolytic disease are anemia and hyperbilirubinemia. The red blood cell count is decreased because the red blood cell production cannot keep pace with red blood cell destruction. Hyperbilirubinemia results from the red blood cell destruction accompanying this disorder as well as from the normally decreased ability of the neonate's liver to conjugate and excrete bilirubin efficiently from the body. Hypoglycemia is associated with hypertrophy of the pancreatic islet cells and increased levels of insulin. White blood cell count is not related to this disorder.

*Test-Taking Strategy:* Focus on the infant's diagnosis. Noting the name *hemolytic* will direct you to option 1. If you had difficulty with this question, review the clinical manifestations associated with hemolytic disease.

*Level of Cognitive Ability:* Analysis
*Client Needs:* Physiological Integrity
*Integrated Concept/Process:* Nursing Process/Analysis
*Content Area:* Child Health

*Reference*
Wong, D. (1999). *Whaley & Wong's Nursing care of infants and children* (6th ed.). St. Louis: Mosby, p. 372.

**17.** A nurse is performing an assessment of a child who is to receive a measles, mumps, and rubella (MMR) vaccine. The nurse notes that the child is allergic to eggs. Which of the following would the nurse anticipate to be prescribed for this child?

1. Administration of diphenhydramine (Benadryl) and acetaminophen (Tylenol) prior to the administration of the MMR vaccine
2. Administration of a killed measles vaccine
3. Eliminating this vaccine from the immunization schedule
4. Administration of epinephrine (Adrenalin) prior to the administration of the MMR

**Answer: 2**

*Rationale:* Live measles vaccine is produced by chick embryo cell culture, so the possibility of an anaphylactic hypersensitivity in children with egg allergies should be considered. If there is a question of sensitivity, children should be tested before the administration of MMR vaccine. If a child tests positive for sensitivity, the killed measles vaccine may be given as an alternative.

*Test-Taking Strategy:* Use the process of elimination. Option 3 can be eliminated first because a vaccine would not be eliminated from the immunization schedule. Options 1 and 4 can be eliminated next because the use of medications prior to a vaccine is not normal procedure. Also, recalling that live measles vaccine is produced by chick embryo cell culture will direct you to option 2. Review the procedures related to the administration of vaccines, if you had difficulty with this question.

*Level of Cognitive Ability:* Analysis
*Client Needs:* Health Promotion and Maintenance
*Integrated Concept/Process:* Nursing Process/Analysis
*Content Area:* Child Health

*Reference*
Clark, J., Queener, S., & Karb, V. (2000). *Pharmacologic basis of nursing practice* (6th ed.). St. Louis: Mosby, p. 450.

**18.** Intravenous immune globulin (IVIG) therapy is prescribed for a child with immune thrombocytopenic purpura (ITP). The nurse determines that this medication is prescribed for the child to:

1   Provide immunity against infection
2   Increase the number of circulating platelets
3   Decrease the production of antiplatelet antibodies
4   Prevent infection following exposure to communicable diseases

**Answer: 2**

*Rationale:* IVIG is usually effective in bringing about a rapid increase in the platelet count. It is thought to act by interfering with the attachment of antibody-coded platelets to receptors on the macrophage cells of the reticuloendothelial system. Corticosteroids may be prescribed to enhance vascular stability and decrease the production of antiplatelet antibodies. Options 1, 3, and 4 are unrelated to the administration of this medication.

*Test-Taking Strategy:* Note the relationship between the name of the diagnosis, *thrombocytopenic purpura,* and the word *platelets* in the correct option. This relationship may assist in directing you to the correct option. If you are unfamiliar with ITP and the purpose of IVIG, review this content.

*Level of Cognitive Ability:* Analysis
*Client Needs:* Physiological Integrity
*Integrated Concept/Process:* Nursing Process/Analysis
*Content Area:* Child Health

*Reference*
Bowden, V., Dickey, S., & Greenberg, C. (1998). *Children and their families: The continuum of care.* Philadelphia: W.B. Saunders, p. 562.

---

**19.** A child has been diagnosed with acute poststreptococcal glomerulonephritis, and renal insufficiency is suspected. Which of the following laboratory results will a nurse expect to note in the child?

1   An elevated white blood cell (WBC) count
2   Negative red blood cells in the urinalysis
3   Negative protein in the urinalysis
4   Elevated blood urea nitrogen (BUN) and creatinine

**Answer: 4**

*Rationale:* In poststreptococcal glomerulonephritis, a urinalysis will reveal hematuria with red cell casts. Proteinuria is also present. If renal insufficiency is severe, the BUN and creatinine levels will be elevated. The WBC is usually within normal limits, and mild anemia is common.

*Test-Taking Strategy:* Use the process of elimination, focusing on the child's diagnosis. Recalling that BUN and creatinine are laboratory studies that relate to the renal system will direct you to option 4. Review the clinical manifestations associated with this disorder, if you had difficulty with this question.

*Level of Cognitive Ability:* Analysis
*Client Needs:* Physiological Integrity
*Integrated Concept/Process:* Nursing Process/Analysis
*Content Area:* Child Health

*Reference*
Wong, D. (1999). *Whaley & Wong's Nursing care of infants and children* (6th ed.). St. Louis: Mosby, p. 1380.

**20.** A nurse is assigned to care for a child with juvenile rheumatoid arthritis (JRA). The nurse reviews the plan of care, knowing that which of the following is a priority nursing diagnosis?

1　Body Image Disturbance related to activity intolerance

2　Potential for Self-Care Deficit related to immobility

3　High Risk for Injury related to impaired physical mobility

4　Pain related to the inflammatory process

**Answer: 4**

*Rationale:* All of the nursing diagnoses are appropriate for the child with JRA; however, pain needs to be managed before other problems can be addressed.

*Test-Taking Strategy:* Note the key word *priority.* Use Maslow's Hierarchy of Needs theory, remembering that physiological needs (option 4) receive highest priority. Option 3 addresses safety and security needs. Option 1 addresses self-esteem needs. Option 2 identifies a potential, not an actual, problem. Review care of a child with JRA if you had difficulty with this question.

*Level of Cognitive Ability:* Analysis
*Client Needs:* Physiological Integrity
*Integrated Concept/Process:* Nursing Process/Analysis
*Content Area:* Child Health

*Reference*
Wong, D. (1999). *Whaley & Wong's Nursing care of infants and children* (6th ed.). St. Louis: Mosby, p. 1951.

**21.** A child is admitted to the hospital with a suspected diagnosis of immune thrombocytopenic purpura (ITP). Diagnostic studies are performed. Which of the following diagnostic results is indicative of this disorder?

1　Bone marrow examination indicating an increased number of immature white blood cells

2　Bone marrow examination showing an increased number of megakaryocytes

3　Elevated platelet count

4　Elevated hemoglobin and hematocrit levels

**Answer: 2**

*Rationale:* The laboratory manifestations of ITP include the presence of a low platelet count, usually less than 50,000 cells/mm$^3$. Thrombocytopenia is the only laboratory abnormality expected with ITP. If there has been significant blood loss, there is evidence of anemia in the blood cell count (CBC). If a bone marrow examination is performed, the results with ITP show a normal or increased number of megakaryocytes, the precursors of platelets. Option 1 indicates the bone marrow result that would be found in leukemia.

*Test-Taking Strategy:* Specific knowledge regarding the laboratory findings in ITP is required to answer this question. If you are unfamiliar with this disorder or the associated clinical manifestations, review this content.

*Level of Cognitive Ability:* Analysis
*Client Needs:* Physiological Integrity
*Integrated Concept/Process:* Nursing Process/Analysis
*Content Area:* Child Health

*Reference*
Bowden, V., Dickey, S., & Greenberg, C. (1998). *Children and their families: The continuum of care.* Philadelphia: W.B. Saunders, p. 1559.

**22.** An infant is brought to a health care clinic, and the mother tells a nurse that the infant has been vomiting after meals. The mother tells the nurse that the vomiting is now becoming more frequent and forceful and that the infant seems to be constipated. On assessment, the nurse notes visible peristaltic waves moving from left to right across the abdomen. On the basis of this finding, the nurse would suspect which of the following?

1 Colic
2 Intussusception
3 Pyloric stenosis
4 Congenital megacolon

**Answer: 3**

*Rationale:* In pyloric stenosis, the vomitus contains sour, undigested food, but no bile, the child is constipated, and visible peristaltic waves move from left to right across the abdomen. A movable, palpable, firm olive-shaped mass in the right upper quadrant may be noted. Crying during the evening hours, appearing to be in pain, but eating well and gaining weight are clinical manifestations of colic. An infant who suddenly becomes pale, cries out, and draws the legs up to chest is demonstrating physical signs of intussusception. Ribbon-like stool, bile-stained emesis, absence of peristalsis, and abdominal distention are symptoms of congenital megacolon (Hirschsprung's disease).

*Test-Taking Strategy:* Focus on the data provided in the question. Consider each condition presented in the options, and think about the clinical manifestations of each. Recalling the manifestations associated with pyloric stenosis will direct you to option 3. If you are unfamiliar with this disorder, review its clinical manifestations.

*Level of Cognitive Ability:* Analysis
*Client Needs:* Physiological Integrity
*Integrated Concept/Process:* Nursing Process/Analysis
*Content Area:* Child Health

*Reference*
Wong, D. (1999). *Whaley & Wong's Nursing care of infants and children* (6th ed.). St. Louis: Mosby, p. 1564.

---

**23.** A nurse is reviewing the laboratory analysis of cerebrospinal fluid (CSF) obtained during a lumbar puncture from a child suspected of having bacterial meningitis. Which of the following results would most likely confirm this diagnosis?

1 Cloudy CSF with low protein and low glucose
2 Cloudy CSF with high protein and low glucose
3 Clear CSF with low protein and low glucose
4 Decreased pressure, cloudy CSF with high protein

**Answer: 2**

*Rationale:* A diagnosis of meningitis is made by testing CSF obtained by lumbar puncture. In the case of bacterial meningitis, findings usually include increased pressure, cloudy CSF, high protein, and low glucose. Options 1, 3, and 4 are incorrect.

*Test-Taking Strategy:* Use the process of elimination. Eliminate options 3 and 4 first because clear CSF and decreased pressure are not likely to be found with an infectious process such as meningitis. From the remaining options, recalling that high protein indicates a possible diagnosis of meningitis will direct you to option 2. If you had difficulty with this question, review this diagnostic test.

*Level of Cognitive Ability:* Analysis
*Client Needs:* Physiological Integrity
*Integrated Concept/Process:* Nursing Process/Analysis
*Content Area:* Child Health

*Reference*
Wong, D. (1999). *Whaley & Wong's Nursing care of infants and children* (6th ed.). St. Louis: Mosby, p. 1799.

**24.** A child is admitted to a pediatric unit with a diagnosis of acute gastroenteritis. A nurse monitors the child for signs of hypovolemic shock as a result of fluid and electrolyte losses that have occurred in the child. Which of the following findings would indicate to the nurse the presence of compensated shock?

1  Bradycardia
2  Hypotension
3  Profuse diarrhea
4  Capillary refill time greater than 2 seconds

**Answer: 4**

*Rationale:* Shock may be classified as compensated or decompensated. In compensated shock, the child becomes tachycardic in an effort to increase the cardiac output. The blood pressure remains normal. Capillary refill time may be prolonged and greater than 2 seconds, and the child may become irritable because of increasing hypoxia. The most prevalent cause of hypovolemic shock is fluid and electrolyte losses associated with gastroenteritis. Diarrhea is not a sign of shock; rather it is a cause of the fluid and electrolyte imbalance.

*Test-Taking Strategy:* Use the process of elimination, focusing on the key words *compensated shock*. Recalling that hypotension is a late sign of shock in children will assist in eliminating option 2. Recalling that tachycardia rather bradycardia occurs in shock will assist in eliminating option 1. From the remaining options, focusing on the issue, signs of shock, will direct you to option 4. If you had difficulty with this question, review the signs of shock in a child.

*Level of Cognitive Ability:* Analysis
*Client Needs:* Physiological Integrity
*Integrated Concept/Process:* Nursing Process/Analysis
*Content Area:* Child Health

*Reference*
Bowden, V., Dickey, S., & Greenberg, C. (1998). *Children and their families: The continuum of care.* Philadelphia: W.B. Saunders, p. 2062.

**25.** A mother brings her child to a health care clinic for a routine examination. The mother tells the nurse that the teacher has reported that the child appears to be daydreaming and starring off into space. The teacher tells the mother that this occurs numerous times throughout the day. The remainder of the day the child is alert and participates in classroom activity. The nurse documents the findings and suspects that which of the following is occurring with this child?

1  The child has attention deficit hyperactivity syndrome and is in need of medication
2  The child probably has school phobia
3  The child is experiencing absence seizures
4  The child is showing signs of a behavioral problem

**Answer: 3**

*Rationale:* Absence seizures are a type of generalized seizure that was formerly known as petit mal seizures. They consist of a sudden, brief (no longer than 30 seconds) arrest of the child's motor activities, accompanied by a blank stare and loss of awareness. The child's posture is maintained at the end of the seizure. The child returns to activity that was in process as though nothing has happened. A child with attention deficit hyperactivity syndrome becomes easily distracted, is fidgety, and has difficulty following directions. School phobia includes physical symptoms that usually occur at home and may prevent the child from attending school. Behavior problems would be characterized by more overt symptoms than described in this question.

*Test-Taking Strategy:* Use the process of elimination, focusing on the information provided in the question to direct you to option 3. If you are unfamiliar with the characteristics associated with absence seizures, review this content.

*Level of Cognitive Ability:* Analysis
*Client Needs:* Physiological Integrity
*Integrated Concept/Process:* Nursing Process/Analysis
*Content Area:* Child Health

*Reference*
Bowden, V., Dickey, S., & Greenberg, C. (1998). *Children and their families: The continuum of care.* Philadelphia: W.B. Saunders, p. 1348.

*1.fenol,kitahijurial*

**26.** A mother of a 3-week-old infant arrives at a well-baby clinic for a rescreening test for phenylketonuria (PKU). A nurse reviews the result and notes that the serum phenyl-alanine level is 1.0 mg/dL. The nurse interprets this level as:

1  Normal
2  Elevated, indicating PKU
3  Inconclusive
4  Requiring a repeat study

**Answer: 1**

*Rationale:* The normal PKU level is less than 2 mg/dL. With early postpartum discharge, screening is often performed at less than 2 days of age because of the concern that the infant will be lost to follow-up. Infants should be rescreened by 14 days of age if the initial screening was done at 24 to 48 hours of age.

*Test-Taking Strategy:* Use the process of elimination and knowledge regarding the normal phenylalanine level. Recalling that the normal level is less than 2 mg/dL will direct you to option 1. If you are unfamiliar with this screening test, review this content.

*Level of Cognitive Ability:* Analysis
*Client Needs:* Physiological Integrity
*Integrated Concept/Process:* Nursing Process/Analysis
*Content Area:* Child Health

*Reference*
Wong, D. (1999). *Whaley & Wong's Nursing care of infants and children* (6th ed.). St. Louis: Mosby, p. 383.

**27.** A child is admitted to the hospital with a suspected diagnosis of bacterial endocarditis. The child has been experiencing fever, malaise, anorexia, and a headache, and diagnostic studies are performed. Which of the following studies will primarily confirm the diagnosis?

1  An electrocardiogram (ECG)
2  A white blood cell count
3  A blood culture
4  A sedimentation rate

**Answer: 3**

*Rationale:* The diagnosis of bacterial endocarditis is primarily established on the basis of a positive blood culture of the organisms and visualization of a vegetation on echocardiographic studies. Other laboratory test results that may help to confirm the diagnosis are elevated sedimentation rate and C-reactive protein level. An ECG is not usually helpful in the diagnosis of bacterial endocarditis.

*Test-Taking Strategy:* Note the key words *primarily confirm* in the stem of the question. Use the process of elimination, recalling that bacterial endocarditis is caused by an organism. The only test that will confirm the presence of an organism is the blood culture. If you are unfamiliar with the diagnostic studies associated with bacterial endocarditis, review this content.

*Level of Cognitive Ability:* Analysis
*Client Needs:* Physiological Integrity
*Integrated Concept/Process:* Nursing Process/Analysis
*Content Area:* Child Health

*Reference*
Wong, D. (1999). *Whaley & Wong's Nursing care of infants and children* (6th ed.). St. Louis: Mosby, p. 1628.

**28.** A nurse is caring for a client with an intracranial aneurysm. The nurse interprets that which of the following is related to dysfunction of cranial nerve III?

**1** Mild drowsiness
**2** Less frequent spontaneous speech
**3** Slight slurring of speech
**4** Ptosis of the left eyelid

**Answer: 4**

*Rationale:* Ptosis of the eyelid is due to pressure on and dysfunction of cranial nerve III. Options 1, 2, and 3 are early signs of a deteriorating level of consciousness.

*Test Taking Strategy:* Note the key words *cranial nerve III*. Recalling the function of this nerve will direct you to option 4. If this question was difficult, review the function of cranial nerve III.

*Level of Cognitive Ability:* Analysis
*Client Needs:* Physiological Integrity
*Integrated Concept/Process:* Nursing Process/Analysis
*Content Area:* Adult Health/Neurological

*Reference*
Monahan, F., & Neighbors, M. (1998). *Medical-surgical nursing: Foundations for clinical practice* (2nd ed.). Philadelphia: W.B. Saunders, p. 745.

---

**29.** A client with thrombotic cerebrovascular accident (CVA) experiences periods of emotional lability. The client alternately laughs and cries, and intermittently becomes irritable and demanding. A nurse interprets that this behavior indicates:

**1** That the problem is likely to get worse before it gets better
**2** That the client is experiencing the usual sequelae of a CVA
**3** That the client is not adapting well to the disability
**4** That the client is experiencing side effects of prescribed anticoagulants

**Answer: 2**

*Rationale:* After a CVA, the client often experiences periods of emotional lability, which are characterized by sudden bouts of laughing or crying, or by irritability, depression, confusion, or being demanding. This is a normal part of the clinical picture for the client with this health problem, although it may be difficult for health care personnel and family members to deal with. The other options are incorrect.

*Test-Taking Strategy:* Use the process of elimination. Eliminate options 1 and 4 first. Anticoagulants do not cause emotional lability, and there are no data in the question to support option 1. From the remaining options, recalling the emotional changes that accompany a CVA will direct you to option 2. Review the effects of a CVA if you had difficulty with this question.

*Level of Cognitive Ability:* Analysis
*Client Needs:* Psychosocial Integrity
*Integrated Concept/Process:* Nursing Process/Analysis
*Content Area:* Adult Health/Neurological

*Reference*
Monahan, F., & Neighbors, M. (1998). *Medical-surgical nursing: Foundations for clinical practice* (2nd ed.). Philadelphia: W.B Saunders, p. 804.

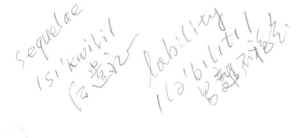

---

**30.** A nurse is caring for a client with myasthenia gravis. The client is vomiting and complaining of abdominal cramps and diarrhea. The nurse also notes that the client is hypotensive and is experiencing facial muscle twitching. The nurse interprets that these symptoms are compatible with:

**1** Systemic infection
**2** A reaction to plasmapheresis
**3** Cholinergic crisis
**4** Myasthenic crisis

**Answer: 3**

*Rationale:* Signs and symptoms of cholinergic crisis include nausea, vomiting, abdominal cramping, diarrhea, blurred vision, pallor, facial muscle twitching, miosis, and hypotension. Cholinergic crisis is due to overmedication with cholinergic (anticholinesterase) medications and is treated by withholding medications. Myasthenic crisis is an exacerbation of myasthenic symptoms and is caused by undermedication with anticholinesterase medications. There are no data in the question to support options 1, 2, and 4.

*Test-Taking Strategy:* Use the process of elimination. Note the lient's diagnosis and think about the treatment for this disorder. Recalling the effects of cholinergic medications and focusing on the data in the question will direct you to option 3. Review the clinical manifestations associated with cholinergic crisis, if you had difficulty with this question.

*Level of Cognitive Ability:* Analysis
*Client Needs:* Physiological Integrity
*Integrated Concept/Process:* Nursing Process/Analysis
*Content Area:* Adult Health/Neurological

*Reference*
Monahan, F., & Neighbors, M. (1998). *Medical-surgical nursing: Foundations for clinical practice* (2nd ed.). Philadelphia: W.B Saunders, p. 782.

# Nursing Process: Planning

**1.** A nurse is caring for a client who is receiving total parental nutrition (TPN). The nurse plans which nursing intervention to prevent infection?
1    Using strict aseptic technique for intravenous site dressing changes
2    Monitoring serum blood urea nitrogen (BUN) daily
3    Weighing the client daily
4    Encouraging increased fluid intake

**Answer: 1**
*Rationale:* Strict aseptic technique is vital during dressing changes because the IV catheter can serve as a direct entry for microorganisms. Options 2, 3, and 4 are not measures that will prevent infection.

*Test-Taking Strategy:* Use the process of elimination. Note the relationship between *infection* in the question and *aseptic* in the correct option. In addition, the only option that will prevent infection is option 1. If you had difficulty with this question, review care of a client receiving TPN.

*Level of Cognitive Ability:* Application
*Client Needs:* Safe, Effective Care Environment
*Integrated Concept/Process:* Nursing Process/Planning
*Content Area:* Fundamental Skills

*Reference*
Smeltzer, S., & Bare, B. (2000). *Brunner & Suddarth's Textbook of medical-surgical nursing* (9th ed.). Philadelphia: Lippincott Williams & Wilkins, p. 853.

**2.** A nurse develops a plan of care for a client with a spica cast that covers a lower extremity and documents a nursing diagnosis of Potential for Altered Elimination. When planning for bowel elimination needs, the nurse includes which of the following in the plan of care?
1    Use a fracture pan for bowel elimination
2    Use a regular bedpan to prevent spilling of contents in the bed
3    Use a bedside commode for all elimination needs
4    Administer an enema daily

**Answer: 1**
*Rationale:* A fracture pan is designed for use in clients with body or leg casts. A client with a spica cast (body cast) that covers a lower extremity cannot bend at the hips to sit up. Therefore, a regular bedpan and a commode would be inappropriate. Daily enemas are not a part of routine care.

*Test-Taking Strategy:* Focus on the key words *covers a lower extremity.* Use the process of elimination, noting the key word *fracture* in the correct option. Review care of the client with a spica cast if you had difficulty with this question.

*Level of Cognitive Ability:* Application
*Client Needs:* Physiological Integrity

*Integrated Concept/Process:* Nursing Process/Planning
*Content Area:* Fundamental Skills

*Reference*
Potter, P., & Perry, A. (2001). *Fundamentals of nursing* (5th ed.). St. Louis: Mosby, p. 1459.

---

**3.** A nurse is caring for a postpartum client with thromboembolitic disease. When planning care to prevent the complication of pulmonary embolism, the nurse prepares specifically to:
1 Administer and monitor anticoagulant therapy as prescribed
2 Assess breath sounds frequently
3 Enforce strict bed rest
4 Monitor vital signs frequently

**Answer: 1**
*Rationale:* The purpose of anticoagulant therapy to treat thromboembolitic disease is to prevent the clot from moving to another area, thus preventing pulmonary embolism. Although options 2, 3, and 4 may be planned for a client with thromboembolitic disease, option 1 will specifically prevent pulmonary embolism.

*Test-Taking Strategy:* Focus on the issue, preventing the complication of pulmonary embolism. Note the key word *specifically* in the stem of the question. Anticoagulant therapy is the only intervention listed that will prevent the clot from traveling to the pulmonary circulation. Review interventions for the client with thromboembolitic disease that will prevent pulmonary embolism if you had difficulty with this question.

*Level of Cognitive Ability:* Application
*Client Needs:* Physiological Integrity
*Integrated Concept/Process:* Nursing Process/Planning
*Content Area:* Maternity

*Reference*
Sherwen, L., Scoloveno, M.A., & Weingarten, C. (1999). *Maternity nursing: Care of the childbearing family* (3rd ed.). Stamford, Conn.: Appleton & Lange, p. 906.

---

**4.** After reviewing a client's serum electrolytes, a physician states that the client would benefit most from an isotonic IV solution. A nurse plans care, anticipating that the order will indicate that which of the following solutions should be administered?
1 0.45% saline
2 5% dextrose in water
3 10% dextrose in water
4 5% dextrose in 0.9% saline

**Answer: 2**
*Rationale:* 5% dextrose in water is an isotonic solution. Another example of an isotonic solution is 0.9% saline. 0.45% saline is a hypotonic solution. 10% dextrose in water and 5% dextrose in 0.9% saline are hypertonic solutions.

*Test-Taking Strategy:* To answer this question accurately, you must be familiar with the tonicity of various IV solutions. Note the key word *isotonic* and recall that 5% dextrose in water and 0.9% saline are isotonic. If this question was difficult, review the tonicity of IV fluids.

*Level of Cognitive Ability:* Analysis
*Client Needs:* Physiological Integrity
*Integrated Concept/Process:* Nursing Process/Planning
*Content Area:* Fundamental Skills

*Reference*
LeMone, P., & Burke, K. (2000). *Medical-surgical nursing: Critical thinking in client care* (2nd ed.). Upper Saddle River, N.J.: Prentice-Hall, p. 110.

**5.** A nurse is admitting to the hospital a client who recently had a bilateral adrenalectomy. Which of the following interventions is essential for the nurse to include in the client's plan of care?
  1   Prevent social isolation
  2   Discuss changes in body image
  3   Consider occupational therapy
  4   Avoid stress-producing situations and procedures

**Answer: 4**
*Rationale:* Adrenalectomy can lead to adrenal insufficiency. Adrenal hormones are essential in maintaining homeostasis in response to stressors. Options 1, 2, and 3 are not essential interventions specific to this client's problem.

*Test-Taking Strategy:* Note the key word *essential* in the stem of the question. This indicates the need to prioritize. Remember that according to Maslow's Hierarchy of Needs theory, physiological needs come first. The stress reaction involves physiological processes. Review the postoperative effects following an adrenalectomy, if you had difficulty with this question.

*Level of Cognitive Ability:* Application
*Client Needs:* Physiological Integrity
*Integrated Concept/Process:* Nursing Process/Planning
*Content Area:* Adult Health/Endocrine

*Reference*
Black, J., Hawks, J., & Keene, A. (2001). *Medical-surgical nursing: Clinical management for positive outcomes* (6th ed.). Philadelphia: W.B. Saunders, p. 1131.

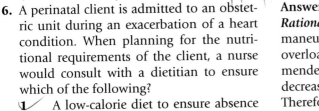

**6.** A perinatal client is admitted to an obstetric unit during an exacerbation of a heart condition. When planning for the nutritional requirements of the client, a nurse would consult with a dietitian to ensure which of the following?
  1   A low-calorie diet to ensure absence of weight gain
  2   A diet low in fluids and fiber to decrease blood volume
  3   A diet high in fluids and fiber to decrease constipation
  4   Unlimited sodium intake to increase circulating blood volume

**Answer: 3**
*Rationale:* Constipation can cause the client to use the Valsalva maneuver. This maneuver can cause blood to rush to the heart and overload the cardiac system. A low-calorie diet is not recommended during pregnancy. Diets low in fluid and fiber can cause a decrease in blood volume that can deprive the fetus of nutrients. Therefore, adequate fluid intake and high-fiber foods are important. Sodium should be restricted to some degree, as prescribed by the physician, because it will cause an overload of the circulating blood volume and contribute to cardiac complications.

*Test Taking Strategy:* Use the process of elimination. Think about the physiology of the cardiac system, the maternal and fetus needs, and the factors that increase the workload on the heart to answer the question. If you had difficulty with this question, review nursing measures for the pregnant client with cardiac disease.

*Level of Cognitive Ability:* Analysis
*Client Needs:* Physiological Integrity
*Integrated Concept/Process:* Nursing Process/Planning
*Content Area:* Maternity

*Reference*
Gorrie, T., McKinney, E., & Murray, S. (1998). *Foundations of maternal newborn nursing* (2nd ed.). Philadelphia: W.B. Saunders, p. 724.

**7.** A nurse is developing a plan of care for a client with a hip spica cast. In the planning, the nurse includes measures to limit complications of prolonged immobility. The nurse includes which essential item in the plan to prevent this complication?

1 Provide a daily fluid intake of 1000 mL

2 Monitor for signs of low serum calcium

3 Maintain the client in a supine position

4 Limit the intake of milk and milk products

**Answer: 4**

*Rationale:* Daily fluid intake should be 2000 mL or greater. The nurse should monitor for signs and symptoms of hypercalcemia, such as nausea, vomiting, polydipsia, polyuria, and lethargy. A supine position increases urinary stasis; therefore it should be limited or avoided. Limiting milk and milk products is the best measure.

*Test-Taking Strategy:* Focus on the issue, a complication of prolonged immobility. Option 3 should be eliminated immediately because it refers to maintaining an immobile client in one position. Eliminate option 1 next, noting the amount of fluid in this option. From the remaining options, recalling the effect of the movement of calcium into the blood from the bones will direct you to option 4. If you had difficulty with this question, review the complications of immobility.

*Level of Cognitive Ability:* Application
*Client Needs:* Physiological Integrity
*Integrated Concept/Process:* Nursing Process/Planning
*Content Area:* Adult Health/Musculoskeletal

**Reference**
Smeltzer, S., & Bare, B. (2000). *Brunner & Suddarth's Textbook of medical-surgical nursing* (9th ed.). Philadelphia: Lippincott Williams & Wilkins, p. 1780.

**8.** A nurse determines that the result of a Mantoux tuberculin skin test is positive. In order to most accurately diagnose tuberculosis (TB), the nurse plans to consult with the physician to follow up the skin test with a:

1 Chest x-ray

2 Computed tomography scan of the chest

3 Sputum culture

4 Complete blood cell count

**Answer: 3**

*Rationale:* Although the findings of a chest x-ray examination are important, it is not possible to make a diagnosis of TB solely on the basis of this examination. This is because other diseases can mimic the appearance of TB. The demonstration of tubercle bacilli bacteriologically is essential for establishing a diagnosis. Microscopic examination of sputum for acid-fast bacilli is usually the first bacteriological evidence of the presence of tubercle bacilli. Options 2 and 4 will not diagnose TB.

*Test-Taking Strategy:* Note the key words *most accurately diagnose tuberculosis*. Recalling that the presence of tubercle bacilli indicates TB will direct you to option 3. Review the tests used in diagnosing tuberculosis, if you had difficulty with this question.

*Level of Cognitive Ability:* Application
*Client Needs:* Physiological Integrity
*Integrated Concept/Process:* Nursing Process/Planning
*Content Area:* Adult Health/Respiratory

**Reference**
Smeltzer, S., & Bare, B. (2000). *Brunner & Suddarth's Textbook of medical-surgical nursing* (9th ed.). Philadelphia: Lippincott Williams & Wilkins, p. 438.

**9.** A home care nurse is preparing a plan of care for a client with Meniere's disease who is experiencing severe vertigo. Which nursing intervention would the nurse include in the plan of care to assist the client in controlling the vertigo?
1 Encourage the client to increase daily fluid intake
2 Encourage the client to avoid sudden head movements
3 Instruct the client to cut down on cigarette smoking
4 Instruct the client to increase sodium in the diet

**Answer: 2**
*Rationale:* The nurse instructs the client to make slow head movements to prevent worsening of the vertigo. Dietary changes, such as salt and fluid restrictions, that reduce the amount of endolymphatic fluid are sometimes prescribed. Clients are advised to stop smoking because of its vasoconstrictive effects.

*Test-Taking Strategy:* Identify the issue of the question, severe vertigo. Note the relationship between vertigo and the correct option, to avoid sudden head movements. Recalling that salt and fluid restrictions are sometimes prescribed will also assist in eliminating options 1 and 4. Noting the words *cut down* in option 3 will assist in eliminating this option. If you had difficulty with this question, review measures that will reduce vertigo in the client with Meniere's disease.

*Level of Cognitive Ability:* Application
*Client Needs:* Health Promotion and Maintenance
*Integrated Concept/Process:* Nursing Process/Planning
*Content Area:* Adult Health/Ear

*Reference*
Ignatavicius, D., Workman, M., & Mishler, M. (1999). *Medical-surgical nursing across the health care continuum* (3rd ed.). Philadelphia: W.B. Saunders, p. 1217.

**10.** An 18-year-old woman is admitted to a mental health unit with the diagnosis of anorexia nervosa. A nurse plans care, knowing that health promotion should focus on:
1 Helping the client identify and examine dysfunctional thoughts and beliefs
2 Emphasizing social interaction with clients who are withdrawn
3 Providing a supportive environment
4 Examining intrapsychic conflicts and past issues

**Answer: 1**
*Rationale:* Health promotion focuses on helping clients identify and examine dysfunctional thoughts as well as identify and examine values and beliefs that maintain these thoughts. Providing a supportive environment is important but is not as primary as option 1 in this client. Emphasizing social interaction is not appropriate at this time. Examining intrapsychic conflicts and past issues is not directly related to the client's problem.

*Test-Taking Strategy:* Use the process of elimination, focusing on the issue of health promotion. Option 1 is the only option that is specifically client centered. This option also focuses on assessment, the first step of the nursing process. Review care of the client with anorexia nervosa if you had difficulty with this question.

*Level of Cognitive Ability:* Application
*Client Needs:* Health Promotion and Maintenance
*Integrated Concept/Process:* Nursing Process/Planning
*Content Area:* Mental Health

*Reference*
Varcarolis, E. (1998). *Foundations of psychiatric mental health nursing* (3rd ed.). Philadelphia: W.B. Saunders, p. 812.

702 UNIT III Integrated Concepts and Processes

**11.** A nurse is preparing discharge plans for a client who has attempted suicide. The nurse includes which of the following in the plan?

1 Weekly follow-up appointments
2 Contracts and immediately available crisis resources
3 Encouraging family and friends always to be present
4 Providing phone numbers for the hospital and the physician

**Answer: 2**

*Rationale:* Crisis times may occur between appointments. Contracts facilitate clients feeling a responsibility for keeping a promise. This gives the client control. Family and friends cannot always be present. Providing phone numbers will not ensure the immediate availability of crisis intervention.

*Test-Taking Strategy:* Focus on the issue, the immediate availability of resources for the client. Eliminate option 3 first because this is unrealistic. Options 1 and 4 will not necessarily provide immediately available resources. Also, note the word *immediately* in the correct option. Review discharge plans for a client who has attempted suicide if you had difficulty with this question.

*Level of Cognitive Ability:* Application
*Client Needs:* Psychosocial Integrity
*Integrated Concept/Process:* Nursing Process/Planning
*Content Area:* Mental Health

*Reference*
Fortinash, K., & Holoday-Worret, P. (2000). *Psychiatric mental health nursing* (2nd ed.). St. Louis: Mosby, p. 672.

**12.** A nurse is developing a plan of care for a newborn infant diagnosed with bilateral club feet. The nurse includes instructions in the plan to tell the parents that:

1 Genetic testing is wise for future pregnancies, since other children born to this couple may also be affected
2 If casting is needed, it will begin at birth and continue for 12 weeks; then the condition will be reevaluated
3 Surgery performed immediately after birth has been found to be most effective in achieving a complete recovery
4 The regimen of manipulation and casting is effective in all cases of bilateral club feet

**Answer: 2**

*Rationale:* Casting should begin at birth and continue for at least 12 weeks or until maximum correction is achieved. At this time, corrective shoes may provide support to maintain alignment or surgery can be performed. Surgery is usually delayed until 4 to 12 months of age. Options 3 and 4 are inaccurate. Option 1 does not address the issue of the question.

*Test-Taking Strategy:* Focus on the issue, parental instructions for a child with bilateral club feet. Eliminate option 1 because this is not the time to discuss the future. Eliminate option 3 because of the word *immediately*. From the remaining options, note that option 2 provides accurate information and that option 4 contains the absolute word *all*. Review the treatment plan for bilateral club feet, if you had difficulty with this question.

*Level of Cognitive Ability:* Application
*Client Needs:* Health Promotion and Maintenance
*Integrated Concept/Process:* Nursing Process/Planning
*Content Area:* Child Health

*Reference*
Wong, D. (1999). *Whaley & Wong's Nursing care of infants and children* (6th ed.). St. Louis: Mosby, p. 511.

**13.** A nurse is planning to assist with obtaining a set of arterial blood gases on a client. In addition to sending the specimen to the laboratory immediately, the nurse plans to provide which of the following items to optimally maintain the integrity of the specimen?

1 A syringe containing a preservative
2 A syringe containing a preservative and a bag of ice
3 A heparinized syringe and a preservative
4 A heparinized syringe and a bag of ice

**Answer: 4**

*Rationale:* The arterial blood gas sample is obtained by using a heparinized syringe. The sample of blood is placed on ice and sent to the laboratory immediately. A preservative is not used.

*Test-Taking Strategy:* Specific knowledge regarding this procedure is needed to answer this question. If you are unfamiliar with this procedure, review this content

*Level of Cognitive Ability:* Application
*Client Needs:* Physiological Integrity
*Integrated Concept/Process:* Nursing Process/Planning
*Content Area:* Adult Health/Respiratory

*Reference*
Black, J., Hawks, J., & Keene, A. (2001). *Medical-surgical nursing: Clinical management for positive outcomes* (6th ed.). Philadelphia: W.B. Saunders, p. 1641.

**14.** A client is experiencing diabetes insipidus secondary to cranial surgery. The nurse who is caring for the client plans to implement which of these anticipated therapies?

1 Fluid restriction
2 IV replacement of fluid losses
3 Increased sodium intake
4 Administering diuretics

**Answer: 2**

*Rationale:* The client with diabetes insipidus excretes large amounts of extremely dilute urine. This usually occurs as a result of decreased synthesis or release of antidiuretic hormone (ADH) in conditions such as head injury, surgery near the hypothalamus, or increased intracranial pressure. Corrective measures include allowing ample oral fluid intake, administering IV fluid as needed to replace sensible and insensible losses, and administering vasopressin (Pitressin). Sodium is not administered because the serum sodium level is usually high, as is the serum osmolality. Option 4 is incorrect.

*Test-Taking Strategy:* Focus on the client's diagnosis, recalling that a large fluid loss is the problem in this client. This will assist in eliminating options 1 and 4. From the remaining options, recalling that the serum sodium level is already elevated in this disorder, or knowing that fluid replacement is the most direct form of therapy for fluid loss, will direct you to option 2. Review the treatment for diabetes insipidus, if you had difficulty with this question.

*Level of Cognitive Ability:* Analysis
*Client Needs:* Physiological Integrity
*Integrated Concept/Process:* Nursing Process/Planning
*Content Area:* Adult Health/Neurological

*Reference*
Monahan, F., & Neighbors, M. (1998). *Medical-surgical nursing: Foundations for clinical practice* (2nd ed.). Philadelphia: W.B Saunders, p. 1275.

**15.** A nurse is planning care for a child with an infectious and communicable disease. The nurse determines that the primary goal is that the:

1 Child will experience only minor complications
2 Child will not spread the infection to others
3 Public health department will be notified
4 Child will experience mild discomfort

**Answer: 2**

*Rationale:* The primary goal is to prevent the spread of the disease to others. The child should experience no complications. Although the health department may need to be notified at some point, it is not the most important primary goal. It is also important to prevent discomfort as much as possible.

*Test-Taking Strategy:* Use the process of elimination. Note the key words *primary goal.* Note the relationship between *infectious and communicable disease* in the question and *infection* in the correct option. Review goals of care for the child with an infectious and communicable disease if you had difficulty with this question.

*Level of Cognitive Ability:* Analysis
*Client Needs:* Safe, Effective Care Environment
*Integrated Concept/Process:* Nursing Process/Planning
*Content Area:* Child Health

*Reference*
Wong, D. (1999). *Whaley & Wong's Nursing care of infants and children* (6th ed.). St. Louis: Mosby, p. 730.

---

**16.** A nurse is preparing to care for an infant with pertussis. In planning care, the nurse addresses which most critical problem first?

1 Ineffective airway clearance
2 Fluid volume excess
3 Sleep pattern disturbance
4 High risk for infection

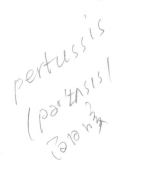

**Answer: 1**

*Rationale:* The most important problem relates to adequate air exchange. Because of the copious, thick secretions that occur with pertussis and the small airways of an infant, air exchange is critical. A fluid volume deficit is more likely to occur in this infant because of the thick secretions and vomiting. Sleep patterns may be disturbed because of the coughing, but sleep pattern disturbance is not the most critical issue. Infection is an important consideration, but airway is the priority.

*Test-Taking Strategy:* Use the process of elimination and the ABCs—airway, breathing, and circulation. Airway is always the most critical concern. This should direct you to option 1. Review care of the infant with pertussis if you had difficulty with this question.

*Level of Cognitive Ability:* Application
*Client Needs:* Physiological Integrity
*Integrated Concept/Process:* Nursing Process/Planning
*Content Area:* Child Health

*Reference*
Wong, D. (1999). *Whaley & Wong's Nursing care of infants and children* (6th ed.). St. Louis: Mosby, p. 726.

**17.** A nurse is planning care for an infant who has pyloric stenosis. In order to most effectively meet the infant's preoperative needs, the nurse includes which of the following in the plan of care?

1 Monitor the IV infusion, intake and output, and weight

2 Provide small, frequent feedings of glucose, water, and electrolytes

3 Administer enemas until returns are clear

4 Provide the mother privacy to breast-feed every 2 hours

**Answer: 1**

*Rationale:* Preoperatively, important nursing responsibilities include monitoring the intravenous infusion, intake and output, and weight, and obtaining urine specific gravity measurements. In addition, weighing the infant's diapers provides information regarding output. Preoperatively, the infant is kept NPO unless the physician prescribes a thickened formula. Enemas until clear would further compromise the fluid volume status.

*Test-Taking Strategy:* Use the process of elimination, noting the key word *preoperative.* Eliminate options 2 and 4 because the infant needs to be NPO in the preoperative period. Eliminate option 3 because enemas would further compromise the fluid balance status. Review preoperative care of the infant with pyloric stenosis, if you had difficulty with this question.

*Level of Cognitive Ability:* Application
*Client Needs:* Physiological Integrity
*Integrated Concept/Process:* Nursing Process/Planning
*Content Area:* Child Health

*Reference*
Wong, D. (1999). *Whaley & Wong's Nursing care of infants and children* (6th ed.). St. Louis: Mosby, p. 1564.

**18.** A client who was a victim of a gunshot incident states, "I feel like I am losing my mind. I keep hearing the gunshots and seeing my friend lying on the ground." A nurse most appropriately plans strategies to formulate a therapeutic relationship that will include:

1 Asking a psychiatrist to order an antianxiety medication

2 Encouraging the client to talk about the incident and feelings related to it

3 Encouraging the client to think about how lucky he or she is to be alive

4 Teaching the client relaxation techniques

**Answer: 2**

*Rationale:* In developing a therapeutic relationship, it is important to acknowledge and validate the client's feelings. Although teaching the client relaxation techniques may be helpful at some point, it is not related to the issue of the question. Options 1 and 3 are nontherapeutic techniques and do not promote a therapeutic relationship.

*Test-Taking Strategy:* Use therapeutic communication techniques. Eliminate options 1 and 3 because they do not encourage further discussion about the client's feelings. Teaching the client how to relax may be helpful at some point, but not in the beginning of the therapeutic relationship. Remember to address the client's feelings. Review therapeutic communication techniques if you had difficulty with this question.

*Level of Cognitive Ability:* Application
*Client Needs:* Psychosocial Integrity
*Integrated Concept/Process:* Nursing Process/Planning
*Content Area:* Mental Health

*Reference*
Varcarolis, E. (1998). *Foundations of psychiatric mental health nursing* (3rd ed.). Philadelphia: W.B. Saunders, pp. 188-189.

**19.** A nurse is caring for a hospitalized child with a diagnosis of rheumatic fever (RF), and the child has developed carditis. The mother asks the nurse to explain the meaning of carditis. The nurse plans to respond, knowing that which of the following most appropriately describes this complication of RF?

1 Tender, painful joints, especially in the elbows, knees, ankles, and wrists

2 Inflammation of all parts of the heart, primarily the mitral valve

3 Involuntary movements affecting the legs, arms, and face

4 Red skin lesions that start as flat or slightly raised macules, usually over the trunk, and spread peripherally

**Answer: 2**

*Rationale:* Carditis is the inflammation of all parts of the heart, primarily the mitral valve, and is a complication of RF. Option 1 describes polyarthritis. Option 3 describes chorea. Option 4 describes erythema marginatum.

*Test-Taking Strategy:* Use the process of elimination. Note the relationship between the word *carditis* in the question and *heart* in the correct option. If you are unfamiliar with this complication that is associated with rheumatic fever, review this content.

*Level of Cognitive Ability:* Application
*Client Needs:* Physiological Integrity
*Integrated Concept/Process:* Nursing Process/Planning
*Content Area:* Child Health

*Reference*
Wong, D. (1999). *Whaley & Wong's Nursing care of infants and children* (6th ed.). St. Louis: Mosby, p. 1629.

**20.** A nurse receives a telephone call from the emergency room and is told that a 7-month-old infant with febrile seizures will be admitted to the pediatric unit. In planning care for the admission of the infant, the nurse would anticipate the need for which of the following?

1 A padded tongue blade taped to the head of the bed

2 A code cart at the bedside

3 Restraints at the bedside

4 Suction equipment at the bedside

**Answer: 4**

*Rationale:* A padded tongue blade should never be used; in fact, nothing should be placed in a client's mouth during a seizure. During a seizure, the infant should be placed in a side-lying position, but should not be restrained. Suctioning may be required during a seizure to remove secretions that obstruct the airway. It is not necessary to place a code cart at the bedside, but a cart should be readily available on the nursing unit.

*Test-Taking Strategy:* Use the process of elimination and the ABCs—airway, breathing, and circulation—to answer the question. Option 4 is the only option that specifically relates to airway. Review nursing interventions for an infant with seizures, if you had difficulty with this question.

*Level of Cognitive Ability:* Application
*Client Needs:* Physiological Integrity
*Integrated Concept/Process:* Nursing Process/Planning
*Content Area:* Child Health

*Reference*
Wong, D. (1999). *Whaley & Wong's Nursing care of infants and children* (6th ed.). St. Louis: Mosby, p. 1813.

**21.** A 10-month-old infant is hospitalized for respiratory syncytial virus (RSV). A nurse develops a plan of care for the infant. On the basis of the developmental stage of the infant, the nurse includes which of the following in the plan of care?

**1** Wash hands, wear a mask when caring for the child, and keep the child as quiet as possible

**2** Follow the home feeding schedule, and allow the infant to be held only when the parents visit

**3** Restrain the infant with a total body restraint to prevent any tubes from being dislodged

**4** Provide a consistent routine, as well as touching, rocking, and cuddling, throughout the hospitalization

**Answer: 4**

*Rationale:* A 10-month-old infant is in the Trust vs. Mistrust stage of psychosocial development (Erik Erikson) and in the sensorimotor period of cognitive development (Piaget). RSV is not airborne (mask is not required) and is usually transmitted by the hands. Touching and holding the infant only when the parents visit will not provide adequate stimulation and interpersonal contact for the infant. Total body restraint is unnecessary and an incorrect action. Hospitalization may have an adverse effect. A consistent routine accompanied by touching, rocking, and cuddling will help the child to develop trust and provide sensory stimulation.

*Test-Taking Strategy:* Note the age and diagnosis of the infant. Focusing on the key words *developmental stage of the infant* will direct you to option 4. Review the psychosocial needs of an infant if you had difficulty with this question.

*Level of Cognitive Ability:* Application
*Client Needs:* Health Promotion and Maintenance
*Integrated Concept/Process:* Nursing Process/Planning
*Content Area:* Child Health

*Reference*
Wong, D. (1999). *Whaley & Wong's Nursing care of infants and children* (6th ed.). St. Louis: Mosby, p. 1479.

**22.** A pediatric nurse receives a telephone call from the admission office and is informed that a child with a diagnosis of Reye's syndrome is being admitted to the hospital. The nurse develops a plan of care for the child and includes which priority nursing action in the plan?

**1** Provide a quiet environment with low, dimmed lighting

**2** Monitor for hearing loss

**3** Monitor intake and output (I & O)

**4** Reposition the child every 2 hours

**Answer: 1**

*Rationale:* Cerebral edema is a progressive part of the disease process in Reye's syndrome. A major component of care for a child with Reye's syndrome is to maintain effective cerebral perfusion and control intracranial pressure. Decreasing stimuli in the environment would decrease the stress on the cerebral tissue and neuron responses. Hearing loss does not occur in this disorder. Although monitoring I & O may be a component of the plan, it is not the priority. Changing the body position every 2 hours would not affect the cerebral edema and intracranial pressure directly. The child should be in a head-elevated position to decrease the progression of cerebral edema and promote drainage of cerebrospinal fluid.

*Test-Taking Strategy:* Note the key words *priority nursing action*. Recalling that increased intracranial pressure is a concern will direct you to option 1. If you had difficulty with this question, review the priorities in the plan of care for a child with Reye's syndrome.

*Level of Cognitive Ability:* Application
*Client Needs:* Physiological Integrity
*Integrated Concept/Process:* Nursing Process/Planning
*Content Area:* Child Health

*Reference*
Wong, D. (1999). *Whaley & Wong's Nursing care of infants and children* (6th ed.). St. Louis: Mosby, p. 1806.

**23.** A nursing student is preparing to conduct a clinical conference on cerebral palsy. Which of the following characteristics related to this disorder will the student plan to include in the discussion?

1. Cerebral palsy is a chronic disability characterized by a difficulty in controlling muscles
2. Cerebral palsy is an infectious disease of the central nervous system
3. Cerebral palsy is an inflammation of the brain as a result of a viral illness
4. Cerebral palsy is a congenital condition that results in moderate to severe retardation

**Answer: 1**

*Rationale:* Cerebral palsy is a chronic disability characterized by a difficulty in controlling muscles as a result of an abnormality in the extrapyramidal or pyramidal motor system. Meningitis is an infectious process of the central nervous system. Encephalitis is an inflammation of the brain that occurs as a result of viral illness or central nervous system infections. Down's syndrome is an example of a congenital condition that results in moderate to severe retardation.

*Test-Taking Strategy:* Use the process of elimination. Eliminate options 2 and 3 first, noting that they are similar and basically stating the same thing. From the remaining options, note the relationship between *palsy* in the question and *muscles* in the correct option. If you had difficulty with this question, review the characteristics associated with cerebral palsy.

*Level of Cognitive Ability:* Application
*Client Needs:* Physiological Integrity
*Integrated Concept/Process:* Nursing Process/Planning
*Content Area:* Child Health

*Reference*
Wong, D. (1999). *Whaley & Wong's Nursing care of infants and children* (6th ed.). St. Louis: Mosby, p. 1966.

---

**24.** A nursing student is asked to conduct a clinical conference on autism. The student plans to include in the discussion that the primary characteristic associated with autism is:

1. The consistent imitation of others' actions
2. Normal social play
3. Lack of social interaction and awareness
4. Normal verbal but abnormal nonverbal communication

**Answer: 3**

*Rationale:* Autism is a severe developmental disorder that begins in infancy or toddlerhood. A primary characteristic is lack of social interaction and awareness. Social behaviors in autism include the lack of or abnormal imitation of others' actions and the lack of or abnormal social play. Additional characteristics include lack of or impaired verbal communication and marked abnormal nonverbal communication.

*Test-Taking Strategy:* Use the process of elimination. Eliminate options 2 and 4 first because they include normal behaviors. From the remaining options, recalling that the autistic child lacks social interaction and awareness will direct you to option 3. If you had difficulty with this question, review the characteristics associated with autism.

*Level of Cognitive Ability:* Analysis
*Client Needs:* Psychosocial Integrity
*Integrated Concept/Process:* Nursing Process/Planning
*Content Area:* Child Health

*Reference*
Wong, D. (1999). *Whaley & Wong's Nursing care of infants and children* (6th ed.). St. Louis: Mosby, p. 657.

**25.** A nurse is developing a plan of care for a child returning from the operating room after a tonsillectomy. The nurse avoids placing which intervention in the plan of care?

**1** Offer clear, cool liquids when the child is awake

**2** Eliminate milk or milk products from the diet

**3** Monitor for bleeding from the surgical site

**4** Suction whenever necessary

**Answer: 4**

*Rationale:* After tonsillectomy, suction equipment should be available, but suctioning is not performed unless there is an airway obstruction. Clear, cool liquids are encouraged. Milk and milk products are avoided initially because they coat the throat, causing the child to clear the throat, thus increasing the risk of bleeding. Option 3 is an important intervention after any type of surgery.

*Test-Taking Strategy:* Use the process of elimination, noting the key word *avoids*. Eliminate option 3 first because this is an expected general nursing procedure. From the remaining options, thinking about the anatomical location of the surgery will direct you to option 4. Suctioning following tonsillectomy will disrupt the integrity of the surgical site and can cause bleeding. Review postoperative care after tonsillectomy, if you had difficulty with this question.

*Level of Cognitive Ability:* Application
*Client Needs:* Physiological Integrity
*Integrated Concept/Process:* Nursing Process/Planning
*Content Area:* Child Health

*Reference*
Wong, D. (1999). *Whaley & Wong's Nursing care of infants and children* (6th ed.). St. Louis: Mosby, p. 1466.

**26.** A nurse is preparing a plan of care for a child being admitted to the hospital with a diagnosis of congestive heart failure (CHF). The nurse avoids including which of the following in the plan?

**1** Limiting the time the child is allowed to bottle-feed

**2** Elevating the head of the bed

**3** Waking the child for feeding to ensure adequate nutrition

**4** Providing oxygen during stressful periods

**Answer: 3**

*Rationale:* Measures that will decrease the workload on the heart include limiting the time the child is allowed to bottle-feed or breast-feed, elevating the head of the bed, allowing for uninterrupted rest periods, and providing oxygen during stressful periods.

*Test-Taking Strategy:* Note the key word *avoids* in the stem of the question. Review each option carefully, recalling that the goal for a child with CHF is to decrease the workload on the heart. Option 3 is the only option that will not provide this measure. If you are unfamiliar with the measures associated with caring for a child with CHF, review this content.

*Level of Cognitive Ability:* Application
*Client Needs:* Physiological Integrity
*Integrated Concept/Process:* Nursing Process/Planning
*Content Area:* Child Health

*Reference*
Wong, D. (1999). *Whaley & Wong's Nursing care of infants and children* (6th ed.). St. Louis: Mosby, p. 1594.

**27.** A nurse is preparing a plan of care for a child with leukemia who is scheduled to receive chemotherapy. Which of the following nursing interventions will be included in the plan of care?
1  Monitor rectal temperatures every 4 hours
2  Monitor mouth and anus each shift for signs of breakdown
3  Provide meticulous mouth care several times daily, using an alcohol-based mouthwash and a toothbrush
4  Encourage the child to consume fresh fruits and vegetables to maintain nutritional status

**Answer: 2**
*Rationale:* When the child is receiving chemotherapy, the nurse should avoid taking rectal temperatures. Oral temperatures are also avoided if mouth ulcers are present. Axillary temperatures should be done to prevent alterations in skin integrity. Meticulous mouth care should be performed, but the nurse should avoid alcohol-based mouthwash and should use a soft-bristled toothbrush. The nurse should assess the mouth and anus each shift for ulcers, erythema, or breakdown. Bland, nonirritating foods and liquids should be provided to the child. Fresh fruits and vegetables need to be avoided because they can harbor organisms. Chemotherapy can cause neutropenia, and the child should be maintained on a low-bacteria diet if the white blood cell count is low.

*Test-Taking Strategy:* Use the process of elimination, reading each option carefully. Thinking about the side effects that can occur with chemotherapy will direct you to option 2. If you had difficulty with this question, review these important nursing measures.

*Level of Cognitive Ability:* Application
*Client Needs:* Physiological Integrity
*Integrated Concept/Process:* Nursing Process/Planning
*Content Area:* Child Health

*Reference*
Wong, D. (1999). *Whaley & Wong's Nursing care of infants and children* (6th ed.). St. Louis: Mosby, p. 1727.

**28.** A nurse is assisting in preparing to admit a client from the post-anesthesia care unit who has had microvascular decompression of the trigeminal nerve. The nurse asks a nursing assistant to make sure that which of the following equipment is at the bedside when the client arrives?
1  Flashlight and pulse oximeter
2  Cardiac monitor and pulse oximeter
3  Padded bed rails and suction equipment
4  Blood pressure cuff and cardiac monitor

**Answer: 1**
*Rationale:* The postoperative care of a client having microvascular decompression of the trigeminal nerve is the same as for a client undergoing craniotomy. This client requires hourly neurological assessment, as well as monitoring of cardiovascular and respiratory status. Cardiac monitoring and padded bed rails are not indicated unless there is a special need based on a client history of cardiac disease or seizures, respectively. Suctioning is done very cautiously and only when necessary after craniotomy, to avoid increasing the intracranial pressure.

*Test-Taking Strategy:* Use the process of elimination, focusing on the data in the question. The client is not necessarily at risk for seizures postoperatively, so option 3 is eliminated first. Knowing that the procedure is done by craniotomy enables you to recall that neurological assessment is needed, which helps you choose option 1 from the remaining options. A flashlight would be required to perform a neurological assessment. Review care of a client following this procedure, if you had difficulty with this question.

*Level of Cognitive Ability:* Application
*Client Needs:* Physiological Integrity
*Integrated Concept/Process:* Nursing Process/Planning
*Content Area:* Adult Health/Neurological

*Reference*
Monahan, F., & Neighbors, M. (1998). *Medical-surgical nursing: Foundations for clinical practice* (2nd ed.). Philadelphia: W.B Saunders, p. 760.

---

**29.** A nurse is receiving a client in transfer from the emergency room; the client has a diagnosis of Guillain-Barré syndrome. The client's chief complaint is an ascending paralysis that has reached the level of the waist. The nurse plans to have which of the following items available for emergency use?
1   Cardiac monitor and intubation tray
2   Blood pressure cuff and flashlight
3   Nebulizer and pulse oximeter
4   Flashlight and incentive spirometer

**Answer: 1**
*Rationale:* A client with Guillain-Barré syndrome is at risk for respiratory failure because of ascending paralysis. An intubation tray should be available for emergency use. Another complication of this syndrome is cardiac dysrhythmias, the risk of which necessitates cardiac monitoring.

*Test-Taking Strategy:* Use the process of elimination. Note the key words *emergency use*, which tell you that the correct answer will be an option that contains equipment that is not routinely used in providing care. With this in mind, eliminate options 2 and 4 first, since a flashlight is needed for routine neurological assessment. From the remaining options, recalling the complications of this syndrome will direct you to option 1. Review nursing care measures for the client with Guillain-Barré syndrome, if you had difficulty with this question.

*Level of Cognitive Ability:* Application
*Client Needs:* Physiological Integrity
*Integrated Concept/Process:* Nursing Process/Planning
*Content Area:* Adult Health/Neurological

*Reference*
Monahan, F., & Neighbors, M. (1998). *Medical-surgical nursing: Foundations for clinical practice* (2nd ed.). Philadelphia: W.B Saunders, p. 774.

---

**30.** A nurse in a newborn nursery receives a telephone call and is informed that a newborn infant whose mother is Rh negative will be admitted to the nursery. In the planning of care for the infant's arrival, the priority nursing action would be to:
1   Obtain the necessary equipment from the blood bank needed for an exchange transfusion
2   Call the maintenance department and ask for a phototherapy unit to be brought to the nursery
3   Obtain the newborn infant's blood type and direct Coombs results from the laboratory
4   Obtain a vial of vitamin K from the pharmacy and prepare to administer an injection to prevent isoimmunization

**Answer: 3**
*Rationale:* To further plan for the newborn infant's care, the infant's blood type and direct Coombs must be known. Umbilical cord blood is taken at the time of delivery to determine blood type, Rh factor, and antibody titer (direct Coombs test) of the newborn infant. The nurse should obtain these results from the laboratory. Options 1 and 2 are inappropriate at this time, and additional data are needed to determine whether these actions are needed. Option 4 is incorrect because vitamin K is given to prevent hemorrhagic disease of the newborn infant.

*Test-Taking Strategy:* Use the process of elimination and focus on the issue, that the mother is Rh negative. Note the relationship between the issue of the question and option 3. Also, note that option 3 is the only option that addresses assessment. Review Rh incompatibilities if you had difficulty with this question.

*Level of Cognitive Ability:* Application
*Client Needs:* Physiological Integrity

*Integrated Concept/Process:* Nursing Process/Planning
*Content Area:* Maternity

**Reference**
Gorrie, T., McKinney, E., & Murray, S. (1998). *Foundations of maternal-newborn nursing* (2nd ed.) Philadelphia: W.B. Saunders, p. 705.

# Nursing Process: Implementation

**1.** A client in late active first stage labor has just reported a gush of vaginal fluid. A nurse observes a fetal monitor pattern of variable decelerations during contractions followed by a brief acceleration. Then there is a return to baseline until the next contraction, when the pattern is repeated. On the basis of these data, the nurse prepares to initially:
1 Take the vital signs
2 Perform a manual sterile vaginal exam
3 Perform Leopold's maneuver
4 Test the vaginal fluid with a nitrazine strip

**Answer: 2**
*Rationale:* Variable deceleration with brief acceleration after a gush of amniotic fluid is a common clinical manifestation of cord compression resulting from occult or frank prolapse of the umbilical cord. A manual vaginal exam can detect the presence of the cord in the vagina, confirming the problem. On the basis of the data in the question, options 1, 3, and 4 are not initial actions.

*Test-Taking Strategy:* Use the process of elimination. Focusing on the data in the question and determining the significance of the data will direct you to option 2. Review the signs of cord compression if you had difficulty with this question.

*Level of Cognitive Ability:* Application
*Client Needs:* Physiological Integrity
*Integrated Concept/Process:* Nursing Process/Implementation
*Content Area:* Maternity

**Reference**
Lowdermilk, D., Perry, S., & Bobak, I. (2000). *Maternity & women's health care* (7th ed.). St. Louis: Mosby, p. 1014.

**2.** A nurse is preparing to administer a feeding to a client who is receiving enteral nutrition through a nasogastric tube. What is the priority nursing action before administering the feeding?
1 Measuring intake and output
2 Weighing the client
3 Adding blue food coloring to the formula
4 Determining tube placement

**Answer: 4**
*Rationale:* Initiating a tube feeding prior to determining tube placement can lead to serious complications, such as aspiration. Options 1 and 2 are part of the total plan of care for a client on enteral feedings. Option 3 is instituted for a client who has been identified as being at high risk for aspiration. Option 4 is the priority nursing action.

*Test-Taking Strategy:* Use the ABCs—airway, breathing, and circulation—and the nursing process to answer the question. Option 4 relates to assessment and to the risk of aspiration. If you had difficulty with this question, review nursing interventions when a tube feeding is initiated.

*Level of Cognitive Ability:* Application
*Client Needs:* Physiological Integrity
*Integrated Concept/Process:* Nursing Process/Implementation
*Content Area:* Fundamental Skills

**Reference**
Lewis, S., Heitkemper, M., & Dirksen, S. (2000). *Medical-surgical nursing: Assessment and management of clinical problems* (5th ed.). St. Louis: Mosby, p. 1058.

**3.** A nurse teaches a client with a rib fracture to cough and deep breathe. The client resists directions by the nurse because of the pain. The nurse most appropriately:

1 Continues to give the client gentle encouragement

2 Requests that the physician perform a nerve block to deaden the pain

3 Explains in detail the potential complications resulting from lack of coughing and deep breathing

4 Premedicates the client and assists the client to splint the area during the coughing and deep-breathing exercises

**Answer: 4**

*Rationale:* The shallow respirations and splinting that occur with rib fracture predispose the client to developing atelectasis and pneumonia. It is essential that the client perform coughing and deep breathing to prevent these complications. The nurse accomplishes this most effectively by premedicating the client with pain medication and assisting the client with splinting during the exercises.

*Test-Taking Strategy:* Use the process of elimination, noting the key words *most appropriately*. Options 2 and 3 are likely to be the most extreme or unrealistic options, respectively, and should be eliminated first. From the remaining options, premedication and assistance are more likely to be effective than continued gentle encouragement. Review care of the client with a rib fracture if you had difficulty with this question.

*Level of Cognitive Ability:* Application
*Client Needs:* Physiological Integrity
*Integrated Concept/Process:* Nursing Process/Implementation
*Content Area:* Adult Health/Respiratory

*Reference*
Smeltzer, S., & Bare, B. (2000). *Brunner & Suddarth's Textbook of medical-surgical nursing* (9th ed.). Philadelphia: Lippincott Williams & Wilkins, p. 323.

**4.** A nurse is caring for a 14-year-old child who is hospitalized and placed in Crutchfield traction. The child is having difficulty adjusting to the length of the hospital confinement. Which nursing action would be most appropriate to meet the child's needs?

1 Allow the child to have his or her hair dyed if the parent agrees

2 Allow the child to play loud music in the hospital room

3 Let the child wear his or her own clothing when friends visit

4 Allow the child to keep the shades closed and the room darkened at all times

**Answer: 3**

*Rationale:* An adolescent needs to identify with peers and has a strong need to belong to a group. The child should be allowed to wear his or her own clothes to feel a sense of belonging to the group. Adolescents like to dress like the group and wear similar hairstyles. Because Crutchfield traction uses skeletal pins, hair dye is not appropriate. Loud music may disturb others in the hospital. A child's request for a darkened room is indicative of a possible problem with depression that may need further evaluation and intervention.

*Test-Taking Strategy:* Use the process of elimination and focus on the issues, Crutchfield traction and a 14-year-old child. Knowledge regarding Crutchfield traction and its limitations, and knowledge of growth and development concepts, will direct you to option 3. Review growth and development and care of the child in traction if you had difficulty with this question.

*Level of Cognitive Ability:* Application
*Client Needs:* Psychosocial integrity
*Integrated Concept/Process:* Nursing Process/Implementation
*Content Area:* Child Health

*Reference*
Potter, P., & Perry, A. (2001). *Fundamentals of nursing* (5th ed.). St. Louis: Mosby, pp. 213, 216.

**5.** A nurse receives a telephone call from the emergency room and is told that a client in leg traction will be admitted to the nursing unit. The nurse prepares for the arrival of the client and asks a certified nursing assistant to obtain which of the following items that will be essential for helping the client move in bed while in the leg traction?

1 An electric bed
2 A bed trapeze
3 Extra pillows
4 A foot board

**Answer: 2**

*Rationale:* A trapeze is essential to allow the client to lift straight up while being moved, so that the amount of pull exerted on the limb in traction is not altered. Either an electric bed or a manual bed can be used for traction but does not specifically assist the client to move in bed. A foot board and extra pillows do not facilitate moving.

*Test-Taking Strategy:* Note the key words *essential* and *move in bed*. Attempt to visualize the items in the options, focusing on the issue, helping the client move in bed. Using the process of elimination will direct you to option 2. Review care of the client in traction if you had difficulty with this question.

*Level of Cognitive Ability:* Application
*Client Needs:* Physiological Integrity
*Integrated Concept/Process:* Nursing Process/Implementation
*Content Area:* Adult Health/Musculoskeletal

*Reference*
Monahan, F., & Neighbors, M. (1998). *Medical-surgical nursing: Foundations for clinical practice* (2nd ed.). Philadelphia: W.B Saunders. p. 862.

---

**6.** A physician's order reads: tobramycin sulfate (Nebcin), 7.5 mg IM bid. The medication label reads: 10 mg/mL. A nurse prepares how many milliliters to administer one dose?

1 0.25 mL
2 0.50 mL
3 0.75 mL
4 1.33 mL

**Answer: 3**

*Rationale:* Use the formula for calculating a medication dose.
Formula:

$$\frac{\text{Desired}}{\text{Available}} \times \text{Volume} = \text{mL per dose}$$

$$\frac{7.5 \text{ mg}}{10 \text{ mg}} \times 1.0 \text{ mL} = 0.75 \text{ mL}$$

*Test-Taking Strategy:* Identify the key components of the question and what the question is asking. In this case, the question asks for the milliliters per dose. Use the formula to determine the correct dose. Review the formula for calculating a medication dose if you had difficulty with this question.

*Level of Cognitive Ability:* Application
*Client Needs:* Physiological Integrity
*Integrated Concept and Process:* Nursing Process/Implementation
*Content Area:* Fundamental Skills

*Reference*
Kee, J., & Marshall, S. (2000). *Clinical calculations: With applications to general and specialty areas* (4th ed.). Philadelphia: W.B. Saunders, p. 78.

**7.** A client in the second trimester of pregnancy is being assessed at a health care clinic. The nurse performing the assessment notes that the fetal heart rate is 100 beats per minute. Which of the following nursing actions would be most appropriate?

**1**   Document the findings

**2**   Inform the mother that the assessment is normal and everything is fine

**3**   Notify the physician

**4**   Instruct the mother to return to the clinic in 1 week for reevaluation of the fetal heart rate

**Answer: 3**

*Rationale:* The fetal heart rate should be between 120 and 160 beats per minute during pregnancy. A fetal heart rate of 100 beats per minute would require that the physician be notified and the client be further evaluated. Options 1 and 2 are similar and can be eliminated first. Option 4 is an inaccurate nursing action.

*Test-Taking Strategy:* Use the process of elimination. Knowing that the limits for the fetal heart rate are 120 and 160 beats per minute will direct you to option 3. If you had difficulty with this question, review the normal findings in the pregnant client.

*Level of Cognitive Ability:* Application
*Client Needs:* Physiological Integrity
*Integrated Concept/Process:* Nursing Process/Implementation
*Content Area:* Maternity

*Reference*
Sherwen, L., Scoloveno, M.A., & Weingarten, C. (1999). *Maternity nursing: Care of the childbearing family* (3rd ed.). Stamford, Conn.: Appleton & Lange, p. 781.

---

**8.** A client is admitted to the hospital with a leaking cerebral aneurysm and is scheduled for surgery. A nurse implements which of the following during the preoperative period?

**1**   Encourages the client to be up at least twice per day

**2**   Allows the client to ambulate to the bathroom

**3**   Obtains a bedside commode for the client's use

**4**   Places the client on strict bed rest

**Answer: 4**

*Rationale:* The client's activity is kept at a minimum to prevent Valsalva maneuver. Clients often hold their breath and strain while pulling up to get out of bed. This exertion may cause a rise in blood pressure, which increases bleeding. Clients who have bleeding aneurysms in any vessel will have activity curtailed.

*Test-Taking Strategy:* Use the process of elimination, focusing on the client's diagnosis and the key words *preoperative period.* Eliminate options 1, 2, and 3 because they are similar in that they all involve out-of-bed activity. If you had difficulty with this question, review aneurysm precautions.

*Level of Cognitive Ability:* Application
*Client Needs:* Physiological Integrity
*Integrated Concept/Process:* Nursing Process/Implementation
*Content Area:* Adult Health/Neurological

*Reference*
Smeltzer, S., & Bare, B. (2000). *Brunner & Suddarth's Textbook of medical-surgical nursing* (9th ed.). Philadelphia: Lippincott Williams & Wilkins, p. 700.

---

**9.** A physician calls a nurse to obtain the daily laboratory results for a client receiving total parenteral nutrition (TPN). Which of the following laboratory results from the client's record would provide the most valuable information regarding the client's status related to the TPN?

**1**   Serum electrolyte levels

**2**   Arterial blood gas (ABG) levels

**3**   White blood cell count (WBC)

**4**   Complete blood cell count (CBC)

**Answer: 1**

*Rationale:* TPN solutions contain amino acid and dextrose solutions, with electrolytes and trace elements added. The physician uses the electrolyte values to determine whether changes are needed in the composition of the TPN solutions that will be administered over the next 24 hours. This prevents the client from developing electrolyte imbalance. Options 2, 3, and 4 are not directly related to evaluating client status related to TPN.

*Test-Taking Strategy:* Use the process of elimination. Eliminate options 3 and 4 first because a CBC includes a WBC count. From the remaining options, focusing on the issue and considering the composition of TPN solutions will direct you to option 1. If you had difficulty with this question, review the composition of TPN.

*Level of Cognitive Ability:* Application
*Client Needs:* Physiological Integrity
*Integrated Concept/Process:* Nursing Process/Implementation
*Content Area:* Fundamental Skills

### Reference

Black, J., Hawks, J., & Keene, A. (2001). *Medical-surgical nursing: Clinical management for positive outcomes* (6th ed.). Philadelphia: W.B. Saunders, p. 668.

---

**10.** A client who has episodes of bronchospasm and a history of tachydysrhythmias is admitted to the hospital. A nurse reviews the physician's orders and contacts the physician to verify which medication, if prescribed by the physician?
1  Metaproterenol (Alupent)
2  Albuterol (Proventil)
3  Epinephrine (Primatene Mist)
4  Salmeterol (Serevent)

**Answer: 3**
*Rationale:* A client with a history of tachydysrhythmias should not be given bronchodilators that contain catecholamines, such as epinephrine and isoproterenol hydrochloride (Isuprel). Sympathomimetics that are noncatecholamines should be used instead. These include metaproterenol, albuterol, and salmeterol.

*Test-Taking Strategy:* Focus on the client's diagnosis, tachydysrhythmias. Use the process of elimination. Recalling that epinephrine is a catecholamine will direct you to this option. Review the effects of epinephrine if you had difficulty with this question.

*Level of Cognitive Ability:* Analysis
*Client Needs:* Safe, Effective Care Environment
*Integrated Concept/Process:* Nursing Process/Implementation
*Content Area:* Pharmacology

### Reference

Hodgson, B., & Kizior, R. (2001). *Saunders nursing drug handbook 2001.* Philadelphia: W.B. Saunders, pp. 366-369.

---

**11.** A client has a compulsive bed making ritual in which the client makes and remakes a bed numerous times. The client often misses breakfast and some of the morning activities because of the ritual. Which of the following nursing actions would be most helpful?
1  Verbalize tactful, mild disapproval of the behavior
2  Help the client to make the bed so that the task can be finished quicker
3  Discuss the ridiculousness of the behavior
4  Offer reflective feedback, such as "I see you have made your bed several times."

**Answer: 4**
*Rationale:* Verbalizing minimal disapproval would increase the client's anxiety and reinforce the need to perform the ritual. Helping with the ritual is nontherapeutic and also reinforces the behavior. The client is usually aware of the irrationality (or ridiculousness) of the behavior. Reflective feedback acknowledges the client's behavior.

*Test-Taking Strategy:* Use the process of elimination. Recalling that the purpose of the ritual is to relieve anxiety would assist to eliminate options 1 and 3 because these actions would increase the anxiety. Eliminate option 2 because there is no therapeutic value in participating in the ritual. Review the appropriate interventions for the client with compulsive behavior, if you had difficulty with this question.

*Level of Cognitive Ability:* Application
*Client Needs:* Psychosocial Integrity
*Integrated Concept/Process:* Nursing Process/Implementation
*Content Area:* Mental Health

*Reference*
Varcarolis, E. (1998). *Foundations of psychiatric mental health nursing* (3rd ed.). Philadelphia: W.B. Saunders, p. 450.

---

**12.** An elderly client who has undergone internal fixation after fracturing a left hip has developed a reddened left heel. A nurse obtains which of the following as a priority item to manage this problem?
1  Bed cradle
2  Sheepskin
3  Trapeze
4  Draw sheet

**Answer: 2**
*Rationale:* The reddened heel results from pressure of the foot against the mattress. The nurse obtains a sheepskin, heel protectors, or an alternating pressure mattress. The bed cradle is unnecessary in managing this problem. A draw sheet and trapeze are of general use for this client but are not specific in dealing with the reddened heel.

*Test-Taking Strategy:* Note the issue of the question, a reddened left heel. Eliminate option 1 first as an unnecessary measure. Eliminate options 3 and 4 next, because although they are generally helpful in aiding the client's mobility, they are not related to the issue of the question. Option 2 addresses the problem stated in the question. Review measures that prevent skin breakdown in the immobile client if you had difficulty with this question.

*Level of Cognitive Ability:* Application
*Client Needs:* Physiological Integrity
*Integrated Concept/Process:* Nursing Process/Implementation
*Content Area:* Adult Health/Musculoskeletal

*Reference*
Monahan, F., & Neighbors, M. (1998). *Medical-surgical nursing: Foundations for clinical practice* (2nd ed.). Philadelphia: W.B Saunders, p. 1622.

---

**13.** A nurse is caring for an infant after pyloromyotomy performed to treat hypertrophic pyloric stenosis. The nurse places the infant in which position following surgery?
1  Flat on the nonoperative side
2  Flat on the operative side
3  Prone with the head of the bed elevated
4  Supine with the head of the bed elevated

**Answer: 3**
*Rationale:* Following pyloromyotomy, the head of the bed is elevated and the infant is placed prone to reduce the risk of aspiration. Options 1, 2, and 4 are incorrect positions after this type of surgery.

*Test-Taking Strategy:* Consider the anatomical location of the surgical procedure and the risks associated with the procedure to answer the question. Visualize each of the positions identified in the options. Keeping in mind that aspiration is a major concern will direct you to option 3. Review nursing care measures following pyloromyotomy, if you had difficulty with this question.

*Level of Cognitive Ability:* Application
*Client Needs:* Physiological Integrity
*Integrated Concept/Process:* Nursing Process/Implementation
*Content Area:* Child Health

*Reference*
Wong, D. (1999). *Whaley & Wong's Nursing care of infants and children* (6th ed.). St. Louis: Mosby, p. 1564.

---

14. A mother of a child with mumps calls a health care clinic to tell the nurse that the child has been very lethargic and has been vomiting. The nurse most appropriately tells the mother:
    1   To continue to monitor the child
    2   That lethargy and vomiting are normal manifestations of mumps
    3   To bring the child to the clinic to be seen by the physician
    4   That as long as there is no fever, there is nothing to be concerned about

**Answer: 3**
*Rationale:* Mumps generally affects the salivary glands, but can also affect multiple organs. The most common complication is meningitis, with the virus being identified in the cerebrospinal fluid. Common signs include nuchal rigidity, lethargy, and vomiting. The child should be seen by the physician.

*Test-Taking Strategy:* Focus on the signs and symptoms presented in the question. Recalling that meningitis is a complication of mumps will direct you to option 3. Review the complications of mumps and the associated clinical manifestations, if you had difficulty with this question.

*Level of Cognitive Ability:* Application
*Client Needs:* Physiological Integrity
*Integrated Concept/Process:* Nursing Process/Implementation
*Content Area:* Child Health

*Reference*
Wong, D. (1999). *Whaley & Wong's Nursing care of infants and children* (6th ed.). St. Louis: Mosby, p. 726.

---

15. A child is admitted to the hospital with a diagnosis of sickle cell crisis. The nurse contacts the physician to question which order documented in the child's record?
    1   Intravenous fluids
    2   Supplemental oxygen
    3   Bed rest
    4   Meperidine hydrochloride (Demerol)

**Answer: 4**
*Rationale:* Meperidine hydrochloride is contraindicated for ongoing pain management because of the increased risk of seizures associated with the use of the medication. Management of severe pain generally includes the use of strong narcotic analgesics such as morphine sulfate or hydromorphone (Dilaudid). These medications are usually most effective when given as a continuous infusion or at regular intervals around the clock. Options 1, 2, and 3 are appropriate prescriptions for treating vaso-occlusive pain crisis.

*Test-Taking Strategy:* Use the process of elimination. Note the key words *orders would the nurse question*. Recalling that oxygen, fluids, and bed rest are components of care will direct you to option 4. Review care of a child with sickle cell anemia, if you had difficulty with this question.

*Level of Cognitive Ability:* Application
*Client Needs:* Safe, Effective Care Environment
*Integrated Concept/Process:* Nursing Process/Implementation
*Content Area:* Child Health

*Reference*
Wong, D. (1999). *Whaley & Wong's Nursing care of infants and children* (6th ed.).
St. Louis: Mosby, p. 1667.

---

**16.** A nurse is caring for an infant with laryngomalacia (congenital laryngeal stridor). In which of the following positions would the nurse place the infant to decrease the incidence of stridor?
**1** Supine
**2** Supine with the neck flexed
**3** Prone
**4** Prone with the neck hyperextended

**Answer: 4**
*Rationale:* The prone position with the neck hyperextended improves the child's breathing. Options 1, 2, and 3 are not appropriate positions.

*Test-Taking Strategy:* Use the process of elimination, noting the key words *decrease the incidence of stridor.* Visualize each of the positions identified in the options to assist in directing you to option 4. If you had difficulty with this question, review this content.

*Level of Cognitive Ability:* Application
*Client Needs:* Physiological Integrity
*Integrated Concept/Process:* Nursing Process/Implementation
*Content Area:* Child Health

*Reference*
Wong, D. (1999). *Whaley & Wong's Nursing care of infants and children* (6th ed.).
St. Louis: Mosby, p. 1334.

---

**17.** A nurse in the newborn nursery prepares to admit a newborn infant with spina bifida, meningomyelocele type. Which of the following is the priority nursing action in the immediate plan of care for this infant?
**1** Monitor blood pressure
**2** Monitor specific gravity of the urine
**3** Inspect the anterior fontanel for bulging
**4** Monitor temperature

**Answer: 3**
*Rationale:* Intracranial pressure is a complication associated with spina bifida. A sign of intracranial pressure in the newborn infant with spina bifida is a bulging or tough anterior fontanel. The newborn infant is at risk for infection before the surgical procedure and closure of the gibbus, and monitoring the temperature is an important intervention; however, assessing the anterior fontanel for bulging is the immediate priority. A normal saline dressing is placed over the affected site to maintain moisture of the gibbus and its contents. This prevents tearing or breakdown of skin integrity at the site. Blood pressure is difficult to assess during the newborn period, and it is not the best indicator of infection or a potential complication. Urine concentration is not well developed in the newborn stage of development.

*Test-Taking Strategy:* Use the process of elimination, focusing on the key words *priority nursing action.* Eliminate options 1 and 2 first because blood pressure and specific gravity are common assessments, but are not as reliable as indicators of changes in the newborn status as they would be for an older child. From the remaining options, focusing on the key words will direct you to option 3. Review care of the infant with spina bifida, if you had difficulty with this question.

*Level of Cognitive Ability:* Application
*Client Needs:* Physiological Integrity
*Integrated Concept/Process:* Nursing Process/Implementation
*Content Area:* Child Health

*Reference*
Wong, D. (1999). *Whaley & Wong's Nursing care of infants and children* (6th ed.). St. Louis: Mosby, p. 485.

---

**18.** On assessment of a child, a nurse notes that the child's genitals are swollen. The nurse suspects that the child is being sexually abused. Which action by the nurse is most appropriate?
  **1** Document the child's physical findings
  **2** Report the case in which the abuse is suspected
  **3** Refer the family to appropriate support groups
  **4** Assist the family in identifying resources and support systems

**Answer: 2**
*Rationale:* The primary legal responsibility of a nurse when child abuse is suspected is to report the case. All 50 states require health care professionals to report all cases of suspected abuse. Although documentation of assessment findings, assisting the family, and referring the family to appropriate resources and support groups are important, the primary legal responsibility is to report the case.

*Test-Taking Strategy:* Use the process of elimination. In addition to the many implications associated with child abuse, recall that abuse is a crime. Keeping this in mind will direct you to option 2. If you had difficulty with this question, review the responsibilities of the nurse when child abuse is suspected.

*Level of Cognitive Ability:* Application
*Client Needs:* Psychosocial Integrity
*Integrated Concept/Process:* Nursing Process/Implementation
*Content Area:* Child Health

*Reference*
Wong, D. (1999). *Whaley & Wong's Nursing care of infants and children* (6th ed.). St. Louis: Mosby, p. 758.

---

**19.** A nurse is planning care for an infant with a diagnosis of encephalocele located in the occipital area. Which of the following items would the nurse use to assist in positioning the child to avoid pressure on the encephalocele?
  **1** Sheepskin
  **2** Foam half-donut
  **3** Feather pillow
  **4** Sandbag

**Answer: 2**
*Rationale:* The infant is positioned to avoid pressure on the lesion. If the encephalocele is in the occipital area, a foam half-donut may be useful in positioning to prevent this pressure. A sheepskin, feather pillow, or sandbag will not protect the encephalocele from pressure.

*Test-Taking Strategy:* Note the key word *occipital* and use the process of elimination. Note the similarities in options 1, 3, and 4 in that they would require the head to remain flat and therefore would not protect the lesion. If you have difficulty with this question, review nursing care associated with a child with an encephalocele.

*Level of Cognitive Ability:* Application
*Client Needs:* Physiological Integrity
*Integrated Concept/Process:* Nursing Process/Implementation
*Content Area:* Child Health

*Reference*
Bowden, V., Dickey, S., & Greenberg, C. (1998). *Children and their families: The continuum of care.* Philadelphia: W.B. Saunders, p. 1369.

**20.** A nurse is caring for a child with a head injury. On review of the record the nurse notes that the physician has documented decorticate posturing. On assessment of the child, the nurse notes extension of the upper extremities and internal rotation of the upper arm and wrist. The nurse also notes that the lower extremities are extended, with some internal rotation noted at the knees and feet. On the basis of these findings, which of the following is the appropriate nursing action?

1 Document the findings
2 Continue to monitor for posturing of the child
3 Attempt to flex the child's lower extremities
4 Notify the physician

**Answer: 4**

*Rationale:* Decorticate posturing refers to flexion of the upper extremities and extension of the lower extremities. Plantar flexion of the feet may also be observed. Decerebrate posturing involves extension of the upper extremities with internal rotation of the upper arm and wrist. The lower extremities will extend, with some internal rotation noted at the knees and feet. The progression from decorticate to decerebrate posturing usually indicates deteriorating neurological function and warrants physician notification.

*Test-Taking Strategy:* Focus on the data in the question, and use knowledge regarding the assessment findings associated with decerebrate and decorticate positioning. It is also necessary to know the neurological assessment findings that indicate deterioration in the condition of the neurological status in the child. If you had difficulty with this question or are unfamiliar with these assessment findings, review this content.

*Level of Cognitive Ability:* Application
*Client Needs:* Physiological Integrity
*Integrated Concept/Process:* Nursing Process/Implementation
*Content Area:* Child Health

*Reference*
Wong, D. (1999). *Whaley & Wong's Nursing care of infants and children* (6th ed.). St. Louis: Mosby, p. 1772.

**21.** A child with a diagnosis of hepatitis B is being cared for at home. The mother of the child calls the health care clinic and tells a nurse that the jaundice seems to be worsening. Which of the following responses to the mother would be most appropriate?

1 "The hepatitis may be spreading."
2 "You need to bring the child to the health care clinic to see the physician."
3 "The jaundice may appear to get worse before it resolves."
4 "It is necessary to isolate the child from others."

**Answer: 3**

*Rationale:* The parents should be instructed that jaundice may appear to get worse before it resolves. The parents of a child with hepatitis should also be taught the danger signs that could indicate a worsening of the child's condition, specifically changes in neurological status, bleeding, and fluid retention.

*Test-Taking Strategy:* Use the process of elimination and knowledge regarding the physiology associated with hepatitis to answer this question. Knowing that the jaundice worsens before is resolves will direct you to the correct option. If you had difficulty with this question, review the instructions to the parents of a child with hepatitis.

*Level of Cognitive Ability:* Application
*Client Needs:* Physiological Integrity
*Integrated Concept/Process:* Nursing Process/Implementation
*Content Area:* Child Health

*Reference*
Wong, D. (1999). *Whaley & Wong's Nursing care of infants and children* (6th ed.). St. Louis: Mosby, pp. 551, 1574.

**22.** A nurse is preparing to suction a tracheostomy in an infant. The nurse prepares the equipment for the procedure and turns the suction to which of the following settings?

1    60 mm Hg
2    90 mm Hg
3    110 mm Hg
4    120 mm Hg

**Answer: 2**

*Rationale:* The suctioning procedure for pediatric clients varies from that which is used in adults. Suctioning in infants and children requires the use of a smaller suction catheter and lower suction settings than in the adult. Suction settings for a neonate are 60 to 80 mm Hg, for an infant are 80 to 100 mm Hg, and for larger children are 100 to 120 mm Hg.

*Test-Taking Strategy:* Use the process of elimination. Noting the key word *infant* and focusing on the procedure will direct you to option 2. If you are unfamiliar with this procedure, review this content.

*Level of Cognitive Ability:* Application
*Client Needs:* Physiological Integrity
*Integrated Concept/Process:* Nursing Process/Implementation
*Content Area:* Child Health

*Reference*
Wong, D. (1999). *Whaley & Wong's Nursing care of infants and children* (6th ed.). St. Louis: Mosby, p. 1438.

**23.** A nurse is caring for a client who begins to experience seizure activity while in bed. The nurse determines that this particular client is at risk for aspiration. Which of the following actions by the nurse would be most helpful to prevent this from occurring?

1    Loosen restrictive clothing
2    Remove the pillow and raise the padded side rails
3    Raise the head of the bed
4    Position the client on the side if possible, with the head flexed forward

**Answer: 4**

*Rationale:* Positioning the client on one side with the head flexed forward allows the tongue to fall forward and facilitates drainage of secretions, which could help prevent aspiration. The nurse would also remove restrictive clothing and the pillow, and raise the padded side rails, but these actions would not decrease the risk of aspiration. Rather, they are general safety measures to use during seizure activity. The nurse would not raise the head of the client's bed.

*Test Taking Strategy:* Note that the key words *most helpful, aspiration,* and *prevent.* Eliminate option 2 first because it is unrelated to the issue of the question. Visualize the effect that each of the remaining options would have on airway and aspiration to direct you to option 4. Review care of the client with seizures who is at risk for aspiration, if you had difficulty with this question.

*Level of Cognitive Ability:* Application
*Client Needs:* Physiological Integrity
*Integrated Concept/Process:* Nursing Process/Implementation
*Content Area:* Adult Health/Neurological

*Reference*
Monahan, F., & Neighbors, M. (1998). *Medical-surgical nursing: Foundations for clinical practice* (2nd ed.). Philadelphia: W.B Saunders, p. 796.

**24.** A client who has had a cerebrovascular accident (CVA) has episodes of coughing while swallowing liquids. The client has developed a temperature of 101.6° F, oxygen saturation of 91% (down from 98% previously), slight confusion, and noticeable dyspnea. The nurse would take which of the following most appropriate actions?

1. Administer a bronchodilator ordered on a PRN basis
2. Administer an acetaminophen (Tylenol) suppository
3. Encourage the client to cough and deep breathe
4. Notify the physician

**Answer: 4**

*Rationale:* The client is exhibiting clinical signs and symptoms of aspiration, which include fever, dyspnea, decreased arterial oxygen levels, and confusion. Other symptoms that occur with this complication are difficulty in managing saliva, and coughing or choking while eating. Since the client has developed a complication requiring medical intervention, the most appropriate action is to contact the physician.

*Test-Taking Strategy:* Use the process of elimination. Focusing on the data in the question will indicate that aspiration has most likely occurred. Eliminate options 1, 2, and 3 because these actions will not assist in alleviating this life-threatening condition. Review the findings in the client who is aspirating and the appropriate nursing interventions, if you had difficulty with this question.

*Level of Cognitive Ability:* Application
*Client Needs:* Physiological Integrity
*Integrated Concept/Process:* Nursing Process/Implementation
*Content Area:* Adult Health/Neurological

*Reference*
Monahan, F., & Neighbors, M. (1998). *Medical-surgical nursing: Foundations for clinical practice* (2nd ed.). Philadelphia: W.B Saunders, p. 809.

**25.** A nurse is providing care to a client after a bone biopsy. Which of the following actions would the nurse take as part of aftercare for this procedure?

1. Keep the area in a dependent position
2. Monitor vitals signs once per day
3. Monitor the site for swelling, bleeding, or hematoma formation
4. Administer intramuscular narcotic analgesics

**Answer: 3**

*Rationale:* Nursing care after bone biopsy includes monitoring the site for swelling, bleeding, or hematoma formation. The biopsy site is elevated for 24 hours to reduce edema. The vital signs are monitored every 4 hours for 24 hours. The client usually requires mild analgesics; more severe pain usually indicates that complications are arising.

*Test-Taking Strategy:* Use the process of elimination. Begin to answer this question by recalling that after this procedure the client must have periodic assessments. With this in mind, eliminate option 2 because the assessments would be too infrequent. Knowing that the procedure is done under local anesthesia helps you to eliminate option 4 next. From the remaining options, recall the principles related to circulation and positioning to direct you to option 3. Review care of a client after bone biopsy, if you had difficulty with this question.

*Level of Cognitive Ability:* Application
*Client Needs:* Physiological Integrity
*Integrated Concept/Process:* Nursing Process/Implementation
*Content Area:* Adult Health/Musculoskeletal

*Reference*
Monahan, F., & Neighbors, M. (1998). *Medical-surgical nursing: Foundations for clinical practice* (2nd ed.). Philadelphia: W.B Saunders. p. 1444.

**26.** A nurse is caring for a client who is scheduled for a diagnostic test requiring the use of a contrast medium. Which of the following actions by the nurse has the highest priority?

1    Determining the presence of client allergies
2    Telling the client that frequent ambulation will be required during the procedure
3    Asking if the client has any last-minute questions
4    Telling the client to try to move the bowels before leaving the unit

**Answer: 1**

*Rationale:* Because of the risk of allergy to contrast medium, the nurse places highest priority on assessing whether the client has an allergy to iodine or shellfish. The nurse reinforces information about the test and reminds the client that he or she will most likely need to remain still during the procedure. There is no special need to ensure that the bowel is empty before the procedure, but it is helpful to have the client void before the procedure for comfort.

*Test-Taking Strategy:* Use the process of elimination, noting the key words *contrast medium* and *highest priority.* Recalling the risk associated with the administration of contrast medium will direct you to option 1. Review preprocedure care for an arthrogram, if you had difficulty with this question.

*Level of Cognitive Ability:* Application
*Client Needs:* Physiological Integrity
*Integrated Concept/Process:* Nursing Process/Implementation
*Content Area:* Adult Health/Musculoskeletal

*Reference*
Black, J., Hawks, J., & Keene, A. (2001). *Medical-surgical nursing: Clinical management for positive outcomes* (6th ed.). Philadelphia: W.B. Saunders, p. 546.

**27.** A nurse responds to a call bell and finds a client lying on the floor after a fall. The nurse suspects that the client's arm may be broken. Which action would the nurse take as the highest priority before moving the client?

1    Tell the client that there is no permanent damage
2    Immobilize the arm
3    Take a set of vital signs
4    Call the radiology department

**Answer: 2**

*Rationale:* When a fracture is suspected, it is imperative that the area is splinted before the client is moved. Emergency help should be called for if the client is external to a hospital, and a physician is called if the client is hospitalized. The nurse should remain with the client and provide realistic reassurance. The client would not be told that there is no permanent damage.

*Test-Taking Strategy:* Use the process of elimination, noting the key words *highest priority.* Eliminate option 4 because the physician will order radiology films. Option 1 is eliminated next because the nurse does not make statements to the client that could provide false reassurance. From the remaining options, noting that a fracture is suspected will direct you to option 2. Review care of the client with a suspected extremity fracture, if you had difficulty with this question.

*Level of Cognitive Ability:* Application
*Client Needs:* Physiological Integrity
*Integrated Concept/Process:* Nursing Process/Implementation
*Content Area:* Adult Health/Musculoskeletal

*Reference*
Black, J., Hawks, J., & Keene, A. (2001). *Medical-surgical nursing: Clinical management for positive outcomes* (6th ed.). Philadelphia: W.B. Saunders, p. 590.

**28.** A nurse in a postpartum unit checks the temperature of a client who delivered a healthy newborn infant 4 hours ago. The mother's temperature is 100.8° F. The nurse provides oral hydration to the mother and encourages fluids. Four hours later the nurse rechecks the temperature and notes that it is still 100.8° F. Which of the following is the most appropriate nursing intervention?

1. Notify the physician
2. Continue hydration and recheck the temperature 4 hours later
3. Document the temperature
4. Increase the IV fluids

**Answer: 1**

*Rationale:* A temperature of greater than 100.4° F in two consecutive readings is considered febrile, and the physician should be notified. Options 2, 3, and 4 are inappropriate actions at this time.

*Test-Taking Strategy:* Use the process of elimination. Option 4 can be eliminated first because this action requires a physician's order. From the remaining options, noting that the temperature has remained unchanged after nursing intervention should provide you with the clue that further intervention is necessary and direct you to option 1. Review normal and abnormal findings in the postpartum period, if you had difficulty with this question.

*Level of Cognitive Ability:* Application
*Client Needs:* Physiological Integrity
*Integrated Concept/Process:* Nursing Process/Implementation
*Content Area:* Maternity

*Reference*
Lowdermilk, D., Perry, S., & Bobak, I. (2000). *Maternity & women's health care* (7th ed.). St. Louis: Mosby, p. 1032.

---

**29.** A nurse is checking the fundus in a postpartum woman. The nurse notes that the uterus is soft and spongy. Which of the following nursing actions is most appropriate initially?

1. Massage the fundus gently until firm
2. Document fundal position and consistency and height
3. Encourage the mother to ambulate
4. Notify the physician

**Answer: 1**

*Rationale:* If the fundus is boggy (soft), the nurse should massage it gently until it is firm, observing for increased bleeding or clots. Option 3 is an inappropriate action at this time. The nurse should document fundal position, consistency and height, the need to perform fundal massage, and the client's response to the intervention. The physician will need to be notified if uterine massage is not helpful.

*Test-Taking Strategy:* Note the key words *most appropriate initially*. Note the relationship between the data in the question (soft and spongy) and the data in the correct option (massage the fundus gently until firm). Review nursing interventions related to this occurrence if you had difficulty with this question.

*Level of Cognitive Ability:* Application
*Client Needs:* Physiological Integrity
*Integrated Concept/Process:* Nursing Process/Implementation
*Content Area:* Maternity

*Reference*
Lowdermilk, D., Perry, S., & Bobak, I. (2000). *Maternity & women's health care* (7th ed.). St. Louis: Mosby, p. 593.

**30.** A primipara is being evaluated in the clinic during her second trimester of pregnancy. The nurse checks the fetal heart rate (FHR) and notes that it is 190 beats per minute. The most appropriate nursing action would be to:

1. Document the finding
2. Consult with the physician
3. Tell the client that the FHR is normal
4. Recheck the FHR with the client in the standing position

**Answer: 2**

*Rationale:* The fetal heart rate should be 120 to 160 beats per minute throughout pregnancy. In this situation, the FHR is above the normal range, and the nurse should most appropriately consult with the physician. The FHR would be documented, but option 2 is the most appropriate action. The nurse would not tell the client that the FHR is normal because this is not true information. Option 4 is an inappropriate action.

*Test-Taking Strategy:* Note the key words *most appropriate* in the stem of the question. Recalling that the normal FHR is 120 to 160 beats per minute will direct you to option 2. If you had difficulty with this question, review the normal FHR.

*Level of Cognitive Ability:* Application
*Client Needs:* Physiological Integrity
*Integrated Concept/Process:* Nursing Process/Implementation
*Content Area:* Maternity

*Reference*
Gorrie, T., McKinney, E., & Murray, S. (1998). *Foundations of maternal-newborn nursing* (2nd ed.). Philadelphia: W.B. Saunders, p. 347.

## Nursing Process: Evaluation

**1.** To improve hydration, a nurse has been encouraging the intake of oral fluids by a woman in labor. Which of the following indicates a successful outcome of this action?

1. A urine specific gravity of 1.020
2. Continued leaking of amniotic fluid during labor
3. Blood pressure of 150/90 mm Hg
4. Ketones in the urine

**Answer: 1**

*Rationale:* Urine specific gravity is an expression of the concentration of the urine. During the first stage of labor, the renal system has a tendency to concentrate urine. Labor and birth require hydration and caloric intake to replenish energy expenditure and promote efficient uterine function. An elevated blood pressure and ketones in the urine are not expected outcomes related to labor and hydration. Once membranes are ruptured, it is expected that amniotic fluid may continue to leak.

*Test-Taking Strategy:* Use the process of elimination, focusing on the issue, a successful outcome related to oral intake. Recalling the relationship of oral intake to urine concentration will direct you to option 1. Review the importance of hydration in the woman in labor if you had difficulty with this question.

*Level of Cognitive Ability:* Analysis
*Client Needs:* Health Promotion and Maintenance
*Integrated Concept/Process:* Nursing Process/Evaluation
*Content Area:* Maternity

*Reference*
Olds, S., London. M., & Ladewig, P. (2000). *Maternal-newborn nursing: A family and community-based approach* (6th ed.). Upper Saddle River, N.J.: Prentice-Hall Health, p. 562.

**2.** A postpartum client has a nursing diagnosis of High Risk for Infection. The following goal has been developed: "The client will not develop an infection during her hospital stay." Which of the following assessment data would support the conclusion that the goal has been met?
1   Presence of chills
2   Abdominal tenderness
3   Absence of fever
4   Loss of appetite

**Answer: 3**
*Rationale:* Fever is the first indication of an infection. Chills, abdominal tenderness, and loss of appetite also indicate the presence of an infection. Therefore, the absence of a fever indicates that an infection is not present.

*Test-Taking Strategy:* Use the process of elimination, noting the key words *that the goal has been met.* The question is asking for a means of recognizing the achievement of a goal that relates to infection. Options 1, 2, and 4 would indicate that the goal had not been met. Review the signs of postpartum infection if you had difficulty with this question.

*Level of Cognitive Ability:* Analysis
*Client Needs:* Physiological Integrity
*Integrated Concept/Process:* Nursing Process/Evaluation
*Content Area:* Maternity

*Reference*
Sherwen, L., Scoloveno, M.A., & Weingarten, C. (1999). *Maternity nursing: Care of the childbearing family* (3rd ed.). Stamford, Conn.: Appleton & Lange, p. 896.

**3.** A nurse is monitoring the nutritional status of a client who is receiving enteral nutrition because of dysphagia resulting from a head injury. The nurse monitors which of the following to best determine the effectiveness of the tube feedings for this client?
1   Calorie count
2   Daily intake and output
3   Daily weight
4   Serum protein level

**Answer: 3**
*Rationale:* The most accurate way of measuring the effectiveness of nutritional management of the client is monitoring of daily weight. This should be done at the same time (preferably early morning), in the same clothes, and with the same scale. Options 1, 2, and 4 assist in monitoring nutrition and hydration status. However, the effectiveness of the diet is evidenced by maintenance of body weight.

*Test-Taking Strategy:* Note the key word *effectiveness,* which tells you that the correct option is an outcome. With this in mind, eliminate options 1 and 2 first because these are tools the nurse uses to monitor nutrition and fluid status. Eliminate option 4 next because it reflects only one component of the diet, namely protein. If you had difficulty with this question, review the methods of monitoring nutritional status.

*Level of Cognitive Ability:* Application
*Client Needs:* Physiological Integrity
*Integrated Concept/Process:* Nursing Process/Evaluation
*Content Area:* Fundamental Skills

*Reference*
Lewis, S., Heitkemper, M., & Dirksen, S. (2000). *Medical-surgical nursing: Assessment and management of clinical problems* (5th ed.). St. Louis: Mosby, p. 1056.

**4.** An adult client with a critically high potassium level has received sodium polystyrene sulfonate (Kayexalate). A nurse concludes that the medication was most effective if the client's repeat serum potassium level is:

1   6.2 mEq/L
2   5.8 mEq/L
3   5.4 mEq/L
4   4.9 mEq/L

**Answer: 4**

*Rationale:* The normal serum potassium level in the adult is 3.5 to 5.1 mEq/L. Option 4 is the only option reflecting a value that has dropped down into the normal range. Options 1, 2, and 3 are elevated potassium levels.

*Test-Taking Strategy:* Use the process of elimination. Note the key words *critically high.* You would expect that this medication is administered to lower the potassium level. Recalling the normal serum potassium level will direct you to option 4. If this question was difficult, review the expected effects of this medication and the normal potassium level.

*Level of Cognitive Ability:* Analysis
*Client Needs:* Physiological Integrity
*Integrated Concept/Process:* Nursing Process/Evaluation
*Content Area:* Fundamental Skills

**References**

Ignatavicius, D., Workman, M., & Mishler, M. (1999). *Medical-surgical nursing across the health care continuum* (3rd ed.). Philadelphia: W.B. Saunders, p. 221.
Hodgson, B., & Kizior, R. (2000). *Saunders nursing drug handbook 2000.* Philadelphia: W.B. Saunders, p. 935.

**5.** A nurse assesses a client who has a nasogastric tube (NG) in place and connected to suction after abdominal surgery. Which observation by the nurse indicates most reliably that the tube is functioning properly?

1   The suction gauge reads low intermittent suction
2   The distal end of the NG tube is pinned to the client's gown
3   The client indicates that pain is a 3 on a scale of 1 to 10
4   The client denies nausea and has 250 mL of fluid in the suction collection container

**Answer: 4**

*Rationale:* An NG tube connected to suction is used postoperatively to decompress and rest the bowel. The gastrointestinal tract lacks peristaltic activity as a result of manipulation during surgery. Although the nurse makes pertinent observations of the tube to ensure that it is secure and connected to suction properly, the client is assessed for the effect. The client should not experience symptoms of ileus (nausea and vomiting) if the tube is functioning properly. A pain indicator of 3 is an expected finding in a postoperative client.

*Test-Taking Strategy:* Use the process of elimination. Focus on the issue, that the tube is functioning properly. Recalling the purpose of the NG tube in a postoperative client will direct you to option 4. Review care of the client with an NG tube, if you had difficulty with this question.

*Level of Cognitive Ability:* Analysis
*Client Needs:* Physiological Integrity
*Integrated Concept/Process:* Nursing Process/Evaluation
*Content Area:* Adult Health/Gastrointestinal

**Reference**

Smeltzer, S., & Bare, B. (2000). *Brunner & Suddarth's Textbook of medical-surgical nursing* (9th ed.). Philadelphia: Lippincott Williams & Wilkins, p. 838.

**6.** A nurse is caring for a client following prostatectomy. The client has a three-way Foley catheter with an infusion of continuous bladder irrigation (CBI). The nurse determines that the flow rate is adequate if the urinary drainage is:

1  Red
2  Concentrated yellow
3  Clear as water
4  Slightly pink

**Answer: 4**

*Rationale:* The bladder irrigant is not infused at a preset rate, but rather the rate is increased or decreased to maintain urine that is a clear pale yellow color, or that has just a slight pink tinge. The infusion rate should be increased if the drainage is cherry colored (red) or if clots are seen. Correspondingly, the rate can be slowed down slightly if the returns are as clear as water.

*Test-Taking Strategy:* Use the process of elimination. Note the issue of the question, an adequate flow rate. With this in mind, eliminate option 2 because clots are not expected. Next, eliminate options 1 and 3 as reflecting inadequate and excessive irrigation flow, respectively. Review care of the client with CBI if you had difficulty with this question.

*Level of Cognitive Ability:* Analysis
*Client Needs:* Physiological Integrity
*Integrated Concept/Process:* Nursing Process/Evaluation
*Content Area:* Adult Health/Renal

*Reference*
Smeltzer, S., & Bare, B. (2000). *Brunner & Suddarth's Textbook of medical-surgical nursing* (9th ed.). Philadelphia: Lippincott Williams & Wilkins, p. 1316.

---

**7.** A nurse who is caring for a client with Graves' disease notes a nursing diagnosis of "Altered Nutrition: Less than Body Requirements, related to the effects of the hypercatabolic state" in the care plan. Which of the following would indicate a successful outcome for this diagnosis?

1  The client maintains his or her normal weight or gradually gains weight if it is below normal
2  The client demonstrates knowledge regarding the need to consume a diet high in fat and low in protein
3  The client verbalizes the need to avoid snacking between meals
4  The client discusses the relationship between mealtime and the blood glucose level

**Answer: 1**

*Rationale:* Graves' disease causes a state of chronic nutritional and caloric deficiency resulting from the metabolic effects of excessive $T_3$ and $T_4$. Clinical manifestations are weight loss and increased appetite. It is therefore a nutritional goal that the client will not lose additional weight and will gradually return to his or her ideal body weight if necessary. To accomplish this, the client must be encouraged to eat frequent high-calorie, high-protein, and high-carbohydrate meals and snacks.

*Test-Taking Strategy:* Use the process of elimination, focusing on the key words *hypercatabolic state*. Options 2 and 3 would not be beneficial for a client in a hypercatabolic state. Option 4 can be eliminated because discussing the fluctuation in the blood glucose level will not assist a client who is hypercatabolic. If you had difficulty with this question, review altered nutrition and Graves' disease.

*Level of Cognitive Ability:* Analysis
*Client Needs:* Health Promotion and Maintenance
*Integrated Concept/Process:* Nursing Process/Evaluation
*Content Area:* Adult Health/Endocrine

*Reference*
Smeltzer, S., & Bare, B. (2000). *Brunner & Suddarth's Textbook of medical-surgical nursing* (9th ed.). Philadelphia: Lippincott Williams & Wilkins, p. 1044.

**8.** A nurse has developed a plan of care for a client who is in traction and documents a nursing diagnosis of Self-Care Deficit. The nurse evaluates the plan of care and determines that which of the following observations indicates a successful outcome?

1 The client allows the nurse to complete the care on a daily basis
2 The client allows the family to assist in the care
3 The client refuses care
4 The client assists in self-care as much as possible

**Answer: 4**

*Rationale:* A successful outcome for the nursing diagnosis of Self-Care Deficit is for the client to do as much of the self-care as possible. The nurse should promote independence in the client and allow the client to perform as much self-care as is optimal, considering the client's condition. The nurse would determine that the outcome is unsuccessful if the client refused care or allows others to do the care.

*Test-Taking Strategy:* Focus on the key words *successful outcome*. Option 3 can be easily eliminated first. Note that options 1 and 2 are similar in that they indicate relying on others to perform care. Review successful outcomes related to the nursing diagnosis of Self-Care Deficit, if you had difficulty with this question.

*Level of Cognitive Ability:* Analysis
*Client Needs:* Health Promotion and Maintenance
*Integrated Concept/Process:* Nursing Process/Evaluation
*Content Area:* Adult Health/Musculoskeletal

*Reference*

Smeltzer, S., & Bare, B. (2000). *Brunner & Suddarth's Textbook of medical-surgical nursing* (9th ed.). Philadelphia: Lippincott Williams & Wilkins, pp. 1791-1792.

**9.** A nurse instructs a parent regarding the appropriate actions to take when a toddler has a temper tantrum. Which statement by the parent indicates a successful outcome of the education?

1 "I will send my child to a room alone for 10 minutes after every tantrum."
2 "I will reward my child with candy at the end of each day without a tantrum."
3 "I will give frequent reminders that only bad children have tantrums."
4 "I will ignore the tantrums as long as there is no physical danger."

**Answer: 4**

*Rationale:* Ignoring a negative attention-seeking behavior is considered the best way to extinguish it, provided the child is safe from injury. Option 1 gives attention to the tantrum and also exceeds the recommended time of 1 minute per year of age for time-out. Providing candy for rewards is unhealthy and unlikely to be effective at the end of a day. Option 3 is untrue and negative.

*Test-Taking Strategy:* Use the process of elimination. Recalling that ignoring a tantrum is the best way to extinguish it will direct you to option 4. If you had difficulty with this question, review interventions for the child who has temper tantrums.

*Level of Cognitive Ability:* Analysis
*Client Needs:* Health Promotion and Maintenance
*Integrated Concept/Process:* Nursing Process/Evaluation
*Content Area:* Child Health

*Reference*

Wong, D. (1999). *Whaley & Wong's Nursing care of infants and children* (6th ed.). St. Louis: Mosby, p. 673.

**10.** A nurse is caring for a client in seclusion. The nurse best determines that it is safe for the client to come out of seclusion when the nurse hears the client say which of the following?

1   "I am no longer a threat to myself or others."
2   "I need to use the rest room right away."
3   "I'd like to go back to my room and be alone for a while."
4   "I can't breathe in here. The walls are closing in on me."

**Answer: 1**
*Rationale:* Option 1 indicates that the client may be safely removed from seclusion. The client in seclusion must be assessed at regular intervals (usually every 15 to 30 minutes) for physical needs, safety, and comfort. Option 2 indicates a physical need that could be met with a urinal, bedpan, or commode. It does not indicate that the client has calmed down enough to leave the seclusion room. Option 3 could be an attempt to manipulate the nurse. It gives no indication that the client will control himself or herself when alone in the room. Option 4 could be handled by supportive communication or a PRN medication, if indicated. It does not necessitate discontinuing seclusion.

*Test-Taking Strategy:* Focus on the issue of the question, removing a client from seclusion. Recalling the purpose and the use of seclusion will direct you to option 1. Review seclusion procedure, if you had difficulty with this question.

*Level of Cognitive Ability:* Analysis
*Client Needs:* Psychosocial Integrity
*Integrated Concept/Process:* Nursing Process/Evaluation
*Content Area:* Mental Health

*Reference*
Stuart, G.W., & Laraia, M.T. (1998). *Principles and practice of psychiatric nursing.* (6th ed.). St. Louis: Mosby, p. 634.

**11.** A client has had a laryngectomy for throat cancer and has started oral intake. A nurse concludes that the client has tolerated the first stage of dietary advancement if the client takes which of the following types of diet without aspiration or choking?

1   Bland
2   Clear liquids
3   Full liquids
4   Semisolid foods

**Answer: 4**
*Rationale:* Oral intake after laryngectomy is started with semi-solid foods. Once the client can manage this type of food, liquids may be introduced. Thin liquids are not given until the risk of aspiration is negligible. A bland diet is not appropriate. The client may not be able to tolerate the texture of some of the solid foods that would be included in a bland diet.

*Test-Taking Strategy:* Use the process of elimination. Eliminate options 2 and 3 first, recalling that a client with swallowing difficulty will be unable to manage liquids. From the remaining options, recall that a bland diet provides no control over the consistency or texture of the food. Review dietary measures for a client who has had a laryngectomy if you had difficulty with this question.

*Level of Cognitive Ability:* Analysis
*Client Needs:* Health Promotion and Maintenance
*Integrated Concept/Process:* Nursing Process/Evaluation
*Content Area:* Adult Health/Oncology

*Reference*
Smeltzer, S., & Bare, B. (2000). *Brunner & Suddarth's Textbook of medical-surgical nursing* (9th ed.). Philadelphia: Lippincott Williams & Wilkins, p. 418.

**12.** An elderly male client who is a victim of elder abuse and the client's family have been seen in a counseling center weekly for the past month. Which of the following statements, if made by the abusive family member, would indicate that he or she has learned more positive coping skills?

  **1** "I will be more careful to make sure that my father's needs are 100% met."

  **2** "I am so sorry and embarrassed that the abusive event occurred. It won't happen again."

  **3** "I feel better equipped to care for my father now that I know where to turn if I need assistance."

  **4** "Now that my father is moving into my home, I will have to stop drinking alcohol."

**Answer: 3**

*Rationale:* Elder abuse is sometimes the result of family members being expected to care for their aging parents. This care can cause the family to become overextended, frustrated, or financially depleted. Knowing where to turn in the community for assistance in caring for an aging family member can bring much-needed relief. Using such alternatives is a positive coping skill that many families learn. Options 1, 2, and 4 are statements of good faith or promises, which may or may not be kept in the future.

*Test-Taking Strategy:* Focus on the issue, positive coping skills, and use the process of elimination. Option 3 is the only option that identifies a means of coping with the issues and outlines a definitive plan for how to handle the pressure associated with the father's care. Review the concepts related to elder abuse if you had difficulty with this question.

*Level of Cognitive Ability:* Analysis
*Client Needs:* Psychosocial Integrity
*Integrated Concept/Process:* Nursing Process/Evaluation
*Content Area:* Mental Health

*Reference*
Fortinash, K., & Holoday-Worret, P. (2000). *Psychiatric mental health nursing* (2nd ed.). St. Louis: Mosby, p. 644.

**13.** A nurse is caring for a term infant who is 24 hours old and who had a confirmed episode of hypoglycemia at 1 hour of age. Which of the following observations by the nurse would indicate the need for further evaluation?

  **1** Blood glucose level of 40 mg/dL before the last feeding

  **2** High-pitched cry; eating 10 to 15 mL of formula per feeding

  **3** Weight loss of 4 ounces and dry, peeling skin

  **4** Breast-feeding for 20 minutes or longer; strong sucking

**Answer: 2**

*Rationale:* At 24 hours of age, a term infant should be able to consume at least 1 ounce (30 mL) of formula per feeding. A high-pitched cry is indicative of neurological involvement. Blood glucose levels are acceptable at 40 mg/dL in the first few days of life. Weight loss over the first few days of life and dry, peeling skin are normal findings for term infants. Breast-feeding for 20 minutes with a strong suck is an excellent finding. Hypoglycemia causes central nervous system symptoms (high-pitched cry), and also is exhibited by lack of strength to eat enough for growth.

*Test-Taking Strategy:* Use the process of elimination, noting the key words *need for further evaluation*. Eliminate options 1, 3, and 4 because these are normal findings. The words *high-pitched cry* should direct you to option 2. If you had difficulty with this question, review normal newborn findings and the indications of hypoglycemia.

*Level of Cognitive Ability:* Analysis
*Client Needs:* Physiological Integrity
*Integrated Concept/Process:* Nursing Process/Evaluation
*Content Area:* Maternity

*References*
Olds, S., London. M., & Ladewig, P. (2000). *Maternal-newborn nursing: A family and community-based approach* (6th ed.). Upper Saddle River, N.J.: Prentice-Hall Health, p. 731.

**14.** A home care nurse visits a child with a diagnosis of celiac disease. Which of these findings would best indicate that a gluten-free diet is being maintained and has been effective?

1   The child is free of diarrhea
2   The child is free of bloody stools
3   The child tolerates dietary wheat and rye
4   A balanced fluid and electrolyte status as noted in the laboratory results

**Answer: 1**
*Rationale:* Watery diarrhea is a frequent clinical manifestation of celiac disease. The absence of diarrhea indicates effective treatment. The grains of wheat and rye contain gluten and are not allowed. A balance in fluids and electrolytes does not necessarily demonstrate improved status of celiac disease.

*Test-Taking Strategy:* Focus on the issue, a lack of signs and symptoms related to celiac disease. Recalling that watery diarrhea is a manifestation of celiac disease will direct you to option 1. If you had difficulty with this question, review the manifestations of this disorder.

*Level of Cognitive Ability:* Analysis
*Client Needs:* Health Promotion and Maintenance
*Integrated Concept/Process:* Nursing Process/Evaluation
*Content Area:* Child Health

*Reference*
Wong, D. (1999). *Whaley & Wong's Nursing care of infants and children* (6th ed.). St. Louis: Mosby, p. 1567.

**15.** A nurse is assisting in caring for a woman in labor who is receiving oxytocin (Pitocin) by intravenous (IV) infusion. The nurse monitors the client, knowing that which of the following indicates an adequate contraction pattern?

1   Three to five contractions in a 10-minute period, with resultant cervical dilatation
2   One contraction per minute, with resultant cervical dilatation
3   Four contractions every 5 minutes, with resultant cervical dilatation
4   One contraction every 10 minutes, without resultant cervical dilatation

**Answer: 1**
*Rationale:* The preferred oxytocin dosage is the minimal amount necessary to maintain an adequate contraction pattern, characterized by three to five contractions in a 10-minute period, with resultant cervical dilatation. If contractions are more frequent than every 2 minutes, contraction quality may be decreased.

*Test-Taking Strategy:* Use the process of elimination. Focusing on the issue, an adequate contraction pattern, will assist in eliminating option 4. Next, eliminate options 2 and 3 because they are similar. If you had difficulty with this question, review the expected effects of this medication.

*Level of Cognitive Ability:* Analysis
*Client Needs:* Physiological Integrity
*Integrated Concept/Process:* Nursing Process/Evaluation
*Content Area:* Maternity

*Reference*
Lowdermilk, D., Perry, S., & Bobak, I. (2000). *Maternity & women's health care* (7th ed.). St. Louis: Mosby, p. 572.

**16.** A home care nurse is assigned to visit a preschooler who has a diagnosis of scarlet fever and is on bed rest. What data obtained by the nurse would indicate that the child is coping with the illness and bed rest?

1. The child is coloring and drawing pictures in a notebook
2. The mother keeps providing new activities for the child to do
3. The child insists that the mother stay in the room
4. The child sucks the thumb whenever the child does not get what is asked for

**Answer: 1**

*Rationale:* According to Piaget, for the preschooler, play is the best way to understand and adjust to life's experiences. Preschoolers are able to use pencils and crayons. They can draw stick figures and other rudimentary things. A child with scarlet fever needs quiet play, and drawing will provide that. Options 2, 3, and 4 do not identify coping behaviors.

*Test-Taking Strategy:* Think about the developmental level of preschoolers. Note the issue, an analysis of data by the nurse to determine if the child is coping with the disease and bed rest. Option 1 is a positive coping behavior for preschoolers. Options 2, 3, and 4 do not identify positive coping behaviors. Review the expected developmental level of a preschooler and the effects of bed rest on the child if you had difficulty with this question.

*Level of Cognitive Ability:* Analysis
*Client Needs:* Psychosocial integrity
*Integrated Concept/Process:* Nursing Process/Evaluation
*Content Area:* Child Health

*Reference*
Wong, D. (1999). *Whaley & Wong's Nursing care of infants and children* (6th ed.). St. Louis: Mosby, p. 1006.

**17.** A client has just taken a dose of trimethobenzamide (Tigan). A nurse concludes that the medication has been effective if the client expresses relief of:

1. Heartburn
2. Constipation
3. Nausea and vomiting
4. Abdominal pain

**Answer: 3**

*Rationale:* Tigan is an antiemetic agent; it is used in the treatment of nausea and vomiting. The medication is not used to treat heartburn, constipation, or abdominal pain.

*Test-Taking Strategy:* Use the process of elimination. Recalling that this medication is an antiemetic will direct you to option 3. Review the action of this medication if you had difficulty with this question.

*Level of Cognitive Ability:* Analysis
*Client Needs:* Physiological Integrity
*Integrated Concept/Process:* Nursing Process/Evaluation
*Content Area:* Pharmacology

*Reference*
Deglin, J., & Vallerand, A. (1999). *Davis's drug guide for nurses* (6th ed.). Philadelphia: F.A. Davis, p. 1008.

**18.** A nurse is providing instructions to the mother of a child with a diagnosis of strabismus of the left eye. The nurse reviews the procedure for patching. The nurse determines that the mother understands the procedure if the mother makes which statement?

1   "I will place the patch on the right eye."
2   "I will place the patch on both eyes."
3   "I will place the patch on the left eye."
4   "I will alternate the patch from the right to the left eye every hour."

**Answer: 1**

*Rationale:* Patching may be used in the treatment of strabismus to strengthen the weak eye. In this treatment, the good eye is patched. This encourages the child to use the weaker eye. Patching is most successful when done during the preschool years. The schedule for patching is individualized and prescribed by the ophthalmologist.

*Test-Taking Strategy:* Use the process of elimination. Remembering that this condition is a lazy eye will direct you to the correct option. It makes sense to patch the unaffected eye in order to strengthen the muscles in the affected eye. Review the procedure for patching, if you had difficulty with this question.

*Level of Cognitive Ability:* Analysis
*Client Needs:* Physiological Integrity
*Integrated Concept/Process:* Nursing Process/Evaluation
*Content Area:* Child Health

*Reference*
Wong, D. (1999). *Whaley & Wong's Nursing care of infants and children* (6th ed.). St. Louis: Mosby, pp. 259, 1098.

---

**19.** A nurse is assessing a client with pregnancy-induced hypertension (PIH) who was admitted to the hospital 48 hours ago. Which of the following data would indicate that the condition has not yet resolved?

1   Blood pressure reading at prenatal baseline
2   Urinary output is increased
3   Client complaints of blurred vision
4   Presence of trace urinary protein

**Answer: 3**

*Rationale:* Client complaints of headache or blurred vision indicate a worsening of the condition and warrant immediate further evaluation. Options 1, 2, and 4 are all signs that the pregnancy-induced hypertension is being resolved.

*Test-Taking Strategy:* Note the key words *has not yet resolved*. This indicates that you need to look for the option that identifies a symptom of PIH. Options 1 and 2 can be eliminated first because they are normal findings. From the remaining options, note that option 4 contains the word *trace* and is the most normal finding of these two options. If you had difficulty with this question, review the clinical manifestations associated with PIH.

*Level of Cognitive Ability:* Analysis
*Client Needs:* Physiological Integrity
*Integrated Concept/Process:* Nursing Process/Evaluation
*Content Area:* Maternity

*Reference*
Gorrie, T., McKinney, E., & Murray, S. (1998). *Foundations of maternal-newborn nursing* (2nd ed.). Philadelphia: W.B. Saunders, p. 690.

**20.** A client has begun medication therapy with betaxolol (Kerlone). A nurse would conclude that the client is experiencing the intended effects of therapy if which of the following is noted?
1  Weight loss of 5 pounds
2  Pulse rate increased to 74 from 58 beats per minute
3  Blood pressure decreased from 142/94 mm Hg to 128/82 mm Hg
4  Edema present at 3+

**Answer: 3**
*Rationale:* Betaxolol is a beta-adrenergic blocking agent used to lower blood pressure, relieve angina, or eliminate dysrhythmias. Side effects include bradycardia and symptoms of congestive heart failure, such as weight gain and increased edema.

*Test-Taking Strategy:* Note that the question asks for the *intended effects* of the medication. Remember that beta-adrenergic blocking agents end with the suffix *-olol.* Recalling the action of the medication will direct you to option 3. Review the intended effects of this medication, if you had difficulty with this question.

*Level of Cognitive Ability:* Analysis
*Client Needs:* Physiological Integrity
*Integrated Concept/Process:* Nursing Process/Evaluation
*Content Area:* Pharmacology

*Reference*
Hodgson, B., & Kizior, R. (2001). *Saunders nursing drug handbook 2001.* Philadelphia: W.B. Saunders, p. 109.

**21.** A nurse has taught a client taking a xanthine bronchodilator about beverages to avoid. The nurse concludes that the client understands the information if the client chooses which of the following beverages from the dietary menu?
1  Chocolate milk
2  Cranberry juice
3  Coffee
4  Cola

**Answer: 2**
*Rationale:* Cola, coffee, and chocolate contain xanthine and should be avoided by a client taking a xanthine bronchodilator. This could lead to an increased incidence of the cardiovascular and central nervous system side effects that can occur with the use of this type of bronchodilator.

*Test-Taking Strategy:* Use the process of elimination. Note the similarity between options 1, 3, and 4 in that they all contain some form of stimulant. Review dietary measures for a client taking a xanthine bronchodilator if the question was difficult.

*Level of Cognitive Ability:* Analysis
*Client Needs:* Health Promotion and Maintenance
*Integrated Concept/Process:* Nursing Process/Evaluation
*Content Area:* Pharmacology

*Reference*
Black, J., Hawks, J., & Keene, A. (2001). *Medical-surgical nursing: Clinical management for positive outcomes* (6th ed.). Philadelphia: W.B. Saunders, p. 1691.

**22.** A client is started on tolbutamide (Orinase) once daily. A nurse observes for which of the following intended effects of this medication?
1  Decreased blood pressure
2  Decreased blood glucose
3  Weight loss
4  Resolution of infection

**Answer: 2**
*Rationale:* Tolbutamide is an oral hypoglycemic agent that is taken in the morning. It is not used to decrease blood pressure, enhance weight loss, or treat infection.

*Test-Taking Strategy:* Note the key words *intended effects.* Recalling that this medication is an oral hypoglycemic will direct you to option 2. Review the action of this medication, if you had difficulty with this question.

*Level of Cognitive Ability:* Analysis
*Client Needs:* Physiological Integrity
*Integrated Concept/Process:* Nursing Process/Evaluation
*Content Area:* Pharmacology

**Reference**
Deglin, J., & Vallerand, A. (1999). *Davis's drug guide for nurses* (6th ed.).
   Philadelphia: F.A. Davis, p. 1143.

---

**23.** A client who chronically uses nonsteroidal antiinflammatory drugs (NSAIDs) has been taking misoprostol (Cytotec). A nurse would monitor the client to see if the client experienced relief of which of the following symptoms?
1   Epigastric pain
2   Diarrhea
3   Bleeding
4   Infection

**Answer: 1**
*Rationale:* The client who chronically uses NSAIDs is prone to gastric mucosal injury, which gives the client epigastric pain as a symptom. Misoprostol is administered to prevent this occurrence. Diarrhea can be a side effect of the medication, but is not an intended effect. Bleeding and infection are unrelated to the question.

*Test-Taking Strategy:* Note key words *NSAIDs* and *relief*. They tell you that the medication is being given to treat or prevent the occurrence of a specific symptom. Recalling that NSAIDs can cause gastric mucosal injury will direct you to option 1. Review the action and indications for the use of misoprostol, if you had difficulty with this question.

*Level of Cognitive Ability:* Analysis
*Client Needs:* Physiological Integrity
*Integrated Concept/Process:* Nursing Process/Evaluation
*Content Area:* Pharmacology

**Reference**
Deglin, J., & Vallerand, A. (1999). *Davis's drug guide for nurses* (6th ed.).
   Philadelphia: F.A. Davis, p. 670.

---

**24.** A client has received a dose of a PRN medication called loperamide (Imodium). A nurse evaluates the client after administration to see if the client has experienced relief of:
1   Constipation
2   Diarrhea
3   Tarry stools
4   Abdominal pain

**Answer: 2**
*Rationale:* Loperamide is an antidiarrheal agent. It is commonly administered after loose stools. It is used in the management of acute diarrhea and also in chronic diarrhea, such as with inflammatory bowel disease. It can also be used to reduce the volume of drainage from an ileostomy.

*Test-Taking Strategy:* Use the process of elimination. Recalling that this medication is an antidiarrheal agent will direct you to option 2. Review the purpose of this medication if you had difficulty with this question.

*Level of Cognitive Ability:* Analysis
*Client Needs:* Physiological Integrity
*Integrated Concept/Process:* Nursing Process/Evaluation
*Content Area:* Pharmacology

**Reference**
Deglin, J., & Vallerand, A. (1999). *Davis's drug guide for nurses* (6th ed.).
   Philadelphia: F.A. Davis. p. 587.

**25.** A nurse has reinforced discharge instructions to the parents of a child who has had heart surgery. Which of the following if stated by the parent would indicate a need for further instructions?

1 "I should call the physician if my child develops faster or harder breathing than normal."
2 "My child can return to school for full days in 3 weeks following discharge."
3 "I should have my child avoid crowds and people for 1 week after discharge."
4 "I should allow my child to play inside but omit play outside at this time."

**Answer: 2**

*Rationale:* The child may return to school 3 weeks after hospital discharge, but the child should go to school for half-days for the first week. Outside play should be omitted for several weeks; inside play should be allowed as tolerated. The child should avoid crowds of people for 1 week after discharge, including crowds at day care centers and churches. If any difficulty with breathing occurs, the parents should notify the physician.

*Test-Taking Strategy:* Note the key words *indicate a need for further instructions.* Recalling the principles related to the prevention of infection and the complications of surgery will direct you to option 2. If you had difficulty with this question, review home care instructions for the parents of a child who has had heart surgery.

*Level of Cognitive Ability:* Analysis
*Client Needs:* Health Promotion and Maintenance
*Integrated Concept/Process:* Nursing Process/Evaluation
*Content Area:* Child Health

*Reference*
Wong, D. (1999). *Whaley & Wong's Nursing care of infants and children* (6th ed.). St. Louis: Mosby, p. 1623.

**26.** A client has been given a prescription for a course of azithromycin (Zithromax). A nurse concludes that the medication is having the intended effect if which of the following is noted?

1 Signs and symptoms of infection are relieved
2 Pain is relieved
3 Joint discomfort is reduced
4 Blood pressure is lower

**Answer: 1**

*Rationale:* Azithromycin is a macrolide antibiotic, which is used to treat infection. It is not ordered for the treatment of pain, joint inflammation, or blood pressure.

*Test-Taking Strategy:* Use the process of elimination. Eliminate options 2 and 3 first because they are similar. From the remaining options, recalling the action of this medication will direct you to option 1. Review the action and purpose of azithromycin if you had difficulty with this question.

*Level of Cognitive Ability:* Analysis
*Client Needs:* Physiological Integrity
*Integrated Concept/Process:* Nursing Process/Evaluation
*Content Area:* Pharmacology

*Reference*
Deglin, J., & Vallerand, A. (1999). *Davis's drug guide for nurses* (6th ed.). Philadelphia: F.A. Davis. p. 91.

**27.** A nurse is assigned to care for a client with acquired immunodeficiency syndrome (AIDS) who is receiving amphotericin B (Fungizone) for a fungal respiratory infection. Which of the following would indicate an adverse reaction to the medication?

   1   Hypocalcemia
   2   Hypokalemia
   3   Hypercalcemia
   4   Hyperkalemia

**Answer: 2**

*Rationale:* Clients receiving amphotericin B may develop hypokalemia, which can be severe and lead to extreme muscle weakness and electrocardiogram (ECG) changes. Distal renal tubular acidosis commonly occurs, contributing to the development of hypokalemia. High potassium levels do not occur. The medication does not cause calcium levels to fluctuate.

*Test-Taking Strategy:* Knowledge that an adverse reaction to amphotericin B is hypokalemia is necessary to answer the question. Review this medication if you had difficulty with this question.

*Level of Cognitive Ability:* Analysis
*Client Needs:* Physiological Integrity
*Integrated Concept/Process:* Nursing Process/Evaluation
*Content Area:* Pharmacology

*Reference*
Hodgson, B., & Kizior, R. (2001). *Saunders nursing drug handbook 2001.* Philadelphia: W.B. Saunders, p. 57.

**28.** A client is seen in a health care clinic, and a diagnosis of conjunctivitis is made. A nurse provides instructions to the client regarding care for the disorder while the client is at home. Which of the following statements if made by the client indicates a need for further education?

   1   "I do not need to be concerned about spreading this infection to others in my family."
   2   "I should apply a warm compress before instilling antibiotic drops if purulent discharge is present in my eye."
   3   "I should perform a saline eye irrigation prior to instilling the antibiotic drops into my eye if purulent discharge is present."
   4   "I can use an ophthalmic analgesic ointment at nighttime if I have eye discomfort."

**Answer: 1**

*Rationale:* Conjunctivitis is highly contagious. Antibiotic drops are usually administered four times a day. When purulent discharge is present, saline eye irrigations or eye applications of warm compresses may be necessary before instillation of the medication. Ophthalmic analgesic ointment or drops may be instilled, especially at bedtime, because discomfort becomes more noticeable when the eyelids are closed.

*Test-Taking Strategy:* Use the process of elimination, noting the key words *need for further education.* Knowing that this disorder is considered highly contagious will direct you to option 1. If you have difficulty with this question, review management of the client with this disorder.

*Level of Cognitive Ability:* Analysis
*Client Needs:* Health Promotion and Maintenance
*Integrated Concept/Process:* Nursing Process/Evaluation
*Content Area:* Adult Health/Eye

*Reference*
Beare, P., & Myers, J. (1998). *Adult Health Nursing* (3rd ed.). St. Louis: Mosby, p. 1143.

**29.** A nurse reviews the nursing care plan for a hospitalized child who is immobilized because of skeletal traction. The nurse notes a nursing diagnosis of Altered Growth and Development related to immobilization and hospitalization. Which of the following evaluative statements indicates a positive outcome for the child?

1 The fracture heals without complications

2 The child displays age-appropriate developmental behaviors

3 The caregivers verbalize safe and effective home care

4 The child maintains normal joint and muscle integrity

**Answer: 2**

*Rationale:* Regression and inappropriate developmental behaviors may be displayed in response to immobilization and hospitalization. With individualized care planning, a positive outcome of age-appropriate behavior can be achieved. Options 1, 3, and 4 are appropriate evaluative statements for an immobilized child but do not directly address the nursing diagnosis, Altered Growth and Development.

*Test-Taking Strategy:* Focus on the issue, altered growth and development. Use the process of elimination. Recalling that altered growth & development is the state in which an individual is not performing age-appropriate tasks will direct you to option 2. All options are evaluative statements, but only option 2 addresses this nursing diagnosis. Review the defining characteristics and the appropriate outcomes for this nursing diagnosis if you had difficulty with this question.

*Level of Cognitive Ability:* Analysis
*Client Needs:* Health Promotion and Maintenance
*Integrated Concept/Process:* Nursing Process/Evaluation
*Content Area:* Child Health

*Reference*
Wong, D. (1999). *Whaley & Wong's Nursing care of infants and children* (6th ed.). St. Louis: Mosby, p. 1919.

**30.** A nurse is evaluating the effects of care for a client with nephrotic syndrome. The nurse determines that the client showed the least amount of improvement if which of the following information was obtained serially over 2 days of care?

1 Initial weight 208 pounds, down to 203 pounds

2 Daily intake and output record of 2100 mL intake and 1900 mL output, and 2000 mL intake and 2900 mL output

3 Blood pressure 160/90 mm Hg, down to 140/80 mm Hg

4 Serum albumin 1.9 g/dL, up to 2.0 g/dL

**Answer: 4**

*Rationale:* The goal of therapy in nephrotic syndrome is to heal the leaking glomerular membrane. This would then control edema by stopping the loss of protein in the urine. Fluid balance and albumin levels are monitored to determine the effectiveness of therapy. Option 1 represents a loss of fluid that slightly exceeds 2 liters and represents a significant improvement. Option 2 represents a total fluid loss of 700 mL over the 2 days, which is also helpful. Option 3 shows improvement because both systolic and diastolic blood pressures are lower. The least amount of improvement is in the serum albumin level, since the normal albumin level is 3.5 to 5.0 g/dL.

*Test-Taking Strategy:* Use the process of elimination, noting the key words *least amount of improvement.* Option 1 illustrates the greatest improvement and is eliminated first. Option 2 is also a significant improvement and is eliminated next. From the remaining options, noting that the blood pressure has reentered the normal range will direct you to option 4. Review care of the client with nephrotic syndrome if you had difficulty with this question.

*Level of Cognitive Ability:* Analysis
*Client Needs:* Physiological Integrity
*Integrated Concept/Process:* Nursing Process/Evaluation
*Content Area:* Adult Health/Renal

**Reference**
Monahan, F., & Neighbors, M. (1998). *Medical-surgical nursing: Foundations for clinical practice* (2nd ed.). Philadelphia: W.B Saunders, p. 1255.

# CARING

1. A woman comes into an emergency room in a severe state of anxiety following a car accident. The most important nursing intervention at this time would be to:
   1 Remain with the client
   2 Put the client in a quiet room
   3 Teach the client deep breathing
   4 Encourage the client to talk about her feelings and concerns

**Answer: 1**
*Rationale:* If the client is left alone with severe anxiety, she may feel abandoned and become overwhelmed. Placing the client in a quiet room is also indicated, but the nurse must stay with the client. It is not possible to teach the client deep breathing or relaxation exercises until the anxiety decreases. Encouraging the client to discuss concerns and feelings would not take place until the anxiety has decreased.

*Test-Taking Strategy:* Note the key words *severe state of anxiety*. Since the anxiety state is severe, eliminate options 3 and 4. From the remaining options, consider the words *most important* in the stem of the question. They should direct you to option 1. Review care of the client with severe anxiety if you had difficulty with this question.

*Level of Cognitive Ability:* Application
*Client Needs:* Psychosocial Integrity
*Integrated Concept/Process:* Caring
*Content Area:* Mental Health

**Reference**
Varcarolis, E. (1998). *Foundations of psychiatric mental health nursing* (3rd ed.). Philadelphia: W.B. Saunders, p. 349.

2. A nurse has cared for a client who died a few minutes ago. The nurse reflects on the care given to the client. Which of the following statements supports the nurse's belief that the client died with dignity?
   1 The family thanks the nurse and states that the client was not in pain and was peaceful at the end
   2 The physician recognizes that all the orders were carried out and that there were no questions
   3 A new nurse states that it is difficult to give that kind of care to a dying client
   4 The nurse gave increasing doses of pain medication to keep the client well sedated

**Answer: 1**
*Rationale:* The family's response is an external perception and is extremely important. Families derive a great deal of comfort from knowing that their loved ones received the best care possible. Option 1 provides external validation that the client received comprehensive, high-quality care. Option 2 focuses on physicians' orders rather than client care. Option 3 focuses on the feelings of a new nurse, who may be expressing his or her own anxiety. Option 4 reflects only one aspect of caring for a dying client.

*Test-Taking Strategy:* Use the process of elimination and focus on the issue, that the client died with dignity. The only option that addresses this issue is option 1. Review the concepts related to death and dying if you had difficulty with this question.

*Level of Cognitive Ability:* Analysis
*Client Needs:* Psychosocial Integrity

*Integrated Concept/Process:* Caring
*Content Area:* Fundamental Skills

*Reference*
Monahan, F., & Neighbors, M. (1998). *Medical-surgical nursing: Foundations for clinical practice* (2nd ed.). Philadelphia: W.B Saunders, pp. 38-29.

---

**3.** The family of a client with Parkinson's disease tells a nurse that the client is having difficulty adjusting to the disorder and that they do not know what to do to help. The nurse advises the family that which of the following would be the most therapeutic in assisting the client to cope with the disease?

1 Encourage and praise client efforts to exercise and perform activities of daily living (ADLs)
2 Cluster activities at the end of the day, when the client is restless and bored
3 Plan only a few activities for the client during the day
4 Assist the client with ADLs as much as possible

**Answer: 1**

*Rationale:* The client with Parkinson's disease has a tendency to become withdrawn and depressed, which can be limited by encouraging the client to be an active participant in his or her own care. The family should also give the client encouragement and praise for perseverance in these efforts. The family should plan activities intermittently throughout the day to inhibit daytime sleeping and boredom.

*Test-Taking Strategy:* Use the process of elimination. Eliminate option 2 first because clustering activities at one time will tire the client. Eliminate option 3 next because of the use of the absolute word *only*. From the remaining options, recalling that the client should be an active participant in his or her own care will direct you to option 1. Review therapeutic techniques for assisting the client with Parkinson's disease with adjustment to the disease, if you had difficulty with this question.

*Level of Cognitive Ability:* Application
*Client Needs:* Psychosocial Integrity
*Integrated Concept/Process:* Caring
*Content Area:* Adult Health/Neurological

*Reference*
Monahan, F., & Neighbors, M. (1998). *Medical-surgical nursing: Foundations for clinical practice* (2nd ed.). Philadelphia: W.B. Saunders, p. 787.

---

**4.** A community health nurse is caring for a group of homeless people in a certain area of a city. In planning for the potential needs of this group, what is the most immediate concern?

1 Peer support through structured groups
2 Setting up a 24-hour crisis center and hotline
3 Meeting the basic needs to ensure that adequate food, shelter, and clothing are available
4 Finding affordable housing for the group

**Answer: 3**

*Rationale:* The question asks about the immediate concern. The ABCs of community health are always attending to peoples basic needs of food, shelter, and clothing. Options 1, 2, and 4 are activities that may be carried out at a later time.

*Test-Taking Strategy:* Use Maslow's Hierarchy of Needs theory to answer the question. Option 3 addresses basic physiological needs. Although options 1, 2, and 4 are also appropriate actions, option 3 is the immediate concern. Review the needs of the homeless population if you had difficulty with this question.

*Level of Cognitive Ability:* Analysis
*Client Needs:* Physiological Integrity
*Integrated Concept/Process:* Caring
*Content Area:* Mental Health

*Reference*
Varcarolis, E. (1998). *Foundations of psychiatric mental health nursing* (3rd ed.). Philadelphia: W.B. Saunders. p. 842.

**5.** A stillborn was delivered a few hours ago. After the birth, the family has remained together, holding and touching the baby. Which statement by the nurse would further assist the family in their initial period of grief?

1  "I feel so bad. I don't understand why this happened either."
2  "You can hold the baby for another 15 minutes; then I need to take the baby away."
3  "What did you name your baby?"
4  "You seem upset. Do you need a tranquilizer?"

**Answer: 3**

*Rationale:* Nurses should be able to explore measures that assist the family to create memories of an infant so that the existence of the child is confirmed and the parents can complete the grieving process. Option 3 identifies such a measure and also demonstrates a caring and empathetic response. Option 1 is inappropriate and reflects a lack of knowledge on the nurse's part. Option 2 is uncaring. Option 4 devalues the parents feelings and is inappropriate.

*Test-Taking Strategy:* Note the key words *further assist the family in their initial period of grief.* Use the process of elimination and therapeutic communication techniques. Choose the option that demonstrates a caring and empathetic response by the nurse and meets the psychosocial needs of the family. Review therapeutic communication techniques and the grief process if you had difficulty with this question.

*Level of Cognitive Ability:* Application
*Client Needs:* Psychosocial Integrity
*Integrated Concept/Process:* Caring
*Content Area:* Maternity

*Reference*
Gorrie, T., McKinney, E., & Murray, S. (1998). *Foundations of maternal-newborn nursing* (2nd ed.) Philadelphia: W. B. Saunders, p. 663.

**6.** While counseling a prenatal client about her dietary and alcohol drinking habits, a nurse observes that the client has difficulty concentrating and appears agitated. The nurse should proceed with the assessment by using which guideline?

1  Discussing the possible consequences of drinking alcohol during pregnancy should be avoided
2  Women respond negatively to a hopeful message of the potential benefits of drinking cessation during pregnancy
3  A nonjudgmental approach may help to gain maternal trust
4  Provoking maternal guilt may help a woman recognize her problem and seek support services

**Answer: 3**

*Rationale:* The potential effects of alcohol abuse during pregnancy for both the mother and the fetus have been well documented. The nurse who expresses genuine concern for suspected abusers may motivate positive behavioral changes during the prenatal period. The maternal behaviors of lack of concentration and agitation are frequently seen in childbearing women who are abusing alcohol. Options 1, 2, and 4 are inappropriate guidelines for the nurse to follow in this situation, and they do not address a caring approach.

*Test-Taking Strategy:* Use therapeutic communication techniques and the process of elimination. Remember that it is important to display a caring and nonjudgmental attitude. Review therapeutic communication techniques if you had difficulty with this question.

*Level of Cognitive Ability:* Application
*Clients Needs:* Psychosocial Integrity
*Integrated Concept/Process:* Caring
*Content Area:* Maternity

*Reference*
Lowdermilk, D., Perry, S., & Bobak, I. (2000). *Maternity & women's health care* (7th ed.). St. Louis: Mosby, p. 945.

**7.** A client was injured in an automobile accident as a result of passing out at the wheel of the car after drinking alcohol. The client's only daughter, who was a passenger in the car, was killed instantly. In a change-of-shift report, a nurse is told that the client is upset and withdrawn. In the care of this client, what is the most appropriate nursing action initially?

1 Let the client have some time alone to grieve over the loss
2 Tell the client that the injury and the daughter's death were a result of alcohol abuse and refer the client for counseling
3 Inform the physician of the client's depression and request medication to assist the client in coping with the loss
4 Reflect back to the client that he or she appears upset

**Answer: 4**

*Rationale:* The nurse needs to encourage the client to express feelings. Reflection statements tend to elicit deeper awareness of feelings. In addition, option 4 validates the perception that the client is upset. A well-timed reflection can reveal an emotion that has escaped the client's notice. Option 2 is inappropriate and is a block to communication. Options 1 and 3 address interventions prior to assessment of the situation.

*Test-Taking Strategy:* Note the key words *most appropriate* and *initially.* Use therapeutic communication techniques and the process of elimination. Select the option that encourages the client to express his or her feelings and talk more. Remember to always address the client's feelings. Review therapeutic communication techniques if you had difficulty with this question.

*Level of Cognitive Ability:* Application
*Client Needs:* Psychosocial Integrity
*Integrated Concept/Process:* Caring
*Content Area:* Mental Health

*Reference*
Varcarolis, E. (1998). *Foundations of psychiatric mental health nursing* (3rd ed.). Philadelphia: W.B. Saunders, p. 189.

**8.** An emergency room nurse is assigned to care for an elderly client who has been identified as a victim of physical abuse. In planning care for this client, the nurse's priority is focused toward:

1 Referring the abusing family member for treatment
2 Adhering to the mandatory abuse reporting laws
3 Encouraging the client to file charges against the abuser
4 Removing the client from any immediate danger

**Answer: 4**

*Rationale:* Whenever the abused client remains in the abusive environment, priority must be placed on ascertaining whether the person is in any immediate danger. If so, emergency action must be taken to remove him or her from the abusing situation. Options 1 and 2 may be appropriate interventions but are not the priority. Option 3 is not an appropriate intervention at this time and may produce increased fear and anxiety in the client.

*Test-Taking Strategy:* Use the process of elimination and eliminate option 3 first, knowing that this action may produce increased fear and anxiety in the client. Use Maslow's Hierarchy of Needs theory to select from the remaining options, remembering that if a physiological need is not present, then safety is the priority. This guide should direct you to option 4, the only option that directly addresses client safety. Review the principles related to caring for the abused client if you had difficulty with this question.

*Level of Cognitive Ability:* Application
*Client Needs:* Safe, Effective Care Environment
*Integrated Concept/Process:* Caring
*Content Area:* Mental Health

*Reference*
Varcarolis, E. (1998). *Foundations of psychiatric mental health nursing* (3rd ed.). Philadelphia: W.B. Saunders, p. 394.

*(handwritten: X  ↗ dispandant! 沮喪)*

**9.** A community health nurse is working with elderly people involved in a recent flood. Many were despondent and refused to leave their homes for days. In planning for the rescue and relocation of these elderly residents, what is the first item that the nurse needs to consider?

1 Attending to their emotional needs
2 Attending to nutritional status and basic needs
3 Contacting the elderly residents' families
4 Arranging for ambulance transportation for the elderly residents

**Answer: 2**
*Rationale:* The question asks about the first thing that the nurse needs to consider. The ABCs of community health are always attending to people's basic needs of food, shelter, and clothing. Options 1, 3, and 4 are activities that may or may not be needed at a later date.

*Test-Taking Strategy:* Use Maslow's Hierarchy of Needs theory to answer the question. Option 2 addresses basic physiological needs. Although options 1, 3, and 4 may be appropriate actions at a later time, option 2 is the immediate concern. Review care of clients experiencing crisis if you had difficulty with this question.

*Level of Cognitive Ability:* Application
*Client Needs:* Physiological Integrity
*Integrated Concept/Process:* Caring
*Content Area:* Mental Health

*Reference*
Varcarolis, E.M. (1998). *Foundations of psychiatric mental health nursing.* (3rd ed.). Philadelphia: W.B. Saunders, pp. 368-370.

**10.** A nurse is assisting in planning care for a newly admitted suicidal client. In order to provide a caring, therapeutic environment, which of the following is included in the nursing care plan?

1 Placing the client in a private room to ensure privacy and confidentiality
2 Establishing a therapeutic relationship and conveying unconditional positive regard
3 Placing the client in charge of a meaningful unit activity, such as the morning chess tournament
4 Maintaining a distance of 12 inches at all times to assure the client that control will be provided

**Answer: 2**
*Rationale:* The establishment of a therapeutic relationship with the suicidal client increases feelings of acceptance. While the suicidal behavior and thinking of the client are unacceptable, the use of unconditional positive regard acknowledges the client in a human-to-human context and increases the client's sense of self-worth. The client would not be placed in a private room because this is an unsafe action and may intensify the client's feelings of worthlessness. Placing the client in charge of the morning chess game is a premature intervention that can overwhelm and cause the client to fail. This can reinforce the client's feelings of worthlessness. Distances of 18 inches or less between two individuals constitute intimate space. Invasion of this space may be misinterpreted by the client and increase the client's tension and feelings of helplessness.

*Test-Taking Strategy:* Use the process of elimination. Eliminate option 1 because isolation (private room) is not the safe and therapeutic intervention. Option 3 may produce feelings of worthlessness. Eliminate option 4 because a distance of 12 inches is restrictive. Option 2 is the only option that addresses a caring and therapeutic environment. Review care of the suicidal client if you had difficulty with this question.

*Level of Cognitive Ability:* Application
*Client Needs:* Safe, Effective Care Environment
*Integrated Concept/Process:* Caring
*Content Area:* Mental Health

*Reference*
Varcarolis, E. (1998). *Foundations of psychiatric mental health nursing* (3rd ed.). Philadelphia: W.B. Saunders, pp. 733-734.

**11.** A client has died, and a nurse asks a family member about the funeral arrangements. The family member refuses to discuss the issue. The nurse's most appropriate action is to:
1 Provide information needed for decision making
2 Assess the risk of self-harm and refer the family member to a mental health professional
3 Demonstrate acceptance of the family member's feelings
4 Remain with the family member without discussing funeral arrangements

**Answer: 4**
*Rationale:* The family member is exhibiting the first stage of grief, denial. Option 1 may be an appropriate intervention for the bargaining stage. Option 2 may be an appropriate intervention for the depression stage. Option 3 is an appropriate intervention for the acceptance or reorganization and restitution stage.

*Test-Taking Strategy:* Note the key words *most appropriate action*. Use therapeutic communication techniques. Eliminate options 1 and 2 because they do not address the issue of the question. From the remaining options, noting the key words *refuses to discuss the issue* will direct you to option 4. Acceptance of feelings is important, but in this situation, remaining with the family member is most appropriate. Review the grieving process and therapeutic communication techniques, if you had difficulty with this question.

*Level of Cognitive Ability:* Application
*Client Needs:* Psychosocial Integrity
*Integrated Concept/Process:* Caring
*Content Area:* Fundamental Skills

*Reference*
Leahy, J., & Kizilay, P. (1998). *Foundations of nursing practice: A nursing process approach.* Philadelphia: W.B. Saunders, p. 226.

**12.** A 39-year-old man learned today that his 36-year-old wife has an incurable cancer and is expected to live not more than a few weeks. A nurse explores the client's feelings and identifies which of these responses by the husband as indicative of effective individual coping?
1 He states that he will not allow his wife to come home to die
2 He immediately arranges for their three teen-aged children to live with relatives in another state
3 He expresses his anger at God and the physicians for allowing this to happen
4 He refuses to visit his wife in the hospital or to discuss her illness

**Answer: 3**
*Rationale:* The expression of anger is known to be a normal response to impending loss, and the anger may be directed toward oneself, the dying person, God or other spiritual being, or the caregivers. Options 1 and 2 indicate possibly rash and unilateral decisions made by the husband, without taking into consideration anyone else's feelings. There is evidence of denial in option 4, as he refuses to visit his wife or discuss her illness. The only response that indicates effective individual coping by the husband is option 3.

*Test-Taking Strategy:* Use the process of elimination. Note the key words *effective individual coping*. Knowledge of the stages of grief associated with loss will easily direct you to option 3. Review effective coping mechanisms if you had difficulty with this question.

*Level of Cognitive Ability:* Analysis
*Client Needs:* Psychosocial Integrity
*Integrated Concept/Process:* Caring
*Content Area:* Fundamental Skills

*Reference*
Harkreader, H. (2000). *Fundamentals of nursing: Caring and clinical judgment.* Philadelphia: W.B. Saunders, p. 1366.

**13.** A nurse is providing care to a Cuban-American client who is terminally ill. Numerous family members are present most of the time, and many of the family members are very emotional. The most appropriate nursing action is to:

1   Restrict the number of family members visiting at one time
2   Inform the family that emotional outbursts are to be avoided
3   Request permission to move the client to a private room, and allow the family members to visit
4   Contact the physician to speak to the family members regarding their behavior

**Answer: 3**

*Rationale:* In the Cuban-American culture, loud crying and other physical manifestations of grief are considered socially acceptable. Of the options provided, option 3 is the only option that represents a culturally sensitive and caring approach on the part of the nurse. Options 1, 2, and 4 are inappropriate nursing interventions.

*Test-Taking Strategy:* Focus on the clients of the question, who are the family members of a Cuban-American client. Use the process of elimination, recalling the characteristics of this culture and the importance of cultural sensitivity. This will easily direct you to option 3. If you had difficulty with this question, review the characteristics of this culture.

*Level of Cognitive Ability:* Application
*Client Needs:* Psychosocial Integrity
*Integrated Concept/Process:* Caring
*Content Area:* Fundamental Skills

*Reference*
Purnell, L., & Paulanka, B. (1998). *Transcultural health care: A culturally competent approach.* Philadelphia: F.A. Davis, p. 203.

---

**14.** A nurse is caring for an elderly client who has been recently admitted from home to a long-term-care facility. The client has a diagnosis of end-stage renal cancer. The nurse recognizes that the resident is coping with many losses. The best way to address the client's psychosocial needs is to:

1   Provide total care for the client
2   Medicate the client for pain every 4 hours as prescribed
3   Sit with the client to allow the client to verbalize feelings
4   Encourage the client to participate in daily social activities

**Answer: 3**

*Rationale:* Clients admitted from home into a long-term-care facility are dealing with losses in independence, privacy, and control over their environment. Providing total care does not facilitate independence. Medicating for pain will keep the client comfortable, but this does not address psychosocial needs. Sitting with the client to allow the client to express feelings is the best way to address psychosocial needs. Participation in daily social activities will not meet the special psychosocial needs of this client.

*Test-Taking Strategy:* Focus on the key words *psychosocial needs.* Eliminate options 1 and 2 first because these options deal with physiological needs. From the remaining options, recall that the client's feelings should be addressed first. This will direct you to option 3. Review care of the client experiencing loss if you had difficulty with this question.

*Level of Cognitive Ability:* Application
*Client Needs:* Psychosocial Integrity
*Integrated Concept/Process:* Caring
*Content Area:* Fundamental Skills

*Reference*
Leahy, J., & Kizilay, P. (1998). *Foundations of nursing practice: A nursing process approach.* Philadelphia: W.B. Saunders, pp. 361-362.

**15.** A client with diabetes mellitus is told that amputation of a leg is necessary to sustain life. The client is very upset and says to a nurse, "This is all the doctor's fault! I have done everything that the doctor has asked me to do!" The nurse interprets the client's statement as:

1   An expected coping mechanism
2   A need to notify the hospital lawyer
3   An expression of guilt on the part of the client
4   An ineffective coping mechanism

**Answer: 1**

*Rationale:* The expression of anger is known to be a normal response to impending loss, and the anger may be directed toward oneself, God or other spiritual being, or the caregivers. The nurse needs to be aware of the effective and ineffective coping mechanisms that can occur in a client when loss is anticipated. Notifying the hospital lawyer is inappropriate. Guilt may or may not be a component of the client's feelings, and the data in the question do not provide an indication that guilt is present.

*Test-Taking Strategy:* Focus on the data provided in the question. Note that options 1 and 4 address coping mechanisms. This may provide you with the clue that one of these may be the correct option. Noting that the client is blaming the doctor and knowledge of the stages of grief associated with loss will direct you to option 1. Review these stages and expected client expressions if you had difficulty with this question.

*Level of Cognitive Ability:* Analysis
*Client Needs:* Psychosocial Integrity
*Integrated Concept/Process:* Caring
*Content Area:* Fundamental Skills

*Reference*
Leahy, J., & Kizilay, P. (1998). *Foundations of nursing practice: A nursing process approach.* Philadelphia: W.B. Saunders, p. 115.

---

**16.** A nurse has been caring for a terminally ill client whose death is imminent. The nurse has developed a close relationship with the family of the client. Which of the following nursing interventions will the nurse avoid in dealing with the family during this difficult time?

1   Making the decisions for the family during the difficult moments
2   Encouraging family discussion of feelings
3   Facilitating the use of spiritual practices identified by the family
4   Accepting the family's expressions of anger

**Answer: 1**

*Rationale:* Maintaining effective and open communication among family members affected by death and grief is of utmost importance. The nurse needs to maintain and enhance communication as well as preserve the family's sense of self-direction and control. Option 2 is likely to enhance communication. Option 3 is also an effective intervention, because spiritual practices give meaning to life and have an impact on how people react to crisis. Option 4 is also an effective technique, and the family needs to know that someone will be there who is supportive and nonjudgmental. Option 1 removes autonomy and decision making from the family members at a time when they are already experiencing feelings of loss of control. This is an ineffective intervention that can impair communication.

*Test-Taking Strategy:* Note the key word *avoid* in the stem of the question. Use the process of elimination, focusing on therapeutic communication techniques. This will direct you to option 1. Review therapeutic techniques for individuals in crisis if you had difficulty with this question.

*Level of Cognitive Ability:* Application
*Client Needs:* Psychosocial Integrity
*Integrated Concept/Process:* Caring
*Content Area:* Fundamental Skills

*Reference*
Leahy, J., & Kizilay, P. (1998). *Foundations of nursing practice: A nursing process approach.* Philadelphia: W.B. Saunders, pp. 1145-1147.

**17.** A client brought to the emergency room is dead on arrival (DOA). The family of the client tells the emergency room physician that the client had terminal cancer. The physician examines the client and asks a nurse to contact the medical examiner regarding an autopsy. The family members tell the nurse that they do not want an autopsy performed. Which of the following responses to the family is most appropriate?

1   "It is required by federal law. Why don't we talk about it, and why don't you tell me how you feel?"
2   "The decision is made by the medical examiner."
3   "I will contact the medical examiner regarding your request."
4   "An autopsy is mandatory for any client who is dead on arrival to the hospital."

**Answer: 3**
*Rationale:* An autopsy is required by state law in certain circumstances, including the sudden death of a client and a death that occurs under suspicious circumstances. It is not a requirement of federal law. It is not mandatory that every client who is DOA have an autopsy. If a family requests not to have an autopsy performed on a family member, then the nurse should contact the medical examiner about the request.

*Test-Taking Strategy:* Note the key words *most appropriate.* Use knowledge regarding therapeutic communication techniques and the laws and issues surrounding autopsy to answer the question. Eliminate options 1 and 4 because these statements are not accurate. From the remaining options, option 3 is the most therapeutic and caring response to the family. Review the issues and laws surrounding autopsy, if you had difficulty with this question.

*Level of Cognitive Ability:* Application
*Client Needs:* Safe, Effective Care Environment
*Integrated Concept/Process:* Caring
*Content Area:* Fundamental Skills

*Reference*
Leahy, J., & Kizilay, P. (1998). *Foundations of nursing practice: A nursing process approach.* Philadelphia: W.B. Saunders, p. 76.

**18.** An elderly client who lives alone is scheduled for hospital discharge. The client states, "I don't know how I'll be able to take care of myself once I get home." The nurse should plan which of the following actions to assist the client?

1   Call an out-of-town relative to come and stay with the client
2   Call the physician to delay the discharge
3   Ask a social worker to follow up with a telephone call after discharge
4   Suggest a referral to a home health agency

**Answer: 4**
*Rationale:* With earlier hospital discharge, clients are returning home with greater acuity of problems than was previously true, and may require support from a home health agency until they are independent in functioning. Option 3 does nothing to actively assist the client, and option 2 is not realistic in the current health care environment. Although option 1 is a viable option, it does not assure the client continued care until the client is able to be independent in managing his or her own care.

*Test-Taking Strategy:* Focus on the issue of the question and the client's concern. Use the process of elimination, noting that option 4 is the only action that will ensure that the client has the necessary assistance until independence is achieved.

*Level of Cognitive Ability:* Application
*Client Needs:* Safe, Effective Care Environment
*Integrated Concept/Process:* Caring
*Content Area:* Fundamental Skills

*Reference*
Potter, P., & Perry, A. (2001). *Fundamentals of nursing* (5th ed.). St. Louis: Mosby, p. 389.

**19.** A nurse is interacting with the family of a client who is unconscious as a result of a head injury. Which of the following approaches would the nurse use to help the family cope with this situation?

1 Enforce adherence to visiting hours to ensure the client's rest
2 Encourage the family not to "give in" to their feelings of grief
3 Discourage the family from touching the client
4 Explain equipment and procedures on an ongoing basis

**Answer: 4**

*Rationale:* Families often need assistance to cope with the sudden severe illness of a loved one. The nurse should explain all equipment, treatments, and procedures, and supplement or reinforce information given by the physician. The family should be encouraged to touch and speak to the client and to become involved in the client's care in some way if they are comfortable with this. The nurse should allow the family to stay with the client whenever possible. The nurse also encourages the family to eat properly and to obtain enough sleep to maintain their strength.

*Test-Taking Strategy:* Use the process of elimination and basic therapeutic communication techniques to answer this question. Each of the incorrect options puts distance between the family and the client. Review therapeutic techniques that assist the family to deal with a sudden illness if you had difficulty with this question.

*Level of Cognitive Ability:* Application
*Client Needs:* Psychosocial Integrity
*Integrated Concept/Process:* Caring
*Content Area:* Adult Health/Neurological

*Reference*
Potter, P., & Perry, A. (2001). *Fundamentals of nursing* (5th ed.). St. Louis: Mosby, p. 151.

**20.** A nurse is performing an assessment on a client being admitted to the hospital. The client has right-sided weakness, aphasia, and urinary incontinence. One of the client's family members states, "If this is a stroke, it's the kiss of death." The nurse's best response would be:

1 "Wait until the doctor gets here to think like that."
2 "A stroke is not the kiss of death."
3 "You feel as if your family member is dying?"
4 "These symptoms may be reversible."

**Answer: 3**

*Rationale:* Option 3 allows the family member to verbalize and begin to cope with and adapt to what is happening. By restating what was said, the nurse is able to clarify the family member's feelings and begin to offer information that will help to ease some of the fears that he or she may face at the moment. Options 1 and 2 offer disapproval and put the family member's feeling on hold. Option 4 provides false hope at this point.

*Test-Taking Strategy:* Use therapeutic communication techniques. Option 3 is the only option that addresses the family member's feelings. Review therapeutic communication techniques if you had difficulty with this question.

*Cognitive Level of Ability:* Application
*Client Needs:* Psychosocial Integrity
*Integrated Concept/Process:* Caring
*Content Area:* Fundamental Skills

*Reference*
Potter, P., & Perry, A. (2001). *Fundamentals of nursing* (5th ed.). St. Louis: Mosby, p. 459.

# COMMUNICATION AND DOCUMENTATION

**1.** A nurse is trying to determine a client's adjustment to a new diagnosis of coronary heart disease before discharge from the hospital. Of the following questions, which one should the nurse ask to elicit the most useful response by the client in determining the client's adjustment?
   1   "Do you have anyone at home to help with housework and shopping?"
   2   "How do you feel about the lifestyle changes you are planning to make?"
   3   "Do you understand the use of your new medications?"
   4   "Are you going to book your follow-up physician visit?"

**Answer: 2**
*Rationale:* All questions relate to aspects of post-hospital care, but only option 2 explores the client's feelings about the disease. Exploring feelings as the initial assessment will assist in determining the individualized plan of care for the client.

*Test-Taking Strategy:* Use therapeutic communication techniques. Open-ended questions are needed to explore the client's reactions or feelings to an identified situation. Closed-ended questions generally elicit a "yes" or "no" response exclusively. All of the incorrect options are closed-ended questions. Review therapeutic communication techniques if you had difficulty with this question.

*Level of Cognitive Ability:* Application
*Client Needs:* Health Promotion and Maintenance
*Integrated Concept/Process:* Communication and Documentation
*Content Area:* Fundamental Skills

*Reference*
Potter, P., & Perry, A. (2001). *Fundamentals of nursing* (5th ed.). St. Louis: Mosby, p. 459.

**2.** A female client with a long leg cast has been using crutches to ambulate for 1 week. She comes to the clinic with complaints of pain, fatigue, and frustration with crutch walking. She states, "I feel like I have a crippled leg." Which of the following responses by the nurse is most appropriate?
   1   "I know how you feel; I had to use crutches before, too."
   2   "Just remember, you'll be done with the crutches in another month."
   3   "Why don't you take a couple of days off work and rest."
   4   "Tell me what is bothersome for you."

**Answer: 4**
*Rationale:* Option 4 is the therapeutic communication technique of clarification and validation and indicates that the nurse is dealing with the client's problem from the client's perspective. Option 1 devalues the client's feelings and thus blocks communication. Option 2 provides false reassurance because the client may not be done with the crutches in another month. In addition, it does not focus on the present problem. Option 3 gives advice and is a communication block.

*Test-Taking Strategy:* Use therapeutic communication techniques. Option 4 is the only response that encourages communication. Review therapeutic communication techniques if you had difficulty with this question.

*Level of Cognitive Ability:* Application
*Client Needs:* Psychosocial Integrity
*Integrated Concept/Process:* Communication and Documentation
*Content Area:* Adult Health/Musculoskeletal

*Reference*
Potter, P., & Perry, A. (2001). *Fundamentals of nursing* (5th ed.). St. Louis: Mosby, p. 459.

**3.** An 18-year-old client is being discharged from the hospital after surgery and will need to ambulate with a cane for the next 6 months. A nurse asks the client which question that will provide data about the psychosocial status of the client regarding the use of the cane?

1   "How do you feel about having to walk with a cane for the next 6 months?"
2   "Do you have any questions about how to walk with the cane?"
3   "Time will pass quickly, don't you think?"
4   "You are not worried about what your friends will think, are you?"

**Answer: 1**
*Rationale:* How a client feels is an important part of the psychosocial assessment. Option 2 deals with a physical issue. Option 3 gives an opinion. Option 4 can be intimidating to the client. In addition, options 2, 3, and 4 are closed-ended responses and are barriers to effective communication.

*Test-Taking Strategy:* Use therapeutic communication techniques. Avoid responses that include communication blocks. Eliminate options 2, 3, and 4 because they are closed-ended responses and are blocks to communication. Remember to address the client's feelings first. Review therapeutic communication techniques if you had difficulty with this question.

*Level of Cognitive Ability:* Application
*Client Needs:* Psychosocial Integrity
*Integrated Concept/Process:* Communication and Documentation
*Content Area:* Fundamental Skills

*Reference*
Kozier, B., Erb, G., Berman, A., & Burke, K. (2000). *Fundamentals of nursing: Concepts, process, and practice* (6th ed.). Upper Saddle River, N.J.: Prentice-Hall, p. 437.

**4.** An 85-year-old client is hospitalized for a right fractured hip. During the postoperative period, the client's appetite is poor and the client refuses to get out of bed. Which nursing statement would be most appropriate to make to the client?

1   "It is important for you to get out of bed to be sure that calcium moves back into the bone."
2   "We need to increase your calcium intake because you are spending too much time in bed."
3   "We need to give you iodine so that it will help in hemoglobin synthesis."
4   "You need to remember to turn yourself in bed every 2 hours to keep from getting so stiff."

**Answer: 1**
*Rationale:* Early ambulation in the postoperative period is important because if a client does not increase activity, the bones will lose calcium. Increasing calcium intake in an immobile client would cause elevated amounts of calcium in the blood, which could lead to kidney stones. Iron, not iodine, is recommended for hemoglobin synthesis. Clients who are not turned in bed will develop pressure ulcers. A client who is immobile and is 85 years old needs to be turned every 2 hours by the nursing staff. The client should not be expected to turn himself or herself.

*Test-Taking Strategy:* Use therapeutic communication techniques and knowledge regarding the effects of immobility. Option 4 is eliminated first because in this statement, the nurse is not accepting any responsibility for the client's care. Next, eliminate option 3 because it is incorrect. From the remaining options, noting the key words *refuses to get out of bed* will direct you to option 1. Review the complications associated with immobility, if you had difficulty with this question.

*Level of Cognitive Ability:* Application
*Client Needs:* Physiological Integrity
*Integrated Concept/Process:* Communication and Documentation
*Content Area:* Fundamental Skills

*Reference*
Leahy, J., & Kizilay, P. (1998). *Foundations of nursing practice: A nursing process approach.* Philadelphia: W.B. Saunders, pp. 749-750.

5. A client is diagnosed with thrombophlebitis of the left leg. A nurse documents in the nursing care plan that the client should be placed on bed rest with:
   1   The left leg kept flat
   2   Elevation of the left leg
   3   The left leg in a dependent position
   4   Bathroom privileges

**Answer: 2**
*Rationale:* Elevation of the affected leg facilitates blood flow by the force of gravity and also decreases venous pressure, which in turn relieves edema and pain. Bed rest is indicated to prevent emboli and to prevent pressure fluctuations in the venous system that occur with walking. Thus, the nurse documents to elevate the left leg. Options 1, 3, and 4 are inappropriate positions and will not facilitate blood flow.

*Test-Taking Strategy:* Use the process of elimination. Focus on the client's diagnosis and think about the principles related to gravity flow and edema to answer the question. If you had difficulty with this question, review nursing care for clients with a venous disorder.

*Level of Cognitive Ability:* Application
*Client Needs:* Physiological Integrity
*Integrated Concept/Process:* Communication and Documentation
*Content Area:* Fundamental Skills

*Reference*
Ignatavicius, D., Workman, M., & Mishler, M. (1999). *Medical-surgical nursing across the health care continuum* (3rd ed.). Philadelphia: W.B. Saunders, p. 873.

---

6. A female client who is experiencing disordered thinking about food being poisoned is admitted to a mental health unit. A nurse uses which communication technique to encourage the client to eat dinner?
   1   Asking open-ended questions followed by silence
   2   Offering opinions about the need to eat
   3   Verbalizing reasons why the client may not choose to eat
   4   Focusing on self-disclosure of own food preferences

**Answer: 1**
*Rationale:* Open-ended questions and silence are strategies used to encourage clients to discuss their problems in a descriptive manner. Options 2 and 3 are not helpful to the client because they do not encourage the client to express feelings. Option 4 is not a client-centered intervention.

*Test-Taking Strategy:* Use the process of elimination and therapeutic communication techniques. Eliminate options 2 and 3 first because they do not support client expression of feelings. Eliminate option 4 next because it is not a client-centered response. Review therapeutic communication techniques if you had difficulty with this question.

*Level of Cognitive Ability:* Application
*Client Needs:* Physiological Integrity
*Integrated Concept/Process:* Communication and Documentation
*Content Area:* Mental Health

*Reference*
Stuart, G.W., & Laraia, M.T. (1998). *Principles and practice of psychiatric nursing.* (6th ed.). St. Louis: Mosby, p. 34.

**7.** A nurse is engaged in preparing a client for electroconvulsive therapy (ECT). After a thorough discussion with the client and family, the client signs the informed consent. Upon departure from the session, a family member states, "I don't know. . . . I don't think that this ECT will be helpful if it is going to make people's memory worse." The nurse would then:

1    Involve the family member in a dialogue to ascertain how the family member arrived at this conclusive statement

2    Inquire with other family members and the client if they thought the same way about ECT making people worse

3    Immediately reassure the client that the decision to receive ECT will help and that memory loss or confusion is minimal and temporary

4    Reinforce with the family member that depression causes more memory impairment than ECT

**Answer: 1**

*Rationale:* In option 1, the nurse is exploring for data to assist in clarifying information about the procedure with the family. Option 2 may place family members on the defensive and promote conflict among family members. Option 3 would not acknowledge the family member's statement and concern. Option 4 offers information but does not assess and is not the most therapeutic action.

*Test-Taking Strategy:* Use therapeutic communication techniques and the nursing process. Remember that assessment is the first step in the nursing process. In option 1, the nurse gathers more data and addresses the family member's thoughts and feelings. Review therapeutic communication techniques if you had difficulty with this question.

*Level of Cognitive Ability:* Application
*Client Needs:* Psychosocial Integrity
*Integrated Concept/Process:* Communication and Documentation
*Content Area:* Mental Health

*Reference*
Varcarolis, E. (1998). *Foundations of psychiatric mental health nursing* (3rd ed.). Philadelphia: W.B. Saunders, p. 597.

**8.** A client with type 2 diabetes mellitus was recently hospitalized for hyperglycemic-hyperosmolar nonketotic syndrome (HHNS). Upon discharge from the hospital, the client expresses concern about the recurrence of HHNS. Which statement by the nurse is the most therapeutic?

1    "Don't worry, your family will help you."

2    "I'm sure this won't happen again."

3    "You have concerns about the treatment for your condition?"

4    "I think you might need to go to the nursing home."

**Answer: 3**

*Rationale:* The nurse should provide time and listen to the client's concerns. In option 3, the nurse is attempting to clarify the client's feelings. Options 1 and 2 provide inappropriate false hope. In addition, a nurse does not tell a client not to worry. Option 4 is not an appropriate nursing response, disregards the client's concerns, and gives advice.

*Test-Taking Strategy:* Use therapeutic communication techniques. Remembering to always address the client's feelings will direct you to option 3. Review these therapeutic techniques, if you had difficulty with this question.

*Level of Cognitive Ability:* Application
*Client Needs:* Psychosocial Integrity
*Integrated Concept/Process:* Communication and Documentation
*Content Area:* Adult Health/Endocrine

*Reference*
Potter, P., & Perry, A. (2001). *Fundamentals of nursing* (5th ed.). St. Louis: Mosby, p. 459.

**9.** The husband of a client who has a Sengstaken-Blakemore tube states to the nurse, "I thought having this tube down her nose the first time would convince my wife to quit drinking." The most appropriate response by the nurse is:
1  "Alcoholism is a disease that affects the whole family."
2  "You sound frustrated in dealing with your wife's drinking problem."
3  "Have you discussed this subject at the Al-Anon meetings?"
4  "I think you are a good person to stay with your wife."

**Answer: 2**
*Rationale:* In option 2, the nurse uses the therapeutic communication techniques of clarifying and focusing in assisting the client (the husband) to express feelings concerning the wife's chronic illness. Stereotyping (option 1), changing the subject (option 3), and showing approval (option 4) are nontherapeutic techniques and block communication.

*Test-Taking Strategy:* Use therapeutic communication techniques. Remembering to always address the client's feelings will direct you to option 2. Review these therapeutic techniques if you had difficulty with this question.

*Level of Cognitive Ability:* Application
*Client Needs:* Psychosocial Integrity
*Integrated Concept/Process:* Communication and Documentation
*Content Area:* Adult Health/Gastrointestinal

*Reference*
Potter, P., & Perry, A. (2001). Fundamentals of nursing (5th ed.). St. Louis: Mosby, p. 459.

**10.** A nurse has an order to institute aneurysm precautions for a client with a cerebral aneurysm. Which of the following items would the nurse document in the plan of care for this client?
1  Instruct the client not to strain with bowel movements
2  Allow the client to read and watch television
3  Limit out-of-bed activities to twice daily
4  Encourage the client to take his or her own daily bath

**Answer: 1**
*Rationale:* Aneurysm precautions include placing the client on bed rest in a quiet setting. Lights are kept dim to minimize environmental stimulation. Any activity that increases the blood pressure (BP) or impedes venous return from the brain is prohibited, such as pushing, pulling, sneezing, coughing, or straining. The nurse provides all physical care to minimize increases in the BP. For the same reason, visitors, radio, television, and reading materials are prohibited or limited. Stimulants such as caffeine and nicotine are prohibited. The nurse documents that the client is instructed to avoid straining with bowel movements.

*Test-Taking Strategy:* Recall that the components of aneurysm precautions are to limit the amount of stimulation (in any form) that the client receives and to prevent increased intracranial pressure (ICP). With this in mind, eliminate options 3 and 4 first. From the remaining options, recall that straining can increase ICP, so it is appropriate to tell the client not to do so. Review the components of aneurysm precautions, if you had difficulty with this question.

*Level of Cognitive Ability:* Application
*Client Needs:* Physiological Integrity
*Integrated Concept/Process:* Communication and Documentation
*Content Area:* Adult Health/Neurological

*Reference*
Monahan, F., & Neighbors, M. (1998). *Medical-surgical nursing: Foundations for clinical practice* (2nd ed.). Philadelphia: W.B Saunders, p. 372.

**11.** A client with myasthenia gravis is having difficulty with the motor aspects of speech. The client has difficulty forming words, and the voice has a nasal tone. A nurse would use which of the following communication strategies when working with this client?
1 Repeat what the client said to verify the message
2 Encourage the client to speak quickly
3 Nod continuously while the client is speaking
4 Engage the client in lengthy discussions to strengthen the voice

**Answer: 1**
*Rationale:* The client has speech that is nasal in tone and dysarthritic because of cranial nerve involvement of the muscles governing speech. The nurse listens attentively and verbally verifies what the client has said. Other helpful techniques are to ask questions requiring a yes or no response, and to develop alternative communication methods (letter board, picture board, pen and paper, flash cards). Encouraging the client to speak quickly is inappropriate and counterproductive. Continuous nodding may be distracting and is unnecessary. Lengthy discussions will tire the client rather than strengthen the voice.

*Test-Taking Strategy:* Use the process of elimination and basic principles of communication techniques to answer this question. This will direct you to option 1. If this question was difficult, review this disorder and effective communication strategies.

*Level of Cognitive Ability:* Application
*Client Needs:* Psychosocial Integrity
*Integrated Concept/Process:* Communication and Documentation
*Content Area:* Adult Health/Neurological

*Reference*
Monahan, F., & Neighbors, M. (1998). *Medical-surgical nursing: Foundations for clinical practice* (2nd ed.). Philadelphia: W.B Saunders, p. 782.

---

**12.** A client with a peripheral intravenous (IV) site calls a nurse to the room and tells the nurse that the IV site is swollen. The nurse inspects the IV site and notes that it is also cool and pale and that the IV has stopped running. The nurse documents in the client's record that which of the following has probably occurred?
1 Infiltration
2 Phlebitis
3 Thrombosis
4 Infection

**Answer: 1**
*Rationale:* An infiltrated IV is one that has dislodged from the vein and is lying in subcutaneous tissue. The pallor, coolness, and swelling are the result of IV fluid being deposited in the subcutaneous tissue. When the pressure in the tissues exceeds the pressure in the tubing, the flow of the IV solution will stop. The corrective action will be to remove the catheter and have a new IV line started. The other three options are likely to be accompanied by warmth at the site, not coolness. The nurse would document that the client's IV has infiltrated.

*Test-Taking Strategy:* Use the process of elimination and knowledge regarding the signs of the complications associated with IV therapy. Focusing on the data in the question and noting the words *swollen, cool,* and *pale* will direct you to option 1. If this question was difficult, review the signs of infiltration.

*Level of Cognitive Ability:* Application
*Client Needs:* Physiological Integrity
*Integrated Concept/Process:* Communication and Documentation
*Content Area:* Fundamental Skills

*Reference*
Leahy, J., & Kizilay, P. (1998). *Foundations of nursing practice: A nursing process approach.* Philadelphia: W.B. Saunders, p. 822.

**13.** A nurse is observing a nursing assistant talking to a client who is hearing impaired. The nurse would intervene if which of the following were performed by the nursing assistant during communication with the client?
1    The nursing assistant is facing the client when speaking
2    The nursing assistant is speaking clearly to the client
3    The nursing assistant is speaking directly into the impaired ear
4    The nursing assistant is speaking in a normal tone

**Answer: 3**
*Rationale:* When communicating with a hearing impaired client, the nursing assistant should speak in a normal tone to the client and should not shout. The nursing assistant should talk directly to the client while facing the client and speak clearly. If the client does not seem to understand what is said, the nursing assistant should express the statement differently. Moving closer to the client and toward the better ear may facilitate communication, but the nursing assistant needs to avoid talking directly into the impaired ear.

*Test-Taking Strategy:* Use the process of elimination, noting the key words *the nurse would intervene.* Knowledge regarding effective communication techniques for the hearing impaired will direct you to option 3. If you had difficulty with this question, review these therapeutic communication techniques.

*Level of Cognitive Ability:* Analysis
*Client Needs:* Safe, Effective Care Environment
*Integrated Concept/Process:* Communication and Documentation
*Content Area:* Adult Health/Ear

*Reference*
Leahy, J., & Kizilay, P. (1998). *Foundations of nursing practice: A nursing process approach.* Philadelphia: W.B. Saunders, p. 216.

**14.** A nurse is caring for a client diagnosed with catatonic stupor. The client is found lying on the bed with the body pulled into a fetal position. The most appropriate nursing action is to:
1    Leave the client alone
2    Take the client into the dayroom
3    Sit beside the client in silence
4    Ask the client direct questions

**Answer: 3**
*Rationale:* Clients who are withdrawn may be immobile and mute (catatonic stupor), and require consistent, repeated approaches. Intervention includes establishment of interpersonal contact. Communication with these clients requires much patience from the nurse. The nurse facilitates communication with the client by sitting in silence, asking open-ended questions, and pausing to provide opportunities for the client to respond. The client would not be left alone. Asking direct questions to the client is not therapeutic. It is not appropriate at this time to place the client in a public place, such as a dayroom.

*Test-Taking Strategy:* Use the process of elimination. Eliminate option 1 because you would not leave the client alone. Eliminate option 2 because it is not appropriate to place the client in a public place. Eliminate option 4 because asking direct questions to this client is not therapeutic. Option 3 is the best action because it provides client supervision and communication with the client. Review care of the client with catatonic stupor, if you had difficulty with this question.

*Level of Cognitive Ability:* Application
*Client Needs:* Psychosocial Integrity
*Integrated Concept/Process:* Communication and Documentation
*Content Area:* Mental Health

*Reference*
Varcarolis, E. (1998). *Foundations of psychiatric mental health nursing* (3rd ed.). Philadelphia: W.B. Saunders, p. 659.

**15.** A nurse is developing a plan of care for an elderly client and includes strategies that will facilitate effective communication. The nurse would include which strategy to accomplish this goal?

1 Use an authoritarian approach
2 Use active listening
3 React enthusiastically during the conversation
4 React only to the facts during conversation

**Answer: 2**

*Rationale:* For effective communication, the nurse uses active listening and creates an environment in which the client feels comfortable expressing feelings. An authoritarian approach is directive and demeaning and will not create an environment for verbal exchange from the client. Reacting only to the facts is an example of inactive listening. Reacting enthusiastically is not the most effective strategy.

*Test-Taking Strategy:* Use the process of elimination and therapeutic communication techniques. This will direct you to option 2. If you had difficulty with this question or are unfamiliar with therapeutic communication techniques, review this content.

*Level of Cognitive Ability:* Application
*Client Needs:* Psychosocial Integrity
*Integrated Concept/Process:* Communication and Documentation
*Content Area:* Fundamental Skills

*Reference*
Leahy, J., & Kizilay, P. (1998). *Foundations of nursing practice: A nursing process approach.* Philadelphia: W.B. Saunders, p. 336.

**16.** A nurse has made an error in documenting vital signs of a client and obtains the client's record to correct the error. The nurse corrects the error by:

1 Using whiteout
2 Erasing the error
3 Documenting a late entry
4 Drawing one line through the error and initialing and dating the correction

**Answer: 4**

*Rationale:* If a nurse makes an error in documenting in the client's record, the nurse should follow agency policy to correct the error. This includes drawing one line through the error, initialing and dating the correction, and then providing the correct information. Erasing data from the client's record and the use of whiteout are prohibited. A late entry is used to document additional information not remembered at the initial time of documentation.

*Test-Taking Strategy:* Use the process of elimination and principles related to documentation. Recalling that alterations to a client's record are avoided will eliminate options 1 and 2. From the remaining options, focusing on the issue of the question will direct you to option 4. Review the principles related to documentation if you had difficulty with this question.

*Level of Cognitive Ability:* Application
*Client Needs:* Safe, Effective Care Environment
*Integrated Concept/Process:* Communication and Documentation
*Content Area:* Fundamental Skills

*Reference*
Leahy, J., & Kizilay, P. (1998). *Foundations of nursing practice: A nursing process approach.* Philadelphia: W.B. Saunders, p. 71.

**17.** A nurse hears a client calling out for help. The nurse hurries down the hallway to the client's room and finds the client lying on the floor. The nurse performs a thorough assessment and assists the client back to bed. The physician is notified of the incident, and the nurse completes an incident report. The nurse documents which of the following on the incident report?

1   The client was found lying on the floor
2   The client climbed over the side rails
3   The client fell out of bed
4   The client became restless and tried to get out of bed

**Answer: 1**
*Rationale:* The incident report should contain the client's name, age, and diagnosis. It should contain a factual description of the incident, any injuries experienced by those involved, and the outcome of the situation. Option 1 is the only option that describes the facts as observed by the nurse. Options 2, 3, and 4 are interpretations of the situation and are not factual data as observed by the nurse.

*Test-Taking Strategy:* Use the process of elimination. Focus on factual information when documenting, and avoid including interpretations. This will direct you to option 1. Review documentation principles related to incident reports if you had difficulty with this question.

*Level of Cognitive Ability:* Application
*Client Needs:* Safe, Effective Care Environment
*Integrated Concept/Process:* Communication and Documentation
*Content Area:* Fundamental Skills

*Reference*
Leahy, J., & Kizilay, P. (1998). *Foundations of nursing practice: A nursing process approach.* Philadelphia: W.B. Saunders, p. 72.

---

**18.** A client diagnosed with angina pectoris appears to be very anxious and states, "So I had a heart attack, right?" Which of the following is the best response for a nurse to make?

1   "No, and we will see to it that you do not have a heart attack."
2   "Yes, this is why you are here."
3   "No, but the doctor wants to monitor you and control or eliminate your pain."
4   "Yes, but there is minimal damage to your heart."

**Answer: 3**
*Rationale:* Angina pectoris is pain that occurs as a result of inadequate blood supply to the myocardium. A myocardial infarction refers to a heart attack. Option 1 provides false reassurance. Neither the nurse nor the physician can guarantee that a heart attack will not occur.

*Test-Taking Strategy:* Use therapeutic communication techniques and knowledge regarding the definition of angina pectoris to eliminate options 2 and 4. From the remaining options, eliminate option 1 because it provides false reassurance. Review the pathophysiology associated with angina pectoris, as well as therapeutic communication techniques, if you had difficulty with this question.

*Level of Cognitive Ability:* Application
*Client Needs:* Psychosocial Integrity
*Integrated Concept/Process:* Communication and Documentation
*Content Area:* Adult Health/Cardiovascular

*Reference*
Monahan, F., & Neighbors, M. (1998). *Medical-surgical nursing: Foundations for clinical practice* (2nd ed.). Philadelphia: W.B Saunders, p. 288.

**19.** A nurse is caring for a hospitalized client who has a diagnosis of depression and who is silent and not communicating. The nurse develops a plan of care and incorporates strategies for communicating with the client. Which of the following statements would be most appropriate for the nurse to make when caring for this client?

1   "Can you tell me how you are feeling today?"
2   "Do you feel like talking today?"
3   "You are wearing your new shoes."
4   "Can you tell me how you slept last night?"

**Answer: 3**

*Rationale:* When a depressed client is mute or silent, a nurse should use the communication technique of making observations. A statement such as "you are wearing your new shoes" is an appropriate statement to make to the client. When the client is not ready to talk, direct questions (options 1, 2, and 4) can raise the client's anxiety level. Pointing to commonalties in the environment draws the client into and reinforces reality.

*Test-Taking Strategy:* Use therapeutic communication techniques. Eliminate options 1, 2, and 4 because they are similar. These options are direct questions requiring a response from the client. Review communication techniques for the depressed client if you had difficulty with this question.

*Level of Cognitive Ability:* Application
*Client Needs:* Psychosocial Integrity
*Integrated Concept/Process:* Communication and Documentation
*Content Area:* Mental Health

*Reference*
Varcarolis, E. (1998). *Foundations of psychiatric mental health nursing* (3rd ed.). Philadelphia: W.B. Saunders, p. 565.

**20.** A nurse is caring for a client with delirium who states, "Look at the spiders on the wall." Which of the following nursing responses is most appropriate?

1   "I can see the spiders on the wall, but they are not going to hurt you."
2   "Would you like me to kill the spiders for you?"
3   "I know you are frightened, but I do not see spiders on the wall."
4   "You're having a hallucination; there are no spiders in this room at all."

**Answer: 3**

*Rationale:* When hallucinations are present, the nurse should reinforce reality with the client. In option 3, the nurse addresses the client's feelings and reinforces reality. Options 1 and 2 do not reinforce reality. Option 4 reinforces reality but does not address the client's feelings.

*Test-Taking Strategy:* Use therapeutic communication techniques. Eliminate options 1 and 2 because they reinforce the client's hallucination. Eliminate option 4 because although it reinforces reality, it diminishes the importance of the client's feelings. Review therapeutic communication techniques for the client experiencing altered thought processes if you had difficulty with this question.

*Level of Cognitive Ability:* Application
*Client Needs:* Psychosocial Integrity
*Integrated Concept/Process:* Communication and Documentation
*Content Area:* Mental Health

*Reference*
Varcarolis, E. (1998). *Foundations of psychiatric mental health nursing* (3rd ed.). Philadelphia: W B. Saunders, p. 660.

# CULTURAL AWARENESS

**1.** A nurse is developing a plan of care for a hospitalized Asian-American client. The nurse avoids including which of the following in the plan of care?
1   Maintaining physical space with the client
2   Limiting eye contact
3   Clarifying responses to questions
4   Providing light touch to the head for comfort

**Answer: 4**

*Rationale:* Avoiding physical closeness, limiting eye contact, avoiding hand gestures, and clarifying responses to questions are all components of the plan of care for an Asian-American client. The head is considered to be sacred; therefore touching the client on the head is disrespectful. Remember, touch the client's head only when necessary, and inform the client before doing so.

*Test-Taking Strategy:* Use the process of elimination, noting the key word *avoids*. Eliminate options 1 and 2 because they are similar in that they both address a lack of physical contact. Eliminate option 3 because it is a therapeutic communication technique. If you had difficulty with this question, review the beliefs associated with this culture.

*Level of Cognitive Ability:* Application
*Client Needs:* Psychosocial Integrity
*Integrated Concept/Process:* Cultural Awareness
*Content Area:* Fundamental Skills

*Reference*
Potter, P., & Perry, A. (2001). *Fundamentals of nursing* (5th ed.). St. Louis: Mosby, p. 129.

**2.** A nurse consults with a nutritionist regarding the dietary preferences of an Asian-American client. Which of the following foods would most appropriately be included in the dietary plan?
1   Red meat
2   Rice
3   Fried foods
4   Chili

**Answer: 2**

*Rationale:* Asian-American food preferences include raw fish, rice, and soy sauce. African-American food preferences include pork, greens, rice, and fried foods. Hispanic Americans prefer beans, fried foods, spicy foods, chili, and carbonated beverages. European-Americans prefer carbohydrates and red meat.

*Test-Taking Strategy:* Use the process of elimination. Correlate rice with Asian-Americans. This may assist in answering other questions similar to this one. If you had difficulty with this question, review the food preferences associated with the Asian-American culture.

*Level of Cognitive Ability:* Application
*Client Needs:* Physiological Integrity
*Integrated Concept/Process:* Cultural Awareness
*Content Area:* Fundamental Skills

*Reference*
Leahy, J., & Kizilay, P. (1998). *Foundations of nursing practice: A nursing process approach.* Philadelphia: W.B. Saunders, p. 1106.

**3.** A European-American client maintains eye contact with a nurse during a conversation regarding a preoperative teaching plan. The nurse interprets this nonverbal communication as:
1   Rudeness
2   Arrogance
3   Indicating uneasiness
4   Indicating trustworthiness

**Answer:** 4
*Rationale:* In the European-American culture, eye contact is viewed as indicating trustworthiness. Eye contact is considered rude in the Asian-American culture. Arrogance and uneasiness are incorrect interpretations of this nonverbal communication in the European-American client.

*Test-Taking Strategy:* Use the process of elimination, noting that options 1, 2, and 3 are similar in that they indicate a negative response. Option 4 is the only option indicating positiveness. If you had difficulty with this question, review the communication practices of the European-American culture.

*Level of Cognitive Ability:* Analysis
*Client Needs:* Psychosocial Integrity
*Integrated Concept/Process:* Cultural Awareness
*Content Area:* Fundamental Skills

*Reference*
Purnell, P., & Paulanka, B. (1998). *Transcultural healthcare: A culturally competent approach.* Philadelphia: F.A. Davis, p. 357.

**4.** A nurse develops a plan of care for a European-American client. The nurse considers the practices and preferences of the culture when planning the care, knowing that which of the following is not a characteristic of this group?
1   Community social organizations are important
2   Health is often viewed as an absence of disease or illness
3   The client will appear stoic when expressing physical concerns
4   The woman is the dominant figure

**Answer:** 4
*Rationale:* In the European-American culture, the man is the dominant figure. Community social organizations are important in this culture. Health is often viewed as the absence of disease or illness. European-Americans tend to be aloof, to avoid physical contact, and to appear stoic when expressing physical concerns.

*Test-Taking Strategy:* Use the process of elimination, noting the key word *not*. Recalling the practices and beliefs associated with the European-American culture will direct you to option 4. If you had difficulty with this question, review the practices and beliefs of the European-American culture.

*Level of Cognitive Ability:* Analysis
*Client Needs:* Psychosocial Integrity
*Integrated Concept/Process:* Cultural Awareness
*Content Area:* Fundamental Skills

*Reference*
Purnell, P., & Paulanka, B. (1998). *Transcultural healthcare: A culturally competent approach.* Philadelphia: F.A. Davis, p. 358.

**5.** A nurse calls the dietary department to obtain a dinner meal for a European-American client who was admitted to the hospital at 4:00 P.M. The physician prescribed a diet "as tolerated." Considering the practices and preferences of the European-American, which of the following foods would the nurse request for the meal?
1   Red meat and potatoes
2   Blue cornmeal
3   Kosher foods
4   Rice

**Answer: 1**

*Rationale:* Food preferences of European-Americans include carbohydrates, such as potatoes and red meat. Native American preferences include blue cornmeal, fish, game, fruits, and berries. Asian-Americans prefer rice and raw fish. Dietary kosher laws are adhered to by members of the Jewish community.

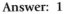

*Test-Taking Strategy:* Use the process of elimination. Remember that kosher foods are important to the Jewish population, blue cornmeal with Native Americans, and rice with Asian-Americans. Review food preferences of the various cultures if you had difficulty with this question.

*Level of Cognitive Ability:* Application
*Client Needs:* Psychosocial Integrity
*Integrated Concept/Process:* Cultural Awareness
*Content Area:* Fundamental Skills

*Reference*
Purnell, P., & Paulanka, B. (1998). *Transcultural healthcare: A culturally competent approach.* Philadelphia: F.A. Davis, p. 363.

**6.** A Hispanic American mother brings her child to a clinic for an examination. Which of the following would be most important during the assessment of the child?
1   Avoiding eye contact
2   Touching the child during the examination
3   Avoiding speaking to the child
4   Using body language only

**Answer: 2**

*Rationale:* In the Hispanic American culture, eye behavior is significant. The "evil eye" can be given to a child if a person looks at and admires a child without touching the child. Therefore, touching the child during the examination is very important. Although avoiding eye contact indicates respect and attentiveness, this is not the most important intervention during the assessment of a child. Avoiding speaking to the child and using body language only are not therapeutic interventions.

*Test-Taking Strategy:* Use the process of elimination. Eliminate options 3 and 4 first because they are similar. From the remaining options, select the intervention that is most therapeutic, that being touch. If you had difficulty with this question, review the characteristics associated with Hispanic Americans.

*Level of Cognitive Ability:* Application
*Client Needs:* Psychosocial Integrity
*Integrated Concept/Process:* Cultural Awareness
*Content Area:* Fundamental Skills

*Reference*
Purnell, P., & Paulanka, B. (1998). *Transcultural healthcare: A culturally competent approach.* Philadelphia: F.A. Davis, p. 400.

**7.** A nurse is caring for a Hispanic American client admitted with a diagnosis of diabetic ketoacidosis. Several family members are present. Which of the following behaviors, if displayed by the family members, would the nurse interpret as characteristic of this cultural group?
   1   Dramatic body language
   2   Consistently expressing negative feelings
   3   Maintaining consistent eye contact
   4   Consistently confronting the nurse directly

**Answer: 1**
*Rationale:* Characteristics of the Hispanic American culture include the use of dramatic body language, such as gestures or facial expressions, to express emotion or pain. The members of this culture believe that direct confrontation is disrespectful and that the expression of negative feelings is impolite. In addition, in this culture, avoiding direct eye contact indicates respect and attentiveness.

*Test-Taking Strategy:* Knowledge regarding the beliefs and traditions of this culture is required to answer this question. Recalling that dramatic body language is a characteristic of this culture will direct you to option 1. If you had difficulty with this question, review the beliefs of the Hispanic American culture.

*Level of Cognitive Ability:* Analysis
*Client Needs:* Psychosocial Integrity
*Integrated Concept/Process:* Cultural Awareness
*Content Area:* Fundamental Skills

*Reference*
Purnell, P., & Paulanka, B. (1998). *Transcultural healthcare: A culturally competent approach.* Philadelphia: F.A. Davis, p. 400.

**8.** A nurse develops a plan of care for a Native American client and considers the practices and preferences of the culture. In developing the plan, the nurse understands that which of the following practices or preferences is not a characteristic of a Native American?
   1   Integration of religion and healing practices
   2   Touching the body of a dead family member
   3   Avoiding eye contact
   4   Use of healing practices

**Answer: 2**
*Rationale:* A Native American is prohibited from touching the body of a dead family member. Religion and healing practices are integrated into health care and illness practices. Eye contact is avoided because it is a sign of disrespect.

*Test-Taking Strategy:* Use the process of elimination, noting the key word *not.* Eliminate options 1 and 4 first because they are similar. Remembering that maintaining eye contact is a sign of disrespect will direct you to option 2. If you had difficulty with this question, review the traditional beliefs of the Native American.

*Level of Cognitive Ability:* Analysis
*Client Needs:* Psychosocial Integrity
*Integrated Concept/Process:* Cultural Awareness
*Content Area:* Fundamental Skills

*Reference*
Clark, M.J. (1999). *Nursing in the community: Dimensions of community health nursing* (3rd ed.). Stamford, Conn.: Appleton & Lange, p. 342.

**9.** A nurse who is caring for an Orthodox Jewish client plans a diet that adheres to the practices of Judaism. The nurse avoids including which of the following in the plan?
1 Eating fish with scales and fins is allowed
2 Meat is allowed if ritually slaughtered
3 Only unleavened bread is eaten during Passover week
4 Meat and milk can be eaten together

**Answer: 4**
*Rationale:* Dietary kosher laws must be adhered to by Orthodox believers. Meats allowed include animals that are vegetable eaters, cloven-hoofed animals, and animals that are ritually slaughtered. Fish that have scales and fins are allowed; however, any combination of meat and milk is prohibited. During Passover week, only unleavened bread is eaten.

*Test-Taking Strategy:* Use the process of elimination, noting the key word *avoids* in the stem of the question. Recalling the dietary practices in Judaism will direct you to option 4. If you had difficulty with the question, review the dietary practices of this cultural group.

*Level of Cognitive Ability:* Application
*Client Needs:* Psychosocial Integrity
*Integrated Concept/Process:* Cultural Awareness
*Content Area:* Fundamental Skills

**Reference**
Kozier, B., Erb, G., Berman, A., & Burke, K. (2000). *Fundamentals of nursing: Concepts, process, and practice* (6th ed.). Upper Saddle River, N.J.: Prentice-Hall, p. 213.

---

**10.** A nurse is caring for an African-American client. The nurse enters the room, and, following a greeting and introduction to the client, the nurse begins to describe the angiogram procedure scheduled for the following day. The client turns away from the nurse. Which of the following nursing actions is most appropriate?
1 Continue with the explanation
2 Ask the client if he or she can hear the nurse
3 Walk around to the client so that the nurse faces the client
4 Leave the room and return later to continue with the explanation

**Answer: 1**
*Rationale:* In the African-American culture, direct eye contact is often viewed as being rude. If the client turns away from the nurse during a conversation, the most appropriate action is to continue with the conversation. Walking around to the client so that the nurse faces the client is in direct conflict with this cultural practice. Asking the client if he or she can hear the nurse or leaving the room and returning later to continue with the explanation may be viewed as a rude gesture by the client.

*Test-Taking Strategy:* Use the process of elimination and therapeutic communication techniques. Eliminate options 2 and 4 first because they are nontherapeutic actions. From the remaining options, option 1 is the most therapeutic. If you had difficulty with this question, review the communication practices of this cultural group.

*Level of Cognitive Ability:* Application
*Client Needs:* Psychosocial Integrity
*Integrated Concept/Process:* Cultural Awareness
*Content Area:* Fundamental Skills

**Reference**
Potter, P. & Perry, A. (2001). *Fundamentals of nursing* (5th ed.). St. Louis: Mosby, p. 122.

**11.** A nurse caring for a Chinese-American client is reviewing the plan of care with the client. The client frequently nods the head during the review. The nurse interprets this behavior as:

1 The client agrees with the plan
2 The client may not necessarily agree with the plan
3 The client would like to hear more about the plan
4 The client is very anxious

**Answer: 2**

*Rationale:* In the Chinese-American culture, head nodding does not necessarily mean that the client is in agreement with the plan, wants to hear more about the plan, or is anxious. The nurse needs to be alert to nonverbal communication and validate the client's nonverbal communication.

*Test-Taking Strategy:* Focus on the issue of the question, interpreting nonverbal communication. Using the process of elimination and recalling the characteristics of this cultural group will direct you to option 2. Review the importance and meaning of nonverbal communication in the Chinese-American culture if you had difficulty with this question.

*Level of Cognitive Ability:* Analysis
*Client Needs:* Psychosocial Integrity
*Integrated Concept/Process:* Cultural Awareness
*Content Area:* Fundamental Skills

*Reference*
Giger, J., & Davidhizar, R. (1999). *Transcultural nursing: Assessment & Intervention* (3rd ed.) St. Louis: Mosby, p. 15.

**12.** A nursing instructor is providing a session on cultural beliefs related to health and illness. After the session, the instructor asks a nursing student to describe the beliefs of an African-American in regard to illness. Which of the following would be the most appropriate response by the student?

1 "Illness is due to an imbalance between yin and yang."
2 "Illness is punishment for sins."
3 "Illness is a disharmonious state that may be caused by demons and spirits."
4 "Illness is due to lack of exercise."

**Answer: 3**

*Rationale:* In the African-American culture, illness is viewed as a disharmonious state that may be caused by demons and spirits. The goal of treatment, from the traditional African perspective, is to remove the harmful spirit from the body of the ill person. Asian-Americans believe that illness is due to an imbalance between yin and yang, to prolonged sitting or lying, or to overexertion. Hispanic Americans believe that illness occurs as a result of punishment for sins.

*Test-Taking Strategy:* Focus on the issue, African-American health beliefs. Recalling the beliefs in this culture will direct you to option 3. If you had difficulty with the question, review the various beliefs of the African-American culture.

*Level of Cognitive Ability:* Analysis
*Client Needs:* Psychosocial Integrity
*Integrated Concept/Process:* Cultural Awareness
*Content Area:* Fundamental Skills

*Reference*
Giger, J., & Davidhizar, R. (1999). *Transcultural nursing: Assessment & Intervention* (3rd ed.) St. Louis: Mosby, p. 178.

*倒入空, 打喷*

**13.** A clinic nurse is performing an admission assessment on an African-American client who is scheduled for cataract removal and intraocular lens implant. Which of the following assessment questions would be inappropriate for the nurse to ask on initial assessment?

1   "Do you have any difficulty breathing?"
2   "Do you have a close family relationship?"
3   "Do you ever experience chest pain?"
4   "Do you frequently have episodes of headache?"

**Answer: 2**
*Rationale:* In the African-American culture, it is considered intrusive to ask personal questions during the initial contact or meeting. African-Americans are highly verbal and express feelings openly to family or friends, but what transpires within the family is viewed as private. In addition, the psychosocial assessment would be the lowest priority during the initial admission assessment. Respiratory, cardiovascular, and neurological assessments are the priority assessments.

*Test-Taking Strategy:* Knowledge regarding the characteristics of the African-American culture will assist in answering the question. Also, use Maslow's Hierarchy of Needs theory noting the key words *inappropriate* and *initial*. Options 1, 3, and 4 address physiological needs. Option 2 addresses a psychosocial need.

*Level of Cognitive Ability:* Application
*Client Needs:* Psychosocial Integrity
*Integrated Concept/Process:* Cultural Awareness
*Content Area:* Fundamental Skills

*Reference*
Purnell, L., & Paulanka, B. (1998). *Transcultural health care: A culturally competent approach.* Philadelphia: F.A. Davis. p. 55.

**14.** A nurse is preparing to deliver a food tray to a client whose religion is Jewish. The nurse checks the food on the tray and notes that the client has received a roast beef dinner with whole milk as a beverage. Which of the following actions will the nurse take?

1   Deliver the food tray to the client
2   Call the dietary department and ask for a new meal tray
3   Replace the whole milk with fat-free milk
4   Ask the dietary department to replace the roast beef with pork

**Answer: 2**
*Rationale:* In the Jewish religion, the dairy-meat combination is not acceptable. Pork and pork products are not allowed in the traditional Jewish religion. The only correct nursing action is to ask the dietary department to deliver a new meal tray.

*Test-Taking Strategy:* Use the process of elimination. Recalling that the dairy-meat combination is not acceptable in this religion will direct you to option 2. Review the dietary rules of this religious group if you had difficulty with this question.

*Level of Cognitive Ability:* Application
*Client Needs:* Psychosocial Integrity
*Integrated Concept/Process:* Cultural Awareness
*Content Area:* Fundamental Skills

*Reference*
Leahy, J., & Kizilay, P. (1998). *Foundations of nursing practice: A nursing process approach.* Philadelphia: W.B. Saunders, pp. 1110-1111.

**15.** A nurse is planning to instruct a Mexican-American client about nutrition and dietary restrictions. When developing the plan, the nurse is aware that this ethnic group:

1 Enjoys foods that lack color, flavor, and texture
2 Primarily eats raw fish
3 Enjoys eating red meat
4 Views food as a primary form of socialization

**Answer: 4**

*Rationale:* Mexican foods are rich in color, flavor, texture, and spiciness. In the Mexican-American culture, any occasion is seen as a time to celebrate with food and enjoy the companionship of family and friends. Because food is a primary form of socialization, Mexican-Americans may have difficulty adhering to a prescribed diet. Asian-Americans eat raw fish, rice, and soy sauce. European-Americans prefer carbohydrates and red meat.

*Test-Taking Strategy:* Knowledge regarding the food practices and preferences and the meaning of food in the Mexican-American culture is required to answer this question. If you had difficulty with this question, review the food preferences associated with this culture.

*Level of Cognitive Ability:* Application
*Client Needs:* Psychosocial Integrity
*Integrated Concept/Process:* Cultural Awareness
*Content Area:* Fundamental Skills

*Reference*
Purnell, L., & Paulanka, B. (1998). *Transcultural health care: A culturally competent approach.* Philadelphia: F.A. Davis, p. 407.

**16.** A community health nurse has volunteered to assist in providing health care instruction to a Navajo Indian community group. The nurse plans instruction based on the common practices and rituals, knowing that which of the following is not a common characteristic associated with this ethnic group?

1 Corn is an important component of the diet
2 Alcohol use is minimal
3 Fried bread and mutton are prepared in lard
4 Vitamin D deficiency is a concern

**Answer: 2**

*Rationale:* American Indian diets may be deficient in vitamin D because many individuals suffer from lactose intolerance or do not drink milk. Corn is an important staple in the diet of the Navajo and other American Indian tribes. Fried bread and mutton are prepared in lard, and these dietary rituals have contributed to the increased risk of gallbladder disease in this population. Alcohol abuse is a concern, and many American Indian tribes exhibit high-risk behaviors related to alcohol abuse.

*Test-Taking Strategy:* Note the key word *not* in the stem of the question. Recalling that alcohol abuse is a concern in American Indian tribes will direct you to option 2. Review these common rituals and health care practices if you had difficulty with this question.

*Level of Cognitive Ability:* Analysis
*Client Needs:* Psychosocial Integrity
*Integrated Concept/Process:* Cultural Awareness
*Content Area:* Fundamental Skills

*Reference*
Purnell, L., & Paulanka, B. (1998). *Transcultural health care: A culturally competent approach.* Philadelphia: F.A. Davis, pp. 434-436.

**17.** A home care nurse is assigned to visit a Mexican-American client to perform an admission assessment. During the initial meeting with the client, the nurse should plan to:
1   Greet the client with a handshake
2   Avoid touching the client
3   Avoid any affirmative nods during the conversations with the client
4   Smile and use humor throughout the entire admission assessment

**Answer: 1**
*Rationale:* To demonstrate respect, compassion, and understanding, health care providers should greet Mexican-American clients with a handshake. On establishing rapport, providers may further demonstrate approval and respect through touch, smiling, and affirmative nods of the head. Given the diversity of dialects and the nuances of language, culturally congruent use of humor is difficult to accomplish and therefore should be avoided.

*Test-Taking Strategy:* Use the process of elimination. Knowledge regarding the cultural communication patterns of the Mexican-American will direct you to option 1. Review the characteristics of this cultural group if you had difficulty with this question.

*Level of Cognitive Ability:* Application
*Client Needs:* Psychosocial Integrity
*Integrated Concept/Process:* Cultural Awareness
*Content Area:* Fundamental Skills

*Reference*
Purnell, L., & Paulanka, B. (1998). *Transcultural health care: A culturally competent approach.* Philadelphia: F.A. Davis, p. 401.

**18.** A nurse is developing a postoperative plan of care for a 40-year-old male Filipino client who is scheduled for an appendectomy. The nurse most appropriately includes in the plan of care to:
1   Inform the client the he will need to ask for pain medication when needed
2   Offer pain medication when nonverbal signs of discomfort are identified
3   Offer pain medication on a regular basis as prescribed
4   Allow the client to maintain control and request pain medication on his own

**Answer: 3**
*Rationale:* Filipinos view pain as part of living an honorable life. The client may appear stoic and be tolerant of a high degree of pain. The nurse needs to offer pain medication on a regular basis, and in fact encourage pain relief interventions for the Filipino client who does not complain of pain, despite physiological indicators. Option 3 is the most appropriate intervention to include in the plan of care.

*Test-Taking Strategy:* Note the key words *most appropriately.* Use the process of elimination and eliminate options 1 and 4 first because they are similar. From the remaining options, recalling the cultural responses to pain in the Filipino client will direct you to option 3. If you had difficulty with this question, review the characteristics of this cultural group.

*Level of Cognitive Ability:* Application
*Client Needs:* Psychosocial Integrity
*Integrated Concept/Process:* Cultural Awareness
*Content Area:* Fundamental Skills

*Reference*
Purnell, L., & Paulanka, B. (1998). *Transcultural health care: A culturally competent approach.* Philadelphia: F.A. Davis, p. 256.

**19.** A nurse is planning the menu for a Chinese client with the hospital dietitian. In collaboration with the dietitian, the meal plan is designed to include which of the following foods that are generally included in the diet of this cultural group?

1  Vegetables
2  Milk
3  A dessert high in sugar content
4  Large portions of meat

**Answer: 1**

*Rationale:* The Chinese diet is generally vegetarian. Native Chinese generally do not drink milk or eat milk products because of a genetic tendency toward lactose intolerance. Most Chinese do not eat desserts high in sugar content.

*Test-Taking Strategy:* Use the process of elimination. Recalling the food rituals related to the Chinese culture will direct you to option 1. If you had difficulty with this question, review the dietary characteristics of this culture.

*Level of Cognitive Ability:* Application
*Client Needs:* Psychosocial Integrity
*Integrated Concept/Process:* Cultural Awareness
*Content Area:* Fundamental Skills

*Reference*
Purnell, L., & Paulanka, B. (1998). *Transcultural health care: A culturally competent approach.* Philadelphia: F.A. Davis, p. 176.

**20.** A clinic nurse is preparing to examine a Hispanic child who was brought to the clinic by the mother. During assessment of the child, the nurse avoids which of the following?

1  Asking the mother questions about the child
2  Admiring the child
3  Taking the child's temperature
4  Obtaining an interpreter if necessary

**Answer: 2**

*Rationale:* Hispanic clients may believe in the "evil eye." They believe that an individual becomes ill as a result of excessive admiration by another. Options 1 and 3 are appropriate interventions. It is appropriate for the nurse to obtain an interpreter if the child or mother does not speak the same language as the nurse.

*Test-Taking Strategy:* Use the process of elimination. Note the key word *avoids* in the stem of the question. Options 1 and 4 can be eliminated because these are therapeutic and appropriate interventions. Eliminate option 3 because there is no reason to avoid taking the child's temperature. If you had difficulty with this question, review the cultural characteristics of the Hispanic population.

*Level of Cognitive Ability:* Application
*Client Needs:* Psychosocial Integrity
*Integrated Concept/Process:* Cultural Awareness
*Content Area:* Fundamental Skills

*Reference*
Purnell, P., & Paulanka, B. (1998). *Transcultural healthcare: A culturally competent approach.* Philadelphia: F.A. Davis, p. 400.

# SELF-CARE

1. A home health care nurse is assessing a client's functional abilities and ability to perform activities of daily living (ADLs). The nurse focuses the assessment on:
   1. Self-care needs, such as toileting, feeding, and ambulating
   2. The normal everyday routine in the home
   3. Ability to do light housework, heavy housework, and pay the bills
   4. Ability to drive a car

**Answer: 1**
*Rationale:* Activities of daily living refer to the client's ability to bathe, toilet, ambulate, dress, and feed himself or herself. These functional abilities are always assessed by the home health care nurse. The normal routine in the home is not a component of functional assessment. The ability to do housework and the ability to drive a car relate to instrumental activities of daily living.

*Test-Taking Strategy:* Use the process of elimination, focusing on the issue, ability to perform ADLs. Recalling that ADLs refer to self-care needs will direct you to option 1. Review the concept of ADLs if you had difficulty with this question.

*Level of Cognitive Ability:* Application
*Client Needs:* Health Promotion and Maintenance
*Integrated Concept/Process:* Self-Care
*Content Area:* Fundamental Skills

*Reference*
Potter, P., & Perry, A. (2001). *Fundamentals of nursing* (5th ed.). St. Louis: Mosby, p. 355.

2. A client with a short leg plaster cast complains of an intense itching under the cast. The nurse provides instructions to the client regarding relief measures for the itching. Which of the following statements if made by the client indicates an understanding of the measures to relieve the itching?
   1. "I can use the blunt part of a ruler to scratch the area."
   2. "I need to obtain assistance when placing an object into the cast for the itching."
   3. "I can use a hair dryer on the low setting and allow the air to blow into the cast."
   4. "I can trickle small amounts of water down inside the cast."

**Answer: 3**
*Rationale:* Itching is a common complaint of clients with casts. Objects should not be put inside a cast because of the risk of scratching the skin and providing a point of entry for bacteria. A plaster cast can break down when wet. Therefore, the best way to relieve itching is with a forceful injection of air inside the cast.

*Test-Taking Strategy:* Use the process of elimination and eliminate options 1 and 2 first because they both involve the use of an object being placed inside the cast. Recalling that water can soften a plaster cast and cause maceration of the skin will easily direct you to option 3. Review client education regarding cast care if you had difficulty with this question.

*Level of Cognitive Ability:* Analysis
*Client Needs:* Health Promotion and Maintenance
*Integrated Concept/Process:* Self-Care
*Content Area:* Adult Health/Musculoskeletal

*Reference*
Monahan, F., & Neighbors, M. (1998). *Medical-surgical nursing: Foundations for clinical practice* (2nd ed.). Philadelphia: W.B Saunders, p. 858.

**3.** A nurse has instructed a female client with chronic vertigo about measures to prevent injury or exacerbation of symptoms. Which statement by the client indicates an understanding of how to care for herself?

1 "I will drive as long as I do not feel dizzy."

2 When I get dizzy, I will go to the bedroom to lie down."

3 "I will remove the throw rugs from my house."

4 "I will turn my head slowly when someone talks to me."

**Answer: 3**

*Rationale:* A client with chronic vertigo should avoid driving and using public transportation. The sudden movements involved in each could precipitate an attack. To further prevent vertigo attacks, the client should change positions slowly and should turn the entire body, not just the head, when spoken to. If vertigo does occur, the client should immediately sit down or grasp the nearest piece of furniture. The client should maintain the home in a state that is free of clutter and should have throw rugs removed, since the effort of trying to regain balance after slipping could trigger the onset of vertigo.

*Test-Taking Strategy:* Use the process of elimination and focus on the issue, safety. Begin to answer this question by eliminating options 1 and 2 first, since they put the client at greatest risk of injury resulting from vertigo. Choose option 3 over option 4, since it is the safer intervention of the remaining options. Review safety measures for the client with vertigo, if you had difficulty with this question.

*Level of Cognitive Ability:* Application
*Client Needs:* Health Promotion and Maintenance
*Integrated Concept/Process:* Self-Care
*Content Area:* Adult Health/Ear

*Reference*
Smeltzer, S., & Bare, B. (2000). *Brunner & Suddarth's Textbook of medical-surgical nursing* (9th ed.). Philadelphia: Lippincott Williams & Wilkins, p. 1597.

**4.** A nurse is caring for a client who has been prescribed disulfiram (Antabuse). Which statement by the client would indicate the need for further health teaching ?

1 "As long as I don't drink alcohol, I'll be fine."

2 "I must be careful taking cold medicines."

3 "I'll have to check my aftershave lotion."

4 "I'll have to be more careful with the ingredients I use for cooking."

**Answer: 1**

*Rationale:* Clients who are taking Antabuse must be taught that substances containing alcohol can trigger an adverse reaction. Sources of hidden alcohol include foods (soups, sauces, vinegars), medicine (cold medicine), mouthwashes, and skin preparations (alcohol rubs, aftershave lotions).

*Test-Taking Strategy:* Note the key words *need for further health teaching.* Remember that Antabuse is used for clients who have alcoholism, and that any form of alcohol needs to be avoided with this medication. If you are unfamiliar with this medication and the health teaching that is indicated when this medication is prescribed, review this content.

*Level of Cognitive Ability:* Analysis
*Client Needs:* Health Promotion and Maintenance
*Integrated Concept/Process:* Self-Care
*Content Area:* Pharmacology

*Reference*
Hodgson, B., & Kizior, R. (2001). *Saunders nursing drug handbook 2001.* Philadelphia: W.B. Saunders, p. 339.

**5.** A nurse has provided instructions to a client who is receiving external radiation therapy. Which of the following if stated by the client would indicate a need for further instructions regarding self-care related to the radiation therapy?

1 "I need to avoid exposure to sunlight."
2 "I need to wash my skin with a mild soap and pat dry."
3 "I need to apply pressure to the irritated area to prevent bleeding."
4 "I need to eat a high-protein diet."

**Answer: 3**

*Rationale:* The client should avoid pressure on the irritated area and should wear loose-fitting clothing. Specific physician instructions would be necessary to obtain if an alteration in skin integrity occurred as a result of the radiation therapy. Options 1, 2, and 4 are accurate measures regarding radiation therapy.

*Test-Taking Strategy:* Use the process of elimination. Note the key words *need for further instructions* in the stem of the question. The word *pressure* in option 3 is an indication that this is an inappropriate measure. Review client teaching points related to skin care and radiation therapy if you had difficulty with this question.

*Level of Cognitive Ability:* Application
*Client Needs:* Health Promotion and Maintenance
*Integrated Concept/Process:* Self-Care
*Content Area:* Adult Health/Oncology

*Reference*
Monahan, F., & Neighbors, M. (1998). *Medical-surgical nursing: Foundations for clinical practice* (2nd ed.). Philadelphia: W. B. Saunders, p. 1523.

**6.** A female client tells a clinic nurse that her skin is very dry and irritated. Which of the following products would the nurse suggest that the client apply to the dry skin?

1 Glycerin emollient
2 Aspercreame
3 Myoflex
4 Acetic acid solution

**Answer: 1**

*Rationale:* Glycerin is an emollient that is used for dry, cracked, and irritated skin. Aspercreame and Myoflex are used to treat muscular aches. Acetic acid solution is used for irrigating, cleansing, and packing wounds infected by *Pseudomonas aeruginosa*.

*Test-Taking Strategy:* Use the process of elimination. Noting the key words *skin is very dry and irritated* will direct you to option 1. Review these products if you had difficulty with this question.

*Level of Cognitive Ability:* Application
*Client Needs:* Health Promotion and Maintenance
*Integrated Concept/Process:* Self-Care
*Content Area:* Pharmacology

*Reference*
Karch, A. (2000). *Focus on nursing pharmacology*. Philadelphia: Lippincott, p. 744.

**7.** A female client being discharged from a mental health unit has a history of anxiety and command hallucinations to harm herself or others. A nurse teaches the client about interventions for hallucinations and anxiety. The nurse determines that the client understands these measures when the client says:

1  "If I take my medication, I won't be anxious."
2  "I can call my clinical specialist when I'm hallucinating, so that I can talk about my feelings and plans and not hurt anyone."
3  "I can go to group and talk about my feelings."
4  "If I get enough sleep and eat well, I won't get anxious and hear things."

**Answer: 2**
*Rationale:* There may be an increased risk for impulsive and/or aggressive behavior if the client is receiving command hallucinations to harm herself or others. Talking with the clinical specialist about auditory hallucinations can interfere with subvocal muscular activity associated with a hallucination. Options 1, 3, and 4 are general interventions but are not specific to anxiety and hallucinations.

*Test-Taking Strategy:* Use the process of elimination. Focus on the issue, anxiety and hallucinations. Options 1, 3, and 4 are all interventions that the client can do to promote wellness. Option 2 is specific to the issue and indicates self-responsible commitment and control over her own behavior. Review interventions for anxiety and hallucinations if you had difficulty with this question.

*Level of Cognitive Ability:* Analysis
*Client Needs:* Health Promotion and Maintenance
*Integrated Concept/Process:* Self-Care
*Content Area:* Mental Health

*Reference*
Stuart, G.W., & Laraia, M.T. (1998). *Principles and practice of psychiatric nursing.* (6th ed.). St. Louis: Mosby, p. 427.

**8.** A nurse has provided instructions to a client regarding testicular self-examination (TSE). Which of the following statements by the client indicates that he needs further teaching regarding TSE?

1  "I feel the spermatic cord in back and going up."
2  "I know to report any small lumps."
3  "I examine myself after I take a warm shower."
4  "I examine myself every 2 months."

**Answer: 4**
*Rationale:* TSE should be performed every month. Small lumps or abnormalities should be reported. The spermatic cord finding is normal. After a warm bath or shower, the scrotum is relaxed, making it easier to perform TSE.

*Test-Taking Strategy:* Use the process of elimination. Remembering that breast self-examination needs to be performed monthly may assist in recalling that TSE is also performed monthly. If you had difficulty with this question, review the procedure for TSE.

*Level of Cognitive Ability:* Analysis
*Client Needs:* Health Promotion and Maintenance
*Integrated Concept/Process:* Self-Care
*Content Area:* Adult Health/Oncology

*Reference*
Smeltzer, S., & Bare, B. (2000). *Brunner & Suddarth's Textbook of medical-surgical nursing* (9th ed.). Philadelphia: Lippincott Williams & Wilkins, p. 1319.

**9.** A male client who initially denied that he drank two six-packs of beer a day is being discharged and is now willing to admit that he has a drinking problem. He states that he will "get some help" in order to will live a healthier lifestyle. A nurse plans for a representative of which of the following groups to meet with the client prior to discharge?
1   Al-Anon — *for families of al*
2   Alcoholics Anonymous
3   Families Anonymous — *parents of children who abuse substances*
4   Fresh Start — *nicotine addicts*

**Answer: 2**
*Rationale:* Alcoholics Anonymous is a major self-help organization for the treatment of alcoholism. Option 1 is a group for families of alcoholics. Option 3 is for parents of children who abuse substances. Option 4 is for nicotine addicts.

*Test-Taking Strategy:* Use the process of elimination. Note the relationship between *drinking* in the question and *Alcoholics* in the correct option. Review the purpose of specific support groups, if you had difficulty with this question.

*Level of Cognitive Ability:* Application
*Client Needs:* Health Promotion and Maintenance
*Integrated Concept/Process:* Self-Care
*Content Area:* Mental Health

*Reference*
Stuart, G.W., & Laraia, M.T. (1998). *Principles and practice of psychiatric nursing.* (6th ed.). St. Louis: Mosby, p. 514.

**10.** A client with acquired immunodeficiency syndrome (AIDS) has a nursing diagnosis of Fatigue. The nurse plans to teach the client which of the following strategies to conserve energy after discharge from the hospital?
1   Stand in the shower instead of taking a bath
2   Bathe before eating breakfast
3   Sit for as many activities as possible
4   Group all tasks to be performed early in the morning

**Answer: 3**
*Rationale:* The client is taught to conserve energy by sitting for as many activities as possible, such as for dressing, shaving, preparing food, and ironing. The client should also sit in a shower chair instead of standing while bathing. The client needs to prioritize activities, such as eating breakfast before bathing, and should intersperse major activities with periods of rest.

*Test-Taking Strategy:* Focus on the issue, conserving energy. Think about the amount of exertion required by the client in performing each of the activities in the options. Options 1 and 4 are obviously taxing for the client and are eliminated first. From the remaining options, recall that bathing may take away energy that could be used for eating, which would not be helpful. Review measures that conserve energy if you had difficulty with this question.

*Level of Cognitive Ability:* Application
*Client Needs:* Health Promotion and Maintenance
*Integrated Concept/Process:* Self-Care
*Content Area:* Adult Health/Immune

*Reference*
Ignatavicius, D., Workman, M., & Mishler, M. (1999). *Medical-surgical nursing across the health care continuum* (3rd ed.). Philadelphia: W.B. Saunders, p. 454.

**11.** A nurse has provided self-care activity instructions to a client after insertion of an automatic internal cardioverter-defibrillator (AICD). The nurse determines that further instruction is needed if the client makes which of the following statements?

**1** "I should try to avoid tight clothing over the AICD insertion site."

**2** "I should keep away from electromagnetic sources such as transformers, large electrical generators, and metal detectors, including not leaning over running motors."

**3** "I can perform activities such as swimming, driving, or operating heavy equipment as I need to."

**4** "I need to avoid doing anything that would involve rough contact with the AICD insertion site."

**Answer:** 3

*Rationale:* Postdischarge instructions typically include avoiding tight clothing or belts over AICD insertion sites, rough contact with the AICD insertion site, and electromagnetic fields such as with electrical transformers, radios, TV, or radar transmitters, metal detectors, and running motors of cars or boats. Clients must also alert physicians or dentists to the presence of the device, because certain procedures such as diathermy, electrocautery, and magnetic resonance imaging may need to be avoided to prevent device malfunction. Clients should follow the specific advice of a physician regarding activities that are potentially hazardous to themselves or others, such as swimming, driving, or operating heavy equipment.

*Test-Taking Strategy:* Use the process of elimination, noting the key words *further instruction is needed*. Options 2 and 4 can be eliminated first, since they are similar to standard post–pacemaker insertion instructions. From the remaining options, noting the words *heavy equipment* in option 3 will direct you to this option. Review client teaching points for an AICD if you had difficulty with this question.

*Level of Cognitive Ability:* Analysis
*Client Needs:* Health Promotion and Maintenance
*Integrated Concept/Process:* Self-Care
*Content Area:* Adult Health/Cardiovascular

*Reference*
Smeltzer, S., & Bare, B. (2000). *Brunner & Suddarth's Textbook of medical-surgical nursing* (9th ed.). Philadelphia: Lippincott Williams & Wilkins, p. 587.

**12.** A perinatal client has been instructed in the prevention of genital tract infections. Which statement by the client indicates an understanding of these preventive measures?

**1** "I should avoid the use of condoms."

**2** "I can douche anytime I want."

**3** "I can wear my tight-fitting jeans."

**4** "I should wear underwear with a cotton panel liner."

**Answer:** 4

*Rationale:* Condoms should be used to minimize the spread of genital tract infections. Wearing tight clothes irritates the genital area and does not allow for air circulation. Douching is to be avoided. Wearing items with a cotton panel liner allows for air movement in and around the genital area.

*Test-Taking Strategy:* Use the process of elimination, noting the key words *indicates an understanding*. Options 1, 2, and 3 are all incorrect statements regarding client self-care. If you had difficulty with this question, review preventive measures associated with genital tract infections.

*Level of Cognitive Ability:* Analysis
*Client Needs:* Health Promotion and Maintenance
*Integrated Concept/Process:* Self-Care
*Content Area:* Maternity

*Reference*
Olds, S., London. M., & Ladewig, P. (2000). *Maternal-newborn nursing: A family and community-based approach* (6th ed.). Upper Saddle River, N.J.: Prentice-Hall Health, p. 996.

**13.** A nurse has given a client information about the use of nitroglycerin sublingual tablets. The client has an order for PRN use if chest pain occurs. The nurse would determine that the client understands how to self-administer the medication if the client stated an intention to:

1  Avoid using the medication until chest pain actually begins and intensifies

2  Take acetylsalicylic acid (aspirin) to treat a headache that occurs with early use

3  Discard unused tablets 6 to 9 months after the bottle is opened

4  Keep the tablets in a shirt pocket close to the body

**Answer: 3**

*Rationale:* Nitroglycerin may be self-administered sublingually 5 to 10 minutes before an activity that triggers chest pain. Tablets should be discarded 6 to 9 months after the bottle is opened, and a new bottle of pills should be obtained from the pharmacy. Nitroglycerin is very unstable and is affected by heat and cold, so it should not be kept close to the body (warmth) in a shirt pocket; rather it should be kept in a jacket pocket or purse. Headache often occurs with early use and diminishes with time. Acetaminophen (Tylenol) may be used to treat headache.

*Test-Taking Strategy:* Use the process of elimination, noting the key words *understands how to self-administer the medication.* Recalling that nitroglycerin loses its potency in 6 to 9 months will direct you to option 3. Review the client teaching points related to nitroglycerin if you had difficulty with this question.

*Level of Cognitive Ability:* Analysis
*Client Needs:* Health Promotion and Maintenance
*Integrated Concept/Process:* Self-Care
*Content Area:* Pharmacology

*Reference*
Hodgson, B., & Kizior, R. (2001). *Saunders nursing drug handbook 2001.* Philadelphia: W.B. Saunders, p. 750.

---

**14.** A client who has had a cerebral vascular accident (CVA) is prepared for discharge from the hospital. The physician has prescribed range-of-motion (ROM) exercises for the client's right side. In planning for the client's care, a home health care nurse:

1  Considers the use of active, passive, or active-assisted exercises in the home

2  Implements range-of-motion exercises to the point of pain for the client

3  Encourages the client to be dependent upon the home health care nurse to complete the exercise program

4  Develops a schedule in which range-of-motion exercises are performed every 2 hours while the client is awake, even if he or she is fatigued

**Answer: 1**

*Rationale:* The home health care nurse must consider all forms of range-of-motion exercises for the client. Even if the client has right hemiplegia, the client can assist in some of his or her own rehabilitative care. In addition, the goal in home health care nursing is for the client to assume as much self-care and independence as possible. The nurse needs to teach so that the client becomes self-reliant. Options 2 and 4 are incorrect from a physiological standpoint.

*Test-Taking Strategy:* Use the process of elimination. Options 2 and 4 can be eliminated first because these actions can be harmful to the client. From the remaining options, recall that dependence is not in the best interest of a client's sense of health promotion, which eliminates option 3. Also, note that option 1 is the global option. Review basic knowledge related to ROM exercises, if you had difficulty with this question.

*Level of Cognitive Ability:* Application
*Client Needs:* Health Promotion and Maintenance
*Integrated Concept/Process:* Self-Care
*Content Area:* Adult Health/Neurological

*Reference*
Smeltzer, S., & Bare, B. (2000). *Brunner & Suddarth's Textbook of medical-surgical nursing* (9th ed.). Philadelphia: Lippincott Williams & Wilkins, p. 1656.

**15.** A nurse plans to instruct a client with candidiasis (thrush) of the oral cavity about how to care for the disorder. The nurse avoids telling the client to:

1 Rinse the mouth four times daily with a commercial mouthwash
2 Eliminate spicy foods from the diet
3 Eliminate citrus juices and hot liquids from the diet
4 Eat foods that are liquid or pureed

**Answer: 1**

*Rationale:* Clients with thrush cannot tolerate commercial mouthwashes because the high alcohol concentration in these products can cause pain and discomfort to the lesions. A solution of warm water or mouthwash formulas without alcohol are better tolerated and may promote healing. A change in diet to liquid or pureed foods often eases the discomfort of eating. The client should avoid spicy foods, citrus juices, and hot liquids.

*Test-Taking Strategy:* Use the process of elimination and note the key word *avoids*. Also, noting the words *commercial mouthwash* in option 1 should direct you to this option. Review the client teaching points related to candidiasis (thrush) if you had difficulty with this question.

*Level of Cognitive Ability:* Application
*Client Needs:* Health Promotion and Maintenance
*Integrated Concept/Process:* Self-Care
*Content Area:* Adult Health/Immune

*Reference*

Ignatavicius, D., Workman, M., & Mishler, M. (1999). *Medical-surgical nursing across the health care continuum* (3rd ed.). Philadelphia: W.B. Saunders, p. 1337.

**16.** A client with a history of hypertension has been prescribed triamterene (Dyrenium). A nurse determines that the client understands the impact of this medication on the diet if the client states an intention to avoid which of the following fruits?

1 Apples
2 Pears
3 Bananas
4 Cranberries

**Answer: 3**

*Rationale:* Triamterene is a potassium-sparing diuretic, and the client should avoid foods high in potassium. Fruits that are naturally high in potassium include avocado, bananas, fresh oranges, mangoes, nectarines, papayas, and dried prunes.

*Test-Taking Strategy:* Recall that triamterene is a potassium-sparing diuretic. Then identify the high-potassium food. If you had difficulty with this question, review this medication and those food items high in potassium.

*Level of Cognitive Ability:* Analysis
*Client Needs:* Health Promotion and Maintenance
*Integrated Concept/Process:* Self-Care
*Content Area:* Adult Health/Cardiovascular

*References*

Peckenpaugh, N., & Poleman, C. (1999). *Nutrition essentials and diet therapy* (8th ed.). Philadelphia: W.B. Saunders, p. 148.
Hodgson, B., & Kizior, R. (2001). *Saunders nursing drug handbook 2001.* Philadelphia: W.B. Saunders, p. 1021.

**17.** Breathing exercises and postural drainage are prescribed for a child with cystic fibrosis (CF). A nurse plans to implement these procedures by telling the child to:

1   Perform the postural drainage, then the breathing exercises
2   Perform the breathing exercises, then the postural drainage
3   Schedule the procedures so they are 4 hours apart
4   Perform postural drainage in the morning and breathing exercises in the evening

**Answer: 1**

*Rationale:* Breathing exercises are recommended for the majority of children with CF, even for those with minimal pulmonary involvement. The exercises are usually performed twice daily, and they are preceded by postural drainage. The postural drainage will mobilize secretions, and the breathing exercises will then assist with expectoration. Exercises to assist with posture and to mobilize the thorax are included, such as swinging the arms and bending and twisting the trunk. The ultimate aim of these exercises is to establish a good habitual breathing pattern.

*Test-Taking Strategy:* Use the process of elimination. Recalling that postural drainage and breathing exercises are most effective when performed together will assist in eliminating options 3 and 4. From the remaining options, consider the effectiveness that each procedure will have on the mobilization of secretions to direct you to option 1. Review these procedures if you had difficulty with this question.

*Level of Cognitive Ability:* Application
*Client Needs:* Health Promotion and Maintenance
*Integrated Concept/Process:* Self-Care
*Content Area:* Child Health

*Reference*
Wong, D. (1999). *Whaley & Wong's Nursing care of infants and children* (6th ed.). St. Louis: Mosby, p. 1522.

---

**18.** A ten-year-old child has been diagnosed with type 1 diabetes mellitus. The nurse prepares to educate the family. The child is very active socially and is often away from the parents. The nurse prepares to teach:

1   The child's schoolteacher to monitor insulin requirements and administer the child's insulin
2   The child to monitor insulin requirements and administer his or her own insulin
3   The parents to always be available to monitor the child's insulin requirements
4   All the friends and family involved with the child's activities to monitor the child's insulin requirements

**Answer: 2**

*Rationale:* Most children 9 years old or older can understand the principles of monitoring their own insulin requirements. They are usually responsible enough to determine the appropriate intervention needed to maintain their health. The schoolteacher will not take responsibility for health care interventions. Parents, friends, and family cannot always be available.

*Test-Taking Strategy:* Noting the age of the child will indicate that the child is able to take control and responsibility regarding the health care situation. Eliminate option 4 first because of the absolute word *all*. From the remaining options, note that options 1 and 3 rely on other individuals to care for the child. If you had difficulty with this question, review growth and development of a ten-year-old.

*Level of Cognitive Ability:* Application
*Client Needs:* Health Promotion and Maintenance
*Integrated Concept/Process:* Self-Care
*Content Area:* Child Health

*Reference*
Wong, D. (1999). *Whaley & Wong's Nursing care of infants and children* (6th ed.). St. Louis: Mosby, p. 1878.

**19.** A client is being discharged to home after application of a plaster leg cast. The nurse would conclude that the client understands proper care of the cast if the client states an intention to:

1    Avoid getting the cast wet
2    Use the fingertips to lift and move the leg
3    Cover the casted leg with warm blankets
4    Use a padded coat hanger end to scratch under the cast

**Answer: 1**

*Rationale:* A plaster cast must remain dry to keep its strength. The cast should be handled by using the palms of the hands, not the fingertips, until it is fully dry. Air should circulate freely around the cast to help it dry. In addition, the cast gives off heat as it dries. The client should never scratch under the cast. A cool hair dryer may be used to relieve an itch.

*Test-Taking Strategy:* Use the process of elimination, noting the key word *plaster*. Option 4 is dangerous to skin integrity and is eliminated first. Knowing that a wet cast can be dented with the fingertips, causing pressure underneath, helps to eliminate option 2. Recalling that the cast needs to dry eliminates option 3. Remember, plaster casts, once they have dried after application, should not become wet. Review home care instructions for a client with a plaster cast if you had difficulty with this question.

*Level of Cognitive Ability:* Analysis
*Client Needs:* Health Promotion and Maintenance
*Integrated Concept/Process:* Self-Care
*Content Area:* Adult Health/Musculoskeletal

*Reference*
Black, J., Hawks, J., & Keene, A. (2001). *Medical-surgical nursing: Clinical management for positive outcomes* (6th ed.). Philadelphia: W.B. Saunders, p. 606.

**20.** A client is being discharged to home while recovering from acute renal failure (ARF). The client indicates an understanding of the therapeutic dietary regimen if the client states an intention to eat foods that are lower in:

1    Vitamins
2    Potassium
3    Carbohydrates
4    Fats

**Answer: 2**

*Rationale:* Most of the excretion of potassium and the control of potassium balance are normal functions of the kidneys. In a client with renal failure, potassium intake must be restricted as much as possible (30 to 50 mEq/day). The primary mechanism of potassium removal during ARF is dialysis. Options 1, 3, and 4 are not normally restricted in the client with ARF unless a secondary health problem warrants the need to do so.

*Test-Taking Strategy:* Noting the diagnosis of the client will assist in answering the question. Recalling that potassium balance and excretion are controlled by the kidney will direct you to option 2. Review the therapeutic diet in the client with ARF if you had difficulty with this question.

*Level of Cognitive Ability:* Analysis
*Client Needs:* Health Promotion and Maintenance
*Integrated Concept/Process:* Self-Care
*Content Area:* Adult Health/Renal

*Reference*
Grodner, M., Anderson, S., & DeYoung, S. (2000). *Foundations and clinical applications of nutrition: A nursing approach.* St. Louis: Mosby, pp. 594-595.

# TEACHING/LEARNING

**1.** A nurse has given instructions on site care to a hemodialysis client who has had an arteriovenous (AV) fistula implanted in the right arm. The nurse determines that the client needs further instructions if the client states an intention to:
1   Avoid carrying heavy objects on the right arm
2   Sleep on the right side
3   Report increased temperature, redness, or drainage at the site
4   Perform range-of-motion exercises routinely on the right arm

**Answer: 2**
*Rationale:* Routine instructions to a client with an AV fistula, graft, or shunt include reporting signs and symptoms of infection, performing routine range-of-motion exercises on the affected extremity, avoiding sleeping with the body weight on the extremity with the access site, and avoiding carrying heavy objects with or compressing the extremity that has the access site.

*Test-Taking Strategy:* Use the process of elimination, noting the key words *needs further instructions.* Recalling the importance of maintaining the patency of the AV fistula will direct you to option 2. Review home care instructions for a client with an AV fistula if you had difficulty with this question.

*Level of Cognitive Ability:* Analysis
*Client Needs:* Health Promotion and Maintenance
*Integrated Concept/Process:* Teaching/Learning
*Content Area:* Adult Health/Renal

*Reference*
Smeltzer, S., & Bare, B. (2000). *Brunner & Suddarth's Textbook of medical-surgical nursing* (9th ed.). Philadelphia: Lippincott Williams & Wilkins, p. 1113.

---

**2.** A nurse provides instructions to a client about administering nitroglycerin ointment (Nitrobid). The nurse determines that the client is using correct technique when applying the ointment if the client:
1   Applies additional ointment if chest pain occurs
2   Applies the ointment directly to the skin, then gently rubs the ointment into the skin
3   Applies the ointment to any non-hairy area of the body
4   Washes the ointment off when bathing and reapplies after the bath

**Answer: 3**
*Rationale:* Nitroglycerin ointment is used on a scheduled basis and is not prescribed specifically for the occurrence of chest pain. The ointment is not rubbed into the skin. It is reapplied only as directed.

*Test-Taking Strategy:* Use the process of elimination and focus on the issue, using correct technique. Recalling medication principles related to the application of ointments will direct you to option 3. Review these client teaching points if you had difficulty with this question.

*Level of Cognitive Ability:* Analysis
*Client Needs:* Health Promotion and Maintenance
*Integrated Concept/Process:* Teaching/Learning
*Content Area:* Pharmacology

*Reference*
Hodgson, B., & Kizior, R. (2001). *Saunders nursing drug handbook 2001.* Philadelphia: W.B. Saunders, pp. 750-753.

**3.** A nurse is giving medication instructions to a client receiving furosemide (Lasix). The nurse determines that further teaching is necessary if the client makes which of the following statements?

1 "I need to avoid the use of salt substitutes."
2 "I need to change positions slowly."
3 "I need to talk to my physician about the use of alcohol."
4 "I need to be careful not to get overheated in warm weather."

**Answer: 1**

*Rationale:* Furosemide is a potassium-losing diuretic, so there is no need to avoid high-potassium products, such as a salt substitute. Orthostatic hypotension is a risk, and the client must use caution with changing positions and with exposure to warm weather. The client needs to discuss the use of alcohol with the physician.

*Test-Taking Strategy:* Use the process of elimination, noting the key words *further teaching is necessary.* Recalling that furosemide is a potassium-losing diuretic, and that diuretic therapy can induce orthostatic hypotension, will direct you to option 1. Review this medication if you had difficulty with this question.

*Level of Cognitive Ability:* Analysis
*Client Needs:* Health Promotion and Maintenance
*Integrated Concept/Process:* Teaching/Learning
*Content Area:* Pharmacology

*Reference*
Hodgson, B., & Kizior, R. (2001). *Saunders nursing drug handbook 2001.* Philadelphia: W.B. Saunders, pp. 452-454.

**4.** A client has been prescribed a clonidine patch (Catapres TTS), and a nurse has instructed the client in the use of the patch. The nurse determines that further instruction is needed if the client:

1 Verbalizes an intention to leave the patch in place during bathing or showering
2 Verbalizes an intention to change the patch every 7 days
3 Trims the patch because one edge becomes loose
4 Selects a hairless site on the torso for application

**Answer: 3**

*Rationale:* The clonidine patch should be applied to a hairless site on the torso or upper arm. It is changed every 7 days and is left in place during bathing or showering. The patch should not be trimmed because doing so will alter the medication dose. If it becomes slightly loose, it should be covered with an adhesive overlay from the medication package. If it becomes very loose or falls off, it should be replaced. The patch is discarded by being folded in half with the adhesive sides together.

*Test-Taking Strategy:* Use the process of elimination, noting the key words *further instruction is needed.* Noting the words *trims the patch* will direct you to this option because this client action would alter the medication dose. Review this medication if you had difficulty with this question.

*Level of Cognitive Ability:* Analysis
*Client Needs:* Health Promotion and Maintenance
*Integrated Concept/Process:* Teaching/Learning
*Content Area:* Pharmacology

*Reference*
Hodgson, B., & Kizior, R. (2001). *Saunders nursing drug handbook 2001.* Philadelphia: W.B. Saunders, pp. 240-242.

**5.** A client is being discharged from the hospital to home and will be taking cholestyramine (Questran). The nurse determines that further teaching is needed if the client makes which of the following statements?
1 "I need to mix the Questran with juice or applesauce."
2 "I should call my doctor immediately if I develop diarrhea."
3 "I should increase my fluid intake while taking this medication."
4 "I should take this medication with meals."

**Answer: 2**
*Rationale:* This medication should not be taken dry and can be mixed in water, juice, carbonated beverage, applesauce, or soup. Common side effects include constipation, nausea, indigestion, and flatulence. Increasing fluids will minimize the constipating effects of the medication. Questran must be administered with food to be effective. Diarrhea is not a concern, but severe constipation is.

*Test-Taking Strategy:* Use the process of elimination, noting the key words *further teaching is needed.* Select option 2 because there are normally measures that can be taken for diarrhea rather than immediately calling the physician. Review this medication, if you are unfamiliar with it.

*Level of Cognitive Ability:* Analysis
*Client Needs:* Health Promotion and Maintenance
*Integrated Concept/Process:* Teaching/Learning
*Content Area:* Pharmacology

*Reference*
Hodgson, B., & Kizior, R. (2001). *Saunders nursing drug handbook 2001.* Philadelphia: W.B. Saunders, pp. 215-217.

**6.** A nurse is preparing written medication instructions for a client receiving colestipol hydrochloride (Colestid). The nurse plans to include instructions about the need for the client to take which of the following to counteract unintended medication effects?
1 Vitamin D
2 All fat-soluble vitamins
3 B-complex vitamins
4 Vitamin C

**Answer: 2**
*Rationale:* Colestipol, a bile-sequestering agent, is used to lower blood cholesterol levels. However, the bile salts (rich in cholesterol) interfere with the absorption of the fat-soluble vitamins A, D, E, and K, as well as folic acid. With ongoing therapy, the client is at risk for deficiency of these vitamins, and is counseled to take supplements of these vitamins.

*Test-Taking Strategy:* Use the process of elimination. Recalling that bile-sequestering agents interfere with the absorption of fat-soluble vitamins will assist in eliminating options 3 and 4. From the remaining options, select option 2 because it is the global option. Review client teaching points regarding this medication if you had difficulty with this question.

*Level of Cognitive Ability:* Application
*Client Needs:* Health Promotion and Maintenance
*Integrated Concept/Process:* Teaching/Learning
*Content Area:* Pharmacology

*Reference*
Hodgson, B., & Kizior, R. (2001). *Saunders nursing drug handbook 2001.* Philadelphia: W.B. Saunders, p. 253.

**7.** A client with tuberculosis (TB) is preparing for discharge from the hospital. Which of the following client statements indicates that further teaching is necessary?

1 "If I miss a dose of medication because of nausea, I just skip that dose and resume my regular schedule."

2 "I need to eat foods that are high in iron, protein, and vitamin C."

3 "I need to place used tissues in a plastic bag when I am home."

4 "I will not need respiratory isolation when I am home."

**Answer: 1**

*Rationale:* Because of the resistant strains of tuberculosis, the nurse must emphasize that noncompliance regarding medication could lead to an infection that is difficult to treat and may cause total drug resistance. Clients may prevent nausea related to the medication by taking the daily dose at bedtime. Antinausea medications may also prevent this symptom. Medication doses should not be skipped. Options 2, 3, and 4 are correct statements.

*Test-Taking Strategy:* Use the process of elimination, noting the key words *further teaching is necessary*. General principles related to medication administration will direct you to option 1. Review medication therapy and its importance in TB if you had difficulty with this question.

*Level of Cognitive Ability:* Analysis
*Client Needs:* Health Promotion and Maintenance
*Integrated Concept/Process:* Teaching/Learning
*Content Area:* Pharmacology

*Reference*
Smeltzer, S., & Bare, B. (2000). *Brunner & Suddarth's Textbook of medical-surgical nursing* (9th ed.). Philadelphia: Lippincott Williams & Wilkins, p. 441.

---

**8.** A nurse is planning to teach a client who is newly diagnosed with tuberculosis (TB) about how to prevent the spread of TB. Which of the following instructions would be least effective in preventing the spread of TB?

1 Teach the client to cover the mouth when coughing

2 Teach the client to sterilize dishes at home

3 Teach the client to properly dispose of Kleenex

4 Teach the client that close contacts should be tested for TB

**Answer: 2**

*Rationale:* Options 1, 3, and 4 would assist in breaking the chain of infection. Not only would option 2 be impractical, but there is no evidence to suggest that sterilizing dishes would break the chain of infection with pulmonary TB.

*Test-Taking Strategy:* Focus on the issue, to prevent the spread of TB. Use the process of elimination, noting the key words *least effective*. Recalling the methods of transmission of TB will direct you to option 2. Review home care principles related to TB, if you had difficulty with this question.

*Level of Cognitive Ability:* Application
*Client Needs:* Safe, Effective Care Environment
*Integrated Concept/Process:* Teaching/Learning
*Content Area:* Adult Health/Respiratory

*Reference*
Smeltzer, S., & Bare, B. (2000). *Brunner & Suddarth's Textbook of medical-surgical nursing* (9th ed.). Philadelphia: Lippincott Williams & Wilkins, p. 442.

**9.** A client is being discharged to home with a heparin lock (intermittent IV catheter) to receive a week of antibiotic IV therapy at home following abdominal surgery. When a nurse is evaluating the discharge teaching, which of the following statements by the client indicates the need for further instruction?
1  "I'll examine the IV site frequently."
2  "If the IV site becomes wet or moist, it can air dry."
3  "Pain, redness, and swelling need to be reported to the physician."
4  "If the lock or catheter accidentally comes out, I'll apply pressure to the site."

**Answer: 2**
*Rationale:* Clients at home with IV sites need to be instructed on site assessment as well as complications to report to the physician. Clients should also know how to treat complications, such as bleeding at the IV site. Clients often are expected to change dressings and need to be aware that if the dressing is wet or soiled, it needs to be changed immediately in order to prevent infection.

*Test-Taking Strategy:* Using the process of elimination and principles related to asepsis will easily direct you to option 2. Review these principles if you had difficulty with this question.

*Level of Cognitive Ability:* Analysis
*Client Needs:* Safe, Effective Care Environment
*Integrated Concept/Process:* Teaching/Learning
*Content Area:* Fundamental Skills

*Reference*
Potter, P., & Perry, A. (2001). *Fundamentals of nursing* (5th ed.). St. Louis: Mosby, p. 1235.

**10.** A home health nurse provides instructions to a client with jaundice who is experiencing pruritus. The nurse avoids telling the client to:
1  Wear loose cotton clothing
2  Use tepid water for bathing
3  Maintain a warm house temperature
4  Take the prescribed antihistamines to relieve the itch

**Answer: 3**
*Rationale:* Pruritus is caused by the accumulation of bile salts in the skin and results from obstructed biliary excretion. Antihistamines may relieve the itching, as will tepid water or emollient baths. The client should avoid the use of alkaline soap and wear loose, soft cotton clothing. The client is instructed to keep the house temperature cool.

*Test-Taking Strategy:* Use the process of elimination, noting the key word *avoids*. Recalling that heat causes vasodilation will assist in answering this question. This principle should direct you to option 3 as the measure to avoid in the treatment of pruritus. If you had difficulty with this question, review the measures that assist in alleviating pruritus.

*Level of Cognitive Ability:* Application
*Client Needs:* Health Promotion and Maintenance
*Integrated Concept/Process:* Teaching/Learning
*Content Area:* Adult Health/Gastrointestinal

*Reference*
Ignatavicius, D., Workman, M., & Mishler, M. (1999). *Medical-surgical nursing across the health care continuum* (3rd ed.). Philadelphia: W.B. Saunders, p. 1711.

**11.** A nurse provides home care instructions to a client hospitalized for a transurethral resection of the prostate (TURP). Which statement by the client indicates the need for further instructions?

1   "I need to avoid strenuous activity for 4 to 6 weeks."
2   "I need to maintain an intake of 6 to 8 glasses of water daily."
3   "I can lift and push objects up to 30 pounds in weight."
4   "I need to include prune juice in my diet."

**Answer: 3**

*Rationale:* The client needs to be advised to avoid strenuous activity for 4 to 6 weeks and to avoid lifting items weighing more than 20 pounds. The client needs to maintain a daily intake of at least 6 to 8 glasses of nonalcoholic fluids to minimize clot formation. Straining during defecation is avoided to prevent bleeding. Prune juice is a satisfactory bowel stimulant.

*Test-Taking Strategy:* Use the process of elimination, noting the key words *need for further instructions.* Options 1 and 2 can be easily eliminated. If you consider the anatomical location of the surgical procedure, it would be reasonable to think that constipation needs to be avoided; therefore, eliminate option 4. Select option 3 because items weighing 30 pounds seems to be rather excessive. Review TURP discharge teaching points, if you had difficulty with this question.

*Level of Cognitive Ability:* Application
*Client Needs:* Health Promotion and Maintenance
*Integrated Concept/Process:* Teaching/Learning
*Content Area:* Adult Health/Renal

*Reference*
Smeltzer, S., & Bare, B. (2000). *Brunner & Suddarth's Textbook of medical-surgical nursing* (9th ed.). Philadelphia: Lippincott Williams & Wilkins, p. 1316.

**12.** A nurse is providing home care instructions to a client who will be receiving intravenous (IV) therapy at home. The nurse teaches the client that the most important action to prevent an infection from the IV site is to:

1   Assess the IV site carefully every day for redness and edema
2   Redress the IV site daily, cleansing it with alcohol
3   Carefully wash hands with antibacterial soap before working with the IV site or equipment
4   Change IV tubing and fluid containers daily

**Answer: 3**

*Rationale:* Although assessment of the IV site is important, it will not actively prevent an infection. IV sites do not need to be redressed daily unless the dressing becomes soiled, wet, or loose. Although IV containers should be changed daily, tubing only needs to be changed every 48 to 72 hours, according to Centers for Disease Control guidelines. It is extremely important for the client to understand the absolute necessity of handwashing prior to working with IV fluids.

*Test-Taking Strategy:* Note the key words *most important* and focus on the issue, preventing infection. Remember, the top priority in infection prevention is proper handwashing technique. Review universal precautions and its role in preventing infection if you had difficulty with this question.

*Level of Cognitive Ability:* Application
*Client Needs:* Safe, Effective Care Environment
*Integrated Concept/Process:* Teaching/Learning
*Content Area:* Fundamental Skills

*Reference*
Potter, P., & Perry, A. (2001). *Fundamentals of nursing* (5th ed.). St. Louis: Mosby, p. 1235.

**13.** A 64-year-old client is being treated for an atrial dysrhythmia with quinidine gluconate (Duraquin). A nurse provides instructions to the client about the medication. Which statement by the client indicates that the instructions have been effective?
1   "If I miss a dose, I take two doses of the medication at the next scheduled time."
2   "If I miss a dose, I should call my doctor."
3   "If I miss a dose, I should take the dose in the evening if I remember."
4   "If I miss a dose, I should take the next prescribed dose as usual."

**Answer: 4**
*Rationale:* The client should be instructed not to take an extra dose. The client should be instructed to take the medication if remembered within 2 hours of the missed dose, or to omit the dose and then resume the normal schedule. Quinidine gluconate needs to be taken exactly as prescribed. There is no need to call the doctor.

*Test-Taking Strategy:* Use the process of elimination and general principles related to medication administration. Eliminate option 1 because this action is inaccurate and could cause toxic effects. There is no need to call the doctor unless toxic effects occur; therefore eliminate option 2. From the remaining options, recalling that a missed dose can be taken within 2 hours if remembered will direct you to option 4. If you had difficulty with this question, review the basic principles associated with medication administration.

*Level of Cognitive Ability:* Analysis
*Client Needs:* Health Promotion and Maintenance
*Integrated Concept/Process:* Teaching/Learning
*Content Area:* Pharmacology

*Reference*
Hodgson, B., & Kizior, R. (2001). *Saunders nursing drug handbook 2001.* Philadelphia: W.B. Saunders, p. 894.

**14.** A client asks a nurse for a recommendation about how to prevent fires and burn injury. The nurse tells the client that the one single intervention that has been shown to decrease the risk of dying in a residential fire is:
1   The installation of a sprinkler system
2   Fire extinguishers placed in key areas such as the kitchen, near the furnace, and near the hot water heater
3   The use of operable smoke detectors
4   Installation of fire-resistant dry-wall panels throughout the house

**Answer: 3**
*Rationale:* Early detection of smoke and, subsequently, immediate evacuation from the house have been shown to significantly reduce mortality. The installation of a sprinkler system is very expensive and not usually done in residential situations. Fire extinguishers are useful to put out small fires, but they are unrealistic and dangerous to use to attempt to extinguish large fires. Although fire-resistant products may help slow down a blaze, fire-resistant products can eventually catch on fire.

*Test-Taking Strategy:* Look for the health prevention measure that is simple to implement and will alert individuals of the need to evacuate a residence. This will direct you to option 3. If you had difficulty with this question, review fire safety.

*Level of Cognitive Ability:* Application
*Client Needs:* Safe, Effective Care Environment
*Integrated Concept/Process:* Teaching/Learning
*Content Area:* Fundamental Skills

*Reference*
Potter, P., & Perry, A. (2001). *Fundamentals of nursing* (5th ed.). St. Louis: Mosby, p. 1021.

**15.** A client has had same-day surgery to insert a ventilating tube into the tympanic membrane. A nurse concludes that the client understands the discharge instructions if the client states an intention to:

1  Use a shower cap if taking a shower
2  Swim only with the head above water
3  Wash the hair quickly, in 2 minutes or less
4  Avoid taking any medication for pain

**Answer: 1**

*Rationale:* After insertion of a tube into the tympanic membrane, it is important to avoid getting water in the ears. For this reason, swimming, showering, or washing the hair is avoided after surgery until the time frame designated for each is identified by the surgeon. A shower cap or earplug may be used by the client when showering, if allowed by the physician. The client should take medication as advised for postoperative discomfort.

*Test-Taking Strategy:* Use the process of elimination, noting the key words *understands the discharge instructions.* Eliminate option 2 because of the absolute word *only* and option 3 because of the word *quickly.* From the remaining options, focusing on the anatomical location of the surgery will direct you to option 1. Review client instructions following this type of surgery, if you had difficulty with this question.

*Level of Cognitive Ability:* Analysis
*Client Needs:* Health Promotion and Maintenance
*Integrated Concept/Process:* Teaching/Learning
*Content Area:* Adult Health/Ear

*Reference*
Beare, P., & Myers, J. (1998). *Adult health nursing* (3rd ed.). St. Louis: Mosby, p. 1177.

**16.** A nurse has completed diet teaching for a client on a low-sodium diet for the treatment of hypertension. The nurse concludes that further teaching is necessary when the client makes which of these statements?

1  "This diet will help to lower my blood pressure."
2  "The reason I need to lower my salt intake is to reduce fluid retention."
3  "This diet is not a replacement for my antihypertensive medications."
4  "Frozen foods are lowest in sodium."

**Answer: 4**

*Rationale:* A low-sodium diet is used as an adjunct to antihypertensive medications for the treatment of hypertension. Sodium retains fluid, which leads to hypertension secondary to increased fluid volume. Frozen foods use salt as a preservative and should not be encouraged as part of a low-sodium diet.

*Test-Taking Strategy:* Note the key words *further teaching is necessary.* Use the process of elimination and eliminate options 1, 2, and 3 because these are accurate statements related to hypertension. If you had difficulty with this question, review the treatment of hypertension and foods high in sodium.

*Level of Cognitive Ability:* Analysis
*Client Needs:* Health Promotion and Maintenance
*Integrated Concept/Process:* Teaching/Learning
*Content Area:* Adult Health/Cardiovascular

*Reference*
Grodner, M., Anderson, S., & DeYoung, S. (2000). *Foundations and clinical applications of nutrition: A nursing approach.* St. Louis: Mosby, p. 226.

**17.** A nurse is preparing a plan regarding home care instructions for the parents of a child with generalized tonic-clonic seizures who is being treated with oral phenytoin (Dilantin). The nurse includes instructions in the plan regarding:
1  Monitoring the child's intake and output daily
2  Checking the child's blood pressure prior to the administration of the medication
3  Providing oral hygiene, especially care of the gums
4  Administering the medication 1 hour before food intake

**Answer: 3**
*Rationale:* Phenytoin causes gum bleeding and hyperplasia, and therefore use of a soft toothbrush and gum massage should be instituted to diminish this complication and prevent trauma. Options 1 and 2 are incorrect because the intake and output and the blood pressure are not affected by this medication. Option 4 is incorrect because directions for administration of this medication include to administer with food to minimize gastrointestinal upset.

*Test-Taking Strategy:* Use the process of elimination. Correlate phenytoin with gum bleeding and hyperplasia. Also, note the word *oral* in the question and in the correct option. Review the side effects and the method of administration of this medication if you had difficulty with this question.

*Level of Cognitive Ability:* Application
*Client Needs:* Health Promotion and Maintenance
*Integrated Concept/Process:* Teaching/Learning
*Content Area:* Pharmacology

*Reference*
Hodgson, B., & Kizior, R. (2000). *Saunders nursing drug handbook 2000.* Philadelphia: W.B. Saunders, pp. 823-824.

**18.** A nurse performs an initial assessment on a pregnant client and determines that the client is at risk for toxoplasmosis. The nurse would teach the client which of the following to prevent exposure to this disease?
1  Wash hands only before meals
2  Eat raw meats
3  Avoid exposure to litter boxes used by cats
4  Use topical corticosteroid treatments prophylactically

**Answer: 3**
*Rationale:* Infected house cats transmit toxoplasmosis through the feces. Handling litter boxes can transmit the disease to the pregnant client. Meats that are undercooked can harbor microorganisms that can cause infection. Hands should be washed frequently throughout the day. The use of topical corticosteroids will not prevent exposure to the disease.

*Test-Taking Strategy:* Use the process of elimination. Eliminate option 1 because of the absolute word *only*. Option 2 represents an extreme statement and can also be eliminated. Focusing on the key words *prevent exposure* will direct you to option 3. Review the causes of toxoplasmosis if you had difficulty with this question.

*Level of Cognitive Ability:* Application
*Client Needs:* Health Promotion and Maintenance
*Integrated Concept/Process:* Teaching/Learning
*Content Area:* Maternity

*Reference*
Gorrie, T., McKinney, E., & Murray, S. (1998). *Foundations of maternal newborn nursing* (2nd ed.) Philadelphia: W.B. Saunders, p. 739.

**19.** A home health nurse is instructing the mother of a child with cystic fibrosis (CF) about the appropriate dietary measures. The nurse tells the mother that the child needs to consume a:

1 Low-calorie, low-fat diet
2 High-calorie, high-protein diet
3 Low-calorie, low-protein diet
4 High-calorie, restricted-fat diet

**Answer: 2**
*Rationale:* Children with CF are managed with a high-calorie, high-protein diet. Pancreatic enzyme replacement therapy and fat-soluble vitamin supplements are administered. Fat restriction is not necessary.

*Test-Taking Strategy:* Use the process of elimination. Eliminate options 1 and 4 first because they are similar. Thinking about the pathophysiology related to CF will direct you to option 2 from the remaining options. If you are unfamiliar with the diet plan for the child with CF, review these measures.

*Level of Cognitive Ability:* Application
*Client Needs:* Physiological Integrity
*Integrated Concept/Process:* Teaching/Learning
*Content Area:* Child Health

*Reference*
Wong, D. (1999). *Whaley & Wong's Nursing care of infants and children* (6th ed.). St. Louis: Mosby, p. 1524.

**20.** A nurse in an ambulatory care unit is reviewing the surgical instructions with a client who will be admitted for knee replacement surgery. The nurse informs the client that crutches will be needed for ambulation after surgery and that the client will be instructed in the use of the crutches:

1 At the time of discharge following surgery
2 Before surgery
3 On the second postoperative day
4 On the first postoperative day

**Answer: 2**
*Rationale:* It is best to assess crutch walking ability and to instruct the client in the use of the crutches prior to surgery because this task can be difficult to learn when the client is in pain and not used to the imbalance that may occur following surgery. Options 1, 3, and 4 are not the appropriate times to teach a client about crutch walking.

*Test-Taking Strategy:* Use the process of elimination. Note the similarity between options 1, 3, and 4 in that they all address the postoperative period. Review preoperative teaching principles if you had difficulty with this question.

*Level of Cognitive Ability:* Application
*Client Needs:* Health Promotion and Maintenance
*Integrated Concept/Process:* Teaching/Learning
*Content Area:* Adult Health/Musculoskeletal

*Reference*
Maher, A., Salmond, S., & Pellino, T. (1998). *Orthopaedic nursing* (2nd ed.). Philadelphia: W.B. Saunders, p. 269.

## CRITICAL THINKING: FREE-TEXT ENTRY

**1.** A 13-year-old female client is adamantly refusing to take the prescribed corticosteroid therapy for the treatment of Crohn's disease. On the basis of these data, a nurse initiates a supportive and caring interaction, knowing that the adolescent is most likely fearful of what effect that can occur with this treatment?

**Answer:** Altered body image
*Rationale:* One of the main concerns in the adolescent population is body image. Corticosteroids can greatly alter the body's appearance by causing weight gain, puffy skin, and a humped back.

*Test-Taking Strategy:* Use the concepts of growth and development and knowledge regarding the side effects of corticosteroids to answer the question. Recalling that body image is a main concern of the adolescent will assist in answering the question. Review these concepts and the side effects of these medications if you had difficulty answering this question.

*Level of Cognitive Ability:* Analysis
*Client Needs:* Health Promotion and Maintenance
*Integrated Concept/Process:* Caring
*Content Area:* Child Health

*Reference*
Wong, D. (1999). *Whaley & Wong's Nursing care of infants and children* (6th ed.). St. Louis: Mosby, p. 1557.

---

**2.** A home care nurse makes a home visit to a client. The client tells the nurse that the physician's instructions state to take ibuprofen (Advil), 0.4 g, for mild pain. The medication bottle states ibuprofen (Advil), 200 mg tablets. How many tablet(s) will the nurse instruct the client to take?

**Answer:** 2 tablets
*Rationale:* Convert 0.4 g to mg. In the metric system, to convert larger to smaller multiply by 1000 or move the decimal 3 places to the right. Then, use the following formula:

$$4 \text{ g} = 400 \text{ mg}$$

$$\frac{400 \text{ mg}}{200 \text{ mg}} \times 1 \text{ tablet} = 2 \text{ tablets}$$

*Test-Taking Strategy:* Knowledge of the formula for the calculation of a medication is required to answer this question. Remember to convert grams to milligrams. Follow the formula and make sure that the calculated dose makes sense. If you had difficulty with this question, review conversions and calculations.

*Level of Cognitive Ability:* Application
*Client Needs:* Physiological Integrity
*Integrated Concept/Process:* Teaching/Learning
*Content Area:* Fundamental Skills

*Reference*
Leahy, J., & Kizilay, P. (1998). *Foundations of nursing practice: A nursing process approach.* Philadelphia: W.B. Saunders, pp. 451-455.

---

**3.** A mother of a 3-year-old child calls a neighbor who is a nurse and tells the nurse that her child just ate the mouse poison that was stored in a cabinet. The nurse would instruct the mother to take what action immediately?

**Answer:** Call the Poison Control Center
*Rationale:* If a poisoning occurs, the Poison Control Center should be contacted immediately. The Poison Control Center will advise the mother regarding the initial action to take. The Poison Control Center may advise the mother to bring the child to the emergency room, and if this is the case, the mother should call an ambulance.

*Test-Taking Strategy:* Note the key word *immediately.* Remember that if a poisoning occurs, the Poison Control Center should be contacted immediately. Any action that delays treatment is avoided. Review poison control measures if you had difficulty with this question.

*Level of Cognitive Ability:* Application
*Client Needs:* Physiological Integrity
*Integrated Concept/Process:* Nursing Process/Implementation
*Content Area:* Child Health

**Reference**

Wong, D. (1999). *Whaley & Wong's Nursing care of infants and children* (6th ed.). St. Louis: Mosby, p. 740.

---

**4.** A client is using diphenhydramine (Benadryl) 1% as a topical agent for allergic dermatosis. A nurse concludes that the medication is having the intended effect if the client reports relief of what complaint?

**Answer:** Urticaria

*Rationale:* Diphenhydramine is an antihistamine medication that has many uses. When used as a topical agent on the skin, it reduces the symptoms of allergic reaction, such as itching or urticaria.

*Test-Taking Strategy:* Note the key words *intended effect.* Recalling that diphenhydramine is an antihistamine medication will assist in answering this question. Review the action of this medication, if you had difficulty with this question.

*Level of Cognitive Ability:* Analysis
*Client Needs:* Health Promotion and Maintenance
*Integrated Concept/Process:* Nursing Process/Evaluation
*Content Area:* Pharmacology

**Reference**

Deglin, J., & Vallerand, A. (1999). *Davis's drug guide for nurses* (6th ed.). Philadelphia: F.A. Davis. p. 291.

---

## REFERENCES

Beare, P., & Myers, J. (1998). *Adult health nursing* (3rd ed.). St. Louis: Mosby.

Black, J., Hawks, J., & Keene, A. (2001). *Medical-surgical nursing: Clinical management for positive outcomes* (6th ed.). Philadelphia: W.B. Saunders.

Bowden, V., Dickey, S., & Greenberg, C. (1998). *Children and their families: The continuum of care.* Philadelphia: W.B. Saunders.

Clark, J., Queener, S., & Karb, V. (2000). *Pharmacologic basis of nursing practice* (6th ed.). St. Louis: Mosby.

Clark, M.J. (1999). *Nursing in the community: Dimensions of community health nursing* (3rd ed.). Stamford, Conn.: Appleton & Lange.

Deglin, J., & Vallerand, A. (2001). *Davis's drug guide for nurses* (7th ed.). Philadelphia: F.A. Davis.

Deglin, J., & Vallerand, A. (1999). *Davis's drug guide for nurses* (6th ed.). Philadelphia: F.A. Davis.

Fischbach, F. (2000). *A manual of laboratory & diagnostic tests* (6th ed.). Philadelphia: Lippincott Williams & Wilkins.

Fortinash, K., & Holoday-Worret, P. (2000). *Psychiatric mental health nursing* (2nd ed.). St. Louis: Mosby.

Giger, J., & Davidhizar, R. (1999). *Transcultural nursing: Assessment & Intervention* (3rd ed.) St. Louis: Mosby.

Gorrie, T., McKinney, E., & Murray, S. (1998). *Foundations of maternal-newborn nursing* (2nd ed.). Philadelphia: W.B. Saunders.

Grodner, M., Anderson, S., & DeYoung, S. (2000). *Foundations and clinical applications of nutrition: A nursing approach.* St. Louis: Mosby.

Harkreader, H. (2000). *Fundamentals of nursing: Caring and clinical judgment.* Philadelphia: W.B. Saunders.

Hodgson, B., & Kizior, R. (2001). *Saunders nursing drug handbook 2001.* Philadelphia: W.B. Saunders.

Ignatavicius, D., Workman, M., & Mishler, M. (1999). *Medical-surgical nursing across the health care continuum* (3rd ed.). Philadelphia: W.B. Saunders.

Karch, A. (2000). *Focus on nursing pharmacology.* Philadelphia: Lippincott.

Kee, J., & Marshall, S. (2000). *Clinical calculations: With applications to general and specialty areas* (4th ed.). Philadelphia: W.B. Saunders.

Kozier, B., Erb, G., Berman, A., & Burke, K. (2000). *Fundamentals of nursing: Concepts, process, and practice* (6th ed.). Upper Saddle River, N.J.: Prentice-Hall.

Leahy, J., & Kizilay, P. (1998). *Foundations of nursing practice: A nursing process approach.* Philadelphia: W.B. Saunders.

LeMone, P., & Burke, K. (2000). *Medical-surgical nursing: Critical thinking in client care* (2nd ed.). Upper Saddle River, N.J.: Prentice-Hall.

Lewis, S., Heitkemper, M., & Dirksen, S. (2000). *Medical-surgical nursing: Assessment and management of clinical problems* (5th ed.). St. Louis: Mosby.

Lowdermilk, D., Perry, S., & Bobak, I. (2000). *Maternity & women's health care* (7th ed.). St. Louis: Mosby.

Maher, A., Salmond, S., & Pellino, T. (1998). *Orthopaedic nursing* (2nd ed.). Philadelphia: W.B. Saunders.

Monahan, F., & Neighbors, M. (1998). *Medical-surgical nursing: Foundations for clinical practice* (2nd ed.). Philadelphia: W.B. Saunders.

Olds, S., London, M., & Ladewig, P. (2000). *Maternal-newborn nursing: A family and community-based approach* (6th ed.). Upper Saddle River, N.J.: Prentice-Hall Health.

Peckenpaugh, N., & Poleman, C. (1999). *Nutrition essentials and diet therapy* (8th ed.). Philadelphia: W.B. Saunders.

Phipps, W., Sands, J., & Marek, J. (1999). *Medical-surgical nursing: Concepts & clinical practice* (6th ed.). St. Louis: Mosby.

Potter, P., & Perry, A. (2001). *Fundamentals of nursing* (5th ed.). St. Louis: Mosby.

Purnell, P., & Paulanka, B. (1998). *Transcultural healthcare: A culturally competent approach.* Philadelphia: F.A. Davis.

Sherwen, L., Scoloveno, M.A., & Weingarten, C. (1999). *Maternity nursing: Care of the childbearing family* (3rd ed.). Stamford, Conn.: Appleton & Lange.

Smeltzer, S., & Bare, B. (2000). *Brunner & Suddarth's Textbook of medical-surgical nursing* (9th ed.). Philadelphia: Lippincott Williams & Wilkins.

Stuart, G.W., & Laraia, M.T. (1998). *Principles and practice of psychiatric nursing* (6th ed.). St. Louis: Mosby.

Varcarolis, E. (1998). *Foundations of psychiatric mental health nursing* (3rd ed.). Philadelphia: W.B. Saunders.

Wong, D. (1999). *Whaley & Wong's Nursing care of infants and children* (6th ed.). St. Louis: Mosby.

# Comprehensive Test

(kəmpri'hɛnsɪv)

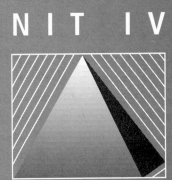

UNIT IV

1. A nurse is performing an assessment on a 6-month-old infant suspected of having hydrocephalus. Which of the following symptoms if noted in the infant is associated with this diagnosis?
   1 The presence of protein in the urine
   2 An elevated apical heart rate
   3 A drop in blood pressure from baseline
   4 A bulging anterior fontanel

**Answer: 4**

*Rationale:* A bulging anterior fontanel indicates increased cerebrospinal fluid collection in the cerebral ventricle, which occurs in hydrocephalus. Proteinuria, an elevated apical pulse, and a drop in blood pressure are not specifically related to increasing cerebrospinal fluid in the brain tissue.

*Test-Taking Strategy:* Use the principles associated with excessive fluid build up in the cranial cavity to answer this question. Remember that fluid accumulation in the cranial cavity will exert pressure on the soft brain tissue. This will cause the anterior fontanel to expand. Additionally, correlate the word *hydrocephalus* in the question with *anterior fontanel* in option 4. If you had difficulty with this question, review the symptoms associated with hydrocephalus.

*Level of Cognitive Ability:* Analysis
*Client Needs:* Physiological Integrity
*Integrated Concept/Process:* Nursing Process/Assessment
*Content Area:* Child Health

*Reference*
Wong, D. (1999). *Whaley & Wong's Nursing care of infants and children* (6th ed.). St. Louis: Mosby, p. 495.

2. Crutchfield tongs have been placed in a child to stabilize a fracture in the cervical area. The nurse is developing a plan of care for a child and avoids including which of the following in the plan?
   1 Log roll the child when positioning
   2 Check the tongs every 24 hours for displacement and looseness
   3 Monitor neurological status
   4 Perform pin care every shift

**Answer: 2**

*Rationale:* The purpose of Crutchfield tongs is to stabilize fractures or displaced vertebrae in cervical and thoracic areas. Tongs are inserted on the sides of the scalp through drill holes. Traction pull is always along the axis of the spine. The nurse should check the tongs at least every 8 hours and PRN for displacement and looseness. The child can be repositioned by log rolling or turned as a unit when repositioning. Neurological status should be checked frequently, because spinal cord injury frequently accompanies a cervical injury. Pin care is done every shift.

*Test-Taking Strategy:* Note the key word *avoids* in the stem of the question. Use the process of elimination. Attempt to visualize the child who is in Crutchfield tongs and note the key words *every 24 hours* in option 2. Review nursing care for a child in Crutchfield tongs if you had difficulty with this question.

*Level of Cognitive Ability:* Application
*Client Needs:* Physiological Integrity
*Integrated Concept/Process:* Nursing Process/Planning
*Content Area:* Child Health

*Reference*
Wong, D. (1999). *Whaley & Wong's Nursing care of infants and children* (6th ed.). St. Louis: Mosby, p. 1919.

3. A client is being given prednisone (Deltasone) as part of anticancer therapy. The nurse avoids giving the client which of the following analgesics while the client is taking this medication?
   1   Oxycodone (Oxycontin)
   2   Propoxyphene (Darvon)
   3   Acetaminophen (Tylenol)
   4   Acetylsalicylic acid (aspirin)

**Answer: 4**
*Rationale:* Prednisone is irritating to the gastrointestinal (GI) tract, which could be worsened by the use of other products that have the same side effect. Therefore, products such as aspirin and nonsteroidal anti-inflammatory drugs are not used during corticosteroid therapy.

*Test-Taking Strategy:* Use the process of elimination and think about the side effects of prednisone. Recalling that aspirin is irritating to the GI tract will assist you in answering the question. If this question was difficult, review the side effects of prednisone.

*Level of Cognitive Ability:* Application
*Client Needs:* Physiological Integrity
*Integrated Concept/Process:* Nursing Process/Planning
*Content Area:* Pharmacology

*Reference*
Hodgson, B., & Kizior, R. (2001). *Saunders Nursing drug handbook 2001.* Philadelphia: W.B. Saunders, p. 855.

4. A nurse is asked to go to a local high school to talk to students about sexually transmitted diseases (STDs). The nurse plans to tell the student that:
   1   Birth control pills are the only way to prevent STDs
   2   A diaphragm provides a barrier to prevent STDs
   3   The use of condoms does not provide any protection at all
   4   The use of condoms and avoiding casual sex with multiple partners prevent STDs

**Answer: 4**
*Rationale:* The use of condoms and avoiding casual sex with multiple partners should be the focus of discussion, because these measures prevent STDs. The use of condoms does provide some protection against STDs. Birth control pills and the use of a diaphragm help to prevent pregnancy but do not provide protection from STDs.

*Test-Taking Strategy:* Use the process of elimination. Focus on the issue, which relates to STDs, not pregnancy. This focus will eliminate options 1, 2, and 3. Review the methods of protection against STDs if you had difficulty with this question.

*Level of Cognitive Ability:* Application
*Client Needs:* Safe, Effective Care Environment
*Integrated Concept/Process:* Teaching/Learning
*Content Area:* Fundamental Skills

*Reference*
Black, J., Hawks, J., & Keene, A. (2001). *Medical-surgical nursing: Clinical management for positive outcomes* (6th ed.). Philadelphia: W.B. Saunders, p. 1043.

**5.** A home care nurse is caring for a client who has just been discharged from the hospital after implantation of a permanent pacemaker. A priority nursing action to maintain a safe environment for the client would be to assess the client's home for the presence of:

1 Hair dryers and electric blankets, which can cause electromagnetic interference
2 Electric toothbrushes, which can cause microshock to occur
3 Electrical items that have strong electric currents or magnetic fields
4 Electrical items, such as a personal computer, which can cause failure to pace

**Answer: 3**

*Rationale:* A pacemaker is shielded from interference from most electrical devices. Radio, TV, electric blankets, toaster, microwave ovens, heating pads, and hair dryers are considered to be safe. Devices to be forewarned about include those with a strong electric current or magnetic field, such as antitheft devices in stores, metal detectors used in airports, and radiation therapy (if applicable and which might require relocation of the pacemaker).

*Test-Taking Strategy:* Use the process of elimination. Note that option 3 is the most global option addressing items with strong electric currents or magnetic fields. Review home care measures for the client with a pacemaker if you had difficulty with this question.

*Level of Cognitive Ability:* Application
*Client Needs:* Safe, Effective Care Environment
*Integrated Concept/Process:* Nursing Process/Assessment
*Content Area:* Adult Health/Cardiovascular

*Reference*
Black, J., Hawks, J., & Keene, A. (2001). *Medical-surgical nursing: Clinical management for positive outcomes* (6th ed.). Philadelphia: W.B. Saunders, p. 1569.

---

**6.** A client with low back pain asks a nurse which type of exercise will best strengthen the lower back muscles. The nurse tells the client to participate in which most beneficial exercise?

1 Tennis
2 Diving
3 Canoeing
4 Swimming

**Answer: 4**

*Rationale:* Walking and swimming are very beneficial in strengthening back muscles for the client with low back pain. The other options involve twisting and pulling of the back muscles, which is not helpful to the client experiencing back pain.

*Test-Taking Strategy:* Use the process of elimination. Recalling that low back pain is aggravated by any activity that twists or turns the spine, evaluate each of the options according to this guideline. This will enable you to eliminate options 1, 2, and 3. Review home care measures for the client with low back pain if you had difficulty with this question.

*Level of Cognitive Ability:* Application
*Client Needs:* Health Promotion and Maintenance
*Integrated Concept/Process:* Teaching/Learning
*Content Area:* Adult Health/Neurological

*Reference*
Monahan, F., & Neighbors, M. (1998). *Medical-surgical nursing: Foundations for clinical practice* (2nd ed.). Philadelphia: W.B Saunders, p. 911.

**7.** A nurse is caring for a child with a diagnosis of Kawasaki disease. The mother of the child asks the nurse about the disorder. The nurse bases the response on which of the following appropriate descriptions of this disorder?
1    It is an acquired cell-mediated immunodeficiency disorder
2    It is an inflammatory autoimmune disease that affects the connective tissue of the heart, joints, and subcutaneous tissues
3    It is a chronic multisystem autoimmune disease characterized by the inflammation of connective tissue
4    Is also called mucocutaneous lymph node syndrome and is a febrile, generalized vasculitis of unknown cause

**Answer: 4**
*Rationale:* Kawasaki disease, also called mucocutaneous lymph node syndrome, is a febrile generalized vasculitis of unknown etiological factors. Option 1 describes human immunodeficiency virus (HIV) infection. Option 2 describes rheumatic fever. Option 3 describes systemic lupus erythematosus.

*Test-Taking Strategy:* Knowledge regarding the description of Kawasaki disease is required to answer this question. If you are unfamiliar with this disorder, review this content.

*Level of Cognitive Ability:* Application
*Client Needs:* Physiological Integrity
*Integrated Concept/Process:* Teaching/Learning
*Content Area:* Child Health

*Reference*
Wong, D. (1999). *Whaley & Wong's Nursing care of infants and children* (6th ed.). St. Louis: Mosby, p. 1631.

**8.** A nurse is preparing to teach the parents of a child with anemia about the dietary sources of iron that are easy for the body to absorb. Which of the following food items would the nurse include in the teaching plan?
1    Cereals
2    Poultry
3    Fruits
4    Vegetables

**Answer: 2**
*Rationale:* Dietary sources of iron that are easy for the body to absorb include meat, poultry, and fish. Vegetables, fruits, cereals and breads are also dietary sources of iron but they are harder for the body to absorb.

*Test-Taking Strategy:* Focus on the issue: food sources that are high in iron and easy to absorb. Options 3 and 4 are similar and should be eliminated first. From the remaining options, recalling that meat, fish, and poultry items are high in iron will assist in eliminating option 1. Review the food items high in iron if you had difficulty with this question.

*Level of Cognitive Ability:* Application
*Client Needs:* Health Promotion and Maintenance
*Integrated Concept/Process:* Teaching/Learning
*Content Area:* Child Health

*Reference*
Wong, D. (1999). *Whaley & Wong's Nursing care of infants and children* (6th ed.). St. Louis: Mosby, p. 1665.

**9.** A nurse is caring for a child with patent ductus arteriosus. The nurse reviews the child's assessment data, knowing that which of the following is characteristic of this disorder?

**1** It involves an opening between the two atria

**2** It involves an opening between the two ventricles

**3** It produces abnormalities in the atrial septum

**4** It involves an artery that connects the aorta and the pulmonary artery during fetal life

**Answer: 4**

*Rationale:* Patent ductus arteriosus is described as an artery that connects the aorta and the pulmonary artery during fetal life. It generally closes spontaneously within a few hours to several days after birth. It allows abnormal blood flow from the high-pressure aorta to the low-pressure pulmonary artery, resulting in a left-to-right shunt. Options 1, 2, and 3 are not characteristics of this cardiac defect.

*Test-Taking Strategy:* Knowledge regarding the characteristics associated with patent ductus arteriosus is required to answer this question. If you are unfamiliar with this cardiac defect, review this content.

*Level of Cognitive Ability:* Analysis
*Client Needs:* Physiological Integrity
*Integrated Concept/Process:* Nursing Process/Analysis
*Content Area:* Child Health

*Reference*
Wong, D. (1999). *Whaley & Wong's Nursing care of infants and children* (6th ed.). St. Louis: Mosby, p. 452.

---

**10.** A nurse is caring for a client who has returned to the physician's office for follow-up following a parathyroidectomy with autotransplantation of some parathyroid tissue into the forearm. The client has been taking oral calcium and vitamin D supplements since discharge 2 weeks ago. Which statement by the client indicates a good understanding of the medical management following this type of surgical procedure?

**1** "Well, I guess the transplant isn't working because my calcium levels are still low."

**2** "The thought of taking these pills for the rest of my life makes me shudder!"

**3** "I can't wait for the transplant to start working. I'm tired of taking all these pills!"

**4** "Do you think I'll always have to take these pills?"

**Answer: 3**

*Rationale:* In autotransplantation of parathyroid tissue, the transplant takes some time to mature. Oral calcium and vitamin D supplements must be taken to prevent hypoparathyroidism, until the transplant matures and becomes an active endocrine gland.

*Test-Taking Strategy:* Use the process of elimination. Options 2 and 4 can be eliminated first because they are similar and both seem to negate the purpose of transplants, that being gaining function of the organ. From the remaining options, eliminate option 1 because the question does not address low calcium levels. If you had difficulty with this question, review the purpose of parathyroid transplant surgery.

*Level of Cognitive Ability:* Analysis
*Client Needs:* Health Promotion and Maintenance
*Integrated Concept/Process:* Teaching/Learning
*Content Area:* Adult Health/Endocrine

*Reference*
Black, J., Hawks, J., & Keene, A. (2001). *Medical-surgical nursing: Clinical management for positive outcomes* (6th ed.). Philadelphia: W.B. Saunders, p. 1113.

**11.** Desmopressin acetate (DDAVP) is prescribed via intranasal route for a child with von Willebrand's disease. The nurse instructs the parents regarding the administration of this medication. Which statement by the parents indicates a need for further instructions?
  1 "We need to restrict our child's fluid intake."
  2 "We need to refrigerate the DDAVP."
  3 "Nausea and abdominal cramps can occur as a side effect of the medication."
  4 "Headache and drowsiness may be a sign of water intoxication that can occur with the medication."

**Answer: 1**
*Rationale:* The parents should be instructed to monitor intake and output and to avoid overhydration, but fluids should not be restricted. The medication should be refrigerated, but freezing should be avoided. Side effects of the medication include facial flushing, nasal congestion, increased blood pressure, nausea, abdominal cramps, decreased urination, and vulval pain. Signs and symptoms of water intoxication include headache, drowsiness and confusion, weight gain, seizures, and coma.

*Test-Taking Strategy:* Focus on the issue: *a need for further instructions*. Noting the word *restrict* in option 1 will direct you to this option. If you are unfamiliar with this medication, review its action, use, and side effects.

*Level of Cognitive Ability:* Analysis
*Client Needs:* Health Promotion and Maintenance
*Integrated Concept/Process:* Teaching/Learning
*Content Area:* Child Health

*Reference*
Bowden, V., Dickey, S., & Greenberg, C. (1998). *Children and their families: The continuum of care.* Philadelphia: W.B. Saunders, p. 1555.

**12.** A child is brought to the emergency department after being bitten in the arm by a neighborhood dog. The nurse performs an initial assessment, cleanses the wound as prescribed, and continues to perform a thorough assessment on the child. Which of the following is the priority question for the nurse to ask the mother of the child?
  1 "Did the dog have rabies?"
  2 "Are the child's immunizations up-to-date?"
  3 "How old is the dog?"
  4 "Did the dog have all of its recommended shots?"

**Answer: 2**
*Rationale:* When a bite occurs, the injury site of the bite should be cleansed carefully, and the child should be given tetanus prophylaxis if immunizations are not up-to-date. Option 2 is the priority consideration. Options 1, 3, and 4 identify information that may have to be obtained, but are not the priority questions, and the mother may not have the answers to these questions.

*Test-Taking Strategy:* Use the process of elimination and note the key word *priority*. Option 2 is the only option that focuses on the needs of the child. If you are unfamiliar with the assessment and care of a child who receives a dog bite, review this content.

*Level of Cognitive Ability:* Analysis
*Client Needs:* Health Promotion and Maintenance
*Integrated Concept/Process:* Nursing Process/Assessment
*Content Area:* Child Health

*Reference*
Wong, D. (1999). *Whaley & Wong's Nursing care of infants and children* (6th ed.). St. Louis: Mosby, p. 860.

**13.** A nurse is providing instructions to the mother of a child who had a myringotomy with insertion of tympanostomy tubes. The nurse tells the mother that if the tubes fall out:
1   It is important to replace the tubes immediately so that the surgical opening does not close
2   To bring the child to the emergency department immediately
3   It is not an emergency, but it is best to call the health care clinic
4   Clean the tubes with half-strength hydrogen peroxide for 30 minutes and then replace them into the child's ears

**Answer: 3**
*Rationale:* The mother should be assured that if the tympanostomy tubes fall out, it is not an emergency, but it is best that the physician or health care clinic be notified. The size and appearance of the tympanostomy tubes should be described to the mother following surgery so she will be familiar with their appearance. Options 1, 2, and 4 are incorrect.

*Test-Taking Strategy:* Use the process of elimination. Option 2 is eliminated first because it will cause concern in the mother. Next eliminate options 1 and 4 because they are similar and relate to replacing the tubes. Review home care instructions following this procedure if you had difficulty with this question.

*Level of Cognitive Ability:* Application
*Client Needs:* Physiological Integrity
*Integrated Concept/Process:* Teaching/Learning
*Content Area:* Child Health

*Reference*
Wong, D. (1999). *Whaley & Wong's Nursing care of infants and children* (6th ed.). St. Louis: Mosby, p. 1472.

**14.** A mother calls the health care clinic and tells a nurse that her child has developed a bloody nose. The nurse instructs the mother to do which of the following?
1   Maintain the child in a sitting position with the head tilted backward
2   Pinch the nostrils for 5 minutes then recheck for bleeding
3   Lay the child down with a pillow tucked under the neck and stay with the child to keep the child calm
4   Have the child sit with the head tilted forward and hold pressure on the soft part of the nose for 10 minutes

**Answer: 4**
*Rationale:* The child should be positioned erect, sitting with the head tilted forward to avoid blood dripping posteriorly to the pharynx. The soft part of the nose should be tightly pinched against the center wall for 10 minutes and the mother should be instructed that this pinch should be timed by a clock, not estimated. The mother should be told not to release pressure for 10 minutes. The child is encouraged to remain calm and quiet and to breathe through the mouth.

*Test-Taking Strategy:* Use the process of elimination, focusing on the issue, controlling a bloody nose. Attempt to visualize the positions presented in the options to direct you to option 4. If you had difficulty with the question, review the interventions used when epistaxis occurs.

*Level of Cognitive Ability:* Application
*Client Needs:* Physiological Integrity
*Integrated Concept/Process:* Nursing Process/Implementation
*Content Area:* Child Health

*Reference*
Bowden, V., Dickey, S., & Greenberg, C. (1998). *Children and their families: The continuum of care.* Philadelphia: W.B. Saunders, p. 2082.

**15.** A nurse is assessing a child admitted to the hospital with a diagnosis of rheumatic fever. The child is accompanied by the mother. The initial nursing question that the nurse would ask during assessment is which of the following?
   **1** "Has the child had difficulty urinating?"
   **2** "Has any family member had a sore throat within the past few weeks?"
   **3** "Has any family member had a gastrointestinal disorder in the past few weeks?"
   **4** "Has the child been exposed to anyone with chickenpox?"

**Answer: 2**
*Rationale:* Rheumatic fever characteristically presents 2 to 6 weeks after an untreated or partially treated group A beta-hemolytic streptococcal infection of the respiratory tract. Initially, the nurse determines whether any family member has had a sore throat or unexplained fever within the past few weeks. Options 1, 3, and 4 are unrelated to the assessment findings of rheumatic fever.

*Test-Taking Strategy:* Use the process of elimination. Recalling that rheumatic fever characteristically presents 2 to 6 weeks following a streptococcal infection of the respiratory tract will direct you to the correct option. If you are unfamiliar with the etiological factors and the pathophysiology associated with this disorder, review this content.

*Level of Cognitive Ability:* Application
*Client Needs:* Physiological Integrity
*Integrated Concept/Process:* Nursing Process/Assessment
*Content Area:* Child Health

**Reference**
Wong, D. (1999). *Whaley & Wong's Nursing care of infants and children* (6th ed.). St. Louis: Mosby, p. 1629.

**16.** The parents of a child with mumps express concern that their child will develop orchitis as a result of having mumps. The parents ask the nurse about the complication and about the signs that may indicate this complication. The nurse responds knowing that which of the following is not a sign of this complication?
   **1** Abrupt onset of pain
   **2** Headache and vomiting
   **3** Fever and chills
   **4** Difficulty urinating

**Answer: 4**
*Rationale:* Unilateral orchitis occurs more frequently than bilateral orchitis. About one week after the appearance of parotitis, there is an abrupt onset of testicular pain, tenderness, fever, chills, headache, and vomiting. The affected testicle becomes red, swollen, and tender. Atrophy resulting in sterility occurs only in a small number of cases. Difficulty urinating is not a sign of this complication.

*Test-Taking Strategy:* Use the process of elimination. Note the key word *not* in the stem of the question. Knowledge regarding the signs associated with orchitis is required to answer this question. If you had difficulty with this question, review the characteristics of orchitis.

*Level of Cognitive Ability:* Application
*Client Needs:* Health Promotion and Maintenance
*Integrated Concept/Process:* Teaching/Learning
*Content Area:* Child Health

**Reference**
Ball, J., & Bindler, R. (1999). *Pediatric nursing: Caring for children* (2nd ed.). Stamford, Conn.: Appleton & Lange, p. 390.

**17.** A maternity nurse is teaching a pregnant woman about the physiological effects and hormone changes that occur in pregnancy. The woman asks the nurse about the purpose of estrogen. The nurse plans to base the response on which of the following purposes of this hormone?

1   It maintains the uterine lining for implantation
2   It stimulates metabolism of glucose and converts the glucose to fat
3   It prevents the involution of the corpus luteum and maintains the production of progesterone until the placenta is formed
4   It stimulates uterine development to provide an environment for the fetus, and stimulates the breasts to prepare for lactation

**Answer: 4**

*Rationale:* Estrogen stimulates uterine development to provide an environment for the fetus, and stimulates the breasts to prepare for lactation. Progesterone maintains the uterine lining for implantation and relaxes all smooth muscle. Human placental lactogen stimulates the metabolism of glucose and converts the glucose to fat. Human chorionic gonadotropin prevents involution of the corpus luteum and maintains the production of progesterone until the placenta is formed.

*Test-Taking Strategy:* Use the process of elimination. Knowledge regarding the functions of various hormones related to pregnancy is required to answer this question. If you had difficulty with this question or are unfamiliar with these hormones, review this content.

*Level of Cognitive Ability:* Application
*Client Needs:* Physiological Integrity
*Integrated Concept/Process:* Teaching/Learning
*Content Area:* Maternity

*Reference*
Olds, S., London. M., & Ladewig, P. (2000). *Maternal-newborn nursing: A family and community-based approach* (6th ed.). Upper Saddle River, N.J.: Prentice-Hall Health, p. 233.

---

**18.** A nurse has explained the reason that the physician has chosen laser surgery to treat a client's cervical cancer. Which statement, if made by the client, indicates a correct understanding?

1   "I have too much cancer to be removed with surgery."
2   "I want to be asleep during my procedure."
3   "The doctor is able to see all the edges of my cancer clearly."
4   "I am young and the laser keeps cervical tissue from regrowing."

**Answer: 3**

*Rationale:* Laser therapy is performed in an outpatient setting and is used when all boundaries of the lesion are visible. Option 1 is not the reason for performing laser surgery. Laser surgery is painless and the client would not receive general anesthesia. Laser therapy does not prevent regrowth.

*Test-Taking Strategy:* Use the process of elimination. Thinking about the procedure involved in laser surgery will direct you to option 3. If you had difficulty with this question, review this type of treatment for cervical cancer.

*Level of Cognitive Ability:* Analysis
*Client Needs:* Physiological Integrity
*Integrated Concept/Process:* Teaching/Learning
*Content Area:* Adult Health/Oncology

*Reference*
Smeltzer, S., & Bare, B. (2000). *Brunner & Suddarth's Textbook of medical-surgical nursing* (9th ed.). Philadelphia: Lippincott Williams & Wilkins, p. 273.

**19.** A 9-year-old male child is newly diagnosed with type 1 diabetes mellitus. The nurse is planning for home care with the child and his family and determines that an age-appropriate activity for this child for health maintenance is:

1   Independently self-administering insulin

2   Making independent decisions regarding sliding scale coverage of insulin

3   Having an adult assist in self-administration of insulin and glucose monitoring

4   Administering insulin drawn up by an adult

**Answer: 1**

*Rationale:* School-aged children have the cognitive and motor skills to independently administer insulin with adult supervision. Developmentally, they do not yet have the maturity to make situational decisions without adult validation. Options 3 and 4 suppress the maximum level of independence appropriate to the level of this child.

*Test-Taking Strategy:* Use the process of elimination. Focusing on the age of the child will assist in eliminating options 3 and 4. From the remaining options, recalling that in this age group, decision making is a cognitive skill that develops later than motor skills will direct you to option 1. If you had difficulty with this question, review growth and development of a 9-year-old child.

*Level of Cognitive Ability:* Analysis
*Client Needs:* Health Promotion and Maintenance
*Integrated Concept/Process:* Self-Care
*Content Area:* Child Health

*Reference*
Wong, D. (1999). *Whaley & Wong's Nursing care of infants and children* (6th ed.). St. Louis: Mosby, p. 781.

---

**20.** A nursing instructor is reviewing a plan of care formulated by a nursing student who is working in the health care clinic and is preparing to instruct a pregnant woman to perform Kegel exercises. The nursing instructor asks the student the purpose of the Kegel exercises. Which response by the student indicates an understanding of the purpose of these types of exercises?

1   "The exercises will help to strengthen the pelvic floor in preparation for delivery."

2   "The exercises will help to prevent urinary tract infections."

3   "The exercises will help reduce backache."

4   "The exercises will help prevent ankle edema."

**Answer: 1**

*Rationale:* Kegel exercises will assist to strengthen the pelvic floor (pubococcygeal muscle). Pelvic tilt exercises will help reduce backaches. Instructing a client to drink 8 oz of fluid six times a day will help prevent urinary tract infections. Leg elevation will assist in preventing ankle edema.

*Test-Taking Strategy:* Focus on the issue of the question and use the process of elimination. Remember that Kegel exercises will help to strengthen the pelvic floor muscles. If you had difficulty with this question, review the purpose of Kegel exercises.

*Level of Cognitive Ability:* Analysis
*Client Needs:* Health Promotion and Maintenance
*Integrated Concept/Process:* Teaching/Learning
*Content Area:* Maternity

*Reference*
Sherwen, L., Scoloveno, M.A., & Weingarten, C. (1999). *Maternity nursing: Care of the childbearing family* (3rd ed.). Stamford, Conn.: Appleton & Lange, p. 244.

**21.** The physician's order reads: piperacillin sodium (Pipracil), 650 mg IV every 6 hours. The medication label reads: 2 g and reconstitute with 5 mL of bacteriostatic water. The nurse prepares to draw up how many mL to administer one dose?

  **1**    0.62 mL
  **2**    1.0 mL
  **3**    1.62 mL
  **4**    5.0 mL

**Answer: 3**

*Rationale:* Convert 2 g to milligrams. In the metric system, to convert larger to smaller, multiply by 1000 or move the decimal three places to the right. Therefore 2 g = 2000 mg. The formula is:

$$\frac{\text{Desired}}{\text{Available}} \times \text{Volume} = \text{Milliliters per dose}$$

$$\frac{650 \text{ mg}}{2000 \text{ mg}} \times 5.0 \text{ mL} = 1.625 \text{ mL} = 1.62 \text{ mL}$$

*Test-Taking Strategy:* Identify the key components of the question and what the question is asking. In this case, the question asks for the milliliters per dose. Convert grams to milligrams first. Next, use the formula to determine the correct dose, knowing that 2000 mg = 5.0 mL.

*Level of Cognitive Ability:* Application
*Client Needs:* Physiological Integrity
*Integrated Concept/Process:* Nursing Process/Planning
*Content Area:* Fundamental Skills

*Reference*
Kee, J., & Marshall, S. (2000). *Clinical calculations: With applications to general and specialty areas* (4th ed.). Philadelphia: W.B. Saunders, p. 78.

---

**22.** A child with sickle cell disease is admitted to the hospital for treatment of vaso-occlusive pain crisis. A nursing student is assigned to care for the child and the nursing instructor reviews the plan of care with the student. Which intervention, if included in the plan of care, indicates a need for further research by the student?

  **1**    IV fluids for rehydration
  **2**    Meperidine hydrochloride (Demerol) for pain management
  **3**    Oxygen
  **4**    Increased fluid intake

**Answer: 2**

*Rationale:* Management of the severe pain that occurs with vaso-occlusive crisis includes the use of strong narcotic analgesics, such as morphine sulfate and hydromorphone hydrochloride (Dilaudid). Meperidine hydrochloride is contraindicated because of its side effects and increased risk of seizures. Oxygen is administered to increase tissue perfusion. Fluids are necessary to promote hydration.

*Test-Taking Strategy:* Use the process of elimination. Note the key words *need for further research*. Eliminate options 1 and 4 first knowing that hydration is necessary, and because these options are similar. From the remaining options, use the ABCs, airway, breathing, and circulation, to direct you to the correct option. Review care of a client with sickle cell disease if you had difficulty with this question.

*Level of Cognitive Ability:* Analysis
*Client Needs:* Physiological Integrity
*Integrated Concept/Process:* Teaching/Learning
*Content Area:* Child Health

*Reference*
Bowden, V., Dickey, S., & Greenberg, C. (1998). *Children and their families: the continuum of care.* Philadelphia: W.B. Saunders, p. 1578.

**23.** A newborn infant receives the first dose of hepatitis B vaccine within 12 hours of birth. The nurse instructs the mother regarding the immunization schedule for this vaccine and tells the mother that the second vaccine is administered at:

1. 1 to 2 months of age, and then 4 months after the initial dose
2. 6 months of age, and then 8 months after the initial dose
3. 8 months of age, and then 1 year after the initial dose
4. 3 years of age, and then during the adolescent years

**Answer: 1**

*Rationale:* The vaccination schedule for an infant whose mother tests negative for hepatitis B consists of a series of three immunizations given at 0 months (birth), 1 to 2 months of age, and then 4 months after the initial dose. An infant whose mother tests positive receives human B immune globulin along with the first dose of the hepatitis vaccine within 12 hours of birth.

*Test-Taking Strategy:* Knowledge regarding the immunization schedule for hepatitis B vaccine is required to answer this question. Review this schedule if you are unfamiliar with it.

*Level of Cognitive Ability:* Application
*Client Needs:* Health Promotion and Maintenance
*Integrated Concept/Process:* Teaching/Learning
*Content Area:* Child Health

*Reference*
Lowdermilk, D., Perry, S., & Bobak, I. (2000). *Maternity & women's health care* (7th ed.). St. Louis: Mosby, p. 742.

---

**24.** A nurse assesses the client with a diagnosis of thyroid storm. Which of the following classic signs and symptoms associated with thyroid storm would indicate the need for immediate nursing intervention?

1. Fever, tachycardia, and systolic hypertension
2. Polyuria, nausea, and severe headaches
3. Profuse diaphoresis, flushing, and constipation
4. Hypotension, translucent skin, and obesity

**Answer: 1**

*Rationale:* The excessive amounts of thyroid hormone cause a rapid increase in the metabolic rate, thereby causing the classic signs and symptoms of thyroid storm such as fever, tachycardia, and hypertension. When these signs present themselves, the nurse must take quick action to prevent deterioration of the client's health since death can ensue. Priority interventions include maintaining a patent airway and stabilizing the hemodynamic status. Options 2, 3, and 4 do not indicate the need for immediate nursing intervention.

*Test-Taking Strategy:* Use the principles associated with prioritizing when answering this question. Tachycardia, hypertension, and a fever indicate hemodynamic instability and take precedence over the signs and symptoms identified in options 2, 3, and 4. Additionally, option 1 is the only option that identifies all the signs and symptoms of thyroid storm. If you had difficulty with this question, review thyroid storm.

*Level of Cognitive Ability:* Analysis
*Client Needs:* Physiological Integrity
*Integrated Concept/Process:* Nursing Process/Assessment
*Content Area:* Adult Health/Endocrine

*Reference*
Black, J., Hawks, J., & Keene, A. (2001). *Medical-surgical nursing: Clinical management for positive outcomes* (6th ed.). Philadelphia: W.B. Saunders, p. 1100.

**25.** A client is hospitalized for ingesting an overdose of acetaminophen (Tylenol). The nurse prepares to administer which specific antidote for this medication overdose?

1　Protamine sulfate
2　Naloxone hydrochloride (Narcan)
3　Acetylcysteine (Mucomyst)
4　Vitamin K (AquaMephyton)

**Answer: 3**
*Rationale:* Acetylcysteine restores sulfhydryl groups that are depleted by acetaminophen metabolism. Vitamin K is the antidote for warfarin sodium (Coumadin). Naloxone hydrochloride reverses respiratory depression. Protamine sulfate is the antidote for heparin.

*Test-Taking Strategy:* Use the process of elimination. Recalling the specific antidotes for both heparin and warfarin sodium will assist in eliminating options 1 and 4. Next, recalling that naloxone hydrochloride reverses respiratory depression will assist in eliminating option 2. Review these antidotes if you had difficulty with this question.

*Level of Cognitive Ability:* Analysis
*Client Needs:* Physiological Integrity
*Integrated Concept/Process:* Nursing Process/Planning
*Content Area:* Pharmacology

*Reference*
Hodgson, B., & Kizior, R. (2001). *Saunders Nursing drug handbook 2001.* Philadelphia: W.B. Saunders, p. 6.

**26.** A nurse is caring for a male client at risk for suicide. Which of the following behaviors is most indicative that the client may be contemplating suicide?

1　The client tells the nurse that he plans to use his shoelaces to strangle himself
2　The client cries for long periods of time
3　The client spends long periods of time alone
4　The client reports sleep disturbances

**Answer: 1**
*Rationale:* If a client displays a suicidal ideation and is able to share a plan, the client should be taken very seriously, and suicide precautions should be implemented. Option 1 clearly states such a plan. Options 2, 3 and 4 are indicative of depression but are not as definitive as option 1 in regard to suicide.

*Test-Taking Strategy:* Note the key words *most indicative* and focus on the issue: suicide. Recalling that a cardinal sign of suicidal ideation is the formulation of a specific suicidal plan will direct you to option 1. If you had difficulty with this question, review assessment of the client at risk for suicide.

*Level of Cognitive Ability:* Analysis
*Client Needs:* Physiological Integrity
*Integrated Concept/Process:* Nursing Process/Analysis
*Content Area:* Mental Health

*Reference*
Stuart, G.W., & Laraia, M.T. (1998). *Principles and practice of psychiatric nursing* (6th ed.). St. Louis: Mosby, p. 354.

**27.** A physical assessment is performed on a suicidal client on admission to the inpatient unit. The nurse understands that this is an important part of the admission process because it provides the nurse with information regarding:

1　The presence of abnormalities
2　Evidence of physical self-harm
3　Existing medical problems
4　Baseline data

**Answer: 2**
*Rationale:* The physical assessment of a suicidal client should be thorough and should focus on the evidence of self-harm or the formulation of a plan for the suicide attempt. Although all of the options are correct, option 2 is most appropriate in the context of the suicidal client. Clients with a history of self-harm are greater suicide risks.

*Test-Taking Strategy:* Use the process of elimination and focus on the client's diagnosis. Remember, assessing for physical evidence of harm is an important component of the assessment process of a suicidal client. If you had difficulty with this question, review the characteristics of the client at risk for suicide.

*Level of Cognitive Ability:* Application
*Client Needs:* Physiological Integrity
*Integrated Concept/Process:* Nursing Process/Assessment
*Content Area:* Mental Health

*Reference*
Stuart, G.W., & Laraia, M.T. (1998). *Principles and practice of psychiatric nursing* (6th ed.). St. Louis: Mosby, p. 354.

---

**28.** A client is admitted to the hospital for a thyroidectomy. While preparing the client for surgery, the nurse assesses the client for any psychosocial problems that may cause preoperative anxiety knowing that a realistic source of anxiety is fear of:
1 Developing gynecomastia and hirsutism postoperatively
2 Sexual dysfunction and infertility
3 Imposed dietary restrictions post discharge
4 Changes in body image secondary to the location of the incision

**Answer: 4**
*Rationale:* Because the incision is in the neck area, the client may be fearful of having a large scar postoperatively. Having all or part of the thyroid gland removed will not cause the client to experience gynecomastia or hirsutism. Sexual dysfunction and infertility could possibly occur if the entire thyroid gland was removed and if the client was not placed on thyroid replacement medications. The client will not have specific dietary restrictions after discharge.

*Test-Taking Strategy:* Use the process of elimination, focusing on the surgical procedure. Recalling the location of the thyroid gland will direct you to option 4. Review the psychosocial concerns of the client following thyroidectomy if you had difficulty with this question.

*Level of Cognitive Ability:* Analysis
*Client Needs:* Psychosocial Integrity
*Integrated Concept/Process:* Nursing Process/Assessment
*Content Area:* Adult Health/Endocrine

*Reference*
Black, J., Hawks, J., & Keene, A. (2001). *Medical-surgical nursing: Clinical management for positive outcomes* (6th ed.). Philadelphia: W.B. Saunders, p. 1105.

---

**29.** A physician prescribes 10% Intralipids fat emulsion intravenously for a client. Before initiating the solution, the nurse should assess which of the following?
1 The client's blood pressure
2 Hypersensitivity to eggs
3 Fingerstick blood glucose level
4 History of seizures

**Answer: 2**
*Rationale:* Before administering any medication, the nurse must assess for allergy or hypersensitivity to substances used in producing the medication. Fat emulsions such as Intralipids contain an emulsifying agent obtained from egg yolks. Clients sensitive to eggs are at risk for developing hypersensitivity reactions.

*Test-Taking Strategy:* Specific knowledge regarding the administration of Intralipids is required to answer this question. If you had difficulty with this question, review the content related to the administration of Intralipids.

*Level of Cognitive Ability:* Application
*Client Needs:* Physiological Integrity
*Integrated Concept/Process:* Nursing Process/Assessment
*Content Area:* Fundamental Skills

*Reference*
Salerno, E. (1999). *Pharmacology for health professionals.* St. Louis: Mosby, p. 1196.

---

**30.** A client is admitted to the hospital with angina pectoris and is experiencing no difficulty at this time. The nurse reviews the electrocardiogram (ECG) rhythm strip and finds that the P-R interval is 0.16 seconds. The nurse determines that this rhythm indicates:

1   First degree AV block
2   An abnormal finding
3   An impending reinfarction
4   A normal finding

**Answer: 4**
*Rationale:* The P-R interval represents the time it takes for the cardiac impulse to spread from the atria to the ventricles. The P-R interval range is 0.12 to 0.20 seconds.

*Test-Taking Strategy:* Use the process of elimination. Eliminate options 1, 2, and 3 because they are similar and all indicate an abnormal finding. Review basic ECG findings if you had difficulty with this question.

*Level of Cognitive Ability:* Analysis
*Client Needs:* Physiological Integrity
*Integrated Concept/Process:* Nursing Process/Analysis
*Content Area:* Adult Health/Cardiovascular

*Reference*
Black, J., Hawks, J., & Keene, A. (2001). *Medical-surgical nursing: Clinical management for positive outcomes* (6th ed.). Philadelphia: W.B. Saunders, p. 1466.

---

**31.** A nurse administers 30 units of NPH insulin at 7:00 A.M. to a client with a blood glucose level of 200 mg/dL. The nurse monitors the client for a hypoglycemic reaction, knowing that NPH insulin peaks in how many hours following administration?

1   2 hours
2   3 to 4 hours
3   4 to 12 hours
4   7 to 15 hours

**Answer: 3**
*Rationale:* NPH is an intermediate-acting insulin with an onset of action in 3 to 4 hours, a peak time in 4 to 12 hours, and a duration time of 18 to 28 hours.

*Test-Taking Strategy:* Knowledge of the onset, peak, and duration of NPH insulin is required. Recalling that NPH is an intermediate-acting insulin will direct you to option 3. If you had difficulty with this question, review the various types of insulin.

*Level of Cognitive Ability:* Application
*Client Needs:* Physiological Integrity
*Integrated Concept/Process:* Nursing Process/Assessment
*Content Area:* Pharmacology

*Reference*
Hodgson, B., & Kizior, R. (2001). *Saunders Nursing drug handbook 2001.* Philadelphia: W.B. Saunders, p. 531.

**32.** A client is brought to the emergency department following a severe burn caused by a fire at home. The burns are extensive covering greater than 25% of the total body surface area (TBSA). The nurse reviews the laboratory results drawn on the client and would most likely expect to note which of the following?

1   White blood cell (WBC) count 6000/μL
2   Hematocrit 65%
3   Albumin 4.0 g/dL
4   Sodium 140 mEq/L

**Answer: 2**

*Rationale:* Extensive burns covering greater than 25% of the TBSA result in generalized body edema in both burned and nonburned tissues and a decrease in circulating intravascular blood volume. Hematocrit levels elevate in the first 24 hours after injury as a result of hemoconcentration from the loss of intravascular fluid. The normal WBC count is 5000 to 10,000/μL. The normal sodium level is 135 to145 mEq/L. The normal albumin is 3.4 to 5 g/dL. The normal hematocrit is 40% to 54% in the male and 38% to 47% in the female.

*Test-Taking Strategy:* Use the process of elimination and knowledge regarding physiological alterations and fluid and electrolyte balance during the first 24 hours after injury of a burn client. Note that the only abnormal laboratory value is option 2, the hematocrit level. If you had difficulty with this question, review normal laboratory values and the immediate postinjury period of burns.

*Level of Cognitive Ability:* Analysis
*Client Needs:* Physiological Integrity
*Integrated Concept/Process:* Nursing Process/Analysis
*Content Area:* Adult Health/Integumentary

*Reference*
Black, J., Hawks, J., & Keene, A. (2001). *Medical-surgical nursing: Clinical management for positive outcomes* (6th ed.). Philadelphia: W.B. Saunders, p. 1344.

**33.** A home health nurse visits an elderly client who has osteoarthritis. Indomethacin (Indocin) has been prescribed for the client and the nurse teaches the client about the medication. Which statement by the client indicates that further teaching is necessary?

1   "I can take a pill whenever I need to for pain."
2   "I need to call the doctor if I notice a rash."
3   "I'll balance rest periods and moderate activity."
4   "I'll watch for any swollen feet or fingers or any stomach distress."

**Answer: 1**

*Rationale:* In osteoarthritis, a noninflammatory disorder of the movable joints, pain is aggravated by joint motion, weight-bearing, and weather changes. The disease course is described as slow and progressive, with no periods of remission or exacerbation. Rest and exercise should be balanced. When pain occurs, the client will usually limit movement. Medications such as indomethacin may be prescribed to alleviate pain but should be administered on a scheduled time frame, not a PRN schedule. A rash should be reported, because it could indicate hypersensitivity to the medication. The client should be instructed to monitor for swelling and gastric distress, which can be caused by this medication.

*Test-Taking Strategy:* Use the process of elimination. Note the key words *further teaching is necessary.* Recalling the action and purpose of indomethacin will direct you to option 1. Review this medication if you had difficulty with this question.

*Level of Cognitive Ability:* Analysis
*Client Needs:* Health Promotion and Maintenance
*Integrated Concept/Process:* Teaching/Learning
*Content Area:* Pharmacology

*Reference*
Hodgson, B., & Kizior, R. (2001). *Saunders Nursing drug handbook 2001.* Philadelphia: W.B. Saunders, p. 528.

**34.** A nurse is teaching a community group about violence in the family. Which of the following statements by a group member would indicate a need for further instruction?
1  "Abusers usually have poor self-esteem."
2  "Abusers use fear and intimidation."
3  "Abusers are often jealous or self-centered."
4  "Abuse occurs mostly in low-income families."

**Answer: 4**
*Rationale:* Personal characteristics of abusers include low self-esteem, immaturity, dependence, insecurity, and jealousy. Abusers will often use fear and intimidation to the point where their victims will do anything just to avoid further abuse. The statement that abuse occurs more in low-income families is a myth.

*Test-Taking Strategy:* Note the key words, *need for further instruction.* Use knowledge regarding the characteristics related to family violence to direct you to option 4. If you had difficulty with this question, review the characteristics of an abuser and family violence.

*Level of Cognitive Ability:* Analysis
*Client Needs:* Psychosocial Integrity
*Integrated Concept/Process:* Teaching/Learning
*Content Area:* Mental Health

*Reference*
Fortinash, K., & Holoday-Worret, P. (2000). *Psychiatric mental health nursing* (2nd ed.). St. Louis: Mosby, p. 624.

**35.** A nurse is caring for a client with possible cholelithiasis who is being prepared for a cholangiogram. The nurse teaches the client about the procedure. Which client statement indicates that the client understands the purpose of this procedure?
1  "They are going to look at my gallbladder and ducts."
2  "This procedure will drain my gallbladder."
3  "My gallbladder will be irrigated."
4  "They will put medication in my gallbladder."

**Answer: 1**
*Rationale:* Intravenous cholangiography is for diagnostic purposes. The cholangiogram outlines both the gallbladder and the ducts, so gallstones that have moved into the ductal system can be detected. X-rays are used to visualize the biliary duct system after IV injection of a radiopaque dye.

*Test-Taking Strategy:* Use the process of elimination and recall the pathophysiology of cholelithiasis and the purpose of the cholangiogram. Note that options 2, 3, and 4 are similar because they involve some form of treatment. Option 1 involves assessment of the gallbladder. If you had difficulty with this question, review the purpose of this procedure.

*Level of Cognitive Ability:* Analysis
*Client Needs:* Physiological Integrity
*Integrated Concept/Process:* Teaching/Learning
*Content Area:* Adult Health/Gastrointestinal

*Reference*
Smeltzer, S., & Bare, B. (2000). *Brunner & Suddarth's Textbook of medical-surgical nursing* (9th ed.). Philadelphia: Lippincott Williams & Wilkins, p. 964.

**36.** A nursing instructor asks a nursing student about suicide and suicide intentions. The instructor determines that the student understands the concepts associated with this topic if the student makes which of the following statements?

1 "Suicide runs in the family, so there is nothing that health care personnel can do about it."
2 "Suicidal attempts are just attention-seeking behaviors."
3 "Many individuals who commit suicide have talked about their suicidal intentions to others."
4 "Only psychotic individuals commit suicide."

**Answer: 3**

*Rationale:* Most people who do commit suicide have given definite clues or warnings about their intentions. Suicide is not an inherited condition. A suicide attempt is not an attention-seeking behavior, and each act should be taken very seriously. The individual who is suicidal is not necessarily psychotic or even mentally ill. Options 1, 2, and 4 are considered myths regarding suicide.

*Test-Taking Strategy:* Use the process of elimination. Eliminate option 1 because of the statement "there is nothing that health care personnel can do about it." Eliminate option 2 because of the statement "just attention-seeking behaviors." Eliminate option 4 because of the word *only*. Review concepts related to suicide if you had difficulty with this question.

*Level of Cognitive Ability:* Analysis
*Client Needs:* Psychosocial Integrity
*Integrated Concept/Process:* Teaching/Learning
*Content Area:* Mental Health

*Reference*
Varcarolis, E. (1998). *Foundations of psychiatric mental health nursing* (3rd ed.). Philadelphia: W.B. Saunders, p. 729.

**37.** A hospitalized 19-year-old famous female pianist wanders in and out of other client rooms, taking their possessions while singing to herself and then giggling for no apparent reason. The nurse, recognizing the severe regression of the client and the difficulty with limit setting, implements which of the following actions?

1 Putting arms around the client, saying, "You're okay. You just need a hug."
2 Taking the client to seclusion until she cooperates with unit rules
3 Saying, "I can see you are very anxious today. Let's go and play the piano."
4 Taking her to the lounge and saying, "Sit here and behave yourself."

**Answer: 3**

*Rationale:* The use of a defense mechanism allows a person to avoid the painful experience of anxiety or to transform it into a more tolerable symptom, such as regression. Regression allows the threatened client to move backward developmentally to a stage in which more security is felt. The recognition of regression is a signal that the client feels anxious. Option 3 will help the client feel less anxious. Options 2 and 4 are restrictive and degrading. Option 1 does not address the client's anxiety.

*Test-Taking Strategy:* Use the process of elimination. Recall that because anxiety consumes energy, it should be redirected into a healthier task. Also, note the relationship between the word *pianist* in the question and the suggestion "Let's go and play the piano" in the correct option. Review defense mechanisms if you had difficulty with this question.

*Level of Cognitive Ability:* Application
*Client Needs:* Psychosocial Integrity
*Integrated Concept/Process:* Nursing Process/Implementation
*Content Area:* Mental Health

*Reference*
Varcarolis, E. (1998). *Foundations of psychiatric mental health nursing* (3rd ed.). Philadelphia: W.B. Saunders, p. 511.

**38.** A nurse is caring for a pregnant client who is positive for human immunodeficiency virus (HIV). To help prevent the transmission of HIV from the woman to her baby during the intrapartum period, the nurse plans to initiate measures to avoid:

1   Cesarean birth
2   Intrauterine pressure catheter insertion
3   Epidural anesthesia
4   Direct (internal) fetal heart rate monitoring

**Answer: 4**

*Rationale:* Health care professionals must use caution during the intrapartal period to reduce the risk of the transmission of HIV to the fetus. Any procedure that exposes blood or body fluids from the mother to the fetus should be avoided. Direct (internal) fetal monitoring is a procedure that may expose the fetus to maternal blood or body fluids and therefore should be avoided. Options 1, 2, and 3 are not measures that place the fetus at risk in the intrapartum period.

*Test-Taking Strategy:* Use the process of elimination and knowledge of how HIV is transmitted from the mother to the fetus. All the options address invasive procedures that may take place during the intrapartum period, but only option 4 is invasive with regard to the fetus. Recalling that transmission of HIV occurs primarily by the exchange of body fluids will direct you to option 4. Review this content area if you had difficulty with this question.

*Level of Cognitive Ability:* Application
*Client Needs:* Safe, Effective Care Environment
*Integrated Concept/Process:* Nursing Process/Implementation
*Content Area:* Maternity

*Reference*
Lowdermilk, D., Perry, S., & Bobak, I. (2000). *Maternity & women's health care* (7th ed.). St. Louis: Mosby, p. 1052.

**39.** During electroconvulsive therapy (ECT), the client is mechanically ventilated. The nurse assisting with this procedure knows that mechanical ventilation is necessary because:

1   Grand mal seizure activity depresses respiration
2   Muscle relaxants given to prevent injury during seizure activity depress respirations
3   Anesthesia is administered during the procedure
4   Decreased oxygen to the brain increases confusion and disorientation

**Answer: 2**

*Rationale:* A short-acting skeletal muscle relaxant such as succinylcholine (Anectine) is administered during this procedure to prevent injuries during the seizure. The client's lungs must be ventilated until the muscle relaxant is metabolized, usually within 2 to 3 minutes. Options 1, 3, and 4 do not address the issue of the question and the specific reason for mechanical ventilation.

*Test-Taking Strategy:* Use the process of elimination and focus on the issue. Recalling that a muscle relaxant is administered will direct you to option 2. If you are unfamiliar with the procedure for ECT, review this content.

*Level of Cognitive Ability:* Analysis
*Client Needs:* Physiological Integrity
*Integrated Concept/Process:* Nursing Process/Analysis
*Content Area:* Mental Health

*Reference*
Varcarolis, E. (1998). *Foundations of psychiatric mental health nursing* (3rd ed.). Philadelphia: W.B. Saunders, p. 578.

**40.** A client is in a coma of unknown cause, and the physician has written several orders for the client, including the need for intubation. Which of the following procedures would the nurse withhold until the client was properly intubated?
1   Gastric feeding
2   Fingerstick for blood glucose level
3   Urethral catheterization
4   Venipuncture for complete blood cell (CBC) count

**Answer: 1**
*Rationale:* Intubation should always precede gastric feeding to prevent pulmonary aspiration. All other options identify procedures that can be initiated before intubation of client.

*Test-Taking Strategy:* Use the process of elimination and the ABCs: airway, breathing, and circulation. Recalling that the comatose client is at risk for aspiration will direct you to option 1. Review care of a comatose client if you had difficulty with this question.

*Level of Cognitive Ability:* Application
*Client Needs:* Physiological Integrity
*Integrated Concept/Process:* Nursing Process/Implementation
*Content Area:* Adult Health/Neurological

*Reference*
Monahan, F., & Neighbors, M. (1998). *Medical-surgical nursing: Foundations for clinical practice* (2nd ed.). Philadelphia: W.B Saunders, p. 559.

**41.** A manic client is being placed in a seclusion room because of an episode of violent behavior. As the client is secluded, the nurse should:
1   Remain silent
2   Tell the client that he or she will be let out when he or she can behave
3   Ask the client to verbalize the reason why the seclusion is necessary
4   Inform the client that he or she is being secluded to help regain control of self

**Answer: 4**
*Rationale:* The client is removed to a nonstimulating environment as a result of behavior. Options 1, 2, and 3 are nontherapeutic. In addition, option 2 implies punishment. It is best to directly inform the client of the purpose of the seclusion.

*Test-Taking Strategy:* Use the process of elimination. Look for the option that presents reality most clearly to the client. Option 4 is the only option that provides a clear and direct purpose of the seclusion. Review care of a client requiring seclusion if you had difficulty with this question.

*Level of Cognitive Ability:* Application
*Client Needs:* Psychosocial Integrity
*Integrated Concept/Process:* Nursing Process/Implementation
*Content Area:* Mental Health

*Reference*
Varcarolis, E. (1998). *Foundations of psychiatric mental health nursing* (3rd ed.). Philadelphia: W.B. Saunders, p. 321.

**42.** A client with a ruptured cerebral aneurysm who also has a history of essential hypertension exhibits a sudden elevation in blood pressure (BP). The nurse immediately contacts the physician and immediate treatment is prescribed for the client. Which of the following medications would the nurse expect to be prescribed?
1   Epinephrine (Adrenaline)
2   Dobutamine (Dobutrex)
3   Sodium nitroprusside (Nipride)
4   Dopamine (Intropin)

**Answer: 3**
*Rationale:* Sodium nitroprusside decreases the BP by vasodilation, thus reducing pressure in the aneurysm. The other medications increase blood pressure, which may disrupt an existing cerebral clot and precipitate bleeding.

*Test-Taking Strategy:* Focus on the issue: a sudden elevation in BP. Remember that nitroglycerin compounds are vasodilators and that they decrease the BP. If you had difficulty with this question, review the actions of these medications.

*Level of Cognitive Ability:* Analysis
*Client Needs:* Physiological Integrity

*Integrated Concept/Process:* Nursing Process/Analysis
*Content Area:* Adult Health/Neurological

*Reference*
Hodgson, B., & Kizior, R. (2001). *Saunders Nursing drug handbook 2001.* Philadelphia: W.B. Saunders, p. 341, 345, 366, 754.

---

**43.** A client has received electroconvulsive therapy (ECT). In the posttreatment area, when the client awakens, the nurse will first engage in which of the following activities?
1   Orient the client and monitor the client's vital signs
2   Offer the client frequent reassurance and repeat orientation statements
3   Assist the client from the stretcher to a wheelchair
4   Assess the return of the gag reflex and then encourage the client to eat breakfast and resume activity

**Answer: 1**
*Rationale:* The nurse would first monitor vital signs, orient the client, and review with the client that the client had just received an ECT treatment. The posttreatment area should include accessibility to the anesthesia staff, oxygen, suction, pulse oximeter, vital sign monitoring, and emergency equipment. The nursing interventions outlined in options 2, 3, and 4 will follow accordingly.

*Test-Taking Strategy:* Use the process of elimination and note the key word *first.* Use the ABCs, airway, breathing, and circulation, remembering that vital signs are a method of assessing the ABCs. Review care of a client following ECT if you had difficulty with this question.

*Level of Cognitive Ability:* Application
*Client Needs:* Physiological Integrity
*Integrated Concept/Process:* Nursing Process/Implementation
*Content Area:* Mental Health

*Reference*
Varcarolis, E. (1998). *Foundations of psychiatric mental health nursing* (3rd ed.). Philadelphia: W.B. Saunders, p. 578.

---

**44.** A nurse is providing emergency treatment for a client in ventricular tachycardia. The nurse is preparing to defibrillate the client. Which nursing action provides for the safest environment during a defibrillation attempt?
1   Placing the charged paddles one at a time on the client's chest
2   Ensuring that no lubricant is on the paddles
3   Holding the client's upper torso stable while the defibrillation is performed
4   Performing a visual and verbal check that all assisting personnel are clear of the client and the client's bed

**Answer: 4**
*Rationale:* Safety during defibrillation is essential for preventing injury to the client and to the personnel assisting with the procedure. The person performing the defibrillation ensures that all personnel are standing clear of the bed by a verbal and visual check of "all clear." For the shock to be effective, some type of conductive medium (lubricant, gel) must be placed between the paddles and the skin. Both paddles are placed on the client's chest.

*Test-Taking Strategy:* Use the process of elimination, focusing on the issue, safest environment. Option 4 involves a verbal and visual check of "all clear" providing for the safety of all involved. Review the procedure for defibrillation if you had difficulty with this question.

*Level of Cognitive Ability:* Application
*Client Needs:* Safe, Effective Care Environment
*Integrated Concept/Process:* Nursing Process/Implementation
*Content Area:* Adult Health/Cardiovascular

*Reference*
Monahan, F., & Neighbors, M. (1998). *Medical-surgical nursing: Foundations for clinical practice* (2nd ed.). Philadelphia: W.B Saunders, p. 260.

**45.** A client is admitted to the emergency department with complaints of severe, radiating chest pain. The client is extremely restless, frightened, and dyspneic. Immediate admission orders include oxygen by nasal cannula at 4 L/min, STAT blood levels of creatinine phosphokinase (CPK) and isoenzymes, a chest x-ray evaluation, and a 12-lead ECG. Which initial action would the nurse take?

**1** Obtain the 12-lead ECG

**2** Call the laboratory to order the STAT blood work

**3** Call radiology to order the chest x-ray evaluation

**4** Apply the oxygen to the client

**Answer: 4**

*Rationale:* The initial action would be to apply the oxygen because the client can be experiencing myocardial ischemia. The ECG can provide evidence of cardiac damage and the location of myocardial ischemia. However, oxygen is the priority to prevent further cardiac damage. The STAT blood work is not priority. The cardiac isoenzymes can help in determining the choice of treatment. However, they don't begin to rise until 1 to 2 hours after the onset of a myocardial infarction. Although the chest x-ray can show cardiac enlargement, having the chest x-ray is not the initial treatment

*Test-Taking Strategy:* Note the key word *initial.* Remember that the immediate goal of therapy is to prevent myocardial ischemia. The only option that will achieve that goal is option 4. Also, use the ABCs, airway, breathing, and circulation, to direct you to option 4. If you had difficulty with this question, review care of a client with a myocardial infarction.

*Level of Cognitive Ability:* Application
*Client Needs:* Physiological Integrity
*Integrated Concept/Process:* Nursing Process/Implementation
*Content Area:* Adult Health/Cardiovascular

*Reference*
Smeltzer, S., & Bare, B. (2000). *Brunner & Suddarth's Textbook of medical-surgical nursing* (9th ed.). Philadelphia: Lippincott Williams & Wilkins, p. 625.

**46.** Chemical cardioversion is prescribed for the client with atrial fibrillation. The nurse who is assisting in preparing the client would expect that which of the following medications specific for chemical cardioversion will be needed?

**1** Verapamil (Calan)

**2** Nifedipine (Procardia)

**3** Quinidine (Quinidex)

**4** Bretylium (Bretylol)

**Answer: 3**

*Rationale:* Quinidine is an antidysrhythmic. Verapamil is generally used to control heart rate. Nifedipine is a vasodilator. Bretylium is generally used for control of ventricular dysrhythmia.

*Test-Taking Strategy:* Note the key words *chemical cardioversion.* Recalling the action of these medications and that quinidine is an antidysrhythmic will direct you to option 3. If you are unfamiliar with these medications or with preprocedure care, review this content.

*Level of Cognitive Ability:* Analysis
*Client Needs:* Physiological Integrity
*Integrated Concept/Process:* Nursing Process/Analysis
*Content Area:* Adult Health/Cardiovascular

*Reference*
Smeltzer, S., & Bare, B. (2000). *Brunner & Suddarth's Textbook of medical-surgical nursing* (9th ed.). Philadelphia: Lippincott Williams & Wilkins, p. 580.

**47.** A nurse is assisting the respiratory therapist in auscultating the breath sounds of a client on the nursing unit. The nurse would avoid doing which of the following, which represents incorrect technique?
1 Ask the client to sit straight up
2 Have the client breathe slowly and deeply through the mouth
3 Place the stethoscope directly on the client's skin
4 Use the bell of the stethoscope

**Answer: 4**
*Rationale:* The bell of the stethoscope is not used to auscultate breath sounds. The client ideally should sit up and breathe slowly and deeply through the mouth. The diaphragm of the stethoscope, which is warmed before use, is placed directly on the client's skin, not over a gown or clothing.

*Test-Taking Strategy:* Use the process of elimination and note the key word *avoid*. Recalling the procedure for auscultating breath sounds will direct you to option 4. If this question was difficult, review auscultation as a basic physical assessment technique.

*Level of Cognitive Ability:* Application
*Client Needs:* Health Promotion and Maintenance
*Integrated Concept/Process:* Nursing Process/Assessment
*Content Area:* Adult Health/Respiratory

*Reference*
Leahy, J., & Kizilay, P. (1998). *Foundations of nursing practice: A nursing process approach.* Philadelphia: W.B. Saunders, p. 848.

**48.** A nurse is caring for an obese adult client who is at home after receiving treatment for a sprained right ankle. The client is using a cane to ambulate but has not exercised for over one week and has missed the last two rehabilitation appointments. The client says, "I'm getting therapy for my ankle, and I do my exercises three times a day." Which nursing response is most therapeutic?
1 "Sounds good to me. Have you kept all of your appointments?"
2 "You say you are following your exercise plan, yet you've missed the last two appointments with the physical therapist?"
3 "Show me how you do your exercises. I want to determine if you're doing them correctly."
4 "You must keep your appointments. I already know that you've missed two appointments with the therapist."

**Answer: 2**
*Rationale:* In option 2, the nurse employs the therapeutic communication technique of sharing perceptions. Sharing perceptions involves asking the client to verify the nurse's understanding of what the client is feeling, thinking, or doing. In this situation, the client is employing avoidance. By sharing perceptions, the nurse is assisting the client to begin problem solving. In option 1, the nurse is nontherapeutic in giving approval and is mirroring the client's avoidance and passivity by not dealing directly with the problem of missed appointments. In option 3, the nurse is therapeutic in the attempt to engage the client in exercises, but this nursing action does not occur in a helpful manner. In this option, the nurse is "telling" the client to perform the exercises, which could lead to resistance and eventually, a regressive struggle. In option 4, the nurse is empathic but does so by giving advice and using inappropriate timing.

*Test-Taking Strategy:* Use therapeutic communication techniques and the process of elimination. Option 2 is the only option that is addressing what the client is feeling, thinking, or doing. Review therapeutic communication techniques if you had difficulty with this question.

*Level of Cognitive Ability:* Application
*Client Needs:* Psychosocial Integrity
*Integrated Concept/Process:* Communication and Documentation
*Content Area:* Fundamental Skills

*Reference*
Varcarolis, E. (1998). *Foundations of psychiatric mental health nursing* (3rd ed.). Philadelphia: W.B. Saunders, p. 188.

**49.** A client with unstable ventricular tachycardia (VT) loses consciousness and becomes pulseless after an initial treatment with a dose of lidocaine intravenously. The nurse who is caring for the client would immediately obtain which of the following needed items?

1    A second dose of lidocaine
2    A pacemaker
3    An electrocardiogram (ECG) machine
4    A defibrillator

**Answer: 4**

*Rationale:* For the client with VT who becomes pulseless, the physician or qualified advanced cardiac life support (ACLS) personnel immediately defibrillates the client. In the absence of this equipment, cardiopulmonary resuscitation (CPR) is initiated immediately. Options 1, 2, and 3 are not items that are needed immediately in this situation.

*Test-Taking Strategy:* Use the process of elimination, noting the key word *immediately* and that the client is in VT. Options 1 and 3 should be eliminated first, because option 1 was unsuccessful and option 3 is of no use. From the remaining options, focusing on the issue will direct you to option 4. Review the immediate measures for VT if you had difficulty with this question.

*Level of Cognitive Ability:* Application
*Client Needs:* Physiological Integrity
*Integrated Concept/Process:* Nursing Process/Implementation
*Content Area:* Adult Health/Cardiovascular

*Reference*
Monahan, F., & Neighbors, M. (1998). *Medical-surgical nursing: Foundations for clinical practice* (2nd ed.). Philadelphia: W.B Saunders, p. 248.

**50.** A nurse has done preoperative teaching with a client scheduled for percutaneous insertion of an inferior vena cava (IVC) filter. The nurse determines that the client needs further clarification if the client states that the procedure:

1    Is rarely associated with complications
2    Eliminates the need for anticoagulant therapy
3    Is performed while the client is under general anesthesia
4    May cause congestion when clots get trapped at the filter

**Answer: 3**

*Rationale:* Complications after insertion of an IVC filter are very rare. When they do occur, they include air embolism, improper placement, and filter migration. The percutaneous approach uses local anesthesia. There is no need for anticoagulant therapy after surgery. Venous congestion can occur from accumulation of thrombi on the filter; however, the process usually occurs gradually.

*Test-Taking Strategy:* Use the process of elimination. Note the key words *needs further clarification*. Also, noting the word *percutaneous* should direct you to option 3. General anesthesia is not used in this procedure. Review this procedure if you had difficulty with this question.

*Level of Cognitive Ability:* Analysis
*Client Needs:* Physiological Integrity
*Integrated Concept/Process:* Teaching/Learning
*Content Area:* Adult Health/Cardiovascular

*Reference*
Monahan, F., & Neighbors, M. (1998). *Medical-surgical nursing: Foundations for clinical practice* (2nd ed.). Philadelphia: W.B Saunders, p. 386.

**51.** A client with a head injury and a feeding tube continuously tries to remove the tube. The nurse contacts the physician who prescribes the use of restraints. After checking the agency's policy and procedure regarding the use of restraints, the nurse uses which of the following methods in restraining the client?
**1** Mitten splints
**2** Wrist restraints
**3** Waist restraint
**4** Vest restraint

**Answer: 1**
*Rationale:* Mitten splints are useful for this client because the client cannot pull against them, creating resistance that could lead to increased intracranial pressure (ICP). Wrist restraints cause resistance. Vest and waist restraints prevent the client from getting up or falling out of bed, but do nothing to limit hand movement.

*Test-Taking Strategy:* Use the process of elimination and focus on the issue: a restraint that safely limits hand movement for this client. Eliminate options 3 and 4 because they do not address this issue. From the remaining options, thinking about the concern of ICP in a client with a head injury will direct you to option 1. Review care of a client with a head injury if you had difficulty with this question.

*Level of Cognitive Ability:* Application
*Client Needs:* Physiological Integrity
*Integrated Concept/Process:* Nursing Process/Implementation
*Content Area:* Adult Health/Neurological

*Reference*
Smeltzer, S., & Bare, B. (2000). *Brunner & Suddarth's Textbook of medical-surgical nursing* (9th ed.). Philadelphia: Lippincott Williams & Wilkins, p. 1636.

**52.** A nurse has oriented a new employee to basic procedures for continuous ECG monitoring. The nurse would need to intervene if the orientee did which of the following while initiating cardiac monitoring on a client?
**1** Cleansed the skin with Betadine (povidone-iodine) before applying the electrodes
**2** Clipped small areas of hair under the area planned for electrode placement
**3** Stated the need to change the electrodes every 24 hours and inspect the skin
**4** Stated the need to use hypoallergenic electrodes for clients who are sensitive

**Answer: 1**
*Rationale:* The skin is cleansed with soap and water (not Betadine), denatured with alcohol, and is allowed to air dry before electrodes are applied. The other three options are correct.

*Test-Taking Strategy:* Use the process of elimination, noting the key word *intervene*. Eliminate options 3 and 4 because they are correct. From the remaining options, remember that Betadine is used to cleanse the skin usually before some type of invasive procedure that breaks the skin barrier. ECG monitoring does not break the skin. Review the procedure for initiating cardiac monitoring if you had difficulty with this question.

*Level of Cognitive Ability:* Application
*Client Needs:* Safe, Effective Care Environment
*Integrated Concept/Process:* Teaching/Learning
*Content Area:* Adult Health/Cardiovascular

*Reference*
Smeltzer, S., & Bare, B. (2000). *Brunner & Suddarth's Textbook of medical-surgical nursing* (9th ed.). Philadelphia: Lippincott Williams & Wilkins, p. 566.

**53.** A client has been defibrillated three times using an automatic external defibrillator (AED). The nurse observes that the attempts to convert the ventricular fibrillation (VF) were unsuccessful. Based on an evaluation of the situation, the nurse determines that which of the following actions would be best?

1    Performing CPR for 1 minute, then defibrillating up to three more times at 360 joules
2    Performing CPR for 5 minutes, then defibrillating three more times at 400 joules
3    Preparing for the administration of sodium bicarbonate intravenously
4    Terminating the resuscitation effort

**Answer: 1**

*Rationale:* After three unsuccessful defibrillation attempts, CPR should be done for 1 minute, followed by three more shocks, each delivered at 360 joules. There is no information in the question to indicate that life support should be terminated. Sodium bicarbonate may be prescribed, but is not the best action. Giving CPR for 5 minutes may not provide adequate oxygenation to the brain and myocardium and is not the best action. It would be best to administer CPR for 1 minute, then resume attempts to convert the rhythm to a viable one.

*Test-Taking Strategy:* Use the process of elimination and knowledge regarding the treatment for VF. There is no information in the question to indicate that life support should be terminated, so option 4 is eliminated first. From the remaining options, focusing on the key word *best* and recalling the treatment for VF will direct you to option 1. Review the treatment for VF if you had difficulty with this question.

*Level of Cognitive Ability:* Analysis
*Client Needs:* Physiological Integrity
*Integrated Concept/Process:* Nursing Process/Analysis
*Content Area:* Adult Health/Cardiovascular

*Reference*
Monahan, F., & Neighbors, M. (1998). *Medical-surgical nursing: Foundations for clinical practice* (2nd ed.). Philadelphia: W.B Saunders, p. 260.

---

**54.** A nurse is inserting an oropharyngeal airway into an assigned client. The nurse plans to use which correct insertion procedure?

1    Leave any dentures in place
2    Flex the client's neck
3    Insert the airway with the tip pointed upward
4    Suction the client's mouth once per shift

**Answer: 3**

*Rationale:* Before insertion of an oropharyngeal airway, any dentures or partial plates should be removed from the client's mouth. An airway should be selected that is an appropriate size. The client should be positioned supine, with the neck hyperextended if possible. The airway is inserted with the tip pointed upward, and is then rotated downward once the flange has reached the client's teeth. Following insertion, the client's mouth is suctioned every hour or as necessary. The airway is removed for inspection of the mouth every 2 to 4 hours.

*Test-Taking Strategy:* Note the key words *correct insertion procedure.* Eliminate option 4, because this is not part of the insertion procedure. Next eliminate option 2, because the neck is hyperextended (unless contraindicated) to open the airway. From the remaining options, recall that dentures should be removed because they are a potential source of airway obstruction. Review this procedure if you had difficulty with this question.

*Level of Cognitive Ability:* Application
*Client Needs:* Physiological Integrity
*Integrated Concept/Process:* Nursing Process/Planning
*Content Area:* Adult Health/Respiratory

*Reference*
Monahan, F., & Neighbors, M. (1998). *Medical-surgical nursing: Foundations for clinical practice* (2nd ed.). Philadelphia: W.B Saunders, pp. 599-600.

**55.** A nurse is caring for an older female adult client at home. The nurse is told that the client was found wandering the highway in her nightgown last night. Her daughter, who lives with her, says to the nurse, "This wandering started last week, but this is the first time she got out of the house. She always seems to do it around 10:00 P.M. What can I do?" Based on an evaluation of the situation, the most appropriate response would be:

1  "This is probably 'sundowners syndrome,' a common occurrence in older adults."
2  "Since this is the first time your mother has gotten away from you, what has worked to prevent this before this time?"
3  "I think you need to consider a nursing home immediately. Put your mother's name in, and when an empty bed comes up let the doctor admit her. You can't handle this alone, and she could get killed!"
4  "Try approaching your mother before it happens so she doesn't wander. This could be seen as neglect, and you could be prosecuted."

**Answer: 2**
**Rationale:** The nurse should first assess the situation and collect data regarding this change in behavior. The best response is the one that focuses on the daughter's problem solving so that the nurse can then suggest strategies to try. Option 1 does not help at this time and other factors may be causing confusion. Option 3 is histrionic and there are no data to indicate that this action is necessary. Option 4 is inappropriate and may cause resentment if the nurse assumes that the caregiver did not think critically.

**Test-Taking Strategy:** Use the steps of the nursing process. Option 2 is the only option that addresses assessment. Review therapeutic communication techniques and interventions for caregivers if you had difficulty with this question.

**Level of Cognitive Ability:** Application
**Client Needs:** Psychosocial Integrity
**Integrated Concept/Process:** Communication and Documentation
**Content Area:** Fundamental Skills

**Reference**
Varcarolis, E. (1998). *Foundations of psychiatric mental health nursing* (3rd ed.). Philadelphia: W.B. Saunders, p. 190.

**56.** A nurse is assigned to visit an older adult client at home. During the visit, the client says to the nurse, "I wonder if you could do a little grocery shopping for me? I usually go but I'm feeling so 'punk' that I don't think I can manage." Which of the following statements, if made by the nurse, would be the most therapeutic response?

1  "I'm sorry, but I'm not allowed to do that; it's against agency policy."
2  "Do you have any family or support systems you can call on when you're feeling 'punk'?"
3  "Nurses don't have the time to do these things with their heavy caseloads. Please call a grocery store with home delivery."
4  "Not having someone to help on those 'punk' days is a problem. Let's discuss how we can solve it."

**Answer: 4**
**Rationale:** The nurse has a commitment to help the client. It is important that the nurse first collect data, then find an immediate solution as well as a solution for the long-term problem. In option 1, the nurse hides behind policy and rules, and this is a very passive approach. In option 2, the nurse asks a closed-ended question. Option 3 is inappropriate and indicates that the nurse thinks more of status than of helping the client. Option 4 reflects the client's situation and begins to work with the client in a mutual way, which preserves the client's locus of control.

**Test-Taking Strategy:** Use the process of elimination and therapeutic communication techniques. Option 4 is the only option that addresses the client's feelings and provides the means to problem-solve. Review therapeutic communication techniques if you had difficulty with this question.

**Level of Cognitive Ability:** Application
**Client Needs:** Psychosocial Integrity
**Integrated Concept/Process:** Communication and Documentation
**Content Area:** Fundamental Skills

**Reference**
Varcarolis, E. (1998). *Foundations of psychiatric mental health nursing* (3rd ed.). Philadelphia: W.B. Saunders, p. 189.

**57.** A nurse is caring for a client who is being treated with an intravenous (IV) bolus of lidocaine hydrochloride (Xylocaine). The nurse understands the actions and the effects of the medication and plans to monitor which of the following?

1   Respiratory status and blood pressure
2   Urinary pH
3   Radial pulse
4   Temperature

**Answer: 1**

*Rationale:* The nurse is responsible for monitoring the client's respiratory status and blood pressure while the client is being treated with an IV bolus of lidocaine hydrochloride. The urinary pH and temperature are not related to this medication. It is best to monitor the apical pulse in this client.

*Test-Taking Strategy:* Use the ABCs, airway, breathing, and circulation, to answer the question. This should direct you to option 1. If you had difficulty with this question, review nursing responsibilities when a client receives lidocaine hydrochloride.

*Level of Cognitive Ability:* Application
*Client Needs:* Physiological Integrity
*Integrated Concept/Process:* Nursing Process/Assessment
*Content Area:* Pharmacology

*Reference*
Hodgson, B., & Kizior, R. (2001). *Saunders Nursing drug handbook 2001.* Philadelphia: W.B. Saunders, pp. 591-594.

---

**58.** A nurse develops a plan of care for a client with chronic anxiety. Which of the following goals would be most appropriate to include in the plan of care?

1   The client maintains contact with a crisis counselor after discharge
2   The client identifies anxiety-producing situations
3   The client ignores feelings of anxiety
4   The client eliminates all anxiety from daily situations

**Answer: 2**

*Rationale:* Recognizing situations that produce anxiety allows the client to prepare to cope with anxiety or avoid specific stimulus. Counselors will not be available for all anxiety-producing situations, and this option does not encourage the development of internal strengths. Ignoring feelings will not resolve anxiety. It is impossible to eliminate all anxiety from life.

*Test-Taking Strategy:* Use the process of elimination. Eliminate option 1 because it promotes dependence on a counselor. Eliminate options 3 and 4 because of the words *ignores* and *all* found in these options. Option 2 is the only realistic option. Review care of a client with chronic anxiety if you had difficulty with this question.

*Level of Cognitive Ability:* Analysis
*Client Needs:* Psychosocial Integrity
*Integrated Concept/Process:* Nursing Process/Planning
*Content Area:* Mental Health

*Reference*
Varcarolis, E. (1998). *Foundations of psychiatric mental health nursing* (3rd ed.). Philadelphia: W.B. Saunders, p. 443.

**59.** A client has an order for seizure precautions. The nurse avoids doing which of the following when planning care for the client?
1   Monitor the client closely while the client is showering
2   Push the lock-out button on the electric bed to keep the bed in the lowest position
3   Keep all the lights on in the room at night
4   Assist the client to ambulate in the hallway

**Answer: 3**
*Rationale:* A quiet, restful environment is provided as part of seizure precautions. This includes undisturbed times for sleep, while using a night light for safety. The client should be accompanied during activities such as bathing and walking, so that assistance is readily available and injury is minimized if a seizure begins. The bed is maintained in low position for safety.

*Test-Taking Strategy:* Note the key word *avoids* and focus on the issue: seizure precautions. Noting the word *all* in option 3 and thinking about the importance of a quiet, restful environment will direct you to this option. Review care of a client on seizure precautions if you had difficulty with this question.

*Level of Cognitive Ability:* Application
*Client Needs:* Safe, Effective Care Environment
*Integrated Concept/Process:* Nursing Process/Implementation
*Content Area:* Adult Health/Neurological

*Reference*
Monahan, F., & Neighbors, M. (1998). *Medical-surgical nursing: Foundations for clinical practice* (2nd ed.). Philadelphia: W.B Saunders, p. 799.

**60.** A nurse is caring for a child who sustained a head injury from a fall. The nurse avoids which of the following in the care of this child?
1   Keeping the child in a sitting up position
2   Forcing fluids
3   Keeping the child awake as much as possible
4   Performing neurological assessments

**Answer: 2**
*Rationale:* A child with a head injury is at risk for increased intracranial pressure (ICP). Sitting up will decrease fluid retention in cerebral tissue and promote drainage. Keeping the child awake will assist in accurate evaluation of any cerebral edema that is present and will detect early coma. Forcing fluids may cause fluid overload and increased ICP. Neurological assessments need to be performed to monitor for increased ICP.

*Test-Taking Strategy:* Note the key word *avoids*. Use the process of elimination and knowledge regarding increased ICP. Eliminate options 1, 3, and 4 because they are correct in terms of monitoring for and preventing increased ICP. Review measures to prevent increased ICP if you had difficulty with this question.

*Level of Cognitive Ability:* Application
*Client Needs:* Physiological Integrity
*Integrated Concept/Process:* Nursing Process/Implementation
*Content Area:* Child Health

*Reference*
Wong, D. (1999). *Whaley & Wong's Nursing care of infants and children* (6th ed.). St. Louis: Mosby, p. 1793.

**61.** A nurse has conducted a stress management seminar for clients in an ambulatory care setting. Which of the following statements, if made by an attendee, would indicate that further instruction is needed?
1  "Biofeedback might be nice, but I don't like the idea of having to use equipment."
2  "I can use guided imagery anywhere and anytime."
3  "The progressive muscle relaxation technique should ease my tension headaches."
4  "Using confrontation with coworkers should solve my problems at work quickly."

**Answer: 4**
*Rationale:* Biofeedback, progressive muscle relaxation, meditation, and guided imagery are techniques that the nurse can teach the client to reduce the physical impact of stress on the body and promote a feeling of self-control for the client. Biofeedback entails electronic equipment, while the others require no adjuncts, such as tapes, once the technique is learned. Confrontation is a communication technique, not a stress-management technique. It may also exacerbate stress, at least in the short term, rather than alleviate it.

*Test-Taking Strategy:* Note the key words *further instruction is needed.* Recalling the methods of stress management techniques guides you to option 4, which is a communication technique rather than a stress management technique. Review stress management techniques if you had difficulty with this question.

*Level of Cognitive Ability:* Analysis
*Client Needs:* Psychosocial Integrity
*Integrated Concept/Process:* Teaching/Learning
*Content Area:* Mental Health

*Reference*
Varcarolis, E. (1998). *Foundations of psychiatric mental health nursing* (3rd ed.). Philadelphia: W.B. Saunders, p. 868.

**62.** A nurse is caring for a client with a peptic ulcer. In assessing the client for gastrointestinal perforation (GI), the nurse monitors for:
1  Increase in bowel sounds
2  Sudden, severe abdominal pain
3  Positive guaiac tests
4  Slow, strong pulses

**Answer: 2**
*Rationale:* Sudden, severe abdominal pain is the most indicative sign of perforation. When perforation of an ulcer occurs, the nurse may be unable to hear bowel sounds at all. When perforation occurs, the pulse will more likely be weak and rapid. Positive guaiac test results indicate the presence of bleeding but are not necessarily indicative of perforation.

*Test-Taking Strategy:* Use the process of elimination, focusing on the issue: the signs of perforation. Correlate perforation with sudden, severe abdominal pain. Remember that the nurse may be unable to hear bowel sounds and that the pulse will most likely be weak and rapid. Positive guaiac tests results are not specific to perforation. If you had difficulty with this question, review the signs of perforation.

*Level of Cognitive Ability:* Application
*Client Needs:* Physiological Integrity
*Integrated Concept/Process:* Nursing Process/Assessment
*Content Area:* Adult Health/Gastrointestinal

*Reference*
Monahan, F., & Neighbors, M. (1998). *Medical-surgical nursing: Foundations for clinical practice* (2nd ed.). Philadelphia: W.B Saunders, p. 1029.

**63.** Human albumin (Albuminar) IV is prescribed for a client with second- and third-degree burns of the anterior chest and both legs. The nurse reviews the client's medical record to identify the presence of any existing conditions, which would be a contraindication in the use of human albumin. The nurse contacts the physician before administering the human albumin if which of the following is noted in the client's record?

1 Lymphocytic leukemia
2 Multiple myeloma
3 Diabetes mellitus
4 Renal insufficiency

**Answer: 4**

*Rationale:* Human albumin (Albuminar) is classified as a blood derivative and is contraindicated in severe anemia, cardiac failure, history of allergic reaction, renal insufficiency, and when no albumin deficiency is present. It is used with caution in clients with low cardiac reserve, pulmonary disease, or hepatic or renal failure.

*Test-Taking Strategy:* Use the process of elimination and focus on the issue: a contraindication. Eliminate options 1 and 2 first because they are similar in that they are both oncological disorders. From the remaining options, recalling that albumin restores intravascular volume will assist in directing you to option 4. Review this blood derivative if you had difficulty with this question.

*Level of Cognitive Ability:* Application
*Client Needs:* Safe, Effective Care Environment
*Integrated Concept/Process:* Nursing Process/Implementation
*Content Area:* Pharmacology

*Reference*
Hodgson, B., & Kizior, R. (2001). *Saunders Nursing drug handbook 2001.* Philadelphia: W.B. Saunders, pp. 16-17.

**64.** A male newborn is in the intensive care unit for respiratory distress syndrome (RDS) and needs mechanical ventilation for support. Surfactant replacement therapy has been given. The nurse evaluates the infant 1 hour after the surfactant therapy and determines that the infant's condition has somewhat improved. Which of the following, if observed by the nurse, indicated improvement?

1 Decreased need for supplemental oxygen
2 Increased work of breathing
3 Unequal breath sounds
4 Increased level of $CO_2$ in the blood gas analysis

**Answer: 1**

*Rationale:* A decreased need for supplemental oxygen indicates an improvement in the infant's ability to use oxygen. The increased work of breathing indicates air hunger and the need for further support. Unequal breath sounds may indicate atelectasis or blocked airways. Increased levels of $CO_2$ would indicate increasing respiratory acidosis, and not improvement of oxygenation.

*Test-Taking Strategy:* Use the process of elimination, focusing on the key word *improvement*. Noting the word *increased* in options 2 and 4 will assist in eliminating these options. From the remaining options, recall that *unequal* does not indicate improvement. Review the expected effects of surfactant therapy if you had difficulty with this question.

*Level of Cognitive Ability:* Analysis
*Client Needs:* Physiological Integrity
*Integrated Concept/Process:* Nursing Process/Evaluation
*Content Area:* Child Health

*Reference*
Lowdermilk, D., Perry, S., & Bobak, I. (2000). *Maternity & women's health care* (7th ed.). St. Louis: Mosby, p. 1119.

**65.** A nurse is evaluating the effectiveness of antimicrobial therapy for a client with infective endocarditis. The nurse determines that which of the following findings documented in the client's health record is the least reliable indicator of effectiveness?

1　Clear breath sounds
2　Systolic heart murmur
3　Temperature, 98.8° F
4　Negative blood culture results

**Answer: 2**

*Rationale:* A systolic heart murmur, once present, will not resolve spontaneously and is therefore the least reliable indicator. Negative blood cultures and normothermia indicate resolution of infection. Clear breath sounds are a normal finding, and in this instance could mean resolution of heart failure, if that was accompanying the endocarditis.

*Test-Taking Strategy:* Note the key words *least reliable indicator.* The question is worded to look for the finding that will not respond to antimicrobial therapy and which is an abnormal finding. The only option that meets these criteria is option 2, which does not resolve once it has developed. Review care of a client with infective endocarditis if you had difficulty with this question.

*Level of Cognitive Ability:* Analysis
*Client Needs:* Physiological Integrity
*Integrated Concept/Process:* Nursing Process/Evaluation
*Content Area:* Adult Health/Cardiovascular

*Reference*
Monahan, F., & Neighbors, M. (1998). *Medical-surgical nursing: Foundations for clinical practice* (2nd ed.). Philadelphia: W.B Saunders, p. 233.

**66.** A nurse is caring for a client with continuous electrocardiogram (ECG) monitoring. The nurse notes that the electrocardiogram complexes are very small and hard to evaluate. The nurse checks which setting on the ECG monitor console?

1　Power button
2　Low rate alarm
3　Amplitude or "gain"
4　High rate alarm

**Answer: 3**

*Rationale:* The power button turns the machine on and off. The high and low rate alarm settings indicate the heart rate limits beyond which an alarm will sound. The amplitude, commonly called "gain," regulates the size of the complex and can be adjusted up and down to some degree.

*Test-Taking Strategy:* Focus on the issue: that the complexes are small and hard to evaluate. Noting the relationship of the issue to the word amplitude (meaning size or strength) in option 3 will direct you to this option. Review the procedure for the use of an ECG monitor if you had difficulty with this question.

*Level of Cognitive Ability:* Application
*Client Needs:* Physiological Integrity
*Integrated Concept/Process:* Nursing Process/Implementation
*Content Area:* Adult Health/Cardiovascular

*Reference*
Smeltzer, S., & Bare, B. (2000). *Brunner & Suddarth's Textbook of medical-surgical nursing* (9th ed.). Philadelphia: Lippincott Williams & Wilkins, p. 566.

**67.** A nurse is monitoring a client who has received antidysrhythmic therapy for the treatment of premature ventricular contractions (PVCs). The nurse would evaluate this therapy as being less than optimal if the client's PVCs continued to:
1   Be fewer than 6/min
2   Be unifocal in appearance
3   Fall after the end of the T wave
4   Occurred in pairs

**Answer: 4**
*Rationale:* PVCs are considered dangerous when they are frequent (more than 6/min), occur in pairs or couplets, are multifocal (multiform), or fall on the T wave.

*Test-Taking Strategy:* Note the key words *less than optimal.* Knowledge regarding the occurrence of PVCs and the situations in which they may be dangerous to the client is necessary to answer this question. Review this basic information if you had difficulty with this question.

*Level of Cognitive Ability:* Analysis
*Client Needs:* Physiological Integrity
*Integrated Concept/Process:* Nursing Process/Evaluation
*Content Area:* Adult Health/Cardiovascular

*Reference*
Smeltzer, S., & Bare, B. (2000). *Brunner & Suddarth's Textbook of medical-surgical nursing* (9th ed.). Philadelphia: Lippincott Williams & Wilkins, p. 574.

**68.** A nurse is reviewing the client's arterial blood gas (ABG) results. Which of these findings would indicate that the client had respiratory acidosis?
1   pH 7.5, $Pco_2$ 30
2   pH 7.3, $Pco_2$ 50
3   pH 7.3, $HCO_3$ 19
4   pH 7.5, $HCO_3$ 30

**Answer: 2**
*Rationale:* In respiratory acidosis, the pH is decreased and an opposite effect is seen in the $Pco_2$ (pH decreased, $Pco_2$ elevated). Option 1 indicates respiratory alkalosis. Option 3 indicates metabolic acidosis, and option 4 indicates metabolic alkalosis.

*Test-Taking Strategy:* Use the process of elimination. Recalling that the pH is decreased in acidosis will assist in eliminating options 1 and 4. Next, remember in respiratory acidosis the $Pco_2$ has an opposite effect from the pH. This will direct you to option 2. Review these basic interpretations if you had difficulty with this question.

*Level of Cognitive Ability:* Analysis
*Client Needs:* Physiological Integrity
*Integrated Concept/Process:* Nursing Process/Analysis
*Content Area:* Adult Health/Respiratory

*Reference*
Monahan, F., & Neighbors, M. (1998). *Medical-surgical nursing: Foundations for clinical practice* (2nd ed.). Philadelphia: W.B Saunders, p. 108.

**69.** A nurse is assigned to care for a client with a chest tube attached to closed chest drainage. The nurse determines that the client's lung has completely expanded if:
1   The oxygen saturation is greater than 92%
2   Fluctuations in the water seal chamber ceased
3   Pleuritic chest pain has resolved
4   Suction in the chest drainage system is no longer needed

**Answer: 2**
*Rationale:* When the lung has completely expanded, there is no longer air or fluid in the pleural space to be drained into the water seal chamber. Thus, an indication that a chest tube is ready for removal is when fluctuations in the water seal chamber ceases and drainage of fluid into the collection bottle/chamber ceases. Adequate oxygen saturation does not imply that the lung has fully reexpanded. Although air is known to be an irritant to pleural tissue, cessation of pleuritic pain does not indicate that the lung is expanded. The chest tube acts as an irritant and therefore contributes to pain. Use or nonuse of suction in the chest drainage system is not necessarily governed by the degree of lung expansion. Suction is indicated when gravity is not sufficient to

drain air and pleural fluid or if the client has a poor respiratory effort and cough. Suction increases the speed at which air and fluid is removed from the pleural space.

*Test-Taking Strategy:* Note the key words *completely expanded.* Eliminate options 1 and 3 because they are not directly related to a chest tube drainage system. From the remaining options, recalling the functioning of chest tubes will direct you to option 2. Review chest tube drainage systems if you had difficulty with this question.

*Level of Cognitive Ability:* Analysis
*Client Needs:* Physiological Integrity
*Integrated Concept/Process:* Nursing Process/Analysis
*Content Area:* Adult Health/Respiratory

*Reference*
Monahan, F., & Neighbors, M. (1998). *Medical-surgical nursing: Foundations for clinical practice* (2nd ed.). Philadelphia: W.B Saunders, p. 579.

---

**70.** A nurse is caring for a child with leukemia. The nurse notes that the platelet count is 20,000/mm³. Based on this finding, the nurse deletes which of the following from the plan of care?
1   Monitor stools for blood
2   Clean oral cavity with a Toothette
3   Administer acetaminophen (Tylenol) suppositories for fever
4   Provide appropriate play activities

**Answer: 3**
*Rationale:* A platelet count of 20,000/mm³ places the child at risk for bleeding. Options 1, 2, and 4 are accurate interventions. The use of suppositories is avoided because of the risk of rectal bleeding.

*Test-Taking Strategy:* Note the key word *deletes.* Noting the issue of the question, bleeding, and using the process of elimination will direct you to option 3. Review interventions for the child at risk for bleeding if you had difficulty with this question.

*Level of Cognitive Ability:* Application
*Client Needs:* Physiological Integrity
*Integrated Concept/Process:* Nursing Process/Planning
*Content Area:* Child Health

*Reference*
Wong, D. (1999). *Whaley & Wong's Nursing care of infants and children* (6th ed.). St. Louis: Mosby, p. 1727.

**71.** A nurse is caring for a client with deep vein thrombosis (DVT) who is on bed rest at home. The nurse has reinforced teaching regarding the signs of pulmonary embolism, a complication of DVT. Which of the following statements, if made by the client, indicates that the client understands the clinical manifestations of pulmonary embolism?

1   "I will notify the doctor immediately if I develop coughing, profuse sweating, difficulty breathing, and/or chest pain."
2   "I will call you if anything unusual occurs."
3   "I will notify the doctor immediately if I become nauseous, start vomiting, and have diarrhea."
4   "I will call you if I begin to get dizzy."

**Answer: 1**
*Rationale:* Of the clinical manifestations of a pulmonary embolism, chest pain is the most common. Coughing, diaphoresis, dyspnea, and apprehension are the other clinical manifestations. Pleuritic chest pain (sudden onset and aggravated by breathing) is caused by an inflammatory reaction of the lung parenchyma or when there is a pulmonary infarction or ischemia caused by an obstruction of small pulmonary arterial branches. Options 2, 3, and 4 are inaccurate clinical descriptions of pulmonary embolism.

*Test-Taking Strategy:* Focus on the issue: the manifestations of pulmonary embolism. Recalling that chest pain is the most common manifestation will direct you to option 1. If you had difficulty with this question, review the clinical manifestations of pulmonary embolism.

*Level of Cognitive Ability:* Analysis
*Client Needs:* Health Promotion and Maintenance
*Integrated Concept/Process:* Teaching/Learning
*Content Area:* Adult Health/Cardiovascular

*Reference*
Smeltzer, S., & Bare, B. (2000). *Brunner & Suddarth's Textbook of medical-surgical nursing* (9th ed.). Philadelphia: Lippincott Williams & Wilkins, p. 706.

**72.** A nurse evaluates the arterial blood gas (ABG) results of a client who is receiving supplemental oxygen. Which of these findings would indicate that the oxygen level was adequate?

1   A $Po_2$ of 60 mm Hg
2   A $Po_2$ of 50 mm Hg
3   A $Po_2$ of 45 mm Hg
4   A $Po_2$ of 32 mm Hg

**Answer: 1**
*Rationale:* Keeping the $Po_2$ at 60 mm Hg will indicate that the hemoglobin is 90% saturated (unless the pH varies). Options 2, 3, and 4 are low values and do not indicate adequate oxygen levels.

*Test-Taking Strategy:* Focus on the issue: oxygen level was adequate. Use the process of elimination and select the option that identifies the highest oxygen level. This will direct you to option 1. Review interpretation of the results of ABGs if you had difficulty with this question.

*Level of Cognitive Ability:* Analysis
*Client Needs:* Health Promotion and Maintenance
*Integrated Concept/Process:* Nursing Process/Evaluation
*Content Area:* Adult Health/Respiratory

*Reference*
Smeltzer, S., & Bare, B. (2000). *Brunner & Suddarth's Textbook of medical-surgical nursing* (9th ed.). Philadelphia: Lippincott Williams & Wilkins, p. 233.

**73.** A nurse assesses a client admitted to the hospital with rib fractures in order to identify the risk for potential complications. The nurse notes that the client has a history of emphysema. Following the assessment, the nurse ensures that which priority intervention is documented in the plan of care?
1. Have the client cough and breathe deeply 20 minutes after pain medication is given
2. Administer low-flow oxygen at 2 L/min as prescribed
3. Assist the client to a position of comfort
4. Administer small, frequent meals with plenty of fluids

**Answer: 2**
*Rationale:* Giving the client with emphysema a high flow of oxygen would affect the respiratory drive and cause apnea. Options 1, 3, and 4 may be appropriate nursing interventions, but option 2 specifically addresses the issue of the question.

*Test-Taking Strategy:* Note the key word *priority*. Focus on the data in the question and note that the client has emphysema. Recalling the care of a client with emphysema and use of the ABCs, airway, breathing, and circulation, will direct you to option 2. Review the complications that can occur in the client with emphysema if you had difficulty with this question.

*Level of Cognitive Ability:* Application
*Client Needs:* Physiological Integrity
*Integrated Concept/Process:* Communication and Documentation
*Content Area:* Adult Health/Respiratory

*Reference*
Monahan, F., & Neighbors, M. (1998). *Medical-surgical nursing: Foundations for clinical practice* (2nd ed.). Philadelphia: W.B Saunders, p. 690.

**74.** A nurse is developing a plan of care for a client with acquired immunodeficiency syndrome (AIDS). The nurse documents which most appropriate goal in the plan of care?
1. The client does not experience respiratory distress
2. The client has no increased platelet aggregation
3. The client has no evidence of dissecting aortic aneurysm
4. The client has a urinary output of 50 mL/hr

**Answer: 1**
*Rationale:* The absence of respiratory distress is one of the goals that the nurse sets as a priority. The most common, life-threatening opportunistic infection that attacks clients with AIDS is pneumocystis carinii pneumonia. Its symptoms include fever, exertional dyspnea, and nonproductive cough. Options 2, 3, and 4 are not specifically related to the issue of the question.

*Test-Taking Strategy:* Note the issue of the question. Option 1 is the only option that is directly related to the client's diagnosis. In addition, use the ABCs, airway, breathing, and circulation, to answer the question. If you had difficulty with this question, review care of a client with AIDS.

*Level of Cognitive Ability:* Application
*Client Needs:* Physiological Integrity
*Integrated Concept/Process:* Communication and Documentation
*Content Area:* Adult Health/Respiratory

*Reference*
Monahan, F., & Neighbors, M. (1998). *Medical-surgical nursing: Foundations for clinical practice* (2nd ed.). Philadelphia: W.B Saunders, p. 1466.

**75.** A client with active tuberculosis (TB) is to be admitted to a medical-surgical unit. When planning a bed assignment, the nurse:

1  Plans to transfer the client to the intensive care unit
2  Assigns the client to a double room, because intravenous antibiotics will be administered
3  Assigns the client to a double room and places a "strict handwashing" sign outside the door
4  Places the client in a private, well-ventilated room

**Answer: 4**

*Rationale:* According to category specific (respiratory) isolation precautions, a client with TB requires a private room. The room needs to be well-ventilated and should have at least 6 exchanges of fresh air per hour and should be ventilated to the outside if possible. Therefore, option 4 is the only correct option.

*Test-Taking Strategy:* Note that the question states "active tuberculosis." Eliminate options 2 and 3 because they are similar in that they involve a double room. From the remaining options, recalling the need for respiratory isolation precautions will direct you to option 4. Review care of a client with active TB if you had difficulty with this question.

*Level of Cognitive Ability:* Application
*Client Needs:* Safe, Effective Care Environment
*Integrated Concept/Process:* Nursing Process/Planning
*Content Area:* Adult Health/Respiratory

*Reference*
Monahan, F., & Neighbors, M. (1998). *Medical-surgical nursing: Foundations for clinical practice* (2nd ed.). Philadelphia: W.B Saunders, pp. 652-653.

**76.** A client has a diagnosis of an irregular heart rate. What question by the client would indicate client teaching should begin?

1  "How is an ECG interpreted?"
2  "What is it like to have a pacemaker?"
3  "Can you tell me what a diagnosis of irregular heart rate means?"
4  "What is wrong with my roommate's heart?"

**Answer: 3**

*Rationale:* Learning depends on two things: physical and emotional readiness to learn. Without one or the other, teaching can occur, but learning may not take place. There is usually a time at which the client will indicate an interest in learning. Option 3 addresses the client's readiness because the client is directly asking about the disorder. At this point, the client's readiness and motivation to learn is present.

*Test-Taking Strategy:* Use the process of elimination. Note that option 3 directly addresses the client's diagnosis. Also note the similarity of "irregular heart rate" in the question and in the correct option. Review teaching/learning principles if you had difficulty with this question.

*Level of Cognitive Ability:* Analysis
*Client Needs:* Psychosocial Integrity
*Integrated Concept/Process:* Nursing Process/Evaluation
*Content Area:* Fundamental Skills

*Reference*
Monahan, F., & Neighbors, M. (1998). *Medical-surgical nursing: Foundations for clinical practice* (2nd ed.). Philadelphia: W.B Saunders, p. 287.

**77.** A physician orders 20% Intralipids, an intravenous fat emulsion, for a client who will be receiving total parenteral nutrition (TPN) for several months. The nurse explains to the client that the fat solution is administered:

1    To increase the amount of fluid given by the intravenous route
2    On a daily basis and must be administered at bedtime
3    To decrease the incidence of phlebitis in the vein where the TPN is administered
4    To provide essential fatty acids and additional calories

**Answer: 4**
*Rationale:* Intralipids is a brand of intravenous fat emulsion. Clients receiving TPN parenterally for a prolonged period of time are at risk for developing essential fatty acid deficiency. Fat emulsions are given to meet client nonprotein caloric needs that cannot be met by glucose administration alone. Fat emulsions are not administered to increase the amount of fluids administered and they do not decrease the incidence of phlebitis. They may be prescribed daily but do not need to be administered at bedtime.

*Test-Taking Strategy:* Focus on the issue: intravenous fat emulsion. Eliminate option 2 because of the absolute word *must.* From the remaining options, note the relationship between *fat emulsion* in the question and *fatty acids* in the correct option. If you had difficulty with this question, review the purpose of administering fat emulsion during TPN therapy.

*Level of Cognitive Ability:* Application
*Client Needs:* Physiological Integrity
*Integrated Concept/Process:* Teaching/Learning
*Content Area:* Fundamental Skills

*Reference*
Deglin, J., & Vallerand, A. (1999). *Davis's Drug guide for nurses* (6th ed.). Philadelphia: F.A. Davis, p.364.

---

**78.** A client with valvular heart disease is at risk for developing congestive heart failure (CHF). The nurse assesses which of the following most closely when monitoring for CHF?

1    Heart rate
2    Blood pressure
3    Breath sounds
4    Activity tolerance

**Answer: 3**
*Rationale:* Breath sounds are the best way to assess for the onset of CHF. The presence of crackles or rales or an increase in crackles is an indicator of fluid in the lungs caused by CHF. Options 1, 2, and 4 are components of the assessment but are less reliable indicators of CHF.

*Test-Taking Strategy:* Use the process of elimination, thinking about the pathophysiology that occurs with CHF. Use of the ABCs, airway, breathing, and circulation, will direct you to option 3. If you had difficulty with this question, review assessment of CHF.

*Level of Cognitive Ability:* Analysis
*Client Needs:* Physiological Integrity
*Integrated Concept/Process:* Nursing Process/Assessment
*Content Area:* Adult Health/Cardiovascular

*Reference*
Monahan, F., & Neighbors, M. (1998). *Medical-surgical nursing: Foundations for clinical practice* (2nd ed.). Philadelphia: W.B Saunders, p. 264.

**79.** A nurse is caring for a client receiving fludrocortisone acetate (Florinef) for the treatment of Addison's disease. The nurse monitors the client for improvement knowing that the anticipated therapeutic effect of this medication is to:

1   Stimulate the immune response
2   Promote electrolyte balance
3   Stimulate thyroid production
4   Stimulate thytrotropin production

**Answer: 2**

*Rationale:* Florinef is a long-acting oral medication with mineralocorticoid and moderate glucocorticoid activity that is used for long-term management of Addison's disease. Mineralocorticoids act on the renal distal tubules to enhance the reabsorption of sodium and chloride ions and the excretion of potassium and hydrogen ions. The client can rapidly develop hypotension and fluid and electrolyte imbalance if the medication is discontinued abruptly. The medication does not affect the immune response or thyroid or thyrotropin production.

*Test-Taking Strategy:* Remember that Addison's disease produces deficiencies of glucocorticoids, mineralocorticoids, and androgens. Eliminate options 3 and 4 first because they are similar. From the remaining options, recalling that Addison's disease is not related to the immune system will direct you to option 2. Review the action of this medication if you had difficulty with this question.

*Level of Cognitive Ability:* Analysis
*Client Needs:* Physiological Integrity
*Integrated Concept/Process:* Nursing Process/Evaluation
*Content Area:* Adult Health/Endocrine

*Reference*
Hodgson, B., & Kizior, R. (2001). *Saunders Nursing drug handbook 2001.* Philadelphia: W.B. Saunders, pp. 422-423.

**80.** A nurse is assessing the leg pain of a client who has just undergone right femoral-popliteal artery bypass grafting. Which of the following questions would be most useful in determining whether the client is experiencing graft occlusion?

1   "Can you rate the pain on a scale of 1 to 10?"
2   "Can you describe what the pain feels like?"
3   "Can you compare this pain to the pain you felt before surgery?"
4   "Did you get any relief from the last dose of pain medication?"

**Answer: 3**

*Rationale:* The most frequent indication that a graft is occluding is the return of pain that is similar to that experienced preoperatively. Standard pain assessment techniques also include the items described in options 1, 2 and 4, but these will not help to differentiate current pain from preoperative pain.

*Test-Taking Strategy:* Focus on the issue: the assessment question that will help differentiate expected postoperative pain from pain that indicates graft occlusion. Eliminate options 1, 2, and 4 because they are similar and are standard pain assessment questions. If this question was difficult, review care of a client following this type of surgery.

*Level of Cognitive Ability:* Application
*Client Needs:* Physiological Integrity
*Integrated Concept/Process:* Nursing Process/Assessment
*Content Area:* Adult Health/Cardiovascular

*Reference*
Monahan, F., & Neighbors, M. (1998). *Medical-surgical nursing: Foundations for clinical practice* (2nd ed.). Philadelphia: W.B Saunders, p. 364.

**81.** A client has implemented dietary and other lifestyle changes to manage hypertension. The nurse evaluates that the lifestyle changes have been most successful if the client has a follow-up blood pressure reading of:

1    156/82 mm Hg
2    128/84 mm Hg
3    164/72 mm Hg
4    140/94 mm Hg

**Answer: 2**

*Rationale:* Hypertension is defined as a systolic blood pressure (BP) of 140 mm Hg or greater, and/or a diastolic BP that is 90 mm Hg or greater. The goal of therapy is to reduce the BP to less than 140/90 mm Hg.

*Test-Taking Strategy:* Use the process of elimination, recalling the parameters of normal blood pressure and the definition of hypertension. Option 2 is the only option that identifies a normal BP. If this question was difficult, review the standard classification system for hypertension.

*Level of Cognitive Ability:* Analysis
*Client Needs:* Physiological Integrity
*Integrated Concept/Process:* Nursing Process/Evaluation
*Content Area:* Adult Health/Cardiovascular

*Reference*
Monahan, F., & Neighbors, M. (1998). *Medical-surgical nursing: Foundations for clinical practice* (2nd ed.). Philadelphia: W.B Saunders, p. 372.

**82.** A client is scheduled to have insertion of an inferior vena cava (IVC) filter. The nurse would place highest priority on determining whether the surgeon wants which of the following medications held in the preoperative period?

1    Famotidine (Pepcid)
2    Multivitamin with minerals
3    Warfarin (Coumadin)
4    Furosemide (Lasix)

**Answer: 3**

*Rationale:* The nurse is careful to question the surgeon about whether warfarin should be administered in the preoperative period before insertion of an IVC filter. This medication is often withheld for a period of time preoperatively to minimize the risk of hemorrhage during surgery. The other medications may also be withheld if specifically ordered, but usually they are discontinued as part of an NPO (nothing by mouth) after midnight order.

*Test-Taking Strategy:* Note the key words *highest priority*. Recalling that warfarin is an anticoagulant and that when a client is taking an anticoagulant a risk for bleeding exists will direct you to option 3. If this question was difficult, review anticoagulant medication concepts at this time.

*Level of Cognitive Ability:* Analysis
*Client Needs:* Safe, Effective Care Environment
*Integrated Concept/Process:* Nursing Process/Analysis
*Content Area:* Adult Health/Cardiovascular

*Reference*
Monahan, F., & Neighbors, M. (1998). *Medical-surgical nursing: Foundations for clinical practice* (2nd ed.). Philadelphia: W.B Saunders, p. 385.

**83.** A client's medical record states a history of intermittent claudication. In collecting data about this symptom, the nurse would ask the client about which of the following symptoms?
1   Chest pain that is sudden and occurs with exertion
2   Chest pain that is dull and feels like heartburn
3   Leg pain that is achy and gets worse as the day progresses
4   Leg pain that is sharp and occurs with exercise

**Answer: 4**
*Rationale:* Intermittent claudication is a symptom that is characterized by a sudden onset of leg pain that occurs with exercise and is relieved by rest. It is the classic symptom of peripheral arterial insufficiency. Venous insufficiency is characterized by an achy type of leg pain that intensifies as the day progresses. Chest pain can occur for a variety of reasons, one of which is angina pectoris (option 1) or indigestion (option 2).

*Test-Taking Strategy:* Use the process of elimination. Focusing on the key word *intermittent* will direct you to option 4. If this question was difficult or if you are unfamiliar with the term *intermittent claudication*, review this content area.

*Level of Cognitive Ability:* Application
*Client Needs:* Physiological Integrity
*Integrated Concept/Process:* Nursing Process/Assessment
*Content Area:* Adult Health/Cardiovascular

*Reference*
Monahan, F., & Neighbors, M. (1998). *Medical-surgical nursing: Foundations for clinical practice* (2nd ed.). Philadelphia: W.B Saunders, p. 332.

---

**84.** A client has just been diagnosed with right leg deep vein thrombosis (DVT). The nurse immediately implements which of the following interventions?
1   Elevation of the right leg
2   Ice packs to the right leg
3   Vigorous range of motion to the right leg
4   Hourly calf measurements

**Answer: 1**
*Rationale:* Standard therapy for DVT consists of bed rest, leg elevation, and application of warm moist heat to the affected leg. The client may have calf measurements ordered once per shift or once per day, but they would not be obtained hourly. Option 2 is incorrect because heat is used, not cold. Option 3 is dangerous to the client, because vigorous activity after clot formation can cause pulmonary embolus.

*Test-Taking Strategy:* Focus on the client's diagnosis and use knowledge of the treatment for DVT as well as concepts related to gravity and the applications of heat and cold to answer the question. If this question was difficult, review the interventions for this disorder.

*Level of Cognitive Ability:* Application
*Client Needs:* Physiological Integrity
*Integrated Concept/Process:* Nursing Process/Implementation
*Content Area:* Adult Health/Cardiovascular

*Reference*
Monahan, F., & Neighbors, M. (1998). *Medical-surgical nursing: Foundations for clinical practice* (2nd ed.). Philadelphia: W.B Saunders, p. 384.

**85.** A client is scheduled to have a serum digoxin (Lanoxin) level obtained and is scheduled to receive digoxin (Lanoxin) 0.25 mg in 1 hour. The nurse would arrange to have the blood sample drawn:

**1** Just before the dose is given
**2** Just after the dose has been given
**3** 1 hour after the dose is given
**4** 3 hours after the dose is given

**Answer: 1**

*Rationale:* Serum digoxin levels are most often drawn immediately before the next dose, although they may be drawn 4 to 10 hours after a previous dose. Recall that the purpose of the sample is to record the serum concentration of the medication to ensure that it is in the therapeutic range. Drawing the medication before the next dose ensures that the level is not falsely elevated.

*Test-Taking Strategy:* Use the process of elimination. Remember that options that are similar are not likely to be correct. Each of the incorrect options requires the blood sample to be drawn within a relatively short period of time after the client has been given the medication. If this question was difficult review this laboratory test.

*Level of Cognitive Ability:* Application
*Client Needs:* Physiological Integrity
*Integrated Concept/Process:* Nursing Process/Planning
*Content Area:* Adult Health/Cardiovascular

*Reference*

Deglin, J., & Vallerand, A. (1999). *Davis's Drug guide for nurses* (6th ed.). Philadelphia: F. A. Davis, p. 278.

**86.** A nurse is collecting data regarding the environmental safety for the client receiving home oxygen therapy. The nurse determines that which of the following observations is not consistent with the principles of safe oxygen use and in need of intervention?

**1** Gas stove lit in another room
**2** Oxygen concentrator placed against wall
**3** Oxygen tank secured in holder
**4** Absence of smoking in the room containing oxygen

**Answer: 2**

*Rationale:* There should be no open flames or smoking within 10 feet of the oxygen source. The tank should remain secured in its holder, and the concentrator should be away from walls or other close quarters (to allow adequate air circulation around the unit). The oxygen source should also be removed from sources of heat or sunlight.

*Test-Taking Strategy:* Note the key word *not*. Use the process of elimination and read each option carefully. Recalling the principles of safe oxygen use will direct you to option 2. Review these safety principles if you had difficulty with this question.

*Level of Cognitive Ability:* Analysis
*Client Needs:* Safe, Effective Care Environment
*Integrated Concept/Process:* Nursing Process/Evaluation
*Content Area:* Fundamental Skills

*Reference*

Leahy, J., & Kizilay, P. (1998). *Foundations of nursing practice: A nursing process approach.* Philadelphia: W.B. Saunders, p. 889.

**87.** A nurse has finished suctioning the tracheostomy of a client. The nurse evaluates the effectiveness of the procedure by monitoring which of the following items?
1   Respiratory rate
2   Oxygen saturation level
3   Breath sounds
4   Capillary refill

**Answer: 3**
*Rationale:* After suctioning a client either with or without an artificial airway, the breath sounds are auscultated to determine the extent to which the airways have been cleared of respiratory secretions. The other methods are not as precise as breath sounds for this purpose.

*Test-Taking Strategy:* Use the process of elimination, focusing on the issue, evaluating the effectiveness of suctioning. Recalling that the purpose of suctioning is to clear the airways of secretions will direct you to option 3. Review the procedure for suctioning if you had difficulty with this question.

*Level of Cognitive Ability:* Analysis
*Client Needs:* Physiological Integrity
*Integrated Concept/Process:* Nursing Process/Evaluation
*Content Area:* Adult Health/Respiratory

*Reference*
Monahan, F., & Neighbors, M. (1998). *Medical-surgical nursing: Foundations for clinical practice* (2nd ed.). Philadelphia: W.B Saunders, p. 728.

---

**88.** A nurse is performing tracheostomy care and has replaced the tracheostomy ties. The nurse ensures that the ties are not too tight by checking to see if:
1   The client nods that they feel comfortable
2   The tracheostomy does not move more than 1/2 inch when coughing
3   Three fingers can slide comfortably under the tie
4   Two fingers can slide comfortably under the tie

**Answer: 4**
*Rationale:* There should be enough room for two fingers to slide comfortably under the tracheostomy tie. This ensures that they are tight enough to prevent tracheostomy dislocation, while preventing excessive constriction around the neck. The other options are incorrect.

*Test-Taking Strategy:* Use the process of elimination, focusing on the issue, that the ties are not too tight. Visualize each of the descriptions in the options to direct you to option 4. If this question was difficult, review the essentials of this fundamental nursing procedure.

*Level of Cognitive Ability:* Analysis
*Client Needs:* Physiological Integrity
*Integrated Concept/Process:* Nursing Process/Evaluation
*Content Area:* Adult Health/Respiratory

*Reference*
Smeltzer, S., & Bare, B. (2000). *Brunner & Suddarth's Textbook of medical-surgical nursing* (9th ed.). Philadelphia: Lippincott Williams & Wilkins, p. 503.

---

**89.** A nurse is checking a client's disposable closed chest drainage system at the beginning of the shift, and notes continuous bubbling in the water seal chamber. The nurse interprets that:
1   There is an air leak somewhere in the system
2   A pneumothorax is resolving
3   The system is intact
4   The suction to the system is shut off

**Answer: 1**
*Rationale:* Continuous bubbling through both inspiration and expiration indicates that there is air leaking into the system. A resolving pneumothorax would show intermittent bubbling with respiration in the water seal chamber. Shutting the suction off to the system stops bubbling in the suction control chamber, but does not affect the water seal chamber.

*Test-Taking Strategy:* Use the process of elimination and focus on the issue: continuous bubbling in the water seal chamber. The words *continuous bubbling* should provide you with the clue that an air leak is present. If this question was difficult, review the concepts associated with a chest tube drainage system.

*Level of Cognitive Ability:* Analysis
*Client Needs:* Physiological Integrity
*Integrated Concept/Process:* Nursing Process/Evaluation
*Content Area:* Adult Health/Respiratory

*Reference*
Monahan, F., & Neighbors, M. (1998). *Medical-surgical nursing: Foundations for clinical practice* (2nd ed.). Philadelphia: W.B Saunders, p. 575.

---

**90.** A client is suspected of having pulmonary tuberculosis (TB). The nurse assesses the client for which of the following signs and symptoms of TB?
1   Weight gain, insomnia, and night sweats
2   Low-grade fever, fatigue, and productive cough
3   High fever, night sweats, and chest pain
4   Increased appetite, dyspnea, and chills

**Answer: 2**
*Rationale:* The client with pulmonary TB generally has a productive or nonproductive cough, anorexia and weight loss, fatigue, low grade fever, chills and night sweats, dyspnea, hemoptysis, and chest pain. Breath sounds may reveal crackles.

*Test-Taking Strategy:* Use the process of elimination. Remember that when an option has more than one part, all of the parts of that option must be correct if the entire option is to be correct. Eliminate options 1 and 4 first because the client will not have an increased appetite or weight gain. From the remaining options, it is necessary to know that the fever will be low grade. Review findings related to TB if you had difficulty with this question.

*Level of Cognitive Ability:* Application
*Client Needs:* Physiological Integrity
*Integrated Concept/Process:* Nursing Process/Assessment
*Content Area:* Adult Health/Respiratory

*Reference*
Monahan, F., & Neighbors, M. (1998). *Medical-surgical nursing: Foundations for clinical practice* (2nd ed.). Philadelphia: W.B Saunders, p. 650.

---

**91.** A client who has a positive sputum culture for *Mycobacterium tuberculosis* (TB) has been started on therapy with streptomycin (Streptomycin). The nurse interprets that the client is experiencing toxic effects of the medication if which of the following results is abnormal?
1   Hemoglobin and hematocrit
2   Blood urea nitrogen (BUN) and creatinine
3   Hepatic enzymes
4   Vision testing

**Answer: 2**
*Rationale:* BUN and creatinine are measured during therapy with streptomycin because the medication is nephrotoxic. The client taking isoniazid (INH) for TB is at risk for hepatotoxicity. Vision testing is done during treatment with ethambutol (Myambutol). Hemoglobin and hematocrit are not specifically related to TB.

*Test-Taking Strategy:* To answer this question accurately, you must be familiar with the various medications that are used to treat TB, and their associated adverse or toxic effects. If this question was difficult, review the adverse effects of streptomycin.

*Level of Cognitive Ability:* Analysis
*Client Needs:* Physiological Integrity
*Integrated Concept/Process:* Nursing Process/Analysis
*Content Area:* Adult Health/Respiratory

*Reference*
Monahan, F., & Neighbors, M. (1998). *Medical-surgical nursing: Foundations for clinical practice* (2nd ed.). Philadelphia: W.B Saunders, p. 653.

**92.** A nurse is preparing to implement emergency care measures for the client who has just experienced pulmonary embolism. The nurse implements which of the following physician orders first?
1  Administer morphine sulfate
2  Apply oxygen
3  Start an intravenous line
4  Obtain an electrocardiogram (ECG)

**Answer: 2**
*Rationale:* The client needs immediate oxygen therapy because of hypoxemia, which is most often accompanied by respiratory distress and cyanosis. The client should have an IV line for the administration of emergency medications, such as morphine sulfate. An ECG is useful in determining the presence of possible right ventricular hypertrophy. All of the interventions listed are appropriate, but the client needs the oxygen first.

*Test-Taking Strategy:* Note the key word *first.* Use the process of elimination and the ABCs: airway, breathing, and circulation. This will direct you to option 2. Review care of a client with pulmonary embolism if you had difficulty with this question.

*Level of Cognitive Ability:* Application
*Client Needs:* Physiological Integrity
*Integrated Concept/Process:* Nursing Process/Implementation
*Content Area:* Adult Health/Respiratory

*Reference*
Monahan, F., & Neighbors, M. (1998). *Medical-surgical nursing: Foundations for clinical practice* (2nd ed.). Philadelphia: W.B Saunders, p. 386.

**93.** A client is scheduled for bronchoscopy. The nurse would avoid which of the following before the procedure?
1  Obtaining a signed informed consent
2  Letting the client eat or drink
3  Removing contact lenses
4  Removing any dentures

**Answer: 2**
*Rationale:* The client is not allowed to eat or drink for 6 hours before the procedure. The client must give informed consent, since the procedure is invasive. If the client has any contact lenses, dentures, or other prostheses, they are removed before sedation is administered to the client.

*Test-Taking Strategy:* Note the key word *avoid.* Recalling that the client must be on nothing by mouth status (NPO) before a bronchoscopy will direct you to option 2. Review care of the client undergoing bronchoscopy if this question was difficult.

*Level of Cognitive Ability:* Application
*Client Needs:* Physiological Integrity
*Integrated Concept/Process:* Nursing Process/Implementation
*Content Area:* Adult Health/Respiratory

*Reference*
Monahan, F., & Neighbors, M. (1998). *Medical-surgical nursing: Foundations for clinical practice* (2nd ed.). Philadelphia: W.B Saunders, p. 537.

**94.** A client who has no history of immunosuppressive disease has a Mantoux test for tuberculosis (TB). The results indicate an area of induration that is 10 mm in size. The nurse interprets that the client:
1  Has active TB
2  Has a history of TB
3  Has been exposed to TB
4  Has no TB

**Answer: 3**
*Rationale:* The client who is not immunosuppressed is considered positive for TB if the test results in an area of induration that measures 10 mm or more. The reading is generally done 48 to 72 hours after being implanted in the forearm. This result indicates that the client has been exposed to TB and requires further diagnostic workup.

*Test-Taking Strategy:* Use the process of elimination. Recalling that an area of induration of 10 mm or greater indicates exposure will direct you to option 3. Review the normal parameters for this test if you had difficulty with this question.

*Level of Cognitive Ability:* Analysis
*Client Needs:* Physiological Integrity
*Integrated Concept/Process:* Nursing Process/Analysis
*Content Area:* Adult Health/Respiratory

*Reference*
Monahan, F., & Neighbors, M. (1998). *Medical-surgical nursing: Foundations for clinical practice* (2nd ed.). Philadelphia: W.B Saunders, p. 653.

---

**95.** A client has an order to have a set of arterial blood gases (ABGs) drawn. The intended site is the radial artery. The nurse ensures that which of the following is positive before the ABGs are drawn?
1    Homans' sign
2    Brudzinski's sign
3    Babinski reflex
4    Allen test

**Answer: 4**
*Rationale:* The Allen test is performed before drawing arterial blood gases. The radial and ulnar arteries are occluded in turn, and then released. Observation is made in the distal circulation. If the results are positive, then the client has adequate circulation, and that site may be used. Homans' sign tests for deep vein thrombosis by dorsiflexion of the foot. Brudzinski's sign tests for nuchal rigidity by bending the head down toward the chest. The Babinski reflex is checked by stroking upward on the sole of the foot.

*Test-Taking Strategy:* Note the key words *radial artery*. Recalling the purpose of each test listed in the options will direct you to option 4. If this question was difficult, review these tests.

*Level of Cognitive Ability:* Analysis
*Client Needs:* Physiological Integrity
*Integrated Concept/Process:* Nursing Process/Analysis
*Content Area:* Adult Health/Respiratory

*Reference*
Smeltzer, S., & Bare, B. (2000). *Brunner & Suddarth's Textbook of medical-surgical nursing* (9th ed.). Philadelphia: Lippincott Williams & Wilkins, p. 561.

---

**96.** A client having a mild panic attack has the following arterial blood gas (ABG) results: pH 7.49, $Paco_2$ 31 mm Hg, $Pao_2$ 97 mm Hg, $HCO_3^-$ 22 mEq/L. The nurse reviews the results and determines that the client has which of the following acid-base disturbances?
1    Respiratory acidosis
2    Respiratory alkalosis
3    Metabolic acidosis
4    Metabolic alkalosis

**Answer: 2**
*Rationale:* Acidosis is defined as a pH of less than 7.35, while alkalosis is defined as a pH of greater than 7.45. Respiratory alkalosis is present when the $Paco_2$ is less than 35, whereas respiratory acidosis is present when the $Paco_2$ is greater than 45. Metabolic acidosis is present when the $HCO_3^-$ is less than 22 mEq/L, while metabolic alkalosis is present when the $HCO_3^-$ is greater than 27 mEq/L. This client's ABGs are consistent with respiratory alkalosis.

*Test-Taking Strategy:* Note the key words *panic attack*. This may help you to anticipate that the client is having an increased respiratory rate, which makes the client prone to respiratory alkalosis. Otherwise, use the steps for interpreting blood gas results to answer the question. Review these steps if you had difficulty with this question.

*Level of Cognitive Ability:* Analysis
*Client Needs:* Physiological Integrity
*Integrated Concept/Process:* Nursing Process/Analysis
*Content Area:* Adult Health/Respiratory

*Reference*
Monahan, F., & Neighbors, M. (1998). *Medical-surgical nursing: Foundations for clinical practice* (2nd ed.). Philadelphia: W.B Saunders, p. 111.

---

**97.** A nurse is assessing a client with a suspected rib fracture. The nurse observes for which of the following typical symptoms?
1 Pain on expiration; deep, rapid respirations
2 Pain on expiration; shallow, guarded respirations
3 Pain on inspiration; deep, rapid respirations
4 Pain on inspiration; shallow, guarded respirations

**Answer: 4**
*Rationale:* The client with fractured ribs typically has pain over the fracture site with inspiration and to palpation. Respirations are shallow, and guarding of the area is often noted. Bruising may or may not be present.

*Test-Taking Strategy:* Focus on the client's diagnosis. Think about the movement of the chest wall on inspiration and expiration. Remember that pain will occur on inspiration and respirations will be shallow. Review the signs related to a rib fracture if you had difficulty with this question.

*Level of Cognitive Ability:* Application
*Client Needs:* Physiological Integrity
*Integrated Concept/Process:* Nursing Process/Assessment
*Content Area:* Adult Health/Respiratory

*Reference*
Monahan, F., & Neighbors, M. (1998). *Medical-surgical nursing: Foundations for clinical practice* (2nd ed.). Philadelphia: W.B Saunders, p. 690.

---

**98.** A client with a flail chest resulting from four fractured rib segments is experiencing severe pain when trying to breathe. The nurse observes for which of the following characteristics of a flail chest?
1 Slight tachypnea with shallow breaths
2 Pallor and paradoxical chest movement
3 Severe dyspnea and paradoxical chest movement
4 Cyanosis and slow respirations

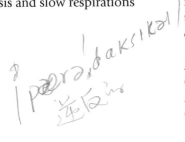

**Answer: 3**
*Rationale:* The client with flail chest is in obvious respiratory distress. The client has severe dyspnea and cyanosis accompanied by paradoxical chest movement. Respirations are shallow, rapid, and grunting in nature.

*Test-Taking Strategy:* Use the process of elimination. Remember that for an option to be correct, all of the parts of that option must also be correct. With this in mind, eliminate options 1 and 2 because of the words *slight* and *pallor*. Choose between the remaining options knowing that this client would be tachypneic, rather than having slow respirations. Review the clinical manifestations associated with flail chest if you had difficulty with this question.

*Level of Cognitive Ability:* Application
*Client Needs:* Physiological Integrity
*Integrated Concept/Process:* Nursing Process/Assessment
*Content Area:* Adult Health/Respiratory

*Reference*
Monahan, F., & Neighbors, M. (1998). *Medical-surgical nursing: Foundations for clinical practice* (2nd ed.). Philadelphia: W.B Saunders, p. 691.

**99.** A nurse is assigned to care for a client with pneumonia. The nurse reviews the nursing care plan and notes documentation of a nursing diagnosis of Activity Intolerance. The nurse implements which of the following in the client's care?

1 Provides stimulation in the environment to maintain client alertness

2 Encourages deep, rapid breathing during activity

3 Schedules activities before giving respiratory medications or treatments

4 Observes vital signs and oxygen saturation periodically during activity

**Answer: 4**

*Rationale:* The nurse monitors vital signs, including oxygen saturation before, during, and after activity to gauge client response. Activities should be planned after giving the client respiratory medications or treatments to increase activity tolerance. The client should use pursed-lip and diaphragmatic breathing to lower oxygen consumption during activity. Finally, the environment should be conducive to rest, since the client is easily fatigued.

*Test-Taking Strategy:* Focus on the issue: activity intolerance, and note the client's diagnosis. Use the ABCs, airway, breathing, and circulation, to direct you to option 4. If you had difficulty with this question, review the interventions for a client with pneumonia and activity intolerance.

*Level of Cognitive Ability:* Application
*Client Needs:* Physiological Integrity
*Integrated Concept/Process:* Nursing Process/Implementation
*Content Area:* Adult Health/Respiratory

*Reference*
Black, J., & Matassarin-Jacobs, E. (1997). *Medical-surgical nursing: Clinical management for continuity of care* (5th ed.). Philadelphia: W.B. Saunders, p. 1138.

**100.** A nurse is assisting in admitting a newborn infant to the nursery and notes that the physician has documented that the newborn has gastroschisis. The nurse plans care, knowing that in this condition the viscera are:

1 Inside the abdominal cavity and under the dermis

2 Inside the abdominal cavity and under the skin

3 Outside the abdominal cavity but inside a translucent sac covered with peritoneum and amniotic membrane

4 Outside the abdominal cavity and not covered with a sac

**Answer: 4**

*Rationale:* Gastroschisis is an abdominal wall defect. Embryonal weakness in the abdominal wall causes herniation of the gut on one side of the umbilical cord during early development. Option 3 describes an omphalocele. Options 1 and 2 describe a umbilical hernia.

*Test-Taking Strategy:* Use the process of elimination. Eliminate options 1 and 2 first because they are similar. From the remaining options, recalling the definition of gastroschisis will direct you to option 4. Review this disorder if you are unfamiliar with it.

*Level of Cognitive Ability:* Application
*Client Needs:* Physiological Integrity
*Integrated Concept/Process:* Nursing Process/Planning
*Content Area:* Maternity

*Reference*
Wong, D. (1999). *Whaley & Wong's Nursing care of infants and children* (6th ed.). St. Louis: Mosby, p. 534.

**101.** A nurse is caring for a client following shoulder arthroplasty for rheumatoid arthritis. The nurse is checking the client for brachial plexus compromise. To assess the status of the median nerve, which of the following would the nurse perform?

1   Have the client move the thumb towards the palm and back to the neutral position
2   Have the client grasp the nurse's hand and the nurse notes the client's strength of the first and the second fingers
3   Have the client spread all the fingers wide and resist pressure
4   Monitor for flexion of the biceps by having the client raise the forearm

**Answer: 2**
*Rationale:* To assess the median nerve status, the client should be instructed to grasp the nurse's hand. The nurse should note the strength of the client's first and second fingers. A weak grip may indicate compromise of the median nerve. Asking the client to move the thumb toward the palm and back to neutral position is assessing the radial nerve status. Asking the client to spread all fingers wide and resisting pressure is assessing the ulnar nerve status. Cutaneous nerve status is assessed by monitoring for flexion of the biceps when the client raises the forearm.

*Test-Taking Strategy:* Use the process of elimination. Recalling the location and function of the median nerve will direct you to option 2. If you are unfamiliar with this procedure, review this assessment technique.

*Level of Cognitive Ability:* Application
*Client Needs:* Health Promotion and Maintenance
*Integrated Concept/Process:* Nursing Process/Assessment
*Content Area:* Adult Health/Musculoskeletal

*Reference*
Monahan, F., & Neighbors, M. (1998). *Medical-surgical nursing: Foundations for clinical practice* (2nd ed.). Philadelphia: W.B Saunders, p. 909.

---

**102.** A nurse is caring for a client who is hospitalized with acute systemic lupus erythematosus (SLE). The nurse monitors the client knowing that which of the following clinical manifestations is not associated with this disease?

1   Fever
2   Muscular aches and pains
3   Butterfly rash on the face
4   Bradycardia

**Answer: 4**
*Rationale:* Manifestations of acute SLE may include fever, musculoskeletal aches and pains, butterfly rash on the face, pleural effusion, basilar pneumonia, generalized lymphadenopathy, pericarditis, tachycardia, hepatosplenomegaly, nephritis, delirium, convulsions, psychosis, and coma.

*Test-Taking Strategy:* Use the process of elimination, noting the key word *not* in the stem of the question. Think about the pathophysiology associated with this disorder to direct you to option 4. If you are unfamiliar with this disorder review its clinical manifestations.

*Level of Cognitive Ability:* Application
*Client Needs:* Physiological Integrity
*Integrated Concept/Process:* Nursing Process/Assessment
*Content Area:* Adult Health/Musculoskeletal

*Reference*
Monahan, F., & Neighbors, M. (1998). *Medical-surgical nursing: Foundations for clinical practice* (2nd ed.). Philadelphia: W.B Saunders, p. 1490.

**103.** A client is seen in the clinic and anemia has been diagnosed. On further assessment, the nurse notes that the client complains of palpitations. The client appears pale and complains of fatigue, weakness, dizziness, headache, and loss of appetite. Based on the client's symptoms, the nurse would expect that the hemoglobin results would indicate which of the following?
1    Hemoglobin of 14 g/dL
2    Hemoglobin of 12 g/dL
3    Hemoglobin of 10 g/dL
4    Hemoglobin of 7 g/dL

**Answer: 4**
*Rationale:* Severely anemic persons (those with a hemoglobin well below 8 g/dL) appear pale and always feel exhausted. They may have severe palpitations, sensitivity to cold, loss of appetite, profound weakness, dizziness, and headaches.

*Test-Taking Strategy:* Use the process of elimination. Focusing on the client's symptoms and recalling the normal hemoglobin level will direct you to option 4. Review the normal hemoglobin level and the signs of anemia if you had difficulty with this question.

*Level of Cognitive Ability:* Analysis
*Client Needs:* Physiological Integrity
*Integrated Concept/Process:* Nursing Process/Analysis
*Content Area:* Fundamental Skills

*Reference*
Monahan, F., & Neighbors, M. (1998). *Medical-surgical nursing: Foundations for clinical practice* (2nd ed.). Philadelphia: W.B Saunders, p. 468.

---

**104.** A nurse in the newborn nursery is performing vital signs on the newborn infant. Which of the following findings would indicate a normal respiratory rate?
1    28 breaths/min
2    50 breaths/min
3    100 breaths/min
4    120 breaths/min

**Answer: 2**
*Rationale:* The normal respiratory rate for a newborn may range from 30 to 80 breaths/min.

*Test-Taking Strategy:* Knowledge regarding the normal respiratory rate of a newborn infant is required to answer this question. If you are unfamiliar with the normal ranges for newborn vital signs, review this content.

*Level of Cognitive Ability:* Analysis
*Client Needs:* Physiological Integrity
*Integrated Concept/Process:* Nursing Process/Assessment
*Content Area:* Maternity

*Reference*
Lowdermilk, D., Perry, S., & Bobak, I. (2000). *Maternity & women's health care* (7th ed.). St. Louis: Mosby, p. 693.

---

**105.** A nurse is assessing a client with a diagnosis of polycythemia vera. Which of the following manifestations would the nurse expect to note in this client?
1    Pallor
2    Hypertension
3    Pale mucous membranes
4    A low hematocrit level

**Answer: 2**
*Rationale:* Manifestations of polycythemia vera include a ruddy complexion, dusky red mucosa, hypertension, dizziness, headache, and a sense of fullness in the head. Signs of congestive heart failure may also be present. The hematocrit level is usually greater than 54% in men and 49% in women.

*Test-Taking Strategy:* Use the process of elimination and focus on the client's diagnosis. Recalling that polycythemia vera is a myeloproliferative disease that causes increased blood viscosity and blood volume will direct you to option 2. If you are unfamiliar with the clinical manifestations associated with this disorder, review this content.

*Level of Cognitive Ability:* Analysis
*Client Needs:* Physiological Integrity
*Integrated Concept/Process:* Nursing Process/Assessment
*Content Area:* Adult Health/Cardiovascular

*Reference*
Monahan, F., & Neighbors, M. (1998). *Medical-surgical nursing: Foundations for clinical practice* (2nd ed.). Philadelphia: W.B Saunders, p. 688.

---

**106.** A nurse is caring for a client with leukemia who is receiving chemotherapy. When reviewing the laboratory results, the nurse notes that the neutrophil count is less than 500/mm³. Based on this laboratory result, the nurse determines that which of the following is not a priority in the plan of care?

1   Padding the side rails and removing all hazardous and sharp objects from the environment
2   Restricting visitors with colds or respiratory infections
3   Removing all live plants, flowers, and stuffed animals in the client's room
4   Placing the client on a low-bacteria diet that excludes raw foods and vegetables

**Answer: 1**
*Rationale:* When the neutrophil count is less than 500/mm³, visitors with potential communicable diseases should be screened for the presence of infection and any visitors or staff with colds or respiratory infections should not be allowed in the client's room. All live plants, flowers, and stuffed animals are removed from the client's room. The client is placed on a low bacteria diet that excludes raw fruits and vegetables. Padding the side rails and removing all hazardous and sharp objects from the environment would be instituted if the client is at risk for bleeding. This client is at risk for infection.

*Test-Taking Strategy:* Use the process of elimination. Note the key word *not* in the stem in the question. Recalling that a low neutrophil count places the client at risk for infection will direct you to option 1. If you are unfamiliar with the normal neutrophil count and the nursing interventions necessary when the count is low, review this content.

*Level of Cognitive Ability:* Application
*Client Needs:* Physiological Integrity
*Integrated Concept/Process:* Nursing Process/Planning
*Content Area:* Adult Health/Oncology

*Reference*
Smeltzer, S., & Bare, B. (2000). *Brunner & Suddarth's Textbook of medical-surgical nursing* (9th ed.). Philadelphia: Lippincott Williams & Wilkins, p. 737.

---

**107.** A nurse is delivering care to a client who was diagnosed with toxic shock syndrome (TSS). The nurse monitors this client for which of the following complications of this syndrome?

1   Pulmonary embolism
2   Disseminated intravascular coagulopathy (DIC)
3   Vitamin K deficiency
4   Factor VIII deficiency

**Answer: 2**
*Rationale:* Toxic shock syndrome is caused by infection and is often associated with tampon use. DIC is a complication of TSS. The nurse monitors the client for signs of this complication, and notifies the physician promptly if signs and symptoms are noted. Options 1, 3, and 4 are not complications of TSS.

*Test-Taking Strategy:* Familiarity with TSS and knowledge that DIC is a complication is needed to answer this question. Review the complications of TTS if you had difficulty with this question.

*Level of Cognitive Ability:* Application
*Client Needs:* Physiological Integrity

*Integrated Concept/Process:* Nursing Process/Assessment
*Content Area:* Adult Health/Cardiovascular

*Reference*
Beare, P., & Myers, J. (1998). *Adult health nursing* (3rd ed.). St. Louis: Mosby, p. 1659.

---

**108.** A nurse is monitoring a client on heparin infusion therapy. The nurse interprets that the client is not experiencing complications of the therapy if which of the following is noted?
1  Bleeding gums
2  Oozing from venipuncture site
3  Dark, tarry stools
4  Hematest negative nasogastric (NG) drainage

**Answer: 4**
*Rationale:* The nurse monitors the client receiving anticoagulant therapy for adverse effects. These would include internal manifestations such as abdominal pain or swelling, backache, dizziness, headache, hematemesis, hemoptysis, hematuria, black or bloody stools, and hematest positive urine, stool, or NG drainage. Overt signs include ecchymoses, petechiae, hematomas, nosebleeds, and bleeding from the gums, wounds, and invasive line insertion sites.

*Test-Taking Strategy:* Use the process of elimination, noting the key words *not experiencing*. Since the greatest risk associated with anticoagulant therapy is hemorrhage, the correct option is the one that indicates no active bleeding. Review the adverse effects related to heparin therapy if you had difficulty with this question.

*Level of Cognitive Ability:* Analysis
*Client Needs:* Physiological Integrity
*Integrated Concept/Process:* Nursing Process/Evaluation
*Content Area:* Adult Health/Cardiovascular

*Reference*
Hodgson, B., & Kizior, R. (2001). *Saunders Nursing drug handbook 2001.* Philadelphia: W.B. Saunders, pp. 489-491.

---

**109.** A client is admitted to the hospital with Cushing's syndrome. The nurse reviews the results of the client's laboratory studies for which of the following manifestations of this disorder?
1  Hypokalemia
2  Hyperglycemia
3  Low white blood cell (WBC) count
4  Decreased plasma cortisol levels

**Answer: 2**
*Rationale:* The client with adrenocorticosteroid excess experiences hyperkalemia, hyperglycemia, elevated WBC count, and elevated plasma cortisol and ACTH levels. These abnormalities are the result of the effects of excess glucocorticoids and mineralocorticoids on the body.

*Test-Taking Strategy:* Recalling that an adrenocorticosteroid excess occurs in Cushing's syndrome will direct you to option 2. Review the manifestations associated with Cushing's syndrome if you had difficulty with this question.

*Level of Cognitive Ability:* Analysis
*Client Needs:* Physiological Integrity
*Integrated Concept/Process:* Nursing Process/Assessment
*Content Area:* Adult Health/Endocrine

*Reference*
Monahan, F., & Neighbors, M. (1998). *Medical-surgical nursing: Foundations for clinical practice* (2nd ed.). Philadelphia: W.B Saunders, p. 1281.

**110.** A nurse is going to suction an adult client with a tracheostomy who has copious amounts of secretions. The nurse does which of the following to accomplish this procedure safely and effectively?

1 Occlude the Y-port of the catheter while advancing it into the tracheostomy
2 Apply continuous suction in the airway for up to 15 seconds
3 Hyperoxygenate the client after the procedure only
4 Set the suction pressure range between 100 and 120 mm Hg

**Answer: 4**

*Rationale:* The safe suction range for an adult is 100 to 120 mm Hg, making option 4 the action that is consistent with safe and effective practice. The nurse should hyperoxygenate the client both before and after suctioning. The nurse should advance the catheter into the tracheostomy without occluding the Y-port to minimize mucosal trauma and aspiration of the client's oxygen. The nurse should use intermittent suction in the airway (not constant) for up to 10 to 15 seconds.

*Test-Taking Strategy:* Use the process of elimination. Eliminate option 3 because of the absolute word *only*. From the remaining options, visualize the procedure to direct you to option 4. Review the procedure for suctioning if you had difficulty with this question.

*Level of Cognitive Ability:* Application
*Client Needs:* Physiological Integrity
*Integrated Concept/Process:* Nursing Process/Implementation
*Content Area:* Adult Health/Respiratory

*Reference*
Monahan, F., & Neighbors, M. (1998). *Medical-surgical nursing: Foundations for clinical practice* (2nd ed.). Philadelphia: W.B Saunders, p. 728.

**111.** A nurse who has just begun the work shift is preparing to do tracheostomy care on a client. The nurse would obtain which of the following tracheostomy care items from the supply area?

1 Tracheostomy care kit, sterile saline and water, and suction kit
2 Bottle of sterile saline and tracheostomy care kit
3 Bottles of sterile saline and water, and tracheostomy dressing
4 Suction kit and tracheostomy dressing

**Answer: 1**

*Rationale:* Equipment needed to perform tracheostomy care includes a tracheostomy care kit, sterile water and saline solutions for cleansing and rinsing, and a suction kit for client suctioning. As part of tracheostomy care, the client's airway should be suctioned before cleansing of the actual tracheostomy. The solutions are changed once per 24 hours, which is often done at the beginning of the work day. A tracheostomy care kit contains the needed supplies for cleaning the tracheostomy, and for changing the dressing and ties.

*Test-Taking Strategy:* Use the process of elimination. Recalling that the key items needed are the tracheostomy kit and suction kit will direct you to option 1. Review the procedure for tracheostomy care if you had difficulty with this question.

*Level of Cognitive Ability:* Application
*Client Needs:* Physiological Integrity
*Integrated Concept/Process:* Nursing Process/Implementation
*Content Area:* Adult Health/Respiratory

*Reference*
Smeltzer, S., & Bare, B. (2000). *Brunner & Suddarth's Textbook of medical-surgical nursing* (9th ed.). Philadelphia: Lippincott Williams & Wilkins, p. 503.

**112.** A nurse is monitoring the function of a client's chest tube. The chest tube is attached to a Pleurevac drainage system. The nurse notes that the fluid in the water seal chamber is below the 2 cm mark. The nurse interprets that:

1   Suction should be added to the system
2   There is a leak in the system
3   This is the result of client pneumothorax
4   Water should be added to the chamber

**Answer: 4**

*Rationale:* The water seal chamber should be filled to the 2 cm mark to provide an adequate water seal between the external environment and the client's pleural cavity. The water seal prevents air from reentering the pleural cavity. Since evaporation of water can occur, the nurse should remedy this problem by adding water until the level is again at the 2 cm mark. The other interpretations are incorrect.

*Test-Taking Strategy:* Focus on the issue: that the water seal chamber is below the 2 cm mark. Recalling that the chamber needs to be filled to the 2 cm mark will direct you to option 4. Review the principles associated with chest tubes if you had difficulty with this question.

*Level of Cognitive Ability:* Analysis
*Client Needs:* Physiological Integrity
*Integrated Concept/Process:* Nursing Process/Analysis
*Content Area:* Adult Health/Respiratory

*Reference*
Smeltzer, S., & Bare, B. (2000). *Brunner & Suddarth's Textbook of medical-surgical nursing* (9th ed.). Philadelphia: Lippincott Williams & Wilkins, p. 1515.

**113.** A nurse is planning care for a client with a chest tube attached to a Pleurevac drainage system. The nurse avoids which of the following actions as part of routine chest tube care?

1   Keeps the collection chamber below the client's waist
2   Clamps the chest tube when the client gets out of bed
3   Monitors for fluctuations in the water seal chamber
4   Monitors the drainage from the chest tube

**Answer: 2**

*Rationale:* To avoid causing tension pneumothorax, the nurse avoids clamping the chest tube for any reason unless specifically ordered. In most instances, clamping of the chest tube is contraindicated by agency policy. The nurse keeps the drainage collection system below the level of the client's waist to prevent fluid or air from reentering the pleural space. The nurse monitors for fluctuations in the water seal chamber and monitors the drainage from the chest tube.

*Test-Taking Strategy:* Note the key word *avoids*. This tells you that the correct option is an incorrect nursing action. Recalling that clamping chest tubes is contraindicated unless specifically ordered will direct you to option 2. Review care of a client with a chest tube if you had difficulty with this question.

*Level of Cognitive Ability:* Application
*Client Needs:* Physiological Integrity
*Integrated Concept/Process:* Nursing Process/Implementation
*Content Area:* Adult Health/Respiratory

*Reference*
Monahan, F., & Neighbors, M. (1998). *Medical-surgical nursing: Foundations for clinical practice* (2nd ed.). Philadelphia: W.B Saunders, p. 578.

**114.** A client is being discharged from the hospital following removal of chest tubes that were inserted following thoracic surgery. The nurse provides home care instructions to the client and determines the need for further instructions if the client states:

1   "I need to remove the chest tube site dressing as soon as I get home."
2   "I need to report any difficulty with breathing to the physician."
3   "I need to avoid heavy lifting for the first 4 to 6 weeks."
4   "I need to take my temperature to detect a possible infection."

**Answer: 1**

*Rationale:* On removal of a chest tube, an occlusive dressing consisting of petrolatum gauze covered by a dry sterile dressing (DSD) is placed over the chest tube site dressing. This is maintained in place until the physician says it may be removed. The client is taught to monitor and report any respiratory difficulty or increased temperature. The client should avoid heavy lifting for the first 4 to 6 weeks after discharge to facilitate continued wound healing.

*Test-Taking Strategy:* Use the process of elimination, noting the key words *need for further instructions.* Recalling that signs of infection and respiratory difficulty should be monitored and reported helps to eliminate options 2 and 4 first. From the remaining options, recalling that either heavy lifting should be avoided postoperatively, or that removal of the chest tube site dressing disturbs the occlusive seal to the site will direct you to option 1. Review teaching points following removal of a chest tube if you had difficulty with this question.

*Level of Cognitive Ability:* Analysis
*Client Needs:* Health Promotion and Maintenance
*Integrated Concept/Process:* Teaching/Learning
*Content Area:* Adult Health/Respiratory

*Reference*
Smeltzer, S., & Bare, B. (2000). *Brunner & Suddarth's Textbook of medical-surgical nursing* (9th ed.). Philadelphia: Lippincott Williams & Wilkins, p. 1515.

**115.** A newborn infant is diagnosed with imperforate anus. The nurse plans care knowing that which of the following most appropriately describes a characteristic of this disorder?

1   Incomplete development of the anus
2   Invagination of a section of the intestine into the distal bowel
3   The infrequent and difficult passage of dry stools
4   The presence of fecal incontinence

**Answer: 1**

*Rationale:* Imperforate anus (anal atresia, anal agenesis) is the incomplete development or absence of the anus in its normal position in the perineum. Option 2 describes intussusception. Option 3 describes constipation. Option 4 describes encopresis. Constipation can affect any child at any time though it peaks at age 2 to 3 years. Encopresis generally affects preschool and school-aged children.

*Test-Taking Strategy:* Use the process of elimination. Noting the relationship between the disorder "imperforate anus" and "incomplete development of the anus" in option 1 should direct you to this option. Review this disorder if you had difficulty with this question.

*Level of Cognitive Ability:* Application
*Client Needs:* Physiological Integrity
*Integrated Concept/Process:* Nursing Process/Planning
*Content Area:* Maternity

*Reference*
Wong, D. (1999). *Whaley & Wong's Nursing care of infants and children* (6th ed.). St. Louis: Mosby, p. 526.

**116.** A nurse is providing bottle-feeding instructions to the mother of a newborn infant. The nurse provides instructions regarding the amount of formula to be given knowing that the stomach capacity for a newborn infant is approximately:

1    5 to 10 mL
2    10 to 20 mL
3    30 to 90 mL
4    75 to 100 mL

**Answer: 2**
*Rationale:* The stomach capacity of a newborn infant is approximately 10 to 20 mL. It is 30 to 90 mL for a 1 week old infant, and 75 to 100 mL for a 2 to 3 week old infant.

*Test-Taking Strategy:* Use the process of elimination. Note the key words *newborn infant*. This should assist in eliminating options 3 and 4. Attempt to visualize the amounts in options 1 and 2. Noting that 5 mL is a very small amount should assist in directing you to option 2. Review these pediatric differences if you had difficulty with this question.

*Level of Cognitive Ability:* Application
*Client Needs:* Health Promotion and Maintenance
*Integrated Concept/Process:* Teaching/Learning
*Content Area:* Maternity

*Reference*
Lowdermilk, D., Perry, S., & Bobak, I. (2000). *Maternity & women's health care* (7th ed.). St. Louis: Mosby, p, 785.

**117.** A mother who is breastfeeding her newborn infant is experiencing nipple soreness and the nurse provides instructions regarding measures to relieve the soreness. Which of the following statements if made by the mother indicates an understanding of the instructions?

1    "I need to avoid rotating breastfeeding positions so that the nipple will toughen."
2    "I need to stop nursing during the period of nipple soreness to allow the nipples to heal."
3    I need to nurse less frequently and substitute a bottle feeding until the nipples become less sore."
4    "I need to position my infant with the ear, shoulder, and hip in straight alignment and place the infant's stomach against me."

**Answer: 4**
*Rationale:* Comfort measures for nipple soreness include positioning the infant with the ear, shoulder, and hip in straight alignment and with the infant's stomach against the mother's. Additional measures include rotating breastfeeding positions; breaking suction with the little finger; nursing frequently; beginning feeding on the less sore nipple; not allowing the infant to chew on the nipple or to sleep holding the nipple in the mouth; and applying tea bags soaked in warm water to the nipple. Options 1, 2, and 3 are incorrect.

*Test-Taking Strategy:* Use the process of elimination, focusing on the key words *indicates an understanding*. Visualize each of the options in terms of how they may or may not lessen the nipple soreness to direct you to option 4. If you had difficulty answering the question, review these measures.

*Level of Cognitive Ability:* Analysis
*Client Needs:* Health Promotion and Maintenance
*Integrated Concept/Process:* Teaching/Learning
*Content Area:* Maternity

*Reference*
Lowdermilk, D., Perry, S., & Bobak, I. (2000). *Maternity & women's health care* (7th ed.). St. Louis: Mosby, p. 779.

**118.** A new breastfeeding mother is seen in the clinic with complaints of breast discomfort. The nurse determines that the mother is experiencing breast engorgement and provides the mother with instructions regarding care for the condition. Which of the following statements if made by the mother indicates an understanding of the measures that will provide comfort for the engorgement?
1   "I will breastfeed using only one breast."
2   "I will apply cold compresses to the breasts."
3   "I will massage the breasts before feeding to stimulate let-down."
4   "I will avoid the use of a bra while the breasts are engorged."

**Answer: 3**
*Rationale:* Comfort measures for breast engorgement include: massaging the breasts before feeding to stimulate let-down; wearing a supportive well-fitting bra at all times; taking a warm shower or applying warm compresses just before feeding; and alternating the breasts during feeding. Options 1, 2, and 4 are incorrect measures.

*Test-Taking Strategy:* Use the process of elimination, noting the key words *indicates an understanding.* Visualize each of the descriptions in the options to assist in directing you to option 3. If you had difficulty answering this question, review the measures to alleviate breast engorgement.

*Level of Cognitive Ability:* Analysis
*Client Needs:* Health Promotion and Maintenance
*Integrated Concept/Process:* Teaching/Learning
*Content Area:* Maternity

*Reference*
Lowdermilk, D., Perry, S., & Bobak, I. (2000). *Maternity & women's health care* (7th ed.). St. Louis: Mosby, p. 586.

---

**119.** A nurse is performing an assessment on a mother who just delivered a healthy newborn infant. The nurse checks the uterine fundus expecting to note that the fundus is positioned:
1   At the level of the umbilicus
2   Above the level of the umbilicus
3   One fingerbreadth above the symphysis pubis
4   To the right of the abdomen

**Answer: 1**
*Rationale:* Immediately after delivery, the uterine fundus should be at the level of the umbilicus or one to three fingerbreadths below it and in the midline of the abdomen. If the fundus is above the umbilicus, this may indicate that there are blood clots in the uterus that need to be expelled by fundal massage. A fundus that is not located in the midline may indicate a full bladder.

*Test-Taking Strategy:* Use the process of elimination, noting the key words *just delivered.* Use knowledge regarding normal anatomy and visualize each description in the options to direct you to option 1. If you had difficulty with this question, review normal postdelivery findings.

*Level of Cognitive Ability:* Analysis
*Client Needs:* Physiological Integrity
*Integrated Concept/Process:* Nursing Process/Assessment
*Content Area:* Maternity

*Reference*
Lowdermilk, D., Perry, S., & Bobak, I. (2000). *Maternity & women's health care* (7th ed.). St. Louis: Mosby, p. 593.

**120.** A nurse obtains the vital signs on a mother who delivered a healthy newborn infant 2 hours ago. The mother's temperature is 102° F. The most appropriate nursing action would be to:

1   Document the finding and recheck the temperature in 4 hours
2   Notify the physician
3   Administer acetaminophen (Tylenol) and recheck the temperature in 4 hours
4   Remove the blanket from the client's bed

**Answer: 2**

*Rationale:* Vital signs return to normal within the first hour postpartum if no complications arise. If the temperature is greater than 2° F above normal, this may indicate infection and the physician should be notified. Options 1, 3, and 4 are inaccurate nursing interventions for a temperature of 102° F 2 hours after delivery.

*Test-Taking Strategy:* Use the process of elimination and think about the normal postpartum findings. It is most appropriate in this situation to report the findings because a temperature of 102° F can indicate infection. Review normal vital signs following delivery and the appropriate nursing interventions if the vital signs are not within the normal range.

*Level of Cognitive Ability:* Application
*Client Needs:* Physiological Integrity
*Integrated Concept/Process:* Nursing Process/Implementation
*Content Area:* Maternity

*Reference*
Lowdermilk, D., Perry, S., & Bobak, I. (2000). *Maternity & women's health care* (7th ed.). St. Louis: Mosby, p. 615.

---

**121.** A nurse in a postpartum unit is caring for a mother after vaginal delivery of a healthy newborn infant. The client received epidural anesthesia for the delivery. Half an hour after the mother's admission to the postpartum unit, the nurse checks the client and suspects the presence of a vaginal hematoma. Which of the following findings would be the best indicator of the presence of this type of hematoma?

1   Client complaints of a tearing sensation
2   Client complaints of intense vaginal pressure
3   Changes in vital signs
4   Signs of vaginal bruising

**Answer: 3**

*Rationale:* Changes in vital signs indicate hypovolemia in the anesthetized postpartum woman with a vaginal hematoma. Because the client received an anesthetic, she would not feel pain or pressure or a tearing sensation. Vaginal bruising may be present, but this may be the result of the delivery process and additionally is not the best indicator of the presence of a hematoma.

*Test-Taking Strategy:* Focus on the data presented in the question. Noting that the client received an epidural anesthetic will assist in eliminating options 1 and 2. From the remaining options, recalling the pathophysiology associated with the development of a hematoma and use of the ABCs, airway, breathing, and circulation, will direct you to option 3. Review the signs of a vaginal hematoma if you had difficulty with this question.

*Level of Cognitive Ability:* Analysis
*Client Needs:* Physiological Integrity
*Integrated Concept/Process:* Nursing Process/Assessment
*Content Area:* Maternity

*Reference*
Lowdermilk, D., Perry, S., & Bobak, I. (2000). *Maternity & women's health care* (7th ed.). St. Louis: Mosby, p. 1023.

**122.** A nurse in the postpartum unit is developing a nursing care plan for a client following <u>cesarean delivery</u>. The nurse documents which intervention in the plan of care that will assist in preventing thrombophlebitis?

1  Frequent ambulation
2  Applying warm moist packs to the legs
3  Remaining on bed rest with the legs elevated
4  Wearing support stockings

**Answer: 1**

*Rationale:* Stasis is believed to be a major predisposing factor in the development of thrombophlebitis. Because cesarean delivery is a risk factor for the development of thrombophlebitis, the mother should ambulate early and frequently to promote circulation and prevent stasis. Bed rest is discouraged. Warm moist packs will not prevent thrombophlebitis. Support stockings may be a helpful measure in treating thrombophlebitis.

*Test-Taking Strategy:* Focus on the issue: to prevent thrombophlebitis. Also, use of basic principles related to nursing care and the prevention of complications following any type of abdominal surgery will direct you to option 1. Recall that thrombophlebitis results from the stasis of blood. Review content related to the prevention of thrombophlebitis in the postoperative period if you had difficulty with this question.

*Level of Cognitive Ability:* Application
*Client Needs:* Physiological Integrity
*Integrated Concept/Process:* Nursing Process/Planning
*Content Area:* Maternity

*Reference*
Lowdermilk, D., Perry, S., & Bobak, I. (2000). *Maternity & women's health care* (7th ed.). St. Louis: Mosby, p. 1031.

**123.** A nurse in the newborn nursery receives a telephone call from the delivery room and is told that a postterm small-for-gestational-age (SGA) newborn will be admitted to the nursery. The nurse develops a plan of care for the newborn and includes that the priority nursing action is to monitor:

1  Urinary output
2  Total bilirubin levels
3  Blood glucose levels
4  Hemoglobin and hematocrit

**Answer: 3**

*Rationale:* The most common metabolic complication in the SGA newborn is hypoglycemia, which can produce central nervous system abnormalities and mental retardation if not corrected immediately. Urinary output, although important, is not the highest priority action, because a postterm SGA newborn is typically dehydrated due to placental dysfunction. Hemoglobin and hematocrit levels are monitored because the postterm SGA newborn exhibits polycythemia, although this also does not require immediate attention. The polycythemia contributes to increased bilirubin levels, usually beginning on the second day after delivery.

*Test-Taking Strategy:* Note the key words *priority nursing action.* Recalling that the most common metabolic complication in the SGA newborn is hypoglycemia will direct you to option 3. Review the SGA newborn content if you had difficulty with this question.

*Level of Cognitive Ability:* Application
*Client Needs:* Physiological Integrity
*Integrated Concept/Process:* Nursing Process/Planning
*Content Area:* Maternity

*Reference*
Gorrie, T., McKinney, E., & Murray, S. (1998). *Foundations of maternal-newborn nursing* (2nd ed.). Philadelphia: W.B. Saunders, p. 841.

**124.** A nurse is caring for a client in the postpartum unit who suddenly exhibits signs of a pulmonary embolism. The nurse immediately prepares to:

1 Administer oxygen by face mask at 8 to 10 L/min
2 Administer pain medication
3 Administer antianxiety medication
4 Monitor the vital signs

**Answer: 1**

*Rationale:* Because pulmonary circulation is compromised in the presence of an embolus, cardiorespiratory support is initiated by oxygen administration. Although option 4 may be a component of care for the client with pulmonary embolism, the immediate action is to prepare to administer oxygen. Options 2 and 3 are not priority interventions.

*Test-Taking Strategy:* Note the key word *immediately.* Use the ABCs: airway, breathing, and circulation. In this case, the airway and breathing may be adequate; but circulation of oxygenated blood can best be supported with oxygen administration. Review immediate care measures for a client with pulmonary embolism if you had difficulty with this question.

*Level of Cognitive Ability:* Application
*Client Needs:* Physiological Integrity
*Integrated Concept/Process:* Nursing Process/Implementation
*Content Area:* Maternity

*Reference*
Gorrie, T., McKinney, E., & Murray, S. (1998). *Foundations of maternal-newborn nursing* (2nd ed.) Philadelphia: W.B. Saunders, p. 796.

---

**125.** A nurse in the newborn nursery receives a telephone call and is informed that a newborn infant with Apgar scores of 1 and 4 will be brought to the nursery. The nurse quickly prepares for the arrival of the newborn and determines that the priority intervention is to:

1 Connect the resuscitation bag to the oxygen
2 Turn on the apnea and cardiorespiratory monitor
3 Prepare for the insertion of an intravenous line with 5% dextrose in water
4 Set up the radiant warmer control temperature at 36.5° C (97.6° F)

**Answer: 1**

*Rationale:* The priority action for a newborn infant with low Apgar scores is airway, which would involve preparing respiratory resuscitation equipment. Options 2, 3, and 4 are also important although they are of lower priority. Setting up an IV with 5% dextrose in water would provide circulatory support. The radiant warmer will provide an external heat source, which is necessary to prevent further respiratory distress. The newborn infant's cardiopulmonary status would be monitored by a cardiorespiratory monitoring device.

*Test-Taking Strategy:* Note the key words *priority intervention.* This question asks you to prioritize care planning based on information about a newborn infant's condition. Use the ABCs, airway, breathing, circulation, to direct you to option 1. Although options 2, 3, and 4 are a component of the plan of care, option 1 is the priority. Review care of a newborn infant with a low Apgar score if you had difficulty with this question.

*Level of Cognitive Ability:* Application
*Client Needs:* Physiological Integrity
*Integrated Concept/Process:* Nursing Process/Implementation
*Content Area:* Maternity

*Reference*
Gorrie, T., McKinney, E., & Murray, S. (1998). *Foundations of maternal-newborn nursing* (2nd ed.). Philadelphia: W.B. Saunders, p. 328.

**126.** A nurse is caring for a client in labor who has butorphanol tartrate (Stadol) prescribed for the relief of labor pain. During the administration of the medication, the nurse would ensure that which of the following priority items were readily available?

1   An intravenous form of an antiemetic
2   Naloxone (Narcan)
3   An intravenous (IV) solution of normal saline
4   Meperidine hydrochloride (Demerol)

**Answer: 2**
*Rationale:* Stadol is an opioid analgesic that provides systemic pain relief during labor. The nurse would ensure that naloxone and resuscitation equipment are readily available to treat respiratory depression, should it occur. Although an antiemetic may be prescribed for vomiting, antiemetics may enhance the respiratory depressant effects of the butorphanol tartrate. Although an IV access may be desirable, option 3 is unrelated to the administration of this medication. Meperidine hydrochloride is also an opioid analgesic that may be used for the relief of pain, but it also causes respiratory depression.

*Test-Taking Strategy:* Use the process of elimination, focusing on the key words *readily available* in the question. Recalling that butorphanol tartrate causes respiratory depression will direct you to option 2. Review this medication and its use during labor if you had difficulty with this question.

*Level of Cognitive Ability:* Application
*Client Needs:* Physiological Integrity
*Integrated Concept/Process:* Nursing Process/Planning
*Content Area:* Maternity

*Reference*
Gorrie, T., McKinney, E., & Murray, S. (1998). *Foundations of maternal-newborn nursing* (2nd ed.) Philadelphia: W.B. Saunders, p. 374.

**127.** Methylergonovine (Methergine) is prescribed for a woman who has just delivered a healthy newborn infant. The priority assessment before administering the medication is to check the client's:

1   Lochia
2   Blood pressure
3   Deep tendon reflexes
4   Uterine tone

**Answer: 2**
*Rationale:* Methergine, an oxytocic, is an agent that is used to prevent or control postpartum hemorrhage by contracting the uterus. The immediate dose is administered intramuscularly, and then if still needed, is administered orally. It causes constant uterine contractions and may elevate the blood pressure. A priority assessment before the administration of methylergonovine is blood pressure. Methylergonovine is to be administered very cautiously in the presence of hypertension and the physician should be notified if hypertension is present. Options 1 and 4 are general components of care in the postpartum period. Option 3 is most specifically related to the administration of magnesium sulfate.

*Test-Taking Strategy:* Use the process of elimination. Options 1 and 4 can be eliminated first because lochia and uterine tone are similar and are general assessments related to the postpartum period. Next, note the key word *priority* and use the ABCs, airway, breathing, circulation, to direct you to option 2. Blood pressure is a method of assessing circulation. Additionally, option 3 can be eliminated because it is most specifically relates to the administration of magnesium sulfate. Review the nursing responsibilities related to the administration of methylergonovine if you had difficulty with this question.

*Level of Cognitive Ability:* Application
*Client's Needs:* Physiological Integrity
*Integrated Concept/Process:* Nursing Process/Assessment
*Content Area:* Maternity

*Reference*
Lowdermilk, D., Perry, S., & Bobak, I. (2000). *Maternity & women's health care* (7th ed.). St. Louis: Mosby, p. 1026.

---

128. A 30-week gestation woman is admitted to the maternity unit in preterm labor. Betamethasone (Celestone) is prescribed to be administered to the mother and the mother asks the nurse about the purpose of the medication. The nurse tells the mother that this medication will:
    1   Stop the premature uterine contractions
    2   Delay delivery for at least 48 hours
    3   Promote fetal lung maturity
    4   Prevent premature closure of the ductus arteriosus

**Answer: 3**
*Rationale:* Betamethasone (Celestone), a corticosteroid, is administered to increase the surfactant level and increase fetal lung maturity reducing the incidence of respiratory distress syndrome in the newborn infant. Surfactant production does not become stable until after 32 weeks' gestation. If adequate amounts of surfactant are not present in the lungs, respiratory distress and death is a possible consequence. Delivery needs to be delayed for at least 48 hours after the administration of betamethasone in order to allow time for the lungs to mature. Options 1, 2, and 4 are incorrect.

*Test-Taking Strategy:* Use the process of elimination. Eliminate options 1 and 2 first because they are similar and both relate to stopping labor. Recalling that respiratory distress syndrome caused by immature lungs is a major concern of prematurity will direct you to option 3 from the remaining options. Review the purpose of this medication if you had difficulty with this question.

*Level of Cognitive Ability:* Application
*Client's Needs:* Physiological Integrity
*Integrated Concept/Process:* Teaching/Learning
*Content Area:* Maternity

*Reference*
Lowdermilk, D., Perry, S., & Bobak, I. (2000). *Maternity & women's health care* (7th ed.). St. Louis: Mosby, p. 975.

---

129. A rubella vaccine is administered to a client who delivered a healthy newborn infant 2 days ago. The nurse provides instructions to the client regarding the potential risks associated with this vaccination. Which of the following statements if made by the client indicates an understanding of the medication?
    1   "I need to stay out of the sunlight for three days."
    2   "The injection site may itch but I can scratch it if I need to."
    3   "I need to prevent becoming pregnant for 2 to 3 months after the vaccination."
    4   "I need to avoid sexual intercourse for 2 to 3 months after the vaccination."

**Answer: 3**
*Rationale:* Rubella vaccine is a live attenuated virus that evokes an antibody response and provides immunity for fifteen years. Because rubella is a live vaccine, it will act as the virus and is potentially teratogenic in the organogenesis phase of fetal development. The client needs to be informed about the potential effects that this vaccine may have and the need to avoid becoming pregnant for a period of 2 to 3 months afterwards. Abstinence from sexual intercourse is not necessary, unless another form of effective contraception is not being used. The vaccine may cause local or systemic reactions but all are mild and short-lived. Sunlight has no effect on the person who is vaccinated.

*Test-Taking Strategy:* Use the process of elimination, recalling the effect of live vaccines on pregnancy and fetal development. Remembering that viruses can cross the placental barrier will direct you to option 3. If you had difficulty with this question, review the potential risks associated with the administration of this vaccine.

*Level of Cognitive Ability:* Analysis
*Client Needs:* Physiological Integrity
*Integrated Concept/Process:* Teaching/Learning
*Content Area:* Maternity

*Reference*
Lowdermilk, D., Perry, S., & Bobak, I. (2000). *Maternity & women's health care* (7th ed.). St. Louis: Mosby, p. 611.

---

**130.** A school nurse is planning to give a class on testicular self-examination (TSE) at a local high school. The nurse plans to include which of the following information on a written handout to be given to the students?

1 Roll the testicle between the thumb and forefinger
2 Perform the self-examination every other month
3 Perform the self-examination after a cold shower
4 Expect the self-examination to be slightly painful

**Answer: 1**

*Rationale:* Testicular self-examination is a self-screening examination for testicular cancer, which predominantly affects men in their late teens and twenties. The self-examination is performed once a month, as is breast-self examination. As an aid to remember to do it, the examination should be done on the same day each month. The scrotum is held in one hand and the testicle is rolled between the thumb and forefinger of the other hand. The self-examination should not be painful. It is easiest to do either during or after a warm shower (or bath) when the scrotum is relaxed.

*Test-Taking Strategy:* Use the process of elimination. Focus on the issue: self-examination, and read each option carefully. Use knowledge of physical examination techniques to direct you to option 1. If you are unfamiliar with the procedure for TSE, review this content.

*Level of Cognitive Ability:* Application
*Client Needs:* Health Promotion and Maintenance
*Integrated Concept/Process:* Teaching/Learning
*Content Area:* Adult Health/Oncology

*Reference*
Black, J., Hawks, J., & Keene, A. (2001). *Medical-surgical nursing: Clinical management for positive outcomes* (6th ed.). Philadelphia: W.B. Saunders, p. 41.

---

**131.** A 32-year-old female client has a history of fibrocystic disorder of the breasts. The nurse determines that the client understands the nature of this disorder if the client states that symptoms are more likely to occur:

1 Before menses
2 After menses
3 In the spring months
4 In the winter months

**Answer: 1**

*Rationale:* The client with fibrocystic breast disorder experiences worsening of symptoms (breast lumps, painful breasts, and possible nipple discharge) before the onset of menses. This is associated with cyclical hormone changes. Clients should understand that this is part of the clinical picture of this disorder. Options 2, 3, and 4 are incorrect.

*Test-Taking Strategy:* Note the key words *more likely*. This implies that there is a predictable variation in symptoms. Focus on the disorder and use knowledge of the effects of the various hormonal changes that occur in the body to direct you to option 1. If you had difficulty with this question, review the cyclical hormonal changes that occur in the female.

*Level of Cognitive Ability:* Analysis
*Client Needs:* Physiological Integrity
*Integrated Concept/Process:* Teaching/Learning
*Content Area:* Adult Health/Oncology

*Reference*
Beare, P., & Myers, J. (1998). *Adult health nursing* (3rd ed.). St. Louis: Mosby, p. 1685.

---

**132.** A client has undergone mastectomy. The nurse interprets that the client is having the most difficulty adjusting to the loss of the breast if which of the following behaviors is observed?
1   Refusing to look at the dressing
2   Asking for pain medication when needed
3   Performing arm exercises
4   Reading the postoperative care booklet

**Answer: 1**
*Rationale:* The client demonstrates the most difficult adjustment to the loss if the client refuses to look at the dressing. This indicates that the client is not ready or willing to begin to acknowledge and cope with the surgery. Asking for pain medication is an action-oriented option that is helpful, although there is no direct connection to adjustment to the loss of the breast. Reading the postoperative care booklet indicates an interest in self-care, and is a positive sign indicating beginning adjustment. Performing arm exercises is also an action-oriented behavior on the part of the client, and is considered a positive sign of adjustment.

*Test-Taking Strategy:* Note the key words *most difficulty* and focus on the issue. Note that options 2, 3, and 4 are similar and indicate a positive client action. Review psychosocial responses related to loss if you had difficulty with this question.

*Level of Cognitive Ability:* Analysis
*Client Needs:* Psychosocial Integrity
*Integrated Concept/Process:* Nursing Process/Evaluation
*Content Area:* Adult Health/Oncology

*Reference*
Beare, P., & Myers, J. (1998). *Adult health nursing* (3rd ed.). St. Louis: Mosby, p. 1692.

---

**133.** A client is preparing for discharge 10 days after a radical vulvectomy. The nurse evaluates that the client has the best understanding of the measures to prevent complications if the client plans to do which of the following after discharge?
1   Sit in a chair all day
2   Drive a car
3   Housework
4   Walking

**Answer: 4**
*Rationale:* The client should resume activity slowly, and walking is a beneficial activity. The client should know to rest when fatigue occurs. Activities to be avoided include driving, heavy housework, wearing tight clothing, crossing the legs, and prolonged standing or sitting. Sexual activity is prohibited for 4 to 6 weeks after surgery.

*Test-Taking Strategy:* Use the process of elimination. Note the key words *prevent complications*. With this in mind, evaluate each of the options in terms of the stress or harm it could cause to the perineal area. This will direct you to option 4. Review teaching points for the client following radical vulvectomy if you had difficulty with this question.

*Level of Cognitive Ability:* Analysis
*Client Needs:* Physiological Integrity
*Integrated Concept/Process:* Teaching/Learning
*Content Area:* Adult Health/Oncology

*Reference*
Beare, P., & Myers, J. (1998). *Adult health nursing* (3rd ed.). St. Louis: Mosby, p. 1684.

**134.** A client has undergone a vaginal hysterectomy. The nurse writes on the nursing care plan for this client that which of the following is to be avoided?
1  Elevating the knee gatch on the bed
2  Using pneumatic compression boots
3  Removing antiembolism stockings twice daily
4  Assisting with range-of-motion leg exercises

**Answer: 1**
*Rationale:* The client is at risk for deep vein thrombosis or thrombophlebitis after this surgery, as for any other major surgery. For this reason, the nurse implements measures that will prevent this complication. Range-of-motion exercises, antiembolism stockings, and pneumatic compression boots are all helpful. The nurse should avoid using the knee gatch in the bed, which inhibits venous return, and places the client more at risk for deep vein thrombosis or thrombophlebitis.

*Test-Taking Strategy:* Note the key word *avoided*. This tells you that the correct answer to the question is an incorrect nursing action. Use basic nursing knowledge of postoperative care to direct you to option 1. Review care of a client following hysterectomy if you had difficulty with this question.

*Level of Cognitive Ability:* Application
*Client Needs:* Physiological Integrity
*Integrated Concept/Process:* Nursing Process/Planning
*Content Area:* Adult Health/Oncology

*Reference*
Beare, P., & Myers, J. (1998). *Adult health nursing* (3rd ed.). St. Louis: Mosby, p. 1669.

**135.** At the beginning of the work shift, a nurse is checking a client who has returned from the postanesthesia care unit following transurethral resection of the prostate (TURP). The client has a bladder irrigation running via a three-way Foley catheter. The nurse would notify the physician if which of the following colors of the urine were noted in the urinary drainage bag?
1  Pale pink
2  Dark pink
3  Bright red
4  Tea colored

**Answer: 3**
*Rationale:* Bright red bleeding should be reported, because it could indicate complications. If the bladder irrigation is infusing at a sufficient rate, the urinary drainage will be pale pink. A dark pink color (sometimes referred to as punch-colored) indicates that the speed of the irrigation should be increased. Tea-colored urine is not seen after TURP, but may be described in the client with renal failure.

*Test-Taking Strategy:* Use the process of elimination, recalling that hemorrhage is a complication following any surgical procedure. Remember also that the purpose of a bladder irrigation is to flush out blood and clots that could otherwise accumulate in the bladder following surgery. With this in mind, select option 3 because bright red drainage would indicate a potential complication. Review care of a client following TURP if you had difficulty with this question.

*Level of Cognitive Ability:* Analysis
*Client Needs:* Physiological Integrity
*Integrated Concept/Process:* Nursing Process/Analysis
*Content Area:* Adult Health/Renal

*Reference*
Monahan, F., & Neighbors, M. (1998). *Medical-surgical nursing: Foundations for clinical practice* (2nd ed.). Philadelphia: W.B Saunders, p. 1711.

---

**136.** A nurse caring for a client immediately following transurethral resection of the prostate (TURP) notices that the client has suddenly become confused and disoriented. The nurse interprets that this may be due to which potential complication of this surgical procedure?
1  Hypernatremia
2  Hyponatremia
3  Hyperchloremia
4  Hypochloremia

**Answer: 2**
*Rationale:* The client who suddenly becomes disoriented and confused following TURP could be experiencing early signs of hyponatremia. This may occur because the flushing solution used during the operative procedure is hypotonic. If enough solution is absorbed through the prostate veins during surgery, the client experiences increased circulating volume and dilutional hyponatremia. The nurse needs to report these symptoms.

*Test-Taking Strategy:* Note the key words *potential complication.* Specific knowledge about the complications of this procedure is needed to answer this question. Review the complications related to TURP if you had difficulty with this question.

*Level of Cognitive Ability:* Analysis
*Client Needs:* Physiological Integrity
*Integrated Concept/Process:* Nursing Process/Analysis
*Content Area:* Adult Health/Renal

*Reference*
Monahan, F., & Neighbors, M. (1998). *Medical-surgical nursing: Foundations for clinical practice* (2nd ed.). Philadelphia: W.B Saunders, p. 1712.

---

**137.** A nurse is caring for a 25-year-old single client who will undergo bilateral orchidectomy for testicular cancer. The nurse would make it a priority to explore which of the following potential psychological concerns with this client?
1  Postoperative pain
2  Postoperative swelling
3  Length of recuperative period
4  Loss of reproductive ability

**Answer: 4**
*Rationale:* Although the client will need factual information about the postoperative period and recuperation, the nurse would place priority on addressing loss of reproductive ability as a psychological concern. The radical effects of this surgery in the reproductive area make it likely that the client may have some difficulty in adjustment to this consequence of surgery.

*Test-Taking Strategy:* Use the process of elimination, focusing on the client's diagnosis and surgical procedure. Eliminate options 1, 2, and 3 because they are general concerns of any surgical procedure. Option 4 is specific to an orchidectomy. Review the psychosocial issues related to an orchidectomy if you had difficulty with this question.

*Level of Cognitive Ability:* Application
*Client Needs:* Psychosocial Integrity
*Integrated Concept/Process:* Caring
*Content Area:* Adult Health/Oncology

*Reference*
Monahan, F., & Neighbors, M. (1998). *Medical-surgical nursing: Foundations for clinical practice* (2nd ed.). Philadelphia: W.B Saunders, p. 1709.

**138.** A nurse is assisting in participating in a prostate screening clinic for men. The nurse questions each client about which of the following signs of prostatism?
1 Excessive force in urinary stream
2 Hesitancy when initiating urinary stream
3 Ability to stop urinating quickly
4 Absence of postvoid dribbling

**Answer: 2**
*Rationale:* Signs of prostatism that may be reported to the nurse are reduced force and size of urinary stream, intermittent stream, hesitancy in beginning the flow of urine, inability to stop urinating quickly, a sensation of incomplete bladder emptying after voiding, and an increase in episodes of nocturia. These symptoms are the result of pressure of the enlarging prostate on the client's urethra.

*Test-Taking Strategy:* Use the process of elimination. Eliminate options 1, 3, and 4 because they are similar and indicate no difficulty with proper emptying of the bladder. Review the signs of prostatism if you had difficulty with this question.

*Level of Cognitive Ability:* Application
*Client Needs:* Health Promotion and Maintenance
*Integrated Concept/Process:* Nursing Process/Assessment
*Content Area:* Adult Health/Renal

*Reference*
Black, J., Hawks, J., & Keene, A. (2001). *Medical-surgical nursing: Clinical management for positive outcomes* (6th ed.). Philadelphia: W.B. Saunders, p. 962.

**139.** A male client being seen in the ambulatory care clinic has a history of being treated for syphilis infection. The nurse interprets that the client has been reinfected if which of the following characteristics is noted in a penile lesion?
1 Multiple vesicles, with some that have ruptured
2 Papular areas and erythema
3 Cauliflower-like appearance
4 Induration and absence of pain

**Answer: 4**
*Rationale:* The characteristic lesion of syphilis is painless and indurated. The lesion is referred to as a chancre. Genital herpes is accompanied by the presence of one or more vesicles that then rupture and heal. Scabies is characterized by erythematous, papular eruptions. Genital warts are characterized by cauliflower-like growths, or growths that are soft and fleshy.

*Test-Taking Strategy:* To answer this question accurately, it is necessary to be familiar with the characteristics of skin lesions of the various sexually transmitted diseases. If you had difficulty with this question, review the appearance of lesions associated with syphilis.

*Level of Cognitive Ability:* Analysis
*Client Needs:* Physiological Integrity
*Integrated Concept/Process:* Nursing Process/Assessment
*Content Area:* Adult Health/Integumentary

*Reference*
Monahan, F., & Neighbors, M. (1998). *Medical-surgical nursing: Foundations for clinical practice* (2nd ed.). Philadelphia: W.B Saunders, p. 1914.

**140.** An adult client has been admitted to the hospital with a 3-day history of uncontrolled vomiting and diarrhea. The nurse assesses for which of the following in this client?
1    Tenting of the skin
2    Bradycardia
3    Hypertension
4    Excitability

**Answer: 1**
*Rationale:* The client described in the question will most likely be dehydrated. The nurse assesses this client for weight loss, lethargy or headache, sunken eyes, poor skin turgor (such as tenting), flat neck and peripheral veins, tachycardia, and low blood pressure.

*Test-Taking Strategy:* Use the process of elimination, focusing on the data in the question. Recalling that a client who has a 3-day episode of uncontrolled vomiting and diarrhea is at risk for dehydration will direct you to option 1. If this question was difficult, review the signs of dehydration.

*Level of Cognitive Ability:* Analysis
*Client Needs:* Physiological Integrity
*Integrated Concept/Process:* Nursing Process/Assessment
*Content Area:* Adult Health/Gastrointestinal

*Reference*
Black, J., Hawks, J., & Keene, A. (2001). *Medical-surgical nursing: Clinical management for positive outcomes* (6th ed.). Philadelphia: W.B. Saunders, p. 222.

---

**141.** An adult client with renal insufficiency has been placed on a fluid restriction of 1200 mL per day. The nurse plans to allow the client to have how many mL of fluid from 7:00 A.M. to 3:00 P.M.?
1    1000
2    800
3    600
4    400

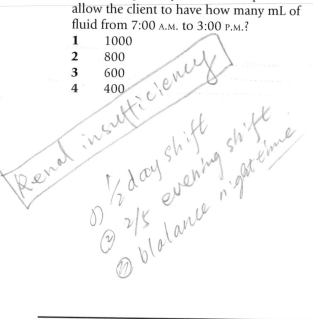

**Answer: 3**
*Rationale:* When calculating how to distribute a fluid restriction, the nurse usually allows half of the daily allotment (600 mL) during the day shift, when the client eats two meals and takes most medications. Another two fifths (480 mL) is allotted to the evening shift, with the balance (120 mL) allowed during the nighttime.

*Test-Taking Strategy:* To answer this question accurately, you must be familiar with fluid restriction and the general principles related to fluid distribution over a 24-hour period. If this question was difficult, review these principles and calculation of fluid distribution in the client with renal insufficiency.

*Level of Cognitive Ability:* Application
*Client Needs:* Physiological Integrity
*Integrated Concept/Process:* Nursing Process/Planning
*Content Area:* Adult Health/Renal

*Reference*
Black, J., Hawks, J., & Keene, A. (2001). *Medical-surgical nursing: Clinical management for positive outcomes* (6th ed.). Philadelphia: W.B. Saunders, p. 879.

**142.** A client with chronic renal failure (CRF) has learned about managing diet and fluid restriction between dialysis treatments. The nurse evaluates that the client is compliant with the therapeutic regimen if the client gains no more than how much weight between hemodialysis treatments?

1   0.5 to 1.0 kg
2   1 to 1.5 kg
3   2 to 4 kg
4   5 to 6 kg

**Answer: 2**

*Rationale:* A limit of 1 to 1.5 kg of weight gain between dialysis treatments helps prevent hypotension that tends to occur during dialysis with the removal of larger fluid loads. The nurse evaluates that the client is compliant with fluid restriction if this weight gain is not exceeded.

*Test-Taking Strategy:* It may be helpful in answering this question to recall that one liter of fluid weighs approximately 1 kg. Recalling that there are approximately 6 L of blood circulating in the body will assist in eliminating options 3 and 4 as being amounts that are too large. Correspondingly, option 1 is eliminated because the amount is too small, representing only 500 to 1000 mL of fluid. Review teaching points for the client with CRF if you had difficulty with this question.

*Level of Cognitive Ability:* Analysis
*Client Needs:* Health Promotion and Maintenance
*Integrated Concept/Process:* Nursing Process/Evaluation
*Content Area:* Adult Health/Renal

*Reference*
Black, J., Hawks, J., & Keene, A. (2001). *Medical-surgical nursing: Clinical management for positive outcomes* (6th ed.). Philadelphia: W.B. Saunders, p. 879.

**143.** A client with chronic renal failure (CRF) has received dietary counseling about potassium restriction in the diet. The nurse determines that the client has learned the information correctly if the client states to do which of the following for preparation of vegetables?

1   Eat only fresh vegetables
2   Buy frozen vegetables whenever possible
3   Use salt substitute on them liberally
4   Boil them and discard the water

**Answer: 4**

*Rationale:* The potassium content of vegetables can be reduced by boiling them and discarding the cooking water. Options 1 and 2 are incorrect. Clients with renal failure should avoid the use of salt substitutes altogether, because they tend to be high in potassium content.

*Test-Taking Strategy:* Use the process of elimination, recalling which foods are high in potassium, and how to reduce their potassium content. Options 2 and 3 can be eliminated first, using basic principles of nutrition. Eliminate option 1 next, noting the word *only* in this option. Review client teaching points related to potassium restrictions if you had difficulty with this question.

*Level of Cognitive Ability:* Analysis
*Client Needs:* Health Promotion and Maintenance
*Integrated Concept/Process:* Teaching/Learning
*Content Area:* Adult Health/Renal

*Reference*
Peckenpaugh, N., & Poleman, C. (1999). *Nutrition essentials and diet therapy* (8th ed.) Philadelphia: W.B. Saunders, p. 147.

**144.** A client with chronic renal failure (CRF) has a protein restriction in the diet. The nurse would include in a teaching plan to avoid which of the following sources of incomplete protein in the diet?

1   Nuts
2   Eggs
3   Milk
4   Fish

**Answer: 1**

*Rationale:* The client whose diet has a protein restriction should be careful to ensure that the proteins eaten are complete proteins with the highest biologic value. Foods such as meat, fish, milk, and eggs are complete proteins, which are optimal for the client with CRF.

*Test-Taking Strategy:* Focus on the issue: protein composition of various foods. Note the key words *avoid* and *incomplete protein* to direct you to option 1. Review foods that are complete and incomplete proteins if you had difficulty with this question.

*Level of Cognitive Ability:* Application
*Client Needs:* Health Promotion and Maintenance
*Integrated Concept/Process:* Teaching/Learning
*Content Area:* Adult Health/Renal

*Reference*
Peckenpaugh, N., & Poleman, C. (1999). *Nutrition essentials and diet therapy* (8th ed.) Philadelphia: W.B. Saunders, p. 146.

---

**145.** A nurse is administering epoetin alfa (Epogen) to a client with chronic renal failure (CRF). The nurse monitors the client for which of the following adverse effects of this therapy?

1   Anemia
2   Hypertension
3   Iron intoxication
4   Bleeding tendencies

**Answer: 2**

*Rationale:* The client taking epoetin alfa is at risk of hypertension and seizure activity as the most serious adverse effects of therapy. This medication is used to treat anemia. The medication does not cause iron intoxication. Bleeding tendencies is not an adverse effect of this medication.

*Test-Taking Strategy:* Knowledge regarding the adverse effects of this medication is needed to answer this question. Review this medication if you had difficulty with this medication.

*Level of Cognitive Ability:* Analysis
*Client Needs:* Physiological Integrity
*Integrated Concept/Process:* Nursing Process/Assessment
*Content Area:* Adult Health/Renal

*Reference*
Hodgson, B., & Kizior, R. (2001). *Saunders Nursing drug handbook 2001*. Philadelphia: W.B. Saunders, p. 359.

---

**146.** A client with chronic renal failure has started receiving epoetin alfa (Epogen). The nurse reminds the client about the importance of taking which of the following prescribed medications to enhance the effects of this therapy?

1   Calcium carbonate (Tums)
2   Aluminum hydroxide gel (Amphogel)
3   Iron supplement
4   Aluminum carbonate (Basaljel)

**Answer: 3**

*Rationale:* In order to form healthy red blood cells, which is the purpose of epoetin alfa, the body needs adequate stores of iron, folic acid, and vitamin $B_{12}$. The client should take these supplements regularly to enhance the hematocrit raising benefit of this medication. The other options are incorrect.

*Test-Taking Strategy:* Use the process of elimination. Recall that this medication is used to stimulate red blood cell formation, and that adequate body stores of vitamins and iron are needed to achieve this effect. Also, note that options 1, 2, and 4 are similar in that they are antacids. Review client teaching points regarding this medication if you had difficulty with this question.

*Level of Cognitive Ability:* Application
*Client Needs:* Physiological Integrity
*Integrated Concept/Process:* Teaching/Learning
*Content Area:* Adult Health/Renal

**Reference**
Hodgson, B., & Kizior, R. (2001). *Saunders Nursing drug handbook 2001.* Philadelphia: W.B. Saunders, p. 359.

---

**147.** A client scheduled for a transurethral prostatectomy (TURP) has listened to the surgeon's explanation of the surgery. The client later asks the nurse to explain again how the prostate is going to be removed. The nurse tells the client that the prostate will be removed through:

1  The urethra using a cutting wire
2  An incision made in the perineal area
3  An upper abdominal incision
4  A lower abdominal incision

**Answer: 1**
*Rationale:* A TURP is done through the urethra. An instrument called a resectoscope is used to cut the tissue using high-frequency current. An incision between the scrotum and anus is made when a perineal prostatectomy is performed. A lower abdominal incision is used for suprapubic or retropubic prostatectomy. An upper abdominal incision is not used.

*Test-Taking Strategy:* Use the process of elimination. Note the relationship between the name of the procedure: *transurethral* in the question and the word *urethra* in the correct option. Review this procedure if you had difficulty with this question.

*Level of Cognitive Ability:* Application
*Client Needs:* Physiological Integrity
*Integrated Concept/Process:* Teaching/Learning
*Content Area:* Adult Health/Renal

**Reference**
Monahan, F., & Neighbors, M. (1998). *Medical-surgical nursing: Foundations for clinical practice* (2nd ed.). Philadelphia: W.B Saunders, p. 1710.

---

**148.** A client is being discharged to home after undergoing a transurethral prostatectomy (TURP). The nurse teaches the client to expect which of the following variations in normal urine color for several days following the procedure?

1  Clear yellow
2  Cloudy amber
3  Pink-tinged
4  Dark red

**Answer: 3**
*Rationale:* The client should expect that the urine will be pink-tinged for several days following this procedure. Dark red urine may be present initially, especially with inadequate bladder irrigation, and if it occurs, it must be corrected. Options 1 and 2 are incorrect, since urine of these colors is not generally expected for several days following surgery.

*Test-Taking Strategy:* Note the issue, a client being discharged to home after a TURP. Eliminate options 1 and 2 because they are similar. From the remaining options, focus on the issue to direct you to option 3. Review assessment of the urine for the client who has had this type of surgery if you had difficulty with this question.

*Level of Cognitive Ability:* Application
*Client Needs:* Health Promotion and Maintenance
*Integrated Concept/Process:* Teaching/Learning
*Content Area:* Adult Health/Renal

**Reference**
Monahan, F., & Neighbors, M. (1998). *Medical-surgical nursing: Foundations for clinical practice* (2nd ed.). Philadelphia: W.B Saunders, p. 1712.

**149.** A nurse is planning to do preoperative teaching with a client scheduled for a transurethral resection of the prostate (TURP). The nurse plans to include in the discussion that the most frequent cause of postoperative pain will be:
1 The lower abdominal incision
2 Bleeding within the bladder
3 Bladder spasms
4 Tension on the Foley catheter

**Answer: 3**

*Rationale:* Bladder spasms can occur after this surgery because of postoperative bladder distention or irritation from the balloon on the indwelling urinary catheter. The nurse administers antispasmodic medications, such as belladonna and opium to treat this type of pain. There is no incision with a TURP (option 1). Options 2 and 4 are not frequent causes of pain. Some surgeons purposefully apply tension to the catheter for a few hours postoperatively to control bleeding.

*Test-Taking Strategy:* Use the process of elimination, focusing on the surgical procedure. Eliminate option 1 knowing that there is no incision with this procedure. Eliminate options 2 and 4 because they are unrelated to the cause of pain. If this question was difficult, review the causes of pain following this type of surgery.

*Level of Cognitive Ability:* Application
*Client Needs:* Physiological Integrity
*Integrated Concept/Process:* Nursing Process/Planning
*Content Area:* Adult Health/Renal

*Reference*
Monahan, F., & Neighbors, M. (1998). *Medical-surgical nursing: Foundations for clinical practice* (2nd ed.). Philadelphia: W.B Saunders, p. 1710.

**150.** A nurse is preparing a poster for a booth at a health fair to promote primary prevention of cervical cancer. The nurse includes which of the following recommendations on the poster?
1 Perform monthly breast self-examination (BSE)
2 Use oral contraceptives as a preferred method of birth control
3 Use a commercial douche on a daily basis
4 Seek treatment promptly for infections of the cervix

**Answer: 4**

*Rationale:* Early treatment of cervical infection can help prevent chronic cervicitis, which can lead to dysplasia of the cervix. Cervical dysplasia is an early cell change that is considered to be premalignant. Oral contraceptives and douches do not decrease the risk for this type of cancer. BSE is useful for early detection of breast cancer, but is unrelated to cervical cancer.

*Test-Taking Strategy:* Note the key words *primary prevention* and *cervical cancer*. Eliminate option 1 because it is unrelated to cervical cancer. From the remaining options, recalling the risk factors associated with this type of cancer will easily direct you to option 4. Review the risk factors associated with cervical cancer if you had difficulty with this question.

*Level of Cognitive Ability:* Application
*Client Needs:* Health Promotion and Maintenance
*Integrated Concept/Process:* Teaching/Learning
*Content Area:* Adult Health/Oncology

*Reference*
Black, J., Hawks, J., & Keene, A. (2001). *Medical-surgical nursing: Clinical management for positive outcomes* (6th ed.). Philadelphia: W.B. Saunders, p. 995.

**151.** A client had a positive Papanicolaou smear and underwent cryosurgery with laser therapy. The nurse would give the client which of the following pieces of information before letting the client go home?

1 There should be no odor or vaginal discharge
2 Vaginal discharge should be clear and watery
3 Sitz baths are soothing to the irritated tissues
4 Pain can be relieved with narcotic analgesics

**Answer: 2**

*Rationale:* Vaginal discharge should be clear and watery following the procedure. The client will then begin to slough off dead cell debris, which may be odorous. This resolves within approximately 8 weeks. Tub and sitz baths are avoided while the area is healing, which takes about 10 weeks. There is mild pain following the procedure and narcotic analgesics would not be required.

*Test-Taking Strategy:* Specific knowledge about the purpose and effects of this procedure is needed to answer the question. Review this surgical procedure and the client teaching points if you had difficulty with this question.

*Level of Cognitive Ability:* Application
*Client Needs:* Physiological Integrity
*Integrated Concept/Process:* Teaching/Learning
*Content Area:* Adult Health/Oncology

*Reference*
Black, J., Hawks, J., & Keene, A. (2001). *Medical-surgical nursing: Clinical management for positive outcomes* (6th ed.). Philadelphia: W.B. Saunders, p. 997.

**152.** A client is admitted to the hospital with a diagnosis of infiltrating ductal carcinoma of the breast. The nurse assesses this client for which of the following expected manifestations?

1 Bilateral palpable masses
2 A fixed, irregularly shaped mass
3 A round-shaped mass that is moveable
4 Pain in the breast and edema

**Answer: 2**

*Rationale:* Infiltrating ductal carcinoma of the breast usually presents as a fixed, irregularly shaped mass. The mass is usually single and unilateral, and is painless, nontender, and hard to the touch.

*Test-Taking Strategy:* Use the process of elimination. Using principles of anatomy and knowledge regarding the characteristics of a cancerous lesion will assist in eliminating options 1 and 3 first. Choose option 2 over option 4, recalling that pain is generally a late sign of this disorder, and that involvement of the ducts makes it more likely that the mass does not move (fixed). Review the characteristics of breast cancer if you had difficulty with this question.

*Level of Cognitive Ability:* Application
*Client Needs:* Physiological Integrity
*Integrated Concept/Process:* Nursing Process/Assessment
*Content Area:* Adult Health/Oncology

*Reference*
Black, J., Hawks, J., & Keene, A. (2001). *Medical-surgical nursing: Clinical management for positive outcomes* (6th ed.). Philadelphia: W.B. Saunders, p. 1011.

**153.** A postmastectomy client has been found to have an estrogen receptor–positive tumor. The nurse interprets after reading this information in the pathology report that the client will most likely have which common follow-up treatment prescribed?
  1  Administration of estrogen
  2  Administration of progesterone
  3  Administration of tamoxifen (Nolvadex)
  4  Removal of the ovaries

**Answer: 3**
*Rationale:* A common treatment for women with estrogen receptor–positive breast tumors is follow-up treatment with tamoxifen. This medication is classified as an antineoplastic agent, and competes with estrogen for binding sites in the breast and other tissues. The medication may be administered for years following surgery. Options 1, 2, and 4 are incorrect.

*Test-Taking Strategy:* Note the key words *estrogen receptor–positive* and *common treatment.* These key words will assist in eliminating option 1. From the remaining options it is necessary to know the action of the tamoxifen. Review the action and use of this medication if you had difficulty with this question.

*Level of Cognitive Ability:* Analysis
*Client Needs:* Physiological Integrity
*Integrated Concept/Process:* Nursing Process/Analysis
*Content Area:* Adult Health/Oncology

*Reference*
Black, J., Hawks, J., & Keene, A. (2001). *Medical-surgical nursing: Clinical management for positive outcomes* (6th ed.). Philadelphia: W.B. Saunders, p. 1020.

**154.** A client has been taking metoclopramide (Reglan) on a long-term basis. A nurse monitors for which potentially irreversible side effect?
  1  Tardive dyskinesia
  2  Irritability
  3  Anxiety
  4  Excitability

**Answer: 1**
*Rationale:* If the client experiences tardive dyskinesia (rhythmic movements of the face or limbs), the nurse should withhold the medication and call the physician. These side effects may be irreversible. Excitability is not a side effect of this medication. Anxiety, irritability, and dry mouth are milder side effects that are not harmful to the client.

*Test-Taking Strategy:* Use the process of elimination. Eliminate options 2, 3, and 4 because they are similar. Review the side effects of this medication and the signs of tardive dyskinesia if you had difficulty with this question.

*Level of Cognitive Ability:* Application
*Client Needs:* Physiological Integrity
*Integrated Concept/Process:* Nursing Process/Assessment
*Content Area:* Pharmacology

*Reference*
Deglin, J., & Vallerand, A. (1999). *Davis's Drug guide for nurses* (6th ed.). Philadelphia: F.A. Davis, p. 643.

**155.** A client has had a left mastectomy with axillary lymph node dissection. The nurse determines that the client understands postoperative restrictions and arm care if the client states to:
1   Use a straight razor to shave under the arms
2   Allow blood pressures to be taken only on the left arm
3   Carry a handbag and heavy objects on the left arm
4   Use gloves when working in the garden

**Answer: 4**
*Rationale:* The client is at risk for edema and infection as a result of lymph node dissection. The client should avoid activities that increase edema such as carrying heavy objects or having blood pressures taken on the affected arm. The client should also use a variety of techniques to avoid trauma to the affected arm. Examples include using an electric razor to shave under the arm, use of gloves when working in the garden, and the use of potholders when cooking.

*Test-Taking Strategy:* Note the surgical procedure and focus on the issue: postoperative restrictions and arm care. Keeping this issue in mind, read each option noting the potential risk related to edema or trauma. This will direct you to option 4. Review teaching points for the client following mastectomy if you had difficulty with this question.

*Level of Cognitive Ability:* Analysis
*Client Needs:* Health Promotion and Maintenance
*Integrated Concept/Process:* Teaching/Learning
*Content Area:* Adult Health/Oncology

*Reference*
Black, J., Hawks, J., & Keene, A. (2001). *Medical-surgical nursing: Clinical management for positive outcomes* (6th ed.). Philadelphia: W.B. Saunders, p. 1020.

**156.** A nurse is teaching a client about the modifiable risk factors that can reduce the risk for colorectal cancer. The nurse places highest priority on discussing which of the following risk factors with this client?
1   Personal history of ulcerative colitis or gastrointestinal (GI) polyps
2   Distant relative with colorectal cancer
3   Age over 30 years
4   High-fat, low-fiber diet

**Answer: 4**
*Rationale:* Common risk factors for colorectal cancer that cannot be changed include age over 40, first-degree relative with colorectal cancer, and history of bowel problems such as ulcerative colitis or familial polyposis. Clients should be aware of modifiable risk factors as part of general health maintenance and primary disease prevention. Modifiable risk factors are those that can be reduced, and include a high-fat and low-fiber diet.

*Test-Taking Strategy:* Focus on the issue: modifiable risk factors related to colorectal cancer. Note the key words *reduce the risk* and *highest priority*. Recalling that modifiable risk factors are those that can be changed will direct you to option 4. Review modifiable and nonmodifiable risk factors related to colorectal cancer if you had difficulty with this question.

*Level of Cognitive Ability:* Application
*Client Needs:* Health Promotion and Maintenance
*Integrated Concept/Process:* Teaching/Learning
*Content Area:* Adult Health/Gastrointestinal

*Reference*
Monahan, F., & Neighbors, M. (1998). *Medical-surgical nursing: Foundations for clinical practice* (2nd ed.). Philadelphia: W.B. Saunders, p. 969.

**157.** A client with gastroesophageal reflux disease (GERD) complains of chest discomfort that feels like heartburn following each meal. After teaching the client to take antacids as prescribed, the nurse suggests that the client lie in which of the following positions to aid in relief?
1 On the left side with the head elevated 30 degrees
2 On the right side with the head elevated 30 degrees
3 Supine with the head of bed flat
4 On the stomach with the head of the bed flat

**Answer: 1**
*Rationale:* The discomfort of reflux is aggravated by positions that compress the abdomen and the stomach. These include lying flat either on the back or stomach after a meal, or lying on the right side. The left side-lying position with the head elevated is most likely to give relief to the client.

*Test-Taking Strategy:* Use the process of elimination and think about the anatomical location of the stomach. Evaluate each of the positions described in terms of their ability to put pressure on the stomach and cause reflux. This will direct you to option 1. Review measures that will reduce discomfort in the client with GERD if you had difficulty with this question.

*Level of Cognitive Ability:* Application
*Client Needs:* Physiological Integrity
*Integrated Concept/Process:* Teaching/Learning
*Content Area:* Adult Health/Gastrointestinal

*Reference*
Beare, P., & Myers, J. (1998). *Adult health nursing* (3rd ed.). St. Louis: Mosby, p. 1485.

**158.** A client with gastroesophageal reflux disease (GERD) has just received a breakfast tray. The nurse setting up the tray for the client notices that which of the following foods is the only one that will increase the lower esophageal sphincter (LES) pressure and thus lessen the client's symptoms?
1 Fresh scrambled eggs
2 Nonfat milk
3 Whole-wheat toast with butter
4 Coffee

**Answer: 2**
*Rationale:* Foods that increase the LES pressure will decrease reflux, and lessen the symptoms of GERD. The food substance that will increase the LES pressure is nonfat milk. The other substances listed decrease the LES pressure, thus increasing reflux symptoms. Aggravating substances include chocolate, coffee, fatty foods, and alcohol.

*Test-Taking Strategy:* Use the process of elimination and recall the effect of various food substances on LES pressure and GERD. Also, noting the key word *nonfat* will assist in directing you to option 2. If you are unfamiliar with the LES pressure and the foods that will increase this pressure, review this content.

*Level of Cognitive Ability:* Analysis
*Client Needs:* Physiological Integrity
*Integrated Concept/Process:* Nursing Process/Analysis
*Content Area:* Adult Health/Gastrointestinal

*Reference*
Beare, P., & Myers, J. (1998). *Adult health nursing* (3rd ed.). St. Louis: Mosby, p. 1484.

**159.** A nurse is preparing to care for a client who has undergone esophagogastroduodenoscopy (EGD). The nurse would do which of the following first after checking the client's vital signs?
1   Monitor for sharp epigastric pain
2   Monitor for complaints of heartburn
3   Check for the return of the gag reflex
4   Give warm gargles for sore throat

**Answer: 3**
*Rationale:* The nurse places highest priority on assessing for the return of the gag reflex, which is part of maintaining the client's airway. The nurse would monitor the client for sharp pain (may indicate a potential complication) and heartburn. The client would also receive warm gargles, but this cannot be done until the gag reflex has returned.

*Test-Taking Strategy:* Note the key word *first.* Use the ABCs, airway, breathing, and circulation, to direct you to option 3. Review postprocedure care following an EGD if you had difficulty with question.

*Level of Cognitive Ability:* Application
*Client Needs:* Physiological Integrity
*Integrated Concept/Process:* Nursing Process/Implementation
*Content Area:* Adult Health/Gastrointestinal

*Reference*
Beare, P., & Myers, J. (1998). *Adult health nursing* (3rd ed.). St. Louis: Mosby, p. 1465.

---

**160.** A nurse plans to teach a client about an upcoming endoscopic retrograde cholangiopancreatography (ERCP) procedure. The nurse avoids telling the client that:
1   A signed informed consent is necessary
2   It is important to lie still during the procedure
3   Medication will be given orally for sedation
4   An anesthetic throat spray will be used

**Answer: 3**
*Rationale:* The client needs to lie still for ERCP, which takes about an hour to perform. The client also has to sign a consent form. IV sedation (not oral) is given to relax the client, and an anesthetic throat spray is used to help keep the client from gagging as the endoscope is passed.

*Test-Taking Strategy:* Note the key word *avoids* in the stem of the question. Recalling that this procedure is endoscopic and noting the word *orally* in option 3 will direct you to this option. Review preprocedure care for an ERCP if you had difficulty with this question.

*Level of Cognitive Ability:* Application
*Client Needs:* Physiological Integrity
*Integrated Concept/Process:* Teaching/Learning
*Content Area:* Adult Health/Gastrointestinal

*Reference*
Beare, P., & Myers, J. (1998). *Adult health nursing* (3rd ed.). St. Louis: Mosby, p. 1472.

**161.** A client has been scheduled for a barium swallow (esophagography) the next day. The nurse determines that the client understands preprocedure instructions if the client states to do which of the following before the test?
1 Take all oral medications as scheduled
2 Monitor own bowel movement pattern for constipation
3 Remove all metal and jewelry
4 Eat a regular breakfast on the day of the test

**Answer: 3**
*Rationale:* A barium swallow, or esophagography, is an x-ray that uses a substance called barium for contrast to highlight abnormalities in the gastrointestinal (GI) tract. The client is told to remove all jewelry before the test, so it won't interfere with x-ray visualization of the field. The client should fast for 8 to 12 hours before the test, depending on physician instructions. Most oral medications are also withheld before the test. It is important after the procedure to monitor for constipation, which can occur as a result of the presence of barium in the GI tract.

*Test-Taking Strategy:* Note the key words *barium swallow* and *before the test*. This tells you that the correct option is an item that the client needs to comply with before the test is done. Eliminate option 2 first, since it is a part of aftercare. Knowing that the procedure is a type of x-ray that involves barium and that the client needs to remain NPO will assist in eliminating options 1 and 4. Review preprocedure care for a barium swallow if you had difficulty with this question.

*Level of Cognitive Ability:* Analysis
*Client Needs:* Physiological Integrity
*Integrated Concept/Process:* Teaching/Learning
*Content Area:* Adult Health/Gastrointestinal

*Reference*
Beare, P., & Myers, J. (1998). *Adult health nursing* (3rd ed.). St. Louis: Mosby, p. 1465.

**162.** A physician orders a chemotherapy medication dose that the nurse believes is too high. The nurse calls the physician but the physician has left the office for the weekend. The nurse most appropriately:
1 Checks with the pharmacist, who agrees the dose is too high, and then reduces the dose accordingly
2 Withholds giving the medication until the physician's partner makes rounds the following day
3 Reschedules the client's chemotherapy until the following week
4 Calls the answering service, and confers with the on-call physician

**Answer: 4**
*Rationale:* If the nurse believes a physician's order to be in error, the nurse is responsible for clarifying the order before carrying out the order. Checking with the pharmacist can assist the nurse in determining whether the dose ordered is incorrect, but the nurse or pharmacist cannot alter the dose without an order from the physician. Withholding the medication until the following day is incorrect. Chemotherapy agents must often be administered in the proper combinations or sequence in order to be effective. Rescheduling the client's chemotherapy is also incorrect. Chemotherapy must be administered on a specific schedule for maximum effect with minimum adverse effects. Additionally, the nurse cannot withhold or reschedule chemotherapy without a physician's order.

*Test-Taking Strategy:* Use the process of elimination and knowledge of the legal responsibilities of the nurse in regard to physician's orders and medication administration. Remember, a nurse cannot alter, withhold, or reschedule a medication dose. Review these legal responsibilities if you had difficulty with this question.

*Level of Cognitive Ability:* Application
*Client Needs:* Safe, Effective Care Environment

*Integrated Concept/Process:* Nursing Process/Implementation
*Content Area:* Fundamental Skills

*Reference*
Leahy, J., & Kizilay, P. (1998). *Foundations of nursing practice: A nursing process approach.* Philadelphia: W.B. Saunders, pp. 198-199.

---

**163.** A nurse working in a long-term care setting has recently attended a workshop on creating a restraint-free environment for the residents. Several coworkers have been employed in this facility for many years, and firmly believe that their current methods are satisfactory. The nurse can be effective in facilitating change by:
1   Informing the nursing supervisor that current restraint policies must be changed and requesting that all staff be required to comply
2   Writing a new restraint policy over the weekend and distributing it to coworkers for immediate implementation on Monday morning
3   Asking coworkers to help gather data comparing the facility's restraint procedures and outcomes with those of others using revised or updated procedures
4   Pointing out to coworkers the various mistakes that they are presently making in adhering to outdated restraint procedures

**Answer: 3**
*Rationale:* To be an effective leader, the nurse must work collaboratively with others to solve common problems. The nurse who works collaboratively with others to facilitate change has a much greater chance of success than one who unilaterally demands or implements change. By enlisting the assistance of others, there is a greater chance that they will support proposed changes in procedures. A punitive atmosphere is not effective in promoting change, because it discourages people from taking risks. To focus on errors (perceived or real), serves only to alienate others and is not effective in promoting change.

*Test-Taking Strategy:* Use the process of elimination, remembering that to facilitate change, collaboration between the nurse and coworkers is important. Additionally, options 1, 2, and 4 focus on unilateral actions by the nurse. Review the change process if you had difficulty with this question.

*Level of Cognitive Ability:* Application
*Client Needs:* Safe, Effective Care Environment
*Integrated Concept/Process:* Nursing Process/Implementation
*Content Area:* Fundamental Skills

*Reference*
Leahy, J., & Kizilay, P. (1998). *Foundations of nursing practice: A nursing process approach.* Philadelphia: W.B. Saunders, p. 104.

---

**164.** A client being discharged from the hospital with a diagnosis of gastric ulcer has an order for sucralfate (Carafate) 1 gram by mouth qid. The nurse interprets that the client understands proper use of the medication if the client states to take it:
1   Every 6 hours around the clock
2   1 hour after meals and at bedtime
3   With meals and at bedtime
4   1 hour before meals and at bedtime

**Answer: 4**
*Rationale:* The medication should be scheduled for administration 1 hour before meals and at bedtime. This timing will allow the medication to form a protective coating over the ulcer before it becomes irritated by food intake, gastric acid production, and mechanical movement. The other options are incorrect.

*Test-Taking Strategy:* Use the process of elimination. Recalling the action of this medication, to form a protective coating, will direct you to option 4. Review client teaching points regarding this medication if you had difficulty with this question.

*Level of Cognitive Ability:* Analysis
*Client Needs:* Physiological Integrity
*Integrated Concept/Process:* Teaching/Learning
*Content Area:* Pharmacology

*Reference*
Deglin, J., & Vallerand, A. (1999). *Davis's Drug guide for nurses* (6th ed.). Philadelphia: F.A. Davis, p. 936.

**165.** A newborn infant is brought to the mother after triple dye has been applied to the infant's umbilical cord. The nurse tells the mother that triple dye is used:

1 For initial cord care because it minimizes bacteria and promotes drying
2 For initial cord care because it makes the cord drop off in 5 to 7 days
3 To prevent the cord from hemorrhaging after birth
4 To prevent *Staphylococcus aureus* colonization

**Answer: 1**
*Rationale:* The umbilical cord begins to dry after delivery. The triple dye prevents bacterial colonization and aids in the drying process. Options 2, 3, and 4 are incorrect.

*Test-Taking Strategy:* Use the process of elimination. Eliminate option 2 because the cord drops off in 7 to 14 days. Option 3 is incorrect because triple dye does not prevent hemorrhaging. From the remaining options, select option 1 because it is the global option. Review the principles of cord care if you had difficulty with this question.

*Level of Cognitive Ability:* Application
*Client Needs:* Physiological Integrity
*Integrated Concept/Process:* Teaching/Learning
*Content Area:* Maternity

*Reference*
Lowdermilk, D., Perry, S., & Bobak, I. (2000). *Maternity & women's health care* (7th ed.). St. Louis: Mosby, p. 725.

---

**166.** A client was admitted to the hospital with a diagnosis of frequent symptomatic premature ventricular contractions (PVCs). After sitting up in a chair for a few minutes, the client complains of feeling lightheaded. On auscultation of the heart beat, the nurse would most likely expect to note:

1 A regular apical pulse
2 An irregular apical pulse
3 A very rapid, regular apical pulse
4 A very slow, regular apical pulse

**Answer: 2**
*Rationale:* The most accurate means of assessing pulse rhythm is by auscultation of the apical pulse. When a client has PVCs, the rate is irregular and if the radial pulse is taken, a true picture of what is happening is not obtained. A very fast regular apical pulse indicates tachycardia. A very slow regular apical pulse indicates bradycardia.

*Test-Taking Strategy:* Use the process of elimination, focusing on the issue, PVCs. Eliminate options 1, 3, and 4 because they are similar and indicate a regular pulse. Review the manifestations associated with PVCs if you had difficulty with this question.

*Level of Cognitive Ability:* Analysis
*Client Needs:* Physiological Integrity
*Integrated Concept/Process:* Nursing Process/Assessment
*Content Area:* Adult Health/Cardiovascular

*Reference*
Monahan, F., & Neighbors, M. (1998). *Medical-surgical nursing: Foundations for clinical practice* (2nd ed.). Philadelphia: W.B Saunders, pp. 248-249.

---

**167.** A client with a history of duodenal ulcer is taking calcium carbonate chewable tablets. The nurse monitors the client for relief of which of the following symptoms?

1 Flatus
2 Rectal pain
3 Muscle twitching
4 Heartburn

**Answer: 4**
*Rationale:* Calcium carbonate is used as an antacid for the relief of heartburn and indigestion. It can also be used as a calcium supplement or to bind phosphorus in the gastrointestinal (GI) tract in clients with renal failure. Options 1, 2, and 3 are unrelated to this medication.

*Test-Taking Strategy:* Use the process of elimination. Focusing on the client's diagnosis will direct you to option 4. Review the action of this medication if you had difficulty with this question.

*Level of Cognitive Ability:* Analysis
*Client Needs:* Physiological Integrity
*Integrated Concept/Process:* Nursing Process/Evaluation
*Content Area:* Pharmacology

*Reference*
Deglin, J., & Vallerand, A. (1999). *Davis's Drug guide for nurses* (6th ed.). Philadelphia: F.A. Davis, p. 144.

---

**168.** A child with Hirschsprung's disease is scheduled for surgery and a temporary colostomy is performed on the child. Postoperatively, the nurse reinforces instructions to the parents about colostomy care at home. Which statement made by the parents indicates their understanding of the instructions?

1   "We will report early evidence of skin breakdown."
2   "We will apply a heat lamp to moist red tissue around the stoma."
3   "We will give antidiarrheal medications."
4   "We will give saline water enemas if stools are absent."

**Answer: 1**
*Rationale:* The parents are instructed to report early evidence of skin breakdown or stomal complications, such as ribbon-like stools, or failure to pass flatus or stools, to the physician or the nurse. Moist, red granulation tissue may grow around an ostomy site and does not require special treatment. Options 3 and 4 are incorrect actions and are contraindicated.

*Test-Taking Strategy:* Use the process of elimination, noting the key words *indicates their understanding of the instructions.* Focusing on the issue: colostomy care, and careful reading of each option will direct you to option 1. If you had difficulty with this question, review parent teaching and colostomy care.

*Level of Cognitive Ability:* Analysis
*Client Needs:* Health Promotion and Maintenance
*Integrated Concept/Process:* Teaching/Learning
*Content Area:* Child Health

*Reference*
Wong, D. (1999). *Whaley & Wong's Nursing care of infants and children* (6th ed.). St. Louis: Mosby, p. 1276.

---

**169.** A female client arrives at the emergency department and states she was just raped. In preparing a plan of care, the priority goal, in addition to medical attention, will include:

1   Providing instructions for medical follow-up
2   Obtaining counseling for the victim
3   Providing anticipatory guidance for police investigations, medical questions, and court proceedings
4   Exploring safety concerns by obtaining permission to notify significant others who can provide shelter

**Answer: 4**
*Rationale:* After the provision of medical treatment, the nurse's next priority would be obtaining support and planning for safety. Options 2 and 3 seek to meet the emotional needs related to the rape and emotional readiness for the process of discovery and legal action. Option 1 is long-term in that it is concerned with ensuring that the victim understands the importance of and commits to the need for medical follow-up.

*Test-Taking Strategy:* Use Maslow's Hierarchy of Needs theory and note the key words *priority goal.* Remember, physiological needs are the priority followed by safety needs. Since medical attention is addressed in the question, select option 4 because it addresses the safety needs. Review care of a rape victim if you had difficulty with this question.

*Level of Cognitive Ability:* Analysis
*Client Needs:* Safe, Effective Care Environment

*Integrated Concept/Process:* Nursing Process/Planning
*Content Area:* Mental Health

*Reference*
Varcarolis, E. (1998). *Foundations of psychiatric mental health nursing* (3rd ed.). Philadelphia: W.B. Saunders, pp. 426-427.

---

**170.** A client has been given a prescription for propantheline (Pro-Banthine) as adjunctive treatment for peptic ulcer disease. The nurse tells the client to take this medication:
1    With antacids
2    30 minutes before meals
3    With meals
4    Just after meals

**Answer: 2**
*Rationale:* Propantheline is an antimuscarinic anticholinergic medication that decreases gastrointestinal secretions. It should be administered 30 minutes before meals. The other options are incorrect.

*Test-Taking Strategy:* Use the process of elimination. Option 1 can be eliminated immediately because most medications cannot be administered with antacids due to interactive effects. Eliminate options 3 and 4 because they are similar and both indicate administering the medication with food. Review this medication if you had difficulty with this question.

*Level of Cognitive Ability:* Application
*Client Needs:* Health Promotion and Maintenance
*Integrated Concept/Process:* Teaching/Learning
*Content Area:* Pharmacology

*Reference*
Deglin, J., & Vallerand, A. (1999). *Davis's Drug guide for nurses* (6th ed.). Philadelphia: F.A. Davis, p. 857.

---

**171.** A nurse is assigned to care for a client who is receiving total parenteral nutrition (TPN). The nurse performs a fingerstick glucose and the result indicates a glucose level of 325 mg/dL. The initial nursing action is to:
1    Change the TPN solution to 5% dextrose
2    Decrease the flow rate of the TPN
3    Increase the flow rate of the TPN
4    Notify the physician

**Answer: 4**
*Rationale:* Hyperglycemia is a complication associated with the administration of TPN. Since the glucose result is elevated, the nurse would immediately notify the physician for further instructions. Options 1, 2, and 3 are not implemented without a physician's order.

*Test-Taking Strategy:* Use the process of elimination. Eliminate options 1, 2, and 3 because they are not within the scope of nursing practice. Additionally, recalling the normal glucose level will easily direct you to option 4. If you are unfamiliar with the care of the client receiving TPN, review this content.

*Level of Cognitive Ability:* Application
*Client Needs:* Physiological Integrity
*Integrated Concept/Process:* Nursing Process/Implementation
*Content Area:* Fundamental Skills

*Reference*
Black, J., Hawks, J., & Keene, A. (2001). *Medical-surgical nursing: Clinical management for positive outcomes* (6th ed.). Philadelphia: W.B. Saunders, p. 676.

**172.** Carbamazepine (Tegretol) is prescribed for a client in the management of generalized tonic-clonic seizures. The nurse provides instructions to the client regarding the side effects associated with the use of the medication. The nurse instructs the client to inform the physician if which of the following occurs?

1 Drowsiness
2 Dizziness
3 Nausea
4 Sore throat

**Answer: 4**
*Rationale:* Drowsiness, dizziness, nausea, and vomiting are frequent side effects associated with the medication. Adverse reactions include blood dyscrasias. If the client developed a fever, sore throat, mouth ulcerations, unusual bleeding or bruising, or joint pain, this may be indicative of a blood dyscrasia and the physician should be notified.

*Test-Taking Strategy:* Recalling that blood dyscrasias can occur with the use of carbamazapine will direct you to option 4. Also, noting the issue, informing the physician, will direct you to option 4 because a sore throat is a sign of infection. If you are unfamiliar with the adverse reactions related to carbamazapine, review this content.

*Level of Cognitive Ability:* Application
*Client Needs:* Health Promotion and Maintenance
*Integrated Concept/Process:* Teaching/Learning
*Content Area:* Pharmacology

*Reference*
Varcarolis, E.M. (1998). *Foundations of psychiatric mental health nursing.* (3rd ed.). Philadelphia: W.B. Saunders, pp. 1006-1007.

**173.** A medication nurse is administering pyridostigmine (Mestinon) PO to a client with myasthenia gravis. Prior to administering the medication, the nurse would ask the client to:

1 Lie down flat
2 Urinate
3 Take sips of water
4 Lie on his or her stomach

**Answer: 3**
*Rationale:* Myasthenia gravis can affect the client's ability to swallow. The primary assessment is to determine the client's ability to swallow. Options 1 and 4 are not appropriate. In this situation, there is no reason for the client to lie down flat or on his or her stomach. There is no specific reason for the client to urinate before taking medication.

*Test-Taking Strategy:* Note the diagnosis of the client and that the question addresses a PO medication. Recalling that myasthenia gravis can affect the client's ability to swallow will direct you to option 3. If you had difficulty with this question, review nursing care of a client with myasthenia gravis.

*Level of Cognitive Ability:* Application
*Client Needs:* Safe, Effective Care Environment
*Integrated Concept/Process:* Nursing Process/Implementation
*Content Area:* Fundamental Skills

*Reference*
Lehne, R. (1998). *Pharmacology for nursing care* (3rd ed.). Philadelphia: W.B. Saunders, p. 132.

**174.** A home care nurse visits a client with chronic obstructive pulmonary disease (COPD) who is on home oxygen at 2 L/min. The client is complaining of increased dyspnea. The nurse would initially:

1  Increase the oxygen
2  Perform a respiratory assessment
3  Call an ambulance
4  Call the physician

**Answer: 2**
*Rationale:* Completing the assessment and collecting additional information regarding the client's respiratory status is the initial nursing action. Once data are obtained, the physician is notified. Calling an ambulance is a premature action. The oxygen is not increased without the approval of the physician, especially since clients with COPD can retain carbon dioxide.

*Test-Taking Strategy:* Use the process of elimination. Remember that assessment is the first step of the nursing process. Also, use the ABCs, airway, breathing, and circulation, to direct you to option 2. Review care of a client with COPD if you had difficulty with this question.

*Level of Cognitive Ability:* Application
*Client Needs:* Physiological Integrity
*Integrated Concept/Process:* Nursing Process/Implementation
*Content Area:* Adult Health/Respiratory

*Reference*
Monahan, F., & Neighbors, M. (1998). *Medical-surgical nursing: Foundations for clinical practice* (2nd ed.). Philadelphia: W.B Saunders, p. 674.

**175.** A client with acute myocardial infarction receives therapy with alteplase recombinant, or tissue plasminogen activator (t-PA). The nurse monitors the client for complications of this treatment. Which finding would indicate a possible complication?

1  Epistaxis
2  Vomiting
3  ECG changes
4  Absent pedal pulses

**Answer: 1**
*Rationale:* Bleeding is a major side effect of t-PA therapy. The bleeding can be superficial or internal, and can be spontaneous. Options 2, 3, and 4 are not side effects of t-PA therapy.

*Test-Taking Strategy:* Use the process of elimination. Recalling that this medication is a thrombolytic and that epistaxis is a bloody nose will direct you to option 1. If you had difficulty with this question, review the side effects of t-PA.

*Level of Cognitive Ability:* Analysis
*Client Needs:* Physiological Integrity
*Integrated Concept/Process:* Nursing Process/Analysis
*Content Area:* Pharmacology

*Reference*
Hodgson, B., & Kizior, R. (2001). *Saunders Nursing drug handbook 2001.* Philadelphia: W.B. Saunders, pp. 30-31.

**176.** A nurse is caring for a postoperative client who is on bed rest. The client needs to urinate and asks to use the commode because the nurse on the previous shift allowed the client to get out of bed. The nurse assists the client to the commode, and as a result, the client sustains an injury at the operative site. The nurse could be liable for his or her action according to the definition of which of the following?

1  Tort
2  Misdemeanor
3  Common law
4  Statutory law

**Answer: 1**
*Rationale:* A tort is a wrongful act intentionally or unintentionally committed against a person or his property. The nurse's action in the situation described is consistent with the definition of a tort offense. Option 2 is an offense under criminal law. Option 3 describes case law that has evolved over time via precedents. Option 4 describes laws that are enacted by State, Federal, or local governments.

*Test-Taking Strategy:* Knowledge regarding the definitions of the items identified in the options is required to answer this question. Review the definitions related to these items if you had difficulty with this question.

*Level of Cognitive Ability:* Analysis
*Client Needs:* Physiological Integrity
*Integrated Concept/Process:* Nursing Process/Analysis
*Content Area:* Fundamental Skills

**Reference**
Potter, P., & Perry, A. (2001). *Fundamentals of nursing* (5th ed.). St. Louis: Mosby, p. 425.

**177.** A mother of a 9-year-old newly diagnosed with diabetes mellitus is very concerned about the child going to school and participating in social events. The nurse assists in developing a plan of care and assists in formulating which goal?
1  The child's normal growth and development will be maintained
2  The child and family will discuss all aspects of the illness and its treatments
3  The child will use effective coping mechanisms to manage anxiety
4  The child and family will integrate diabetes care into patterns of daily living

**Answer: 4**
*Rationale:* In order to effectively manage social events in the child's life, the family and the child need to integrate the care and management of diabetes into their daily living. The other options are all goals for the family; however, they do not deal with social issues.

*Test-Taking Strategy:* Use the process of elimination and focus on the issue: social events. Noting the relationship of this issue and the words *into patterns of daily living* will direct you to option 4. Review goals of care for a child with diabetes mellitus if you had difficulty with this question.

*Level of Cognitive Ability:* Application
*Client Needs:* Psychosocial Integrity
*Integrated Concept/Process:* Nursing Process/Planning
*Content Area:* Child Health

**Reference**
Wong, D. (1999). *Whaley & Wong's Nursing care of infants and children* (6th ed.). St. Louis: Mosby, p. 1867.

**178.** A nurse reviews the client's health care record and notes that the client is taking donepezil hydrochloride (Aricept). Which of the following disorders does the nurse suspect that this client may have based on the use of this medication?
1  Dementia
2  Obsessive compulsive disorder
3  Seizure disorder
4  History of schizophrenia

**Answer: 1**
*Rationale:* Aricept is a cholinergic agent that is used in the treatment of mild to moderate dementia of the Alzheimer's type. It enhances cholinergic functions by increasing the concentration of acetylcholine. It slows the progression of Alzheimer's disease. Options 2, 3, and 4 are incorrect.

*Test-Taking Strategy:* Specific knowledge regarding the use of donepezil hydrochloride is required to answer this question. If you are unfamiliar with this medication, review its action and use.

*Level of Cognitive Ability:* Analysis
*Client Needs:* Physiological Integrity
*Integrated Concept/Process:* Nursing Process/Analysis
*Content Area:* Pharmacology

**Reference**
Varcarolis, E.M. (1998). *Foundations of psychiatric mental health nursing.* (3rd ed.). Philadelphia: W.B. Saunders, p 1012.

**179.** A registered nurse (RN) is supervising a licensed practical nurse (LPN) providing care to a client with end-stage heart failure. The client is withdrawn, reluctant to talk, and shows little interest in participating in hygienic care or activities. Which statement made by the LPN to the client indicates that the LPN needs further teaching in the use of therapeutic communication skills?

1 "You are very quiet today."
2 "Why don't you feel like getting up for your bath?"
3 "What are your feelings right now?"
4 "These dreams you mentioned, what are they like?"

**Answer: 2**

*Rationale:* When a "why" question is made to the client, an explanation for feelings and behaviors is requested and the client may not know the reason. Requesting an explanation is a nontherapeutic communication technique. In option 1, the LPN is using the therapeutic communication technique of acknowledging the client's behavior. In option 3, the LPN is encouraging identification of emotions or feelings. In option 4, the LPN is using the therapeutic communication technique of exploring. Exploring is asking the client to describe something in more detail or to discuss it more fully.

*Test-Taking Strategy:* Note the key words *needs further teaching in the use of therapeutic communication skills.* Use the process of elimination, seeking the option that is a block to communication. The word *why* in option 2 should easily guide you to this option. Review therapeutic communication techniques if you had difficulty with this question.

*Level of Cognitive Ability:* Analysis
*Client Needs:* Safe, Effective Care Environment
*Integrated Concept/Process:* Teaching/Learning
*Content Area:* Adult Health/Cardiovascular

*Reference*
Potter, P., & Perry, A. (2001). *Fundamentals of nursing* (5th ed.). St. Louis: Mosby, p. 459.

**180.** A nurse is administering a dose of prochlorperazine (Compazine) to a client for nausea and vomiting. The nurse tells the client to report which common side effect of this medication?

1 Excessive tearing
2 Blurred vision
3 Diarrhea
4 Drooling

**Answer: 2**

*Rationale:* Prochlorperazine is a phenothiazine-type antiemetic and antipsychotic agent. A frequent side effect is blurred vision. Other frequent side effects of this medication are dry eyes, dry mouth, and constipation.

*Test-Taking Strategy:* To answer this question accurately, it is necessary to know the common side effects of phenothiazines. If you had difficulty with this question and are unfamiliar with the side effects associated with the use of this medication, review this content.

*Level of Cognitive Ability:* Application
*Client Needs:* Physiological Integrity
*Integrated Concept/Process:* Nursing Process/Implementation
*Content Area:* Pharmacology

*Reference*
Deglin, J., & Vallerand, A. (1999). *Davis's Drug guide for nurses* (6th ed.). Philadelphia: F.A. Davis, p. 847.

**181.** A nurse is reviewing a urinalysis report for a client with acute renal failure (ARF). The results are highly positive for proteinuria. The nurse interprets that this client has which of the following types of renal failure?

1 Postrenal failure
2 Prerenal failure
3 Intrinsic renal failure
4 Atypical renal failure

**Answer: 3**
*Rationale:* With intrinsic renal failure, there a fixed specific gravity and the urine tests positive for proteinuria. In postrenal failure, there is a fixed specific gravity and little or no proteinuria. In prerenal failure, the specific gravity is high, and there is very little or no proteinuria. There is no such classification as atypical renal failure.

*Test-Taking Strategy:* Specific knowledge regarding the types of renal failure is required to answer this question. Review the manifestations associated with the classifications of renal failure if you had difficulty with this question.

*Level of Cognitive Ability:* Analysis
*Client Needs:* Physiological Integrity
*Integrated Concept/Process:* Nursing Process/Analysis
*Content Area:* Adult Health/Renal

*Reference*
Black, J., Hawks, J., & Keene, A. (2001). *Medical-surgical nursing: Clinical management for positive outcomes* (6th ed.). Philadelphia: W.B. Saunders, p. 876.

**182.** A nurse is caring for the client with silicosis who has massive pulmonary fibrosis. The nurse monitors the client for emotional reactions related to the chronic respiratory disease. Which of the following emotional reactions if expressed by the client would indicate a need for immediate intervention?

1 Anxiety
2 Ineffective coping
3 Depression
4 Suicidal ideation

**Answer: 4**
*Rationale:* Common emotional reactions to advanced silicosis may be the same as for chronic airflow limitation and include anxiety, ineffective coping, and depression. Suicidal ideation is not a normal emotional reaction with this condition. If it is expressed, it warrants immediate intervention.

*Test-Taking Strategy:* Use the process of elimination. Noting the key word *immediate* will direct you to option 4. If this question was difficult, review the common emotional reactions that occur in chronic diseases and nursing interventions if suicidal ideation is expressed by the client.

*Level of Cognitive Ability:* Analysis
*Client Needs:* Psychosocial Integrity
*Integrated Concept/Process:* Nursing Process/Analysis
*Content Area:* Adult Health/Respiratory

*Reference*
Leahy, J., & Kizilay, P. (1998). *Foundations of nursing practice: A nursing process approach.* Philadelphia: W.B. Saunders, p. 109.

**183.** Sertraline (Zoloft) is prescribed for a client in the treatment of depression. Before administering the medication, the nurse reviews the client's record and consults with the physician if which of the following were noted?

1 Use of phenelzine sulfate (Nardil)
2 A history of myocardial infarction
3 A history of irritable bowel syndrome
4 A history of diabetes mellitus

**Answer: 1**
*Rationale:* Serious potentially fatal reactions may occur if sertraline is administered concurrently with an monoamine oxidase (MAO) inhibitor. Phenelzine sulfate is a MAO inhibitor. MAO inhibitors should be stopped at least 14 days before sertraline therapy. Sertraline should also be stopped at least 14 days before MAO inhibitor therapy. Options 2, 3, and 4 are not concerns with the administration of this medication.

*Test-Taking Strategy:* Knowledge regarding the interactions and contraindications associated with the use of sertraline is required to answer this question. If you are unfamiliar with the medication interactions and contraindications, review this content.

*Level of Cognitive Ability:* Application
*Client Needs:* Safe, Effective Care Environment
*Integrated Concept/Process:* Nursing Process/Implementation
*Content Area:* Pharmacology

*Reference*
Deglin, J., & Vallerand, A. (1999). *Davis's Drug guide for nurses* (6th ed.). Philadelphia: F.A. Davis, p. 914.

---

**184.** A nurse reinforces instructions to a client who is taking allopurinol (Zyloprim) for the treatment of gout. Which statement by the client indicates an understanding of the medication?
1   "I can use an antihistamine lotion if I get a rash that is itchy."
2   "I need to drink at least 8 glasses of fluid every day."
3   "I need to take the medication 1 hour before I eat."
4   "I should put ice on my lips if they swell."

**Answer: 2**
*Rationale:* Clients taking allopurinol are encouraged to drink 3000 mL of fluid a day. Allopurinol is to be given with or immediately following meals or milk. If the client develops a rash, irritation of the eyes, or swelling of the lips or mouth, they should contact the physician because this may indicate hypersensitivity.

*Test-Taking Strategy:* Use the process of elimination, noting the key words *indicates an understanding*. Options 1 and 4 can be easily eliminated because they indicate a hypersensitivity, which is not a normal expected response. From the remaining options, recalling that the medication should be taken with food or milk will direct you to option 2. If you had difficulty with this question, review client instructions related to allopurinol.

*Level of Cognitive Ability:* Analysis
*Client Needs:* Health Promotion and Maintenance
*Integrated Concept/Process:* Teaching/Learning
*Content Area:* Pharmacology

*Reference*
Hodgson, B., & Kizior, R. (2001). *Saunders Nursing drug handbook 2001*. Philadelphia: W.B. Saunders, p. 25.

---

**185.** A nurse provides dietary instructions to a client who is taking probenecid (Benemid) for the treatment of gout. The client has been instructed to restrict high purine foods in the diet. Which of the following foods if selected by the client would indicate an understanding of this dietary restriction?
1   Shrimp
2   Liver
3   Spinach
4   Scallops

**Answer: 3**
*Rationale:* Probenecid (Benemid) is a medication used for clients with gout to inhibit the reabsorption of uric acid by the kidney and promote excretion of uric acid in the urine. Clients are instructed to modify their diets and limit excessive purine intake. High purine foods to avoid or limit include organ meats, roe, sardines, scallops, anchovies, broth, mincemeat, herring, shrimp, mackerel, gravy, and yeast.

*Test-Taking Strategy:* Use the process of elimination. Options 1 and 4 are similar foods and should be eliminated first. Recalling that organ meats are high in purines will direct you to option 3. If you had difficulty with this question, review foods that are high in purine.

*Level of Cognitive Ability:* Analysis
*Client Needs:* Health Promotion and Maintenance

*Integrated Concept/Process:* Teaching/Learning
*Content Area:* Pharmacology

**Reference**
Hodgson, B., & Kizior, R. (2001). *Saunders Nursing drug handbook 2001.* Philadelphia: W.B. Saunders, p. 859.

---

**186.** Auranofin (Ridaura) is prescribed for a client with rheumatoid arthritis. The nurse instructs the client about the early signs of toxicity related to the medication. Which of the following if identified by the client as a sign of toxicity would indicate a need for further teaching?
1  Pruritus
2  Complaints of a metallic taste in the mouth
3  Ringing in the ears
4  Mouth lesions

**Answer: 3**
*Rationale:* Auranofin (Ridaura) is the one gold preparation that is given orally rather than by injection. Gastrointestinal reactions including diarrhea, abdominal pain, nausea, and loss of appetite are common early in therapy, but usually subside during the first three months. Early symptoms of toxic reactions include a rash, purple blotches, pruritus, mouth lesions, and a metallic taste in the mouth. Ringing in the ears is not associated with this medication.

*Test-Taking Strategy:* Note the key words *need for further teaching.* Knowledge that auranofin (Ridaura) is a gold preparation will assist in eliminating option 2. From the remaining options, it is necessary to know the early signs of toxicity to assist in eliminating options 1 and 4. If you had difficulty with this question, review toxicity related to gold compounds.

*Level of Cognitive Ability:* Analysis
*Client Needs:* Physiological Integrity
*Integrated Concept/Process:* Teaching/Learning
*Content Area:* Pharmacology

**Reference**
Hodgson, B., & Kizior, R. (2001). *Saunders Nursing drug handbook 2001.* Philadelphia: W.B. Saunders, p. 85.

---

**187.** A client has decided to use a transcutaneous electrical nerve stimulation (TENS) as prescribed by the physician for the relief of chronic pain. The nurse has provided instructions to the client regarding the TENS unit. Which of the following statements if made by the client would indicate a need for further instruction regarding this pain relief measure?
1  "I'm not sure that I am going to like those electrodes attached to my skin."
2  "I am not real happy that I have to stay in the hospital for this treatment."
3  "This unit will eliminate the need for taking so many pain medications."
4  "I understand that this will help relieve the pain."

**Answer: 2**
*Rationale:* The TENS unit is a portable unit and the client controls the system for relieving pain and reducing the need for analgesics. It is attached to the skin of the body by electrodes. It is not necessary that the client remain in the hospital for this treatment.

*Test-Taking Strategy:* Note the words *need for further instruction* in the stem of the question. Options 3 and 4 can be eliminated first because they are similar. From the remaining options, select option 2, because it would not be a very cost effective pain management technique if the client required hospitalization. Review the principles related to the TENS unit if you had difficulty with this question.

*Level of Cognitive Ability:* Analysis
*Client Needs:* Physiological Integrity
*Integrated Concept/Process:* Teaching/Learning
*Content Area:* Pharmacology

**Reference**
Monahan, F., & Neighbors, M. (1998). *Medical-surgical nursing: Foundations for clinical practice* (2nd ed.). Philadelphia: W.B. Saunders, p. 892.

**188.** Ibuprofen (Motrin) 300 mg PO four times daily has been prescribed for an elderly client with a diagnosis of rheumatoid arthritis. The client asks the nurse about the amount of medication prescribed. The nurse responds based on the understanding that this prescribed dosage is:

1   The normal adult dose
2   Lower than the normal adult dose
3   Higher than the normal adult dose
4   An unusual dosage for this diagnosis

**Answer: 1**

*Rationale:* For acute or chronic rheumatoid arthritis or osteoarthritis, the normal oral adult dose for an elderly client is 300 to 800 mg 3 to 4 times daily. Therefore, options 2, 3, and 4 are incorrect.

*Test-Taking Strategy:* Knowledge of the normal dosage for ibuprofen is required to answer this question. Review the normal dosage for this medication if you had difficulty with this question.

*Level of Cognitive Ability:* Analysis
*Client Needs:* Physiological Integrity
*Integrated Concept/Process:* Nursing Process/Implementation
*Content Area:* Pharmacology

*Reference*
Hodgson, B., & Kizior, R. (2001). *Saunders Nursing drug handbook 2001.* Philadelphia: W.B. Saunders, p. 512.

**189.** A nurse is monitoring a client with multiple sclerosis who is receiving baclofen (Lioresal). Which of the following assessment findings would indicate a therapeutic response from the medication?

1   Increased muscle tone and strength
2   Decreased nausea
3   Decreased muscle spasms
4   Increased range of motion of all extremities

**Answer: 3**

*Rationale:* Baclofen is a skeletal muscle relaxant and acts at the spinal cord level to decrease the frequency and amplitude of muscle spasms in clients with spinal cord injuries or diseases, or multiple sclerosis. Options 1, 2, and 4 are unrelated to the effects of this medication.

*Test-Taking Strategy:* Recalling that this medication is a skeletal muscle relaxant will direct you to option 3. Review the action of this medication if you had difficulty with this question.

*Level of Cognitive Ability:* Analysis
*Client Needs:* Physiological Integrity
*Integrated Concept/Process:* Nursing Process/Evaluation
*Content Area:* Pharmacology

*Reference*
Lehne, R. (1998). *Pharmacology for nursing care* (3rd ed.). Philadelphia: W.B. Saunders, pp. 222-223.

**190.** Lorazepam (Ativan) is prescribed for a client for the management of anxiety. Which of the following if noted on the client's record would indicate the need to consult with the physician before administering the medication?

1   History of glaucoma
2   History of diabetes mellitus
3   History of hypothyroidism
4   History of coronary artery disease

**Answer: 1**

*Rationale:* Ativan is contraindicated if hypersensitivity or cross-sensitivity with other benzodiazepines exist. It is also contraindicated in clients who are comatose, with preexisting central nervous system (CNS) depression, with uncontrolled severe pain, and those with narrow angle glaucoma. It is also not prescribed for clients who are pregnant or breast-feeding.

*Test-Taking Strategy:* Knowledge regarding the contraindications associated with the use of lorazepam is required to answer this question. If you are unfamiliar with these contraindications, review this content.

*Level of Cognitive Ability:* Analysis
*Client Needs:* Safe, Effective Care Environment
*Integrated Concept/Process:* Nursing Process/Implementation
*Content Area:* Pharmacology

*Reference*
Varcarolis, E.M. (1998). *Foundations of psychiatric mental health nursing.* (3rd ed.). Philadelphia: W.B. Saunders, pp. 1018-1019.

**191.** Nefazodone (Serzone) is prescribed for a client in the treatment of depression. The nurse reviews the client's record to determine a history of any present medication use or medical disorders. Which of the following if documented in the client's record would indicate a contraindication associated with the use of nefazodone?
1   Use of astemizole (Hismanal)
2   History of diabetes mellitus
3   History of hyperthyroidism
4   History of coronary artery disease

**Answer: 1**
*Rationale:* To avoid potentially life-threatening cardiotoxicity, the nonsedating antihistamines terfenadine (Seldane) and astemizole (Hismanal) should not be taken by clients on nefazodone. Also, medications such as alprazolam (Xanax) and triazolam (Halcion) require dosage reduction when used concurrently with nefazodone. Nefazodone should not be used in combination with monoamine oxidase inhibitors (MAOI) or within 2 weeks of terminating treatment with an MAOI.

*Test-Taking Strategy:* Knowledge regarding the use of this medication and its contraindications is required to answer this question. If you are unfamiliar with this medication and its contraindications, review this content.

*Level of Cognitive Ability:* Analysis
*Client Needs:* Safe, Effective Care Environment
*Integrated Concept/Process:* Nursing Process/Analysis
*Content Area:* Pharmacology

*Reference*
Varcarolis, E.M. (1998). *Foundations of psychiatric mental health nursing.* (3rd ed.). Philadelphia: W.B. Saunders, p. 1021.

**192.** Phenelzine sulfate (Nardil) is being administered to a client with depression. The client suddenly complains of a severe occipital headache radiating frontally, neck stiffness and soreness, and is vomiting. On further assessment, the client exhibits signs of hypertensive crisis. Which of the following medications would the nurse prepare anticipating that it will be prescribed as the antidote for hypertensive crisis?
1   Phentolamine (Regitine)
2   Vitamin K
3   Protamine sulfate
4   Calcium gluconate

**Answer: 1**
*Rationale:* The antidote for hypertensive crisis is phentolamine (Regitine) and a dosage by IV injection is administered. The manifestations of hypertensive crisis include hypertension, occipital headache radiating frontally, neck stiffness and soreness, nausea, vomiting, sweating, fever and chills, clammy skin, dilated pupils, and palpitations. Tachycardia or bradycardia, and constricting chest pain may also be present. Protamine sulfate is the antidote for heparin and vitamin K is the antidote for warfarin (Coumadin) overdose. Calcium gluconate is used for magnesium overdose.

*Test-Taking Strategy:* Knowledge regarding the antidotes for various medications and disorders is required to answer this question. If you are unfamiliar with the antidotes associated with the use of certain medications and conditions, review this content.

*Level of Cognitive Ability:* Analysis
*Client Needs:* Physiological Integrity
*Integrated Concept/Process:* Nursing Process/Planning
*Content Area:* Pharmacology

*Reference*
Hodgson, B., & Kizior, R. (2001). *Saunders Nursing drug handbook 2001.* Philadelphia: W.B. Saunders, p. 813.

---

**193.** A nurse is assessing a client hospitalized with a diagnosis of schizophrenia. Risperidone (Risperdal) is prescribed for the client for the treatment of this disorder. Which of the following laboratory studies would the nurse anticipate to be prescribed before the initiation of this medication therapy?

1    Complete blood count
2    Liver function studies
3    Blood clotting tests
4    Platelet count

**Answer: 2**
*Rationale:* Baseline assessment includes renal and liver function tests and these studies should be done before the initiation of treatment. This medication is used with caution in clients with renal or hepatic impairment, clients with underlying cardiovascular disorders, and in geriatric or debilitative clients. Options 1, 3, and 4 are unrelated to the administration of this medication.

*Test-Taking Strategy:* Use the process of elimination. Recalling that this medication is used cautiously in clients with renal or hepatic impairment will direct you to option 2. If you are unfamiliar with the contraindications associated with the use of this medication, review this content.

*Level of Cognitive Ability:* Analysis
*Client Needs:* Physiological Integrity
*Integrated Concept/Process:* Nursing Process/Analysis
*Content Area:* Pharmacology

*Reference*
Hodgson, B., & Kizior, R. (2001). *Saunders Nursing drug handbook 2001.* Philadelphia: W.B. Saunders, p. 909.

---

**194.** A nurse has been working with an obese man and is evaluating a weight reduction plan designed for the client. Which of the following statements, if made by the client, indicates the need for additional teaching?

1    "I wish my mother could have seen me lose the 60 pounds in the last 9 months."
2    "It is so difficult to find food exchanges that taste good and fill me up."
3    "My wife was kidding me the other night about my being a whole new husband."
4    "This diet doesn't let me go out for lunch with my friends at work anymore."

**Answer: 4**
*Rationale:* Both options 1 and 3 are responses indicating a positive perception of self. In the absence of other data, option 2 is a normal response to the changes in eating habits. Option 4 indicates that the client may be having difficulty in making appropriate dietary choices when going out for lunch or that he may perceive his coworkers are uncomfortable with his need to eat differently. A sense of not fitting in can leave the obese individual isolated and therefore make it more difficult for him to maintain his diet at work.

*Test-Taking Strategy:* Use the process of elimination, noting the key words *need for additional teaching.* Read each option carefully and determine whether it is a positive indicator or a negative one. This will assist in eliminating options 1 and 3 first. Option 2 is a common response by persons who have had to make dietary changes. Option 4 clearly states that the client perceives a definite barrier in pursuing his lifestyle changes. Review dietary principles related to weight reduction if you had difficulty with this question.

*Level of Cognitive Ability:* Analysis
*Client Needs:* Health Promotion and Maintenance
*Integrated Concept/Process:* Nursing Process/Evaluation
*Content Area:* Fundamental Skills

**Reference**
Potter, P., & Perry, A. (2001). *Fundamentals of nursing* (5th ed.). St. Louis: Mosby, p. 1348.

---

**195.** A client is complaining of skin irritation from the edges of a cast applied the previous day. The skin edges are pink and irritated. The nurse plans to do which of the following as a corrective action?
1   Use a hair dryer set on cool high setting to soothe the irritation
2   Petal the edges of the cast with tape
3   Massage the skin at the rim of the cast
4   Shake a small amount of powder under the cast rim

**Answer: 2**
*Rationale:* The nurse should petal the edges of the cast with tape to minimize skin irritation. A hair dryer is used on a cool low setting if a nonplaster cast becomes wet, or if the client's skin itches under a cast. Massaging the skin will not alleviate the problem. Powder should not be shaken under the cast, because it could clump, become moist, and cause skin breakdown.

*Test-Taking Strategy:* Focus on the issue and note the cause of the client's skin irritation. Since the question tells you that the cast edges are the cause, you can easily eliminate options 1, 3, and 4. If this question was difficult, review the principles of cast care.

*Level of Cognitive Ability:* Application
*Client Needs:* Physiological Integrity
*Integrated Concept/Process:* Nursing Process/Planning
*Content Area:* Adult Health/Musculoskeletal

**Reference**
Monahan, F., & Neighbors, M. (1998). *Medical-surgical nursing: Foundations for clinical practice* (2nd ed.). Philadelphia: W.B Saunders, p. 857.

---

**196.** A nurse is caring for a hospitalized client who has been taking clozapine (Clozaril) for the treatment of a schizophrenic disorder. The nurse reviews the laboratory studies that have been prescribed for the client. Which laboratory study will the nurse specifically review to monitor for an adverse reaction associated with the use of this medication?
1   White blood cell count
2   Platelet count
3   Cholesterol level
4   Blood urea nitrogen

**Answer: 1**
*Rationale:* Hematological reactions can occur in the client taking clozapine, and include agranulocytosis and mild leukopenia. The white blood cell count should be assessed before initiating treatment and should be monitored closely during the use of this medication. The client should also be monitored for signs indicating agranulocytosis, which may include sore throat, malaise, and fever. Options 2, 3, and 4 are unrelated to the use of this medication.

*Test-Taking Strategy:* Recalling that clozapine causes agranulocytosis will direct you to option 1. If you are unfamiliar with these adverse reactions and the laboratory studies that need to be monitored, review this information.

*Level of Cognitive Ability:* Analysis
*Client Needs:* Physiological Integrity
*Integrated Concept/Process:* Nursing Process/Assessment
*Content Area:* Pharmacology

**Reference**
Varcarolis, E.M. (1998). *Foundations of psychiatric mental health nursing.* (3rd ed.). Philadelphia: W.B. Saunders, pp. 1009-1010.

**197.** A nurse is caring for a postoperative client following a thoracotomy. In planning nursing care, the nurse avoids which of the following to minimize the chance for injury?

1 Keeping the call bell within reach
2 Answering the call bell promptly
3 Leaving the side rails down
4 Ensuring that the night-light is working

**Answer: 3**

*Rationale:* Safe nursing actions intended to prevent injury to the client include keeping the side rails up, bed in low position, and providing a call bell that is within the client's reach. Responding promptly to the client's use of the call bell minimizes the chance that the client will try to get up alone, which could result in a fall. Night-lights are built into the lighting systems of most facilities, and these bulbs should be routinely checked to see that they are functional.

*Test-Taking Strategy:* Use the process of elimination, noting the key word *avoids*. Since options 1 and 2 are standard safety measures, they are eliminated first. Use of a night-light would help prevent falls, which is also helpful, and can be eliminated next. Review basic safety measures if you had difficulty with this question.

*Level of Cognitive Ability:* Application
*Client Needs:* Safe, Effective Care Environment
*Integrated Concept/Process:* Nursing Process/Planning
*Content Area:* Adult Health/Respiratory

*Reference*
Leahy, J., & Kizilay, P. (1998). *Foundations of nursing practice: A nursing process approach.* Philadelphia: W.B. Saunders, p. 519.

**198.** A client was admitted to the surgical unit following right total knee replacement (TKR) performed 2 hours earlier. Which of the following observations, if made by the nurse, would indicate the need to contact the surgeon?

1 Ability to flex and extend the right foot
2 Pain relieved by a narcotic analgesic
3 Pale pink and warm right foot
4 Hemovac wound suction drainage of 175 mL/hr

**Answer: 4**

*Rationale:* Following total knee replacement, the neurovascular status of the affected leg is assessed, and findings should be within normal limits. The client should have intact capillary refill, and adequate color, temperature, sensation, and motion to the limb. Incisional pain should be relieved by narcotic analgesic administration. The knee incision has a wound suction drain in place, which is expected to drain up to 200 mL in the first 8 hours after surgery. Drainage of 175 mL in 2 hours is excessive and should be reported.

*Test-Taking Strategy:* Use the process of elimination. Note the key words *need to contact the surgeon*. Options 1 and 3 represent normal neurovascular status and are eliminated first. Knowing that surgery causes the client pain, which is then relieved by analgesics, will assist in eliminating option 2. This leaves option 4 as the correct option given the wording of this question. Review expected findings following a TKR if you had difficulty with this question.

*Level of Cognitive Ability:* Analysis
*Client Needs:* Physiological Integrity
*Integrated Concept/Process:* Nursing Process/Assessment
*Content Area:* Adult Health/Musculoskeletal

*Reference*
Monahan, F., & Neighbors, M. (1998). *Medical-surgical nursing: Foundations for clinical practice* (2nd ed.). Philadelphia: W.B Saunders, p. 869.

**199.** A client is taking lansoprazole (Prevacid) for the chronic management of Zollinger-Ellison syndrome. The nurse determines that the client best understands this disorder and the medication regimen if the client states to take which of the following products for pain?
1  Naprosyn (Aleve)
2  Acetylsalicylic acid (aspirin)
3  Acetaminophen (Tylenol)
4  Ibuprofen (Motrin)

**Answer: 3**
*Rationale:* Zollinger-Ellison syndrome is a hypersecretory condition of the stomach. The client should avoid taking medications that are irritating to the stomach lining. Irritants would include aspirin and nonsteroidal antiinflammatory medications (naprosyn and ibuprofen). The client should take acetaminophen for pain relief.

*Test-Taking Strategy:* Use the process of elimination. Eliminate options 1 and 4 first because they are both nonsteroidal anti-inflammatory medications. From the remaining options, select acetaminophen over aspirin because it is least irritating to the stomach. Review these medications if you had difficulty with this question.

*Level of Cognitive Ability:* Analysis
*Client Needs:* Physiological Integrity
*Integrated Concept/Process:* Self-Care
*Content Area:* Pharmacology

*Reference*
Deglin, J., & Vallerand, A. (1999). *Davis's Drug guide for nurses* (6th ed.). Philadelphia: F.A. Davis, p. 563.

**200.** A client has just been diagnosed with acute renal failure (ARF). The laboratory calls the nurse to report a serum potassium level of 6.1 mEq/L on the client. The nurse takes which of the following actions first?
1  Calls the physician
2  Checks the sodium level
3  Encourages an extra 500 mL of fluid intake
4  Encourages increased vegetables in the diet

**Answer: 1**
*Rationale:* The client with hyperkalemia is at risk of developing cardiac dysrhythmias and resultant cardiac arrest. Because of this, the physician must be notified at once so that the client may receive definitive treatment. Fluid intake would not be increased because it would contribute to fluid overload, and wouldn't effectively lower the serum potassium level. Vegetables are a natural source of potassium in the diet, and their intake would not be increased. The nurse might also check the result of a serum sodium level, but this is not a priority action of the nurse.

*Test-Taking Strategy:* Use the process of elimination, noting the key word *first*. Recalling the normal potassium level and noting that the level identified in the question is elevated will direct you to option 1. Review the normal potassium level if you had difficulty with this question.

*Level of Cognitive Ability:* Application
*Client Needs:* Physiological Integrity
*Integrated Concept/Process:* Nursing Process/Implementation
*Content Area:* Adult Health/Renal

*Reference*
Black, J., Hawks, J., & Keene, A. (2001). *Medical-surgical nursing: Clinical management for positive outcomes* (6th ed.). Philadelphia: W.B. Saunders, p. 878.

**201.** A client with acute renal failure (ARF) has an elevated blood urea nitrogen (BUN). The client is experiencing difficulty remembering information due to uremia. Which of the following would the nurse plan to avoid to enhance communication with this client?

1    Include the family in discussions related to care
2    Give thorough, lengthy explanations of procedures
3    Give simple, clear directions
4    Explain treatments using understandable language

**Answer: 2**

*Rationale:* The client with ARF may have difficulty remembering information and instructions due to anxiety and due to the increased level of the BUN. The nurse should avoid giving lengthy explanations about procedures because this information may not be remembered by the client and could increase client anxiety. Communications should be clear, simple, and understandable. The family should be included whenever possible.

*Test-Taking Strategy:* Use the process of elimination and note the key word *avoid*. Use knowledge of the basic principles of effective communication to eliminate each of the incorrect options. If this question was difficult, review basic communication techniques.

*Level of Cognitive Ability:* Application
*Client Needs:* Psychosocial Integrity
*Integrated Concept/Process:* Nursing Process/Implementation
*Content Area:* Adult Health/Renal

*Reference*
Black, J., Hawks, J., & Keene, A. (2001). *Medical-surgical nursing: Clinical management for positive outcomes* (6th ed.). Philadelphia: W.B. Saunders, p. 409.

**202.** A client with glomerulonephritis is at risk of developing acute renal failure (ARF). The nurse monitors this client for which sign of this complication?

1    Excitability
2    Decreased central venous pressure
3    Hypertension
4    Bradycardia

**Answer: 3**

*Rationale:* ARF caused by glomerulonephritis is classified as intrinsic or intrarenal failure. This form of ARF is commonly manifested by hypertension, tachycardia, oliguria, lethargy, edema, and other signs of fluid overload. ARF from prerenal causes is characterized by decreased blood pressure or a recent history of the same, tachycardia, and decreased cardiac output and central venous pressure. Bradycardia is not part of the clinical picture for any form of renal failure.

*Test-Taking Strategy:* Use the process of elimination, focusing on the client's diagnosis. Eliminate option 4 first because bradycardia will not occur. Remember that renal failure is accompanied by fluid overload. This will help you to eliminate option 2 next. From the remaining options, recall that hypertension and lethargy accompany ARF. Review the manifestations associated with ARF if you had difficulty with this question.

*Level of Cognitive Ability:* Application
*Client Needs:* Physiological Integrity
*Integrated Concept/Process:* Nursing Process/Assessment
*Content Area:* Adult Health/Renal

*Reference*
Monahan, F., & Neighbors, M. (1998). *Medical-surgical nursing: Foundations for clinical practice* (2nd ed.). Philadelphia: W.B Saunders, p. 1376.

**203.** A nurse is caring for a young adult diagnosed with testicular cancer. The client is angry and tells the nurse that there is no point in learning disease management, because there is no possibility of ever being cured. Based on the client's statement, the nurse determines that the client is experiencing which potential problem?

1    Impaired thought processes
2    Altered health maintenance
3    Anxiety
4    Powerlessness

**Answer: 4**

*Rationale:* The client with powerlessness expresses feelings of having no control over a situation or outcome. Altered health maintenance involves the inability to seek out help that is needed to maintain health. Anxiety is a vague sense of unease. Impaired thought processes involves disruption in cognitive abilities or thought.

*Test-Taking Strategy:* Focus on the data in the question. Use the process of elimination noting the key words *no point in learning disease management.* This will direct you to option 4. Review the defining characteristics of powerlessness if you had difficulty with this question.

*Level of Cognitive Ability:* Analysis
*Client Needs:* Psychosocial Integrity
*Integrated Concept/Process:* Nursing Process/Analysis
*Content Area:* Adult Health/Oncology

*Reference*
Leahy, J., & Kizilay, P. (1998). *Foundations of nursing practice: A nursing process approach.* Philadelphia: W.B. Saunders, p. 917.

---

**204.** A nurse is caring for a client with cancer of the lung. The client is receiving chemotherapy. The nurse reviews the laboratory results and notes that the platelet count is 18,000/mm$^3$. Based on this laboratory result, which of the following would the nurse implement?

1    Protective isolation procedures
2    Bleeding precautions
3    Contact isolation
4    Respiratory isolation

**Answer: 2**

*Rationale:* When the platelet count is less than 20,000/mm$^3$, the client is at risk for bleeding and the nurse would institute bleeding precautions. Protective isolation precautions would be instituted for a client with a low neutrophil count. Contact isolation is initiated in a client who has drainage from wounds that may be infectious. Respiratory precautions are instituted for a client with a respiratory infection that is transmitted by the airborne route.

*Test-Taking Strategy:* Use the process of elimination. Recalling that when the platelet count is low, the client is at risk for bleeding will direct you to option 2. Review the normal platelet count and the nursing interventions necessary when the platelet count is low if you had difficulty with this question.

*Level of Cognitive Ability:* Application
*Client Needs:* Physiological Integrity
*Integrated Concept/Process:* Nursing Process/Implementation
*Content Area:* Adult Health/Oncology

*Reference*
Monahan, F., & Neighbors, M. (1998). *Medical-surgical nursing: Foundations for clinical practice* (2nd ed.). Philadelphia: W.B Saunders, p. 1420.

**205.** A client with a leaking intracranial aneurysm has been placed on aneurysm precautions. A visiting family member wants to take the client to the unit lounge for "just a few minutes." The nurse would use which of the following concepts when explaining why the client must remain in the room?
1 Clients with aneurysms need isolation to cope with photosensitivity
2 Reduced environmental stimuli is needed to prevent aneurysm rupture
3 A quiet environment promotes more rapid healing of the aneurysm
4 The client has altered thought processes and needs reduced stimulation

**Answer: 2**
*Rationale:* Subarachnoid precautions (or aneurysm precautions) are intended to minimize environmental stimuli, which could increase intracranial pressure and trigger bleeding or rupture of the aneurysm. The client does not need isolation to "cope" with photosensitivity (although photosensitivity may be a problem). The aneurysm will not heal more rapidly with reduced stimuli, and the client does not necessarily have altered thought processes.

*Test-Taking Strategy:* Focus on the issue: the purpose of aneurysm precautions. Recalling that the concern in this client is rupture will direct you to option 2. If you are unfamiliar with aneurysm precautions and their purpose, review this content.

*Level of Cognitive Ability:* Application
*Client Needs:* Psychosocial Integrity
*Integrated Concept/Process:* Nursing Process/Implementation
*Content Area:* Adult Health/Neurological

*Reference*
Monahan, F., & Neighbors, M. (1998). *Medical-surgical nursing: Foundations for clinical practice* (2nd ed.). Philadelphia: W.B Saunders, p. 372.

**206.** A client with a ruptured intracranial aneurysm has surgery delayed and is maintained on bed rest. Subarachnoid precautions are still in place. The nurse would question an order for which of the following medications if prescribed for this client?
1 Aminocaproic acid (Amicar)
2 Heparin sodium (Heparin)
3 Nimodipine (Nimotop)
4 Docusate sodium (Colace)

**Answer: 2**
*Rationale:* The nurse should question an order for heparin sodium, which is an anticoagulant. This medication could place the client at risk for rebleeding. Aminocaproic acid is an antifibrinolytic agent that prevents clot breakdown or dissolution. It is commonly prescribed after ruptured intracranial aneurysm and subarachnoid hemorrhage if surgery is delayed or contraindicated. Nimodipine is a calcium channel-blocking agent that is useful in the management of vasospasm associated with cerebral hemorrhage. Colace is a stool softener, which helps prevent straining. Straining would raise intracranial pressure.

*Test-Taking Strategy:* Use the process of elimination. Noting the key word *ruptured* in the question suggests that hemorrhage is occurring. It makes sense, knowing the action of heparin sodium, that this medication would be contraindicated. Review care of a client with a ruptured intracranial aneurysm if you had difficulty with this question.

*Level of Cognitive Ability:* Application
*Client Needs:* Safe, Effective Care Environment
*Integrated Concept/Process:* Nursing Process/Implementation
*Content Area:* Adult Health/Neurological

*Reference*
Hodgson, B., & Kizior, R. (2001). *Saunders Nursing drug handbook 2001.* Philadelphia: W.B. Saunders, p. 489.

**207.** A physician has prescribed nimodipine (Nimotop) for a client with subarachnoid hemorrhage. The nurse administering the first dose tells the client that this medication is a:

1   Calcium-channel blocker used to decrease the blood pressure
2   Calcium-channel blocker used to decrease cerebral blood vessel spasm
3   Beta-adrenergic blocker used to decrease blood pressure
4   Vasodilator that has an affinity for cerebral blood vessels

**Answer: 2**

*Rationale:* Nimodipine is a calcium channel-blocking agent that has an affinity for cerebral blood vessels. It is used to prevent or control vasospasm in cerebral blood vessels, thereby reducing the chance for rebleeding of the aneurysm. Options 1, 3, and 4 are incorrect.

*Test-Taking Strategy:* Use the process of elimination. Recalling that nimodipine is a calcium channel blocking agent (ends with the suffix "-dipine") eliminates options 3 and 4. Recalling that calcium channel blockers decrease vasospasm helps you select option 2 from the remaining options. Review the action of this medication if you had difficulty with this question.

*Level of Cognitive Ability:* Application
*Client Needs:* Physiological Integrity
*Integrated Concept/Process:* Teaching/Learning
*Content Area:* Adult Health/Neurological

**Reference**
Hodgson, B., & Kizior, R. (2001). *Saunders Nursing drug handbook 2001*. Philadelphia: W.B. Saunders, p. 746.

---

**208.** A nurse is in the room with a client when a seizure begins. The client's entire body becomes rigid, and the muscles in all four extremities alternate between relaxation and contraction. Following the seizure, the nurse documents that the client has experienced a(n):

1   Absence seizure
2   Generalized tonic-clonic seizure
3   Simple partial seizure
4   Complex partial seizure

**Answer: 2**

*Rationale:* Generalized seizures are seizures that are bilaterally symmetric, and have no focal point of onset. The tonic-clonic pattern is as described in the question. Partial seizures are seizures that begin locally. Absence seizures are characterized by a sudden lapse of consciousness for 2 to 10 seconds and a blank facial expression. No convulsion occurs in an absence seizure.

*Test-Taking Strategy:* Focus on the data in the question. Note the key words *entire body*. This will assist in eliminating options 3 and 4. From the remaining options, recalling that no convulsion occurs in an absence seizure will direct you to option 2. Review the characteristics of the various types of seizures if you had difficulty with this question.

*Level of Cognitive Ability:* Application
*Client Needs:* Physiological Integrity
*Integrated Concept/Process:* Communication and Documentation
*Content Area:* Adult Health/Neurological

**Reference**
Monahan, F., & Neighbors, M. (1998). *Medical-surgical nursing: Foundations for clinical practice* (2nd ed.). Philadelphia: W.B Saunders, p. 796.

**209.** A nurse is reviewing the nursing care plan for a client with a right cerebrovascular accident (CVA) who has left-sided deficits. The nurse notes a nursing diagnosis of Unilateral Neglect. The nurse would tell a family member who is assisting the client that it would ultimately be least helpful to do which of the following?

1 Approach the client from the right side
2 Teach the client to scan the environment
3 Move the commode and chair to the left side
4 Place bedside articles on the left side

**Answer: 1**

*Rationale:* Unilateral neglect is an unawareness of the paralyzed side of the body, which increases the client's risk for injury. The nurse's role is to refocus the client's attention to the affected side. Personal care items, belongings, a bedside chair, and a commode are all placed on the affected side. The client is taught to scan the environment to become aware of that half of the body, and is approached on that side by family and caregivers as well.

*Test-Taking Strategy:* Use the process of elimination, noting the key words *left-sided deficits*. Eliminate options 3 and 4 first because they are similar. From the remaining options note the key words *least helpful* to direct you to option 1. Review care of a client with unilateral neglect if you had difficulty with this question.

*Level of Cognitive Ability:* Application
*Client Needs:* Safe, Effective Care Environment
*Integrated Concept/Process:* Teaching/Learning
*Content Area:* Adult Health/Neurological

*Reference*
Monahan, F., & Neighbors, M. (1998). *Medical-surgical nursing: Foundations for clinical practice* (2nd ed.). Philadelphia: W.B Saunders, p. 813.

---

**210.** A nurse is evaluating the status of a client with myasthenia gravis. The nurse interprets that the client's medication regimen may not be optimal if the client continues to experience fatigue that occurs:

1 Before meals and at the end of the day
2 Early in the morning and late in the day
3 Following exertion and at the end of the day
4 Following exertion and before meals

**Answer: 3**

*Rationale:* The client with myasthenia gravis has weakness after periods of exertion and near the end of the day. The nurse works with the client to space out activities to conserve energy and regain muscle strength by resting between activities. The client is also instructed to take medication as prescribed.

*Test-Taking Strategy:* Use the process of elimination. Remember that clients with any form of chronic condition characterized by fatigue experience the greatest amount of fatigue after exertion and at the end of the day. With this global concept in mind, eliminate options 1, 2, and 4. Review care of a client with myasthenia gravis if you had difficulty with this question.

*Level of Cognitive Ability:* Analysis
*Client Needs:* Physiological Integrity
*Integrated Concept/Process:* Nursing Process/Evaluation
*Content Area:* Adult Health/Neurological

*Reference*
Monahan, F., & Neighbors, M. (1998). *Medical-surgical nursing: Foundations for clinical practice* (2nd ed.). Philadelphia: W.B Saunders, p. 782.

**211.** A nurse has just been told by a physician that an order has been written to administer an iron injection to an adult client. The nurse plans to administer the medication in which of the following locations?

1　In the gluteal muscle using Z-track technique

2　In the deltoid muscle using an air lock

3　In the subcutaneous tissue of the abdomen

4　In the anterolateral thigh using a $\frac{5}{8}$ inch needle

**Answer: 1**

*Rationale:* The correct technique for administering parenteral iron is deep in the gluteal muscle using Z-track technique. This method minimizes the possibility that the injection will stain the skin a dark color. The medication is not given by the subcutaneous route (options 3 and 4), nor is it given in the arms, abdomen, or thighs (options 2, 3, 4).

*Test-Taking Strategy:* Use principles of medication administration by the parenteral route and focus on the issue: an iron injection. Recalling that iron stains the skin will direct you to option 1. Review the procedure for the administration of iron if you had difficulty with this question.

*Level of Cognitive Ability:* Application
*Client Needs:* Physiological Integrity
*Integrated Concept/Process:* Nursing Process/Planning
*Content Area:* Fundamental Skills

*Reference*
Hodgson, B., & Kizior, R. (2001). *Saunders Nursing drug handbook 2001.* Philadelphia: W.B. Saunders, p. 547.

**212.** A client who has never had gastric surgery is diagnosed with pernicious anemia. The nurse reviews the client's health history for disorders involving which organ responsible for vitamin $B_{12}$ absorption?

1　Stomach

2　Duodenum

3　Ileum

4　Colon

**Answer: 3**

*Rationale:* Pernicious anemia can occur in a client who has not had gastric surgery, such as when the client has disease that involves the ileum, where vitamin $B_{12}$ is absorbed. The nurse checks the client's history for small bowel disorders to detect this risk factor.

*Test-Taking Strategy:* Focus on the issue: vitamin $B_{12}$ absorption. Recalling that vitamin $B_{12}$ is absorbed in the small intestine will direct you to option 3. If this question was difficult, review the physiology associated with the gastrointestinal tract.

*Level of Cognitive Ability:* Analysis
*Client Needs:* Physiological Integrity
*Integrated Concept/Process:* Nursing Process/Assessment
*Content Area:* Fundamental Skills

*Reference*
Monahan, F., & Neighbors, M. (1998). *Medical-surgical nursing: Foundations for clinical practice* (2nd ed.). Philadelphia: W.B Saunders, p. 476.

**213.** One unit of packed red blood cells has been prescribed for a client postoperatively because the client's hemoglobin level is low. The physician prescribes diphenhydramine (Benadryl) to be administered before the administration of the transfusion. The nurse determines that this medication has been prescribed to:

1 Prevent a urticaria reaction
2 Prevent a fever
3 Assist in the absorption of the blood product
4 Promote movement of the red blood cells into the bone marrow

**Answer: 1**

*Rationale:* A urticaria reaction is characterized by a rash accompanied by pruritis. This type of transfusion reaction is prevented by pretreating the client with an antihistamine, such as diphenhydramine. Options 2, 3, and 4 are incorrect. Acetaminophen (Tylenol) however, may be prescribed before the administration of blood to assist in preventing an elevated temperature.

*Test-Taking Strategy:* Use the process of elimination, focusing on the issue, the purpose of the diphenhydramine. Eliminate options 3 and 4 first because blood does not absorb or move into the bone marrow. From the remaining options, recalling the classification of diphenhydramine will direct you to option 1. Review the purpose of diphenhydramine if you had difficulty with this question.

*Level of Cognitive Ability:* Analysis
*Client Needs:* Physiological Integrity
*Integrated Concept/Process:* Nursing Process/Analysis
*Content Area:* Fundamental Skills

*Reference*
Hodgson, B., & Kizior, R. (2001). *Saunders Nursing drug handbook 2001.* Philadelphia: W.B. Saunders, pp. 331-333.

**214.** A client is taking amiloride (Midamor) 10 mg po daily for the treatment of hypertension. The nurse gives the client which of the following instructions regarding its use?

1 Take the medication in the morning
2 Take the medication on an empty stomach
3 Eat foods with extra sodium while taking this medication
4 Withhold the medication if the blood pressure is high

**Answer: 1**

*Rationale:* Amiloride is a potassium-sparing diuretic used to treat edema or hypertension. A daily dose should be taken in the morning to avoid nocturia. The dose should be taken with food to increase bioavailability. Sodium should be restricted if used as an antihypertensive. Increased blood pressure is not a reason to hold the medication and it may be an indication for its use.

*Test-Taking Strategy:* Use the process of elimination. Noting the client's diagnosis will direct you to option 1. Review client teaching points related to this medication if you had difficulty with this question.

*Level of Cognitive Ability:* Application
*Client Needs:* Health Promotion and Maintenance
*Integrated Concept/Process:* Teaching/Learning
*Content Area:* Pharmacology

*Reference*
Hodgson, B., & Kizior, R. (2001). *Saunders Nursing drug handbook 2001.* Philadelphia: W.B. Saunders, p. 41.

**215.** A nurse is providing instructions to a female client regarding the procedure for collecting a midstream urine sample. Which of the following statements if made by the client indicates an understanding of the procedure?
1   "I need to douche before collecting the specimen."
2   "I need to cleanse the perineum from front to back."
3   "I need to collect the urine in the cup as soon as I begin to urinate."
4   "I can collect the specimen tonight and drop it off at the clinic in the morning."

**Answer: 2**

*Rationale:* As part of correct procedure, the client should cleanse the perineum from front to back with the antiseptic swabs that are packaged with the specimen kit. The client should begin the flow of urine and collect the sample after starting the flow of urine. The specimen should be sent to the laboratory as soon as possible and not allowed to stand. Improper specimen handling can yield inaccurate test results. It is not normal procedure to douche before collecting the specimen.

*Test-Taking Strategy:* Use the process of elimination. Noting the name of the type of sample "midstream" will assist in eliminating option 3. Recalling that the specimen should be brought to the laboratory after collection will assist in eliminating option 4. From the remaining options, use basic principles related to hygiene to assist in directing you to option 2. If this question was difficult, review this procedure.

*Level of Cognitive Ability:* Analysis
*Client Needs:* Physiological Integrity
*Integrated Concept/Process:* Teaching/Learning
*Content Area:* Fundamental Skills

*Reference*
Potter, P., & Perry, A. (2001). *Fundamentals of nursing* (5th ed.). St. Louis: Mosby, p. 863.

**216.** A nurse is reviewing the serum laboratory test results for a client with sickle cell anemia. The nurse anticipates finding that which of the following values is elevated?
1   Hemoglobin F
2   Hemoglobin S
3   Hemoglobin C
4   Hemoglobin $A_1$

**Answer: 2**

*Rationale:* Sickle cell anemia is a severe anemia that predominantly affects African-Americans. It is characterized by the presence of only hemoglobin S. The client must have two abnormal genes yielding hemoglobin S to have sickle cell anemia. A client could have sickle cell trait by carrying one hemoglobin A gene and one hemoglobin S gene.

*Test-Taking Strategy:* To answer this question accurately, you must know the pathophysiology of sickle cell anemia and how it is reflected in common laboratory studies. If needed, review the pathophysiology of sickle cell anemia.

*Level of Cognitive Ability:* Analysis
*Client Needs:* Physiological Integrity
*Integrated Concept/Process:* Nursing Process/Assessment
*Content Area:* Fundamental Skills

*Reference*
Monahan, F., & Neighbors, M. (1998). *Medical-surgical nursing: Foundations for clinical practice* (2nd ed.). Philadelphia: W.B Saunders, p. 484.

**217.** A client wishes to donate blood for a family member for an upcoming surgery and asks the nurse, "How will I know if our blood types will match?" In formulating a response, the nurse incorporates that which of the following tests will be used to test compatibility?

1    Eosinophil count
2    Monocyte count
3    Direct Coombs'
4    Indirect Coombs'

**Answer: 4**

*Rationale:* The indirect Coombs' test detects circulating antibodies against red blood cells (RBCs), and is the "screening" component of the order to "type and screen" a client's blood. This test is used in addition to the ABO typing, which is normally done to determine blood type. The direct Coombs' test is used to detect idiopathic hemolytic anemia, by detecting the presence of autoantibodies against the client's RBCs. Eosinophil and monocyte counts are part of a complete blood count, a routine hematologic screening test.

*Test-Taking Strategy:* Use the process of elimination. Eliminate options 1 and 2 because they are part of routine laboratory work. From the remaining options, it is necessary to know the difference between the two tests. Review the purpose of the direct and indirect Coombs' test if you had difficulty with this question.

*Level of Cognitive Ability:* Analysis
*Client Needs:* Physiological Integrity
*Integrated Concept/Process:* Nursing Process/Implementation
*Content Area:* Fundamental Skills

*Reference*
Fischbach, F. (2000). *A manual of laboratory & diagnostic tests* (6th ed.). Philadelphia: Lippincott Williams & Wilkins, p. 672.

---

**218.** A client scheduled for a bone marrow aspiration asks the nurse about possible sites that could be used to perform the procedure. The nurse tells the client that, in addition to the iliac crest, the test may be done in which of the following areas?

1    Femur
2    Sternum
3    Scapula
4    Ribs

**Answer: 2**

*Rationale:* The most common sites for bone marrow aspiration in the adult are the iliac crest and the sternum. These areas are rich in bone marrow and are easily accessible for testing. The femur, scapula, and ribs are incorrect options.

*Test-Taking Strategy:* Focus on the issue: a bone marrow aspiration. Recalling the anatomy and physiology related to the bones and bone marrow will direct you to option 2. Review the procedure for a bone marrow aspiration if you had difficulty with this question.

*Level of Cognitive Ability:* Application
*Client Needs:* Physiological Integrity
*Integrated Concept/Process:* Teaching/Learning
*Content Area:* Fundamental Skills

*Reference*
Monahan, F., & Neighbors, M. (1998). *Medical-surgical nursing: Foundations for clinical practice* (2nd ed.). Philadelphia: W.B Saunders, p. 451.

**219.** A client is admitted to the hospital with sickle cell crisis. The nurse monitors this client for which of the following most frequent symptoms of the disorder?

1 Bradycardia
2 Pain
3 Diarrhea
4 Blurred vision

**Answer: 2**

*Rationale:* Sickle cell crisis often causes pain in the bones and joints, accompanied by joint swelling. Pain is a classic symptom and may require large doses of narcotic analgesics when it is severe. The symptoms listed in the other options are not associated with this disorder.

*Test-Taking Strategy:* Note the client's diagnosis. Recalling that the primary treatment of sickle cell crisis focuses of the administration of fluids and on management of pain will direct you to option 2. If this question was difficult, review the manifestations associated with sickle cell crisis.

*Level of Cognitive Ability:* Application
*Client Needs:* Physiological Integrity
*Integrated Concept/Process:* Nursing Process/Assessment
*Content Area:* Fundamental Skills

*Reference*
Black, J., Hawks, J., & Keene, A. (2001). *Medical-surgical nursing: Clinical management for positive outcomes* (6th ed.). Philadelphia: W.B. Saunders, p. 2104.

---

**220.** Quinidine gluconate (Duraquin) is prescribed for a client. The nurse reviews the client's medical record knowing that which of the following is a contraindication in the use of this medication?

1 Complete atrioventricular (AV) block
2 Muscle weakness
3 Asthma
4 Infection

**Answer: 1**

*Rationale:* Quinidine gluconate is an antidysrhythmic medication used as prophylactic therapy to maintain normal sinus rhythm after conversion of atrial fibrillation and/or atrial flutter. It is contraindicated in complete AV block, intraventricular conduction defects, abnormal impulses and rhythms due to escape mechanisms, and in myasthenia gravis. It is used with caution in clients with preexisting asthma, muscle weakness, infection with fever, and hepatic or renal insufficiency.

*Test-Taking Strategy:* Note the key word *contraindicated*. Recalling that this medication has a direct cardiac effect will direct you to option 1. If you are unfamiliar with this medication and its contraindications, review this content.

*Level of Cognitive Ability:* Analysis
*Client Needs:* Safe, Effective Care Environment
*Integrated Concept/Process:* Nursing Process/Analysis
*Content Area:* Pharmacology

*Reference*
Hodgson, B., & Kizior, R. (2001). *Saunders Nursing drug handbook 2001.* Philadelphia: W.B. Saunders, pp. 894-896.

**221.** A postoperative client is anemic from blood loss during a recent surgery. The nurse interprets that which of the following signs and symptoms exhibited by the client is most likely associated with the anemia?

1 Bradycardia
2 Fatigue
3 Increased respiratory rate
4 Muscle cramps

**Answer: 2**

*Rationale:* The client with anemia is likely to complain of fatigue, due to decreased ability of the body to carry oxygen to tissues to meet metabolic demands. The client is likely to have tachycardia, not bradycardia due to efforts by the body to compensate for the effects of anemia. Increased respiratory rate is not an associated finding, although some clients may have shortness of breath. Muscle cramps is an unrelated finding.

*Test-Taking Strategy:* Use the process of elimination, focusing on the issue, the signs and symptoms associated with anemia. Recalling that anemia causes a reduction in the oxygen-carrying capacity to the tissues will direct you to option 2. Review the manifestations associated with anemia if you had difficulty with this question.

*Level of Cognitive Ability:* Analysis
*Client Needs:* Physiological Integrity
*Integrated Concept/Process:* Nursing Process/Analysis
*Content Area:* Fundamental Skills

*Reference*
Monahan, F., & Neighbors, M. (1998). *Medical-surgical nursing: Foundations for clinical practice* (2nd ed.). Philadelphia: W.B Saunders, p. 468.

**222.** A client who has a history of chronic ulcerative colitis is diagnosed with anemia. The nurse interprets that which of the following factors is most likely responsible for the anemia?

1 Decreased intake of dietary iron
2 Intestinal malabsorption
3 Blood loss
4 Intestinal hookworm

**Answer: 3**

*Rationale:* The client with ulcerative colitis is most likely anemic due to chronic blood loss in small amounts that occurs with exacerbations of the disease. These clients often have bloody stools and are at increased risk for anemia. There is no information in the question to support options 1 or 4. In ulcerative colitis, the large intestine is involved, not the small intestine where vitamin $B_{12}$ and folic acid are absorbed (option 2).

*Test-Taking Strategy:* Note the issue, the cause of the anemia. Focusing on the client's diagnosis and recalling the pathophysiology that occurs in this disorder will direct you to option 3. Review the manifestations in ulcerative colitis if you had difficulty with this question.

*Level of Cognitive Ability:* Analysis
*Client Needs:* Physiological Integrity
*Integrated Concept/Process:* Nursing Process/Analysis
*Content Area:* Fundamental Skills

*Reference*
Black, J., Hawks, J., & Keene, A. (2001). *Medical-surgical nursing: Clinical management for positive outcomes* (6th ed.). Philadelphia: W.B. Saunders, p. 772.

**223.** A nurse employed in a rehabilitation center is planning the client assignments for the day. Which of the following clients would the nurse assign to the nursing assistant?
1 A client who had a below-the-knee amputation
2 A client on a 24-hour urine collection who is also on strict bed rest
3 A client scheduled for transfer to the hospital for coronary artery bypass surgery
4 A client scheduled for transfer to the hospital for an invasive diagnostic procedure

**Answer: 2**
*Rationale:* The nurse must assign tasks based on the guidelines of nursing practice acts and the job description of the employing agency. A client who had a below-the-knee amputation, a client scheduled to be transferred to the hospital for coronary artery bypass surgery, and a client scheduled for an invasive diagnostic procedure will have both physiological and psychosocial needs. The nursing assistant has been trained to care for a client on bed rest and on urine collections. The nurse would provide instructions to the nursing assistant regarding the tasks, but the tasks required for this client are within the role description of a nursing assistant.

*Test-Taking Strategy:* Note that the question asks for the assignment to be delegated to the nursing assistant. When asked questions related to delegation, think about the role description of the employee and the needs of the client. By the process of elimination, you will be directed to option 2. Review the responsibilities related to delegation and the job description of the nursing assistant if you had difficulty with this question

*Level of Cognitive Ability:* Application
*Client Needs:* Safe, Effective Care Environment
*Integrated Concept/Process:* Nursing Process/Planning
*Content Area:* Fundamental Skills

*Reference*
Rocchiccioli, J., & Tilbury, M. (1998). *Clinical leadership in nursing.* Philadelphia: W.B. Saunders, p. 140.

**224.** A nurse is monitoring a client who is receiving a blood transfusion. The client begins to complain of a sweaty and warm feeling and a backache. The nurse notes that the client's skin is flushed and suspects that the client is having a transfusion reaction. The nurse anticipates that the immediate action to be prescribed would be to stop the blood transfusion and then:
1 Discontinue the IV line
2 Change the continuous IV to an intermittent needle device
3 Hang an IV bag of 5% dextrose in water
4 Hang an IV bag of normal saline solution

**Answer: 4**
*Rationale:* If a transfusion reaction is suspected, the transfusion is stopped and then normal saline is infused pending further physician orders. This maintains a patent IV access line, and aids in maintaining the client's intravascular volume. The IV line would not be discontinued, because there would be no IV access route. Normal saline is the solution of choice over solutions containing dextrose because saline does not cause clumping of red blood cells.

*Test-Taking Strategy:* Use the process of elimination and knowledge regarding blood transfusions to answer the question. Recalling that normal saline is the solution that is compatible with blood will direct you to option 4. Review interventions if a blood transfusion occurs if you had difficulty with this question.

*Level of Cognitive Ability:* Application
*Client Needs:* Physiological Integrity
*Integrated Concept/Process:* Nursing Process/Implementation
*Content Area:* Fundamental Skills

*Reference*
Monahan, F., & Neighbors, M. (1998). *Medical-surgical nursing: Foundations for clinical practice* (2nd ed.). Philadelphia: W.B Saunders, p. 458.

**225.** A client has been taking lisinopril (Prinivil) for three months. The client complains to the nurse of a persistent dry cough that began about one month ago. The nurse interprets that this is most likely:

1   Caused by a concurrent upper respiratory infection
2   Caused by neutropenia as a result of therapy
3   An expected, although bothersome, side effect of therapy
4   An indication that the client will show signs of heart failure

**Answer: 3**

*Rationale:* A frequent side effect of therapy with any of the angiotensin-converting enzyme (ACE) inhibitors, such as lisinopril, is the appearance of a persistent, dry cough. The cough generally does not improve while the client is taking the medication. Clients are advised to notify the physician if the cough becomes very troublesome to them. The other options are incorrect.

*Test-Taking Strategy:* Use the process of elimination. Eliminate options 1 and 2 first, because they are similar and both focus on infection. From the remaining options, it is necessary to know the frequent side effects of this medication to direct you to option 3. Review the side effects of ACE inhibitor therapy if you had difficulty with this question.

*Level of Cognitive Ability:* Analysis
*Client Needs:* Physiological Integrity
*Integrated Concept/Process:* Nursing Process/Analysis
*Content Area:* Pharmacology

*Reference*
Hodgson, B., & Kizior, R. (2001). *Saunders Nursing drug handbook 2001.* Philadelphia: W.B. Saunders, p. 596.

---

**226.** A client has been given a prescription to begin using nitroglycerin transdermal patches in the management of angina pectoris. The nurse instructs the client about this medication administration system and tells the client to:

1   Apply a new system every 7 days
2   Apply the system in the morning and leave it in place for 12 to 16 hours as directed
3   Place the system in the area of a skinfold to promote better adherence
4   Wait 1 day to apply a new system if it becomes dislodged

**Answer: 2**

*Rationale:* Nitroglycerin is a coronary vasodilator used in the management of coronary artery disease. The client is generally advised to apply a new system each morning and leave it in place for 12 to 16 hours as per physician directions. This prevents the client from developing tolerance (as happens with 24-hour use). The client should avoid placing the system in skin folds or excoriated areas. The client can apply a new system if it becomes dislodged because the dose is released continuously in small amounts through the skin.

*Test-Taking Strategy:* Specific information related to this type of medication administration system is needed to answer this question. Recalling that tolerance can occur with this medication will direct you to option 2. Review the procedures related to transdermal medication systems if you had difficulty with this question.

*Level of Cognitive Ability:* Application
*Client Needs:* Health Promotion and Maintenance
*Integrated Concept/Process:* Teaching/Learning
*Content Area:* Pharmacology

*Reference*
Hodgson, B., & Kizior, R. (2001). *Saunders Nursing drug handbook 2001.* Philadelphia: W.B. Saunders, p. 750.

**227.** A nurse is visiting a client who has been started on therapy with clotrimazole (Lotrimin). The nurse tells the client that this medication will alleviate:

1 Sneezing
2 Rash
3 Fever
4 Pain

**Answer: 2**

*Rationale:* Clotrimazole is a topical antifungal used in the treatment of cutaneous fungal infections. The nurse teaches the client that it is used for this purpose. It is not used for sneezing, fever, or pain.

*Test-Taking Strategy:* Use the process of elimination. Recalling that this medication is an antifungal will direct you to option 2. Review the purpose of this anti-infective if you had difficulty with this question.

*Level of Cognitive Ability:* Application
*Client Needs:* Physiological Integrity
*Integrated Concept/Process:* Teaching/Learning
*Content Area:* Pharmacology

*Reference*
Deglin, J., & Vallerand, A. (1999). *Davis's Drug guide for nurses* (6th ed.). Philadelphia: F.A. Davis, p. 69.

---

**228.** A nurse is providing care to a client who has received medication therapy with tissue plasminogen activator (t-PA, Activase). As part of standard nursing care for this client, the nurse plans to have which of the following items available for use?

1 Pulse oximeter
2 Suction equipment
3 Flashlight
4 Occult blood test strips

**Answer: 4**

*Rationale:* Tissue plasminogen activator is a thrombolytic medication that is used to dissolve thrombi or emboli due to thrombus. A frequent and potentially severe side effect of therapy is bleeding. The nurse monitors for signs of bleeding in clients receiving this therapy. Equipment needed by the nurse would include occult blood test strips to monitor for occult blood in the urine, stool, or nasogastric drainage. Pulse oximeter and suction equipment would be needed if the client had evidence of respiratory problems. A flashlight may be used for pupil assessment as part of the neurological exam in the client who is neurologically impaired.

*Test-Taking Strategy:* Use the process of elimination. Recalling that this medication is a thrombolytic and that bleeding is a side effect of this therapy will direct you to option 4. If this question was difficult, review this medication and its side effects.

*Level of Cognitive Ability:* Application
*Client Needs:* Physiological Integrity
*Integrated Concept/Process:* Nursing Process/Planning
*Content Area:* Pharmacology

*Reference*
Hodgson, B., & Kizior, R. (2001). *Saunders Nursing drug handbook 2001.* Philadelphia: W.B. Saunders, p. 30.

**229.** A client newly diagnosed with angina pectoris has taken two sublingual nitroglycerin tablets for chest pain. The chest pain is relieved, but the client complains of a headache. The nurse interprets that this symptom most likely represents:

1   An allergic reaction to the nitroglycerin
2   An expected side effect of the medication
3   An early sign of medication tolerance
4   A warning that the medication should not be used again

**Answer: 2**

*Rationale:* Headache is a frequent side effect of nitroglycerin, due to the vasodilating action of the medication. It usually diminishes in frequency as the client becomes accustomed to the medication, and is effectively treated with acetaminophen. The other options are incorrect.

*Test-Taking Strategy:* Use the process of elimination. Eliminate options 1 and 4 because they are similar and imply that the medication can no longer be used by the client. From the remaining options, recalling that the medication vasodilates will direct you to option 2. Review the effect of this medication if you had difficulty with question.

*Level of Cognitive Ability:* Analysis
*Client Needs:* Physiological Integrity
*Integrated Concept/Process:* Nursing Process/Analysis
*Content Area:* Pharmacology

*Reference*
Hodgson, B., & Kizior, R. (2001). *Saunders Nursing drug handbook 2001.* Philadelphia: W.B. Saunders, p. 750.

---

**230.** A nurse is caring for a client with atrial fibrillation. The physician has prescribed verapamil (Calan) 5 mg intravenous (IV). The nurse ensures that which of the following most essential items is present when the administering this medication?

1   Pulse oximeter
2   Oxygen
3   Noninvasive blood pressure monitor
4   Cardiac monitor

**Answer: 4**

*Rationale:* Verapamil is a calcium-channel blocking agent that may be used to treat rapid rate supraventricular tachydysrhythmias, such as atrial flutter or atrial fibrillation. The client must be placed on a cardiac monitor to evaluate the effectiveness of the medication. A noninvasive blood pressure monitor is also helpful, but is not as essential as the cardiac monitor. Pulse oximeter and oxygen are related to respiratory care, and are not directly related to the use of this medication.

*Test-Taking Strategy:* Note the key words *most essential.* Eliminate options 1 and 2 first because there is no information about respiratory difficulty in the case situation. From the remaining options, noting the client's diagnosis will direct you to option 4. Review nursing interventions related to the administration of this medication if you had difficulty with this question.

*Level of Cognitive Ability:* Application
*Client Needs:* Physiological Integrity
*Integrated Concept/Process:* Nursing Process/Planning
*Content Area:* Pharmacology

*Reference*
Hodgson, B., & Kizior, R. (2001). *Saunders Nursing drug handbook 2001.* Philadelphia: W.B. Saunders, p. 1082.

**231.** A client is taking albuterol (Ventolin) by inhalation but cannot cough up secretions. The nurse teaches the client to do which of the following to best help clear the bronchial secretions?
1    Administer an extra dose before bedtime
2    Take in increased amounts of fluids every day
3    Get more exercise each day
4    Use a dehumidifier in the home

**Answer: 2**
*Rationale:* The client should take in increased fluids (2000 to 3000 mL/day) to make secretions less viscous. This may help the client to expectorate secretions. This is standard advice given to clients receiving any of the adrenergic bronchodilators, such as albuterol, unless the client has another health problem that could be worsened by increased fluid intake. A dehumidifier will dry secretions. The client would not be advised to take additional medication. Additional exercise will not effectively clear bronchial secretions.

*Test-Taking Strategy:* Focus on the issue: clearing bronchial secretions. Recalling basic respiratory principles will direct you to option 2. Review client teaching points related to this medication if you had difficulty with this question.

*Level of Cognitive Ability:* Application
*Client Needs:* Health Promotion and Maintenance
*Integrated Concept/Process:* Teaching/Learning
*Content Area:* Pharmacology

*Reference*
Hodgson, B., & Kizior, R. (2001). *Saunders Nursing drug handbook 2001.* Philadelphia: W.B. Saunders, p. 18.

**232.** A nurse reviews the serum laboratory results for the client taking chlorothiazide (Diuril). The nurse specifically monitors for which of the following most frequent medication side effect on a regular basis?
1    Hyperphosphatemia
2    Hypocalcemia
3    Hypernatremia
4    Hypokalemia

**Answer: 4**
*Rationale:* The client taking a potassium-wasting diuretic such as chlorothiazide (Diuril) needs to be monitored for decreased potassium levels. Other fluid and electrolyte imbalances that occur with the use of this medication include hyponatremia, hypercalcemia, hypomagnesemia, and hypophosphatemia.

*Test-Taking Strategy:* Focus on the name of the medication and recall that this medication is a potassium-wasting diuretic. Remember that hypokalemia is a concern when a client is taking a potassium wasting diuretic. Review the side effects of this medication if you had difficulty with this medication.

*Level of Cognitive Ability:* Application
*Client Needs:* Physiological Integrity
*Integrated Concept/Process:* Nursing Process/Assessment
*Content Area:* Pharmacology

*Reference*
Hodgson, B., & Kizior, R. (2001). *Saunders Nursing drug handbook 2001.* Philadelphia: W.B. Saunders, p. 208.

**233.** A nurse has administered a dose of diazepam (Valium) to a male client. The nurse would take which of the following most important actions before leaving the client's room?

1 Drawing the shades closed
2 Putting up the side rails on the bed
3 Giving the client a bedpan
4 Turning the volume on the television set down

**Answer: 2**

*Rationale:* Diazepam is a sedative/hypnotic with anticonvulsant and skeletal muscle relaxant properties. The nurse should institute safety measures before leaving the client's room to ensure that the client does not injure himself. The most frequent side effects of this medication are dizziness, drowsiness, and lethargy. For this reason, the nurse puts the side rails up on the bed before leaving the room to prevent falls. Options 1, 3, and 4 may be helpful measures that provide a comfortable, restful environment. However, option 2 is the one that provides for the client's safety needs.

*Test-Taking Strategy:* Note the key words *most important* and *before leaving the client's room.* Recalling that diazepam is a sedative/hypnotic and that safety is an issue will direct you to option 2. Review care of a client receiving this medication if you had difficulty with this question.

*Level of Cognitive Ability:* Application
*Client Needs:* Safe, Effective Care Environment
*Integrated Concept/Process:* Nursing Process/Implementation
*Content Area:* Pharmacology

*Reference*
Deglin, J., & Vallerand, A. (1999). *Davis's Drug guide for nurses* (6th ed.). Philadelphia: F.A. Davis, p. 263.

**234.** A nurse provides home care instructions to a client who is taking lithium carbonate (Eskalith). Which statement by the client indicates a need for further teaching?

1 "Lithium blood levels must be monitored very closely."
2 "I need to stop taking the medication if excessive diarrhea, vomiting, or diaphoresis occurs."
3 "I need to take the lithium with meals."
4 "I need to decrease my salt and fluid intake while taking the lithium."

**Answer: 4**

*Rationale:* Because therapeutic and toxic dosage ranges are so close, lithium blood levels must be monitored very closely, more frequently at first, then once every several months after that. The client should be instructed to stop taking the medication if excessive diarrhea, vomiting, or diaphoresis occurs, and to inform the physician if any of these problems occur. Lithium is irritating to the gastric mucosa therefore lithium should be taken with meals. A normal diet and normal salt and fluid intake (1500 to 3000 mL per day, or six 12-oz glasses) should be maintained because lithium decreases sodium reabsorption by the renal tubules, which could cause sodium depletion. A low sodium intake causes a relative increase in lithium retention and could lead to toxicity.

*Test-Taking Strategy:* Note the key words *need for further teaching.* Remember that generally, it is important that clients be taught to maintain an adequate fluid intake. This principle will easily direct you to option 4. Review the client teaching points related to the administration of this medication if you had difficulty with this question.

*Level of Cognitive Ability:* Analysis
*Client Needs:* Health Promotion and Maintenance
*Integrated Concept/Process:* Teaching/Learning
*Content Area:* Pharmacology

*Reference*
Hodgson, B., & Kizior, R. (2001). *Saunders Nursing drug handbook 2001.* Philadelphia: W.B. Saunders, p. 598.

**235.** A client with a psychotic disorder is being treated with haloperidol (Haldol). The nurse monitors the client for which of the following that indicates the presence of a toxic effect of this medication?
1   Hypotension
2   Nausea
3   Excessive salivation
4   Blurred vision

**Answer: 3**
*Rationale:* Toxic effects of this medication include extrapyramidal symptoms such as marked drowsiness and lethargy, excessive salivation, a fixed stare, akathisia, acute dystonias, and tardive dyskinesia. Hypotension, nausea, and blurred vision are occasional side effects.

*Test-Taking Strategy:* Focus on the issue: toxic effect. Using the process of elimination, select option 3 because of the word *excessive* in this option. If you had difficulty with this question, review the toxic effects of this medication.

*Level of Cognitive Ability:* Application
*Client Needs:* Physiological Integrity
*Integrated Concept/Process:* Nursing Process/Assessment
*Content Area:* Pharmacology

*Reference*
Hodgson, B., & Kizior, R. (2001). *Saunders Nursing drug handbook 2001.* Philadelphia: W.B. Saunders, p. 488

---

**236.** A nurse is caring for a client with Parkinson's disease. The client is taking benztropine mesylate (Cogentin) daily. The nurse assesses the client for side effects of this medication and specifically monitors:
1   Hemoglobin and hematocrit
2   Respiratory status
3   Intake and output
4   Prothrombin time

**Answer: 3**
*Rationale:* Urinary retention is a side effect of benztropine mesylate. The nurse needs to observe for dysuria, distended abdomen, voiding in small amounts, and overflow incontinence. Options 1, 2, and 4 are not specific to this medication.

*Test-Taking Strategy:* Use the process of elimination, recalling that urinary retention is a concern with this medication. Review this medication and its side effects if you had difficulty with this question.

*Level of Cognitive Ability:* Application
*Client Needs:* Physiological Integrity
*Integrated Concept/Process:* Nursing Process/Assessment
*Content Area:* Pharmacology

*Reference*
Hodgson, B., & Kizior, R. (2001). *Saunders Nursing drug handbook 2001.* Philadelphia: W.B. Saunders, pp. 102-104.

---

**237.** A nurse is providing instructions to a client regarding quinapril hydrochloride (Accupril). The nurse tells the client:
1   To take the medication with food only
2   To rise slowly from a lying to a sitting position
3   To discontinue the medication if nausea occurs
4   That a therapeutic effect will be noted immediately

**Answer: 2**
*Rationale:* Accupril is an angiotensin-converting enzyme (ACE) inhibitor. It is used in the treatment of hypertension. The client should be instructed to rise slowly from a lying to sitting position and to permit the legs to dangle from the bed momentarily before standing, to reduce the hypotensive effect. The medication does not need to be taken with meals. It may be given without regard to food. If nausea occurs, the client should be instructed to take a noncola carbonated beverage and salted crackers or dry toast. A full therapeutic effect may be noted in 1 to 2 weeks.

*Test-Taking Strategy:* Use the process of elimination. Focus on the medication classification. Recalling that this medication is an ACE inhibitor used in the treatment of hypertension will direct you to option 2. If you had difficulty with this question, review the action of this medication and the associated client teaching points.

*Level of Cognitive Ability:* Application
*Client Needs:* Health Promotion and Maintenance
*Integrated Concept/Process:* Teaching/Learning
*Content Area:* Pharmacology

*Reference*
Hodgson, B., & Kizior, R. (2001). *Saunders Nursing drug handbook 2001.* Philadelphia: W.B. Saunders, pp. 892-894.

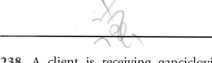

**238.** A client is receiving ganciclovir (Cytovene). The nurse plans to do which of the following while the client is taking this medication?
1 Monitor for bleeding
2 Apply pressure to venipuncture sites for at least 2 minutes
3 Monitor blood glucose levels for elevation
4 Administer the medication on an empty stomach only

**Answer: 1**
*Rationale:* Ganciclovir causes neutropenia and thrombocytopenia as the most frequent side effects. For this reason, the nurse monitors the client for signs and symptoms of bleeding, and implements the same precautions that are used for a client receiving anticoagulant therapy. These include providing a soft toothbrush and electric razor to minimize the risk of trauma that could result in bleeding. Venipuncture sites should be held for approximately 10 minutes. The medication does not have to be taken on an empty stomach. The medication may cause hypoglycemia, but not hyperglycemia.

*Test-Taking Strategy:* Use the process of elimination. Recalling that ganciclovir causes thrombocytopenia will direct you to option 1. Review the side effects of this medication if you had difficulty with this question.

*Level of Cognitive Ability:* Application
*Client Needs:* Safe, Effective Care Environment
*Integrated Concept/Process:* Nursing Process/Planning
*Content Area:* Pharmacology

*Reference*
Deglin, J., & Vallerand, A. (1999). *Davis's Drug guide for nurses* (6th ed.). Philadelphia: F.A. Davis, p. 419.

**239.** A client is to be discharged from the hospital on quinidine gluconate (Quinaglute) to control ventricular ectopy. Which statement by the client would indicate the need for further teaching?
1 "I need to take this medication regularly, even if my heart feels strong."
2 "The best time to schedule this medication is with my meals."
3 "If I get diarrhea, nausea, or vomiting, I need to stop the medication and then call my doctor."
4 "I should avoid alcohol, caffeine, and cigarettes while on this medication."

**Answer: 3**
*Rationale:* Diarrhea, nausea, vomiting, loss of appetite, and dizziness are all common side effects of quinidine. If these should occur, the physician or nurse should be notified; however, the medication should never be stopped by the client. A rapid decrease in the medication level of an antidysrhythmic could precipitate dysrhythmia. Options 1, 2, and 4 are accurate client statements.

*Test-Taking Strategy:* Note the key words *need for further teaching.* Noting that quinidine is used to control ectopy will direct you to option 3. It is reasonable that a client would not stop the medication without first consulting the physician. Review client teaching points related to this medication if you had difficulty with this question.

*Level of Cognitive Ability:* Analysis
*Client Needs:* Physiological Integrity
*Integrated Concept/Process:* Teaching/Learning
*Content Area:* Pharmacology

**Reference**
Deglin, J., & Vallerand, A. (1999). *Davis's Drug guide for nurses* (6th ed.). Philadelphia: F.A. Davis, p. 880.

---

**240.** A client has been taking benzonatate (Tessalon) as ordered. The nurse tells the client that this medication should do which of the following?
1  Take away nausea and vomiting
2  Calm the persistent cough
3  Decrease anxiety level
4  Increase comfort level

**Answer: 2**
*Rationale:* Benzonatate is a locally acting antitussive. Its effectiveness is measured by the degree to which it decreases the intensity and frequency of cough, without eliminating the cough reflex. Options 1, 3, and 4 are not intended effects of this medication.

*Test-Taking Strategy:* Use the process of elimination. Recalling that benzonatate is a locally acting antitussive will easily direct you to option 2. If the question was difficult or if you are unfamiliar with this medication, review this content.

*Level of Cognitive Ability:* Application
*Client Needs:* Physiological Integrity
*Integrated Concept/Process:* Teaching/Learning
*Content Area:* Pharmacology

**Reference**
Deglin, J., & Vallerand, A. (1999). *Davis's Drug guide for nurses* (6th ed.). Philadelphia: F.A. Davis, p. 1131.

---

**241.** Vasopressin (Pitressin) is prescribed for a client with diabetes insipidus. The client asks the nurse about the purpose of the medication. The nurse responds knowing that the action of the medication is to:
1  Inhibit contraction of smooth muscle
2  Produce vasodilation
3  Decrease urinary output
4  Decrease peristalsis

**Answer: 3**
*Rationale:* Vasopressin is a vasopressor and an antidiuretic. It directly stimulates contraction of smooth muscle, causes vasoconstriction, stimulates peristalsis, and increases reabsorption of water by the renal tubules resulting in decreased urinary flow rate.

*Test-Taking Strategy:* Use the process of elimination. Eliminate options 1 and 4 first because they are similar. From the remaining options, recalling the pathophysiology associated with diabetes insipidus will direct you to option 3. Review the actions of this medication if you had difficulty with this question.

*Level of Cognitive Ability:* Application
*Client Needs:* Physiological Integrity
*Integrated Concept/Process:* Teaching/Learning
*Content Area:* Pharmacology

**Reference**
Hodgson, B., & Kizior, R. (2001). *Saunders Nursing drug handbook 2001.* Philadelphia: W.B. Saunders, pp. 1043-1045.

**242.** A client is seen in the health care clinic. The client has diabetes mellitus that has been well controlled with glyburide (Diabeta), but recently, the client's fasting blood glucose has been reported to be 180 to 200 mg/dL. Which of the following medications, if noted in the client's record, may be contributing to the elevated blood glucose level?
1   Cimetidine (Tagamet)
2   Ranitidine (Zantac)
3   Ciprofloxacin hydrochloride (Cipro)
4   Prednisone (Deltasone)

**Answer: 4**
*Rationale:* Corticosteroids, thiazide diuretics, and lithium may decrease the effect of glyburide causing hyperglycemia. Options 1, 2, and 3 may increase the effect of glyburide leading to hypoglycemia.

*Test-Taking Strategy:* Knowledge regarding the medications that have an adverse effect if taken concurrently with glyburide is required to answer this question. If you are unfamiliar with these medications, review this content.

*Level of Cognitive Ability:* Analysis
*Client Needs:* Physiological integrity
*Integrated Concept/Process:* Nursing Process/Analysis
*Content Area:* Pharmacology

*Reference*
Hodgson, B., & Kizior, R. (2001). *Saunders Nursing drug handbook 2001.* Philadelphia: W.B. Saunders, p. 471.

**243.** A nurse in the postpartum unit reviews a client's record and notes that a new mother was administered methylergonovine (Methergine) intramuscularly following delivery. The nurse determines that this medication was administered to:
1   Decrease uterine contractions
2   Maintain a normal blood pressure
3   Prevent postpartum hemorrhage
4   Reduce the amount of lochia drainage

**Answer: 3**
*Rationale:* Methylergonovine, an oxytocic, is an agent that is used to prevent or control postpartum hemorrhage by contracting the uterus. The first dose is usually administered intramuscularly, and then if it needs to be continued, it is given by mouth. It increases the strength and frequency of contractions and may elevate blood pressure. There is no relationship between the action of this medication and lochial drainage.

*Test-Taking Strategy:* Use the process of elimination. Recalling that this medication is an oxytocic agent, will direct you to option 3. If you are unfamiliar with this medication, review its action and use.

*Level of Cognitive Ability:* Analysis
*Client's Needs:* Physiological Integrity
*Integrated Concept/Process:* Nursing Process/Analysis
*Content Area:* Pharmacology

*Reference*
Lowdermilk, D., Perry, S., & Bobak, I. (2000). *Maternity & women's health care* (7th ed.). St. Louis: Mosby, p. 1026.

**244.** Buspirone hydrochloride (BuSpar) is prescribed for a client with an anxiety disorder. The nurse instructs the client regarding the medication and tells the client that:
1   The medication can produce a sedating effect
2   Tolerance can occur with the medication
3   The medication is addicting
4   Dizziness and nervousness may occur

**Answer: 4**
*Rationale:* Buspirone hydrochloride is used in the management of anxiety disorders. The advantages of this medication is that it is not sedating, tolerance does not develop, and it is not addicting. The medication has a more favorable side effect profile than do the benzodiazepines. Dizziness, nausea, headaches, nervousness, lightheadedness, and excitement, which generally are not major problems, are side effects of the medication.

*Test-Taking Strategy:* Knowledge regarding the side effects and the advantages of buspirone hydrochloride is required to answer this question. If you are unfamiliar with this medication and its use, review its characteristics.

*Level of Cognitive Ability:* Application
*Client Needs:* Physiological Integrity
*Integrated Concept/Process:* Teaching/Learning
*Content Area:* Pharmacology

**Reference**
Varcarolis, E.M. (1998). *Foundations of psychiatric mental health nursing.* (3rd ed.). Philadelphia: W.B. Saunders, p. 1005.

---

**245.** Neuroleptic malignant syndrome is suspected in a client who is taking chlorpromazine (Thorazine). Which of the following medications would the nurse prepare in anticipation of being prescribed to treat this adverse reaction related to the use of Thorazine?
1   Phytonadione (vitamin K)
2   Bromocriptine (Parlodel)
3   Enalapril maleate (Vasotec)
4   Protamine sulfate

**Answer: 2**
*Rationale:* Bromocriptine is an antiparkinson prolactin inhibitor used in the treatment of neuroleptic malignant syndrome. Vitamin K is the antidote for warfarin (Coumadin) overdose. Protamine sulfate is the antidote for heparin overdose. Enalapril maleate is an angiotensen converting enzyme (ACE inhibitor) and an antihypertensive that is used in the treatment of hypertension.

*Test-Taking Strategy:* Use the process of elimination. Recalling that option 1 is the antidote for warfarin overdose and option 4 is the antidote for heparin will assist in eliminating these options. From the remaining options, focus on the medication classifications and eliminate option 3 because it is an antihypertensive. Review neuroleptic malignant syndrome if you had difficulty with this question.

*Level of Cognitive Ability:* Application
*Client Needs:* Physiological Integrity
*Integrated Concept/Process:* Nursing Process/Planning
*Content Area:* Pharmacology

**Reference**
Varcarolis, E.M. (1998). *Foundations of psychiatric mental health nursing.* (3rd ed.). Philadelphia: W.B. Saunders, p. 1008.

---

**246.** A client with a fractured leg has learned how to use crutches to assist in ambulation. The nurse evaluates that the client misunderstood the information if the client states to:
1   Keep spare crutch tips available
2   Keep crutch tips dry so they don't slip
3   Keep the set of crutches found in the basement of the home as a spare pair
4   Inspect the crutch tips for wear from time to time

**Answer: 3**
*Rationale:* The client should use only crutches measured for the client. Crutches belonging to another person should not be used unless they have been adjusted to fit the client. Crutch tips should remain dry. Water could cause slipping by decreasing the surface friction of the rubber tip on the floor. If crutch tips get wet, the client should dry them with a cloth or paper towel. The tips should be inspected for wear, and spare tips and crutches fitted to the client should be available if needed.

*Test-Taking Strategy:* Note the key words *misunderstood the information.* Option 2 relates to safety and is eliminated first. Eliminate options 1 and 4 next because they are similar. Review client teaching points related to the use of crutches if you had difficulty with this question.

*Level of Cognitive Ability:* Analysis
*Client Needs:* Health Promotion and Maintenance
*Integrated Concept/Process:* Teaching/Learning
*Content Area:* Adult Health/Musculoskeletal

*Reference*
Potter, P., & Perry, A. (2001). *Fundamentals of nursing* (5th ed.). St. Louis: Mosby, p. 1008.

---

**247.** Disulfiram (Antabuse) is prescribed for a client who is seen in the psychiatric health care clinic. The nurse is collecting data from the client and is providing instructions regarding the use of this medication. Which of the following data are most important for the nurse to obtain before beginning the administration of this medication?

1 When the last alcoholic drink was consumed
2 If the client has a history of diabetes insipidus
3 If the client has a history of hyperthyroidism
4 When the last full meal was consumed

**Answer: 1**
*Rationale:* Disulfiram is used an adjunct treatment for selected clients with chronic alcoholism who want to remain in a state of enforced sobriety. Clients must abstain from alcohol intake for at least 12 hours before the initial dose of the medication is administered. The most important assessment is to determine when the last alcoholic drink was consumed. The medication is used with caution in clients with diabetes mellitus, hypothyroidism, epilepsy, cerebral damage, nephritis, and hepatic disease. It is also contraindicated in severe heart disease, psychosis, or hypersensitivity related to the medication.

*Test-Taking Strategy:* Use the process of elimination. Recalling that this medication is used as an adjunct treatment for chronic alcoholism will direct you to option 1. Review this medication if you are unfamiliar with it.

*Level of Cognitive Ability:* Analysis
*Client Needs:* Physiological integrity
*Integrated Concept/Process:* Nursing Process/Assessment
*Content Area:* Pharmacology

*Reference*
Varcarolis, E.M. (1998). *Foundations of psychiatric mental health nursing.* (3rd ed.). Philadelphia: W.B. Saunders, p. 1012.

---

**248.** A client with breast cancer who has metastasis to the bone states to the nurse, "Why should I even bother to take care of myself? I'll never be cured. It doesn't really matter what I do." Based on the client's statement, the nurse addresses which potential client problem?

1 Powerlessness
2 Ineffective individual coping
3 Anxiety
4 Body image disturbance

**Answer: 1**
*Rationale:* Powerlessness is a problem when the client believes that personal actions will not affect an outcome in any significant way. Ineffective individual coping indicates that the client has impaired adaptive abilities or behaviors in meeting the demands or roles expected from the individual. Anxiety occurs when the client has a feeling of unease with a vague or undefined source. Body image disturbance occurs when there is an alteration in the way the client perceives body image.

*Test-Taking Strategy:* Use the process of elimination, focusing on the data in the question. Note the statement, "It doesn't really matter what I do." This implies the client has a sense of no control of the situation. This will direct you to option 1. Review the defining characteristics of powerlessness if you had difficulty with this question.

*Level of Cognitive Ability:* Analysis
*Client Needs:* Psychosocial Integrity
*Integrated Concept/Process:* Nursing Process/Analysis
*Content Area:* Adult Health/Renal

**Reference**
Leahy, J., & Kizilay, P. (1998). *Foundations of nursing practice: A nursing process approach.* Philadelphia: W.B. Saunders, p. 917.

---

**249.** Fluoxetine hydrochloride (Prozac) is prescribed for a client. The nurse provides instructions to the client regarding the administration of the medication. Which of the following statements if made by the client indicates an understanding regarding the administration of the medication?
1    "I should take the medication with a bed time snack."
2    "I should take the medication with my evening meal."
3    "I should take the medication at noon time with an antacid."
4    "I should take the medication in the morning when I first arise."

**Answer: 4**
*Rationale:* Prozac is administered in the early morning. Options 1, 2, and 3 are incorrect.

*Test-Taking Strategy:* Use the process of elimination. Eliminate options 1, 2, and 3 because they are similar and all indicate taking the medication with food or another item (antacid). If you are unfamiliar with the use of this medication and the client teaching points, review this content.

*Level of Cognitive Ability:* Analysis
*Client Needs:* Health Promotion and Maintenance
*Integrated Concept/Process:* Teaching/Learning
*Content Area:* Pharmacology

**Reference**
Varcarolis, E.M. (1998). *Foundations of psychiatric mental health nursing.* (3rd ed.). Philadelphia: W.B. Saunders, pp. 1013-1014.

---

**250.** A nursing student is assigned to care for a client with a diagnosis of schizophrenia. Haloperidol (Haldol) is prescribed for the client. The nursing instructor asks the student to describe the action of the medication. The student responds correctly by stating that this medication:
1    Blocks the uptake of norepinephrine and serotonin
2    Blocks the binding of dopamine to the postsynaptic dopamine receptors in the brain
3    Is a serotonin reuptake blocker
4    Inhibits the breakdown of released acetylcholine

**Answer: 2**
*Rationale:* Haldol acts by blocking the binding of dopamine to the postsynaptic dopamine receptors in the brain. Imipramine hydrochloride (Tofranil) blocks the reuptake of norepinephrine and serotonin. Donepezil hydrochloride (Aricept) inhibits the breakdown of released acetylcholine. Fluoxetine hydrochloride (Prozac) is a potent serotonin reuptake blocker.

*Test-Taking Strategy:* Knowledge regarding the action of haloperidol is required to answer this question. if you are unfamiliar with this medication, review its action and use.

*Level of Cognitive Ability:* Analysis
*Client Needs:* Physiological Integrity
*Integrated Concept/Process:* Teaching/Learning
*Content Area:* Pharmacology

**Reference**
Varcarolis, E.M. (1998). *Foundations of psychiatric mental health nursing.* (3rd ed.). Philadelphia: W.B. Saunders, pp. 1012-1015.

**251.** A nurse is preparing to teach a client how to mix Regular insulin and NPH insulin in the same syringe. The nurse tells the client to:

1 Take all of the air out of the insulin bottle before mixing
2 Draw up the NPH insulin into the syringe first
3 Keep both bottles in the refrigerator at all times
4 Rotate the NPH insulin bottle in the hands before mixing

**Answer: 4**

*Rationale:* The NPH insulin bottle needs to be rotated for at least one minute between both hands. This resuspends the insulin. The nurse should not shake the bottles. Shaking causes foaming and bubbles to form, which may trap particles of insulin and alter the dosage. Insulin may be maintained at room temperature. Additional bottles of insulin for future use should be stored in the refrigerator. Regular insulin is drawn up before NPH insulin. Air does not need to be removed from the insulin bottle.

*Test-Taking Strategy:* Use the process of elimination. Visualize the procedure for preparing the insulin as you read each option. This will direct you to option 4. Review this procedure if you had difficulty with this question.

*Level of Cognitive Ability:* Application
*Client Needs:* Health Promotion and Maintenance
*Integrated Concept/Process:* Teaching/Learning
*Content Area:* Pharmacology

*Reference*
Lehne, R. (1998). *Pharmacology for nursing care.* (3rd ed.). Philadelphia: W.B. Saunders, pp. 583-583.

**252.** A client has received a dose of dimenhydrinate (Dramamine). The nurse determines that the medication is effective if the client obtains relief of:

1 Nausea and vomiting
2 Ringing in the ears
3 Headache
4 Chills

**Answer: 1**

*Rationale:* Dimenhydrinate is used to treat and prevent the symptoms of dizziness, vertigo, and nausea and vomiting that accompany motion sickness. The other options are incorrect.

*Test-Taking Strategy:* Knowledge regarding the action of this medication is required to answer this question. If the medication is unfamiliar to you, review its action and uses.

*Level of Cognitive Ability:* Analysis
*Client Needs:* Physiological Integrity
*Integrated Concept/Process:* Nursing Process/Evaluation
*Content Area:* Pharmacology

*Reference*
Deglin, J., & Vallerand, A. (1999). *Davis's Drug guide for nurses* (6th ed.). Philadelphia: F.A. Davis, p. 287.

**253.** A client has been taking omeprazole (Prilosec) for 4 weeks. The nurse monitors the client for relief of which of the following symptoms?

1 Constipation
2 Diarrhea
3 Flatulence
4 Heartburn

**Answer: 4**

*Rationale:* Omeprazole is a gastric pump inhibitor and is classified as an antiulcer agent. The intended effect of the medication is relief of pain from gastric irritation, often referred to as heartburn by clients. The medication does not improve the other symptoms listed.

*Test-Taking Strategy:* Specific knowledge of the action of this medication and its uses is needed to answer this question. Recalling that omeprazole is a gastric pump inhibitor will direct you to option 4. If you are unfamiliar with this medication, review its actions and use.

*Level of Cognitive Ability:* Application
*Client Needs:* Physiological Integrity
*Integrated Concept/Process:* Nursing Process/Assessment
*Content Area:* Pharmacology

*Reference*
Deglin, J., & Vallerand, A. (1999). *Davis's Drug guide for nurses* (6th ed.). Philadelphia: F.A. Davis, p. 744.

---

**254.** A nurse is preparing a client who had a total knee replacement (TKR) with a metal prosthesis for discharge to home. Which statement by the client indicates a need for further discharge instructions?
1  "I need to report bleeding gums or tarry stools to the physician."
2  "I need to tell any future caregivers about the metal implant."
3  "I need to report fever, redness, or increased pain to the physician."
4  "I can expect that changes in the shape of the knee will occur."

**Answer: 4**
*Rationale:* After TKR, the client should be taught to report any changes in the shape of the knee. This is not an expected event during recuperation from surgery. Fever, redness, or increased pain may indicate infection. With a metal implant, the client must be on anticoagulant therapy, and should report adverse effects of this therapy, such as evidence of bleeding from a variety of sources. The client must also notify caregivers of the metal implant, because the client will need antibiotic prophylaxis for invasive procedures, and because the client will be ineligible for magnetic resonance imaging as a diagnostic procedure.

*Test-Taking Strategy:* Note the key words *metal prosthesis* and *need for further discharge instructions*. Recalling that the client will be on prophylactic anticoagulant therapy will assist in eliminating option 1. Eliminate options 2 and 3 next because these are standard postoperative guidelines. Review client teaching points following TKR with metal prosthesis if you had difficulty with this question.

*Level of Cognitive Ability:* Analysis
*Client Needs:* Health Promotion and Maintenance
*Integrated Concept/Process:* Teaching/Learning
*Content Area:* Adult Health/Musculoskeletal

*Reference*
Black, J., Hawks, J., & Keene, A. (2001). *Medical-surgical nursing: Clinical management for positive outcomes* (6th ed.). Philadelphia: W.B. Saunders, p. 564.

---

**255.** A nurse in the preoperative holding unit administers a dose of scopolamine to a client. The nurse monitors the client for which of the following common side effects of the medication?
1  Dry mouth
2  Pupillary constriction
3  Excessive urination
4  Diaphoresis

**Answer: 1**
*Rationale:* Scopolamine is an anticholinergic medication that causes the frequent side effects of dry mouth, urinary retention, decreased sweating, and dilation of the pupils. Each of the incorrect options is the opposite of a side effect of this medication.

*Test-Taking Strategy:* Use the process of elimination. Recalling that this medication is an anticholinergic will direct you to option 1. If the medication is unfamiliar to you, review its side effects.

*Level of Cognitive Ability:* Application
*Client Needs:* Physiological Integrity

*Integrated Concept/Process:* Nursing Process/Assessment
*Content Area:* Pharmacology

*Reference*
Deglin, J., & Vallerand, A. (1999). *Davis's Drug guide for nurses* (6th ed.). Philadelphia: F.A. Davis, p. 909.

---

**256.** A nurse is providing medication instructions to a client who is taking imipramine (Tofranil) daily. Which statement by the client indicates a need for further instructions?

1    "If I miss a dose, I need to take it as soon as possible unless it is almost time for the next dose."
2    "I need to take the medication in the morning before breakfast."
3    "The effects of the medication may not be noticed for at least 2 weeks."
4    "I need to avoid alcohol while taking the medication."

**Answer: 2**
*Rationale:* The client should be instructed to take the medication (a single dose) at bed time and not in the morning because of its side effects. The client is instructed to take the medication exactly as directed and if a dose is missed to take it as soon as possible unless almost time for another dose. The client is told that medication effects may not be noticed for at least 2 weeks, and to avoid alcohol or other central nervous system (CNS) depressants during therapy.

*Test-Taking Strategy:* Note the key words *need for further instructions*. General principles related to medication administration will eliminate options 1 and 4. From the remaining options, recalling that this medication is an antidepressant will eliminate option 3. If you are unfamiliar with this medication, review these client teaching points.

*Level of Cognitive Ability:* Analysis
*Client Needs:* Health Promotion and Maintenance
*Integrated Concept/Process:* Teaching/Learning
*Content Area:* Pharmacology

*Reference*
Deglin, J., & Vallerand, A. (1999). *Davis's Drug guide for nurses* (6th ed.). Philadelphia: F.A. Davis, p. 511.

---

**257.** A nurse is preparing to assess a client who was admitted to the hospital with a diagnosis of trigeminal neuralgia (Tic Douloureux). On review of the client's record, the nurse would expect to note that the client experienced:

1    Chronic, intermittent pain in the seventh cranial nerve
2    Abrupt onset of pain in the fifth cranial nerve
3    Bilateral pain in the sixth cranial nerve
4    Unilateral pain in the sixth cranial nerve

**Answer: 2**
*Rationale:* Trigeminal neuralgia is a chronic syndrome characterized by an abrupt onset of pain. It involves one or more divisions of the trigeminal nerve or cranial nerve V. Options 1, 3, and 4 are incorrect.

*Test-Taking Strategy:* Use the process of elimination. Recalling that trigeminal neuralgia affects the fifth cranial nerve will assist in eliminating options 1, 3, and 4. Review the pathophysiology associated with trigeminal neuralgia if you had difficulty with this question.

*Level of Cognitive Ability:* Analysis
*Client Needs:* Physiological Integrity
*Integrated Concept/Process:* Nursing Process/Assessment
*Content Area:* Adult Health /Neurological

*Reference*
Black, J., Hawks, J., & Keene, A. (2001). *Medical-surgical nursing: Clinical management for positive outcomes* (6th ed.). Philadelphia: W.B. Saunders, p. 1995.

**258.** A client is taking docusate (Colace). The nurse tells the client to monitor for which of the following to ensure that the medication has the intended effect?
1  Decrease in fatty stools
2  Regular bowel movements
3  Abdominal pain
4  Decreased heartburn

**Answer: 2**
*Rationale:* Docusate is a stool softener that promotes absorption of water into the stool, producing a softer consistency of stool. The intended effect is relief or prevention of constipation. The medication does not relieve abdominal pain, relieve heartburn, or decrease the amount of fat in the stools.

*Test-Taking Strategy:* Use the process of elimination. Recalling that this medication is a stool softener will direct you to option 2. Review the action of this medication if you had difficulty with this question.

*Level of Cognitive Ability:* Application
*Client Needs:* Health Promotion and Maintenance
*Integrated Concept/Process:* Teaching/Learning
*Content Area:* Pharmacology

*Reference*
Deglin, J., & Vallerand, A. (1999). *Davis's Drug guide for nurses* (6th ed.). Philadelphia: F.A. Davis, p. 307.

**259.** A client's laboratory test results reveal a decreased serum transferrin and total iron binding capacity (TIBC). The nurse interprets that this laboratory finding is compatible with anemia due to which of the following problems?
1  Malnutrition
2  Infection
3  Sickle cell disease
4  Iron deficiency

**Answer: 1**
*Rationale:* Malnutrition can cause reductions in both the serum transferrin and the TIBC. Infection is an unrelated option. Sickle cell disease is diagnosed by determining that the client has hemoglobin S. Iron deficiency anemia is usually characterized by decreased iron-binding capacity but increased transferrin levels. Furthermore, in the actual clinical practice, the hemoglobin level is routinely used to detect iron-deficiency anemia.

*Test-Taking Strategy:* Focus on the laboratory tests identified in the question. Use these data and your knowledge of the findings in a client with malnutrition to direct you to this option. Review the findings in malnutrition if you had difficulty with this question.

*Level of Cognitive Ability:* Analysis
*Client Needs:* Physiological Integrity
*Integrated Concept/Process:* Nursing Process/Analysis
*Content Area:* Fundamental Skills

*Reference*
Fischbach, F. (2000). *A manual of laboratory & diagnostic tests* (6th ed.). Philadelphia: Lippincott Williams & Wilkins, p. 79.

**260.** A nurse notes that the client has an order to have a Schilling test performed. The nurse reads the client's progress notes looking for a tentative diagnosis of which of the following types of anemias?
1  Pernicious
2  Megaloblastic
3  Iron-deficiency
4  Aplastic

**Answer: 1**
*Rationale:* The Schilling test is used to determine the cause of vitamin $B_{12}$ deficiency, which leads to pernicious anemia. This test involves the use of a small oral dose of radioactive $B_{12}$, and a large nonradioactive intramuscular (IM) dose. A 24-hour urine is then collected to measure the amount of radioactivity in the urine.

*Test-Taking Strategy:* Specific knowledge regarding the Schilling test and its purpose is needed to answer this question. If this question was difficult, review this test and the diagnostic tests associated with pernicious anemia.

*Level of Cognitive Ability:* Analysis
*Client Needs:* Physiological Integrity
*Integrated Concept/Process:* Nursing Process/Analysis
*Content Area:* Fundamental Skills

*Reference*

Monahan, F., & Neighbors, M. (1998). *Medical-surgical nursing: Foundations for clinical practice* (2nd ed.). Philadelphia: W.B Saunders, p. 443.

---

**261.** A physician has written an order for a client with diabetic gastroparesis to receive metoclopramide (Reglan) four times a day. The nurse schedules this medication to be given at which of the following times?

**1** 1 hour after each meal and at bedtime

**2** Every 6 hours spaced evenly around the clock

**3** 30 minutes before meals and at bedtime

**4** With each meal and at bedtime

**Answer: 3**

*Rationale:* The client should be taught to take this medication 30 minutes before meals and at bedtime. Before-meals administration allows the medication time to begin working before the client consumes food requiring digestion. The other options are incorrect.

*Test-Taking Strategy:* Use the process of elimination. Focus on the client's diagnosis. Noting that the medication is used to treat gastroparesis will direct you to option 3. Remember, it must be taken before meals to enhance digestion. Review the procedure for the administration of this medication if you had difficulty with this question.

*Level of Cognitive Ability:* Application
*Client Needs:* Physiological Integrity
*Integrated Concept/Process:* Nursing Process/Implementation
*Content Area:* Pharmacology

*Reference*

Deglin, J., & Vallerand, A. (1999). *Davis's Drug guide for nurses* (6th ed.). Philadelphia: F.A. Davis, p. 643.

---

**262.** A nurse is caring for a client who has just had a mastectomy. The nurse assists the client in doing which of the following exercises during the first 24 hours following surgery?

**1** Elbow flexion and extension

**2** Shoulder abduction and external rotation

**3** Pendulum arm swings

**4** Hand wall climbing

**Answer: 1**

*Rationale:* During the first 24 hours following surgery, the client is assisted to move the fingers and hands, and to flex and extend the elbow. The client may also use the arm for self-care provided that the client does not raise the arm above shoulder level or abduct the shoulder. The exercises identified in options 2, 3, and 4 are done once surgical drains are removed and wound healing is well established.

*Test-Taking Strategy:* Note the key words *during the first 24 hours* and use the process of elimination. Remember that options that are similar are not likely to be correct. In this situation, each of the incorrect options involves movement of the shoulder joint. Review appropriate exercises for the client following mastectomy if you had difficulty with this question.

*Level of Cognitive Ability:* Application
*Client Needs:* Physiological Integrity

*Integrated Concept/Process:* Nursing Process/Implementation
*Content Area:* Adult Health/Oncology

*Reference*
Black, J., Hawks, J., & Keene, A. (2001). *Medical-surgical nursing: Clinical management for positive outcomes* (6th ed.). Philadelphia: W.B. Saunders, p. 1027.

---

**263.** Methylphenidate (Ritalin) is prescribed for a child with a diagnosis of attention deficit hyperactivity disorder (ADHD). The nurse provides instructions to the mother regarding the administration of the medication and tells the mother to administer the medication:
1 At bedtime
2 Just before the noon meal
3 In the morning after breakfast
4 At the evening meal

**Answer: 2**
*Rationale:* Methylphenidate should be taken shortly before the noontime meal. It should not be taken after 1:00 P.M. in children or 6:00 P.M. in adults, since the stimulating effect may keep the client awake. Options 1, 3, and 4 are incorrect.

*Test-Taking Strategy:* Use the process of elimination. Noting the name of the medication and the disorder will eliminate options 1 and 4. From the remaining options, recalling that it should be taken before the meal will direct you to option 2. If you had difficulty with this question, review the client teaching points related to the administration of this medication.

*Level of Cognitive Ability:* Application
*Client Needs:* Health Promotion and Maintenance
*Integrated Concept/Process:* Teaching/Learning
*Content Area:* Pharmacology

*Reference*
Varcarolis, E.M. (1998). *Foundations of psychiatric mental health nursing.* (3rd ed.). Philadelphia: W.B. Saunders, p. 1020.

---

**264.** A client has an order to take magnesium citrate to prevent constipation following upper and lower gastrointestinal (GI) barium studies. The nurse tells the client that this medication is best taken:
1 On ice
2 At room temperature
3 With a full glass of water
4 With fruit juice only

**Answer: 1**
*Rationale:* Magnesium citrate is available as an oral solution. It is commonly used as a laxative following certain studies of the GI tract. It should be served on ice, and should not be allowed to stand for prolonged periods. Allowing the medication to stand would reduce the carbonation and make the solution even less palatable. Options 2, 3, and 4 are incorrect.

*Test-Taking Strategy:* Use the process of elimination. Eliminate options 3 and 4 first knowing that magnesium citrate is itself a liquid. From the remaining options, it is necessary to know that it should be given cold to enhance palatability. Review the procedure for administering this medication if you had difficulty with this question.

*Level of Cognitive Ability:* Application
*Client Needs:* Physiological Integrity
*Integrated Concept/Process:* Nursing Process/Implementation
*Content Area:* Pharmacology

*Reference*
Deglin, J., & Vallerand, A. (1999). *Davis's Drug guide for nurses* (6th ed.). Philadelphia: F.A. Davis, p. 596.

**265.** A nurse is planning care for a client with carbon monoxide poisoning from a suicide attempt. The nurse speaks with the physician regarding a consult to which most-needed service?
1   Cardiac rehabilitation
2   Physical therapy
3   Mental health consult
4   Neurological consult

**Answer: 3**

*Rationale:* The client with carbon monoxide poisoning as a result of a suicide attempt should have a mental health consult. The necessity of a neurological consult would depend on the sequelae to the nervous system from the carbon monoxide poisoning. Physical therapy and cardiac rehabilitation are not indicated.

*Test-Taking Strategy:* Note the key words *most needed* in the stem of the question. Eliminate physical therapy first because there is no indication of the need for that service. The client will not need cardiac rehabilitation, so option 1 is eliminated next. A neurological consult could be beneficial, but only if the client suffers long-term central nervous system (CNS) damage from this suicide attempt. This client is most in need of a mental health consult at this time. Review care of a client who attempted suicide if you had difficulty with this question.

*Level of Cognitive Ability:* Application
*Client Needs:* Psychosocial Integrity
*Integrated Concept/Process:* Nursing Process/Implementation
*Content Area:* Mental Health

*Reference*
Leahy, J., & Kizilay, P. (1998). *Foundations of nursing practice: A nursing process approach.* Philadelphia: W.B. Saunders, p. 327.

**266.** A client has begun medication therapy with pancrelipase (Pancrease). The nurse teaches the client that this medication should:
1   Relieve heartburn
2   Help regulate blood glucose
3   Decrease the amount of fat in the stools
4   Eliminate abdominal pain

**Answer: 3**

*Rationale:* Pancrelipase is a pancreatic enzyme used in clients with pancreatitis as a digestive aid. The medication should reduce the amount of fatty stools (steatorrhea). Another intended effect could be improved nutritional status. It is not used to treat abdominal pain or heartburn. It does not regulate blood glucose; blood glucose regulation is a function of insulin, a hormone produced in the beta cells of the pancreas.

*Test-Taking Strategy:* Focus on the name of the medication. The name of the medication gives an indication of the possible uses of this medication. Also use knowledge of the physiology of the pancreas and recall that the suffix "-ase" indicates an enzyme. This will assist in directing you to option 3. Review the action of this medication if you had difficulty with this question.

*Level of Cognitive Ability:* Application
*Client Needs:* Physiological Integrity
*Integrated Concept/Process:* Teaching/Learning
*Content Area:* Pharmacology

*Reference*
Deglin, J., & Vallerand, A. (1999). *Davis's Drug guide for nurses* (6th ed.). Philadelphia: F.A. Davis, p. 764.

**267.** A nurse has given a client directions for proper use of aluminum hydroxide tablets (Alu-Caps). The client indicates an understanding of the medication if which statement is made?
1   "I should take the tablet at the same time as an antacid."
2   "I should take each dose with a laxative to prevent constipation."
3   "I should chew the tablet thoroughly and then drink 4 oz. of water."
4   "I should swallow the tablet whole with a full glass of water."

**Answer: 3**
*Rationale:* Aluminum hydroxide tablets should be chewed thoroughly before swallowing. This prevents them from entering the small intestine undissolved. They should not be swallowed whole. Antacids should be taken at least 2 hours apart from other medications to prevent interactive effects. Constipation is a side effect of use of aluminum products, but the client should not take a laxative with each dose. This promotes laxative abuse. The client should first try other means to prevent constipation.

*Test-Taking Strategy:* Use the process of elimination. Eliminate option 2 first since it does not promote healthy bowel function. Next, eliminate option 1 using general knowledge of antacid interactive effects. From the remaining options, use principles of digestion and medication use to direct you to option 3. Review client teaching points related to the use of this medication if you had difficulty with this question.

*Level of Cognitive Ability:* Analysis
*Client Needs:* Physiological Integrity
*Integrated Concept/Process:* Teaching/Learning
*Content Area:* Pharmacology

*Reference*
Deglin, J., & Vallerand, A. (1999). *Davis's Drug guide for nurses* (6th ed.). Philadelphia: F.A. Davis, p. 27.

**268.** A nurse has assisted the physician in placing a central (subclavian) catheter. Which of the following is the priority action following the procedure?
1   Obtain a temperature reading to monitor for infection
2   Monitor the blood pressure (BP) to check for fluid volume overload
3   Label the dressing with the date and time of catheter insertion
4   Check the results of the prescribed chest x-ray examination

**Answer: 4**
*Rationale:* A major risk associated with central line placement is the possibility of a pneumothorax developing from an accidental puncture of the lung. Assessing the chest x-ray is the best method to determine if this complication has occurred and to verify catheter tip placement before initiating intravenous (IV) therapy. While a client may develop an infection at the central line site, a temperature elevation would not likely occur immediately after placement. While BP assessment is always important in checking a client's status after an invasive procedure, fluid volume overload is not a concern until IV fluids are started. Labeling the dressing site is important, but it is not a priority action in this situation.

*Test-Taking Strategy:* Use the process of elimination. Noting the key words *following the procedure* will assist in eliminating options 1 and 2. Next, noting the words *priority action* will direct you to option 4 from the remaining options. Review postprocedure care following central catheter insertion if you had difficulty with this question.

*Level of Cognitive Ability:* Application
*Clinical Needs:* Physiological Integrity
*Integrated Concept/Process:* Nursing Process/Implementation
*Content Area:* Fundamental Skills

*Reference*
Monahan, F., & Neighbors, M. (1998). *Medical-surgical nursing: Foundations for clinical practice* (2nd ed.). Philadelphia: W.B Saunders, p. 987.

**269.** A client is complaining of gas pains following surgery and requests medication. The nurse reviews the medication order sheet to see if which of the following medications is ordered?
1 Acetaminophen (Tylenol)
2 Simethicone (Mylicon)
3 Magnesium hydroxide (MOM)
4 Droperidol (Inapsine)

**Answer: 2**
*Rationale:* Simethicone is an antiflatulent used in the relief of pain due to excessive gas in the gastrointestinal (GI) tract. Acetaminophen is a nonnarcotic analgesic. Magnesium hydroxide is an antacid and laxative. Droperidol is used to treat postoperative nausea and vomiting.

*Test-Taking Strategy:* Focus on the key words *gas pains*. Recalling the classifications of each of the medications listed in the options will direct you to option 2. If this question was difficult, review the action and purpose of each of the medications listed in the options.

*Level of Cognitive Ability:* Analysis
*Client Needs:* Physiological Integrity
*Integrated Concept/Process:* Nursing Process/Analysis
*Content Area:* Pharmacology

*Reference*
Deglin, J., & Vallerand, A. (1999). *Davis's Drug guide for nurses* (6th ed.). Philadelphia: F.A. Davis, p. 917.

**270.** An elderly client has recently been started on cimetidine (Tagamet). The nurse tells a family member to be alert for which of the following most frequent central nervous system (CNS) side effect of this medication?
1 Headache
2 Hallucinations
3 Confusion
4 Dizziness

**Answer: 3**
*Rationale:* Elderly clients are especially susceptible to the central nervous system (CNS) side effects of cimetidine. The most frequent of these is confusion. Less common CNS side effects include headache, dizziness, drowsiness, and hallucinations.

*Test-Taking Strategy:* Focus on the issue: an elderly client. Noting the key words *most frequent* will direct you to option 3. Review the most frequent CNS side effect of this medication if you had difficulty with this question.

*Level of Cognitive Ability:* Application
*Client Needs:* Health Promotion and Maintenance
*Integrated Concept/Process:* Teaching/Learning
*Content Area:* Pharmacology

*Reference*
Deglin, J., & Vallerand, A. (1999). *Davis's Drug guide for nurses* (6th ed.). Philadelphia: F.A. Davis, p. 477.

**271.** An African-American client with a diagnosis of cerebral hemorrhage is being evaluated for the possibility of a need for a craniotomy. To determine the client's level of anxiety about the possible surgery, the native American Caucasian nurse most appropriately:

1   Interviews the client alone without the presence of the family

2   Avoids questions concerning the risk of death

3   Arranges to have an African-American colleague be assigned to care for the client

4   Minimizes open-ended questioning concerning finances

**Answer: 3**

*Rationale:* A number of fears are common to all clients anticipating surgery. Assessment of these is critical to a successful outcome. African-American clients may have difficulty communicating their feelings to white doctors and nurses. Family members are rarely excluded from discussions. The subjects of death and finances are considered critical to the assessment. Option 3 is most appropriate to the ethnic/cultural aspect of care, especially when psychosocial needs are threatened.

*Test-Taking Strategy:* Focus on the issue: cultural awareness. Noting the key words *most appropriately* will direct you to option 3. If you had difficulty with this question, review the cultural considerations related to the care of the African-American population.

*Level of Cognitive Ability:* Application
*Client Needs:* Psychosocial Integrity
*Integrated Concept/Process:* Cultural Awareness
*Content Area:* Fundamental Skills

*Reference*
Black, J., Hawks, J., & Keene, A. (2001). *Medical-surgical nursing: Clinical management for positive outcomes* (6th ed.). Philadelphia: W.B. Saunders, p. 145.

**272.** A nurse is reviewing the record of a client who was admitted to the hospital for diagnostic studies following a fainting spell. The nurse notes that the client is receiving olanzapine (Zyprexia). Which of the following disorders or conditions would the nurse suspect in the client?

1   History of schizophrenia

2   History of diabetes mellitus

3   History of diabetes insipidus

4   History of coronary artery disease

**Answer: 1**

*Rationale:* Zyprexia is an antipsychotic medication used in the management of manifestations associated with psychotic disorders. It is the first-line treatment for schizophrenia, targeting both the positive and the negative symptoms. Options 2, 3, and 4 are not indicated uses for this medication.

*Test-Taking Strategy:* Use the process of elimination. Recalling that this medication is an antipsychotic will direct you to option 1. If you are unfamiliar with the action and use of this medication, review this content.

*Level of Cognitive Ability:* Analysis
*Client Needs:* Physiological Integrity
*Integrated Concept/Process:* Nursing Process/Analysis
*Content Area:* Pharmacology

*Reference*
Varcarolis, E.M. (1998). *Foundations of psychiatric mental health nursing.* (3rd ed.). Philadelphia: W.B. Saunders, p. 1021.

**273.** A postoperative client who unexpectedly required mechanical ventilation is visibly anxious. To relieve the anxiety, the best nursing action is to:
1 Ask a nursing assistant to sit with the client
2 Ask a family member to stay with the client
3 Administer an antianxiety medication
4 Remain with the client and provide reassurance

**Answer: 4**
*Rationale:* The nurse should remain with the client and provide reassurance. It is not appropriate to ask the family to take on the burden of remaining with the client. Asking a nursing assistant to sit with the client and administering an antianxiety medication are not the best actions.

*Test-Taking Strategy:* Note the key words *best nursing action*. Use the process of elimination, remembering that it is most important to address the client's feelings. Review care of a client who is anxious if you had difficulty with this question.

*Level of Cognitive Ability:* Application
*Client Needs:* Psychosocial Integrity
*Integrated Concept/Process:* Caring
*Content Area:* Adult Health/Respiratory

*Reference*
Monahan, F., & Neighbors, M. (1998). *Medical-surgical nursing: Foundations for clinical practice* (2nd ed.). Philadelphia: W.B Saunders, p. 933.

**274.** A nurse is caring for a client who is receiving colchicine. The nurse plans to monitor for a decrease in which of the following to determine the effectiveness of this medication?
1 Headaches
2 Blood glucose level
3 Serum triglyceride level
4 Joint inflammation

**Answer: 4**
*Rationale:* Colchicine is classified as an anti-gout agent. It interferes with the ability of the white blood cells (WBCs) to initiate and maintain an inflammatory response to monosodium urate crystals. The client should report a decrease in pain and inflammation in affected joints, as well as a decrease in the number of gout attacks. The other options are not related to the use of this medication.

*Test-Taking Strategy:* Use the process of elimination. Recalling that this medication is used in the treatment of gout will direct you to option 4. Review the action of this medication if you had difficulty with this question.

*Level of Cognitive Ability:* Analysis
*Client Needs:* Physiological Integrity
*Integrated Concept/Process:* Nursing Process/Evaluation
*Content Area:* Pharmacology

*Reference*
Deglin, J., & Vallerand, A. (1999). *Davis's Drug guide for nurses* (6th ed.). Philadelphia: F.A. Davis, p. 223.

**275.** A client has an order to begin short-term therapy with enoxaparin (Lovenox). The nurse explains to the client that this medication is being ordered to:
1 Dissolve urinary calculi
2 Reduce the risk of deep vein thrombosis
3 Relieve migraine headaches
4 Stop progression of multiple sclerosis

**Answer: 2**
*Rationale:* Enoxaparin is an anticoagulant that is administered to prevent deep vein thrombosis and thromboembolism in selected clients at risk. It is not used to treat urinary calculi, migraine headaches, or multiple sclerosis.

*Test-Taking Strategy:* Use the process of elimination. Recalling that this medication is an anticoagulant will direct you to option 2. Review the action of this medication if you had difficulty with this question.

*Level of Cognitive Ability:* Application
*Client Needs:* Physiological Integrity
*Integrated Concept/Process:* Teaching/Learning
*Content Area:* Pharmacology

**Reference**
Deglin, J., & Vallerand, A. (1999). *Davis's Drug guide for nurses* (6th ed.). Philadelphia: F.A. Davis, p. 473.

---

**276.** A client takes aluminum hydroxide (Amphojel) as needed for heartburn. The nurse teaches the client that the most common side effect of this medication is:
1 Constipation
2 Excitability
3 Muscle pain
4 Dizziness

**Answer: 1**
*Rationale:* Because of the antacid's aluminum base, aluminum hydroxide causes constipation as a side effect. The other side effect is hypophosphatemia, which is noted by monitoring serum laboratory studies. The other options are incorrect.

*Test-Taking Strategy:* Use the process of elimination. Recalling that aluminum-based antacids cause constipation will direct you to option 1. If this question was difficult, review the side effects associated with this medication.

*Level of Cognitive Ability:* Application
*Client Needs:* Health Promotion and Maintenance
*Integrated Concept/Process:* Teaching/Learning
*Content Area:* Pharmacology

**Reference**
Deglin, J., & Vallerand, A. (1999). *Davis's Drug guide for nurses* (6th ed.). Philadelphia: F.A. Davis, p. 27.

---

**277.** A client has been prescribed metoprolol (Lopressor) for hypertension. The nurse monitors client compliance carefully, due to which common side effect of the medication?
1 Increased appetite
2 Impotence
3 Difficulty swallowing
4 Mood swings

**Answer: 2**
*Rationale:* A common side effect of beta-adrenergic blocking agents, such as metoprolol is impotence. Other common side effects include fatigue and weakness. Central nervous system side effects occur rarely and include mental status changes, nervousness, depression, and insomnia. Increased appetite, difficulty swallowing, and mood swings are not reported side effects.

*Test-Taking Strategy:* Focus on the issue: monitoring compliance, and the key words *common side effect* to direct you to option 2. Review the expected side effects of this group of medications if you had difficulty with this question.

*Level of Cognitive Ability:* Application
*Client Needs:* Physiological Integrity
*Integrated Concept/Process:* Nursing Process/Assessment
*Content Area:* Pharmacology

**Reference**
Deglin, J., & Vallerand, A. (1999). *Davis's Drug guide for nurses* (6th ed.). Philadelphia: F.A. Davis, p. 1067.

**278.** A nurse is providing instructions to the spouse of a client who is taking tacrine (Cognex) for the management of moderate dementia associated with Alzheimer's disease. The nurse tells the spouse:

1 If flu-like symptoms occur it is necessary to notify the physician immediately

2 If a dose is missed, double up on the next dose

3 If a change in the color of the stools occurs, notify the physician

4 Not to administer the medication with food

**Answer: 3**

*Rationale:* Cognex may be administered between meals on an empty stomach and if gastrointestinal upset occurs, it may be administered with meals. Flu-like symptoms without fever is a frequent side effect that may occur with the use of the medication. The client or spouse should never be instructed to double the dose of any medication if it was missed, and the client and caregiver is instructed to notify the physician if nausea, vomiting, diarrhea, rash, jaundice, or changes in the color of the stool occur. This may be indicative of the potential occurrence of hepatitis.

*Test-Taking Strategy:* Use the process of elimination. Recalling that an adverse effect associated with the use of the medication is hepatitis will direct you to option 3. If you are unfamiliar with the use of this medication and its potential adverse effects, review this medication.

*Level of Cognitive Ability:* Application
*Client Needs:* Health Promotion and Maintenance
*Integrated Concept/Process:* Teaching/Learning
*Content Area:* Pharmacology

*Reference*
Deglin, J., & Vallerand, A. (1999). *Davis's Drug guide for nurses* (6th ed.). Philadelphia: F.A. Davis, p. 944.

---

**279.** An elderly client has been using casanthrol (cascara sagrada) on a long-term basis to treat constipation. The nurse interprets that which of the following laboratory results is due to the side effects of this medication?

1 Sodium 135 mEq/L
2 Sodium 145 mEq/L
3 Potassium 3.1 mEq/L
4 Potassium 5.0 mEq/L

**Answer: 3**

*Rationale:* Hypokalemia can result from long-term use of casanthrol (cascara sagrada), which is a laxative. The medication stimulates peristalsis and alters fluid and electrolyte transport, thus helping fluid to accumulate in the colon. The normal range for potassium is 3.6 to 5.1 mEq/L. The normal range for sodium is 135 to 145 mEq/L. Options 1, 2, and 4 are normal values.

*Test-Taking Strategy:* Use the process of elimination and knowledge regarding the normal laboratory values for sodium and potassium. The only abnormal value is option 3. Review the effects of this medication if you had difficulty with this question.

*Level of Cognitive Ability:* Analysis
*Client Needs:* Physiological Integrity
*Integrated Concept/Process:* Nursing Process/Analysis
*Content Area:* Pharmacology

*Reference*
Deglin, J., & Vallerand, A. (1999). *Davis's Drug guide for nurses* (6th ed.). Philadelphia: F.A. Davis, p. 165.

**280.** A client has been started on cyclobenza-prine (Flexeril) for the management of muscle spasms. The nurse teaches the client to observe for which of the following most common central nervous system (CNS) side effects of this medication?
1  Drowsiness
2  Fatigue
3  Irritability
4  Excitability

**Answer: 1**
*Rationale:* The most common side effects of cyclobenzaprine are drowsiness, dizziness, and dry mouth. This medication is a centrally-acting skeletal muscle relaxant used in the management of muscle spasms that accompany a variety of conditions. Fatigue, nervousness, and confusion are less frequent central nervous system (CNS) side effects of the medication.

*Test-Taking Strategy:* Note the key words *most common*. Eliminate options 3 and 4 because they are similar. Recalling that this medication is a centrally-acting skeletal muscle relaxant will direct you to option 1 from the remaining options. Review this medication if this question was difficult.

*Level of Cognitive Ability:* Application
*Client Needs:* Physiological Integrity
*Integrated Concept/Process:* Teaching/Learning
*Content Area:* Pharmacology

*Reference*
Deglin, J., & Vallerand, A. (1999). *Davis's Drug guide for nurses* (6th ed.). Philadelphia: F.A. Davis, p. 229.

**281.** A nurse is providing instructions to a client who is taking zolpidem (Ambien) for the treatment of insomnia. To pro-duce a maximal effect of the medication, the nurse tells the client to take the medication:
1  With a full glass of water
2  Following the evening meal
3  At bed time with a snack
4  With milk or an antacid

**Answer: 1**
*Rationale:* The client should be instructed to take the medication at bed time and to swallow the medication whole with a full glass of water. For faster onset of sleep, the client should be instructed not to administer the medication with milk or food, or immediately after a meal. Antacids should be avoided with the administration of the medication.

*Test-Taking Strategy:* Use the process of elimination. Note the key words *maximal effect* in the question. For maximal effectiveness of medications, medications should be taken on an empty stomach with water only. If you had difficulty with this question, review the principles related to the administration of zolpidem.

*Level of Cognitive Ability:* Application
*Client Needs:* Physiological Integrity
*Integrated Concept/Process:* Teaching/Learning
*Content Area:* Pharmacology

*Reference*
Deglin, J., & Vallerand, A. (1999). *Davis's Drug guide for nurses* (6th ed.). Philadelphia: F.A. Davis, p. 1056.

**282.** A nurse is preparing to administer heparin sodium (Liquaemin) 5000 units subcutaneously (SC). Which of the following indicates the accurate procedure for administering the medication?
1    Injecting the medication at least 2 inches from the umbilicus
2    Massaging the injection site following administration
3    Injecting the medication in the outer aspect of the upper arm
4    Administering the medication below the iliac crest

**Answer: 1**

*Rationale:* The injection site for heparin is above the iliac crest or in the abdominal fat layer. It is injected at least 2 inches from the umbilicus. The needle is withdrawn rapidly, prolonged pressure is applied at the injection site, and the site is not massaged. Injection sites are rotated. After withdrawal of heparin from the vial, the needle is changed before injection to prevent leakage of the heparin along the needle tract, which can cause bruising and bleeding.

*Test-Taking Strategy:* Use the process of elimination, focusing on the issue, accurate procedure. Visualize the procedure as you read each option. This will direct you to option 1. Review this procedure if you had difficulty with this question.

*Level of Cognitive Ability:* Application
*Client Needs:* Physiological Integrity
*Integrated Concept/Process:* Nursing Process/Implementation
*Content Area:* Pharmacology

*Reference*
Hodgson, B., & Kizior, R. (2001). *Saunders Nursing drug handbook 2001.* Philadelphia: W.B. Saunders, p. 489

---

**283.** A client is admitted to the hospital with a tentative diagnosis of pernicious anemia. The nurse assesses the client for which sign associated with this disorder?
1    Constipation
2    Dusky, mucous membranes
3    Red tongue that is smooth and sore
4    Shortness of breath

**Answer: 3**

*Rationale:* Classic signs of pernicious anemia include weakness, mild diarrhea, and a smooth, sore red tongue. The client may also have nervous system symptoms, such as paresthesias, difficulty with balance, and occasional confusion. The mucous membranes do not become dusky and the client does not exhibit shortness of breath.

*Test-Taking Strategy:* To answer this question accurately, you must be familiar with the signs and symptoms that characterize pernicious anemia. Review the assessment data related to this disorder if the question was difficult.

*Level of Cognitive Ability:* Application
*Client Needs:* Physiological Integrity
*Integrated Concept/Process:* Nursing Process/Assessment
*Content Area:* Fundamental Skills

*Reference*
Monahan, F., & Neighbors, M. (1998). *Medical-surgical nursing: Foundations for clinical practice* (2nd ed.). Philadelphia: W.B Saunders, p. 476.

**284.** Benztropine mesylate (Cogentin) is prescribed for a client with a diagnosis of Parkinson's disease. The clinic nurse is reinforcing instructions to the client regarding the medication and tells the client to:

1 Avoid driving if drowsiness or dizziness occurs

2 Expect difficulty swallowing while taking this medication

3 Spend 1 hour a day during rest periods sitting in the sun to enhance the effectiveness of the medication

4 Expect episodes of vomiting and constipation while taking this medication

**Answer: 1**

*Rationale:* The client taking benztropine mesylate should be instructed to avoid driving or operating hazardous equipment if drowsy or dizzy. The client's tolerance to heat may be reduced owing to the diminished ability to sweat, and the client should be instructed to plan rest periods in cool places during the day. The client should be instructed to stop taking the medication if difficulty swallowing or speaking, or vomiting occurs. The client should also inform the physician if central nervous system effects occur. The client is instructed to monitor urinary output and to watch for signs of constipation.

*Test-Taking Strategy:* Use the process of elimination. General principles related to safety and medications will direct you to option 1. If you had difficulty with this question, review client teaching points related to this medication.

*Level of Cognitive Ability:* Application
*Client Needs:* Health Promotion and Maintenance
*Integrated Concept/Process:* Teaching/Learning
*Content Area:* Pharmacology

*Reference*
Varcarolis, E.M. (1998). *Foundations of psychiatric mental health nursing.* (3rd ed.). Philadelphia: W.B. Saunders, p. 1005.

**285.** A nurse is preparing to implement a preoperative teaching plan for a client scheduled for abdominal surgery. The nurse initially focuses on:

1 The client's ability to change the abdominal dressing

2 The client's coping behaviors

3 The client's support systems

4 What the client knows about the surgery

**Answer: 4**

*Rationale:* The first step in client education is establishing what the client already knows. This allows the nurse to not only correct any misinformation, but to determine the starting point for teaching and to implement the education at the client's level.

*Test-Taking Strategy:* Note the key word *initially*. Remember, in the teaching/learning process, client motivation and readiness to learn along with what the client knows are initial assessment items. Review teaching/learning process if you had difficulty with this question.

*Level of Cognitive Ability:* Application
*Client Needs:* Psychosocial Integrity
*Integrated Concept/Process:* Nursing Process/Implementation
*Content Area:* Fundamental Skills

*Reference*
Monahan, F., & Neighbors, M. (1998). *Medical-surgical nursing: Foundations for clinical practice* (2nd ed.). Philadelphia: W.B Saunders, p. 632.

**286.** A client with refractory myasthenia gravis is told by the physician that plasmapheresis therapy is indicated. After the physician leaves the room, the client asks the nurse to repeat the physician's reason for ordering this treatment. The nurse tells the client that this therapy will most likely improve which of the client's symptoms?

1 Urinary incontinence
2 Pins and needles sensation in the legs
3 Double vision
4 Difficulty breathing

**Answer: 4**

*Rationale:* Plasmapheresis is a process that separates the plasma from the blood elements, so that plasma proteins that contain antibodies can be removed. It is used as an adjunct therapy in myasthenia gravis, and may give temporary relief to clients with actual or impending respiratory failure. Usually 3 to 5 treatments are required. This therapy is not indicated for the other reasons listed in options 1, 2, and 3.

*Test-Taking Strategy:* Note the key word *refractory*. This tells you that the client with myasthenia gravis has severe disease, which is not adequately controlled with medication and other measures. Recalling the purpose of plasmapheresis and knowledge of the complications of this disease will direct you to option 4. Review the purpose of this procedure if you had difficulty with this question.

*Level of Cognitive Ability:* Application
*Client Needs:* Physiological Integrity
*Integrated Concept/Process:* Nursing Process/Implementation
*Content Area:* Adult Health/Neurological

*Reference*
Black, J., Hawks, J., & Keene, A. (2001). *Medical-surgical nursing: Clinical management for positive outcomes* (6th ed.). Philadelphia: W.B. Saunders, p. 2020.

**287.** A client is admitted to the hospital in myasthenic crisis. A nurse questions the family about the occurrence of which of the following precipitating factors for this event?

1 Not taking prescribed medication
2 Taking excess prescribed medication
3 Getting more sleep than usual
4 A decrease in food intake recently

**Answer: 1**

*Rationale:* Myasthenic crisis is often caused by undermedication, and responds to the administration of cholinergic medications such as neostigmine (Prostigmin) and pyridostigmine (Mestinon). Cholinergic crisis (the opposite problem) is caused by excess medication and responds to withholding of medications. Change in diet and increased sleep are not precipitating factors. However, overexertion and overeating could possibly trigger myasthenic crisis.

*Test-Taking Strategy:* Focus on the issue: myasthenic crisis. Recalling that myasthenia gravis is treated with medication will direct you to option 1. Review the causes of myasthenia gravis if you had difficulty with this question.

*Level of Cognitive Ability:* Application
*Client Needs:* Physiological Integrity
*Integrated Concept/Process:* Nursing Process/Assessment
*Content Area:* Adult Health/Neurological

*Reference*
Monahan, F., & Neighbors, M. (1998). *Medical-surgical nursing: Foundations for clinical practice* (2nd ed.). Philadelphia: W.B Saunders, p. 782.

**288.** A client with trigeminal neuralgia asks the nurse what can be done to minimize the episodes of pain. The nurse's response is based on an understanding that the symptoms can be triggered by:
1   Infection or stress
2   Excessive watering of the eyes or nasal stuffiness
3   Sensations of pressure or extreme temperature
4   Hypoglycemia and fatigue

**Answer: 3**
*Rationale:* The paroxysms of pain that accompany this neuralgia are triggered by stimulation of the terminal branches of the trigeminal nerve. Symptoms can be triggered by pressure from washing the face, brushing the teeth, shaving, eating, and drinking. Symptoms can also be triggered by thermal stimuli such as a draft of cold air. The items listed in the other options do not trigger the spasm.

*Test-Taking Strategy:* Recalling the pathophysiology of this disorder and precipitating factors will direct you to option 3. Review this cranial nerve disorder if you had difficulty with this question.

*Level of Cognitive Ability:* Analysis
*Client Needs:* Physiological Integrity
*Integrated Concept/Process:* Nursing Process/Analysis
*Content Area:* Adult Health/Neurological

*Reference*
Monahan, F., & Neighbors, M. (1998). *Medical-surgical nursing: Foundations for clinical practice* (2nd ed.). Philadelphia: W.B Saunders, p. 829.

**289.** A client has been diagnosed with Bell's palsy. The nurse assesses the client to see if which of the following signs and symptoms is visible?
1   Speech difficulties and one-sided facial droop
2   Twitching of one side of the face and ruddy cheeks
3   Eye paralysis and ptosis of the eyelid
4   Fixed pupil and an elevated eyelid on one side

**Answer: 1**
*Rationale:* Bell's palsy is a one-sided facial paralysis from compression of the facial nerve (CN VII). There is facial droop from paralysis of the facial muscles, increased lacrimation, painful sensations in the eye, face, or behind the ear, and speech or chewing difficulties. The other items listed are not associated with this disorder.

*Test-Taking Strategy:* Remember that a palsy is a type of paralysis. This will assist in eliminating option 2. Recalling that Bell's palsy results from dysfunction of the facial nerve (CN VII), not the nerves that govern eye movements (CN III, IV, VI) will eliminate options 3 and 4. Review the characteristics associated with Bell's palsy if you had difficulty with this question.

*Level of Cognitive Ability:* Application
*Client Needs:* Physiological Integrity
*Integrated Concept/Process:* Nursing Process/Assessment
*Content Area:* Adult Health/Neurological

*Reference*
Monahan, F., & Neighbors, M. (1998). *Medical-surgical nursing: Foundations for clinical practice* (2nd ed.). Philadelphia: W.B Saunders, p. 829.

**290.** A client with Bell's palsy is distressed about the change in facial appearance. The nurse tells the client about which of the following characteristics of Bell's palsy to help the client cope with the disorder?

1 The symptoms will completely go away once the tumor is removed
2 It usually resolves when treated with vasodilator medications
3 It is similar to stroke, but all symptoms will go away eventually
4 It is not caused by stroke, and many clients recover in 3 to 5 weeks

**Answer: 4**

*Rationale:* Clients with Bell's palsy should be reassured that they have not experienced a stroke, and that symptoms often disappear spontaneously in 3 to 5 weeks. The client is given supportive treatment for symptoms. It is not usually caused by a tumor, and the treatment does not involve administering vasodilators.

*Test-Taking Strategy:* Focus on the issue: helping the client cope with the disorder. Recalling that Bell's palsy is not a stroke and is not caused by a tumor or vasoconstriction will eliminate options 1, 2, and 3. Review the characteristics associated with Bell's palsy if you had difficulty with this question.

*Level of Cognitive Ability:* Application
*Client Needs:* Psychosocial Integrity
*Integrated Concept/Process:* Caring
*Content Area:* Adult Health/Neurological

**Reference**
Monahan, F., & Neighbors, M. (1998). *Medical-surgical nursing: Foundations for clinical practice* (2nd ed.). Philadelphia: W.B Saunders, p. 829.

**291.** A physician is writing medication orders for a client with Bell's palsy. The nurse reviews the client's record for an order for which of the following medications commonly used to decrease edema of nerve tissue?

1 Naprosyn (Aleve)
2 Prednisone (Deltasone)
3 Acetylsalicylic acid (aspirin)
4 Ibuprofen (Motrin)

**Answer: 2**

*Rationale:* Bell's palsy is typically treated with prednisone. The medication reduces inflammation and edema, allowing return of normal circulation to the nerve. If given early, the medication reduces the severity of the palsy, reduces pain, and preserves substantial, if not all, nerve function.

*Test-Taking Strategy:* Use the process of elimination. Eliminate options 1 and 4 first because they are similar and are both nonsteroidal antiinflammatory medications. Recalling that corticosteroid medication is useful in this disorder will direct you to option 2 from the remaining options. Review the management of this disorder if you had difficulty with this question.

*Level of Cognitive Ability:* Analysis
*Client Needs:* Physiological Integrity
*Integrated Concept/Process:* Nursing Process/Analysis
*Content Area:* Adult Health/Neurological

**Reference**
Monahan, F., & Neighbors, M. (1998). *Medical-surgical nursing: Foundations for clinical practice* (2nd ed.). Philadelphia: W.B Saunders, p. 829.

**292.** A nurse is admitting a client to the hospital who has a diagnosis of Guillain-Barré syndrome (polyradiculitis). After ensuring that the client is comfortable in bed, the nurse asks a family member if the client has recently had:

1.  A respiratory or gastrointestinal (GI) infection
2.  Meningitis
3.  A back injury or spinal cord trauma
4.  Seizures or head trauma

**Answer: 1**

*Rationale:* Guillain-Barré syndrome is a clinical syndrome of unknown origin and involves cranial and peripheral nerves. Many clients report a history of respiratory or GI infection in the one to 4 weeks before the onset of neurological deficits. Occasionally, it has been triggered by vaccination or surgery. The other options are not associated with an incidence of this syndrome.

*Test-Taking Strategy:* Use the process of elimination. Eliminate options 2, 3, and 4 because they are similar and relate to neurological problems. Review the etiology associated with Guillain-Barré syndrome if you had difficulty with this question.

*Level of Cognitive Ability:* Application
*Client Needs:* Physiological Integrity
*Integrated Concept/Process:* Nursing Process/Assessment
*Content Area:* Adult Health/Neurological

*Reference*
Monahan, F., & Neighbors, M. (1998). *Medical-surgical nursing: Foundations for clinical practice* (2nd ed.). Philadelphia: W.B Saunders, p. 773.

**293.** A client has fallen and sustained a leg injury. Which of the following questions would the nurse ask the client to help determine if the pain is due to muscle strain?

1.  "Does the pain feel intense, achy, and cramplike?"
2.  "Does the pain feel like pins and needles?"
3.  "Is the pain gripping and viselike?"
4.  "Is the pain sharp and piercing?"

**Answer: 1**

*Rationale:* Pain of muscle origin is often described as a strong aching or cramping pain. Fracture pain is generally described as sharp and piercing. Altered sensations, such as paresthesias (pins and needles) indicate there is pressure on nerves or impairment of circulation. Pain in the extremities is usually not described as gripping or vicelike. These terms (gripping and viselike) are used to describe pain of myocardial infarction, however.

*Test-Taking Strategy:* Use the process of elimination, focusing on the issue, a muscle strain. Eliminate options 2, 3, and 4 since they best describe pain that is either neurological or cardiac in origin. Review the pain characteristics of a muscle strain if you had difficulty with this question.

*Level of Cognitive Ability:* Application
*Client Needs:* Physiological Integrity
*Integrated Concept/Process:* Nursing Process/Assessment
*Content Area:* Adult Health/Musculoskeletal

*Reference*
Monahan, F., & Neighbors, M. (1998). *Medical-surgical nursing: Foundations for clinical practice* (2nd ed.). Philadelphia: W.B Saunders, p. 913.

**294.** A client is treated in the ambulatory clinic for a sprained ankle. Before releasing the client home, the nurse instructs the client to do which of the following during the next 24 hours?

1  Apply ice to the site intermittently
2  Cover the foot with heavy blankets
3  Sit with the foot flat on the floor
4  Walk on the foot for 20 minutes out of each hour

**Answer: 1**

*Rationale:* Soft tissue injuries such as sprains are treated by RICE (Rest, Ice, Compression, Elevation) for the first 24 hours after the injury. Ice is applied intermittently for 20 to 30 minutes at a time. Heat (such as with heavy blankets) is not used in the first 24 hours because it could increase venous congestion, which would increase edema and pain. The client should rest the foot and not walk around on it. The foot should be elevated, and not placed in a dependent position.

*Test-Taking Strategy:* Use the process of elimination. Recalling that sprains should not be aggravated eliminates options 3 and 4. From the remaining options, recall that ice is applied to an injury in the first 24 hours rather than heat. Also, remember that heavy blankets would be uncomfortable on an injured foot. Review measures related to treatment of a sprained ankle if you had difficulty with this question.

*Level of Cognitive Ability:* Application
*Client Needs:* Health Promotion and Maintenance
*Integrated Concept/Process:* Self-Care
*Content Area:* Adult Health/Musculoskeletal

*Reference*
Monahan, F., & Neighbors, M. (1998). *Medical-surgical nursing: Foundations for clinical practice* (2nd ed.). Philadelphia: W.B Saunders, p. 913.

**295.** A client who is being evaluated for tuberculosis has never had a chest x-ray. The nurse instructs the client about which of the following items before the procedure?

1  It is necessary to breathe slowly and deeply while the film is taken
2  The client must void in the bathroom before the procedure
3  The x-ray examination will cause only a small amount of pain
4  A metal neck chain must be removed while the film is taken

**Answer: 4**

*Rationale:* An x-ray film is a photographic image of a part of the body on a special film, which is used to diagnose a wide variety of conditions. The x-ray itself is painless; any discomfort would arise from repositioning a painful part for filming. The nurse may want to premedicate a client who is at risk for pain. Any radiopaque objects such as jewelry or other metal must be removed. The client is asked to breathe in deeply, and then hold the breath while the chest x-ray film is taken. The client is not required to void before the procedure, but may do so to enhance comfort during the procedure.

*Test-Taking Strategy:* Use the process of elimination and focus on the issue: a chest x-ray examination. Note the relationship between the anatomical location of this diagnostic test and the words *metal neck chain* in option 4. Review client teaching points related to a chest x-ray examination if you had difficulty with this question.

*Level of Cognitive Ability:* Application
*Client Needs:* Physiological Integrity
*Integrated Concept/Process:* Nursing Process/Implementation
*Content Area:* Adult Health/Respiratory

*Reference*
Monahan, F., & Neighbors, M. (1998). *Medical-surgical nursing: Foundations for clinical practice* (2nd ed.). Philadelphia: W.B Saunders, p. 652.

**296.** A client is being treated in the emergency department for a fractured tibia. The skin is not broken, but the nurse can see on the x-ray viewer that the bone is completely fractured across the shaft and has small splintered pieces around it. The nurse interprets that this client's fracture is a:

1 Compound fracture
2 Simple fracture
3 Greenstick fracture
4 Comminuted fracture

**Answer: 4**

*Rationale:* A comminuted fracture is a complete fracture across the shaft of a bone, with splintering of the bone into fragments. A compound fracture, also called an open or complex fracture, is one in which the skin or mucous membrane has been broken, and the wound extends to the depth of the fractured bone. A simple fracture is a fracture of the bone across its entire shaft with some possible displacement but without breaking the skin. A greenstick fracture is an incomplete fracture, which occurs through part of the cross section of a bone. One side of the bone is fractured, and the other side is bent.

*Test-Taking Strategy:* Use the process of elimination, focusing on the key words *small splintered pieces.* Remember that a *comminuted* fracture is broken into *minute* (small) pieces. Review the characteristics of the types of fractures if you had difficulty with this question.

*Level of Cognitive Ability:* Analysis
*Client Needs:* Physiological Integrity
*Integrated Concept/Process:* Nursing Process/Analysis
*Content Area:* Adult Health/Musculoskeletal

*Reference*
Monahan, F., & Neighbors, M. (1998). *Medical-surgical nursing: Foundations for clinical practice* (2nd ed.). Philadelphia: W.B Saunders. p. 818.

**297.** A nurse in the emergency department is providing care to a client with a leg fracture. The nurse would determine that which of the following essential items is done before the fracture is reduced in the casting room?

1 Obtain an anesthesia consent
2 Ensure that the client has signed a consent for treatment
3 Notify the operating room staff
4 Administer a narcotic analgesic

**Answer: 2**

*Rationale:* Before a fracture is reduced, a consent for treatment is needed. The nurse would give the client explanations according to the client's needs and ability to understand. An analgesic would be administered as prescribed, because the procedure is painful, but the consent form needs to be obtained before administering the medication. Administration of anesthesia would only be done in the operating room for open reduction of fractures. Closed reductions may be done in the emergency department without anesthesia.

*Test-Taking Strategy:* Note the key word *essential* in the stem of the question. Note that the question specifically states that the procedure is going to be done in the casting room. This will assist in eliminating options 1 and 3. Recalling that a consent form must be obtained before administering sedating medication will direct you to option 2. Review the procedure related to a closed reduction if you had difficulty with this question.

*Level of Cognitive Ability:* Analysis
*Client Needs:* Physiological Integrity
*Integrated Concept/Process:* Nursing Process/Analysis
*Content Area:* Adult Health/Musculoskeletal

*Reference*
Monahan, F., & Neighbors, M. (1998). *Medical-surgical nursing: Foundations for clinical practice* (2nd ed.). Philadelphia: W.B Saunders, p. 919.

**298.** A nurse is monitoring a client with a fracture to the left arm. Which of the following signs observed by the nurse is consistent with impaired venous return in the area?

1   Weakened distal pulse
2   Continued pain despite medication
3   Pallor or blotchy cyanosis
4   Increasing edema

**Answer: 4**

*Rationale:* Impaired venous return is characterized by increasing edema. In the client with a fracture, this is most often prevented by elevating the limb. The other options identify signs of arterial damage, which can occur if the artery is contused, thrombosed, lacerated, or becomes spastic.

*Test-Taking Strategy:* Note the key words *impaired venous return.* Use principles of blood flow to answer the question. Each of the incorrect options identifies difficulty with circulation to the extremity, and are arterial signs. The correct option identifies a sign that is consistent with impaired venous return. Review the signs noted in impaired venous return if you had difficulty with this question.

*Level of Cognitive Ability:* Analysis
*Client Needs:* Physiological Integrity
*Integrated Concept/Process:* Nursing Process/Analysis
*Content Area:* Adult Health/Musculoskeletal

*Reference*

Black, J., Hawks, J., & Keene, A. (2001). *Medical-surgical nursing: Clinical management for positive outcomes* (6th ed.). Philadelphia: W.B. Saunders, p. 599.

**299.** The nurse receives in transfer from the postanesthesia care unit a client who has had skeletal traction applied in the operating room. The nurse takes action to correct which of the following problems noted with the traction setup?

1   Weights are resting against the foot of the bed
2   Knots are secured tightly
3   Ropes are centered in the wheel grooves of the pulleys
4   Ropes are free of frays or shredding

**Answer: 1**

*Rationale:* The traction setup is checked routinely to ensure that the ropes are in the grooves of the pulleys; ropes are not frayed; knots are tied securely; and weights are hanging freely from the ropes. Problems with any of these can interfere with maintenance of proper traction. If any problems are noted, they should be fixed immediately.

*Test-Taking Strategy:* Use the process of elimination, noting the key words *takes action to correct.* Recalling that weights exert the pulling force needed in a traction set-up will direct you to option 1. If this question was difficult, review the principles of setting up traction.

*Level of Cognitive Ability:* Application
*Client Needs:* Physiological Integrity
*Integrated Concept/Process:* Nursing Process/Implementation
*Content Area:* Adult Health/Musculoskeletal

*Reference*

Monahan, F., & Neighbors, M. (1998). *Medical-surgical nursing: Foundations for clinical practice* (2nd ed.). Philadelphia: W.B Saunders, p. 859.

**300.** A client is admitted to the nursing unit after a fall from a roof. The client has multiple lacerations and a right leg fracture, which has been treated with a plaster cast. The nurse positions the leg in which manner to promote optimal circulation?

1　Elevate the right leg on pillows continuously for 24 to 48 hours

2　Elevate the right leg for 3 hours and place it flat for 1 hour

3　Keep the right leg in a flat or level position

4　Keep the right leg flat for 3 hours and elevate it for 1 hour

**Answer: 1**

*Rationale:* A casted extremity is elevated continuously for the first 24 to 48 hours to minimize swelling and to promote venous drainage. The other options are not part of standard positioning of the newly casted extremity.

*Test-Taking Strategy:* Focus on the issue: to promote optimal circulation. Recalling that edema occurs after a fracture and can be increased by casting, and use of the principles of gravity will direct you to option 1. Review appropriate positioning following casting of an extremity if you had difficulty with this question.

*Level of Cognitive Ability:* Application
*Client Needs:* Physiological Integrity
*Integrated Concept/Process:* Nursing Process/Implementation
*Content Area:* Adult Health/Musculoskeletal

*Reference*
Monahan, F., & Neighbors, M. (1998). *Medical-surgical nursing: Foundations for clinical practice* (2nd ed.). Philadelphia: W.B Saunders. p. 853.

# CRITICAL THINKING: FREE-TEXT ENTRY

**1.** A nurse is monitoring for the presence of pitting edema in the prenatal client. The nurse presses the fingertips of the middle and index finger against the shin and holds pressure for 2 to 3 seconds. The nurse notes that the indentation is approximately 1 inch deep. The nurse documents that the client has which level of pitting edema?

**Answer:** 4+ edema

*Rationale:* When evaluating the presence of pitting edema, the nurse presses the fingertips of the index and middle fingers against the shin and holds pressure for 2 to 3 seconds. An indentation of approximately 1-inch deep would be indicative of 4+ edema. A slight indentation would indicate 1+ edema. An indentation of approximately ¼ inch deep indicates 2+ edema. An indentation of approximately ½ inch deep indicates 3+ edema.

*Test-Taking Strategy:* Focus on the words *indentation is approximately 1 inch*. Knowledge regarding this technique and the interpretation of the findings will assist in answering the question. If you are unfamiliar with this technique, review this content.

*Level of Cognitive Ability:* Application
*Client Needs:* Health Promotion and Maintenance
*Integrated Concept/Process:* Communication and Documentation
*Content Area:* Maternity

*Reference*
Lowdermilk, D., Perry, S., & Bobak, I. (2000). *Maternity & women's health care* (7th ed.). St. Louis: Mosby, p. 823.

**2.** A nurse caring for a small for gestational age (SGA) infant reviews the results of a total serum calcium level. The results are reported as 5.9 mg/dL. The nurse documents that the result of this test reflects what finding as compared to the normal serum calcium level?

**Answer:** Lower than normal

*Rationale:* SGA infants are at risk for developing hypocalcemia. The normal range for a total serum calcium is 7.0 mg/dL to 8.5 mg/dL. A value of 5.9 mg/dL is lower than the normal level.

*Test-Taking Strategy:* Knowledge regarding the normal total serum calcium level is required to answer this question. If you are unfamiliar with this laboratory test or the significant findings in a SGA infant, review this content.

*Level of Cognitive Ability:* Analysis
*Client Needs:* Physiological Integrity
*Integrated Concept/Process:* Communication and Documentation
*Content Area:* Maternity

**Reference**
Lowdermilk, D., Perry, S., & Bobak, I. (2000). *Maternity & women's health care* (7th ed.). St. Louis: Mosby, p. 1127.

---

**3.** A nurse is preparing to administer captopril (Capoten), an angiotensin-converting enzyme (ACE) inhibitor. Before administering the medication, the nurse would assess which most important vital sign in the client?

**Answer:** Blood pressure
*Rationale:* ACE inhibitors are potent antihypertensive medications. A baseline blood pressure is needed for comparison to evaluate the effectiveness of this therapy.

*Test-Taking Strategy:* Recalling that ACE inhibitors are most often used to treat hypertension will assist in answering this question. If you are unfamiliar with the action of this medication, review this content.

*Level of Cognitive Ability:* Application
*Client Needs:* Physiological Integrity
*Integrated Concept/Process:* Nursing Process/Assessment
*Content Area:* Pharmacology

**Reference**
Hodgson, B., & Kizior, R. (2001). *Saunders Nursing drug handbook 2001.* Philadelphia: W.B. Saunders, p. 142.

---

**4.** A nurse is assisting a physician with abdominal paracentesis. The nurse assists the client to what position for this procedure?

**Answer:** Upright, or high-Fowler's position
*Rationale:* For abdominal paracentesis, the nurse should position the client in an upright, or a high-Fowler's position. This position allows the intestine to float posteriorly and helps prevent laceration during catheter insertion.

*Test-Taking Strategy:* Focus on the name and the purpose of the procedure. Visualize this procedure to answer the question. If you had difficulty with this question, review the procedure for abdominal paracentesis.

*Level of Cognitive Ability:* Application
*Client Needs:* Physiological Integrity
*Integrated Concept/Process:* Nursing Process/Implementation
*Content Area:* Adult Health/Gastrointestinal

**Reference**
Black, J., Hawks, J., & Keene, A. (2001). *Medical-surgical nursing: Clinical management for positive outcomes* (6th ed.). Philadelphia: W.B. Saunders, p. 1086.

**5.** A nurse is preparing to insert a nasogastric (NG) tube into a client. The nurse determines the appropriate length of the tube needed for insertion by performing what assessment procedure?

**Answer:** Places the tube at the tip of the nose and measures by extending the tube to the earlobe, and then down to the xiphoid process.

*Rationale:* The appropriate method of measuring the length of a tube needed for NG tube insertion is to place the tube at the tip of the nose and to measure by extending the tube to the earlobe and then down to the xiphoid process. The tube should be marked at that length.

*Test-Taking Strategy:* Knowledge regarding the appropriate procedure for measuring the length of an NG tube for insertion is required to answer this question. Attempt to visualize this procedure to answer the question. If you are unfamiliar with this procedure, review this content.

*Level of Cognitive Ability:* Analysis
*Client Needs:* Physiological Integrity
*Integrated Concept/Process:* Nursing Process/Assessment
*Content Area:* Adult Health/Gastrointestinal

*Reference*
Black, J., Hawks, J., & Keene, A. (2001). *Medical-surgical nursing: Clinical management for positive outcomes* (6th ed.). Philadelphia: W.B. Saunders, p. 722.

# REFERENCES

Ball, J., & Bindler, R. (1999). *Pediatric nursing: Caring for children* (2nd ed.). Stamford, Conn.: Appleton & Lange.

Beare, P., & Myers, J. (1998). *Adult health nursing* (3rd ed.). St. Louis: Mosby.

Black, J., Hawks, J., & Keene, A. (2001). *Medical-surgical nursing: Clinical management for positive outcomes* (6th ed.). Philadelphia: W.B. Saunders,

Bowden, V., Dickey, S, & Greenberg, C. (1998). *Children and their families: The continuum of care.* Philadelphia: W.B. Saunders.

Deglin, J., & Vallerand, A. (2001). *Davis's Drug guide for nurses* (7th ed.). Philadelphia: F.A. Davis.

Deglin, J., & Vallerand, A. (1999). *Davis's Drug guide for nurses* (6th ed.). Philadelphia: F.A. Davis.

Fischbach, F. (2000). *A manual of laboratory & diagnostic tests* (6th ed.). Philadelphia: Lippincott Williams & Wilkins.

Fortinash, K., & Holoday-Worret, P. (2000). *Psychiatric mental health nursing* (2nd ed.). St. Louis: Mosby.

Gorrie, T., McKinney, E., & Murray, S. (1998). *Foundations of maternal-newborn nursing* (2nd ed.). Philadelphia: W.B. Saunders.

Hodgson, B., & Kizior, R. (2001). *Saunders Nursing drug handbook 2001.* Philadelphia: W.B. Saunders.

Kee, J., & Marshall, S. (2000). *Clinical calculations: With applications to general and specialty areas* (4th ed.). Philadelphia: W.B. Saunders.

Leahy, J., & Kizilay, P. (1998). *Foundations of nursing practice: A nursing process approach.* Philadelphia: W.B. Saunders.

Lehne, R. (1998). *Pharmacology for nursing care* (3rd ed.). Philadelphia: W.B. Saunders.

Lowdermilk, D., Perry, S., & Bobak, I. (2000). *Maternity & women's health care* (7th ed.). St. Louis: Mosby.

Monahan, F., & Neighbors, M. (1998). *Medical-surgical nursing: Foundations for clinical practice* (2nd ed.). Philadelphia: W.B. Saunders.

Olds, S., London. M., & Ladewig, P. (2000). *Maternal-newborn nursing: A family and community-based approach* (6th ed.). Upper Saddle River, N.J.: Prentice-Hall Health.

Peckenpaugh, N., & Poleman, C. (1999). *Nutrition essentials and diet therapy* (8th ed.). Philadelphia: W.B. Saunders.

Potter, P., & Perry, A. (2001). *Fundamentals of nursing* (5th ed.). St. Louis: Mosby.

Rocchiccioli, J., & Tilbury, M. (1998). *Clinical leadership in nursing.* Philadelphia: W.B. Saunders.

Salerno, E. (1999). *Pharmacology for health professionals.* St. Louis: Mosby.

Sherwen, L., Scoloveno, M.A., & Weingarten, C. (1999). *Maternity nursing: Care of the childbearing family* (3rd ed.). Stamford, Conn.: Appleton & Lange.

Smeltzer, S., & Bare, B. (2000). *Brunner & Suddarth's Textbook of medical-surgical nursing* (9th ed.). Philadelphia: Lippincott Williams & Wilkins.

Stuart, G.W., & Laraia, M.T. (1998). *Principles and practice of psychiatric nursing.* (6th ed.). St. Louis: Mosby.

Varcarolis, E. (1998). *Foundations of psychiatric mental health nursing* (3rd ed.). Philadelphia: W.B. Saunders.

Wong, D. (1999). *Whaley & Wong's Nursing care of infants and children* (6th ed.). St. Louis: Mosby.